Essentials in Ophthalmology

Series Editor

Arun D. Singh, Cleveland Clinic Foundation
Cole Eye Institute, Cleveland, OH, USA

Essentials in Ophthalmology aims to promote the rapid and efficient transfer of medical research into clinical practice. It is published in four volumes per year. Covering new developments and innovations in all fields of clinical ophthalmology, it provides the clinician with a review and summary of recent research and its implications for clinical practice. Each volume is focused on a clinically relevant topic and explains how research results impact diagnostics, treatment options and procedures as well as patient management.

The reader-friendly volumes are highly structured with core messages, summaries, tables, diagrams and illustrations and are written by internationally well-known experts in the field. A volume editor supervises the authors in his/her field of expertise in order to ensure that each volume provides cutting-edge information most relevant and useful for clinical ophthalmologists. Contributions to the series are peer reviewed by an editorial board.

Jaime Aramberri • Kenneth J. Hoffer
Thomas Olsen • Giacomo Savini
H. John Shammas
Editors

Intraocular Lens Calculations

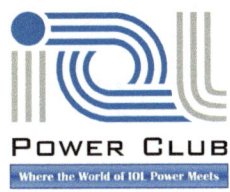

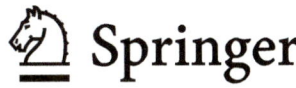

Editors
Jaime Aramberri
Clínica Miranza Ókular
Vitoria-Gasteiz, Alava, Spain

Thomas Olsen
University Eye Clinic
Aarhus University
Aarhus, Denmark

H. John Shammas
The Keck School of Medicine
University of Southern California
Los Angeles, CA, USA

Kenneth J. Hoffer
St. Mary's Eye Center
Santa Monica, CA, USA

Stein Eye Institute, UCLA
Los Angeles, CA, USA

Giacomo Savini
G.B. Bietti Foundation
I.R.C.C.S., Rome
Rome, Italy

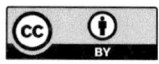

ISSN 1612-3212   ISSN 2196-890X   (electronic)
Essentials in Ophthalmology
ISBN 978-3-031-50665-9   ISBN 978-3-031-50666-6   (eBook)
https://doi.org/10.1007/978-3-031-50666-6

The IOL Power Club

This Springer imprint is published by the registered company Springer Nature Switzerland AG
The registered company address is: Gewerbestrasse 11, 6330 Cham, Switzerland

If disposing of this product, please recycle the paper.

Foreword

As an ophthalmology resident, I hated optics. It was confusing, abstract, and positively boring compared to the excitement of restoring sight through microsurgery. Little did I appreciate at that time how critical those mathematical concepts would be to my success as a cataract surgeon.

Advances in surgical techniques and technology have made cataract surgery the safest and most successful procedures in all of medicine. Performing sutureless surgery under topical anesthesia or a femtosecond laser capsulotomy were unimaginable when I trained. The irony is that being unable to appreciate my technical skills, most of my patients judge the success of their cataract surgery by how well they can see without glasses. So, although we rightfully laud the impressive advances in small incision cataract surgery and IOL designs, we tend to overlook the crucial third pillar of our success—the formulas and technology to calculate each patient's IOL power and cylinder. If the preponderance of lectures, videos, chapters, and papers devoted to surgical techniques and IOL technology is any indication, the importance of IOL power calculations remains relatively unsung [1]. And yet the promise of the most expensive and latest refractive IOL designs will not be fulfilled unless the refractive target is achieved.

To further advance the science of IOL power calculation, several leading international experts founded the IOL Power Club (IPC) in 2005. Their annual scientific meetings spanned the globe and spurred greater scientific rigor, collaboration, and innovation within this important discipline. The IPC decided to undertake the audacious challenge of compiling a definitive textbook on IOL power calculation. The result—**Intraocular Lens Calculations**—is an encyclopedic treasure chest of more than 70 different chapters chronicling the history, science, and current clinical state-of-the-art of this field. The table of contents features an international *who's who* of authorities on this subject. Each chapter is a deep dive into topics of clinical importance to all of us. The format provides us with a balanced and practical guide that covers the entire spectrum of technologies and formulas. The developer of nearly every important formula has written the corresponding chapter, which will add to the historical legacy of this textbook.

I would particularly like to commend Ken Hoffer for being a driving force behind both the IPC and this textbook. It takes uncommon passion and determination to create a new medical society or a definitive textbook. Ken and his IPC colleagues and associate editors have now accomplished both for the betterment of our profession. This is not the first time Ken has done this. As an unknown ophthalmologist in private practice, and just 2 years out of residency, Ken founded the American Intra-Ocular Implant Society in 1974. As its first president, he grew this fledgling society into what eventually was renamed the American Society of Cataract and Refractive Surgery (ASCRS) in 1983. In addition to creating the first scientific meeting devoted to IOLs, Ken launched what is now the *Journal of Cataract and Refractive Surgery* as its first editor in 1975. The very first article published was one he wrote on mathematics and computers in IOL power calculation [2]. Completion of this textbook nearly 50 years later further cements Ken's legacy as one of the founding fathers of this indispensable discipline that has benefited every cataract patient for the past five decades.

I would encourage every IOL surgeon to make use of this authoritative, open access resource. Because the need to be proficient with phacoemulsification and IOL designs seems foremost, many surgeons have neglected to invest much time, study, or interest in IOL power calculations. As I noted earlier, this is ironic because the most common reason that patients are unhappy with flawless cataract surgery is that they don't see well without glasses. That so many patients now pay a premium for better refractive outcomes makes mastery of IOL power calculations more important than ever.

My own career has given me the context to truly appreciate the significance of modern biometry and formulas. I performed nearly 20 intracapsular cataract extractions as a resident and prescribed aphakic spectacles and contact lenses. Those experiences made our first posterior chamber IOL implantations seem miraculous. Because we didn't yet have biometry at our Veterans Administration Hospital, we gave most patients a 19.5 diopter IOL and raised or lowered the power based on the patient's preoperative spectacle prescription. For my first 15 years in practice (until commercial approval of optical biometry), I personally performed applanation A-scan biometry on every patient, knowing that I couldn't trust my staff to avoid corneal compression. I dutifully optimized my personal A-constants with 2-variable formulas for which we manually entered data into a rudimentary software program.

So it is from this perspective that I'd like to salute the editors and authors of this textbook whose collective contributions have been no less important than our best surgical and IOL technologies in achieving patient satisfaction. These individuals who have quietly committed their efforts to the science and betterment of IOL power calculations are the unsung heroes of modern cataract surgery. Remember this every time that your grateful cataract patients thank you because they are thrilled by how well they see without glasses.

References

1. Kane JX, Chang DF. Intraocular lens power formulas, biometry, and intraoperative aberrometry: a review. Ophthalmology. 2021;128:e94–e114.
2. Hoffer KJ. Mathematics and computers in intraocular lens calculation. J Cataract Refract Surg (AIOIS J). 1975;1(1):3.

Los Altos, CA, USA   David F. Chang

Preface

What started in 2005 as a chance meeting of four formula authors (Aramberri, Haigis, Hoffer and Olsen) immediately grew to six (Norrby and Shammas) and led to annual bicontinental meetings in unique settings that combined intense scientific discussion, great camaraderie and friendship and a powerful zeal to improve the accuracy of IOL power calculation. This subject can be intense and complicated and often not a pastime for most of the eye surgeons of the world, but the subject is the essence of successful cataract/IOL surgery for all of our patients.

The IOL Power Club (IPC) has considered several methods to foster dissemination of information to inform our colleagues of the best and most up-to-date methods to improve accuracy in IOL power calculation such as scientific meetings, IPC didactic courses at ASCRS and ESCRS and collaborative studies by international colleagues. It became obvious to us that it would be beneficial to produce a textbook covering every aspect of this subject from all experts in the field as well as industry which could be immediately available Open Access (free) to any eye surgeon anywhere in the world at the touch of a button.

We have to thank the many people who have aided us in our efforts over the years, especially the many colleagues that have contributed their time and ideas to our meetings, those who felt an obligation to sponsor our efforts, especially Jim Mazzo of AMO/Zeiss who kept us going in the early days, Joerg Iwanczuk of Oculus who remained faithful and reminded us of our goals as well as the many corporate sponsors who have supported us, not only financially but by contributing pertinent scientific input and collaborattion.

We hope anyone interested in this subject or in need of information will find something of value and perhaps it will stimulate some to help contribute to this half-century goal of perfection in IOL power prediction.

Santa Monica, CA, USA   Kenneth J. Hoffer

Acknowledgments

By Kenneth J Hoffer MD FACS

Wolfgang Haigis PhD at the IOL Power Club Scientific Meeting in Haarlem, Netherlands, in 2013.

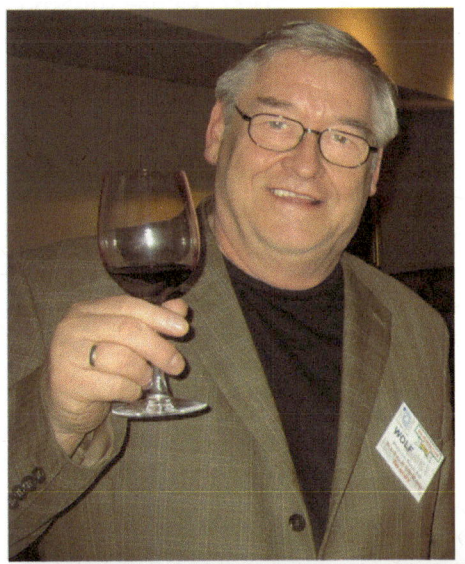

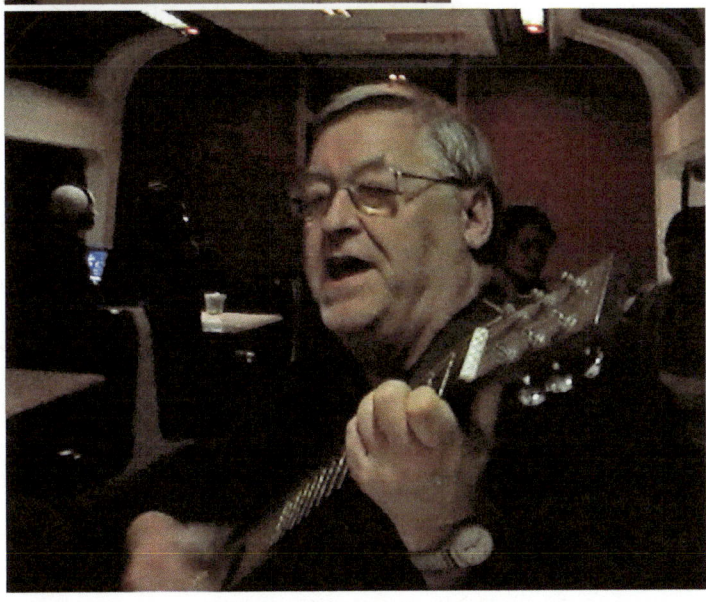

Wolfgang Haigis was born in Stuttgart, Germany on May 30, 1947. He attended Schillerschule in Stuttgart-Bad Cannstatt from 1954 to 1958 and Gottlieb-Daimler Gymnasium in the same city from 1958 to 1962. He then moved to Würzburg to attend High School at the Naturwissenschaftlich-Neusprachliches Röntgengymnasium from 1962 to 1967.

In 1968, he began his academic studies at the Julius-Maximilians-University in Würzburg receiving his PhD diploma on July 5, 1974. He began his work at the Eye Clinic at the University of Würzburg on June 1, 1977 and received a promotion at the university on July 19, 1980. He became a Professor of Ophthalmology at the university's eye department.

Few knew that when Wolf was a student and also at the beginning of his career, he worked as a DJ in a disco in the little village of Eibelstadt just outside Würzburg (Photo: Wolff singing on the train from Chicago to Memphis in 2012 during the IPC Meeting). He was very popular, especially with the girls.

Wolf married Katharina Haigis on May 8, 1987. Katrine still works as a lawyer in a small law office in Hassfurt (her birthplace) practicing family and criminal law.

Wolf, as a physicist, began working on immersion ultrasound measurements of the eye prior to cataract surgery at the clinic. When he was approached in the mid-1990s by Carl Zeiss Meditech to help them set up the first optical biometer (the IOLMaster), he recognized that the instrument results for axial eye length had to match that of immersion ultrasound to allow its use with conventional formulas. His concept worked smoothly and led to the IOLMaster becoming the Gold Standard for biometry. All subsequent optical biometers followed his standard.

Wolf gave over 490 lectures on these subjects all over the world and put on over 158 courses, many at the European Society of Cataract and Refractive Surgery (ESCRS) meetings and of the latter he was most proud of them. He was the author of 188 scientific publications. He was a founding member of Technology in Medicine and Healthcare (TIMUG) and in 2009 was awarded the first Science Prize by the German-speaking Society for Intraocular Lens Implantation, Interventional and Refractive Surgery (DGII). He was inducted as a member of the International Intraocular Implant Club (IIIC) in 2008.

Because there was a need for cataract/IOL surgeons to have access to the latest intraocular lens (IOL) constants when calculating IOL powers, in October 1999, Wolf set up a website with these values that he personally calculated from series of cases sent to him by surgeons from around the world. He called the site the ULIB (User Group for Laser Interference Biometry), and it became used by all surgeons and manufacturers around the world. He did this for no financial reward.

In 2000, he published his formula for IOL power which eschewed the use of corneal power, replacing it with preoperative anterior chamber depth and using three lens constants. The results using his formula have been excellent over these past 20 years. He also developed the Haigis L formula for calculations in eyes that have had previous laser refractive surgery which has also been very successful.

In 2005, he joined five colleagues (Aramberri, Hoffer, Norrby, Olsen, Shammas) to form the IOL Power Club (IPC) and served as its Treasurer from 2005 to 2013. He was elected President for his 2013 to 2015 tenure. He participated in all the activities of the club until his illness began and he missed his first meeting in 2017. At great difficulty, he attended his last meeting in St. Pete Beach, FL in 2018. The IPC has always been very important and dear to him and the club instituted the Haigis Lecture at its annual meetings; the first being given in Napa, CA by David Chang MD only 5 days before he passed away in his sleep on October 15, 2019. The lecture has since been renamed the Haigis Memorial Lecture.

Wolf was a very warm individual and paid attention to everyone who wished to talk to him. He loved anything Italian (including his ancient Fiat he called his "bella la machina") as well as red wine but especially Irish coffees. He was a close personal friend of mine for the past 25 years and I will miss him very much. He is survived by his lovely wife Katharina and his son Michael.

Here are the personal thoughts of what Wolfgang Haigis meant to us.

Giacomo Savini MD:

Having the opportunity to know Wolfgang has been one of the greatest gifts I have received from the IPC. From the very first time I met him in 2007 to the last time I helped him fly back from Florida to Germany in 2018, I realized I had a new friend that was available to teach me his monumental knowledge with no secrets and in a very kind manner. And, when we were not talking about IOL power, he always loved to share social moments with me and all other IPC members. One of the sweetest persons I ever met.

Thomas Olsen MD:

Wolfgang was something special. I first met Wolfgang when he invited me to join his biometry course at the German Congress of Ophthalmic Surgeons (DOC) in Nuremberg. This was the time of ultrasound biometry, and the subject was perhaps not as sexy as it is today. As we all now know, he would become the mastermind of the clinical implementation of optical biometry. His background in physics made him a solid figure in the ophthalmic world, and we are deeply grateful to him for his scientific work. He impressed me with his scientific approach, showing no compromise as to what he felt was the optimal solution. If he disagreed, he often would say "it's rubbish" and shake his head in a convincing way. Although he was a proud person, he was also a very sociable and gentle person, who cared very much for his family. Apart from flying (as a pilot), he had a soft spot for music. Some of us have had the privilege to enjoy Wolfgang playing the guitar singing Bob Dylan and Beatles evergreens all night long. The most enjoyable time.

Jaime Aramberri MD:

Professor Haigis was one of my scientific references as I was a young ophthalmologist interested in ocular biometry and IOL power calculations. His work was fundamental for the implementation of optical biometry, and his formula has been one of my favorites for many years. It made my surgeries much better as the refractive goal was very accurate. Then in 2004, I met Wolfgang when I was introduced by Ken Hoffer and he turned out to be an enthusiastic, friendly, and open scientist who spread his knowledge selflessly, always making an extra effort to make me fully understand. He was patient and comprehensive with me knowing that I did not have his background in physics. Over the many years, I knew Wolf to be a warm person to share some drinks with, listen to good music and chat about life. We both liked the British pop and the American rock of the 1960s. Sometimes he was not in the mood and looked a bit grumpy. But it was just a pose. He had a big heart and everyone who knew him well will miss him forever.

H. John Shammas MD:

I first met Wolf at the 12th SIDUO Congress held in Iguazú Falls, Argentina in 1988. He was a young scientist on his honeymoon. We socialized together the entire week and got to know his lovely bride, Katharina. It was the meeting of the International Society of Ophthalmic Ultrasound. At that meeting, he presented his work on the performance of different transducers in biometry, and he discussed the clinical usefulness of linking biometry systems to personal computers. He was definitely ahead of his time.

Through the years, we got to know him better. He was a pioneer and a driving force in developing optical biometry. His deep knowledge of human optics led him to develop his famous Haigis formula. He even contributed a chapter on the subject for my book on IOL Power Calculation which turned out to be the only place where you can note all the details of his formula. Wolfgang was a gentle person and full of life. He was a dear friend... God rest his soul.

Sverker Norrby PhD:

I first met Wolfgang in 1985, when he came to see me at what was then Medical Workshop, Groningen, Netherlands which had just been acquired by Pharmacia, Uppsala, Sweden. His quest was to obtain IOL design data for the purpose of IOL power calculation by means of optical calculation. The nonoptical SRK regression formula was widely in use at the time. After that visit, I was convinced that optical calculation was the way to go. Sometime later, I went to see Wolfgang in his lab at Würzburg University. He taught me the ins-and-outs of ultrasound sonography of the eye, and also in-depth keratometry. I learned how to distinguish good data from bad. In 1999, when the IOLMaster appeared, I once again went to see Wolfgang to learn exactly how it worked. When the ACMaster appeared, he again patiently explained its mode of action and how to avoid its pitfalls. I am deeply indebted to Wolfgang for all this knowledge. And even more for our friendship through all these years.

Kenneth J Hoffer MD:

I had developed a very early fond relationship with Wolf, and it was always a pleasure when we had the chance to get together. I remember him trying to unsuccessfully teach me matrix math and taking such special care of Marcia and I when we visited them in Würzburg. His genuine warmth to me is what I most remember and he comes into my thoughts every time I am doing something related to the IPC. I can't think of anyone else like him and I miss him very much.

Contents

Part VI Special Situations

Part I

Introduction

The History of the IOL Power Club: 2005–2025

1

Kenneth J. Hoffer

2004: The Origins of the IOL Power Club—How It All Started

The IOL Power Club began because of a happenstance meeting on the last day of the ASCRS meeting in San Diego on May 4, 2004. Thomas Olsen, MD (Århus, Denmark), had visited me in Santa Monica for 2 days prior to the meeting. On the last day of the meeting, he asked me to meet him in the large conference area to discuss the study we were working on. While we were chatting, Jaime Aramberri, MD (San Sebastian, Spain), was passing by and I called him over to introduce him to Dr. Olsen. A remarkably interesting discussion ensued regarding ELP determination. Ten minutes later, Wolfgang Haigis, PhD (Würzburg, Germany), was lugging his bags across the other side of the large room and waved goodbye to me. I waved him over and introductions were made, and then the discussion by the four of us became even more interesting.

I sat back for a moment and realized that this was an amazing interaction among us four IOL power fanatics that was a unique opportunity. But since everyone was on their way home, I suggested that we continue this discussion at some future time when we would have more opportunity to fully discuss these subjects. Since the next ESCRS meeting (that I would be attending) was going to be held in Lisbon, Portugal, in September 2005, I suggested that we might meet somewhere prior to that. Since I love San Sebastian (I first visited in 2001), I asked Dr. Aramberri if he would be willing to host the get-together in his city. He embraced the idea wholeheartedly.

After we returned home, we had all exchanged email addresses and subsequent correspondence led to Dr. Olsen inviting Sverker Norrby, PhD (Groningen, Holland), and me inviting H John Shammas, MD (Los Angeles, CA), to join the meeting if they were interested. They both said they were and they made plans to take part. Being very busy, I did very little to get things moving over the remainder of 2004 and even into 2005. My wife, Marcia, continuously asked me if I had done anything to follow up on this meeting, but I just never got to it. It was only due to her constant persistence and reminders that I finally restarted the email correspondence to get things rolling again. Marcia felt this was a very special idea and it should definitely come to pass; for some reason, this seemed important in her mind. I must admit, without her perseverance, we might never have gotten together. Through email, the dates for the first meeting were set for September 6–8, 2005.

K. J. Hoffer (✉)
St. Mary's Eye Center, Santa Monica, CA, USA

Stein Eye Institute, UCLA, Los Angeles, CA, USA
e-mail: KHofferMD@StartMail.com

© The Author(s) 2024
J. Aramberri et al. (eds.), *Intraocular Lens Calculations*, Essentials in Ophthalmology,
https://doi.org/10.1007/978-3-031-50666-6_1

The Club and By-Laws

The following year, Marcia and I were traveling in France for 3 months prior to the ESCRS meeting. Two weeks before driving to San Sebastian, I had thought it might be of interest to form a private club to have an organizational structure to continue such meetings in the future. In the city of Vézelay, France, I had to stay up very late on August 9, 2005, to make a 4 a.m. tele-conference meeting in the USA. In a nearby restaurant called Le Cheval Blanc (below), I wrote a potential set of by-laws, which we later called the "Rules of Vézelay".

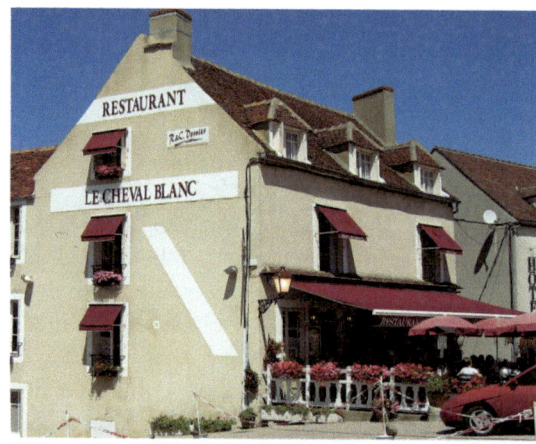

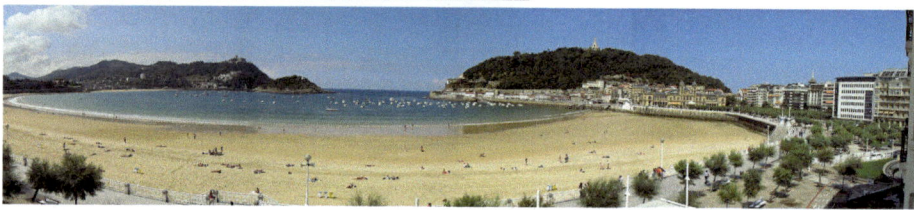

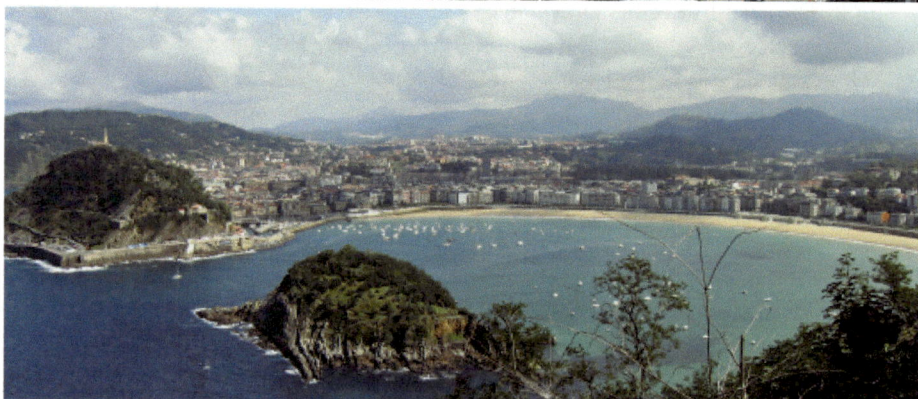

2005: First IPC Meeting—San Sebastian, Spain, September 6–8, Abba Londres y de Inglaterra Hotel

First Meeting

We all arrived in San Sebastian on September 6, 2005. Below are photos of the very first IPC get-together in the lobby of the Londres Hotel and Jaime then showed us his beautiful city (especially the Old Town) and we had an evening of eating tapas (pinxtos in Basque language).

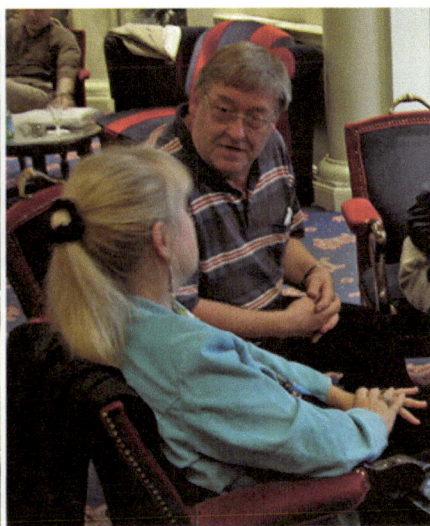

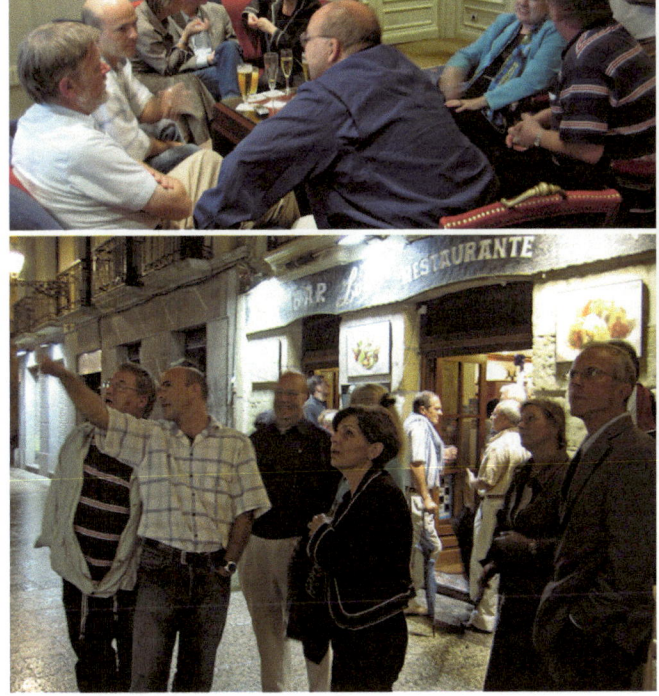

The next day, we held our first scientific meeting at Dr. Aramberri's BegiTeck Clinica which was an easy walk from the hotel. We held an organizational session, discussed, and carefully edited the proposed by-laws I had submitted, printed them out, and all six of us agreed and signed them. Thus, the IOL Power Club was officially formed, not by any planned or preconceived intention, but purely by happenstance.

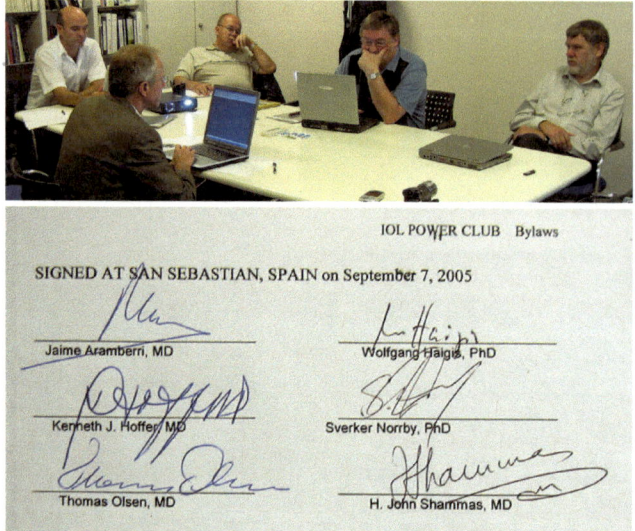

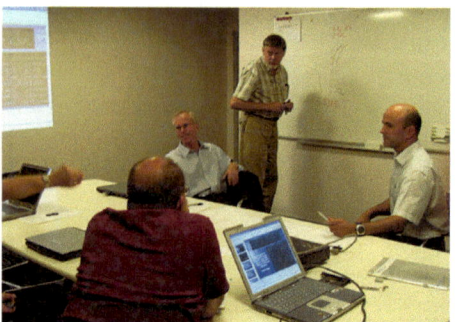

First Officers: Per our new by-laws, we elected officers for a 2-year term: Jaime Aramberri as Vice-President, Thomas Olsen as Secretary, Wolfgang Haigis as Treasurer, and they forced me to be President. We agreed that Executive Committee (EC) members could invite new members, but there was no interest or intention that the Club grow into some large Society; this was heavily stressed by both Haigis and I. The requirements for membership were an MD or PhD degree, long-term interest in IOL Power calculation, and ample evidence of publications, research, and teaching in this subject. It was also agreed, because of the importance of the social interactions of the Club, that if a minimum of one member of the EC did not approve a new member, they would not be admitted. The EC decided that it would hold annual scientific sessions alternating between the USA and the EU. We elected Syvatoslav Fyodorov, MD (Moscow, Russia, deceased), Hermann Gernet, MD (Germany), and John Retzlaff, MD (Medford, OR USA), as Honorary members.

The next day, we participated in a taped video interview session (below) requested by Alcon, Spain, which they wanted to use for educational purposes. In return, they became the very first Sponsor of IPC. We began the session with Dr. Aramberri (as host) moderating and each of us made presentations.

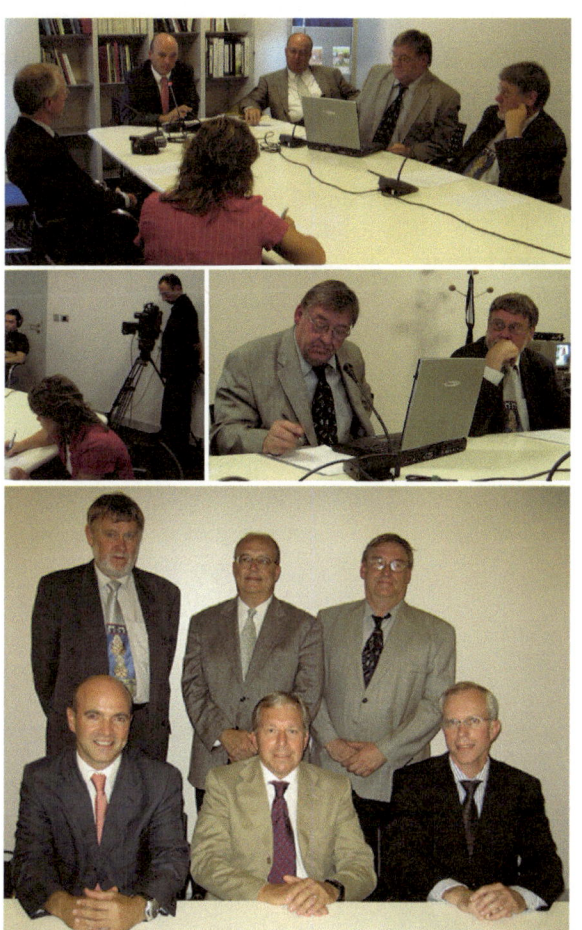

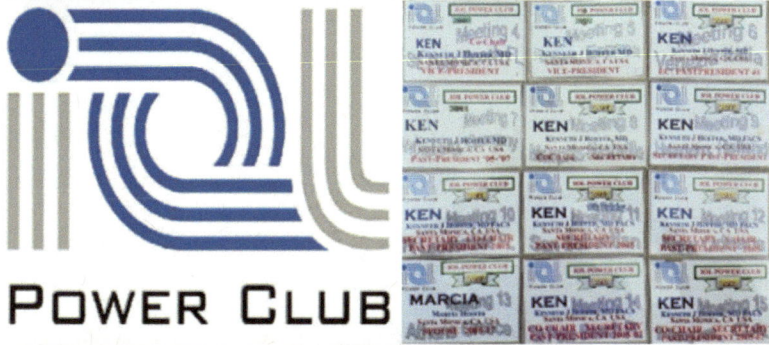

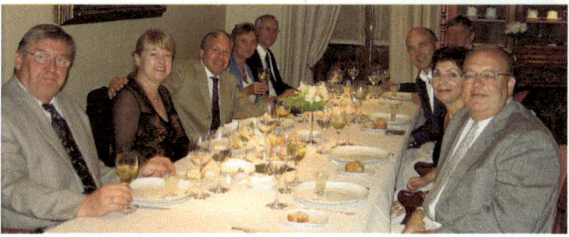

Since we were all professionally dressed, they asked us to take a group photograph (above). This was a once-in-a-lifetime event. We ended the meeting with a celebratory dinner Jamie arranged at Arzak restaurant (above). The best part was the great sense of trust and camaraderie that developed among the six of us. We all agreed not to "borrow" each other's ideas. Jaime had successfully arranged a wonderful meeting that would be very hard to repeat. Over the following year, Jaime engaged an artist to produce a logo for the Club (above). We used it to create name badges, which we have used ever since our second meeting (above right, badges of 12 meetings).

2006: Second IPC Meeting—Carmel, CA, March 22–25, Pine Inn Hotel

Our next meeting was scheduled for Carmel, CA, after the ASCRS meeting in San Francisco. Dr. Shammas and I agreed to Co-Chair our first US meeting, and we held our scientific sessions on the second floor deck room of the Pine Inn Hotel. John Retzlaff attended with his wife, Tommi. Unbeknownst to any of us, Dr. Norrby had informed Han Bor Fam, MD (Singapore) about the meeting and to my surprise, he showed up. He has attended every single IPC meeting (except 2) since then. Below is the schedule for this meeting (the first time we ever prepared one). There were not many of us so, we only had one large table to sit at and make our presentations (photo of Shammas, Hoffer and Aramberri).

	WED Mar 22	THUR Mar 23	FRI Mar 24	SAT Mar 25	SUN Mar 26
8:00	ASCRS SF MAR 18-22 Last Day	Breakfast: Little Swiss Café	Breakfast: Katy's	Open Breakfast: Your Choice	Open Breakfast: Your Choice
9:30		Session I** Industry Standards 1 1) US Biometry 2) Optical Biometry	Session III Industry Standards 3 4) Keratometry	Session V Finalization of Physiologic Eye Model 2 / Carmel Tour: Tor House	Session VII Plenary Session Preferred Practice Patterns
12:30		Lunch*	Lunch*	Lunch*	*Recommended Lunch Places
2:00	DRIVE to Carmel 2-3 Hours PINE INN Ocean Ave See MAP	Session II*** Industry Standards 2 3) IOL Power Labeling	Session IV**** Physiologic Eye Model 1 / Trip to MacDonald Foundry	Session VI Business Mtg / Monterey Movie Tour By Bus	Village Corner O'Faherity's Fish Little Swiss Café Jack London's Hog's Breath Il Forniao
5:00	Check in before 5:30 Pine Inn	FREE			

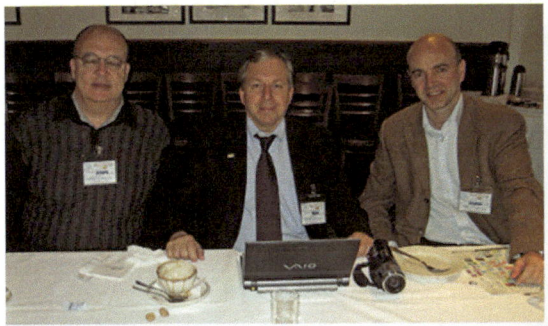
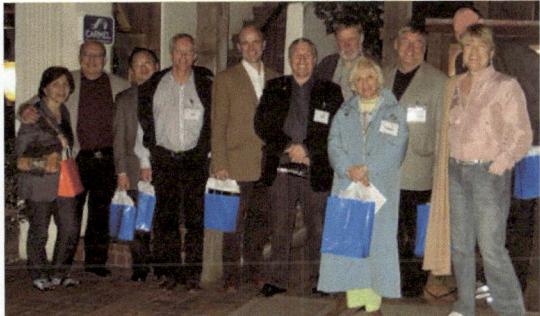
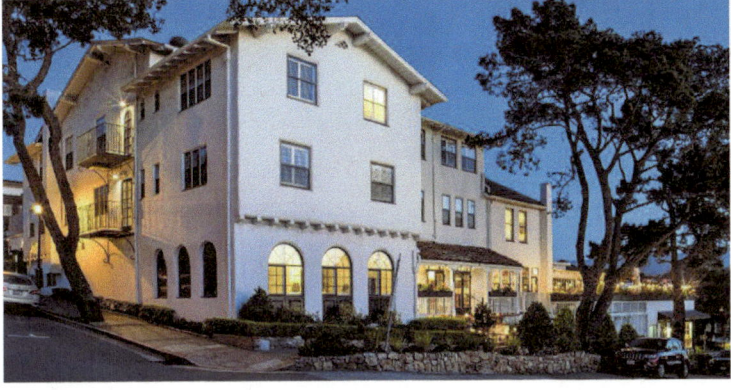
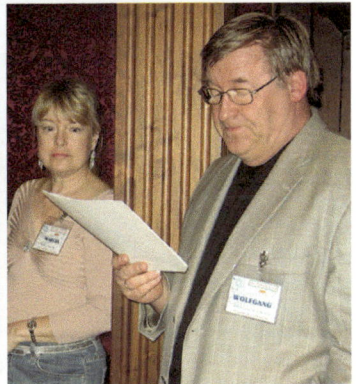

Above is the Pine Inn. Attendees: For the first time, we invited more people from the industry including from Alcon: Shane Dunne, PhD, Charlie Campbell, Eric Storne, and Steve Van Noy as well as Claus Dreher from Carl Zeiss Meditec that joined as Sponsors. The meeting was of high caliber and very successful. The EC got a group photo in front of the famous "Lone Pine" (EC with John & Tommi Retzlaff and Han Bor Fam).

2007: First Independent IPC EC Meeting—San Diego, CA April 28 Croce's Restaurant

The EC decided to hold their first independent meeting in San Diego prior to the 2007 Aarhus meeting. It was there that we invited Jean-Philippe Colliac (Paris, France) for the first time and our new member Scott McClatchey (San Diego) (below left) joined us.

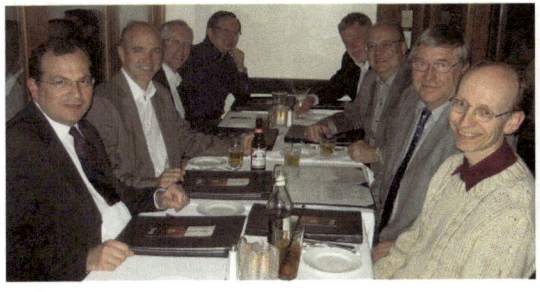
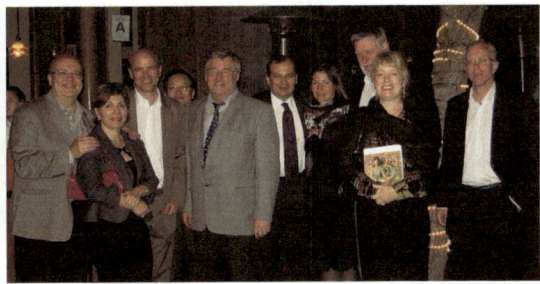

2007: Third IPC Meeting—Århus, Denmark, September 4–6, Hotel Royal

Our next meeting was to be near the September 2007 ESCRS meeting in Stockholm, Sweden. We decided to have our meeting in Århus, Denmark, with Drs. Olsen and Norrby as Co-Chairmen. They chose our venue at the Hotel Royal. We were pleased to have AMO join Alcon and Zeiss in participating in the meeting, thanks to its CEO, Jim Mazzo. Dr. Olsen scheduled an excellent meeting. Invited speakers for the first time were Gabor Koranyi, MD (Växjö, Sweden), Oliver Findl, MD (Vienna, Austria), and Giacomo Savini, MD (Bologna, Italy, below right). Wolfgang brought his wife Katrine and son Michael (below center).

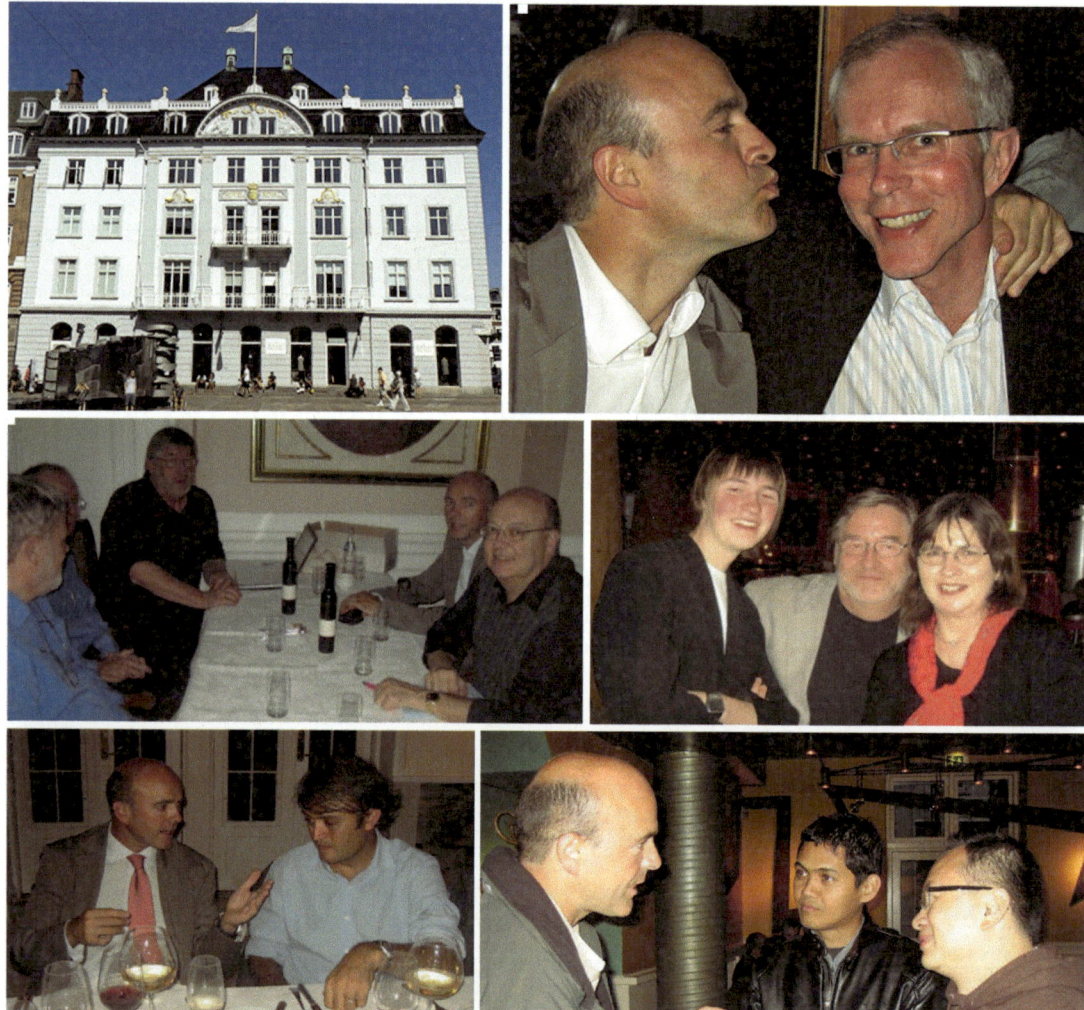

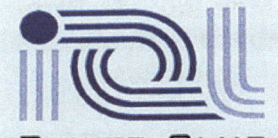

IOL Power Club meeting

September 4 - 7, 2007 in Aarhus, Denmark

Scientific Programme

Program	TUE SEP 4	WED SEP 5	THUR SEP 6	FRI SEP 7	SAT SEP 8
8:00		Breakfast at	Breakfast at	Breakfast at	Breakfast at
8:30		hotel	hotel	hotel	hotel (if wanted)
9:00		**Session I:**	**Session III:**	**Session V**	
9:30		Arni Sicam:	S Norrby: Power	Gabor Koranyi:	
10:00		Aspects of the	calculation	Another	Departure for
10:30		Oliver Stachs:	Oliver Findl:		ESCRS
11:00		Exploring the	Optical biometry	member	Stockholm
11:30		member	member	presentations	
12:00		presentations	presentations		
12:30		Lunch at hotel	Lunch at hotel	Lunch at hotel	
1:00					
1:30		**Session II:**	**Session IV:**	**Business**	
2:00				**Mtg**	
2:30	Arrival and	member			
3:00	Check in Hotel	presentations	member		
3:30	Royal before		presentations		
4:00	5:30 PM			departure for	
4:30				ESCRS	
5:00		Social event	Grand dinner		
06:00:00 +	Get together		EC members		

The titles and timing are subject to change

Suggested themes for remaining time:
How to rid of A-constants
Surgically induced astigmatism
Optimization
ACD methods
Ray tracing
Comparison of formulas
Post-LASIK methods

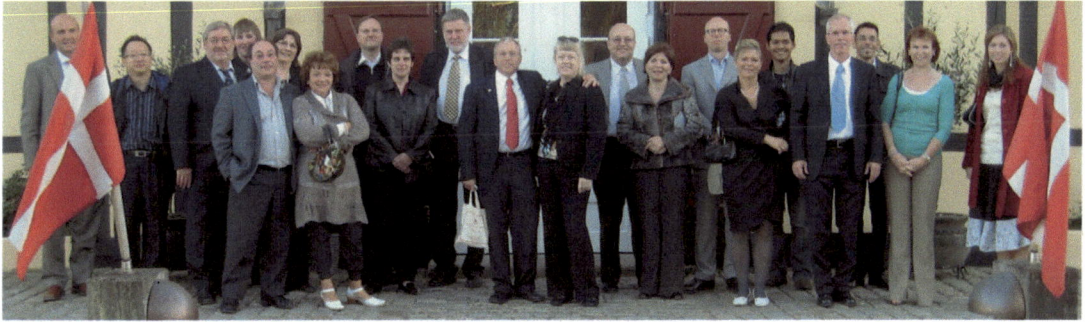

We had a group shot taken of all the attendees (above). Arnie Sicam PhD and Han Bor Fam joined us. After 2 years in office, it was time for an election. We finally cajoled Aramberri to agree to be elected President, and I agreed to serve as Vice-President. Olsen was again elected Secretary as was Haigis as Treasurer. We unanimously elected Oliver Findl, Gabor Koranyi, and Giacomo Savini as members and Rob Van der Heijde, PhD (Amsterdam, Holland), as an Honorary Member. Jaime thanked Tom for organizing an excellent meeting.

2008: Fourth IPC Meeting—St. Pete Beach, FL, November 12–16, Tradewinds Island Grand Resort

Our fourth Scientific Meeting was held after the AAO Meeting in Atlanta, GA. This became our longest and largest meeting thus far. This is the first year we had sign posters made for our meeting Sponsors.

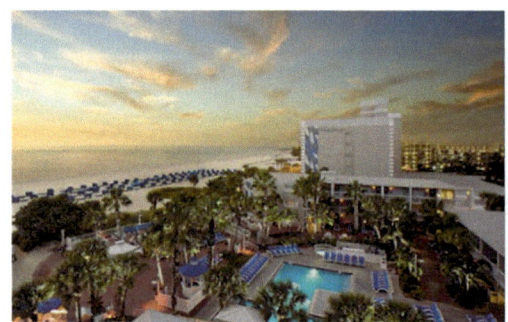
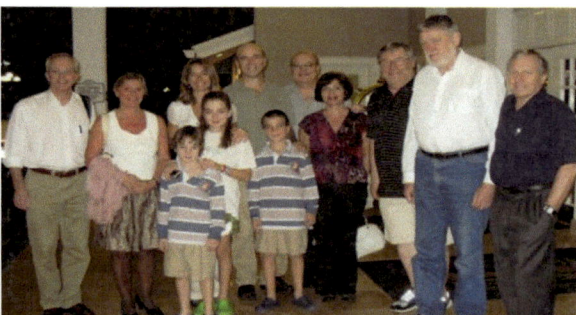
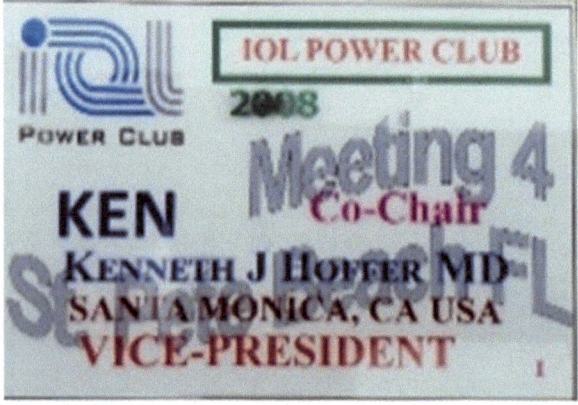

We welcomed our newest Honorary Member, Rob Van der Heijde, PhD (Netherlands), our other new members, Claudio Carbonara, MD (Roma, Italy), Jean-Philippe Colliac, MD (Paris, France), Douglas Koch, MD (Houston, TX), and members Gabor Koranyi, MD (Sweden), John Moran, MD, PhD (Houston, TX), Giacomo Savini, MD, Scott McClatchey, MD, and Han Bor Fam, MD. Our members Oliver Findl, MD (Vienna, Austria), and Massimo Camellin, MD (Rovigo, Italy), were not able to attend.

Below (L-R): Haigis, Aramberri, Norrby, Fam, Van der Heijde, Koch, McClatchey, Moran, He and Wang.

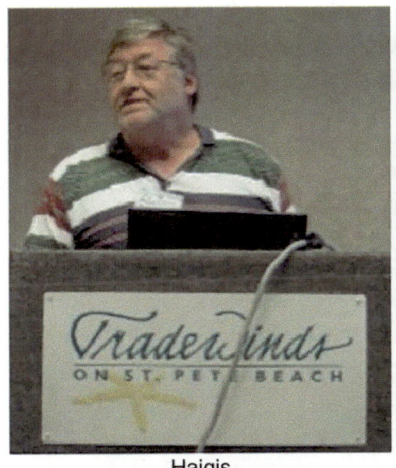

Haigis

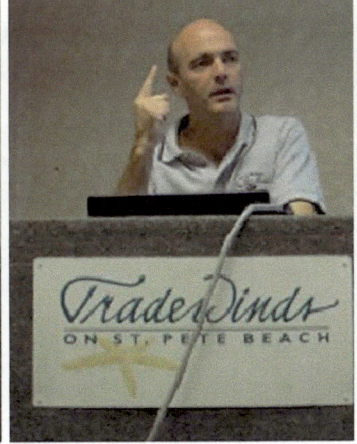

Aramberri

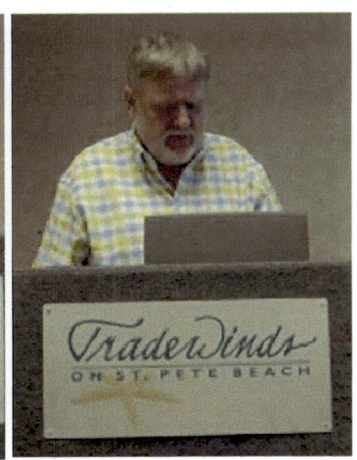

Norrby

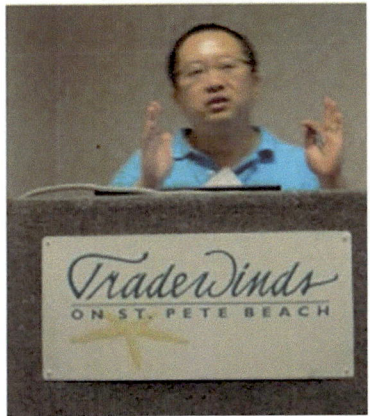

Han Bor Fam

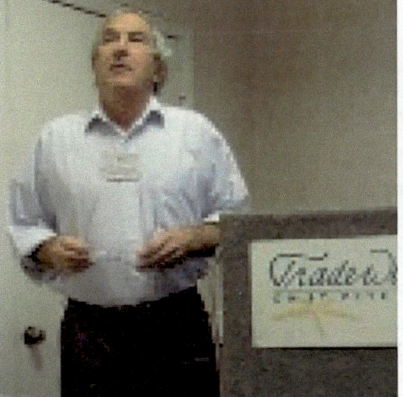

Van der Heidje

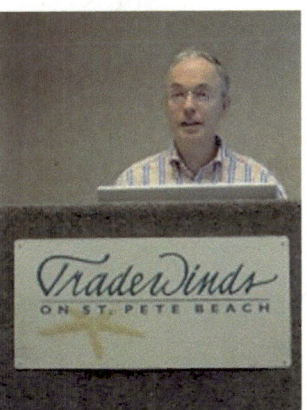

Koch

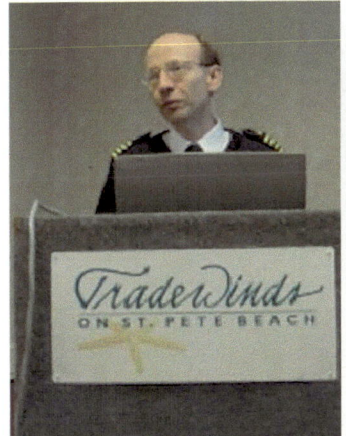

McClatchey

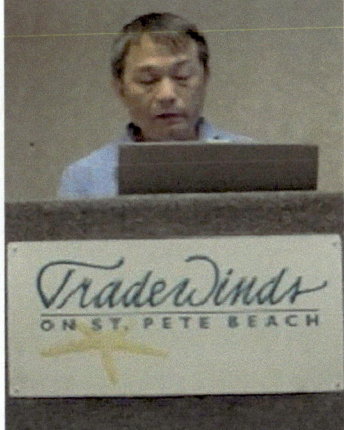

He

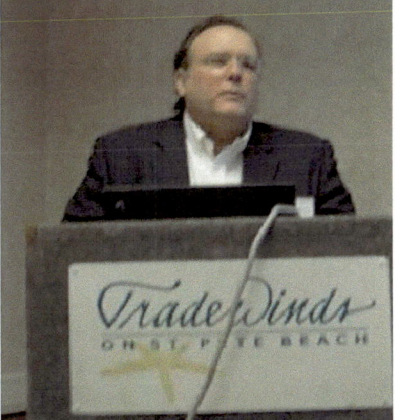

Moran

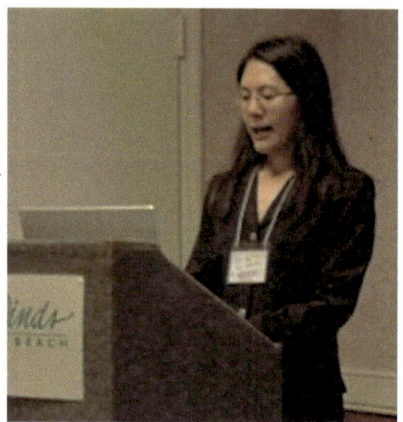

Wang

lent scientific presentations. Invited lecturers this year were Li Wang, MD, PhD (Houston, TX, left) and Ji He, PhD (Boston, MA).

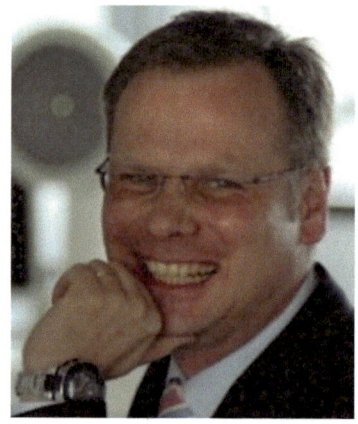

We had return representation from active meeting Sponsors such as **AMO** (Dan Neal, PhD), **Alcon** (Mike Simpson, MD, PhD, and George Pettit, MD, PhD), **Carl Zeiss Meditec** (Claus Dreher and Rudolf Von Buenau), first-time participants **Bausch and Lomb** (Griffith Altman and Gerhard Youssefi), **Haag-Streit** (Ruedi Wätli, PhD), **Ziemer** (Arnoud Snepvangers, Roger Cattin, Cindy Roberts, PhD), and **Oculus** (Jörg Iwanczuk, right). Jörg has participated and sponsored every meeting ever since, even though the EC gave him a hard time at this meeting. Many of them made excel-

Our meetings developed a tradition of treating all physicians, scientists, and members of the industry as equals, eschewing competition, at least during this meeting. Sverker Norrby presented on ACD prediction, and Ken Hoffer presented the first paper on the new Haag-Streit LenStar 900.

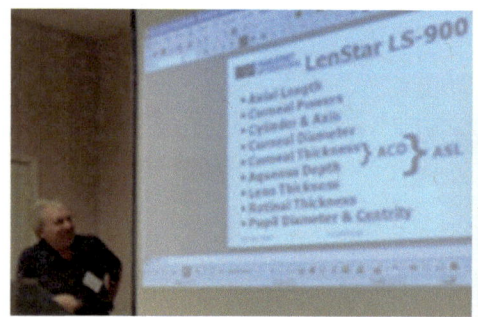

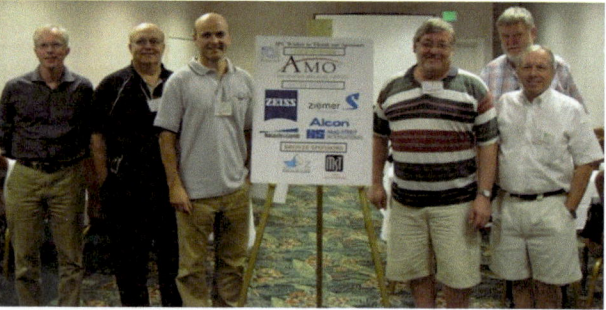

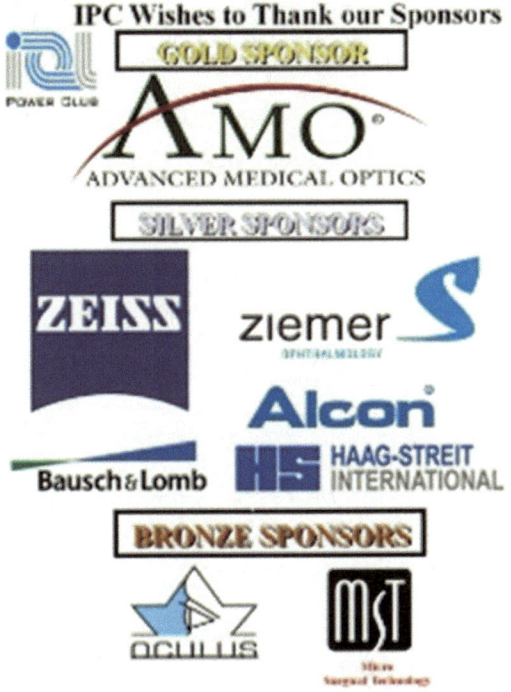

2009: Second IPC Executive Committee Independant Meeting— St. Helena, CA, April 7–9

We had grown in membership and interaction capabilities, so an EC planning session was held in the Napa Valley town of St. Helena after the ASCRS meeting in San Francisco. Dr. Aramberri was unable to attend.

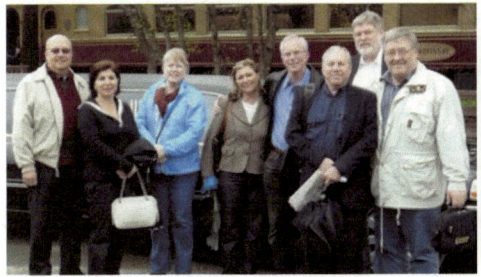
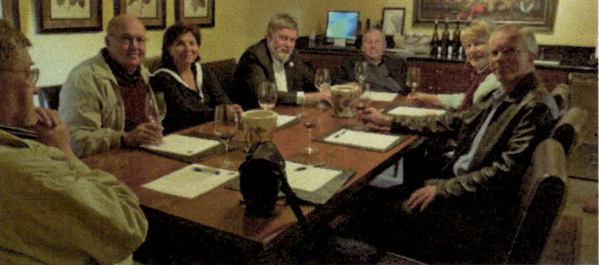

2009: Fifth IPC Meeting—Roses, Spain, September 8–11, Vistabella Hotel

The fifth Scientific Meeting was held at the Vistabell Hotel in the coastal town of Roses, Spain, prior to the ESCRS in Barcelona.

Attendees: New member Massimo Camellin (and his son Umberto), members Claudio Carbonara, Han Bor Fam, Oliver Findl, and Giacomo Savini. **Industry**: Dan Neal (AMO), Rudolf Wätli (Haag-Streit), Claus Dreher (Zeiss), Burkhard Wagner (Zeiss), Steve Van Noy (Alcon), Jörg Iwanczuk (Oculus), and first timer Francesco Versaci (CSO, Italy). Giacomo Savini and I ended the meeting by continuing the work on our collaborative studies.

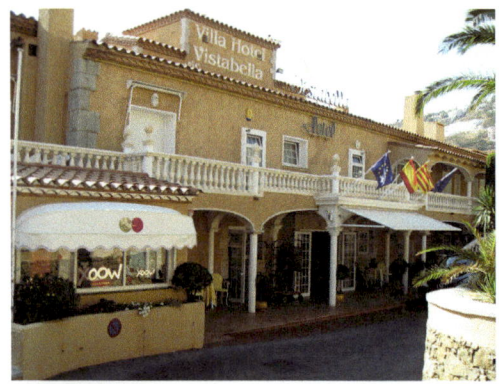
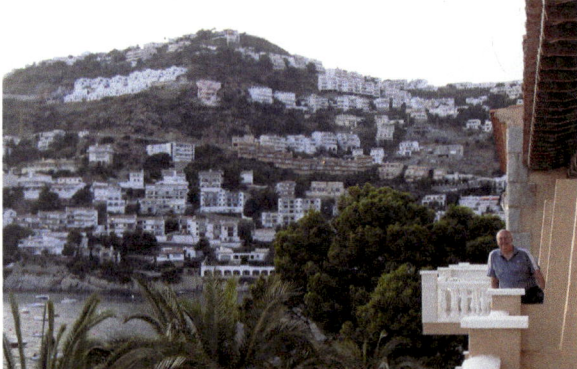
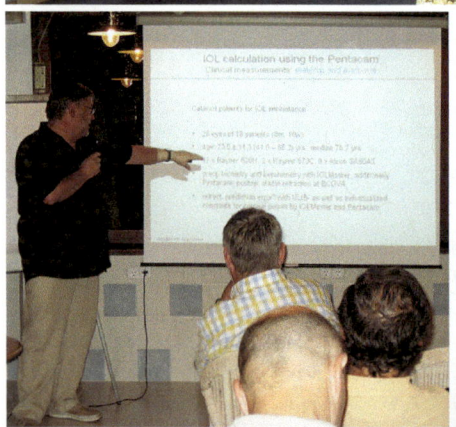
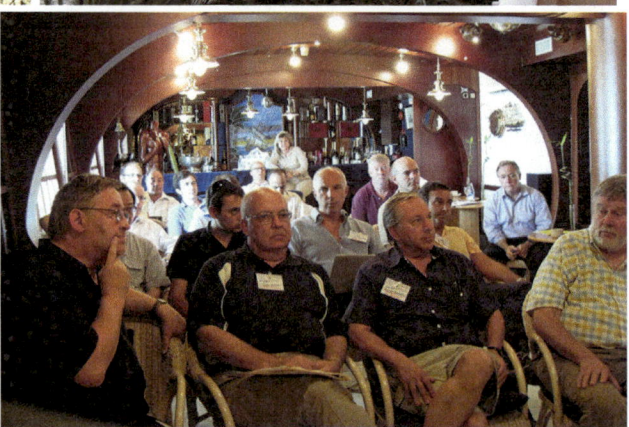
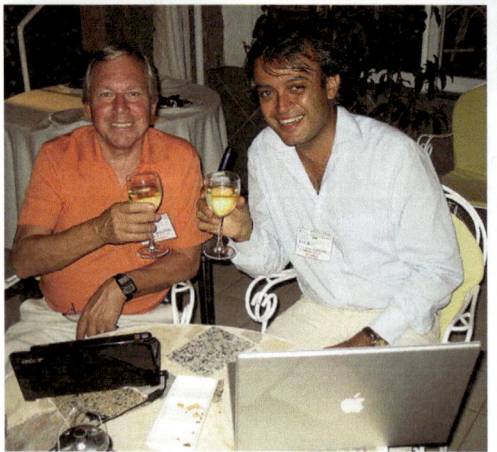

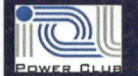 **2009 MEETING PROGRAM**
ROSES, GIRONA, SPAIN
SEPTEMBER 9TH – 11TH

WEDNESDAY, SEPTEMBER 9TH, 2009

9:00-09:15	JAIME ARAMBERRI	OPENING CEREMONY - INTRO OF MEMBERS AND GUESTS
	BIOMETRY SESSION	MODERATOR: KEN HOFFER, V-P
9:15-09:30	JOHN SHAMMAS	LENSTAR 900
9:30-09:45	CLAUDIO CARBONARA	LENSTAR 900 VS IOL MASTER
9:45-10:00	JAIME ARAMBERRI	LENSTAR 900 VS IOL MASTER
0:00-10:15	KEN HOFFER	LENSTAR 900 vs IOL MASTER
0:15-10:30	TOM OLSEN	LENSTAR 900
0:30-10:45	JAIME ARAMBERRI	WHO´S THE FASTEST?
0:45-11:00	RUDOLF WÄLTI	LENSTAR 900: NEW SOFTWARE FEATURES
1:00-11:15	CLAUS DREHER	IOL MASTER: NEW SOFTWARE FEATURES
1:15-11:30	DISCUSSION	

Our third election resulted in Shammas as President, Norrby as Vice-President, Olsen as Secretary, and Haigis as Treasurer. There was discussion by Haigis as to limiting the membership to 20, but it was not passed.

2010: Sixth IPC Meeting—Venice, Italy, August 30 to September 2 Splendid Hotel

This meeting was chaired by Massimo Camellin and Sverker Norrby. The EC Business meeting was fully attended.

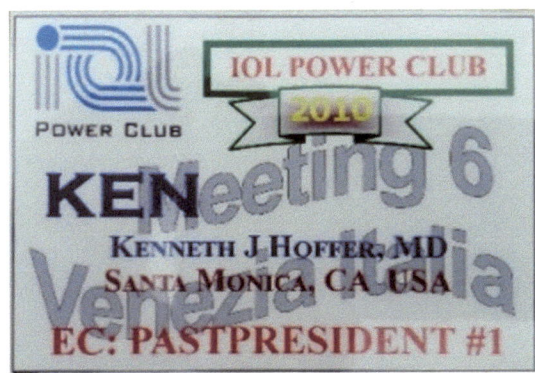

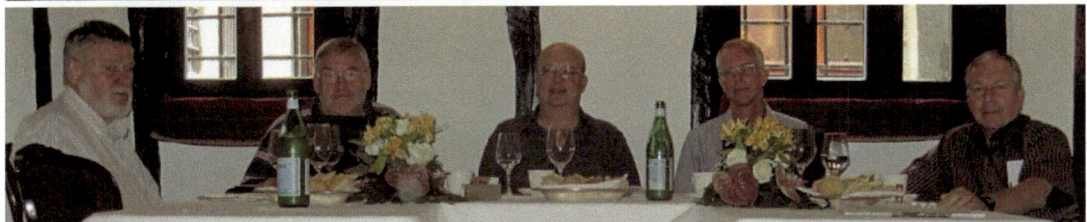

Attendees: **Members**: Edmondo Borasio, Massimo Camellin, Claudio Carbonara, Nino Hirnschall, and Giacomo Savini. **Invited Speakers:** Carmen Canovas, PhD (AMO), and Sean Ianchulev, MD. **Industry**: Jörg Iwanzcuk (Oculus), Jennifer Lewis, PhD (Ziemer), Burkhard Wagner and Tobias Bühren (Zeiss), Rudolf Wätli (Haag-Streit), and Francesco Versaci (CSO).

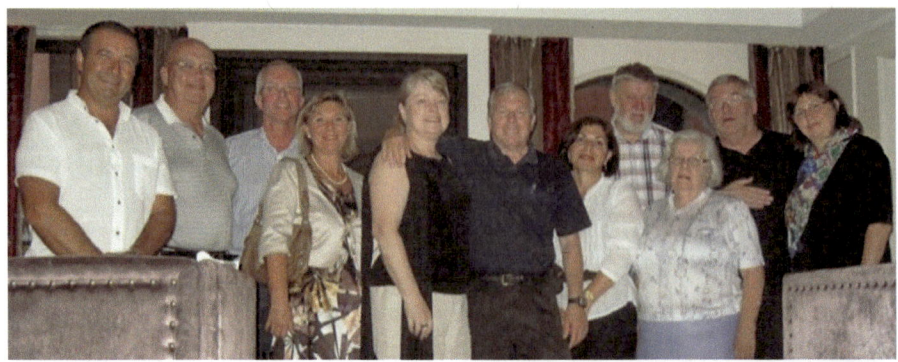

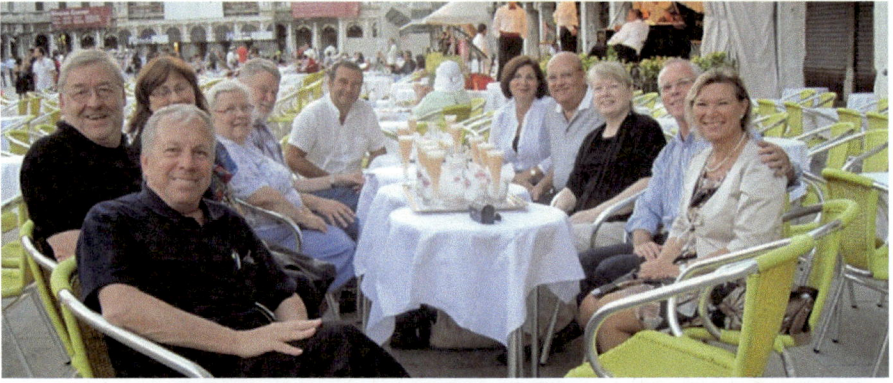

2010 6th IPC MEETING PROGRAM

Chairs:
Massimo Camellin, MD
Sverker Norrby, PhD

MONDAY, AUGUST 30th, 2010

| 18:00-21:00 | IPC WELCOME RECEPTION | Hotel Splendid |
| | All Attendees | Light Hors d'Oeuvres   Not Full dinner   Dinner on your own |

TUESDAY, AUGUST 31st, 2010 DAY #1

9:00-09:15	JOHN SHAMMAS	OPENING CEREMONY - INTRO OF MEMBERS AND GUESTS
	WELCOME	Co-Chairs: Massimo Camellin & Sverker Norrby
	BIOMETRY	**MODERATOR: Wolfgang Haigis**
9:15-09:30	KENNETH HOFFER	COMPARISON OF IOLMASTER AND LENSTAR
9:30-09:45	RUDOLF WÄLTI	LENSTAR KERATOMETRY AND BIOMETRY
9:45-10:00	JÖRG IWANZCUK	LATEST FEATURES OF OCULUS PENTACAM
10:00-10:15	JENNIFER LEWIS	ZIEMER GALILEI FOR POWER CALCULATION
10:15-10:30	BURKHARD WAGNER	ZEISS TORIC IOL WORKFLOW SOLUTION
10:30-10:45	CLAUDIO CARBONARA	THE NEW IOLMASTER 500: MAKE-UP OR UPGRADE?
10:45-11:00	JOHN SHAMMAS	PRECISION OF IOLMASTER MEASUREMENTS
11:00-11:15	GIACOMO SAVINI	TOMEY TMS-5: EVALUATION OF A NEW SCHEIMPFLUG CAMERA
11:15-11:45	**COFFEE BREAK**	

I did my usual introduction of industry attendees which has become a tradition, followed by Session IA "Biometry" moderated by Wolfgang Haigis (below right).

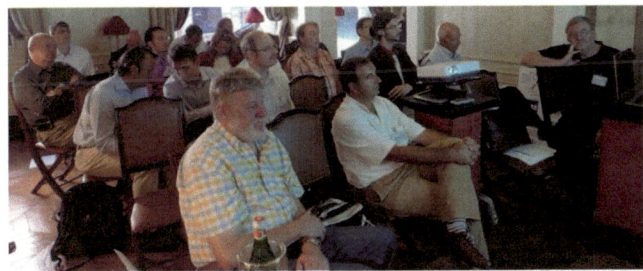 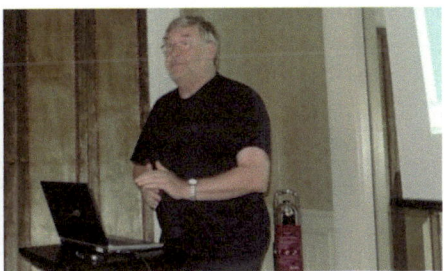

Nino Hirnschall (below left) presented "Influence of IOL Design/Orientation on Decentration and Tilt Measured With A Clinical Purkinjemeter" and Jaime Aramberri (right) on "Lens Thickness Importance In ELP Prediction."

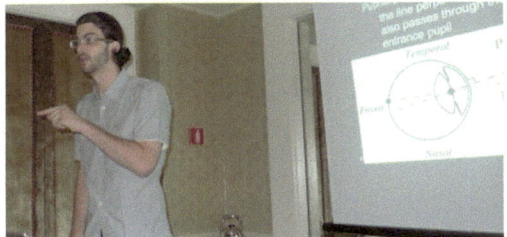 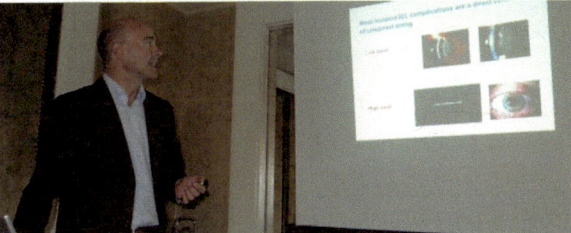

2011: Third EC Independent Meeting Santa Monica, CA March 29-April 2 Le Merigot Hotel

The EC held a Scientific Session following the ASCRS meeting in San Deigo. Jaime Aramberri and Sverker Norrb were not able to attend.

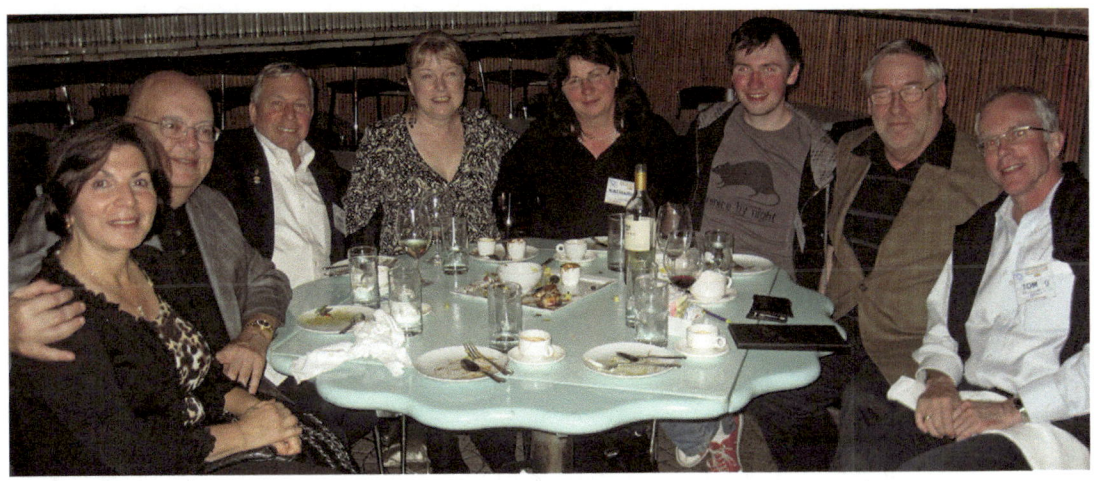

2011: Seventh IPC Meeting— Würzburg, Germany, September 22–25 Steinberg Schloss Hotel

The Meeting was held at the Steinberg Castle and Chaired by Wolfgang Haigis. Our EC Business meeting was held (below left), and our Officers election for 2011–2013 resulted in Norrby as our next President, Olsen as Vice-President, Hoffer as Secretary, and Haigis as Treasurer. Below right are our **Honorary Members**, Drs. Hermann Gernet (left, deceased) and John Retzlaff with his wife Tommi.

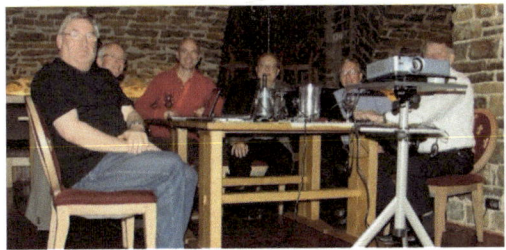

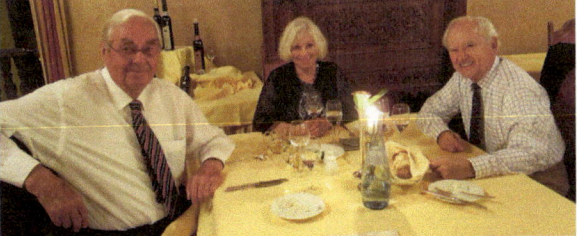

Wolf took the EC for tours (below) before the meeting began. Wolfgang Haigis (below left) opened the meeting welcoming everyone to his city, and then I did my introduction of industry representatives. The lecture room was genuinely nice except for the very large stone column in the center.

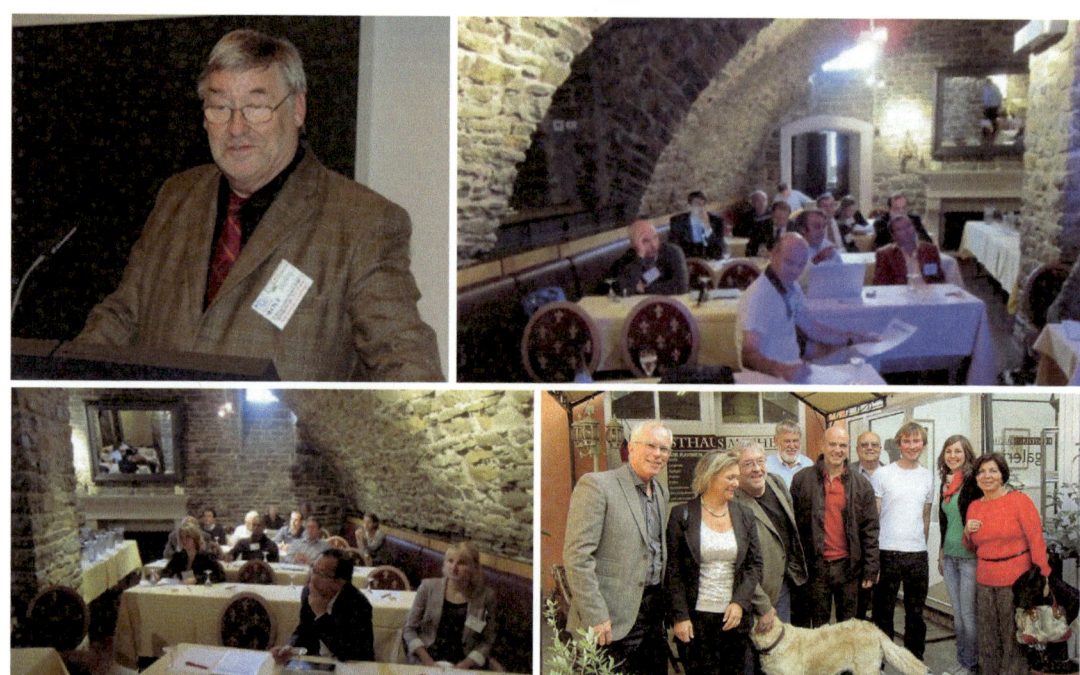

I gave a talk on "A New Take on Corneal Curvatures in RK Eyes," and we welcomed our guest speaker, Thomas Kohnen MD.

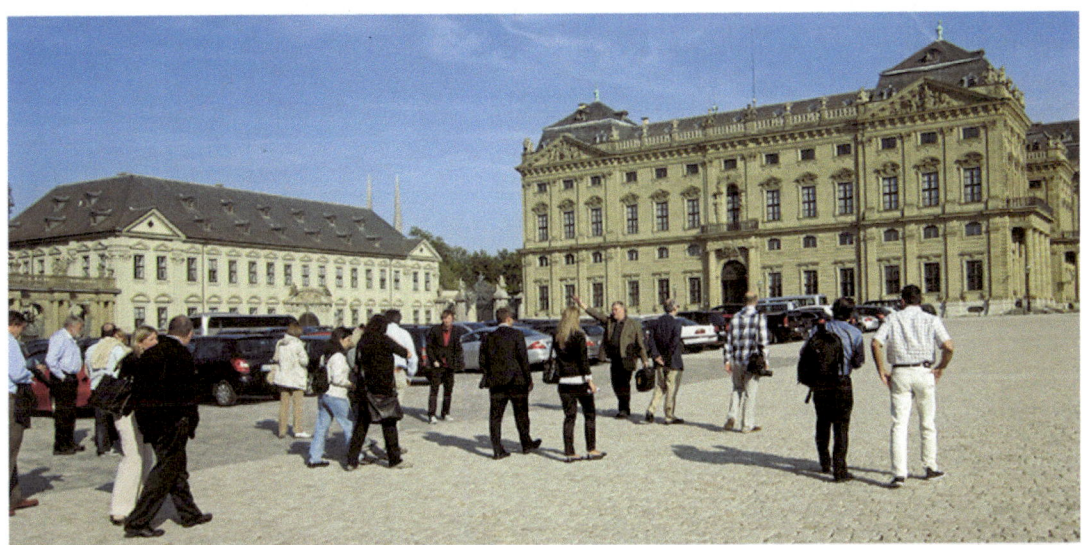

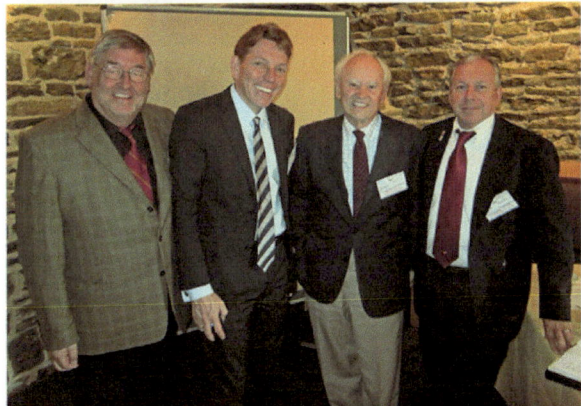 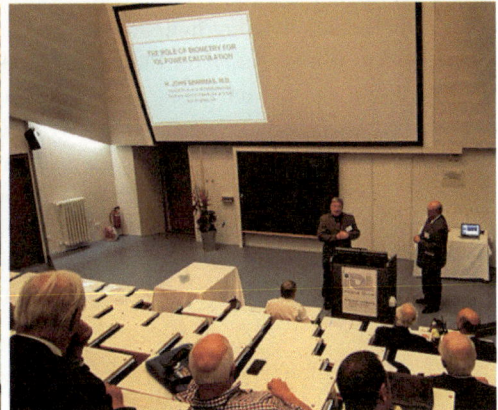

Special Event: Public Honorary Session at the Würzburg University Eye Clinic (Augenklinik) Lecture hall (above right).

At 1:30 p.m., we all took a bus trip to the Würzburg University Augenklinik (Eye Clinic) lecture hall for an Honorary Session with residents and staff of the University attending. This was a very big deal for Wolfgang, in that he was bringing world-renowned authorities to his university. Its purpose was to honor the IPC Honorary members, Gernet and Retzlaff, followed by special lectures given by them and members of the EC. The Session was moderated by John Shammas.

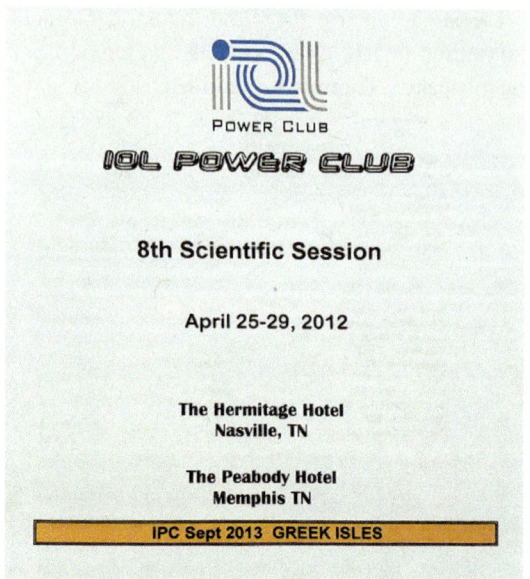

2012: Eighth IPC Meeting— Memphis and Nashville, TN, April 25–29, The Hermitage Hotel, Nashville, The Peabody Hotel, Memphis

Our eighth Scientific Meeting was held in the two cities of Memphis and Nashville, Tennessee, following the ASCRS meeting in Chicago.

Attendees: **Members**: Jean-Philippe Colliac, Han Bor Fam, Scott McClatchey, John Moran, and Giacomo Savini. **Industry**: Wilfried Bissmann, PhD (Zeiss), Tobias Bühren, PhD (Zeiss), Peter Fedor, MD (Zeiss), Reiner Herrmann (Haag-Streit), Jörg Iwanzcuk (Oculus), Jennifer Lewis, PhD (Ziemer), Kai Mothes (Oculus), and Thomas Padrick, PhD (Wavetec).

The EC took an Amtrak overnight train from Chicago to Memphis (below left), a first-time experience for all of them (having dinner on the train). That evening on the train, Wolfgang and I were in the lounge where there was a group playing music. One of them gave Wolf his guitar and he began singing "Eve of Destruction" (he was a DJ while working his way through college). We then took a bus to Nashville and met in the lobby of the historic Hermitage Hotel (below right).

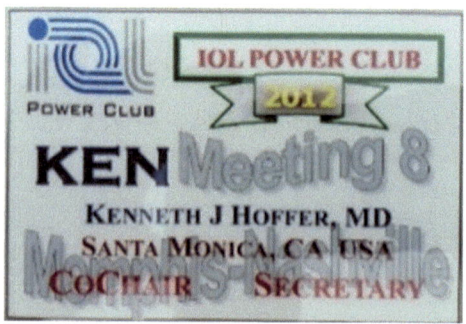

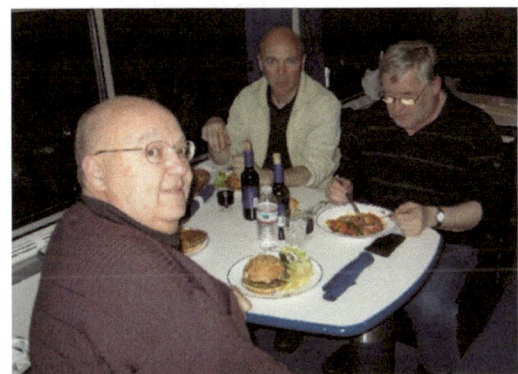
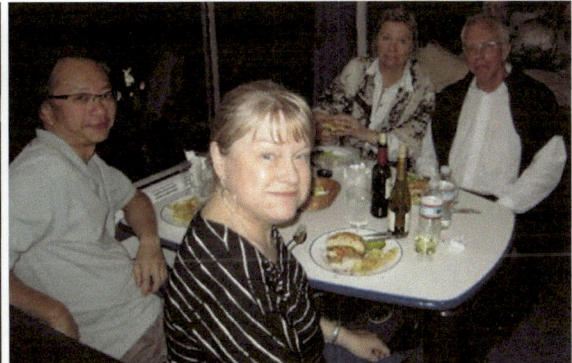
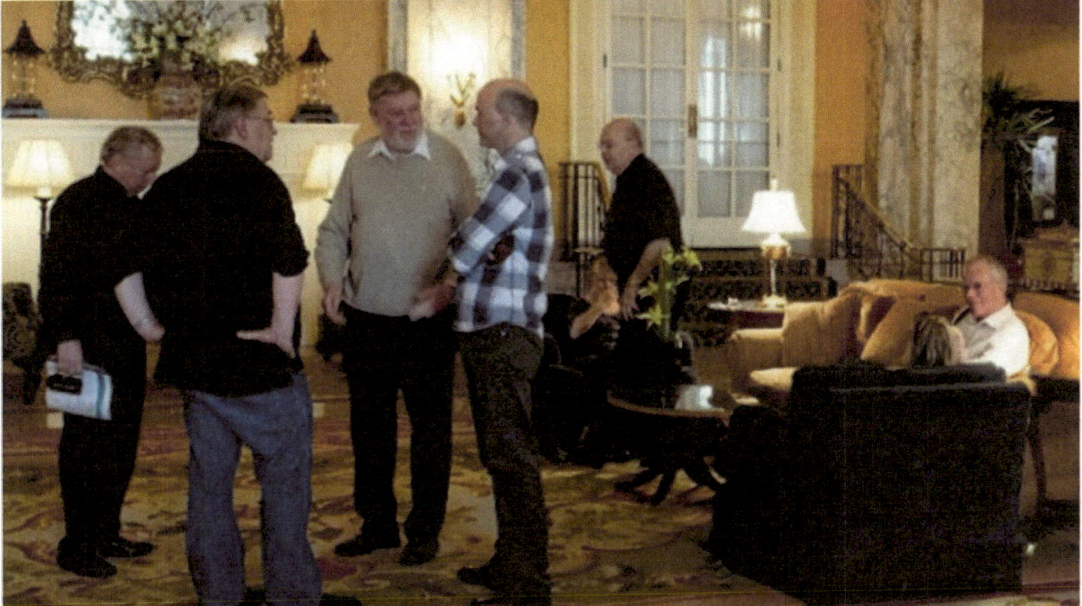
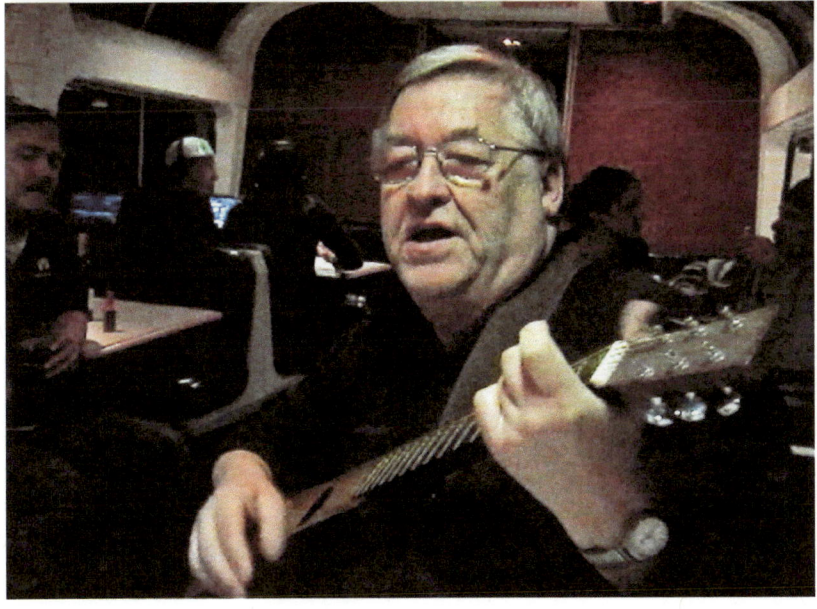

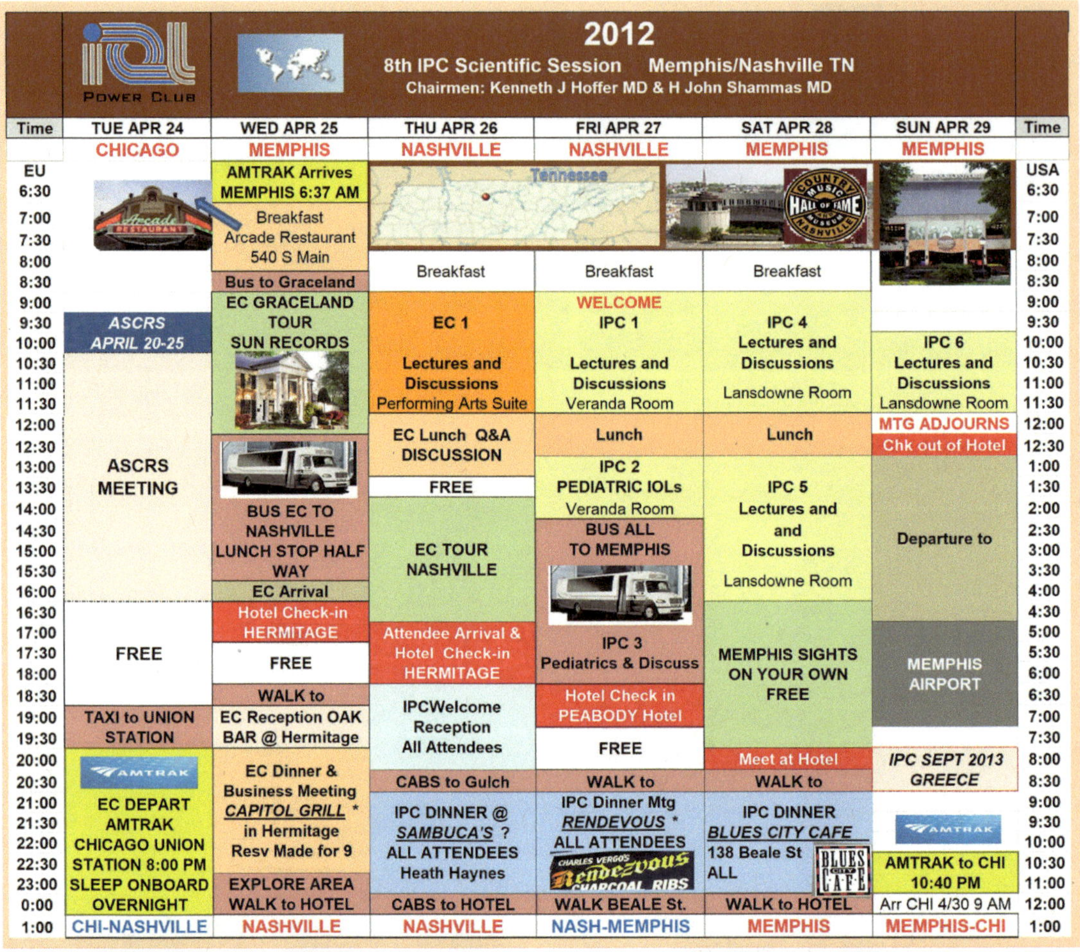

				2012		
			8th IPC Scientific Session Memphis/Nashville TN			
			Chairmen: Kenneth J Hoffer MD & H John Shammas MD			
Time	TUE APR 24	WED APR 25	THU APR 26	FRI APR 27	SAT APR 28	SUN APR 29	Time
	CHICAGO	MEMPHIS	NASHVILLE	NASHVILLE	MEMPHIS	MEMPHIS	
EU 6:30		AMTRAK Arrives MEMPHIS 6:37 AM		Tennessee			USA 6:30
7:00		Breakfast					7:00
7:30		Arcade Restaurant 540 S Main					7:30
8:00			Breakfast	Breakfast	Breakfast		8:00
8:30		Bus to Graceland					8:30
9:00		EC GRACELAND TOUR		WELCOME			9:00
9:30	ASCRS APRIL 20-25	SUN RECORDS	EC 1	IPC 1	IPC 4 Lectures and		9:30
10:00					Discussions	IPC 6	10:00
10:30			Lectures and	Lectures and		Lectures and	10:30
11:00			Discussions	Discussions	Lansdowne Room	Discussions	11:00
11:30			Performing Arts Suite	Veranda Room		Lansdowne Room	11:30
12:00			EC Lunch Q&A	Lunch	Lunch	MTG ADJOURNS	12:00
12:30			DISCUSSION			Chk out of Hotel	12:30
13:00	ASCRS MEETING			IPC 2	IPC 5		1:00
13:30			FREE	PEDIATRIC IOLs	Lectures and		1:30
14:00		BUS EC TO		Veranda Room	and		2:00
14:30		NASHVILLE		BUS ALL	Discussions	Departure to	2:30
15:00		LUNCH STOP HALF	EC TOUR	TO MEMPHIS			3:00
15:30		WAY	NASHVILLE		Lansdowne Room		3:30
16:00		EC Arrival					4:00
16:30		Hotel Check-in					4:30
17:00		HERMITAGE	Attendee Arrival &	IPC 3			5:00
17:30	FREE	FREE	Hotel Check-in	Pediatrics & Discuss	MEMPHIS SIGHTS	MEMPHIS	5:30
18:00			HERMITAGE		ON YOUR OWN	AIRPORT	6:00
18:30		WALK to		Hotel Check in	FREE		6:30
19:00	TAXI to UNION	EC Reception OAK	IPCWelcome	PEABODY Hotel			7:00
19:30	STATION	BAR @ Hermitage	Reception All Attendees	FREE			7:30
20:00	AMTRAK	EC Dinner &			Meet at Hotel	IPC SEPT 2013	8:00
20:30		Business Meeting	CABS to Gulch	WALK to	WALK to	GREECE	8:30
21:00	EC DEPART	CAPITOL GRILL *		IPC Dinner Mtg			9:00
21:30	AMTRAK	in Hermitage	IPC DINNER @	RENDEVOUS *	IPC DINNER	AMTRAK	9:30
22:00	CHICAGO UNION	Resv Made for 9	SAMBUCA'S ?	ALL ATTENDEES	BLUES CITY CAFE		10:00
22:30	STATION 8:00 PM		ALL ATTENDEES	Rendezvous CHARCOAL RIBS	138 Beale St ALL BLUES CAFE	AMTRAK to CHI	10:30
23:00	SLEEP ONBOARD	EXPLORE AREA	Heath Haynes			10:40 PM	11:00
0:00	OVERNIGHT	WALK to HOTEL	CABS to HOTEL	WALK BEALE St.	WALK to HOTEL	Arr CHI 4/30 9 AM	12:00
1:00	CHI-NASHVILLE	NASHVILLE	NASHVILLE	NASH-MEMPHIS	MEMPHIS	MEMPHIS-CHI	1:00

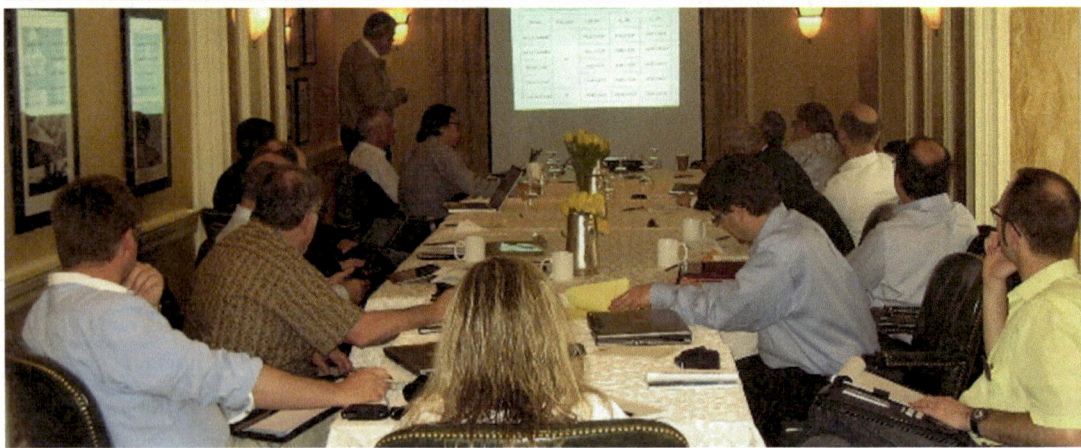

The first 2 days would be in Nashville and the 3rd in Memphis. It was a first-time session for us on "Pediatric IOL Powers" which I moderated. I made the first presentation "Problems with Pediatric IOL Power" (left) followed by Scott McClatchey (right). We continued it while on the bus back to Memphis, a Session 3 "Pediatric IOLs" on improving IOL power in children led by Scott and I. We then arrived at the Memphis Peabody Hotel where we continued the 3rd day of the meeting and we also had a tour of the Elvis Presley Mansion and Sun Records Studio.

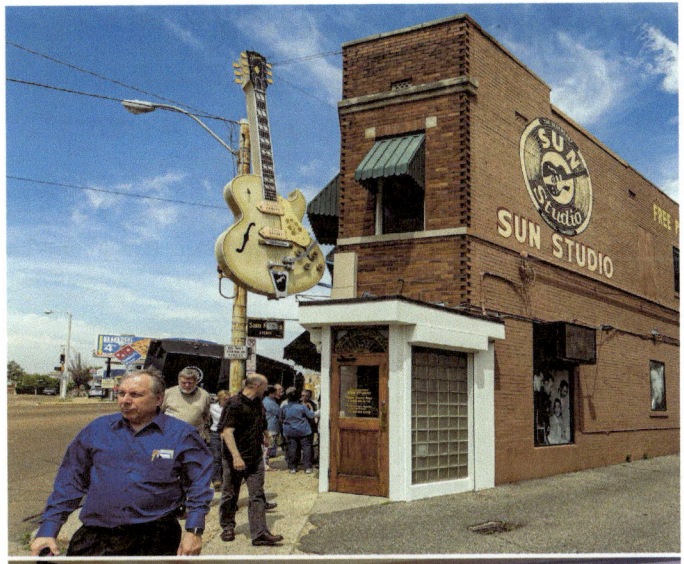

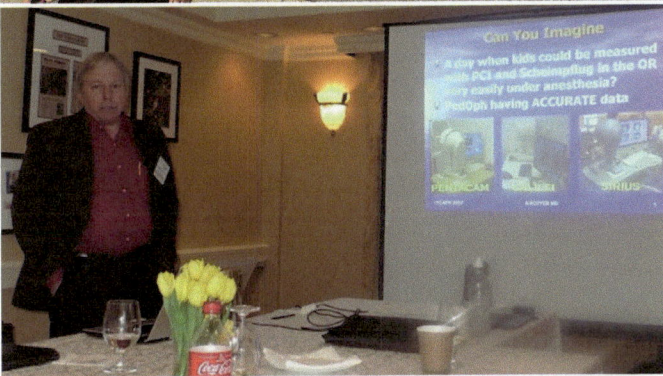

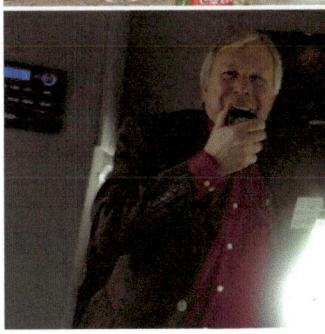
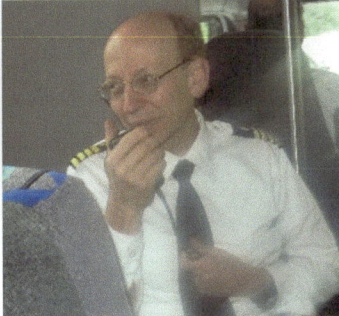

EDITORIALS

The Final Frontier: Pediatric Intraocular Lens Power

KENNETH J. HOFFER, JAIME ARAMBERRI, WOLFGANG HAIGIS, SVERKER NORRBY, THOMAS OLSEN, AND
H. JOHN SHAMMAS, ON BEHALF OF THE IOL POWER CLUB EXECUTIVE COMMITTEE

FOR MORE THAN A HALF A CENTURY SINCE SIR HAR-
old Ridley implanted the first intraocular lens (IOL),
many have worked hard to improve and perfect the
calculation of the correct power of the implant. In 1974

more accurate immersion technique. We know this
introduces a shortening error on average of 0.25 mm²
in adults, and recent excellent studies by Trevidi and
Wilson[] show that 0.37

This discussion later led to our EC *American Journal of Ophthalmology* Editor-requested Editorial on this subject (Amer J Ophthalmol. 2012;154(1):1–2). We held a day and half of lectures before adjourning.

2013: Ninth IPC Meeting—Haarlem, the Netherlands, October 9–12, Amrâth Grand Hotel Frans Hals

The ninth IPC Scientific Meeting was held in Haarlem, the Netherlands at the Amrâth Grand Hotel Frans Hals, after the ESCRS Meeting in Amsterdam with Sverker Norrby and Thomas Olsen as Co-Chairmen.

Attendees: **Members**: Edmondo Borasio, Massimo Camellin, Claudio Carbonara, Jean-Philippe Colliac, Han Bor Fam, Oliver Findl, Gabor Koranyi, and Rob Van der Heijde.

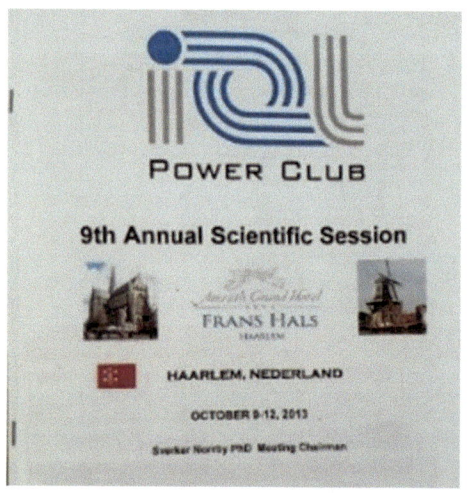

Industry: Stan Bentow, PhD (AMO), Theo Bogaert (AMO), Thomas Bütler (Heyer-Schulte), Carmen Canovas, PhD (AMO), Alessandro Foggi (Topcon/Visia Imaging), Mario Gerlach (Zeiss), Pierre Giessen (Topcon EU), Jörg Iwanczuk (Oculus), Luc Johannes, PhD (Lambda-X), Tom Padrick (WaveTec), Balz Schlund (Ziemer), and Gabriele Vestri (CSO). **Invited Speakers**: Nino Hirnschall MD, Peter Fedor MD, Arni Sicam PhD (iOptics).

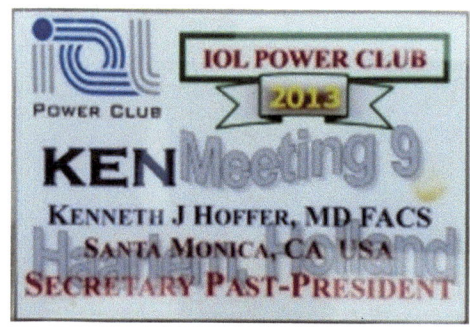

Above is the program cover (left) and an example of our badges (right).

Below is the overall program schedule including the EC sessions.

2013
IPC Scientific Session #9   Haarlem, Netherlands
Chairmen: Sverker Norrby PhD

Time	TUE OCT 8	WED OCT 9	THU OCT 10	FRI OCT 11	SAT OCT 12	Time
EU	AMSTERDAM	HAARLEM	HAARLEM	HAARLEM	HAARLEM	USA
6:30				BUS to		6:30
7:00				Aalsmeer Flower		7:00
7:30				Auction		7:30
8:00			Breakfast	RETURN	Breakfast	8:00
8:30		Breakfast		Breakfast was served		8:30
9:00			WELCOME	on the Bus		9:00
9:30		EC 1	IPC 1-A	IPC 3-A	IPC 5	9:30
10:00	ESCRS MTG	What is the Future	Optics and	Toric IOLs	Instrumentation	10:00
10:30	AMSTERDAM	of IOL Calculation?	Statistics	Coffee Break	and	10:30
11:00	OCT 5-9	Lectures and	Coffee Break	IPC 3-B	Manufacturers	11:00
11:30		Discussions	IPC 1-B	Special	ADJOURN	11:30
12:00			New Approches	Situations		12:00
12:30		EC Lunch Q&A	Lunch Q&A			12:30
13:00	TRAVEL	DISCUSSION	DISCUSSION	Lunch Q&A		1:00
13:30			IPC 2	DISCUSSION		1:30
14:00	EC Arrival	EC 2	Biometry	IPC 4-A		2:00
14:30	& Hotel Check-in	What is the Future	Discussions	Biometry		2:30
15:00	Amrath Grand	of IOL Calculation?	FREE	Coffee Break	Departure	3:00
15:30		Lectures and	FRANS HALS	IPC 4-B		3:30
16:00		Discussions	MUSEUM	Cornea		4:00
16:30	FREE			Calculations		4:30
17:00		Non-EC Arrival &	FREE	Discussions		5:00

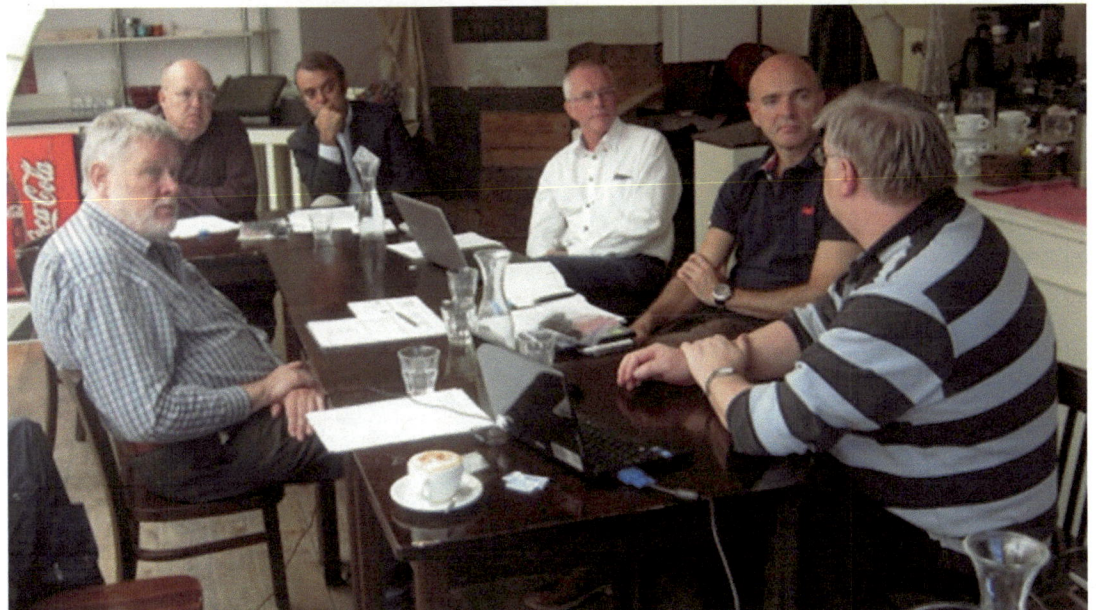

At the EC Business meeting (above), Norrby reminded us of his retirement from the IPC at the end of this meeting. Our elections resulted in Olsen as our next President, Haigis as Vice-President, Hoffer as Secretary and Savini as our new Treasurer. Sverker thanked Wolfgang for his tedious work as Treasurer for the past 8 years. It was unanimous that Norrby be made an Honorary Member.

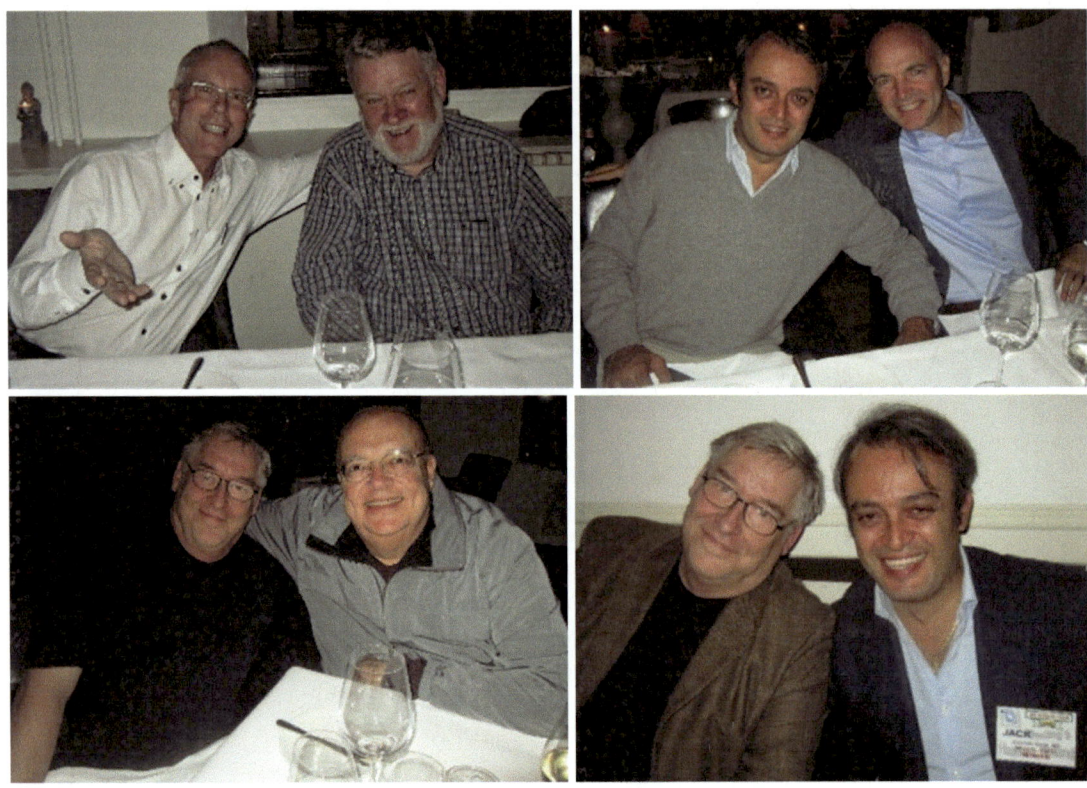

Norrby chaired the meeting and started with an introductory lecture.

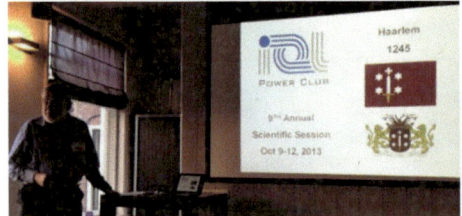 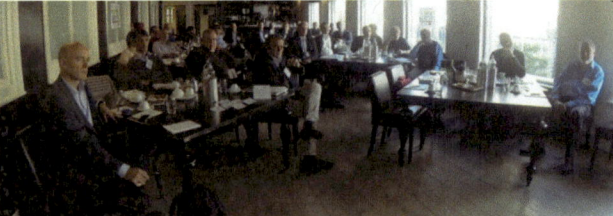

We had a special *Statistics Session*. The EC had invited Stan Bentow, PhD (AMO) (below), to give a full 30-min lecture, as a statistician, on how IOL power results should be accurately reported.

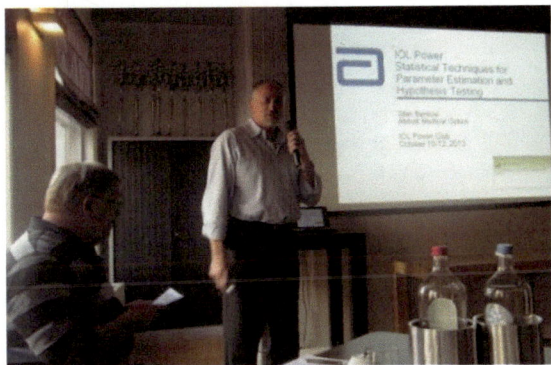
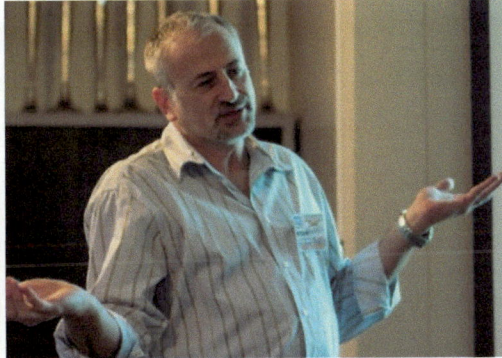

The Bootstrap Algorithm

Given a dataset $\underline{X} = (x_1, x_2, ..., x_n)$

1. Select a random sample of size n drawn with replacement from $\underline{X}$
This is a single bootstrap sample, $\underline{x}^{*1} = x_1^{*1}, x_2^{*1}, ..., x_n^{*1}$ Do this B times yielding B bootstrap samples, each of size n

2. Calculate the parameter of interest for each bootstrap sample. For the mean we would end up with B bootstrap means $\overline{X}^{*} = (\overline{x}_1^{*}, \overline{x}_2^{*}, ..., \overline{x}_B^{*})$

3. Estimate the mean and standard deviation of the B bootstrap means using the usual equations
- The bootstrap mean is the original sample mean
- The bootstrap standard deviation is the standard error of the mean

4. Use the bootstrap mean and standard error for hypothesis testing, calculating confidence intervals, etc. Note: confidence intervals may be calculated empirically using percentiles (95% confidence interval (2.5th, 97.5th))

EDITORIALS

Protocols for Studies of Intraocular Lens Formula Accuracy

KENNETH J. HOFFER, JAIME ARAMBERRI, WOLFGANG HAIGIS, THOMAS OLSEN, GIACOMO SAVINI, H. JOHN SHAMMAS, AND STANLEY BENTOW

MANY STUDIES HAVE BEEN PUBLISHED ASSESSING the accuracy of intraocular lens (IOL) power calculation. Since the formation of the IOL Power Club in 2005, errors have been noted in the proto-values. This may be more difficult with the Haigis formula (see below). It is then appropriate to compare the median absolute error (MedAE) of each formula. The ME being the lowest merely means the lens factor chosen for that

He reiterated the opinions of Haigis and Norrby that using the MAE was inappropriate since absolute errors are not a normal Gaussian distribution and that MedAE is more legitimate. However, he detailed methods such as bootstrapping which can be used so that MAE would be legitimate. (This resulted in the IOL Power Club's accepting an invitation for an Editorial in the *American Journal of Ophthalmology* in 2015. (Protocols for studies of intraocular lens formula accuracy. *Amer J Ophthalm. 2015;160(3): 403–405*)).

First IPC Member Business Meeting

Since the membership had grown over the past decade, the EC decided to have a Membership Business Meeting to allow the members to participate and vote on EC decisions. It was the intention of the EC that these official member business meetings continue. During the meeting, Hoffer made a special tribute to Sverker Norrby for his 8 years of service to this Club as a Founder, an EC Member, and a scientific contributor.

2014: Tenth IPC Meeting—Fort Lauderdale, FL, October 8–11, Il Lugano Hotel and Pelican Grand Hotel

The tenth Scientific Meeting was held at the Il Lugano Hotel in Ft. Lauderdale, FL, prior to the AAO Meeting in Chicago.

Attendees: **Members**: Edmondo Borasio, Jean-Philippe Colliac, Han Bor Fam, Scott McClatchey, and Sabong Srivannaboon. **Honorary Member**: John Retzlaff. **Invited Speaker**: Sean Ianchulev, MD.

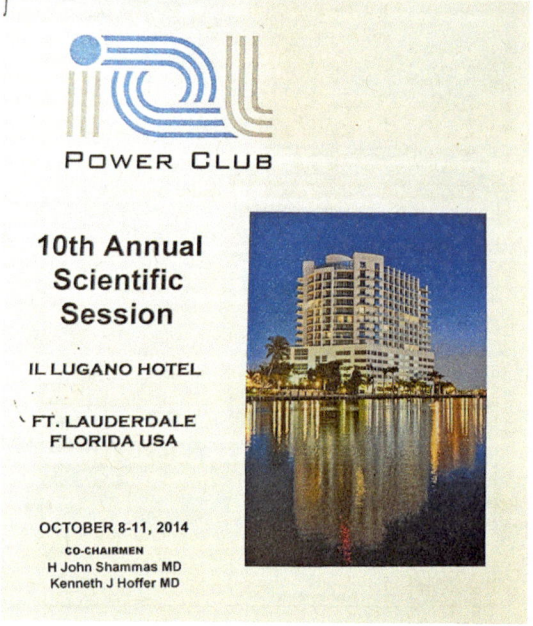

Industry: Kaspar Baltzer (Haag-Streit), Stan Bentow, PhD (AMO), Tobias Bühren, PhD (Zeiss), Changho Chong, PhD (MOVU), Alessandro Foggi and Pierre Gelissen (Topcon EU), Martin Gründig, PhD (Alcon), Hiryuki Hiramatsu (Nidek), Jörg Iwanczuk (Oculus), Chihiro Kato, Koki Nishiwaki, and Hisashi Onizaki (all Tomey), Thomas Padrick, PhD (WaveTec), Gregor Schmid, PhD (Ziemer), and Francesco Versaci (CSO).

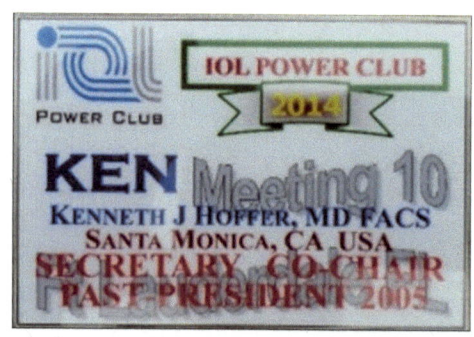

Time	WED OCT 8	THU OCT 9	FRI OCT 10	SAT OCT 11	Time
EU	Ft LAUDERDALE	Ft LAUDERDALE	Ft LAUDERDALE	Ft LAUDERDALE	USA
8:00	ESCRS MTG LONDON	Breakfast	Breakfast	Breakfast	8:00
8:30	SEP 13-17				8:30
9:00		WELCOME		IPC 5	9:00
9:30		IPC 1-A	IPC 3-A	UPDATES	9:30
10:00		BIOMETRY 1	CORNEA		10:00
10:30		Coffee Break	Coffee Break	Coffee Break	10:30
11:00	EXECUTIVE	IPC 1-B	IOL POWER 1		11:00
11:30	COMMITTEE	BIOMETRY 2	IPC 3-B		11:30
12:00	SCIENTIFIC			ADJOURN	12:00
12:30	AND	Lunch			12:30
1:00	BUSINESS		Lunch		13:00
1:30	MEETING	IPC 2			13:30
2:00		VARIOUS	IPC 4-A		14:00
2:30		TOPICS	IOL POWER 2		14:30
3:00					15:00
3:30	ALL TRAVEL TO	FREE TIME	Coffee Break	Departure	15:30
4:00	FT LAUDERDALE	ENJOY THE BEACH	IPC 4-B		16:00
4:30	IL LUGANO HOTEL	OR THE POOL	IOL POWER 3		16:30
5:00					17:00

The EC Business meeting was held as usual and the election resulted in for 2015–2017, Haigis as President, Aramberri as Vice-President, Hoffer as Secretary, and Savini as Treasurer.

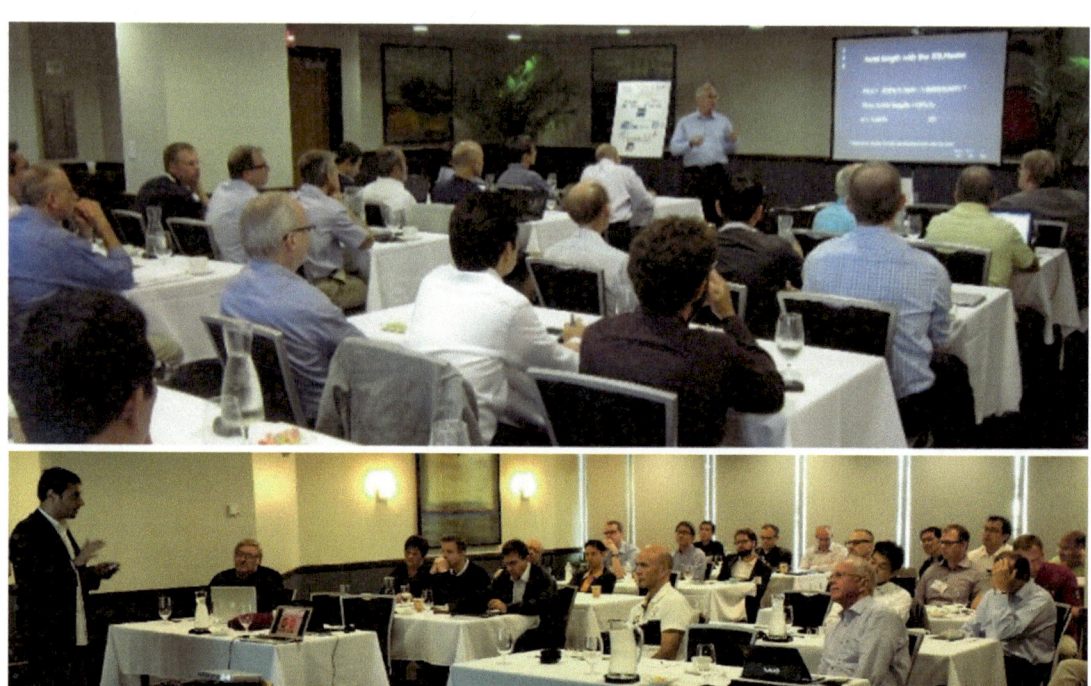

2015: 11th IPC Meeting—San Sebastian, Spain, September 9–12, Londres Hotel

After a decade of existence, the IPC celebrated its 10th birthday by returning to the city of its birth, San Sebastian, Spain.

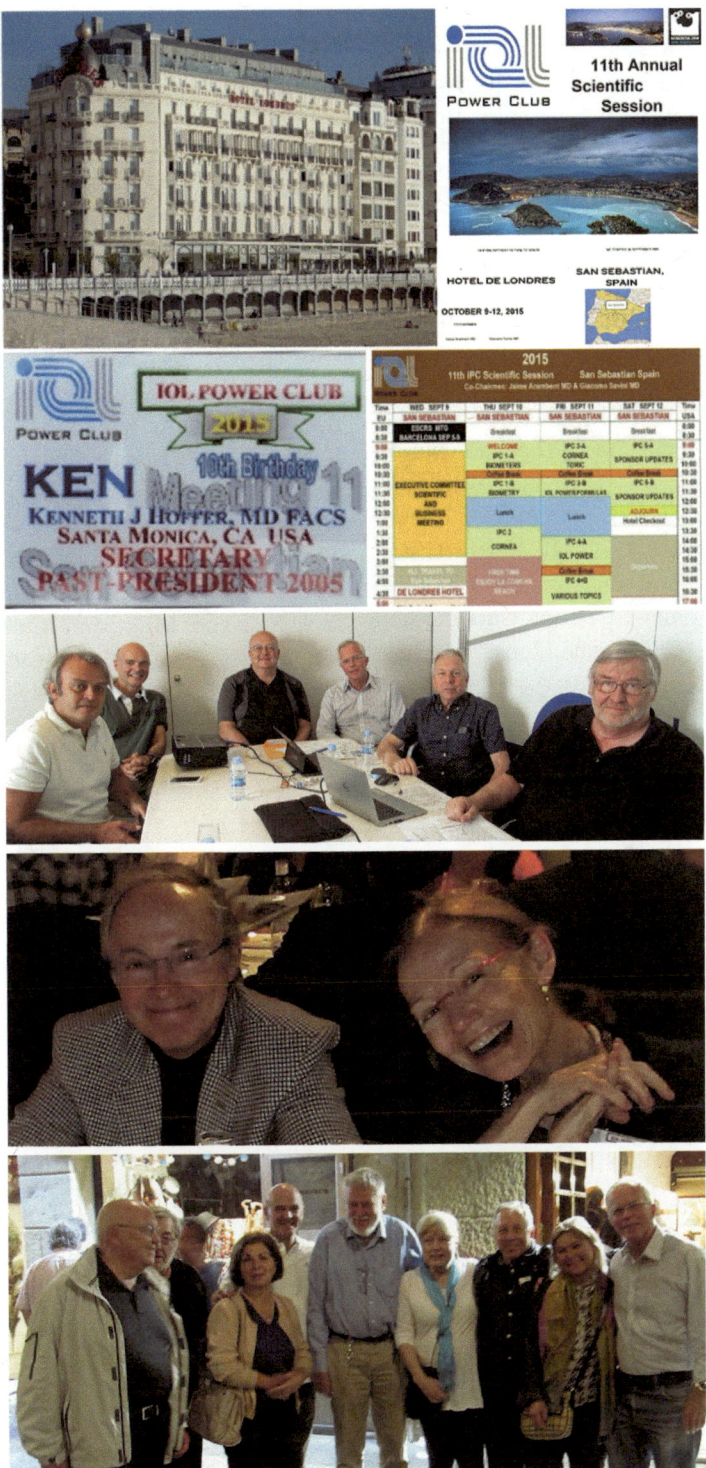

It was held after the ESCRS Meeting in Barcelona and again held at the same Hotel Londres (above L) where we met in 2005.

Attendees: **Members**: Edmondo Borasio, MD, Massimo Camellin, MD, Claudio Carbonara, MD, Jean-Philippe Colliac, MD, Han Bor Fam, MD, Nino Hirnschall, MD, and Douglas Koch, MD. **Guest**: Umberto Camellin, MD. **Invited Speaker**: Jos Rozema, PhD (Antwerp, Belgium). **Industry Representatives**: Kaspar Baltzer (Haag-Streit), Stan Bentow, PhD (AMO), Tobias Bühren, PhD (Zeiss), Carmen Canovas, PhD (AMO), Changho Chong, PhD (MOVU), Alessandro Foggi (Topcon), Martin Gründig, PhD (Alcon), Hiroyuki Hiramatsu (Nidek), Jörg Iwanczuk (Oculus), Gregor Schmid, PhD (Ziemer), Gabrielle Vestri (CSO), Naoko Hara, Hirofumi Owaki, and Keiichiro Okamoto (all of Tomey), Cristina Curatolo and Gianluca Stivale (CSO), and Jonas Haehnle (Haag-Streit).

The meeting was excellent with many new introductions, such as the new MOVU Argos biometer by Shammas.

2016: 12th IPC Meeting—New Orleans, LA, May 10–13 Royal Sonesta Hotel

The 12th meeting was held in New Orleans, LA, after the ASCRS meeting there in May 5–9.

The venue was the Royal Sonesta Hotel on Bourbon St. in the French Quarter with Kenneth J. Hoffer and H. John Shammas as Co-Chairs. John and Najwa Shammas were unable to attend; it is the only IPC Meeting they have ever missed. The Welcome Reception was held in the Sonesta garden court. The EC had the opportunity to meet Jack X. Kane, MD, from Melbourne, Australia, for the first time after I heard his lecture and invited him to meet the IPC EC.

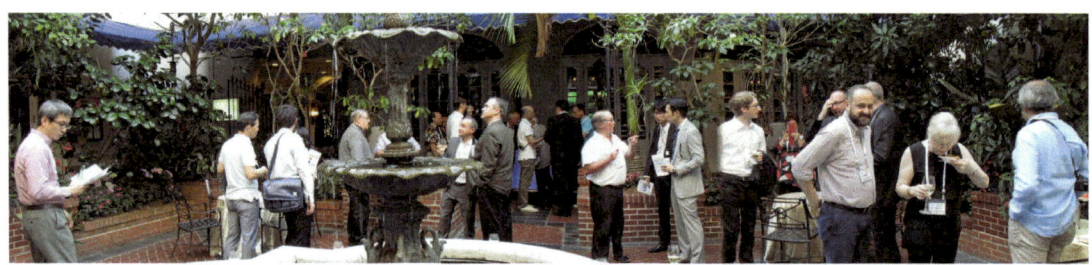

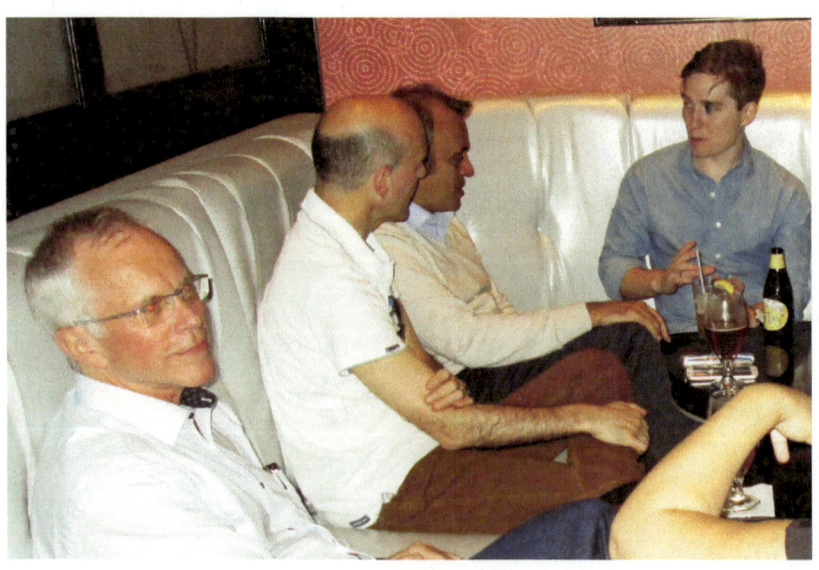

During the meeting I presented a tribute to Larry Laks (owner of Microsurgical Technologies) for his annual support of IPC for the past 10 years after selling his company.

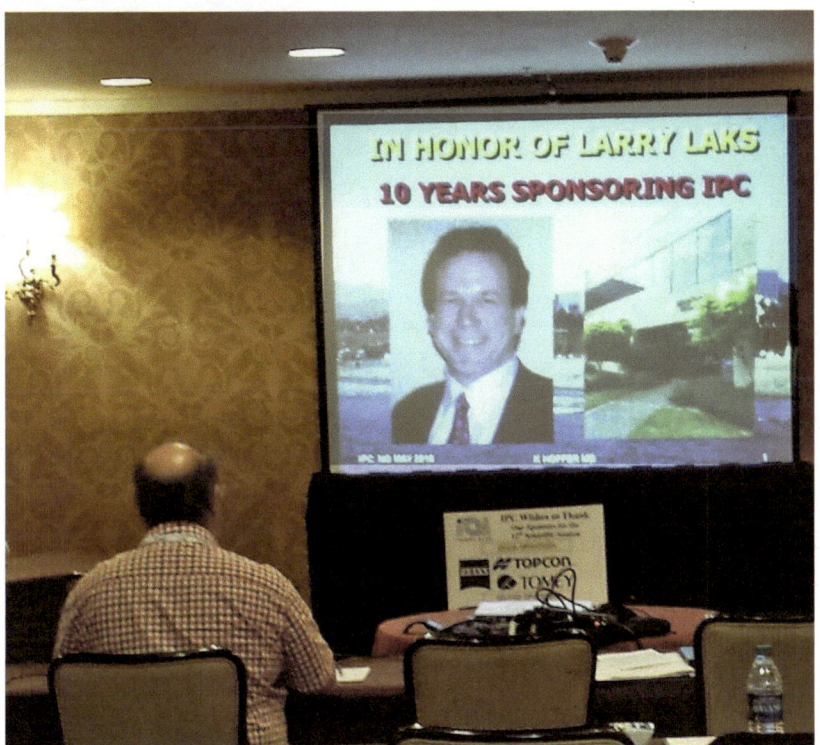

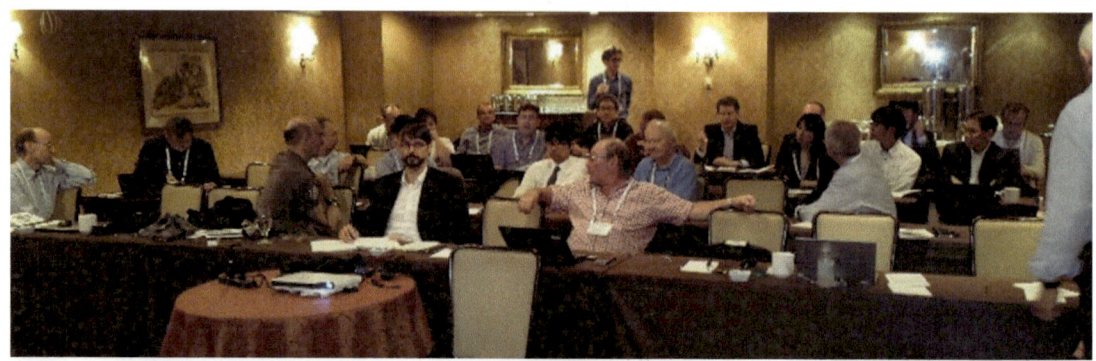

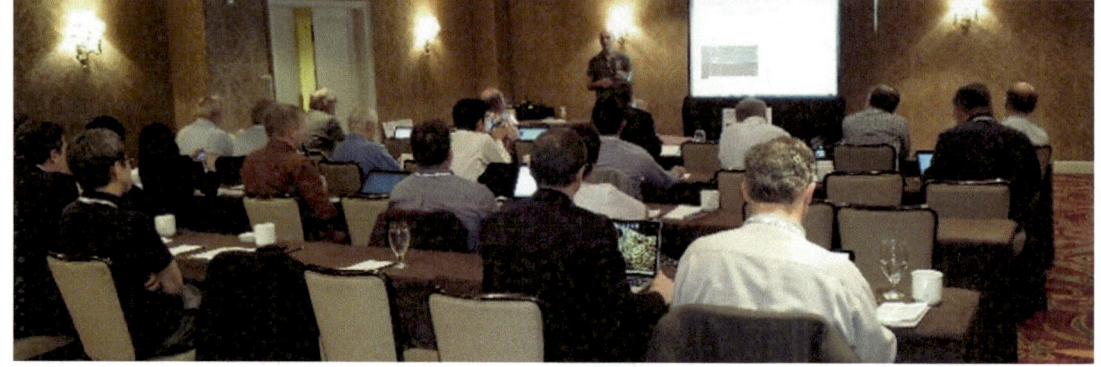

We held our usual EC Business meeting.

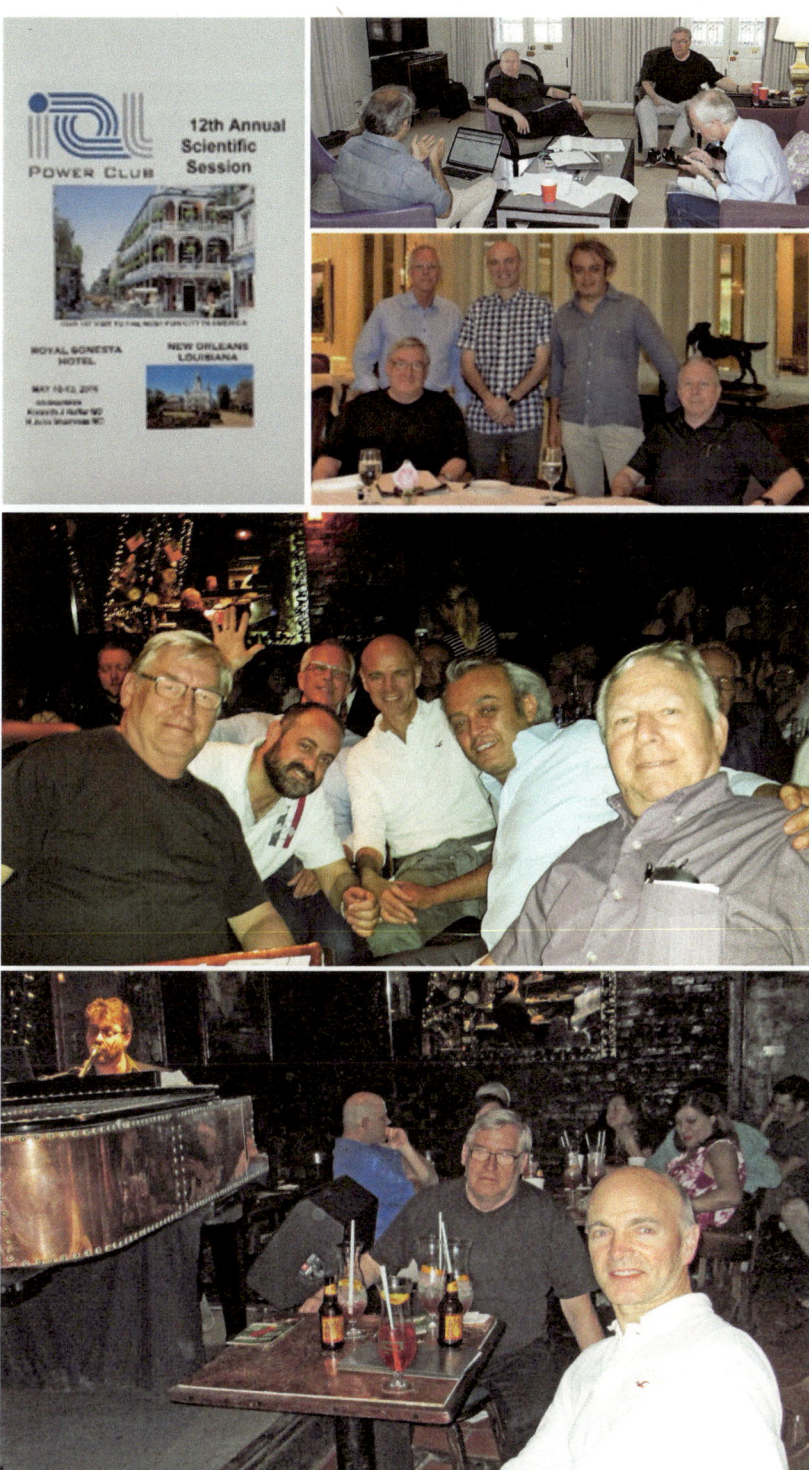

Attendees: **Members**: Claudio Carbonara, MD, Han Bor Fam, MD, Gabor Koranyi, MD, Scott McClatchey, MD, and John Retzlaff, MD. **Industry**: Kaspar Baltzer (Haag-Streit), Christian Brandt, PhD (Heidelberg), Tobias Bühren, PhD (Zeiss), Changho Chong, PhD (MOVU), Alessandro Foggi (Topcon EU), Jörg Iwanzcuk (Oculus), Hiroyuki Hiramatsu (Nidek), Chihiro Kato (Tomey), Gregor Schmid, PhD (Ziemer), and first timer Rosario Occhipinti (SiFi). Several of us had the chance to visit O'Brien's and try their Hurricanes.

On the way back, Wolf made friends with the Bourbon Street Lucky Dog vendor.

Jaime and Giacomo visited Jackson Square.

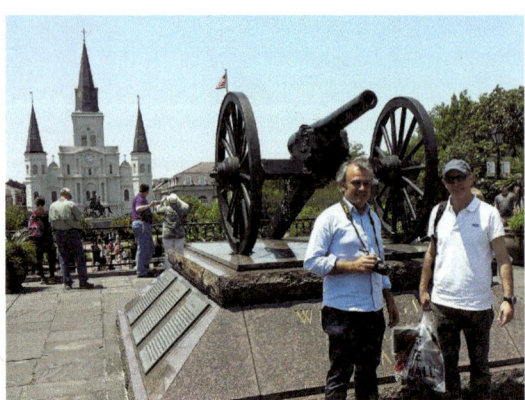

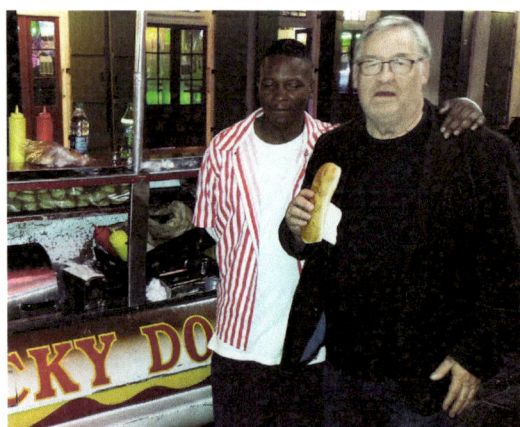

Everyone was invited for a cruise on the Natchez paddlewheel boat on the Mississippi River.

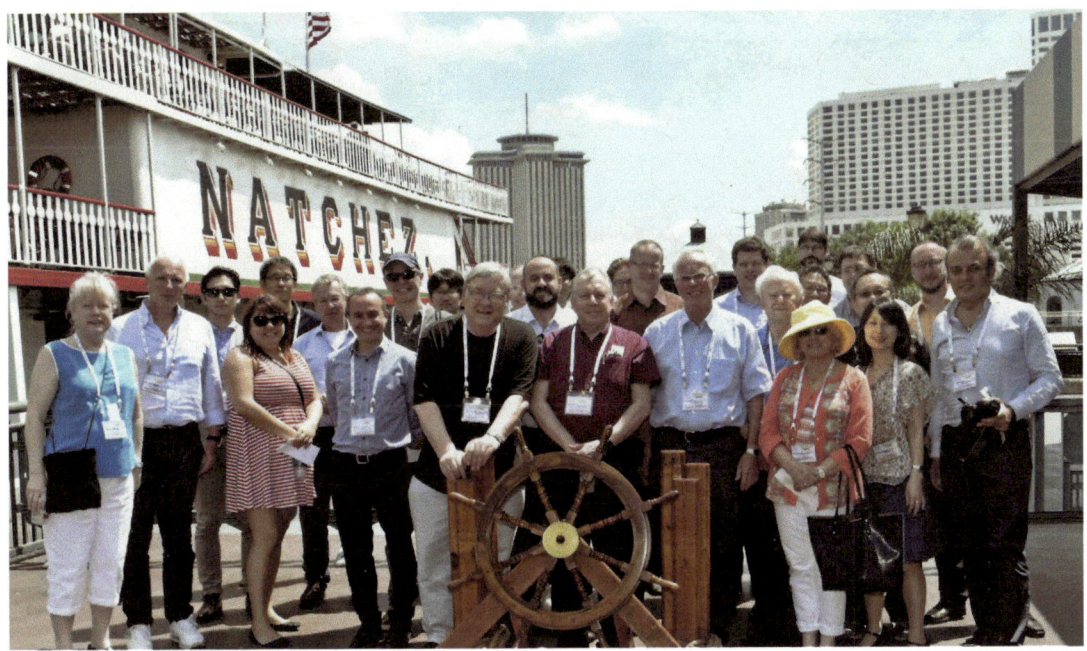

2017: 13th IPC Meeting—Athens, Greece, September 8–16 Grand Britannia Hotel

At the Spring ASCRS meeting in Los Angeles, we had the chance to toast Wolfgang who could not be there with his favorite Irish Coffee. This 13th meeting was the farthest East we have been, in the center of the city of Athens, Greece. The EC held their Business/Lecture Meeting in Crete.

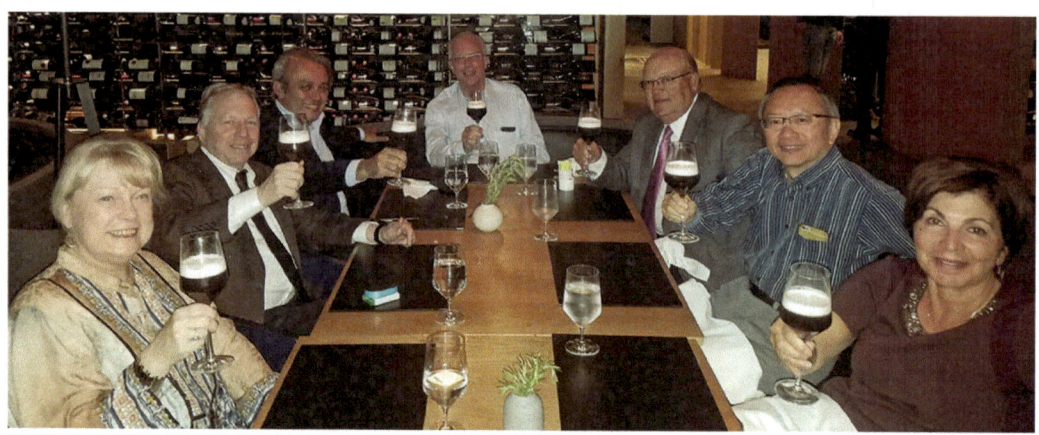

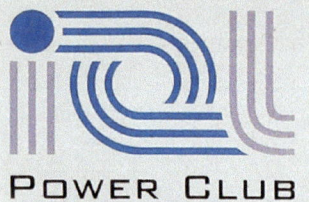

13th Annual Scientific Session

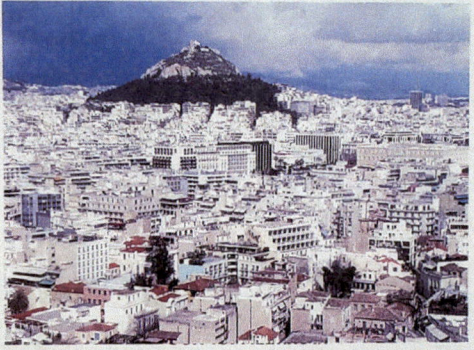

ATHENS, GREECE

GRANDE BRETAGNE HOTEL

SEP 15-16, 2017

CO-CHAIRMEN
Kenneth J Hoffer MD
Giacomo Savini MD

IOL POWER CLUB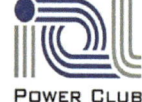

13th Scientific
Session, Part A
Harmony G Ship
September 8-15, 2017

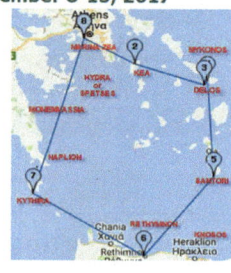

DAY #1 FRI SEPT 8: Embarkation
2-3 PM. Depart via Cape Sounion to Kea.
explore Kea's tiny port, Korrisia after dinner.

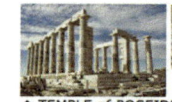 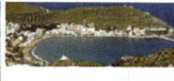

↑ TEMPLE of POSEIDEN   KEA ↑

DAY #2 SAT SEPT 9: Arrive
overnight to Delos – tour sites

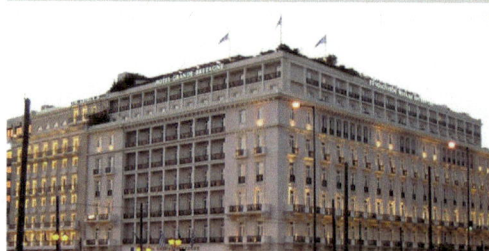

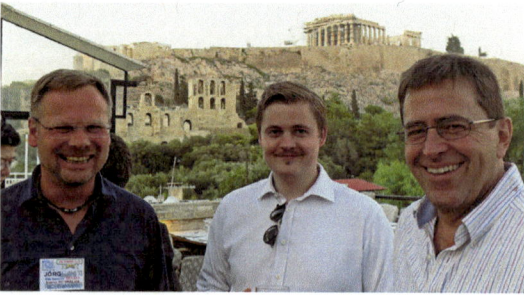

Attendees: **Members**: Jean-Philippe Colliac, MD, Han Bor Fam, MD, Nino Hirnschall, MD, and Jack X. Kane, MD. **Invited Lecturers**: Naoyuki Maeda, MD (Osaka, Japan), Dimitrii Dementiev, MD (Milan, Italy), and Peter Fedor, MD (Traverse City, MI). Haigis was unable to attend. **Industry**: Changho Chong, PhD (MOVU), Alessandro Foggi (Topcon EU/Visia), Owaki Hirofumi (Tomey), Jörg Iwanzcuk (Oculus), Oliver Klaproth (Zeiss), Melanie Polzner (Heidelberg), Gregor Schmid, PhD (Ziemer), Joris Snellenberg, PhD (Cassini), and Gabriel Vestri (CSO).

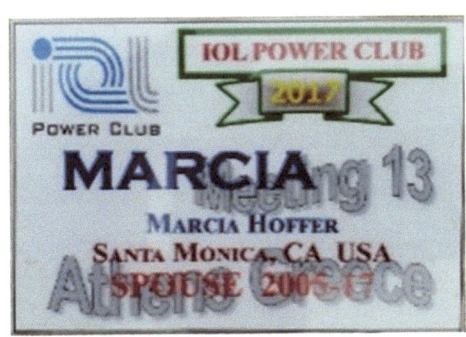

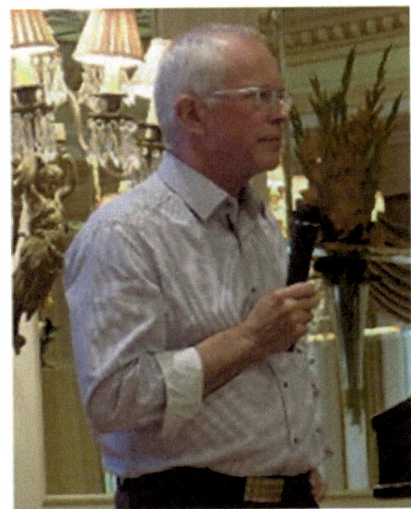

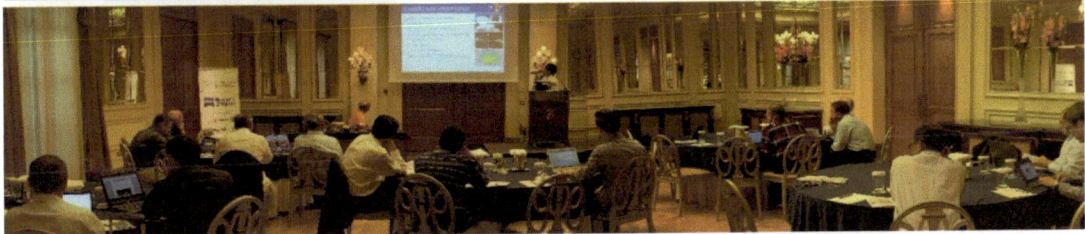

Here is a photo of Joerg Iwanczuk (Oculus), Oliver Klaproth (Zeiss) and Gregor Schmidt (Ziemer) with the Parthenon in the background in Athens. Our 7th Election voted Aramberri as President, Shammas as Vice-President, Hoffer as Secretary, and Savini as Treasurer. The meeting was very productive for everyone.

2018: 14th IPC Meeting—St. Pete Beach, FL, October 22–25 Tradewinds Island Grand Resort

This meeting was our return to the city where we held our fourth meeting in 2008. It wound up being uniquely different, in that I had persuaded Wolfgang Haigis to get to this meeting, which he wanted to very badly even though things were not going well for him. It turned out to be his last meeting.

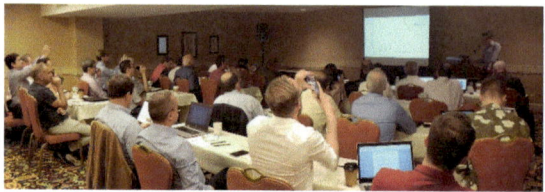
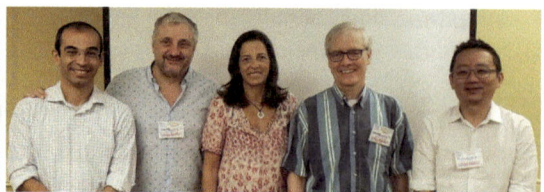

Attendees: **Members**: Edmondo Borasio, MD, Massimo Camellin, MD, Claudio Carbonara, MD, Jean-Philippe Colliac, MD, Han Bor Fam, MD, and Jack X. Kane, MD. **Honorary Member:** John Retzlaff, MD. **Invited speakers** (above L-R): Petros Aristodemou*, MD (Cyprus), David Flikier*, MD (Costa Rica), Filomena Ribeiro*, MD (Lisbon), David Cooke*, MD (Berrien Springs, MI), and Tun Kuan Yeo*, MD (Singapore).

Industry: Changho Chong, PhD (MOVU), Steven Frisken* (Cylite), Sandro Gunkel* (Heidelberg), Jonas Haehnle (Haag-Streit), Naoko Hara (Tomey), Jörg Iwanzcuk (Oculus), Oliver Klaproth (Zeiss), Gregor Schmid, PhD (Ziemer), and Francesco Versaci (CSO) (*first-timers).

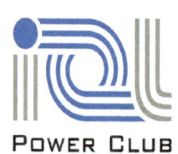

14th Annual Scientific Session

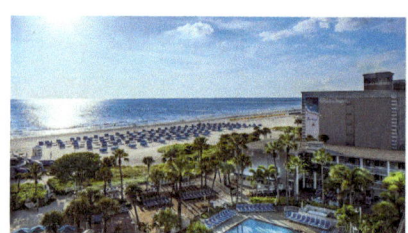

OUR RETURN TO ST. PETE BEACH AFTER A DECADE

TRADEWINDS GRAND   **ST. PETE BEACH FLORIDA**

CO-CHAIRMEN
KENNETH J HOFFER MD
H JOHN SHAMMAS MD

OCTOBER 22-25, 2018

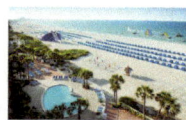

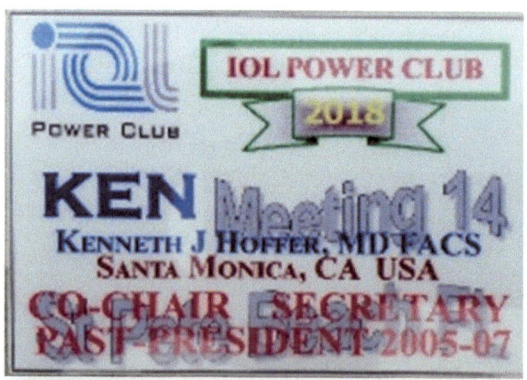

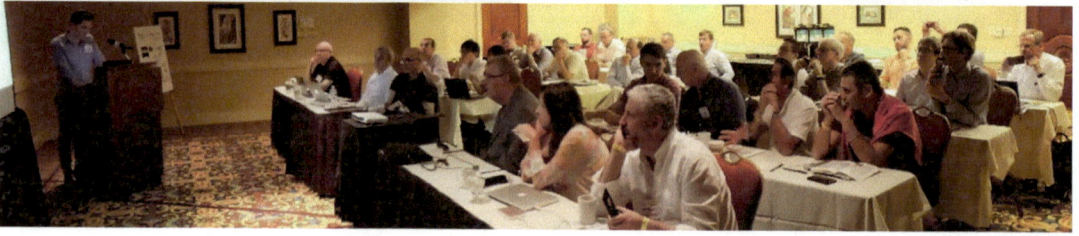

A group shot of all the attendees with Wolfgang Haigis in the center (black shirt).

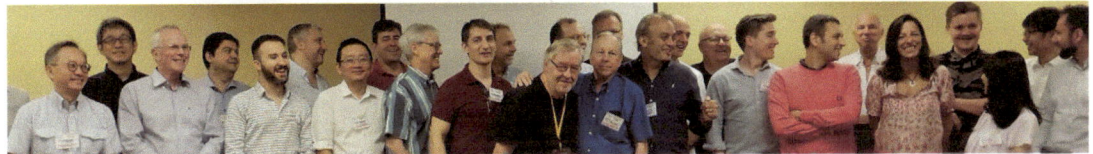

Due to his declining condition, this became Wolfgang's last IPC meeting, to our collective sadness. Below is the last EC Business Meeting Wolfgang attended and the last lecture he ever gave (right). A loss to all of ophthalmology.

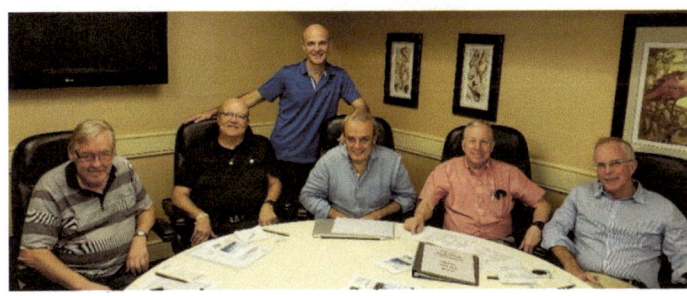
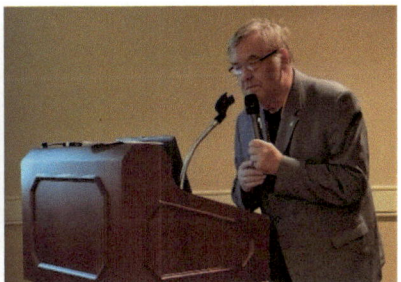

2018: ESCRS—IPC IOL Power Calculation Course, September 23, Vienna, Austria

For several years now, IPC has been putting on IOL Power courses at the ASCRS and ESCRS meetings. There was a standing-room-only audience to attend the 2018 "IPC IOL Power Course" at the ESCRS Meeting.

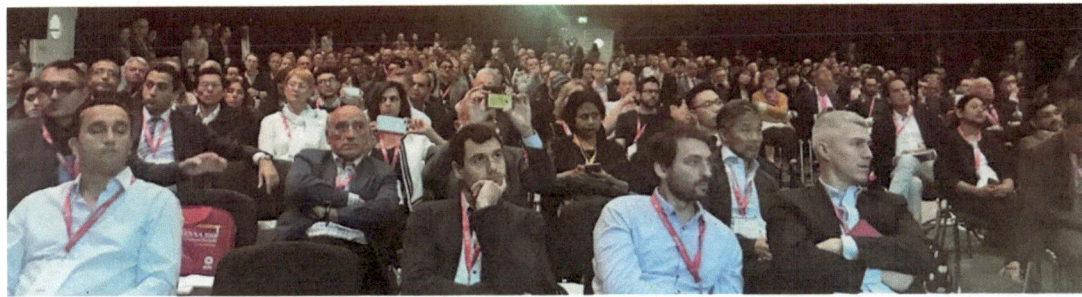

2019: IPC EC Fourth Independant Meeting—La Jolla, CA, May 6–7 La Valencia Hotel

The EC held its fourth separate business meeting at the La Valencia Hotel in La Jolla after the ASCRS meeting to make plans for the upcoming meeting in Napa. Aramberri and Haigis were unable to attend.

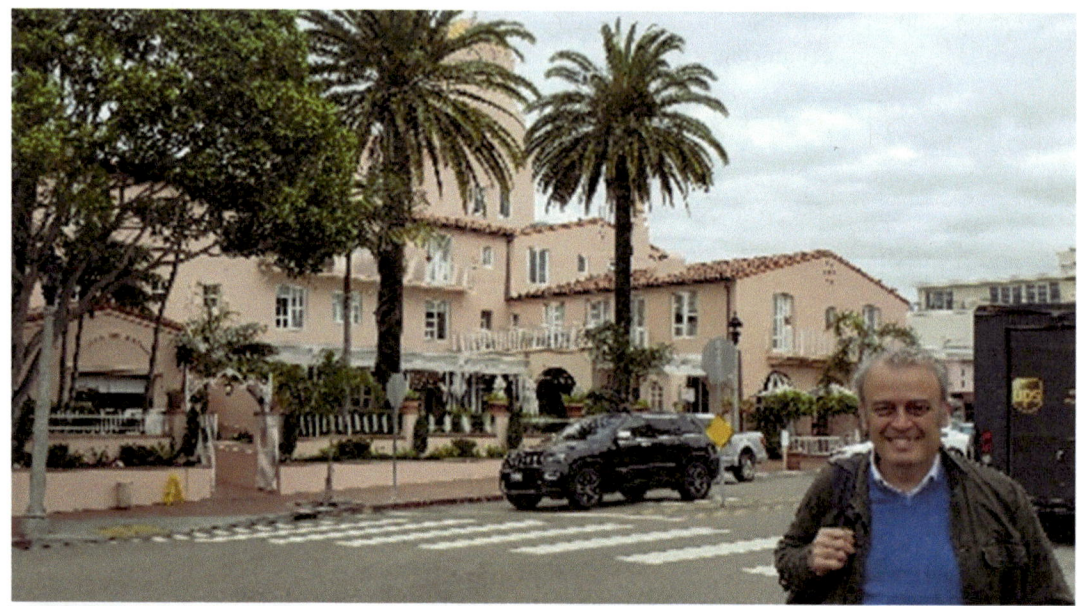

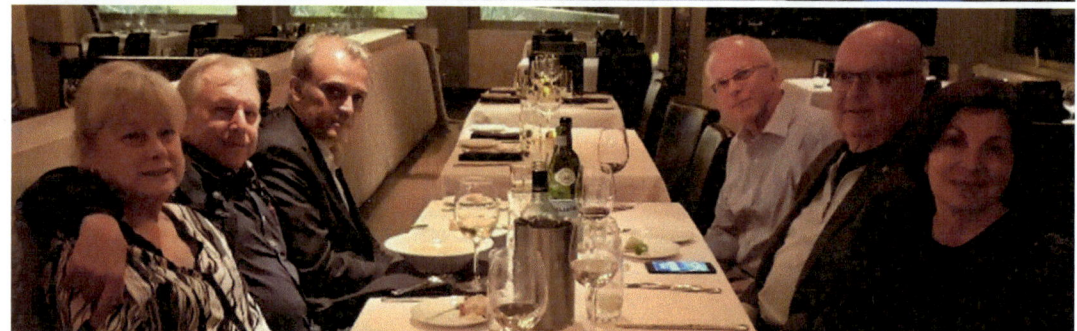

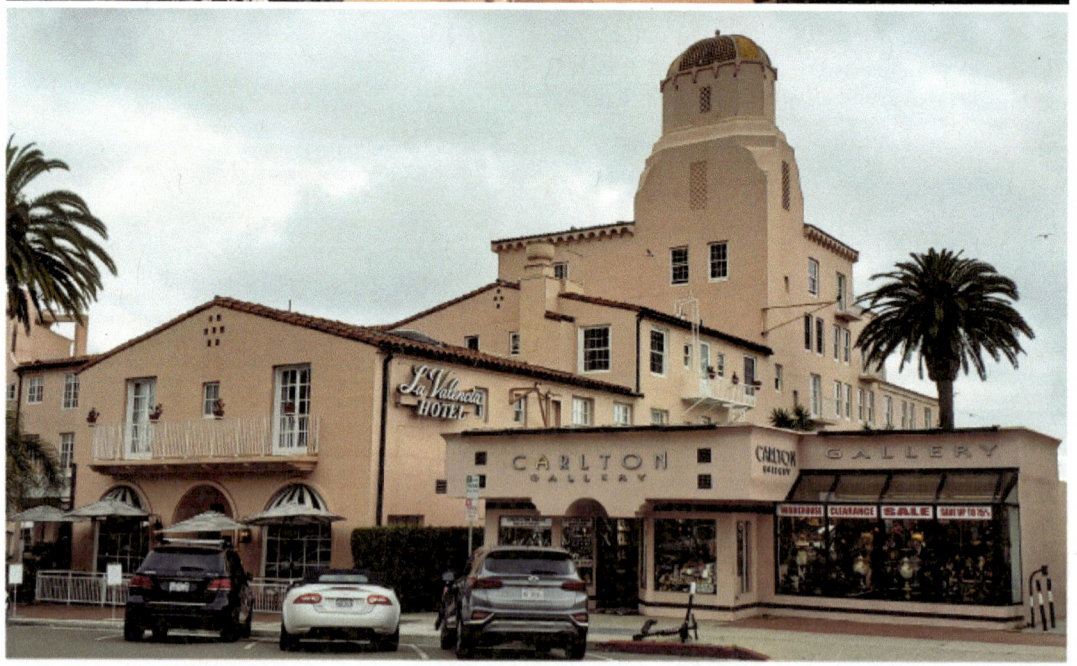

2019: 15th IPC Meeting—Napa, CA, October 8–11, Archer Hotel

The 15th Scientific meeting was held at the Archer Hotel in downtown Napa prior to the AAO Meeting in San Francisco. It was obvious from the last meeting that our dear friend and colleague, Wolfgang Haigis, would not be attending future IPC meetings, so the EC instituted an annual **Haigis Lecture** in his honor. The 30-min two-part inaugural lecture was given on the morning of October 10, 2019, by David Chang, MD, of Los Altos, CA (below, third from left).

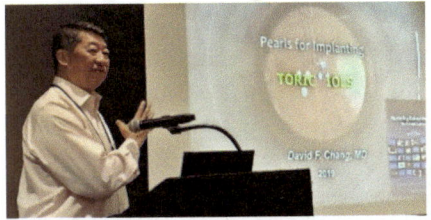
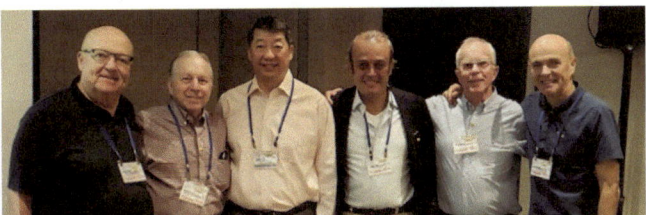

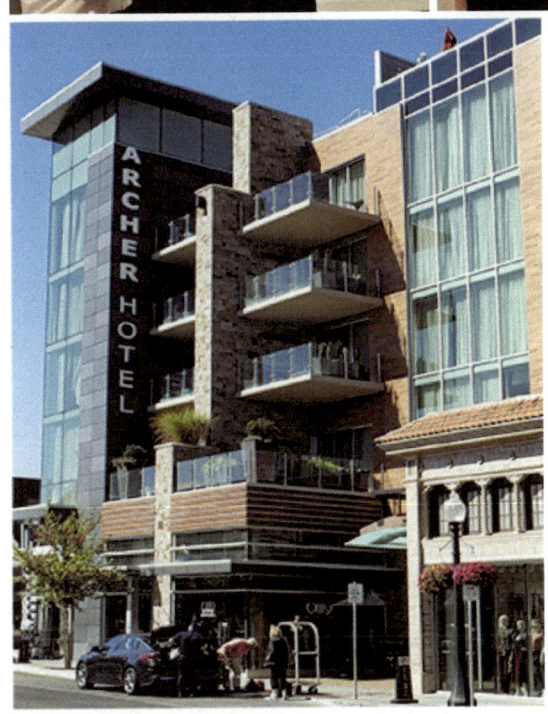

Attendees: **Members**: Edmondo Borasio, MD, Jean-Philippe Colliac, MD, Massimo Camellin, MD, Claudio Carbonara, MD, Han Bor Fam, MD, David Flikier, MD, Oliver Findl, MD, Nino Hirnschall, MD, Jack X. Kane, MD, Scott McClatchy, MD, Sabong Srivannaboon, MD, and Tun Kuan Yeo, MD. **Honorary Member:** John Retzlaff, MD. **Invited speakers**: David Chang*, MD (Los Altos, CA), Damien Gatinel* (Paris), Ron Melles*, MD (Redwood City, CA), Pablo Perez, PhD (Madrid), and Woong-Joo Whang*, MD (Seoul, South Korea) as well as the previous guests who also gave presentations: David Cooke, MD (Berrien Springs, MI), and Peter Fedor, MD (Traverse City, MI).

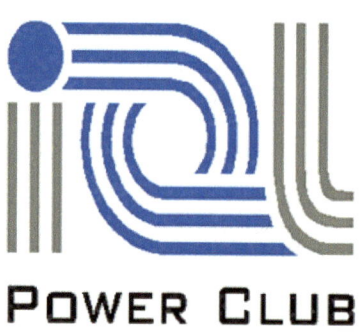

15th
Annual
Scientific
Session

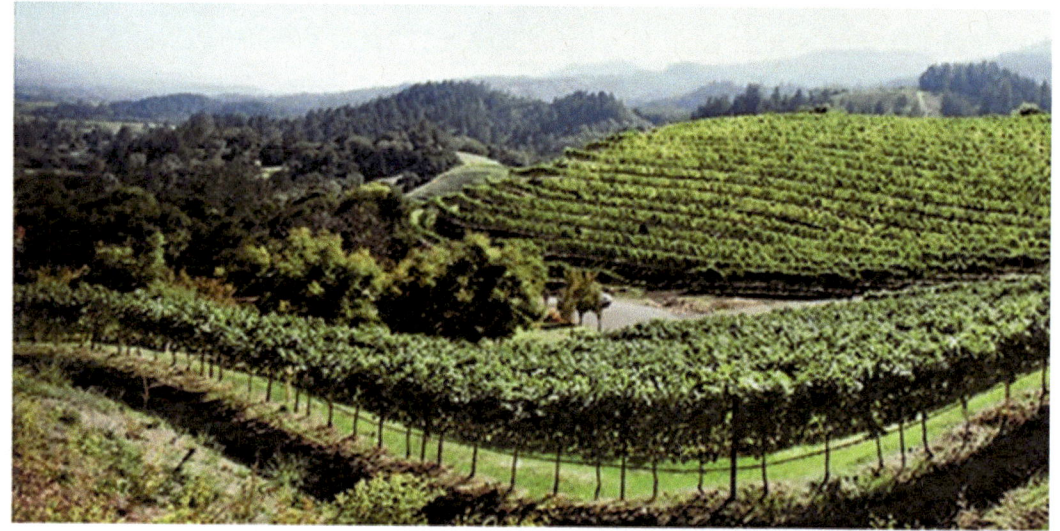

OUR FIRST VISIT TO AMERICA'S FAMOUS WINE REGION

ARCHER HOTEL

CO-CHAIRMEN

H JOHN SHAMMAS MD
KENNETH J HOFFER MD

OCTOBER 8-11, 2019

NAPA VALLEY
CALIFORNIA

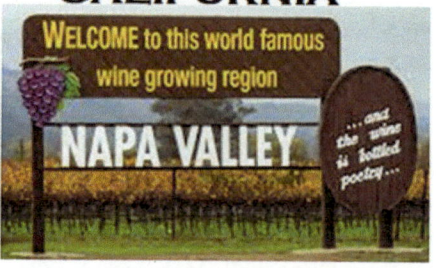

Industry: Jacqueline Asam*, MD (Heidelberg), Thomas Bütler (Haag-Streit), Arkadiusz Chalecki* (Optopol), Naoko Hara (Tomey), Keith Holliday* (Staar), Jörg Iwanzcuk (Oculus), Oliver Klaproth (Zeiss), Thomas Padrick, PhD (Alcon), Gregor Schmid, PhD (Ziemer), Simon Schroeder, PhD (Zeiss), Michael Trost* (Zeiss), and Francesco Versaci (CSO).

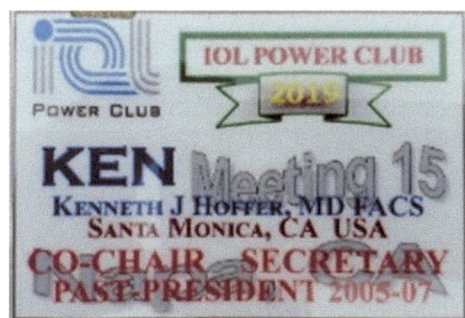

At this meeting, we welcomed new participation by STAAR Surgical (Keith Holliday) and Optopol (Arek Chalecki) from Poland.

At our EC Business meeting, the eighth Election voted in Shammas as President, Olsen as Vice-President, Hoffer as Secretary, and Savini as Treasurer.

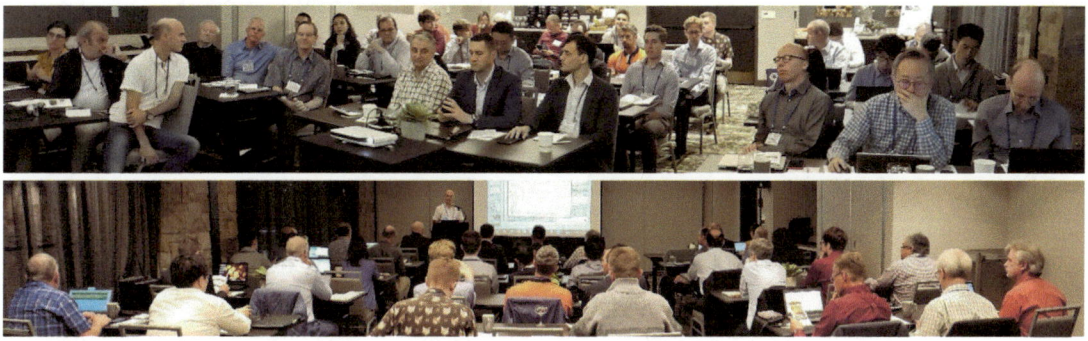

Kristin Hoffer (below left) had been hired as Administrator and did an excellent job with our new policy of having all presentations put on one computer in advance of the session. This made it go much more smoothly than previous meetings. Thanks to Jim Mazzo (AMO, Zeiss) below left, we were invited for a Welcome Reception at his Jessup Cellars winery in Yountville, north of Napa. Mazzos's strong support of IPC as AMO Gold Sponsor had a immense effect on the quality and success of our meetings over these past years.

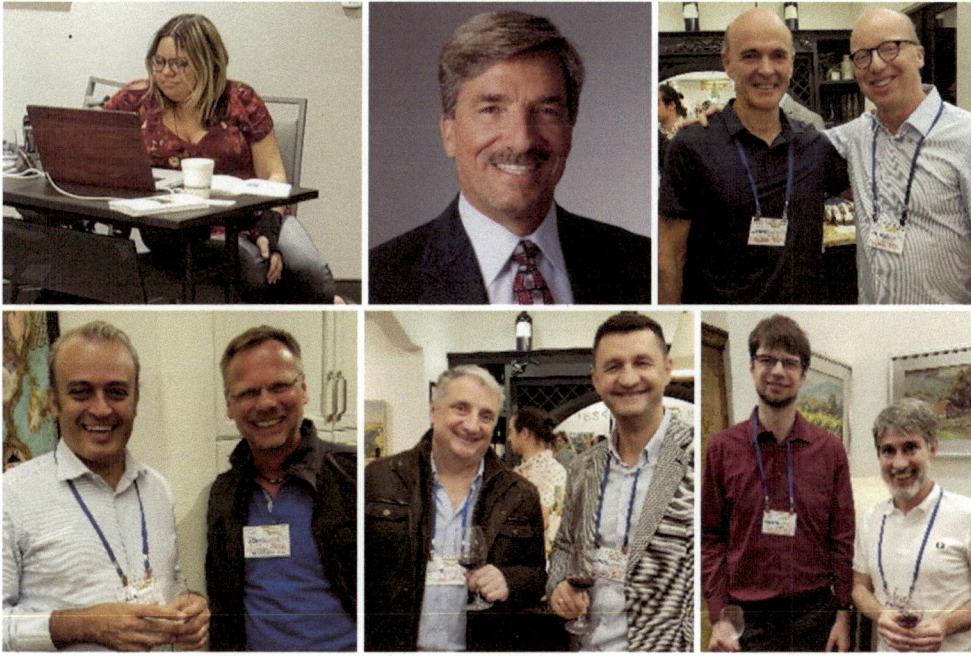

Above (L-R): Jaime and Oliver Findl (Vienna); Giacomo Savini and Jörg Iwanczuk (Oculus); David Flikier, MD (Costa Rica), and Arkadiusz (Arek) Chalecki* (Optopol); Simon Schröder, PhD (Zeiss), and Pablo Pérez, PhD (Madrid) (*first-timers).

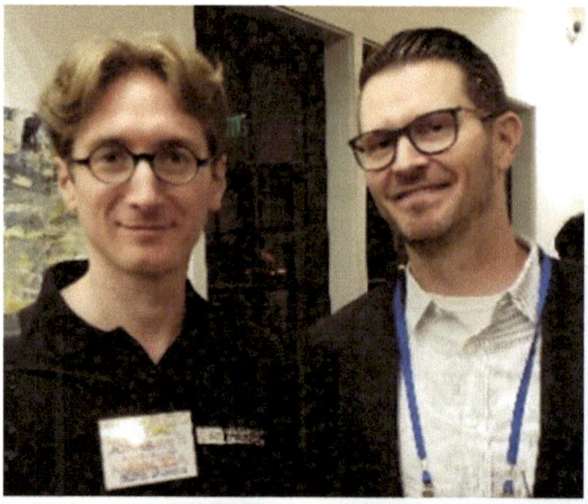

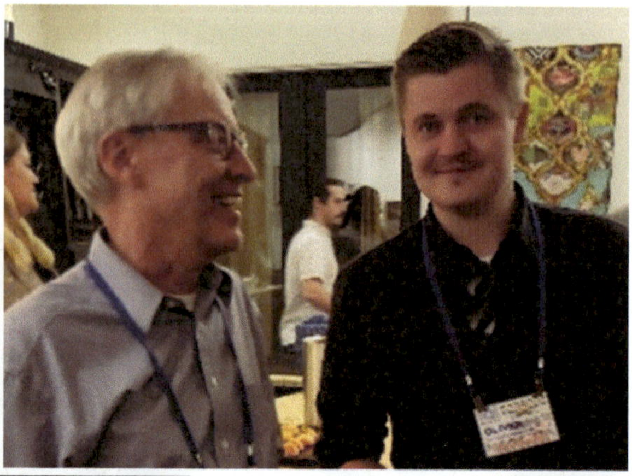

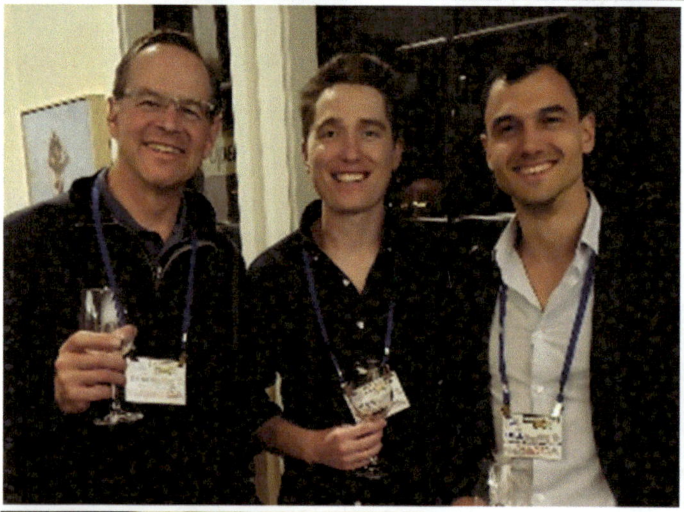

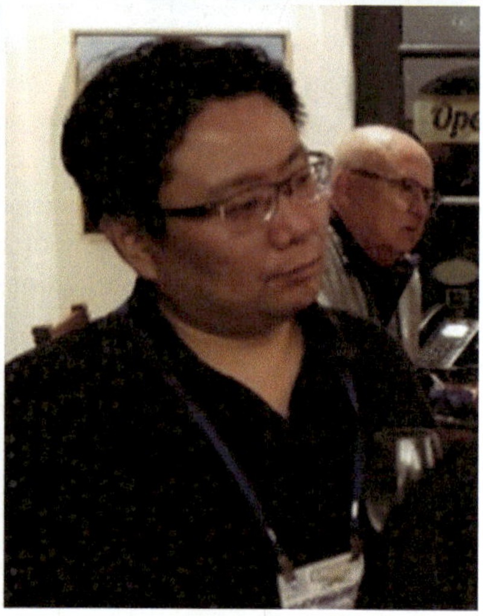

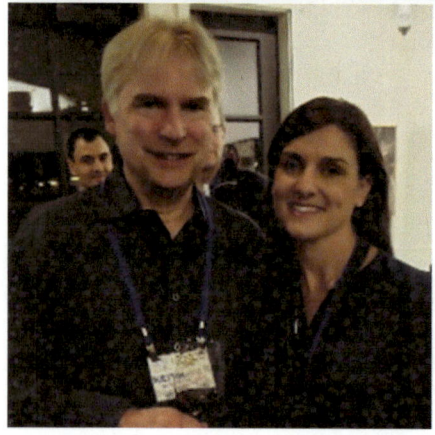

Above (L-R): Jonas Haehnle (Haag-Streit) and Rich Cornwell* (Heidelberg); David Cooke MD and Oliver Klaproth (Zeiss);

Ron Melles* MD (Redwood City, CA), Jack Kane MD (Melbourne) and Guillaume Debellemaniere* MD (Paris); Whong-Joo Whang* MD (Seoul, South Korea): and Keith Holliday* (STAAR Surgical).

Four days after the meeting, Wolfgang Haigis died peacefully in his sleep at home on October 15, and his funeral was held in Würzburg on November 8. The three European EC members visited his wife Katrine and the gravesite the next day. The lecture has been renamed the **Haigis Memorial Lecture**. Below left is the robust Wolfgang Haigis I remember (1999), the Würzburg Cemetery where he is buried and the IPC's final tribute to him at his funeral.

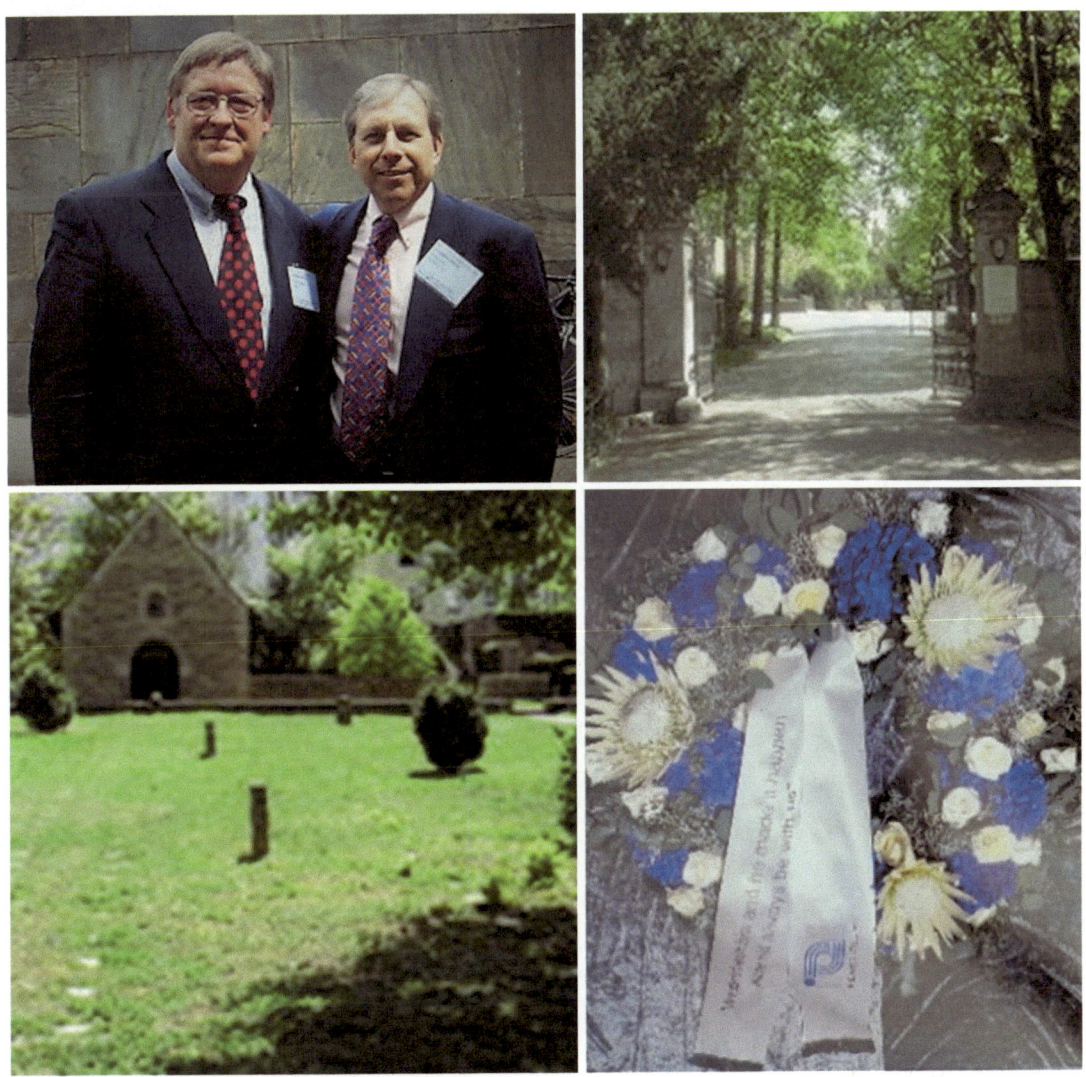

2020 16th IPC Meeting: Rockland, ME, May, Rockland Harbor Hotel and Farnsworth Museum was cancelled due to the pandemic.

2021: 16th IPC Meeting—Carmel, CA, July 28–31 Pine Inn Hotel (Site of our Second Meeting in 2006)

We were able to hold the meeting in August 2021 in Carmel after the live San Francisco ASCRS meeting. The venue was the Pine Inn on Ocean Ave (below left) where the second IPC Meeting was held in 2006 (15 years previously). Because of the continued pandemic travel restrictions we had less attendees and had to do our EC Business meeting on Zoom.

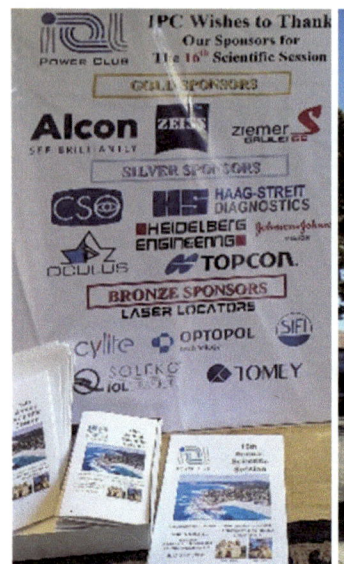
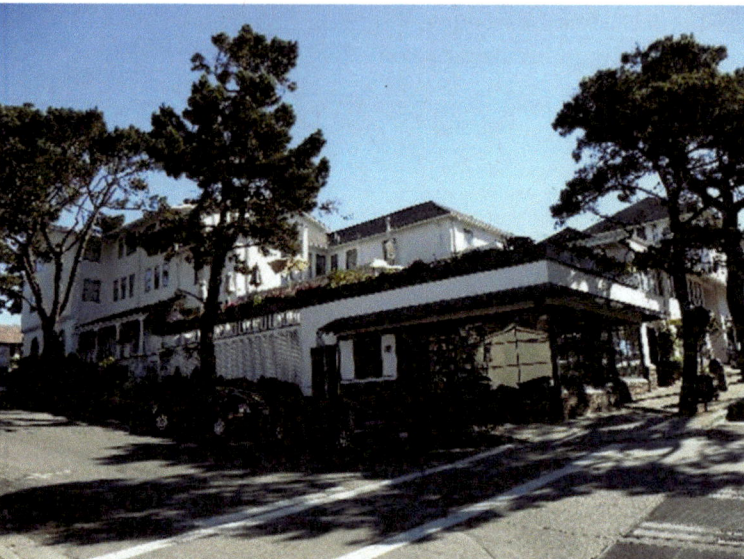
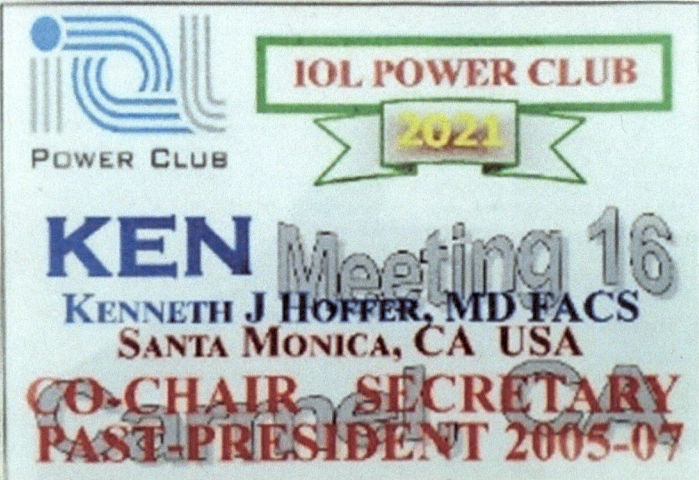
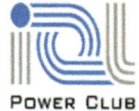
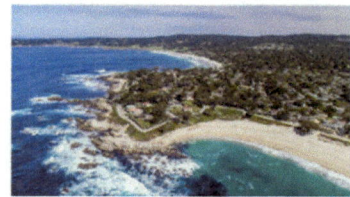
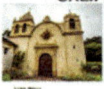

We toured the MacDonald Sculpture Foundry (Famed artist/sculptor Richard MacDonald center)

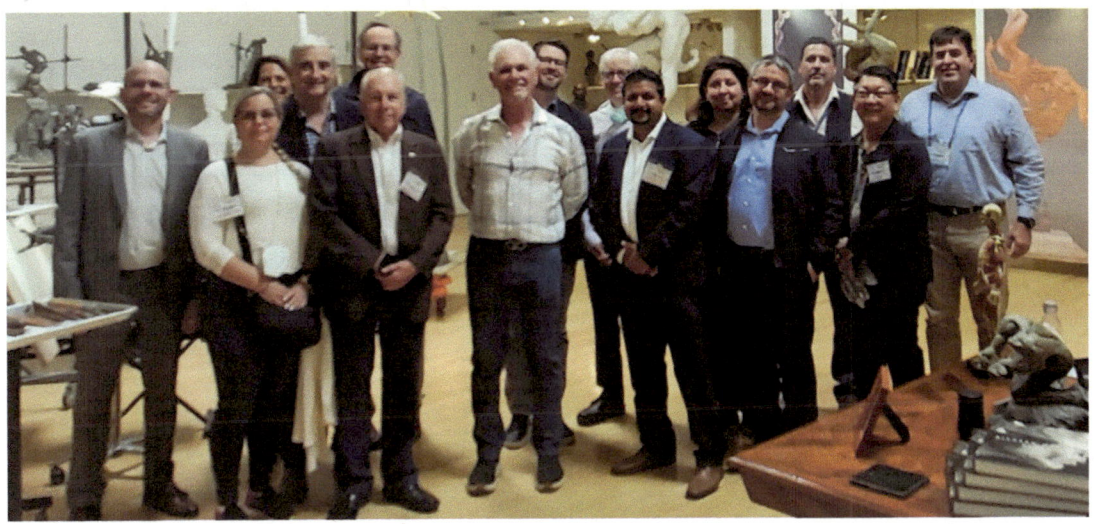

and used their gallery in Carmel for the Welcome Reception (below). Our main dinner was at the Spanish Bay Country Club.

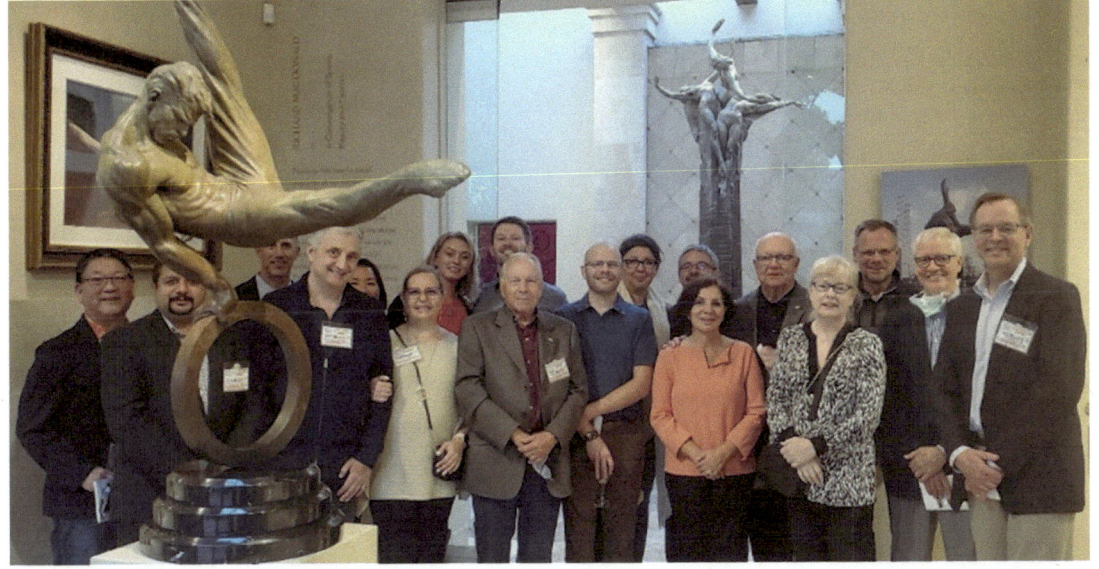

IOL Power Club 16th Scientific Session Agenda DAY #1 THU			
July 29th Pine Inn Hotel, Carmel, CA USA			
IPC SESSION 1-A	**EU TOPICS**	**Moderator**	**SHAMMAS**
TITLE	**Speaker**	**Time**	**Duration**
WELCOME Meeting Co-Chairman	*H John Shammas MD	9:00 AM	0:05
IPC President: Introductions of EC & GUESTS	*H John Shammas MD	9:05 AM	0:10
Effect of Immersion AL on Lens Constants	*David L Cooke MD	9:15 AM	0:10
DISCUSSION	ALL	9:25 AM	0:05
Comparing Biometers for Ant Segment Analysis	*Thomas Olsen MD	9:30 AM	0:10
DISCUSSION	ALL	9:40 AM	0:05
AL in Long Eyes: Argos vs IOLM700 vs Optimiz	*Giacomo Savini MD	9:45 AM	0:10
DISCUSSION	ALL	9:55 AM	0:05
Post-LASIK Exact Ray-Tracing Calculations	*Jaime Aramberri MD	10:00 AM	0:10
DISCUSSION	ALL	10:10 AM	0:05
Standard K vs TK in PO Myopic Femto LASIK	*Giacomo Savini MD	10:15 AM	0:10
DISCUSSION	ALL	10:25 AM	0:05
COFFEE BREAK & DISCUSSION	ALL	10:30 AM	0:30

We didn't really schedule it as a remote virtual meeting but because all our European members and speakers (in Red in the Program) were not allowed into the USA, we had 20 participants live (L) and 20 on Zoom (R), mainly in the early parts of the day due to the time difference.

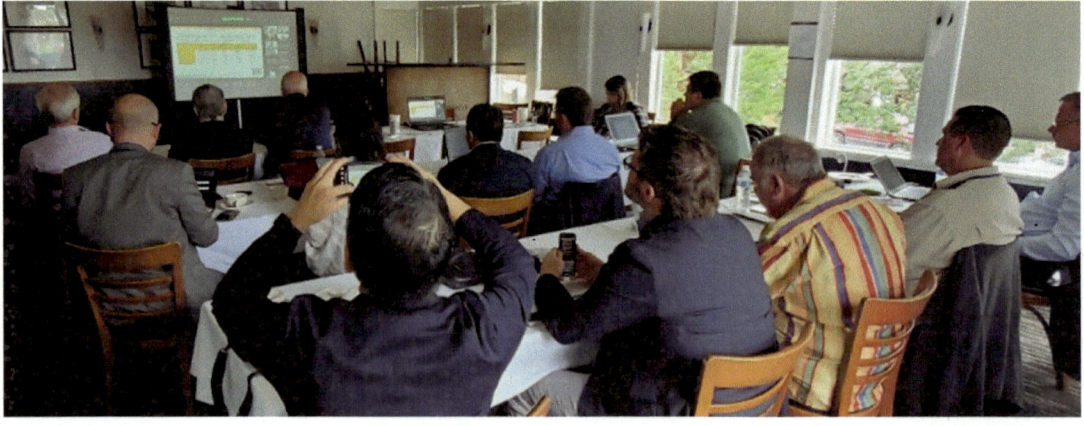

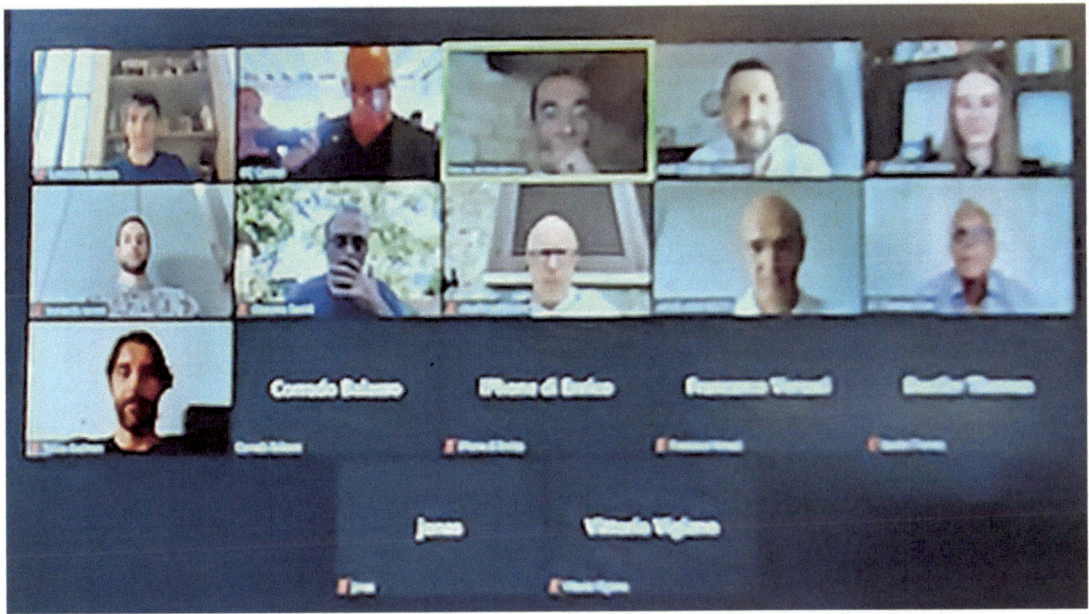

It turned out better than we had expected. It was there that we approved the publication of a **new 72 chapter IPC textbook on IOL Power Calculation** with Open Access to all including all aspects of all biometers and all formula authors. Over the ensuing year, members of the IPC helped foster the development of the free <u>ECSRS All Formula Website Calculator</u> developed by Dante Buosanti, MD, of Buenos Aries, Argentina which is a great benefit to ophthalmologists all over the world.

2022: 17th IPC Meeting—Stresa, Italy, September 21–24 Princess Regina Hotel

The 17th Meeting was held in Stresa on Lago (Lake) Maggiore in the Italian Northern Lakes region after the ESCRS Meeting in Milano, Italy, in September 2022.

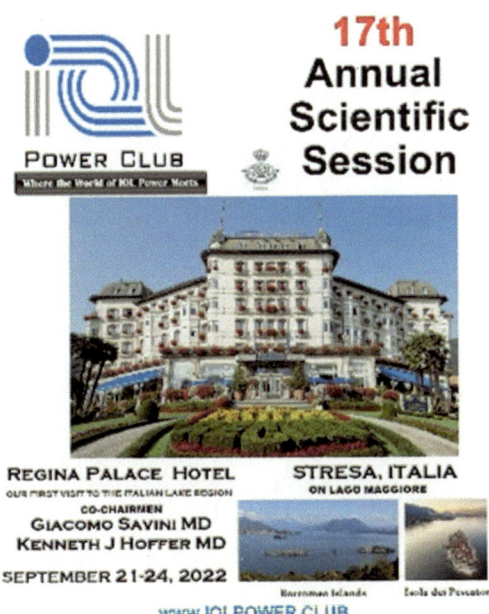

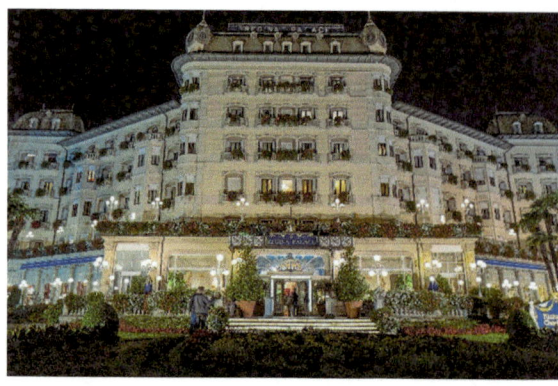 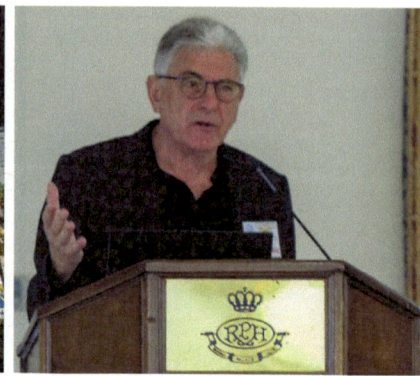

There was an overwhelming response, and it was the largest meeting we have ever had with 75 attendees and many new people from around the world. The second **Haigis Memorial Lecture** was given by Graham Barrett, MD (above right), of Perth, Australia (below).

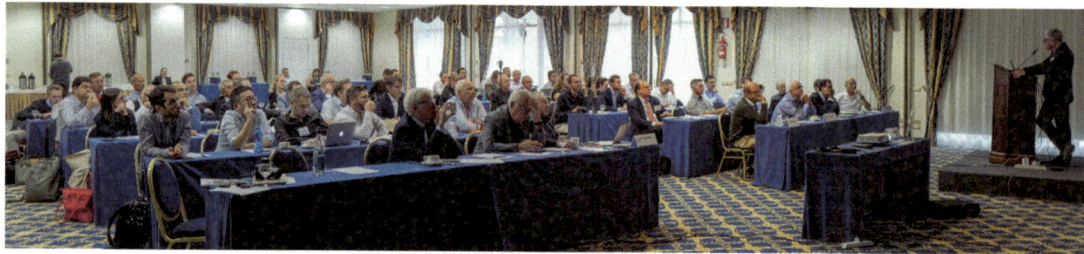

The Membership requested the President appoint a Subcommittee to prepare a general statement by the IPC requesting that all manufacturers comply with publicizing their IOL structural dimensions for the benefit of IOL power accuracy for patients around the world. This was done and led to a special publication in *JCRS* in 2023 [J Cataract Refract Surg 2023;49(6):556-557]. There was a boat tour of the Borromeo Islands and an ancient winery tour in a nearby town. Everyone was pleased to have a live meeting again.

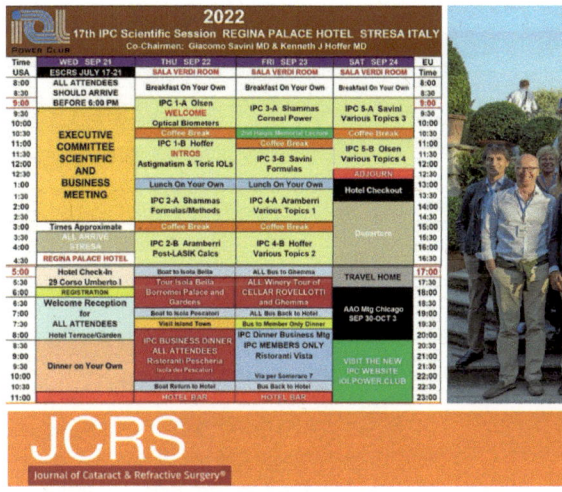
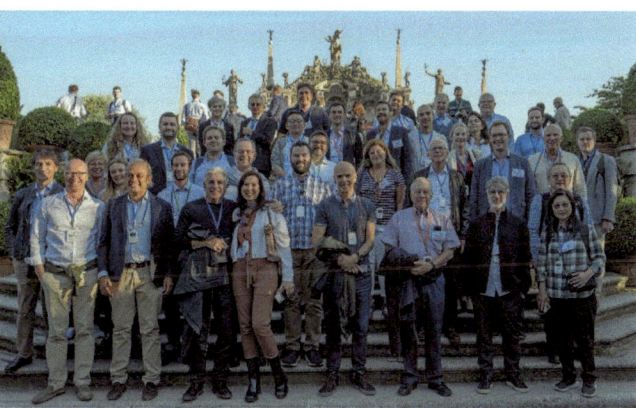

JCRS
Journal of Cataract & Refractive Surgery®

SPECIAL REPORT

Surgeons need to know more about intraocular lens design for accurate power calculation

Olsen, Thomas MD; Cooke, David L. MD; Findl, Oliver MD; Gatinel, Damien MD; Koch, Douglas MD; Langenbucher, Achim MD; Melles, Ronald B. MD; Yeo, Tun K. MD

Journal of Cataract & Refractive Surgery 49(6):p 556-557, june 2023. | *DOI:* 10.1097/j.jcrs.0000000000001159

Acknowledgments

This article was authored by a subcommittee of the IOL Power Club: David L. Cooke, USA; Oliver Findl, Austria; Damien Gatinel, France; Douglas Koch, USA; Achim Langenbucher, Germany; Ronald B. Melles, USA; Thomas Olsen, Denmark; and Tun Kuan Yeo, Singapore.

This meeting really felt like the "world of IOL Power" had gotten together; it was inspiring for everyone who attended and bodes well for the future collaborative efforts of ophthalmologists, scientists, and industry to perfcct the calculation of IOL power. I am not sure Wolfgang would be so happy seeing it become this big, but he sure should be proud of what has been accomplished.

2023: 18th IPC Meeting—Palm Springs, CA, November 8–11 Hotel Zoso Palm Springs

This meeting was held right after the AAO meeting in San Francisco and for the first time in the famed desert city of Palm Springs at the Hotel Zoso (below L). The EC held their usual Business Meeting. There were 65 attendees and for the first time topic discussion groups were help on specific controversies; Savini moderated one on "When to Optimize Constants" and Koch moderated the other on "Best Method to Optimize". Douglas Koch presented the 3rd Haigis Memorial Lecture. The Membership meeting allowed a group photo (EC, Graham Barrett, Han Bor Fam, Doug Koch, David Flikier, David Cooke, Ron Melles, Jean-Philippe Colliac, and Pablo Perez.). It was extremely successful. The meeting led to the JCRS Special Report publication of a new system to classify IOL power formulas (see diagram).

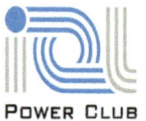

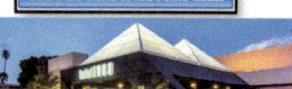

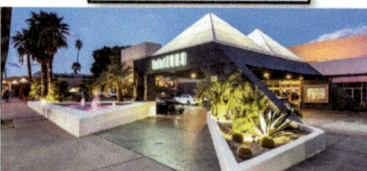

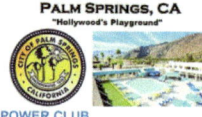

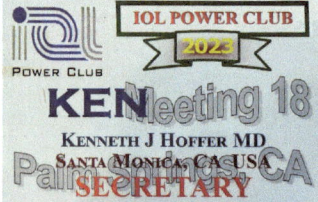

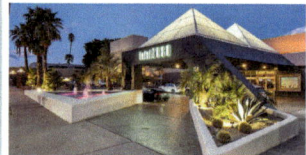

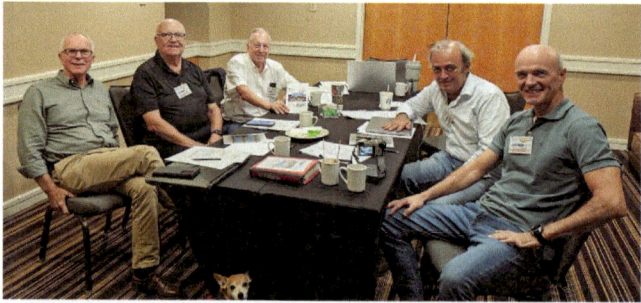

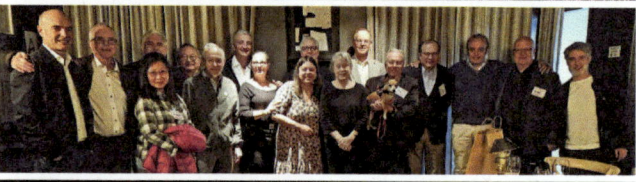

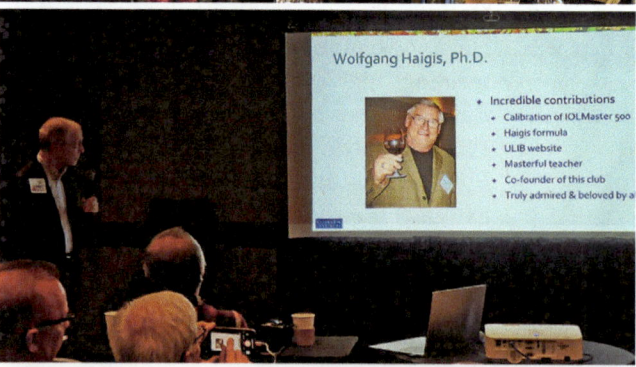

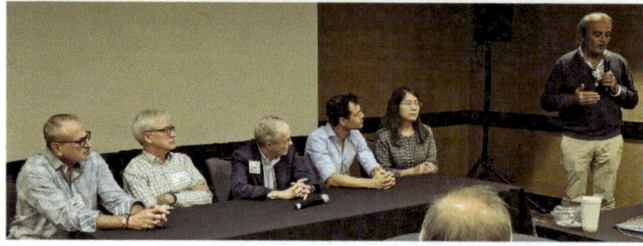

2024: 19th IPC Meeting—Rockland, ME, April 9–12 Rockland Harbor Hotel , Maine Lighthouse Museum and Farnsworth Museum

We held our 19th meeting, where we had originally planned our 16th 4 years ago (cancelled by the pandemic), in Rockland, ME, the "Lobster Capitol of America".

Member Attendees: 6 EC Members, Jean-Philippe Colliac MD, David L Cooke MD, Damien Gatinel MD, Peter Hoffmann MD, Ronald Melles MD, Pablo Perez MD, Jascha Wendelstein MD and Tun Kuan Yeo MD.

Invited Speakers: Catarina Coutinho MSc (Bologna, Italy), Achim Langenbucher PhD (Homberg, German), Peter Fedor MD (Traverse City, MI), Enrico Lupardi MD (Bologna, Italy), Susana Marcos PhD (Rochester, NY), Seonghwan Kim MD (Seoul, Korea) and Woong-Joo Whang MD (Seoul, Korea).

New Attendees: Sutmei Chan MD (Kuala Lumpur, Malaysia), Timothy Cooke (Berrien Springs, MI), Xiansong Dai MSc (Shenzhen, China, Moptim), Kamal Das PhD (Arlington, TX, Alcon), J Christopher Freeman (Oklahoma City, OK, J&J), Daniela Nicolosi (Sant'Antonio, Italy, SIFI), Brian Schwam MD (Jacksonville, FL, J&J). Patrick Shurk (Munich, Germany, Zeiss), Bryan Stanfill PhD (Mansfield, TX, Alcon), Martina Vacalebre (Sant'Antonio, Italy, SIFI), Sid Wei PhD (Irvine, CA, Medennium), Chris Wilcox (Irvine, CA, Medennium), Mengmeng Yang (Shenzhen, China, Moptim) and Peter Zieger PhD (Alcon).

Industry Attendees: Nicolas Bensaid PhD (Berlin, Germany, Zeiss), Thomas Bütler (Köniz, Switzerland, Haag-Streit), Arkadiusz Chalecki (Optopol), Richard Cornwell (Seattle, WA, Heidelberg), Alessandro Foggi (San Giovanni Valdarno, Italy, Visia Imaging/Topcon), Jörg Iwanczuk (Oculus), Gregor Schmid (Ziemer) and Steven Thomson (North Berwick, UK, Heidelberg).

A Program cover and a name badge.

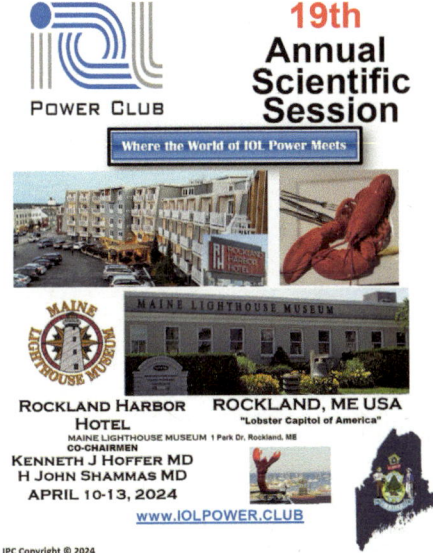

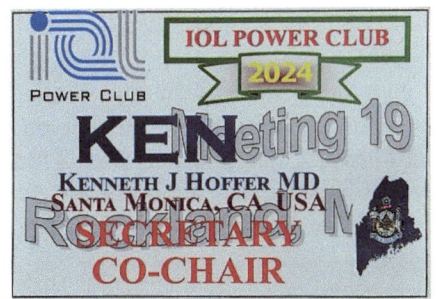

We stayed at the Rockland Harbor Hotel (Below Top) and our Scientific Sessions were all held at the Maine Lighthouse Museum about 6 blocks away (Below Bottom).

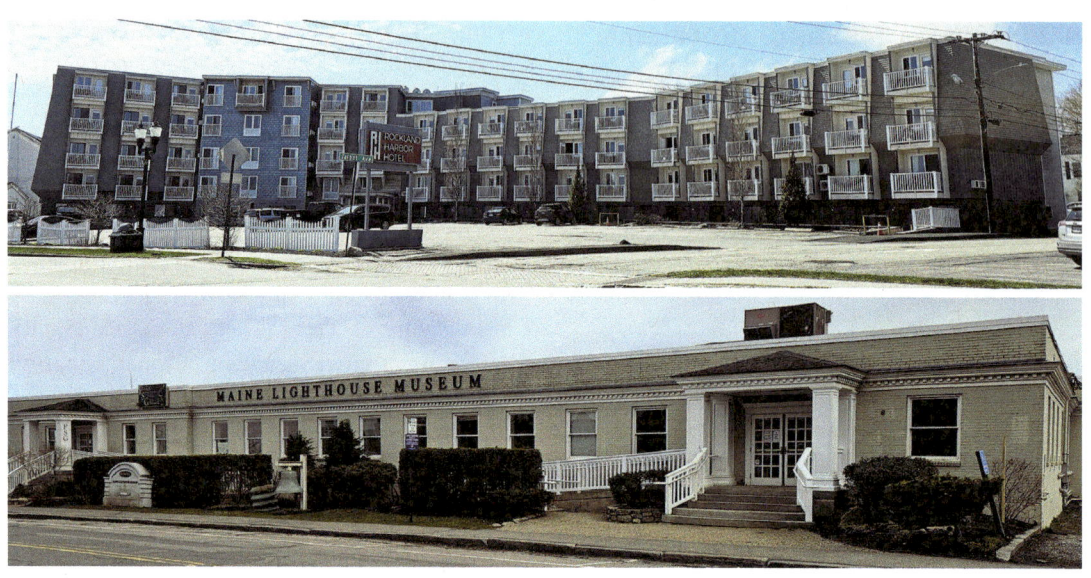

Our Welcome Reception was at the noted Farnsworth Museum (of Andrew Wyeth fame) with a guided tour by its Director (Below). Everyone had the chance to view some of Wyeth's works.

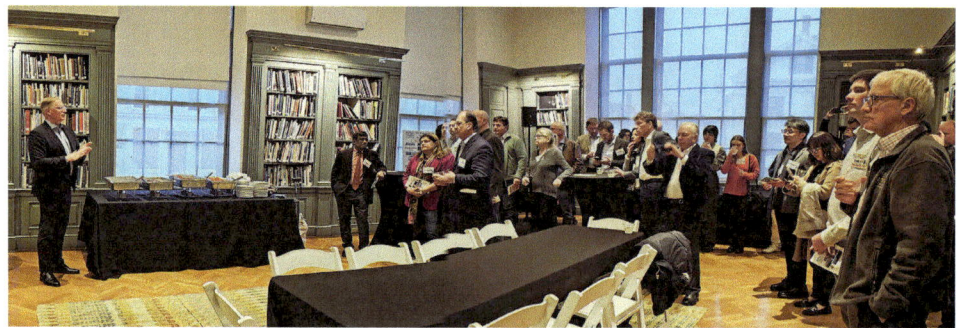

At the start of the first scientific session, Marcia Hoffer (below left) welcomed everyone to Rockland where she was born and raised. I had the pleasure of showing the attendees the 1st mockup of our new 5.5 lb 1,000 page IPC textbook. The EC took a group shot in front of the Museum near the metal lobster sculpture.

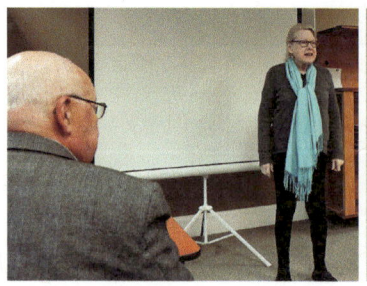 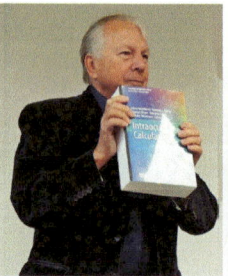 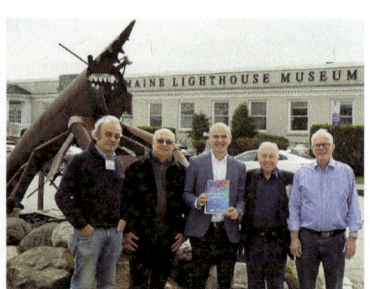

Lectures were held continuously for 2 ½ days. The 4th Haigis Memorial Lecture was given by Thomas Kohnen MD (Frankfurt, Germany) (below right) as part of a special session on Phakic IOLs.

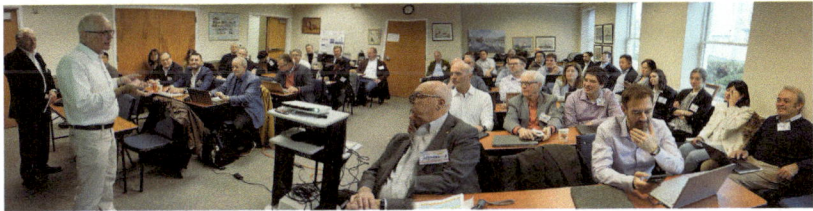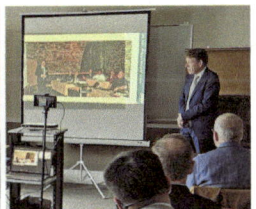

Filomena Ribeiro MD (Lisbon, Portugal) attended her 1st IPC EC business meetings since elected to fill Wolfgang Haigis' seat.

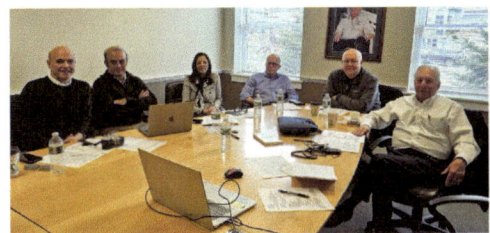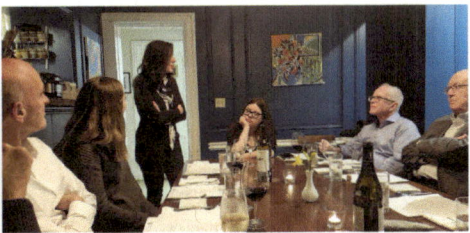

The ALL Dinner was a classical "Maine Lobster Bake" at Archer's on the Pier. Lynn Archer took care of everyone (Below right, with Dr. Wei). The weather was not ideal but improved with time. The Membership Meeting was held at the Camden Harbour Inn.

The person to the left of Jaime is his daughter who is now a practicing ophthalmologist; her photo as a child can also be seen in the photos at the 2008 IPC meeting in St. Pete Beach.

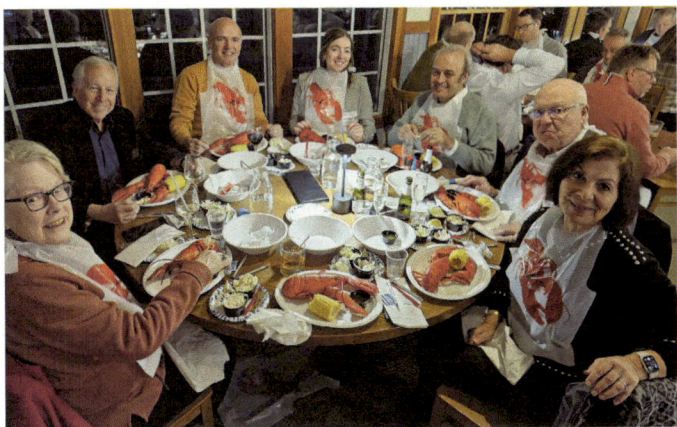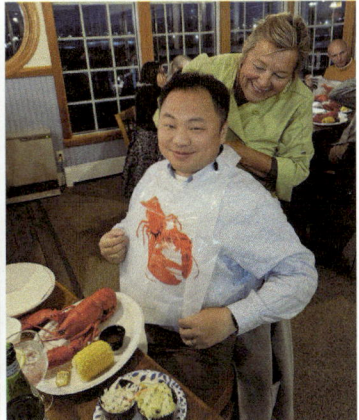

Carl Woodman (left), a lifelong lobsterman (and Marcia's high school classmate), gave an optional tour of his son's lobster processing and shipping facility which was something quite different for many, especially for Dr. Chan (right) from Malaysia.

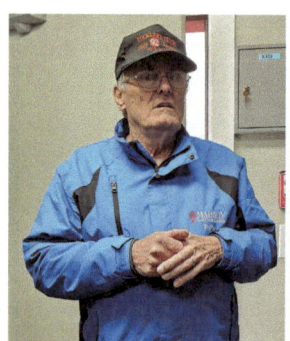
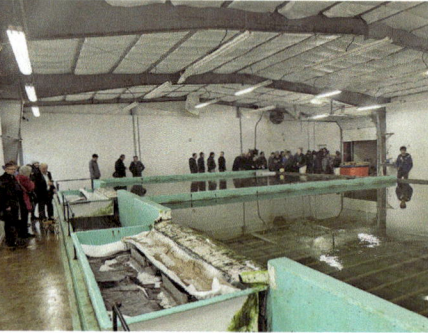
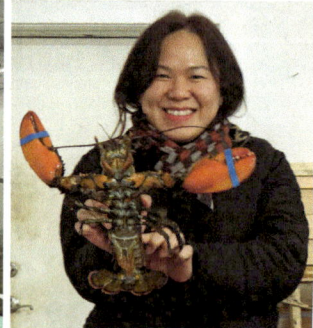

A Panel was held on the possibilities and complexities of the IPC setting up a collaborative data base of PO cases for any Member to use for future studies. We heard the 1st presentations on the new Colombo II optical biometer from Moptim, Shenzhen, China. The caliber of the presentations and interactions were exceptional, maybe one of our best. To our surprise the meeting turned out to be an overwhelming success, even with the cold and rain. A group shot of everyone (in the rain).

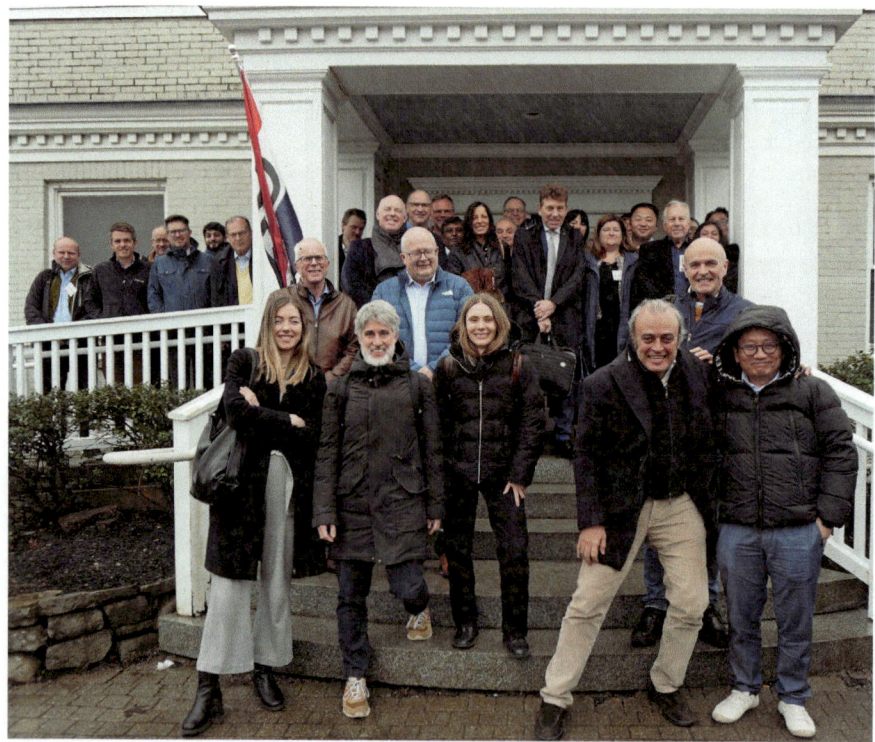

2025: 20th Anniversary IPC Meeting—Santa Barbara, CA, April 29-May 2

We will celebrate our 20th Anniversary Meeting in the coastal beach city of Santa Barbara, CA right after the ASCRS Meeting in Los Angeles.

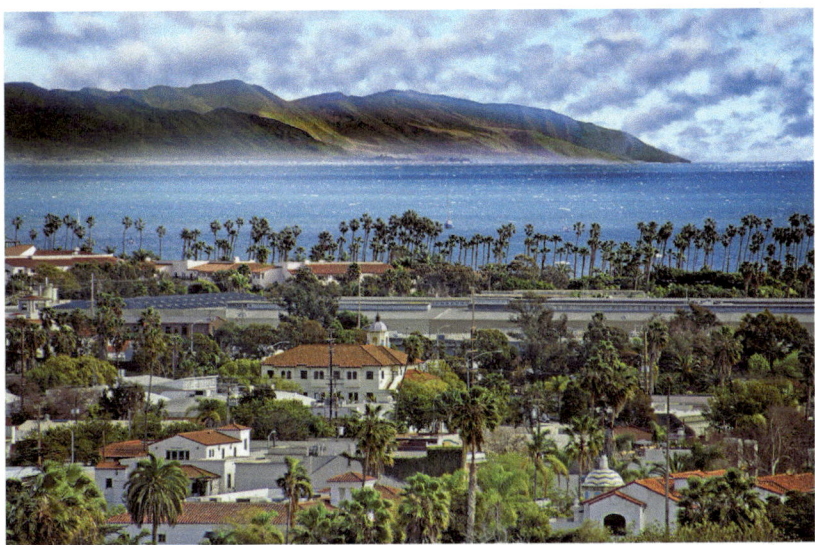

We are ever indebted to Wolfgang Haigis, PhD, and Sverker Norrby, PhD, for helping all this get started in 2005 and their many years of efforts in bringing us to where we are now.

The IPC will endeavor to continue fostering development in IOL power prediction accuracy.

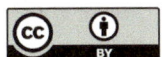

American History of IOL Power Calculation

Kenneth J. Hoffer

Introduction

Without the ability to accurately calculate its desired power, the intraocular lens (IOL) would never have become the revolution in eye surgery that it has. Many pioneers contributed to the development of accurate IOL power calculation, and I merely borrowed from most of them to arrive at methods and systems that would provide the greatest accuracy for my patients. My interest in teaching led me to share these procedures with my colleagues over this past half century. I have also enjoyed the challenge of trying to develop improvements and on occasion these endeavors have been fruitful. I will, therefore, present a personal history of these events as I remember them.

Prior to my first IOL implantation on April 22, 1974, I realized I needed to measure the axial length (AL) of the eye with ultrasound (US), measure the corneal power (K), and use an optical formula to obtain the IOL power needed for the patient.

Personal Ultrasound History

The first time I had ever heard of ultrasound in ophthalmology was from lectures given by Dr. Michael Weinstock during my residency at Kresge Eye Institute (Wayne State University) in Detroit (1969–1972), and I personally found the subject rather uninteresting. The next time the subject arose was in my first year of practice at an Eye Staff meeting at St. John's Hospital in Santa Monica in 1972. Robert Sinskey, the Chairman, asked the staff who would volunteer to fly to New York City and attend a course on how to use the new Sonometrics Coleman B-scan ultrasound diagnostic unit the hospital was purchasing. No one wanted to go and since I had relatives in New York, I volunteered. This decision changed my professional career.

The faculty at the 2-day course in Southampton consisted of Drs. Nathaniel Bronson, Jackson Coleman, and Karl Ossoinig (Fig. 2.1). Karl was a young A-scan pioneer and guru that Dr. Fred Blodi had brought from Vienna, Austria to Iowa City to teach at the university there. Karl gave a lecture on the techniques to accurately measure the axial length of the eye, and I distinctly remember wondering how often that would be of any clinical use and laughing about it with a fellow participant. That evening, the course sponsored a cocktail party at a local eatery and after dinner, Karl and I sampled at least five or six of their various brews. The conversation waxed until closing time, and a friendship started that night that has lasted all these years. What a totally fortuitous event!

K. J. Hoffer (✉)
St. Mary's Eye Center, Santa Monica, CA, USA

Stein Eye Institute, UCLA, Los Angeles, CA, USA
e-mail: KHofferMD@StartMail.com

© The Author(s) 2024
J. Aramberri et al. (eds.), *Intraocular Lens Calculations*, Essentials in Ophthalmology,
https://doi.org/10.1007/978-3-031-50666-6_2

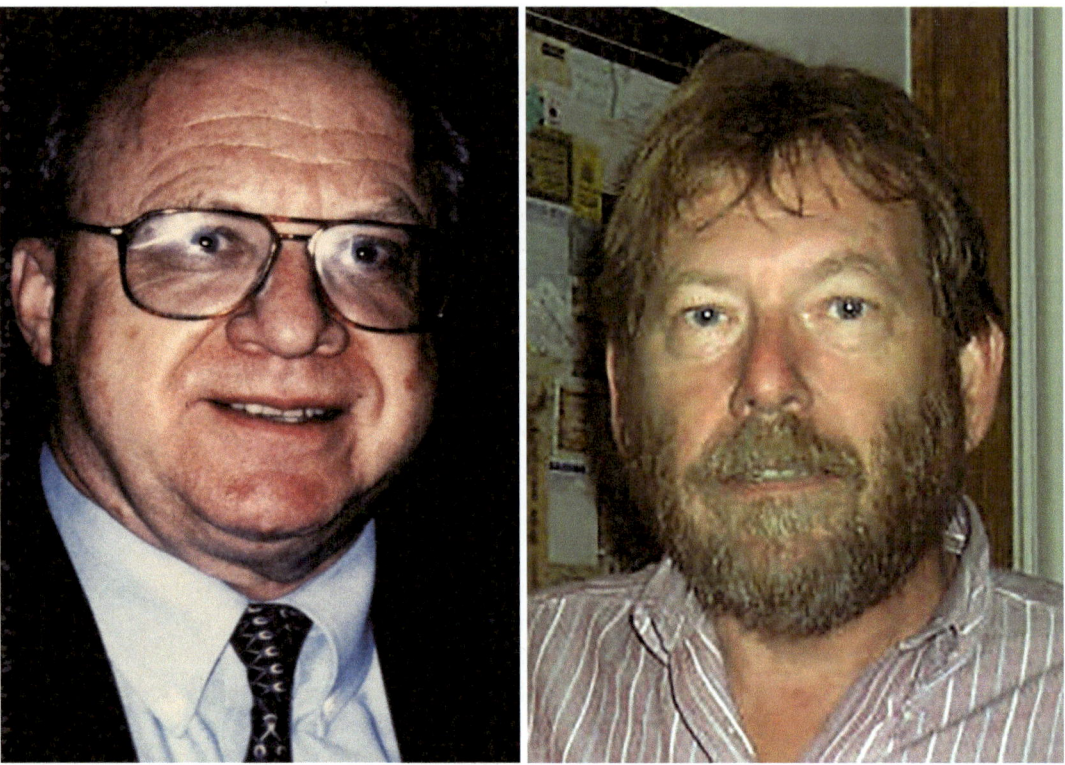

Fig. 2.1 Karl Ossoinig, MD (left), aided in the first ultrasound IOL power calculation in America; Gary G Hoffer, the author's brother

First American Ultrasound IOL Power Calculation

In early 1974, while planning my first IOL implantation on Mrs. Phoebe Miller (deceased), I had learned that Jan Worst (of Groningen, Holland) was using a little A-scan ultrasound unit to obtain an AL for IOL power calculation. I had remembered Ossoinig's lectures and called him for advice on the instrument I should use. Santa Monica Hospital (SMH) subsequently agreed to purchase the recommended Kretz 7200-MA unit (Fig. 2.2) from Austria along with a keratometer and provide a facility where I could perform the tests. They gave me the use of the hospital's old Intensive Care Unit, and I called the new facility the EyeLab. They soon hired a supervisor, Maryanne Hooper RN, and a photographer, Don Allen, who was to begin performing fluorescein angiograms.

I performed the first A-scan IOL power calculation with Dr. Ossoinig [Fig. 2.1] (on the phone from Iowa) talking me through the calibration of the Kretz unit and how to measure the Polaroid camera photo-

graphs using precision calipers. For his willingness to help me, I will be eternally grateful. It worked!

Prior to this time, American lens implanters used a standard 18.0 D IOL for all eyes, expecting the patient to be as myopic or hyperopic as they were before surgery. In the mid-70s, Dennis Shepard devised a nomogram (Fig. 2.3) based on the patient's preoperative refractive error. It was distributed in the syllabus to all those attending the SMH monthly lens implant courses that began in May 1974 and trained 2,600 surgeons over the ensuing years. After the word got out about our EyeLab, many colleagues sent their patients to us for IOL power calculations, including Henry Hirschman, who limousined his patients to Santa Monica from Long Beach. After months of performing the exam myself, I finally decided that I had to train a technician to do it. Our photographer, Don Allen, was the closest at hand and after 2 months he picked it up easily and became the first IOL power calculation technician in America and he trained many others to follow him. Don died 30 years ago and I honor him for his pioneering work.

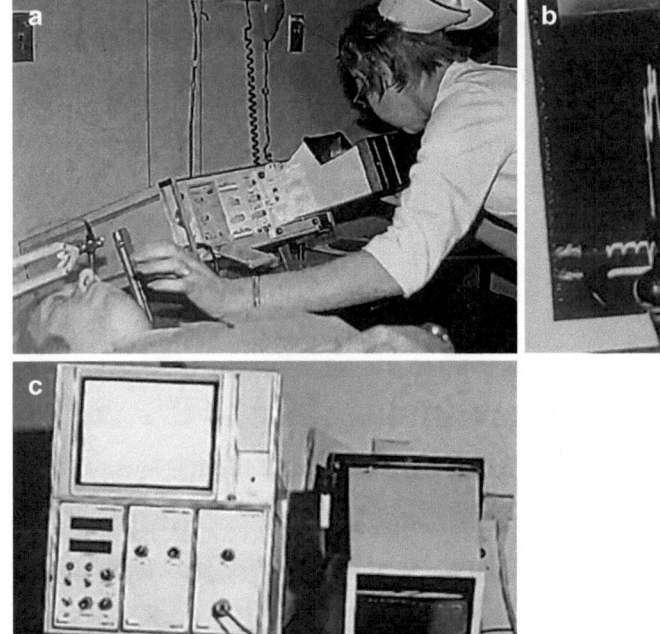

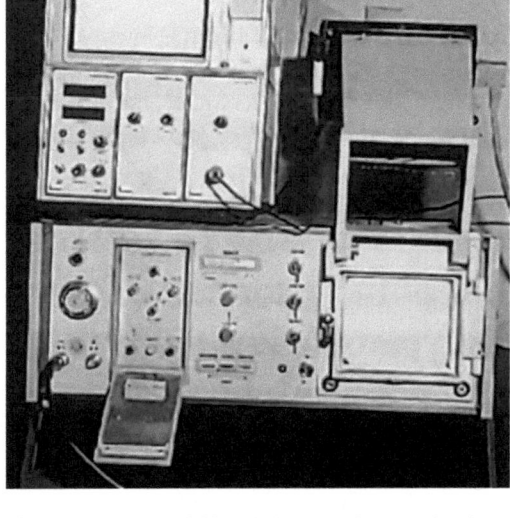

Fig. 2.2 A Kretz 7200-MA A-scan ultrasound unit used for the first IOL power calculation in America 1974. (**a**) Performing an immersion exam on Gary Hoffer (deceased). (**b**) Caliper measurement of the axial length on a Polaroid photograph of the A-scan. (**c**) A Kretz instrument (below) with its Xenotec replacement on top of it.

Fig. 2.3 A Dennis Shepard IOL power prediction nomogram distributed at all early Santa Monica Hospital IOL courses

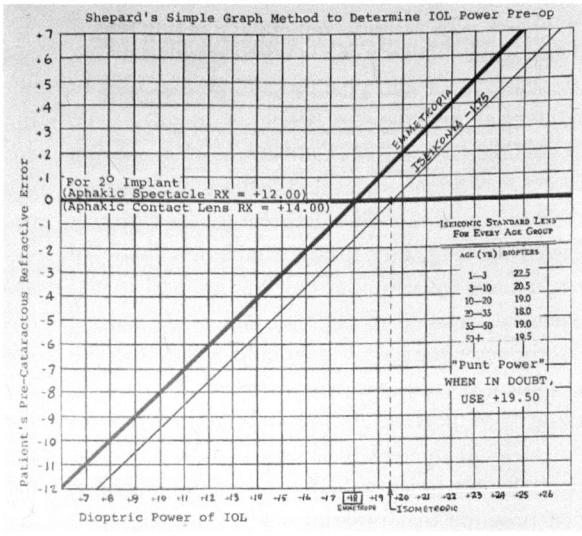

Personal Formula History

See Chapter 43 on Hoffer Formula History.

Earliest Calculators and Computers

At first, I used my new Hoffer formula in longhand with paper and pencil for each patient, which was quite tedious. By July 1974, my brother Gary (patient in Fig. 2.1), who was a computer programmer before there were personal computers, now deceased) convinced me to let him program the formula on the mainframe computer he used at his work (TransAmerica Insurance Co., Los Angeles). The biometric data from each exam was phoned in to him by our nurse, Maryanne, and Gary would later call back with the IOL power result. Often, however, the computer would be tied up and we would have to wait for hours or until the next day for the results. Gary also helped make history by recommending in 1974 that I have the membership list of my fledgling American Intra-Ocular Implant Society (now ASCRS) programmed on a micro computer (years before PCs) making ASCRS the first medical society to do so.

For many years, SMH implant courses usually had from 25 to 40 attendees. Dr. Shepard would implant an intracapsular IOL in three to four cases, and I would do one case of phacoemulsification using a Binkhorst two-loop iridocapsular lens placed in the bag. Most surgeons wanting to learn lens implantation were not using phacoemulsification. During the didactic sessions, I always gave a talk on IOL power calculation and afterward we would give the attendees a tour of the EyeLab. In August of 1974, an attendee from Oklahoma, Dr. Ralph Dahlstrom, after seeing what I was doing, suggested that I get a Hewlett Packard programmable calculator for the formula. The HP-65 (Fig. 2.4) was one of the first handheld programmable consumer calculators, and it was expensive at $880 ($5,653 in 2024). Because it was the only one I knew available at the time, the hospital was willing to buy it for me. It was soon followed by the more affordable Texas Instruments unit at $250 ($1,517 in 2024). It took days and nights for me to learn its programming language, then program the formula, correct the bugs and finally have a working program which we pub-

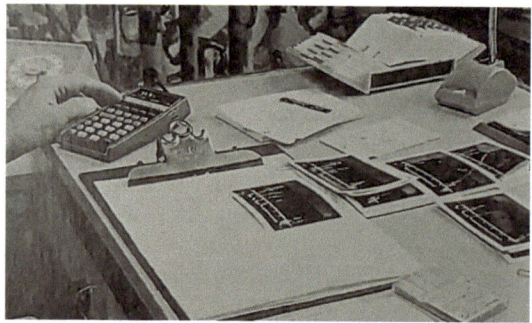

Fig. 2.4 An HP-65-programmed calculator with the first Hoffer formula for IOL power calculation in America 1974

lished [2] so others could use it. Now, we were free of the mainframe computer and the delays. We were on our way, thanks to Ralph Dahlstrom.

In 1978, I started the EyeLab, Inc. to provide accurate lens power calculation for my colleagues and their patients in Southern California since SMH had no interest in doing so. The idea came to me from the old expression "If you can't bring Mohammed to the mountain, bring the mountain to Mohammed." We needed to set up offices in various locations throughout the area (Sherman Oaks, Hollywood, Long Beach, Garden Grove, and a Mobile unit) and would need to equip and staff them. In doing so, we had to find a less expensive method to allow each of the five units to have their own calculator. I discovered the new Casio 4000P unit costing only about $100 ($607 in 2024) and learned its language and programmed the Hoffer formula on it. Over the years, I would update to more powerful Casio units as they came out, including the fx-8500G (Fig. 2.5) which allowed an optional printout using a module and finally the fx-9700GE. These latter units had enough memory to allow me to subsequently program the Holladay 1, the SRK/T and in 1993, the new Hoffer Q formula as well as add their individual personalization programs. I would not be able to program one of these calculators today; I have no idea how I did it. Holladay later came out with his own calculators with the Holladay formula on them which were available for purchase. Due to physician requests, we sold the programmed calculators through the EyeLab under the name "Hoffer® Programs" for many years.

In 1993, due to a colleague's request, I had the Hoffer® Programs (Fig. 2.6) system programmed

Fig. 2.5 Hoffer®
Programs on a Casio
fx-8500G with a user
manual

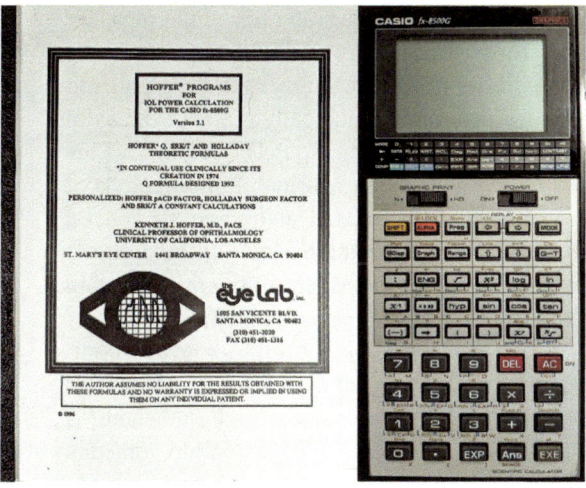

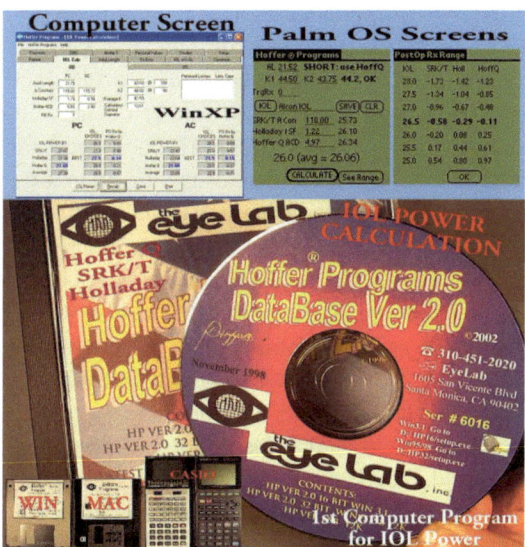

Fig. 2.6 Hoffer® Programs on floppy disks and CDs for
Windows, DOS, MAC, Palm, and Casio fx-8500G and fx-
9700GE calculators

The First Dedicated IOL Power A-Scan: The Invention of the Applanation Method

In 1974, because we were the only facility in California using the Coleman water bath ophthalmic diagnostic B-scan, patients were being referred to my St. John's Clinic from all over Southern California. I soon realized that I did not enjoy doing the time-consuming, tedious water-bath procedures and I did not feel particularly secure with my findings. I could not get out of the job until I trained someone else to do it. Gratefully, Dr. Jerry Pierce took it off my hands.

But before that, in late 1974, I decided that it would be wise if we had an aluminum calibration rod for the Coleman unit. I called the manufacturer, Sonometrics, in New York and reached its president, Mr. Lou Katz. After ordering the rod, I told him of the difficulties I was having with the Kretz 7200 A-scan unit for AL. I mentioned how tedious it was calibrating the unit for each exam, taking the screen Polaroid photographs and most of all, measuring the A-scan Polaroid photos with calipers. I brought up some ideas I had and asked him if his company would consider developing a dedicated A-scan instrument specifically for AL measurement. I told him the new instrument would need to use an immersion method with a water back-off of the probe from the cornea and that it might be more accurate if the patient could sit up rather than lying supine. My theory was

for personal computer use which became the first IOL power calculation program for use on any personal or office computer. First on Microsoft DOS and Windows-based computers and later on Macs and even the Palm handheld PDA phone. It was first on floppy disks and later on CDs. It was used by thousands of ophthalmologists but due to the very high expense to maintain the upgrades for each new rendition of the Windows operating system and the fact that most formulas were becoming available on ultrasound units and optical biometers, Hoffer® Programs ceased in the early 2000s.

that the eye and internal structures might measure differently in the two positions: the upright being more physiologic. Katz suggested using gates to allow the unit to automatically read out the axial length, which I thought would be fantastic. This would eliminate the measuring of photographs of the oscilloscope screen. I also suggested a red fixation light located at the center of the probe to make it easier for the patient to fixate and obtain axiality (which really never worked).

Katz was extremely doubtful about the commercial success of such a device because he had heard that lens implants were "going nowhere." I strenuously argued that implants would someday be routine and that every ophthalmologist would need a dedicated A-scan unit even though I was not sure of that statement. I was willing to say anything to convince him to consider my idea. He said he needed to check with his colleagues in New York and with Dr. Coleman, his chief consultant. I pestered him for months and finally he told me that they were planning to proceed with the development of such a device. I was on the phone with him constantly as production proceeded.

I obviously waited with great anticipation to finally see the device and try it out. Because of this, I lifted the rule I had established for our upcoming first "ASCRS" meeting and allowed Katz to demonstrate the prototype unit just outside the doorway of the first Scientific Meeting of the American Intra-Ocular Implant Society (AIOIS, now ASCRS) at the Statler Hilton Hotel in Dallas, TX, on September 21, 1975 (Fig. 2.7). I had organized and chaired this first meeting and had not made any plans for exhibits by commercial interests. But this was just too exciting for ophthalmology (and for me). During that meeting, I gave a presentation [3] on IOL power calculation and told the attendees about this new instrument I had persuaded Sonometrics to create and that it could be viewed in the hallway after the meeting. At the end of the meeting, I eagerly went out to see the new Sonometrics DBR-100 (Digital Biometric Ruler) instrument (Fig. 2.8) for the first time and proudly demonstrate it to my colleagues. As I approached it, there was a huge crowd surrounding it. I soon noticed that it was being demonstrated by a gentleman I did not

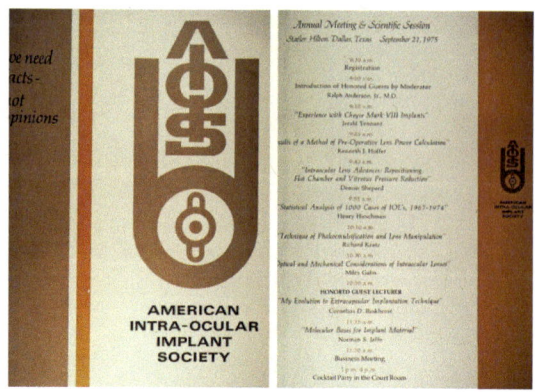

Fig. 2.7 A program for the very first ASCRS meeting in Dallas TX, September 21, 1975

recognize. He was also demonstrating his new IOL power formula which was programmed on a $250 Texas Instruments programmable calculator. Katz then introduced me to Richard D. Binkhorst of New York (brother of the well-known Cornelius Binkhorst of Holland), and, the rest, as they say, is history. If anyone bought the instrument, they would be persuaded to buy the calculator with the Binkhorst formula and that became the world standard for the next decade.

I was obviously put off by this sudden switch without any fore-warning and let my feelings be known to Katz. I asked when the instrument would be delivered to Santa Monica so that I could test it out, and I was told it was first going to Florida for evaluation by Dr. Norman Jaffe (second ASCRS President). This was an excellent scientific, political, and marketing decision but not a fair one. I was never given the opportunity to work with it, evaluate it, or comment on it until it was well on the open market. I would have many occasions to mention my displeasure on how I was treated by Sonometrics to anyone who would listen, including Jaffe. As the major force behind my fledgling "Implant Society" (ASCRS), Jaffe had many occasions to converse with me since I was the Past-President and now the Secretary. He got so sick of hearing about it that he finally contacted Sonometrics and asked them to show me the DBR-100 and "get things straight with me." He also told me that the unit that I had designed was "not especially useful" and that the changes he had recommended made the unit

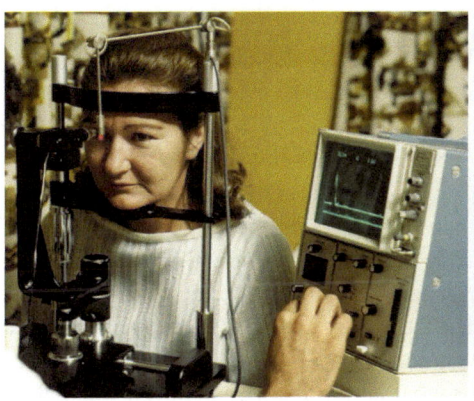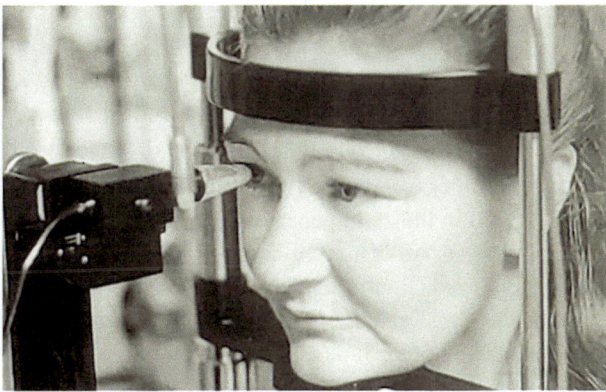

Fig. 2.8 A Sonometrics DBR-100 A-scan applanation ultrasound unit in 1975

functional, even though I told him that I had nothing to do with those negative aspects.

Because of Jaffe, Katz flew to SMH with a DBR-100 unit. He was accompanied by the son of Charles Schepens (Boston), who was president of Medical Instrument Research Associates (MIRA), the company that marketed all Sonometrics products worldwide at the time. After I asked for an explanation as to why I had been treated as I had, Mr. Schepens came clean and explained that it was "purely business." He told me my name was unknown at the time and because of his famous brother, Richard Binkhorst (of NY City) would promote the unit more successfully. I also got the impression that Coleman was happier with that arrangement as well. Regardless of what I said about fairness, it made little difference to them. They had no plans to acknowledge my development of the DBR-100, but, to "shut me up," they offered to give me a unit for free if I would keep quiet. I refused the offer on principle but did recommend they could donate the unit to SMH, which they did. I never agreed to keep quiet. To this day, I have never received any credit for any involvement in the development of the first dedicated IOL power A-scan instrument. Many years later, while negotiating a Sonometrics license for the Hoffer® Q formula, Katz (now deceased) specifically promised that he would make a public notice of my invention of the unit but that never happened. He stayed true to form. This may be a lesson to young naïve ophthalmologists with new ideas.

Early IOL Power Studies

In those first 2 years (1974–1976), we had been performing several studies of our results and I realized that it was not at all clinically useful to report the mean error for IOL power prediction because a +10 D error would cancel out a −10 D error giving a mean error result of 0 while hiding two clinical disasters. I recommended (in a publication [4]) that all future IOL power study results should consist of the following factors: the mean absolute error (MAE) (preventing plus and minus errors from canceling each other out), the percentage of eyes within ±1.00 and ±2.00 D of prediction, and the range of errors from the highest plus to the highest minus. It took several years to catch on, but this became the way most early studies were reported. As accuracy became more precise, I added the reporting of ±0.50 D errors. Today, we are down to reporting ±0.25 D and perhaps soon even ±0.13 D.

Using these principles, I determined that my early results on the very first 127 eyes using the Kretz immersion A-scan done by me personally were 70% (±1.00 D) and 96% (±2.00 D) with a range from +2.50 to −3.80 (6.20 D). A later study using the DOC attachment to the Kretz unit (which used gates to automatically measure the AL) performed by Don Allen on 239 eyes resulted in 72% (±1.00 D) and 98% (±2.00 D) with a range from +2.00 to −3.00 (5.0 D)—not dramatic but an improvement. When we switched to the newer Storz Compuscan 20/20 immersion unit, we saw a definite increase in accuracy. In 63 eyes, we obtained 81% (±1.00 D) and 100% (±2.00 D) with a range from +1.87 to −1.76 (3.63 D)—a dramatic improvement.

In 1974, I attempted to determine whether adding a retinal thickness factor (RTF) to the AL as recommended in the 1973 paper by Colenbrander [5] (but was not a part of his written formula) would improve my prediction accuracy. After reviewing several ophthalmic anatomy sources, I concluded that the thickness of the retina in the fovea was best estimated as 0.26 mm. The theory is that the ultrasound wave bounces off the internal limiting membrane of the retina, whereas the light needs to travel that distance as well as the additional distance from the retinal surface to the visual receptors at the pigment epithelial layer. I analyzed my prediction accuracy without the RTF [70% (±1.00 D), 96% (±2.00 D) range +2.50 to −3.80 (6.20 D)] and then with the 0.26-mm RTF added to each of the ALs. The latter results [45% (±1.00 D), 83% (±2.00 D) range +2.00 to −4.50 (6.50 D)] were much worse and caused a definite shift of the error curve to the hyperopic side (85% hyperopic errors). If the AL is made longer, it will result in a lower power IOL which if incorrect will result in hyperopia, the least desired error. Since it did not improve the accuracy but only created more hyperopia, I have never used an RTF. Richard Binkhorst used an RTF (he said to make up for the corneal flattening that he felt occurred after cataract surgery). I later proved that corneal flattening does not occur and I theorized he may have offset the AL shortening caused by the applanation method.

We also compared the difference between using the measured preoperative ACD [70% (±1.00 D), 96% (±2.00 D) range +2.50 to −3.80 (6.20 D)] and using a standard 3.5-mm ACD for all eyes as recommended by Cornelius Binkhorst [63% (±1.00 D), 90% (±2.00 D) range +3.00 to −4.50 (6.50 D)]. Thus, we were the first to prove that using the preoperative measured ACD with phacoemulsification and an iridocapsular lens fixed in the capsule was more accurate than using a standard ACD value for all eyes. This was ultimately substantiated by Olsen, Haigis, and Holladay. Unfortunately, I was so busy with running ASCRS, the ASCRS meeting, the *JCRS*

journal and my practice, I never published any of these results. So here they are now.

Not to ignore the Richard Binkhorst formula [6], in 1976, I performed a study to analyze the difference in results between the R. Binkhorst, Hoffer, and other formulas. I found that the R Binkhorst always recommended a power 0.50 D stronger compared to all the other theoretic formulas. After analyzing his formula, I understood why. He artificially changed the refractive index of the cornea from 1.375 to 4/3 (1.333…) to correct for what he erroneously believed was a flattening of the cornea that occurs after "all cataract surgery." We proved that this flattening was not true [7]. He based this on a small study of less than 100 eyes that had large incision intracapsular surgery. I felt that this was not very scientific for the following reasons: no definite studies showed that corneas uniformly flatten a specific amount after all types of cataract surgery, and even if it were the case, it would be far better to simply subtract 0.50 D (or the average flattening, X) from all ALs input to the formula rather than changing the refractive index of the cornea which theoretically is a known constant. I warned about this error in publications [8, 9] in 1981 and was severely criticized for it in print [10] in four pages by Katz, R Binkhorst ("The more than 2,000 users of the Binkhorst IOL Power Module should not be misled by Hoffer's false conclusions.") and Coleman ("It is disappointing that the Archives would support Hoffer's unsubstantiated endorsement by including the article in its pages"). I responded accordingly [10–12]. It is interesting to look back 40 years ago.

When we finally received the Sonometrics DBR-100 in the SMH's EyeLab (Fig. 2.8), we performed a study with it. We found it very easy to use the gates rather than measuring photographs but much more difficult to get a measurement without compressing the cornea. In the early 1980s, we did the first study to compare applanation to immersion. We used the same eyes, the same technician, and the same A-scan and probe, leaving the only difference the method of the exam. Our results on 20 eyes showed an average 0.33-mm shortening of the AL using the applanation method. I never found time to publish the results, but when Shammas repeated our study on a larger series of 180 eyes, he found a resultant shortening of 0.25 mm with applanation and included the results of our study in his excellent paper [13]. Several studies since have corroborated this effect. The problem is not that a shortening occurs since, if it were consistent in every case, it could be easily corrected by merely adding that factor to the AL result or by personalizing the formula. The problem is that it occurs sporadically, i.e., not shortening some eyes and extensively shortening others. It is not possible for the examiner to tell which eyes are or are not being shortened. The disatisfaction caused by these errors as well as those due to the R. Binkhorst formula led to the development of regression formulas to improve results.

I warned the ophthalmic community of these drawbacks in courses and publications, but they were little heeded. Clinicians did not want to purchase the more cumbersome and expensive Kretz unit using the "messier" immersion method and the more expensive HP-65 calculator with the Hoffer formula. The DBR, using applanation, combined with the R Binkhorst formula on the TI calculator, became the standard in America and ultimately around the world. Incidentally, the red light I had invented in the DBR's probe was totally useless because the patient could not really see it at such a close distance compounded by the cataract and the probe on the cornea. Our side-by-side study was the first to show the DBR to be clinically less accurate due to probe-compression causing artificial AL shortening.

We therefore continued to use the Kretz immersion unit, which was later aided by a "black box" attachment called the DOC (Digital Ocular Computer) that added gates and an automatic measuring device that would give an AL readout. It was made for us by John McAdams of Instruments for Medicine. Several years went by before competition to the DBR was achieved by the introduction of the Storz Compuscan and the Xenotec Ultrscan. It was then I met John Weymouth of Xenotec who became a major force in convincing ophthalmologists to use the immersion method. What is paradoxical is that I helped invent the DBR and spent most of my career lecturing against its use.

For years, we did side-by-side comparisons of various A-scans as they were introduced and reported our results to the profession [14]. Unfortunately, it was soon obvious to the manufacturers that I would truthfully report if the results were not optimal (as in the case of the Storz Echo-Oculometer) and soon no one asked us to evaluate their equipment—a negative aspect of being publicly honest.

In 1978, Dr. Leo Bores of Detroit asked me to start doing radial keratotomy (RK) so that I could study the effect of RK on AL and endothelial cell counts. I did the first RK on the West Coast in November 1979 and instigated the UCLA Myopia Study with the approval of Bradley Straatsma, the UCLA Stein Eye Institute Chairman. I reported our results at the 1980 American Academy of Ophthalmology (AAO) meeting (first corneal refractive surgery presentation at the AAO), and we published the first RK paper [15] in the American literature. We found an average 0.15 mm shortening of the AL from 25.45 to 25.30 mm after a 16-incision metal-blade RK which could be due to flattening of the cornea, but the change was not consistent or statistically significant.

During my 1982 invention of the first multifocal IOL (the Hoffer Split Bifocal [the U.S. FDA just approved the Lenstec version in 2022]), I devised the method to calculate the exact power needed for the additional power in the near vision optic. This was first published in Maxwell and Nordan's textbook on Multifocal IOLs [16], and later in a 1992 AJO publication [17] by Holladay and I as well as in Jorge Alio's textbook *Multifocal Intraocular Lenses* [18]. It was also included in a Focal Points issue [19] the AAO asked me to write on the subject of IOL power calculation in 1995.

For many years, I have stressed the importance of early (24 hour) IOL exchange to correct IOL power errors [20]. In 2008, we performed the first precision study of the improved accuracy of exact-power-labeled IOLs (made by TechnoMed, Germany) with the US Food and Drug Administration (FDA) proving there was an improvement in IOL Power prediction using them [21]. This was scoffed at as inconsequential by Lindstrom in print.

The EyeLab

In 1978, I started the EyeLab, Inc. to provide accurate lens power calculation for my colleagues and their patients in Southern California. This was done with the help of our technicians Greg Phillippi, Larry Margules, and Dee Zigmund. At that time, Medicare had not approved the examination for reimbursement because very few were being done. I spent 4 months making daily phone calls to the federal officials in the Medicare Administration until we finally received notice that it had been approved with a fee higher than we had requested at that time, i.e., $350 per eye ($2,124 in 2024). This was a feat for which I was personally quite proud. This meant that ultrasound lens power calculation would now be more readily available to the American public. I later successfully fought with them to pay for both eyes being done rather than only the eye being operated on, It is a shame that later, in the 1990s, the valiant attempts by the American Society of Cataract & Refractive Surgery (ASCRS) to prevent Medicare decreases in cataract surgery reimbursement led Stephen Obstbaum and the leaders of ASCRS to offer them instead a reduction in IOL power calculation fees as a compromise. Medicare responded by not only lowering cataract fees but in addition, slashing the power calculation fee drastically.

Over the years, the EyeLab examined well over 10,000 eyes. In 1979, I asked William Link, then president of Heyer-Schulte (later AMO, now J&J), if we could be able to get our data analyzed using their mainframe computers. He agreed and with the help of Ginger Silva, the biometry of 7,500 eyes were entered and analyzed. These results were published in the *American Journal of Ophthalmology* [7] in 1980, the first such large series on human eye biometry. We showed that the average AL of the human cataractous eye by immersion ultrasound was 23.65 mm (±1.35) and the average K reading was 43.81 D (±1.60). We also showed the average cylinder in this cataract age group was 1.00 D (±1.00) and that only 10% of eyes had a cylinder of 2.00 D or greater. We reported that the mean difference between the two eyes of a given patient was 0.34 mm (±0.70) for AL, 0.87 D (±0.83) for K, and 0.23 mm (±0.27) for ACD. This study resulted in my defi-

nition of Short Eyes as <22 mm; Medium Long Eyes as 24.5–26 mm; Very Long Eyes as >26 mm and Normal Length Eyes as 22–24.5 mm. These definitions have been used by many ever since. The data was later used by Holladay in the development of his second formula (unpublished) as well as his recommendations for when to recheck biometry results. This study was also the first to statistically prove that myopic eyes develop cataracts at an earlier age than hyperopes ($p < 0.002$).

To better access the thickness of the cataractous lens, I performed a study in 1993 on 600 eyes using a crystalline lens sound velocity of 1641 m/s which was published in the *Archives of Ophthalmology* [22] (now *JAMA Ophthalmology*). The mean thickness of the lens for the entire series was 4.63 mm (±0.68) with a range of 2.27–6.86 mm. We proved that the lens thickens with age (which makes sense), in that it measured an average of 3.78 mm (±0.21) in the third decade of life and 5.03 mm (±0.46) in the tenth decade. We showed hyperopic ALs (<22 mm) measured 5.03 mm (±0.63) while myopic ALs (>27 mm) measured 4.24 mm (±0.58). This proved that the shorter the eye, the thicker the lens. Younger eyes under age 65 ($n = 158$) had a mean AL of 24.08 mm (±1.53); ages 65–75 ($n = 252$) were 23.67 mm (±1.19), and older eyes over 75 ($n = 190$) were 23.26 mm (±1.03). This again statistically confirmed ($p > 0.0001$) that myopic eyes require cataract surgery at an earlier age than hyperopes.

In the mid-1980s, with the first declines in cataract reimbursement by Medicare, more ophthalmologists purchased an A-scan unit to help offset these decreases which ultimately led to the closure of the EyeLab offices. The EyeLab was revived as an entity in 1990 when the request for Hoffer® Programs calculators and later computer programs became evident and again in 2020 as a structure for the new Hoffer QST free website.

Ultrasound Velocities for Axial Length Measurement

In 1974, I needed to develop a more accurate average sound velocity for the human eye. To do this, I postulated an eye of a given AL of 23.50 mm, a corneal thickness of 0.50 mm, and a crystalline lens thickness of 5.00 mm. Knowing that the velocity of sound through both the cornea and lens was accepted to be 1641 m/s and using the velocity formula $V = d/t$ ($t = d/V$), I was able to calculate the time it took for the sound to travel through the solid parts of the eye (5.00 + 0.50 = 5.5; 5.5 mm/1.641 mm/s = 3.35 μs). Similarly, with the velocity of 1532 m/s through both aqueous and vitreous, the time to traverse the liquid parts of the eye could also be determined (23.50–5.50 = 18; 18 mm/1.532 mm/s = 11.75 μs). Adding the solid and liquid time spans yields the total time for the sound to traverse the entire eye (3.35 + 11.75 = 15.1 μs). Again, using the velocity formula, I simply divided the given 23.50-mm AL by the total time of 15.1 μs to arrive at an average velocity of 1556 m/s. When this process was repeated for an aphakic eye, the result was 1534 m/s. Unfortunately, I was never able to publish this information except in periodicals [23] but only discuss it in my many lectures and courses and thus it never changed the general use of 1550 m/s as the velocity for the average eye.

In 1994, I repeated this work [24] using a more correct 0.55 mm for corneal thickness and the 4.63 mm I obtained from my previous study of lens thickness and obtained an average velocity of 1555 m/s. This schema was repeated for 20- and 30-mm eyes, and we discovered that the longer the eye, the thinner the lens and the slower the average velocity (1550); the shorter the eye, the thicker the lens and the faster the average velocity (1560). I developed formulas to correct for this change in average velocity due to AL, but it is only clinically important in the very extremes of AL. Measuring an eye that contains an IOL (pseudophakic) creates a different situation depending on what material the implant is made of and how thick the IOL is. This concept was first brought to light by Albert Milauskas [25] of Palm Springs, when he discovered the errors obtained measuring eyes containing silicone implants. He proposed that the extremely low sound velocity through silicone was the reason. I used my previously described schema to determine average velocities through eyes with IOLs of PMMA, silicone, glass, acrylic, and collamer. Holladay proposed a different method he termed the CALF factor that may be more precise,

but it requires knowing the thickness of the implant in the eye which is not always easy to obtain. In 2003, I published [20, 21] a method to measure the AL of phakic eyes which contain phakic IOLs (biphakic) when the material and thickness of the phakic IOL is known [26, 27].

Getting the Word Out

Once my colleagues heard about the EyeLab at SMH, I was asked to speak on the subject at the first American scientific meeting on lens implantation which was to be held on November 16, 1974 at the Long Beach Memorial Hospital by its organizer, Dr. Francis ("Red") Hertzog, Jr. Because I had never spoken before any group before, I was a little apprehensive and felt a need to gain "credibility," so I flew to Holland in early November to visit with Dr. Jan Worst and Prof. Colenbrander. I also visited Cornelius Binkhorst in Terneuzen, Holland, and Hermann Gernet in Münster, Germany, who had written several papers on iseikonic IOL power. They were all truly kind to me. Cornelius Binkhorst did excoriate me somewhat for forming this "American Implant Society," which he felt would someday usurp his International Implant Club (IIC, now IIIC). Months later at an ASCRS meeting, he kept on me about this quite emotionally and so to calm him down I recommended he get each EU country's implant society to join a broad European Implant Lens Council that he could preside over as President. I even contacted Leo Amar, the French society's founder and president (I had given him advice on forming it), to get him to agree. Later, Binkhorst did just that and it ultimately became the European Society of Cataract & Refractive Surgery (ESCRS).

In meeting with Prof. Colenbrander at his home for dinner, each and every time I tried to discuss his formula during dinner, he immediately changed the subject. This left me with the impression that perhaps he did not write it. My time with Worst was always hectic, but he was always very helpful to me. Gernet was very kind and showed me his voluminous printout reports from his huge mainframe computer. Because of its extreme complexity (meaning I could not figure out what he was doing), I realized that this would receive little interest in the United States.

After visiting Zurich and Rome (for the very first time), I returned home and was prepared to give my very first lecture on IOL power calculation at the Long Beach meeting. I brought the Kretz 7200 A-scan unit with me to demonstrate it to those who might be interested to see it. The lecture went well and after the meeting, one local ophthalmologist (Ron Jensen of Glendale, CA) spent a lot of time with me learning how to perform the procedure. After months of turning down the many requests for newspaper interviews about our unique EyeLab from Jean Harris, the Public Relations director of SMH, I read the front-page headlines of the LA Herald Examiner to discover that the "first ultrasound IOL power calculations done in Southern California" were done by that same Ron Jensen I had taught that day in Long Beach. I learned early on that not every colleague plays fairly or honestly. Another lesson learned.

My next lectures were at the Southern California Section of the American College of Surgeons Meeting in Santa Barbara and then at the Mexican Ophthalmological Society in Mexicali, Mexico. I got over my shyness. I continued to give these presentations at our SMH courses, ASCRS courses, and Dr. Hirschman's IOL courses in Long Beach as well as at the IOL courses started by Bradley Straatsma, Murry Weber, and I at the UCLA Stein Eye Institute. After applying several times (but I think with the influence of Dr. Jaffe), my IOL power course was finally accepted by the AAO. In the early years, I did it alone, but as I saw others developing an interest in the subject, I invited them to join me. John Shammas of Los Angeles was the very first in 1975.

When I was invited to give a named lecture at the University of Oregon Ophthalmology Meeting in Portland in March 1979, I heard a presentation by a local ophthalmologist, John Retzlaff, on a regression formula he had developed. I was aware of the first regression formula that had been developed by Thomas Lloyd [28], a technician with James Gills in Florida. I pressured the shy and reluctant Retzlaff, to present his formula at my AAO course and at the next Annual ASCRS Meeting at the Century Plaza Hotel in Los Angeles. I also begged him to publish it in the JCRS Journal, all of which he ultimately did [29]. I had told him I was putting his name on the program and if he didn't show up I would present it as "my work." I had also invited Donald Sanders and Manus Kraff of Chicago who had also developed a regression formula [30]. They agreed and after all three of their presentations, collaboration developed between them that led to the amalgamation of their individual formulas into what they termed the SRK regression formula [31]. Over the years, because of its sheer simplicity, it became the formula used throughout the world. Why? Because it was so easy ($P = A - 2.5*AL - 0.9*K$, where A is the lens constant) and it could be done by hand.

In those same years, I met a young ophthalmologist from Houston, Texas, who had an engineering background, tons of enthusiasm, and agreed with me that theoretic formulas were superior to regression. Jack Holladay became a permanent member of my AAO and ASCRS course faculty joining Kraff, Retzlaff, Sanders, and Shammas. Many years later, after one of these courses, Kraff suggested that we were all tired of giving them and everyone who wanted to has probably already attended. Because of that, I stupidly dropped the course the next year. Soon after the next AAO Meeting I received so many irate phone calls from ophthalmologists and technicians who expected the course to be given that I reapplied with one speaker initially for 1 hour. It was soon increased to 2 hours, and I have been giving them ever since. My similar courses at ASCRS paralleled those at the Academy, always presenting the latest unbiased information. Since starting our 3-month European trips in 1997, I have given these courses at the ESCRS meetings in Europe as well. In the past 16 years, I have been joined by Giacomo Savini of Bologna, Italy to discuss toric calculations which I never had much interest in. By the latest count, I have lectured on IOL power over 500 times since that day in November 1974.

A life-altering event occurred in 1999 upon meeting Wolfgang Haigis (Fig. 2.9) for the first

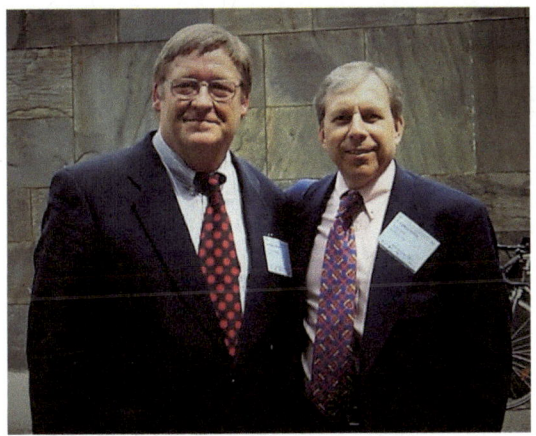

Fig. 2.9 Wolfgang Haigis, PhD (left), with the author in 1999

ing the latest instruments: the German Heidelberg Anterion and the Optopol Revo NX from Poland and the Chinese Colombo II from Moptim. Many new formulas have been made available which show excellent results (see other Chapters).

Conclusion

The events recounted here are based on my personal vivid memory of them. They are not meant to offend anyone or ignore the work of those not mentioned. I am humbly grateful and appreciative of all those who have helped me in these endeavors. I have enjoyed working in this field for these 50 years and hope for a few more years to continue the effort to gain the ultimate goal we all seek; the elimination of all errors in predicting postoperative IOL refractive error.

time. Zeiss asked him to join the team that flew in to install the first American IOLMaster optical biometer in my office in Santa Monica. The company wanted my opinion on the instrument and to check the accuracy of their programming of the Hoffer Q formula in the biometer. I recommended that they change the corneal power readings from radius of curvature (r) to diopters (D) for an American consumer, which they did. Haigis was an expert in immersion ultrasound and had helped set the standards for their optical biometer and all the others that followed. He developed the Haigis formula in 2000 that replaced the K with the preop ACD in predicting the ELP, but it used three lens constants: a_0 (IOL constant), a_1 (based on AL), and a_2 (based on ACD), which required a more cumbersome triple optimization of the lens constants. In all studies, his formula was very accurate. We became very good friends over the years, especially during the 15 years of the IOL Power Club, and I deeply miss him since his passing in October 2019.

Many new optical biometers and corneal biometry measuring devices have been brought to the market since 2009 with the introduction by Haag-Streit of their Lenstar LS-900. Due to my receiving the first Lenstar in the U.S., Giacomo Savini, John Shammas, and I had the opportunity to test it and later compare the accuracy of most all of the new biometers as they appeared and have published our results [32–36]. We are presently test-

References

1. Ossoinig KC. Standardized echography: basic principles, clinical applications and results. Int Ophthalmol Clin. 1979;19:127–210.
2. Hoffer KJ, Allen DR. A simple lens power calculation program for the HP-67 and HP-97 calculators. J Cataract Refract Surg. 1978;4:197.
3. Hoffer KJ. Mathematics and computers in intraocular lens calculation. J Cataract Refract Surg. 1975;1(1):3.
4. Hoffer KJ. Intraocular lens calculation: the problem of the short eye. Ophthalmic Surg. 1981;12:269–72.
5. Colenbrander MC. Calculation of the power of an iris-clip lens for distance vision. Brit J Ophthalmol. 1973;57:735–40.
6. Binkhorst RD. The optical design of intraocular lens implants. Ophthalmic Surg. 1975;6(3):17–31.
7. Hoffer KJ. Biometry of 7,500 Cataractous eyes. Am J of Ophthalmol. 1980;90:360–8.
8. Hoffer KJ. Power formulas for intraocular lenses. Am J of Ophthalmol. 1981;91(1):138.
9. Hoffer KJ. Accuracy of intraocular lens calculation. Arch Ophthalmol. 1981;99:1819–23.
10. Katz L, Coleman DJ, Binkhorst RD. Letters to editor and Hoffer KJ response. Arch Ophthalmol. 1982;100(10):1679–83.
11. Hoffer KJ. Response to Binkhorst letter: IOL power calculation. (letter to the editor). Ophthalmic Surg. 1982;13:419–20.
12. Hoffer KJ. Accuracy of IOL power calculations debated. Ophthalmol Times. 1981.
13. Shammas HJF. A comparison of immersion and contact techniques for axial length measurements. J Cataract Refract Surg. 1984;10:444–7.

14. Hoffer KJ. Comparison of the Storz Compuscan and the Jedmed Axiosonic II ultrasound instruments (chapter 75). In: Emery JM, Jacobson AC, editors. Current concepts in cataract surgery (8th congress). New York: Appleton-Century Crofts; 1983. p. 229–31.

15. Hoffer KJ, Darin JJ, Pettit TH, Hofbauer JA, Elander R, Levenson JE. UCLA clinical trial of radial keratotomy: preliminary report. Ophthalmol. 1981;88:729–36.

16. Hoffer KJ. Lens power calculation for multifocal IOLs, (chapter 17). In: Maxwell A, Nordan LT, editors. Current concepts of multifocal intraocular lenses. Thorofare, NJ: Slack, Inc.; 1991. p. 193–208.

17. Holladay JT, Hoffer KJ. Intraocular lens power calculations for multifocal intraocular lenses. Am J Ophthalmol. 1992;114:405–8.

18. Hoffer KJ, Savini G. (chapter 2), multifocal intraocular lenses: historical perspective. In: Alio J, Pikkel J, editors. Multifocal intraocular lenses: the art and the practice. Switzerland: Springer International Publishing; 2014. p. 5–28.

19. Hoffer KJ. A-scan biometry and IOL implant power calculation. Focal Points (AAO). 1995;XIII:10–14.

20. Hoffer KJ. Early lens exchange for power calculation error. J Cataract Refract Surg. 1995;21:486–7.

21. Hoffer KJ, Calogero D, Faaland RW, Ilev IK. Testing the dioptric power accuracy of exact-power-labeled intraocular lenses. J Cataract Refract Surg. 2009;35(11):1995–9.

22. Hoffer KJ. Axial dimension of the human cataractous lens. Arch Ophthalmol. 1993;111:914–8, Erratum 1993;111:1626.

23. Hoffer KJ. Sound speeds in finding axial lengths. IOL Ocular Surgery News. 1984;2:4.

24. Hoffer KJ. Ultrasound speeds for axial length measurement. J Cataract Refract Surg. 1994;20:554–62.

25. Milauskas AT, Marny S. Pseudo axial length increase after silicone lens implantation as determined by ultrasonic scans. J Cataract Refract Surg. 1988;14:400–2.

26. Hoffer KJ. Ultrasound axial length measurement in biphakic eyes. J Cataract Refract Surg. 2003;29(5):961–5.

27. Hoffer KJ. Addendum to ultrasound axial length measurement in biphakic eyes: factors for Alcon L12500–L14000 anterior chamber phakic IOLs. J Cataract Refract Surg. 2007;33(4):751–2.

28. Gills JP. Regression formula (editorial). J Cataract Refract Surg. 1978;4:163.

29. Retzlaff J. A new intraocular lens calculation formula. J Cataract Refract Surg. 1980;6:148.

30. Sanders DR, Kraff MC. Improvement of intraocular lens power calculation: regression formula. J Cataract Refract Surg. 1980;6:263.

31. Sanders DR, Retzlaff J, Kraff MC, et al. Comparison of the accuracy of the Binkhorst, Colenbrander and SRK implant power prediction formulas. J Cataract Refract Surg. 1981;7:337–40.

32. Hoffer KJ, Shammas HJ, Savini G. Comparison of 2 laser instruments for measuring axial length. J Cataract Refract Surg. 2010;36(4):644–8, Erratum 2010;36(6):1066.

33. Shammas HJ, Hoffer KJ. Repeatability and reproducibility of biometry and keratometry measurements using a noncontact optical low-coherence reflectometer and keratometer. Am J Ophthalmol. 2012;153(1):55–61.

34. Hoffer KJ, Shammas HJ, Savini G, Huang J. Multicenter study of optical low-coherence interferometry and partial-coherence interferometry optical biometers with patients from the United States and China. J Cataract Refract Surg. 2016;42(1):62–7.

35. Hoffer KJ, Hoffmann PC, Savini G. Comparison of a new optical biometer using swept source OCT to one using optical low-coherence reflectometry. J Cataract Refract Surg. 2016;42(8):1165–72.

36. Hoffer KJ, Savini G. Comparison of AL-scan and IOLMaster 500 partial coherence interferometry optical biometers. J Refract Surg. 2016;32(10):694–8.

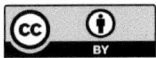

Part II

Basic Science

Gaussian Optics

3

Basic Optics

Jean-Philippe Colliac

Fundamental Hypotheses

Let us retain that in an *isotropic* medium, the *ray of light* is defined by the *ideal line normal to the wave surface* in which the light energy spreads when diffraction is neglected. The experiment shows that, for the *very low wave lengths*, the wave phenomena can be neglected: geometrical optics appears as the approximation of the *very low wave lengths* of wave optics. *Fermat's principle*, also called the *principle of least time*, states that *the path taken by a ray of light between two given points is the path that can be traversed in the least time*. In order to be true on all the cases, "least" must be replaced by "stationary" with respect to variations of the path: *the path taking by the optics ray between two points* A *and* B *is stationary*. The equivalence between the Snell–Descartes law and the Fermat principle in the case of refraction is proved with an *analytical demonstration*.

Gaussian approximation (from the German mathematician and physicist, Carl Friedrich Gauss, 1777–1855) or *paraxial approximation* is the linear approximation of the geometrical optics. The rays of light make small angles with the optical axis, and the distance between the rays and the optical axis is short.

Classical Study in Paraxial Optics

Paraxial Trace Through a Spherical Surface

If the angle of incidence i and the angle of refraction i' remain small enough so that we can assume the cosine to be unity. We obtain the classic *equation of conjugation* (Fig. 3.1):

$$\frac{n'}{x'} = \frac{n}{x} + \frac{n'-n}{r} \tag{3.1}$$

By definition, the *dioptric power* or *vergence* of a spherical surface, which separates two media with indices n and n', is

$$D \equiv \frac{n'-n}{r},$$

where $r = \overline{SC}$ is the radius of curvature in algebraical value of which the sign is *linked to the direction of the incident light*. When r is expressed in meter, the unity for the dioptric power is the *diopter* (δ). Because the angles of incidence i and the angle of refraction i' remain small, their sines may be replaced with their values in radians and the *Snell–Descartes law*:

$$n \sin i = n' \sin i' \tag{3.2}$$

becomes the *Kepler law*:

$$ni = n'i' \tag{3.3}$$

J.-P. Colliac (✉)
Colliac Eye Clinic, Paris, France
e-mail: jpcolliac@aol.com

© The Author(s) 2024
J. Aramberri et al. (eds.), *Intraocular Lens Calculations*, Essentials in Ophthalmology,
https://doi.org/10.1007/978-3-031-50666-6_3

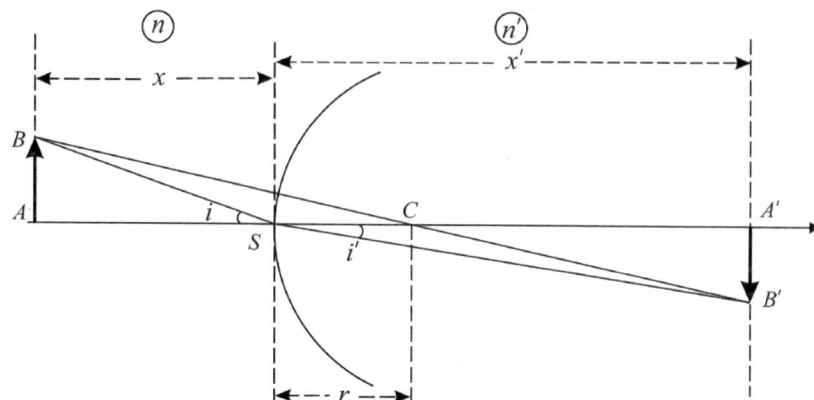

Fig. 3.1 Paraxial trace through a spherical surface with center C

In the paraxial approximation the spherical aberration is not considered. Also in this approximation, a plane perpendicular to the axis at A has as image of all its points a plane perpendicular to the axis at A'. The *transverse magnification* M_T is the ratio of any image length to its corresponding object length. If $y = \overline{AB}$ and $y' = \overline{A'B'}$, we have

$$y' = x'i', y = xi,$$

$$M_T = \frac{y'}{y} = \frac{x'i'}{xi} = \frac{x'n}{xn'}.$$

Consequently,

$$M_T = \frac{y'}{y} = \frac{x'n}{n'x} \qquad (3.4)$$

A positive magnification corresponds to an erect image and a negative magnification to an inverted image.

Rays in object space, parallel to the axis and crossing a refractive spherical surface or a lens, intersect in the image space the axis at the *rear focal point* or *image focal point* F'. Rays in image space, parallel to the axis, intersect in the object space the axis at the *front focal point* or *object focal point* F. The principal focal planes are the planes perpendicular to the axis at the focal points. An object on the axis whose image is located on the image focal plane is at the infinity; its abscissa is the image focal distance f'. An object on the

axis whose image is at the infinity is located on the object focal plane; its abscissa is the object focal distance f. The abscissae of the focal distances f and f' are relative to the apex as the origin. Thus using the classic equation of conjugation (3.1), we obtain this fundamental relation:

$$\frac{n'}{f'} = -\frac{n}{f} = \frac{n'-n}{r} \qquad (3.5)$$

or

$$\frac{f}{f'} = -\frac{n}{n'} \qquad (3.6)$$

Lagrange–Helmholtz Relation

Let a spherical interface between a first medium with a refractive index n and a second medium with a greater refractive index n', with a center of curvature C, a radius r, and an apex S. The size of the object AB and of its image A'B' is y and y', respectively. After a refraction at M with an incident angle i and a refraction angle i', the incident ray $\overline{AM}$ goes to the direction of $\overline{MA'}$. The incident ray $\overline{BC}$ goes through the interface without deviation. The angles of the rays CAM and CA'M with the axis are α and α', respectively. By sign convention α is positive and α' is negative. Since the triangles CAB and CA'B' are similar (Fig. 3.2),

$$\overline{SM} = -\overline{SA}\tan\alpha = -\overline{SA'}\tan\alpha',$$

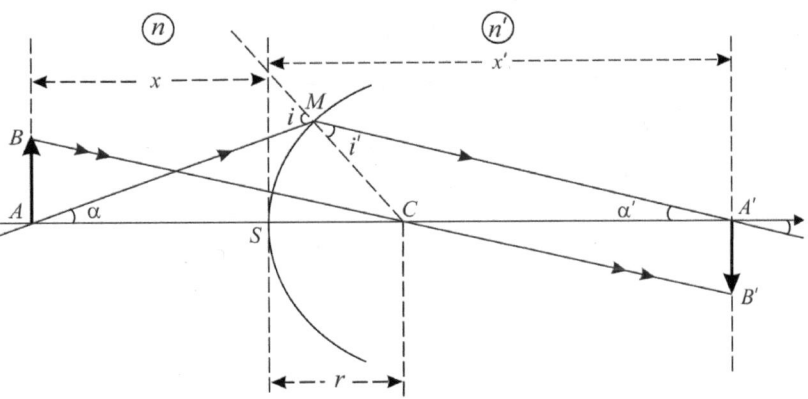

Fig. 3.2 Refraction at a single spherical surface and Lagrange–Helmholtz relation. In the case pictured, α and α' have opposite signs, so the transverse magnification is negative

as we are in paraxial approximation the angles are small and the small-angle approximation is applied: tangents of the angles equal their values expressed in radians:

$$\overline{SA}\,\alpha = \overline{SA'}\,\alpha' \text{ and according to the Eq. (3.4)}$$

$$\frac{y'}{y} = -\frac{n}{n'}\frac{\overline{SA'}}{\overline{SA}} = \frac{\overline{A'B'}}{\overline{AB}} \text{ or } n\,\overline{AB}\,\overline{SA'} = n'\,\overline{A'B'}\,\overline{SA},$$

we obtain the *Lagrange–Helmholtz relation*:

$$n\,y\,\alpha = n'\,y'\,\alpha' \tag{3.7}$$

The Lagrange–Helmholtz relation is important and expresses the fact that the quantity $n\,y\,\alpha$ or *paraxial invariant* remains constant when light passes through any refracting surface. The formula gives the relationship between transverse magnification, angular magnification, and axial magnification.

Centered System

A centered system is a succession of refractive surfaces that have the same axis. Their centers are all situated on the same straight line which is the axis of revolution of the system. For each refractive surface the image serves as the object of the following refractive surface. Each refractive surface establishes a homographic conjugation between the object and its image.

Principal Points and Focal Lengths

An incident ray parallel to the axis (Fig. 3.3) is refracted so as to pass through the *image focal point F'*. Point P' is the intersection of this incident ray and of the refracted ray. The plane tangent to the point P' is called the *image principal plane*. This plane is the locus of all the points P' of which the orthogonal projection on the axis is the point H'. This intersection point H' on the axis is the *image principal point*. The quantity $f' = \overline{H'F'}$ is called the *image focal length* (Fig. 3.3).

We define in an identical manner the object principal plane. The point P is located at the intersection of an incident ray which goes through the *object focal point F* and of the ray which refracts at the point P' parallel to the axis. The plane tangent to the point P is called the *object principal plane*. This plane is the locus of all the points P of which the orthogonal projection on the axis is the point H. This intersection H on the axis is the *object principal point*. The quantity $f = \overline{HF}$ is called the *object focal length* (Fig. 3.3).

Given an object $\overline{FG}$, the incident ray $\overline{GH}$ which intersects the axis at the point H makes with the axis the angle α. This ray $\overline{GH}$ emerges at the point H' making an angle α' with the axis. The incident ray $\overline{GH}$, parallel to the axis, which intersects the principal image plane at K', emerges at the point K' along $\overline{K'F'}$ making an angle α' with the axis (Fig. 3.4). Applying the

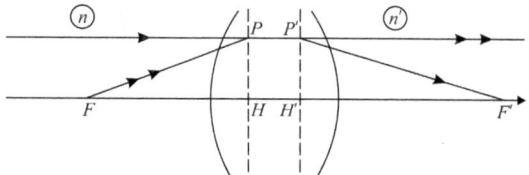

Fig. 3.3 Focal points and principal planes

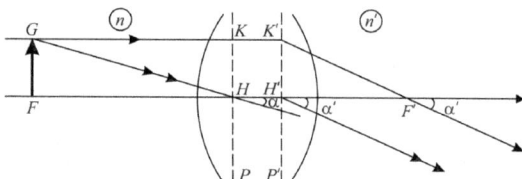

Fig. 3.4 Focal lengths

Lagrange–Helmholtz relation (3.7) and noting that $\overline{FG} = \overline{H'K'}$ or $y = y'$, we obtain

$$n\alpha = n'\alpha' \qquad (3.8)$$

Moreover as

$$\alpha = \frac{\overline{FG}}{f}, \text{ and } \alpha' = \frac{\overline{H'K'}}{f'}, \text{ we get } n\frac{\overline{FG}}{f}$$
$$= n'\frac{\overline{H'K'}}{f'},$$

and we obtain

$$\frac{f}{n} = \frac{-f'}{n'} \qquad (3.9)$$

The object and image focal lenghts are always of the opposite sign.

Nodal Points

The object nodal point N and the image nodal point N' are cardinal points located on the axis. They are such that each incident ray that passes through the object nodal point N emerges from the image nodal point N' as a ray parallel to the incident ray. This output ray has the same direction as the input ray with a parallel offset (Fig. 3.5). So the incident ray going through N and emerging at N' forms with the axis the same angles α.

Let us take a point G on the object focal plane. An incident ray going through G and parallel to the axis emerges at a point P' and then through

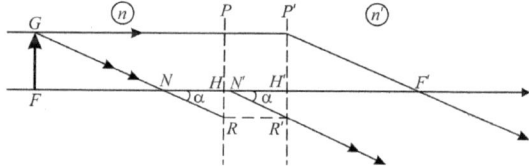

Fig. 3.5 Nodal points

the image point F' with a direction parallel to an incident ray going through G and the nodal point N.

The triangles GFN and $P'H'F'$ are equal and $RNN'R'$ is a parallelogram, and therefore

$$\overline{FN} = \overline{H'F'} = f', \quad \overline{F'N'} = \overline{HF} = f,$$
$$\overline{NH} = \overline{N'H'}, \quad \overline{NN'} = \overline{HH'}.$$

In the frequently encountered situation where the refractive index is the same in front of and behind the optical system, the nodal points coincide with the principal points. In a spherical refractive surface, the distance HH' between the two principal points is nil and both object and image nodal points are coincident with the center of the spherical refractive surface.

Relation of Conjugation and Transverse Magnification

Knowledge of the focal points and of the focal lengths completely determines the system. The principal points and nodal points result immediately from it. The abscissas of any two conjugate points and the magnification can be put in various forms, all of which are various cases of the general homographic relation.

1. Origin at the focal points
   Let ζ be the abscissa of the object point A when we place the origin at the object focal point F, $\overline{FA} = \zeta$. Let ζ' be the abscissa of the image point A' measured from the image focal point F', $\overline{F'A'} = \zeta'$. Moreover $\overline{HF} = f$, $\overline{H'F'} = f'$, $\overline{AB} = y$, and $\overline{A'B'} = y'$.

   The triangles ABF and HSF are similar as well as the triangles $A'B'F'$ and $H'TF'$. The ratio of their sides is therefore equal.

Figure 3.6 can also be used to show that $\overline{AB} = \overline{H'T}$ and $\overline{A'B'} = \overline{HS}$

$$-\frac{\overline{HS}}{\overline{AB}} = -\frac{\overline{A'B'}}{\overline{AB}} = -\frac{\overline{FH}}{\overline{FA}} \quad \text{or} \quad \frac{y'}{y} = -\frac{f}{\zeta},$$

$$-\frac{\overline{A'B'}}{\overline{H'T}} = -\frac{\overline{A'B'}}{\overline{AB}} = -\frac{\overline{F'A'}}{\overline{F'H'}} \quad \text{or} \quad \frac{y'}{y} = -\frac{\zeta'}{f'}.$$

The transverse magnification is

$$M_T = \frac{y'}{y} = -\frac{f}{\zeta} = -\frac{\zeta'}{f'} \tag{3.10}$$

Thus we obtain *Newton's conjugation relation*:

$$\zeta\zeta' = ff' \tag{3.11}$$

Positive and negative values of y/y' characterize, respectively, an erect or an inverted image, relative to the object.

2. Origin at the principal points

   Let $x = \overline{HA} = f + \zeta$ and $x' = \overline{H'A'} = f' + \zeta'$. By replacing in the *Newton relation* (3–11) ζ by $x - f$ and ζ' by $x' - f'$, we get

   $$fx' + f'x = xx',$$

   and dividing by xx', we obtain

   $$\frac{f}{x} + \frac{f'}{x'} = 1 \tag{3.12}$$

or

$$\frac{f}{f'} = -\frac{n}{n'},$$

$$D = -\frac{n}{f} = \frac{n'}{f'}.$$

The *conjugation relation* is

$$\frac{n'}{x'} = \frac{n}{x} + D \tag{3.13}$$

The transverse magnification is obtained using the Lagrange–Helmholtz relation (3–7)

$$ny\alpha = n'y'\alpha'.$$

The transverse magnification is

$$M_T = \frac{y'}{y} = \frac{\alpha'x'}{\alpha x} = \frac{n\,x'}{n'\,x} \tag{3.14}$$

Dioptric Power

The *dioptric power* is defined by

$$D = -\frac{n}{f} = \frac{n'}{f'} \tag{3.15}$$

A positive or convergent system (positive D) thus possesses a negative object focal length and a positive image focal length. For a negative or divergent system (negative D), the object focal length is positive and the image focal length is negative. Instead of power, in the optics books "*D*" is called "*V*" or "*vergence,*" but this term has another meaning in binocular vision, and thus, in ophthalmology, it is better to use the term of "*dioptric power.*"

Magnification

In optics, the magnification γ is the ratio of the size of an image to the size of the object creating it. There are four types of magnification: the transverse magnification (also called linear or lateral), the angular magnification, the longitudinal magnification, and the pupillary magnification (Fig. 3.7 and Table 3.1).

Fig. 3.6 Relation of conjugation, $\overline{AB} = y$ and $\overline{A'B'} = y'$

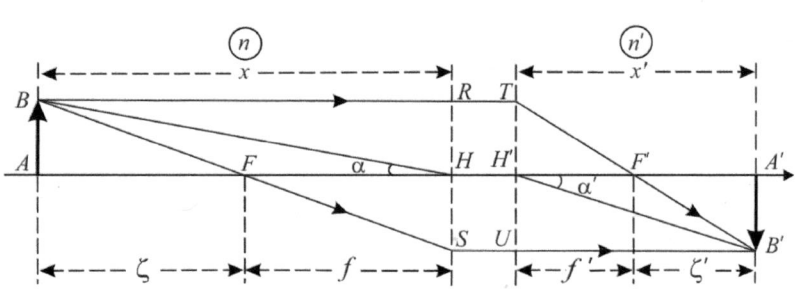

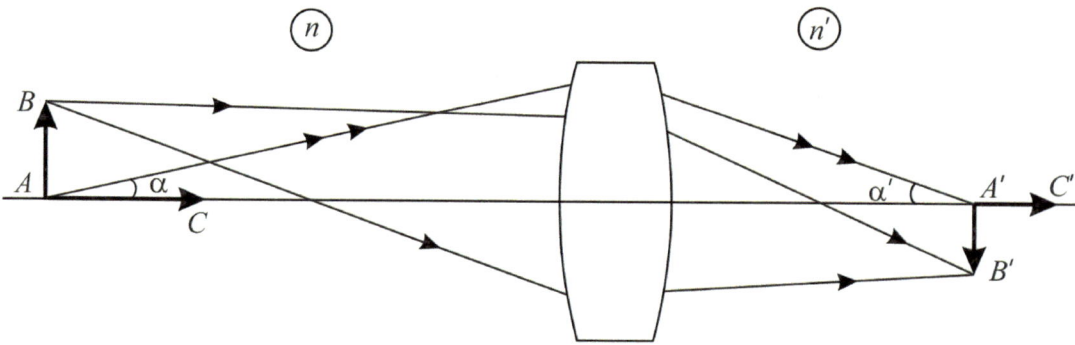

Fig. 3.7 Magnification

Table 3.1 Magnification

	Descartes	Newton
Position of the object	$x = \overline{HA}$	$\zeta = \overline{FA}$
Position of the image	$x' = \overline{H'A'}$	$\zeta' = \overline{F'A'}$
Relation of conjugation	$\dfrac{n'}{x'} - \dfrac{n}{x} = \dfrac{n'}{f'}$	$\zeta\zeta' = ff' = -f'^2$
Transverse magnification	$M_T = \dfrac{y'}{y} = \dfrac{nx'}{n'x}$	$M_T = \dfrac{y'}{y} = -\dfrac{\zeta'}{f'} = -\dfrac{f}{\zeta}$
Angular magnification	$M_\alpha = \dfrac{\alpha'}{\alpha} = \dfrac{x}{x'}$	$M_\alpha = \dfrac{\alpha'}{\alpha} = -\dfrac{\zeta}{f} = -\dfrac{f'}{\zeta'}$
Longitudinal magnification	$M_L = \dfrac{n'M_T^2}{n}$	$M_L = \dfrac{n'M_T^2}{n}$

1. Transverse magnification has been described above.

   If the origins of the optical system are at the focal points, transverse magnification M_T is

$$M_T = \frac{\overline{A'B'}}{\overline{AB}} = \frac{y'}{y} = -\frac{f}{\zeta} = -\frac{\zeta'}{f'} \qquad (3.16)$$

If the origins of the optical system are at the principal points, transverse magnification M_T is

$$M_T = \frac{\overline{A'B'}}{\overline{AB}} = \frac{y'}{y} = \frac{n}{n'}\frac{x'}{x} \qquad (3.17)$$

2. Angular magnification

   The *Abbe sine condition* in mathematical terms is

$$n\overline{AB}\sin\alpha = n'\overline{A'B'}\sin\alpha' \qquad (3.18)$$

Introducing the transverse magnification M_T in the Abbe sine equation,

$$\frac{\sin\alpha}{\sin\alpha'} = \frac{n'}{n}M_T.$$

In the Gaussian approximation the angles are small and we get the angular magnification M_α:

$$M_\alpha = \frac{\sin\alpha}{\sin\alpha'} = \frac{\alpha'}{\alpha} \qquad (3.19)$$

From the two previous equations, we get the *Lagrange–Helmholtz relation*:

$$\frac{n'}{n}M_T = \frac{1}{M_\alpha} \quad \text{or} \quad \frac{n'}{n}M_T M_\alpha = 1 \qquad (3.20)$$

so

$$M_\alpha = \frac{n}{n'M_T} = \frac{x}{x'} = -\frac{\zeta}{f} = -\frac{f'}{\zeta'} \qquad (3.21)$$

3. Longitudinal magnification

   The *Herschell condition* in mathematical terms is

$$n\overline{AC}\sin^2\frac{\alpha}{2} = n'\overline{A'C'}\sin^2\frac{\alpha'}{2} \qquad (3.22)$$

Introducing the longitudinal magnification M_L,

$$M_L = \frac{\overline{A'C'}}{\overline{AC}} \qquad (3.23)$$

The Herschell condition is written as

$$\frac{\sin^2 \dfrac{\alpha}{2}}{\sin^2 \dfrac{\alpha'}{2}} = \frac{n'}{n} M_L.$$

In the Gaussian approximation the angles are small and we get

$$\frac{\sin^2 \dfrac{\alpha}{2}}{\sin^2 \dfrac{\alpha'}{2}} = \left(\frac{\alpha}{\alpha'}\right)^2 = \frac{n'}{n} M_L = \left(\frac{n'}{n}\right)^2 M_T^2.$$

Let the longitudinal magnification M_L be

$$M_L = \frac{n'}{n} M_T^2 \qquad (3.24)$$

4. The pupillary magnification is the ratio of the diameter of the entrance pupil to the diameter of the exit pupil.

Combination of Two Systems

Let there be a first centered system with object and image principal points H_1 and H_1', with refractive indices (object and image) n_1 and n_1', with object and image focal points F_1 and F_1', with object and image focal lengths $f_1 = \overline{H_1 F_1}$ and $f_1' = \overline{H_1' F_1'}$, and with power D_1.

Let there be likewise a second centered system with object and image principal points H_2 and H_2', with refractive indices (object and image) n_2 and n_2', with object and image focal points F_2 and F_2', with object and image focal lengths $f_2 = \overline{H_2 F_2}$ and $f_2' = \overline{H_2' F_2'}$, and with power D_2.

The two systems are placed end to end, on a common axis with the same medium between the two systems, so $n_1' = n_2$. The combination of the two systems has for object index $n = n_1$ and for image index $n' = n_2'$. Optics Interval is defined by $\Delta = \overline{F_1' F_2}$ (Fig 3.8).

(a) Determination of the object focal point
    If we need to get an emerging ray of the second system which emerges parallel to the axis, the incident ray of the second system must go through the object focal point F_2. The object focal point F of the combination of the two systems will be defined as being the object having the image F_2 through the first system. Applying *Newton's formula* to the first system, we get

$$\overline{F_1 F}\, \overline{F_1' F_2} = f_1 f_1'. \qquad (3.25)$$

The **position of the object focal point** F of the combination of the two systems is

$$\overline{F_1 F} = \frac{f_1 f_1'}{\Delta} \qquad (3.26)$$

(b) Determination of the image focal point
    An incident ray on the first system, parallel to the axis, emerges from the first system going through the image focal point F_1'. The image focal point F' of the combination of the two systems is none other than the image of F_1' through the second system. Applying *Newton's formula* to the second system, we get

$$\overline{F_2 F_1'}\, \overline{F_2' F'} = f_2\, f_2'. \qquad (3.27)$$

The **position of the image focal point** F' of the combination of the two systems is

$$\overline{F_2' F'} = -\frac{f_2 f_2'}{\Delta} \qquad (3.28)$$

(c) Determination of the object focal length
    The object principal plane is the locus of all the K points of which the projection on the axis is the image principal point H. Applying the *Thales theorem* which says that if a straight line is drawn parallel to a side of a triangle, then it divides the other two sides proportionally (Fig. 3.8):

$$\frac{\overline{FH}}{\overline{FH_1}} = \frac{\overline{HK}}{\overline{H_1 I_1}} = \frac{\overline{H_2 I_2}}{\overline{H_1' I_1'}} = \frac{\overline{F_2 H_2}}{\overline{F_2 H_1'}},$$

hether

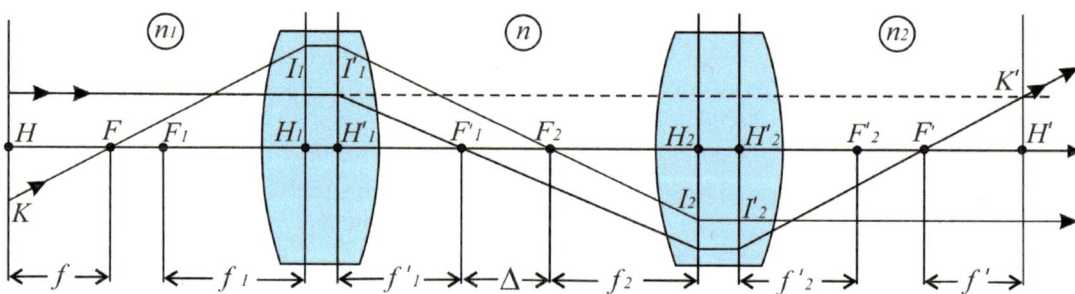

Fig. 3.8 Compound thick lens

$$\frac{\overline{HF}}{H_1F_1+\overline{F_1F}}=\frac{f}{f_1+\dfrac{f_1f_1'}{\Delta}}=\frac{\overline{H_2F_2}}{\overline{H_1'F_1'}+\overline{F_1'F_2}}=\frac{f_2}{f_1'+\Delta}.$$

The object focal length is

$$f=\overline{HF}=\frac{f_1f_2}{\Delta} \qquad (3.29)$$

(d) Determination of the image focal length

The image principal plane is the locus of all the K' points of which the projection on the axis is the image principal point H'. Applying the *Thales theorem* (Fig. 3.8),

$$\frac{\overline{F'H'}}{\overline{F'H_2'}}=\frac{\overline{H'K'}}{\overline{H_2'I_2'}}=\frac{\overline{H_1'I_1'}}{\overline{H_2I_2}}=\frac{\overline{F_1'H_1'}}{\overline{F_1'H_2'}},$$

hether

$$\frac{\overline{H'F'}}{H_2'F_2'+\overline{F_2'F''}}=\frac{f^1}{f_2'+\dfrac{f_2f_2'}{\Delta}}=\frac{\overline{H_1'F_1'}}{\overline{H_2F_2}+\overline{F_2F_1'}}=\frac{f_1'}{f_2-\Delta}.$$

The image focal length is

$$f'=\overline{H'F'}=-\frac{f_1'f_2'}{\Delta} \qquad (3.30)$$

Through the combination of two systems, F_1 and F_2' are conjugated. Furthermore wet get these other relations:

$$\frac{f_1'}{f_1}=-\frac{n_1'}{n} \text{ and } \frac{f_2'}{f_2}=-\frac{n'}{n_2},$$

$$\frac{f'}{f}=-\frac{n'}{n} \qquad (3.31)$$

(e) Determination of dioptric power for a compound of two systems

The dioptric power or vergence of each system is given by

$$D_1=-\frac{n_1}{f_1}=\frac{n}{f_1'}, \qquad (3.32)$$

$$D_2=-\frac{n}{f_2}=\frac{n_2}{f_2'}, \qquad (3.33)$$

and the power of the two systems is given by

$$D=-\frac{n_1}{f}=\frac{n_2}{f'}=-\frac{n_2.\Delta}{f_1'f_2'}. \qquad (3.34)$$

The optics interval can be break down as

$$\Delta=\overline{F_1'F_2}=\overline{F_1'H_1'}+\overline{H_1'H_2}\,\overline{H_1'H_2}+\overline{H_2F_2}$$
$$=-f_1'+f_2+\overline{H_1'H_2},$$

hence

$$D \quad =-\frac{-n_2f_1'+n_2f_2+n_2\overline{H_1'H_2}}{f_1'f_2'},$$

$$D \quad =\frac{n_2}{f_2'}-\frac{n}{f_1'}\frac{n_2}{f_2'}\frac{f_2}{n}-\frac{n}{f_1'}\frac{n_2}{f_2'}\frac{\overline{H_1'H_2}}{n},$$

$$D \quad =D_2+(D_1D_2\frac{1}{D_2})-D_1D_2\overline{H_1'H_2},$$

and we get the *Gullstrand relation*:

$$D=D_1+D_2-\frac{H_1'H_2}{n}D_1D_2 \qquad (3.35)$$

Single Lens

After the refracting surface where there is only one interface, the simplest centered system is the lens. The lens has two spherical refractive surfaces. The cornea is a meniscus lens, and the crystalline lens is biconvex. For the first refractive surface, the refractive indices of the object and image media are n_1 and n_1', and the radius of curvature is r_1.

$$D_1 = \frac{n_1' - n_1}{r_1} \qquad (3.36)$$

For the second refractive surface, the refractives indices of the object and image media are n_2 and n_2', and the radius of curvature is r_2.

$$D_2 = \frac{n_2' - n_2}{r_2} \qquad (3.37)$$

If the lens of index n is placed in a medium with an index n_0, we have $n = n_1' = n_2$ and $n_0 = n_1 = n_2'$. If the lens thickness on the optical axis is t, and according to the *formula of combination*, we get the power of the lens

$$D = (n - n_0)\left(\frac{1}{r_1} - \frac{1}{r_2}\right) + \frac{(n - n_0)^2}{n} \frac{t}{r_1 r_2} \quad (3.38)$$

For a biconvex lens with radii r_1 and r_2 and diameter d, the thickness of the lens t is calculated with the *formula of coupola* (Figs. 3.9, 3.10). The height of each coupola of the lens is h_1 and h_2, and the thickness at the border of the lens is t_0. The thickness of the lens is $t = h_1 + t_0 + h_2$ with

$$h_1 = r_1 - \left(r_1^2 - \frac{d^2}{4}\right)^{1/2} \text{ and } h_2 = r_2 - \left(r_2^2 - \frac{d^2}{4}\right)^{1/2} \quad (3.39)$$

Entrance and Exit Pupils

The pupil is the surface limited by the inner border of the iris. The pupil of the human eye acts as the aperture stop of the eye. When the real pupil is seen from outside, an observer sees the *entrance pupil* which is a virtual image of the real pupil as seen through the corneal refraction. In the example below, entrance and exit pupils of the human eye are calculated with the values of Le Grand's theoretical eye.

1. The *entrance pupil* Δ_0 is conjugated to the real pupil Δ in the object space when the light beam goes through the sub-optical system which is anterior to the pupil (cornea). In this example we calculate the position and the diameter of the entrance pupil of the theoretical eye. We assume that the anterior surface of the iris is in a frontal plane tangent to the cristalline lens apex. The pupil is at the distance of 3.60 mm from the corneal apex S. The position of the principal planes of the cornea is at 0.06 mm in front of the cornea.

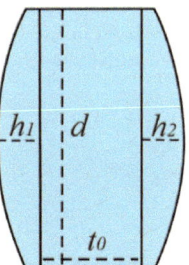

Fig. 3.10 Design of a biconvex lens

Fig. 3.9 Biconvex lens

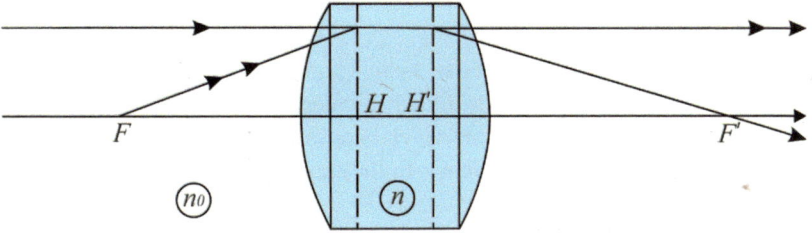

Thus the real pupil is at the distance of $3.60 + 0.06 = 3.66$ mm from the image principal plane of the cornea. The refractive index of aqueous humor is 1.3374 and the corneal power is D_c. According to the equation of conjugation (3.1):

$$\frac{n'}{x'} = \frac{n}{x} + \frac{n'-n}{r},$$

we get

$$\frac{1}{x} = \frac{n'}{x'} - D_c = \left[1.3374/\left(3.66 * 10^{-3}\right)\right] - 42.36$$
$$= 323.05,$$

$$x = \frac{1}{323.05} = 0.0031 \text{ m},$$

and $x = 3.10$ mm.

The distance between the apex of the cornea and the entrance pupil is $3.10 - 0.06 = 3.04$ mm. The entrance pupil is located in front of the real pupil and slightly enlarged. Applying the equation of transverse magnification (3.14), where Δ_0 is the size of the entrance pupil and Δ the diameter of the real pupil:

$$M_T = \frac{y'}{y} = \frac{nx'}{n'x} \quad \text{and} \quad \frac{\Delta_o}{\Delta} = \frac{n'x}{nx'} \frac{1.3374}{1} \frac{3.10}{3.66}$$
$$= 1.13,$$

thus

$$\Delta_o = \Delta * 1.13.$$

For a real pupil with a 6 mm diameter (scotopic vision), the entrance pupil diameter is $6 * 1.13 = 6.78$ mm, for a real pupil with a 4 mm diameter (mesopic vision), the entrance pupil diameter is $4 * 1.13 = 4.52$ mm, and for a real pupil with a 2 mm diameter (photopic vision), the entrance pupil diameter is $2 * 1.13 = 2.26$ mm.

2. The *exit pupil* Δ_i is conjugated to the real pupil Δ in the image space when the light beam goes through the sub-optical system which is posterior to the pupil (crystalline lens). In the same way we calculte the position and the diameter of the exit pupil of the theoretical eye. The refractive index of aqueous humor is 1.3374 and the crystalline lens power is D_{cl}. The pupil is at the distance of 3.60 mm from the vertex. The distance x between the corneal apex and the object principal plane of the crystalline lens is 6.02 mm. The distance between the real pupil and the object principal plane of the crystalline lens x is $6.02 - 3.60 = 2.42$ mm. The distance between the image principal plane of the crystalline lens and the image of the real pupil after passing through the crystalline lens is x'. According to the equation of conjugation (3.1):

$$\frac{n'}{x'} = \frac{n}{x} + \frac{n'-n}{r},$$

we get

$$\frac{n'}{x'} = \frac{n}{x} + D_{cl} = -\left[1.3374/(2.42 * 10^{-3})\right] + 21.78$$
$$= 530.86,$$

$$x' = \frac{1.336}{530,86} = 0.00252 \, m,$$

and $x' = 2.52$ mm.

The distance between the corneal apex and the image principal plane of the crystalline lens is 6.20 mm. The distance between the apex of the cornea and the exit pupil is $6.20 - 2.52 = 3.68$ mm.

The exit pupil is located behind the true pupil and slightly enlarged. Applying the equation of transverse magnification (3.14), where Δ_i is the diameter of the exit pupil and Δ the diameter of the real pupil, the diameter of the exit pupil Δ_i is obtained as

$$M_T = \frac{y'}{y} = \frac{nx'}{n'x} \quad \text{and} \quad \frac{\Delta_i}{\Delta} = \frac{nx'}{n'x} = \frac{1.3374}{1.336} \frac{2.52}{2.42}$$
$$= 1.04,$$

thus

$$\Delta_i = \Delta * 1.04.$$

Fig. 3.11 Entrance and exit pupils of the eye. AB (Δ_o) is the entrance pupil, and $A'B'$ (Δ_i) is the exit pupil

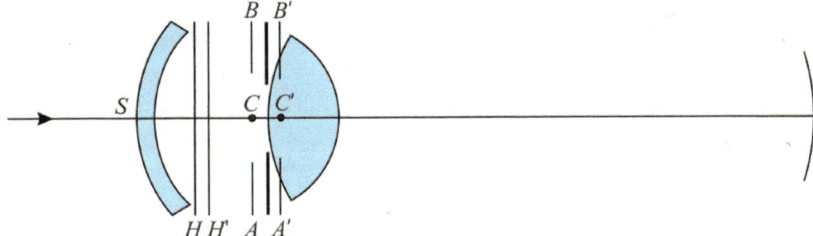

To calculate the diameter of the exit pupil based on the diameter of the entrance pupil, we have

$$\Delta = \frac{\Delta_o}{1.13} \text{ and we get } \Delta_i = \frac{\Delta_o}{1.13} * 1.04,$$

thus

$$\Delta_i = \Delta_o * 0.92.$$

Consequently, the diameter of the exit pupil is equal to the diameter of the entrance pupil multiplied by 0.92. Thus, for a real pupil with a 6 mm diameter (scotopic vision), the exit pupil diameter is $6.78 * 0.92 = 6.24$ mm, for a real pupil with a 4 mm diameter (mesopic vision), the exit pupil diameter is $4.52 * 0.92 = 4.16$ mm, and for a real pupil with a 2 mm diameter (photopic vision), the exit pupil diameter is $2.26 * 0.92 = 2.08$ mm.

The pupil magnification is the ratio of the diameter of the exit pupil to the diameter of the entrance pupil (Fig. 3.11):

$$M_P = \frac{\Delta_i}{\Delta_o}.$$

Matrix Method in Paraxial Optics

The matrix method provides an alternative way for solving paraxial optics problems. Matrices are a mathematical tool designed to deal with linear equations, so that it is natural to apply matrices to paraxial ray tracing. The matrix method will be used to find the first-order properties of the schematic eye and to calculate its cardinal elements.

Elementary Matrices

(a) Vergence of a Spherical Surface

By definition, the *vergence* or *dioptric power* of a spherical surface, which separates two media with indices n_1 and n_2, is

$$V \equiv \frac{n_2 - n_1}{\overline{R}},$$

where $\overline{R} \equiv \overline{SC}$ is the radius of curvature in algebraical value of which the sign is *linked to the direction of the incident light*. When R is expressed in meter, the unity for the vergence is the *diopter* (δ).

(b) Refraction Matrix

In the Gaussian approximation, the linearity of the equations of crossing a spherical surface suggests to use the matrix calculation. The column matrix is defined with the first element $\underline{X}$ which is the *position* x of the crossing point of the ray with the interface and the second element $n\underline{\alpha}$ or *optical angle* which is the product of the index by the tilt angle of the ray with the optical axis:

$$\underline{X} \equiv \begin{bmatrix} x \\ n\underline{\alpha} \end{bmatrix}.$$

The crossing of a spherical surface is written as

$$\begin{bmatrix} x \\ n\underline{\alpha} \end{bmatrix}_2 = \begin{bmatrix} 1 & 0 \\ -V & 1 \end{bmatrix} \begin{bmatrix} x \\ n\underline{\alpha} \end{bmatrix}_1$$

in a condensed form, $\underline{X}_2 = \mathcal{R}(S)\underline{X}_1$, where

$$R = \begin{bmatrix} 1 & 0 \\ -V & 1 \end{bmatrix}$$

is the *refraction matrix* of the spherical surface.

The value of the determinant of $\mathcal{R}(S)$ is 1: det $\mathcal{R} = 1$.

(c) Translation Matrix

The translation matrix is the transformation matrix of the column matrix X between two frontal planes $A_1 xy$ and $A_2 xy$ located in the same homogeneous medium. Using the complex notation and introducing the index, the equations of transformation are

$$\underline{x}_2 = \underline{x}_1 + \frac{\overline{A_1 A_2}}{n}(n\underline{\alpha})_1 \qquad \text{and} \qquad (n\underline{\alpha})_2 = (n\underline{\alpha})_1.$$

Matrix-wise, this is written as

$$\begin{bmatrix} x \\ n\underline{\alpha} \end{bmatrix}_2 = \begin{bmatrix} 1 & \overline{A_1 A_2}/n \\ 0 & 1 \end{bmatrix} \begin{bmatrix} x \\ n\underline{\alpha} \end{bmatrix}_1.$$

In a condensed form, $\underline{X}_2 = \mathcal{T}(\overline{A_1 A_2})\underline{X}_1$ with

$$\tau(\overline{A_1 A_2}) = \begin{bmatrix} 1 & \overline{A_1 A_2}/n \\ 0 & 1 \end{bmatrix}$$

The effective length that characterizes the translation matrix is the *reduced length* $\overline{A_1 A_2}/n$. The value of the determinant of $\mathcal{T}(\overline{A_1 A_2})$ is 1: det $\mathcal{T}(\overline{A_1 A_2}) = 1$.

Centered Systems

A centered system is composed of many refractive or reflective surfaces, usually spherical, such that the set has a symmetry around the same axis of Oz. The centered optical systems, composed of a series of homogeneous media, separated by spherical interfaces, are characterized in the Gaussian approximation by a linear relationship. Two methods are used to get the image of an object. The first is *algebraical*, and it is based on the *conjugate relationships* between the positions of the objects and the corresponding images. The second is *geometrical*, and it visualizes the particular rays of light.

(a) Transfer Matrix of a Centered System

Let us consider a centered system made up of p refractive spherical surfaces separated by homogeneous media. E is the first interface and S is the last interface of the system. Let $T(\overline{ES})$ be the transfer matrix of the system. The parameters that define the ray of light in all the frontal plane are the following complex numbers: the abscissa $\underline{x} = x + iy$ and the optical angle $\underline{\alpha} = n(\alpha + i\beta)$. Therefore the entrance and exit matrices are written as

$$\underline{X}_e = \begin{bmatrix} x \\ n\underline{\alpha} \end{bmatrix}_e \qquad \text{and} \qquad \underline{X}_s = \begin{bmatrix} x \\ n\underline{\alpha} \end{bmatrix}_s.$$

The product of elementary matrices of translation $\mathcal{T}$ and of refraction $\mathcal{R}$, writen from *right to left* following the succession of the spherical surfaces crossed by light, is a matrix $T(\overline{ES})$ with four elements. By definition

$$T(\overline{ES}) \equiv \mathcal{T}(\overline{S_p S})\mathcal{R}(S_p)\cdots\mathcal{T}(\overline{S_1 S_2})\mathcal{R}(S_1)\mathcal{T}(\overline{ES_1})$$

is the *transfer matrix* of the centered system. It is written as

$$T(\overline{ES}) = \begin{bmatrix} a & b \\ c & d \end{bmatrix}.$$

The relationship $\underline{X}_s = T(\overline{ES})\underline{X}_e$ is explained as follows:

$$\underline{X}_s = a\underline{x}_e + b(n\underline{\alpha})_e \quad \text{and} \quad (n\underline{\alpha})_s = c\underline{x}_e + d(n\underline{\alpha})_e.$$

The four elements a, b, c, and d, callled *Gaussian constants*, are linked by a relationship because the determinant of $T(\overline{ES})$, the product of matrices of determinants equal to 1, is also equal to 1.

(b) Vergence of a Centered System

The transfer matrix $T(\overline{A_1 A_2})$ between two frontal planes $A_1 xy$ and $A_2 xy$, respectively, located in the object space and in the image space, with the indices n_o and n_i, is expressed as

$$T(\overline{A_1 A_2}) = \mathcal{T}(\overline{SA_2})T(\overline{ES})\mathcal{T}(\overline{A_1 E}).$$

This matrix transfer of the total system which takes a ray from the object to the image is named *conjugate matrix*. For the couple of points A_1 and A_2, with $z_1 \equiv \overline{EA_1}$ and $z_2 \equiv \overline{SA_2}$ and with $T_{ij}(A)$ the elements of the conjugate matrix, the previous relationship is written as

$$\begin{bmatrix} T_{11}(A) & T_{12}(A) \\ T_{21}(A) & T_{22}(A) \end{bmatrix} = \begin{bmatrix} 1 & z_2/n_i \\ 0 & 1 \end{bmatrix} \begin{bmatrix} a & b \\ c & d \end{bmatrix} \begin{bmatrix} 1 & -z_1/n_o \\ 0 & 1 \end{bmatrix},$$

which gives in performing and in identifying

$$T_{11}(A) = a + c\frac{z_2}{n_i}$$

$$T_{12}(A) = -a\frac{z_1}{n_o} + b + \frac{z_2}{n_i}(-c\frac{z_1}{n_o} + d)$$

$$T_{21}(A) = c$$

$$T_{22}(A) = d - c\frac{z_1}{n_o}.$$

By definition the *vergence* of a system is the opposite of c:

$$V \equiv -c.$$

Matrix-wise, we write

$$\begin{bmatrix} \underline{x} \\ n\underline{\alpha} \end{bmatrix}_s = \begin{bmatrix} a & b \\ -V & d \end{bmatrix} \begin{bmatrix} x \\ 0 \end{bmatrix}_e,$$

or in a condensed form, $\underline{X}_s = T(\overline{ES})\underline{X}_e$, from where $n_i\alpha_s = -Vx_e$.

If $V > 0$, the system is *converging*. If , the system is *diverging*. If $V = 0$, the system is *afocal*.

(c) Conjugate Matrix

Let us consider a centered system and two conjugates planes which are perpendicular to the optical axis and which contain the points A_o, A_i, B_o, and B_i. We write $z_o \equiv \overline{EA_o}$ and $z_i \equiv \overline{SA_i}$. Each element of the transfer matrix of the system between these two conjugate planes or a conjugate matrix is written as

$$T_{11}(A) = a - V\frac{z_i}{n_i}$$

$$T_{12}(A) = -a\frac{z_o}{n_o} + b + \frac{z_i}{n_i}(V\frac{z_o}{n_o} + d)$$

$$T_{21}(A) = -V$$

$$T_{22}(A) = d + V\frac{z_o}{n_o}.$$

Explaining the matrix relationship $\underline{X}_i = T(\overline{A_oA_i})\underline{X}_o$, it becomes

$$\underline{x}_i = T_{11}(A)\underline{x}_o + T_{12}(A)n_o\underline{\alpha}_o \quad \text{and}$$
$$n_i\underline{\alpha}_i = -V\underline{x}_o + T_{22}(A)n_o\underline{\alpha}_o.$$

As the position $\underline{x}_i$ of the image B_i is *independent* of the tilt $\underline{\alpha}_o$ of the rays coming from A_o, we obtain the conjugate relationship which is given $T_{12}(A) \equiv 0$ and let

$$-a\frac{z_o}{n_o} + b + \frac{z_i}{n_i}(V\frac{z_o}{n_o} + d) = 0$$

The transverse magnification M_t, in the case of the Gaussian approximation, is given by the formula:

$$M_t = \frac{\overline{A_iB_i}}{\overline{A_oB_o}}.$$

$T_{11}(A)$ is identified to the *transverse magnification* M_t.

The *angular magnification* is defined by $M_a \equiv (\underline{\alpha}_i/\underline{\alpha}_o)_{x_o} = 0$.

$T_{22}(A)$ is worth:

$$T_{22}(A) = (\frac{n_i\alpha_i}{n_o\alpha_o})_{x_o=0} = 0,$$

$$T_{22}(A) = \frac{n_i}{n_o}M_a.$$

The transfer matrix between two *conjugate planes* is written as

$$T(\overline{A_oA_i}) = \begin{bmatrix} M_t & 0 \\ -V & (n_i/n_o)M_a \end{bmatrix}$$

The determinant of $T(\overline{A_oA_i})$ being equal to 1, we get the *Lagrange and Helmholtz relation*:

$$\frac{n_i}{n_o}M_tM_a = 1$$

Which is also written as

$$n_ox_o\alpha_o = n_ix_i\alpha_i.$$

(d) Homographic Relation

By definition a homographic function is represented in the form of a quotient of affine functions which can be written as

$$y = \frac{ax+b}{cx+d}.$$

This function determines a bijection if $(ad-bc) \neq 0$. Every object point and its image point form a conjugate pair, and by the *principle of inverse return of the light*, the pair persists when the image becomes object and vice versa. This relation is easily obtained with the help of the matrices $T(\overline{ES})$ and $T(\overline{A_oA_i})$. With the usual notations ($z_o = \overline{EA_o}$, $z_i = \overline{SA_i}$, etc.), as A_o and A_i are conjugated, we get

$$T_{12}(A) = -a\frac{z_0}{n_o} + b + \frac{z_i}{n_i}(V\frac{z_o}{n_o} + d) = 0$$

It results the following *homographic relation*:

$$\frac{z_i'}{n_i} = \frac{az_o/n_o - b}{Vz_o/n_o + d}$$

Cardinal Elements

In the Gaussian optics or paraxial approximation, the cardinal elements are sufficient to calculate the position and the size of the image of an object. These elements are the *focal lengths* (and the *focal planes*), the *principal planes*, and the *nodal points* (Fig. 3.12).

(a) Focal lengths

By definition, the *image* and *object focal lengths* are the following *algebraical* quantities:

$$f_i \equiv \frac{n_i}{V} \quad \text{and} \quad f_o \equiv -\frac{n_o}{V}$$

If $V > 0, f_i > 0$ and $f_o < 0$. On the other side, if $V < 0, f_i < 0$ and $f_o > 0$. If the extreme media are identical, $f_i = -f_o$.

(b) Principal planes

Principal planes are frontal conjugate planes $H_o xy$ and $H_i xy$ such that the *transverse magnification* M_t is equal to *unity*. It results that the transfer matrix $T(\overline{H_oH_i})$ between the principal planes has for expression

$$T(\overline{H_oH_i}) = \begin{bmatrix} 1 & 0 \\ -V & 1 \end{bmatrix},$$

and we can write

$$T_{11}(H) = 1 = a - V\frac{\overline{SH_i}}{n_i} \quad \text{and} \quad T_{22}(H) = 1$$
$$= d + V\frac{\overline{EH_o}}{n_o}.$$

Therefore, the positions of the principal planes of a centered system, in function of the transfer matrix $T(\overline{ES})$ of this system, are given by the relations:

$$\overline{SH_i} = f_i(a-1) \quad \text{and} \quad \overline{EH_o} = f_o(d-1)$$

Fig. 3.12 Cardinal elements

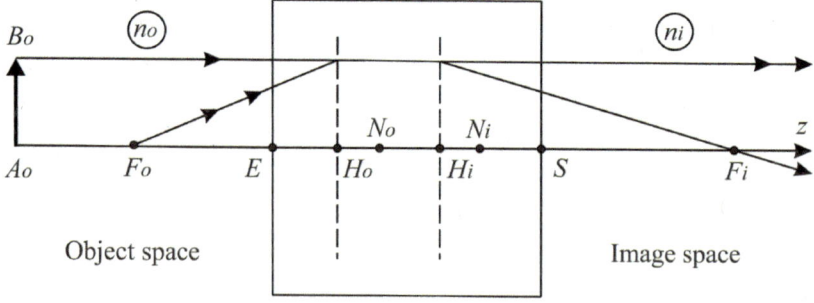

B_o $\quad$ (n_o) $\qquad\qquad\qquad\qquad\qquad\qquad$ (n_i)

$\qquad\qquad\qquad\qquad N_o \quad N_i$

$A_o \qquad F_o \qquad E \qquad |H_o \quad |H_i \qquad S \qquad\qquad F_i$

Object space $\qquad\qquad\qquad\qquad\qquad\qquad$ Image space

(c) **Nodal points**

The two nodal points, N_o and N_i, are two conjugate points located on the optical axis such that all incident rays going through N_o emerge from N_i in parallel to its incident direction. Therefore

$$M_a = 1 = \left(\frac{\alpha_i}{\alpha_o} \right)_{x_o = 0} = 1$$

The transfer matrix $T(\overline{N_o N_i})$ is written as

$$T(\overline{N_o N_i}) = \begin{bmatrix} n_o/n_i & 0 \\ -V & n_i/n_o \end{bmatrix}.$$

From where the following relationships,

$$T_{11}(N) = \frac{n_o}{n_i} = a - V\frac{\overline{SN_1}}{n_i} \quad \text{and} \quad T_{22}(N) = \frac{n_i}{n_o}$$

$$= d + V\frac{\overline{EN_o}}{n_o}$$

and the positions of these points from E and S:

$$\overline{EN_o} = f_o\left(d - \frac{n_i}{n_o}\right) \quad \text{and} \quad \overline{SN_i} = f_i\left(a - \frac{n_o}{n_i}\right)$$

similarly from the principal planes H_i and H_o,

$$\overline{H_i N_i} = \overline{H_o N_o} = f_o + f_i$$

Thus the distances $\overline{H_o H_i}$ and $\overline{N_o N_i}$ are equal.

(d) **Focal planes**

These frontal planes in the object space and in the image space are written as $F_o xy$ and $F_i xy$ and are defined as follows:

All the incident rays of light, *coming* from F_o, emerge *parallel* to the optical axis.

All the incident rays of light, *parallel* to the optical axis, emerge *converging* to F_i.

Object focal point F_o

To locate F_o, the relationship between the entrance and exit parameters is written as

$$x_s = ax_e + bn_o\alpha_e \quad \text{and} \quad n_i\alpha_s = -Vx_e + dn_o\alpha_e.$$

As $\alpha_s = 0$, whatever x_e and α_e, it becomes

$$\frac{x_e}{\alpha_e} = \frac{n_o}{V}d.$$

So, the incident rays of light come from a point F_o such that, *algebraically*,

$$-\overline{EF_o} = \frac{x_e}{\alpha_e} = \frac{n_o}{V}d.$$

It results

$$\overline{EF_o} = f_o d \quad \text{and} \quad \overline{H_o F_o} = \overline{H_o E} + \overline{EF_o} = f_o$$

Image focal point F_i

As in this case $\alpha_e = 0$ whatever x_s and α_s, it becomes

$$x_s = ax_e \quad \text{and} \quad n_i\alpha_s = -Vx_e,$$

hence

$$\frac{x_s}{\alpha_s} = -n_i\frac{a}{V}.$$

So, the rays of light emerge at the point F_i such that, *algebraically*,

$$-\overline{SF_i} = -\frac{x_s}{\alpha_s} = \frac{n_i}{V}a.$$

It results:

$$\overline{SF_i} = f_i a \quad \text{and} \quad \overline{H_i F_i} = \overline{H_i S} + \overline{SF_i} = f_i$$

In summary, the cardinal elements calculated with the Gaussian constants $a, b, -V$, and d of the transfer matrix $\begin{bmatrix} a & b \\ -V & d \end{bmatrix}$ of a centered system are

object focal length :	$f_o = -\dfrac{n_o}{V}$
image focal length :	$f_i = \dfrac{n_i}{V}$
position of the object principal point :	$\overline{EH_o} = f_o\,(d-1)$
position of the image principal point :	$\overline{SH_i} = f_i\,(a-1)$
position of the object focal point :	$\overline{EF_o} = -\dfrac{n_o}{V}d$
position of the image focal point :	$\overline{SF_i} = \dfrac{n_i}{V}a$
position of the object nodal point :	$\overline{EN_o} = f_o\,(d - \dfrac{n_i}{n_o})$
position of the image nodal point :	$\overline{SN_i} = f_i\,(a - \dfrac{n_o}{n_i})$
transverse magnification :	$M_t = a$
angular magnification :	$M_a = \dfrac{n_o}{n_i}d.$

Limits of Paraxial Approximation for the Eye

Two preliminary questions arise: Is the eye a centered system and can we use the paraxial approximation under normal conditions of vision? Strictly, the eye is not a centered system. The four diopters of the eye, anterior and posterior corneal surfaces and anterior and posterior surfaces of the crystalline lens, are not surfaces of revolution. The eye has at least eight surfaces with discontinuity of indices: two for the cornea (epithelium and cornea) and six for the cristalline lens (nucleus and cortex). The surfaces of the cornea and the cristalline lens are not spherical. The axis of the cristalline lens does not go through the axis of the cornea. This gap can be higher than 0.1 mm which is equivalent to an imprecision of $1°$ to $2°$ on the definition of the optical axis.

With a pupil diameter of 4 mm and a mean radius of corneal curvature of 8 mm, the sine of an angle of incidence i of a ray of light parallel to the axis and going through the border of the pupille is 0.25 or about $i = 14.5°$, that is to say $i = 0.253$ rad. There is a difference of more than 1% between i and $\sin i$.

For the posterior surface of the crystalline lens, the differences between the angles of incidence and their sine are even higher; so all in all a difference of more than 2% is likely between the paraxial way and the true way of the ray of light. For an ocular vergence of about 60 δ, this 2% difference is more than one diopter. Strictly speaking, we must study the formation of the images on the retina only in thinking about the true propagation of the ray of light from the corneal vertex to the retina.

Moreover the optical axis, pupil axis, line of sight, and visual axis are not aligned.

Despite that, the paraxial approximation can be used to study the optics of the vision and the corrections of the ametropia with the glasses or with the shaping of the cornea with an excimer laser, because the analysis of the difference between the true ray tracing and the paraxial approximation involves little in the correction. Indeed in first analysing, the paraxial approximation can be used for the eye because on the one hand the cornea flattens from the center to the periphery, and on the other hand the aberrations of the eye are a constant data for the non-corrected eye as for the corrected eye.

However for the intraocular lens correction of cataract surgery, the clinical studies show that the expected results of the formulas using only the paraxial approximation differ from the achieved results with a standard deviation of ± 1 diopter. These formulas must be adjusted including a correcting factor which is calculated usually with a statistical regression formula.

Schematic Eye

The eye is a complex optical system having a succession of spherical interfaces which are not perfectly spherical, of which media are differents and the index of the cristalline lens is not a constant. The schematic eye is an optical system obtained by taking into account the succession of the four spherical diopters centered on the same axis for which we calculate, in the Gaussian approximation, the cardinal elements and the ocular optical constants. The human theoretical eye is a fictitious eye which represents a mean of the dimensions of the adult eye for which we calculate in the Gaussian approximation the cardinal elements and the ocular optical constants (Fig. 3.13).

The matrix calculation has been applied to the eye for the first time by Le Grand and Bourdy (Table 3.2). The use of the matrices, applied to Colliac's theoretical eye, allows to find right away the formulas of association of a combination of optical systems and to calculate the cardinal elements (Fig. 3.14 and Table 3.3).

Fig. 3.13 Interfaces of the schematic eye

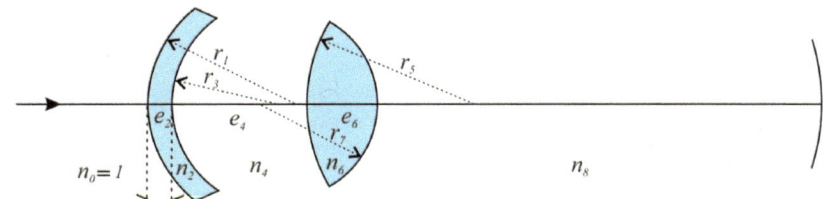

Table 3.2 Gaussian elements of the transfer matrix of the eye

	Gullstrand	Legrand	Colliac
$A = T_{11}$	0.756	0.7446	0.7415
$B = T_{12}$	0.0052	0.0054	0.0054
$C = T_{21}$	-58.5849	-59.940	-61.1514
$D = T_{22}$	0.9198	0.9044	0.8992

Fig. 3.14 Principal planes of a schematic eye

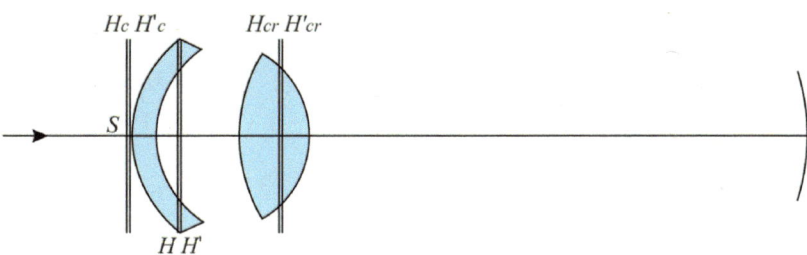

Table 3.3 Theoretical eye

	Gullstrand	Legrand	Colliac
Refractive indices			
Cornea	1.376	1.3771	1.376
Aqueous humor	1.336	1.3374	1.336
Crystalline lens (lens total index)	1.4085	1.42	1.42
Vitreous body	1.336	1.336	1.336
Abscissas (from the corneal apex)			
Posterior surface of the cornea	0.5	0.55	0.55
Anterior surface of the lens	3.60	3.60	3.60
Posterior surface of the lens	7.20	7.60	7.60
Radii of curvature			
Anterior surface of the cornea	7.70	7.80	7.75
Posterior surface of the cornea	6.8	6.5	6.89
Anterior surface of the lens	10	10.2	10.10
Posterior surface of the lens	-6	-6	-5.67
Vergences			
Anterior surface of the cornea	48.83	48.35	48.52
Posterior surface of the cornea	-5.88	-6.11	-5.81
Anterior surface of the lens	5	8.10	8.32
Posterior surface of the lens	8.33	14	14.81
Nucleus of the crystalline lens	5.985		
Cornea			
Vergence	43.053	42.36	42.52
Position of the object principal point	-0.0496	-0.06	-0.05
Position of the image principal point	-0.0506	-0.06	-0.06
Object focal length	-23.227	-23.61	-23.35
Image focal length	31.031	31.57	31.2
Crystalline lens			
Vergence	19.11	21.78	22.78
Position of the object principal point	5.678	6.02	6.05
Position of the image principal point	5.807	6.20	6.23
Object focal length	-69.908	-61.41	-58.64
Image focal length	69.908	61.34	58.64
Total eye			
Vergence	58.636	59.94	61.15
Position of the object principal point	1.348	1.59	1.65
Position of the image principal point	1.602	1.91	1.95
Position of the object focal point	-15.707	-15.09	-14.71
Position of the image focal point	24.387	24.20	23.80
Object focal length	-17.055	-16.68	-16.35
Image focal length	22.785	22.29	21.85
Position of the nodal object point	7.078	7.20	7.14
Position of the nodal image point	7.332	7.51	7.45
Position of the entrance pupil	3.045	3.04	3.04
Position of the exit pupil	3.664	3.68	3.67
Magnification at the pupil	0.909	0.92	0.92

$$\underbrace{\begin{bmatrix} A & B \\ C & D \end{bmatrix}}_{\text{eye}} = \underbrace{\begin{bmatrix} 1 & 0 \\ -V_7 & 1 \end{bmatrix} \begin{bmatrix} 1 & t_6/n_6 \\ 0 & 1 \end{bmatrix} \begin{bmatrix} 1 & 0 \\ -V_5 & 1 \end{bmatrix}}_{\text{crystalline lens}} \underbrace{\begin{bmatrix} 1 & t_4/n_4 \\ 0 & 1 \end{bmatrix}}_{\text{aqueous humor}} \underbrace{\begin{bmatrix} 1 & 0 \\ -V_3 & 1 \end{bmatrix} \begin{bmatrix} 1 & t_2/n_2 \\ 0 & 1 \end{bmatrix} \begin{bmatrix} 1 & 0 \\ -V1 & 1 \end{bmatrix}}_{\text{cornea}}$$

For our Colliac's schematic eye, we get the system matrix of the eye with the four Gaussian constants A, B, C, and D ($C = -V$):

$$\underbrace{\begin{bmatrix} A & B \\ C & D \end{bmatrix}}_{\text{eye}} = \underbrace{\begin{bmatrix} 1 & 0 \\ -14.81 & 1 \end{bmatrix} \begin{bmatrix} 1 & 2.8169 \\ 0 & 1 \end{bmatrix} \begin{bmatrix} 1 & 0 \\ -8.32 & 1 \end{bmatrix}}_{\text{crystalline lens}} \underbrace{\begin{bmatrix} 1 & 2.2829 \\ 0 & 1 \end{bmatrix}}_{\text{aqueous humor}} \underbrace{\begin{bmatrix} 1 & 0 \\ 5.81 & 1 \end{bmatrix} \begin{bmatrix} 1 & 0.3997 \\ 0 & 1 \end{bmatrix} \begin{bmatrix} 1 & 0 \\ -48.52 & 1 \end{bmatrix}}_{\text{cornea}}$$

$$\underbrace{\begin{bmatrix} A & B \\ C & D \end{bmatrix}}_{\text{eye}} = \underbrace{\begin{bmatrix} 0.7415 & 0.0054 \\ -61.1514 & 0.8992 \end{bmatrix}}_{\text{eye}}$$

The dimensions of the human eye vary from person to person. The mean values of the dimension of an adult eye are indicated in Table 3.2. The crystalline lens index of the crystalline lens is not a constant and varies in the thickness of the lens. We admit that the value of the total index of the crystalline lens is the value of 1.42 used by Tscherning and Le Grand.

References

1. Bourdy C. Calcul matriciel et optique paraxiale: application à l'optique ophtalmique. Rev Opt Theor Inst. 1962;4:295–308.

2. Le Grand Y. Optique physiologique, Tome I, La dioptrique de l'œil et sa correction. Paris: Éditions de la revue d'Optique; 1965.

3. Le Grand Y, El Hage SG. Physiological optics. Berlin: Springer; 1980.

4. Bass M, Van Stryland EW, Williams DR, Wolf WL. Handbook of optics, fundamentals, techniques and design, 2nd ed., vol. I. New York: McGraw-Hill; 1995.

5. Ditteon R. Modern geometrical optics. New York: John Wiley and Sons; 1998.

6. Hecht E. Optics. Reading: Addison Wesley Longman; 1998.

7. Pérez J-Ph, Anterrieu E. Optique : fondements et applications. Paris: Dunod; 2004

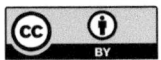

Exact Optics

4

Javier Alda

Introduction

Optics is one of the rare gems of physics where some principles and ideas developed in the ancient times, from Euclid to al-Haytham, still sustain part of the current models of how light behaves [1–4]. These ideas made possible to build simple optical instruments such as glasses and telescopes [5–7]. A few 100 years ago, the advances and ideas presented by a collection of great experimentalists, such as Grimaldi, Young, Fresnel, and Arago, prevailed against Newton's supporters to build the concept of light as a wave. This image of light as a wave was fully understood by Maxwell, who is recognized as the father of electromagnetism. A few decades later, the beginning of the twentieth century saw light as a flux of particles, as Newton postulated, but now is escorted by a sound robust model in the form of the quantum theories of light and flanked by the brilliant minds of Planck, Einstein, and so many others. Actually, all these models are well-recognized in colleges and universities because they predict how light interacts with matter and with itself. Even more, geometrical, electromagnetic, and quantum optics live together in peaceful harmony. Every optics and Photonics book contains these three models [8–12].

Within the scope of this chapter, we will mostly remain within the comfort zone of geometrical optics. When necessary, we will jump to wave optics to understand better those notions about wavefront aberrations and how they describe the deviation from the perfect object-image representation. Every optical system designed to generate an image from a given object requires interfaces and materials where light behaves differently. These image-forming systems collect the light coming from the object and deliver it to the detection area, where it is registered by a variety of mechanisms—from the chemical reactions caused in photographic films to the bio-chemical response given by the specialized light-sensitive cells in the retina. In the very first approach, this process can be described by considering how light travels along geometrical paths or light rays. These rays are bent by the optical system to finally reach their destination such that, ideally, every ray departing from a point in the object arrives at a single corresponding point in the image. One of the key elements in electromagnetic optics is the definition of the electromagnetic spectrum, where light is modeled as an electromagnetic wave. The electromagnetic spectrum classifies electromagnetic waves in terms of their wavelength, λ, given as the spatial distance between equivalent oscillatory states, and frequency, ν, related to the temporal rhythm of oscillation. The relation between them is $\lambda = v/\nu$, where v is the speed of propagation of the electromagnetic wave. This means that a

J. Alda (✉)
Applied Optics Complutense Group, Faculty of Optics and Optometry, Madrid, Spain
e-mail: javier.alda@ucm.es

J. Aramberri et al. (eds.), *Intraocular Lens Calculations*, Essentials in Ophthalmology,
https://doi.org/10.1007/978-3-031-50666-6_4

shorter wavelength corresponds to a higher frequency. At this point, it is interesting to note that, within the quantum model of light, an electromagnetic wave having a frequency ν can be represented by a collection of photons. Each photon carries a tiny amount of energy that obeys the Planck's relation: $E = h\nu$, where h is the Planck's constant ($h = 6.6261 \times 10^{-34}$ m^2 kg/s), meaning that the higher the frequency, the higher the energy is carried by each associated photon. The visible optical range covers the values of $\lambda \in (380, 780)$ nm, where the lower limit corresponds to the violet color and the upper limit to red. In between them, we have the spectral chromatic gamut seen in the rainbow. The visible wavelengths correspond to frequency values in hundreds of terahertz ($'10^{14}$ Hz). The visible range is limited by the ultraviolet ($\lambda \in [100, 380]$ nm) and the infrared ($\lambda \in [0.78, 100]$ μm) ranges.

As a final comment in this Introduction section, we wonder how exact is exact? The correct definitions of approximations, boundary conditions, and limitations are deeply woven into the fabric of Physics, and therefore into optics too. Guided by the scientific method, Physics has developed models and theories to understand how nature behaves. The scientific method is continuously challenging the current theories to find cracks and exceptions in order to build a more complete model that, one more time, requires scrutiny and discussion from scientists. So, an exact quantity is always accompanied by an error bar (and most of the times, even error bars are affected by uncertainties). Our purpose here is to present how optics helps to build a clearer picture of what light is and how optical image-forming systems behave. The certainty of the models should be confronted with the needs in accuracy of the given application. We will also peek at what lies beyond a given approximation—only with the necessary math and formalisms—to improve the understanding of optics and image-forming systems.

Optical Materials and Geometry

The first and the simplest approach to optics is made using geometry. Here, light travels along spatial trajectories known as light rays, and the problem is how to use these rays to describe the image-forming capabilities of optical systems. Very little attention is paid to the energy carried by light and some other important characteristics, such as wavelength and polarization, unless they actually impact the trajectories of the light ray. Geometry also requires some help from materials physics when defining optical parameters, such as the index of refraction or the Abbe number, and also borrows the wavelength concept from electromagnetism to explain the chromatic behavior of optical system. In any case, geometry governs the propagation of light in such a manner that it becomes the first approach to any optical analysis to obtain the location and characteristics of an image given an optical system.

The Index of Refraction

When considering image-forming systems, the materials used to build optical instruments should be as transparent as possible to minimize the amount of energy lost along the light trajectories. Still, they interact with light in a more subtle manner, modifying the speed of light within them. We all know that light travels at the highest possible velocity, $c = 299,792,458$ m/s, when propagating in vacuum. However, when passing through transparent media, light slows down significantly. Actually, one of the optical parameters that defines the light–matter interaction is the ratio between c and the speed of light in the material, v, that is well-known as the index of refraction:

$$n = \frac{c}{v}. \qquad (4.1)$$

Every optical material is characterized by its index of refraction. The lowest possible value is $n = 1$ that corresponds to the case of vacuum when $v = c$. The value of n depends on the composition of the material. For example, because of its low density, gases (including air) have an index of refraction very close to 1. The index of refraction of water is $n_{water}' = 1.333$, and most of the optical glasses are in the range $n \in (1.4, 1.8)$. Moreover, the index of refraction is wavelength-dependent: $n = n(\lambda)$. This means that different spectral colors will behave differently when propagating through optical media. To parameterize this dependence, we define another important variable, the Abbe number, that is given as:

$$V = \frac{n_d - 1}{n_F - n_C} V = \frac{n_d - 1}{n_F - n_C}, \qquad (4.2)$$

where n_d is the index of refraction for a wavelength, $\lambda_d = 587.6$ nm, close to the location where the human eye is more sensitive ($\lambda = 555$ nm), and n_F and n_C are the index of refraction for two wavelengths ($\lambda_F = 486.1$ nm, $\lambda_C = 656.3$ nm) located in the blue and red regions of the visible spectrum, respectively. The Abbe number helps to understand how large the change of the index of refraction is with respect to the wavelength. Then, by providing the index of refraction and the Abbe number of a material, we have quite a good idea of how an optical material behaves in the visible spectrum. Actually, the human lens is not an exception to this and presents a value of the Abbe number that varies between $V_{lens,min} = 45.6$ and $V_{lens,max} = 47.3$, corresponding to the low and high index of refraction of the human lens, $n_{lens} \in (1.386, 1.406)$, respectively [13].

If the material is not transparent, the index of refraction becomes an imaginary number, $\tilde{n} = n - ik$. The value k in its imaginary part describes the absorption of light that is produced along the propagation. Also, this absorption is a function of λ, giving rise to colored filters and some other very interesting mechanism of interaction. For example, the human lens shows a very large absorption coefficient in the ultraviolet region, meaning that a tiny portion of the UV light reaches the retina. This fact also means that this portion of the optical spectrum is strongly absorbed by the cornea and lens where it can produce some other unwanted effects.

The index of refraction is of paramount importance when describing how the straight trajectories observed for homogeneous media bend when passing from one material to another (see Fig. 4.1a). This behavior is well-described by Snell's law:

$$n \sin \epsilon = n' \sin \epsilon', \qquad (4.3)$$

where n and n' are the index of refraction of the involved materials on both sides of the interface, and ϵ and ϵ' are the incidence and refraction angles, respectively. In Fig. 4.1b, we can see how this bending, or angular deviation, is given as $\delta = \epsilon - \epsilon'$, works in an optical prism.

Also, when considering the amount of light (the power budget) that goes through a given separation between materials, the index of refraction appears in the equations and describes how much energy is reflected and how much is transmitted by the interface (see Fig. 4.1c). These relations are known as Fresnel equations, which take quite a simple form in the case of normal incidence ($\epsilon = \epsilon' = 0$)

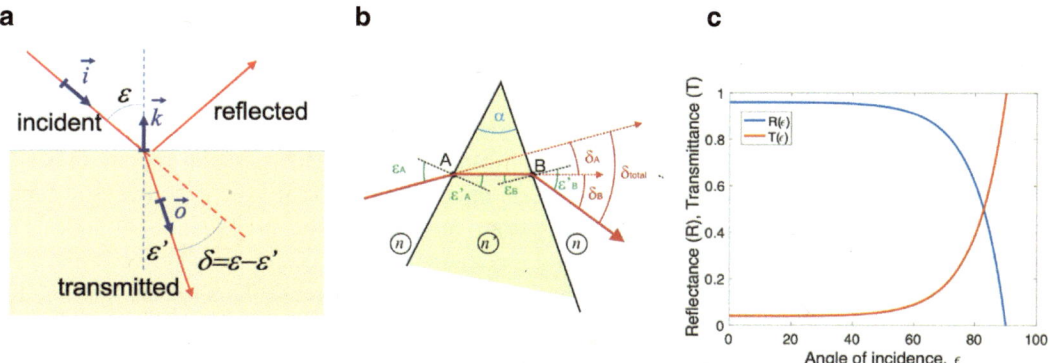

Fig. 4.1 (a) A graphical arrangement of Snell's law (Eq. 4.3), where we represent the incident, the reflected, and the transmitted rays. The vectors *i*, *o*, and *k* are those included in the three-dimensional form of Snell's law (Eq. 4.5). (b) An example of the application of Snell's law to the angular deviation of a prism. (c) Power budget between the transmitted and reflected beams, represented through transmittance (*T*) and reflectance (*R*) as a function of the angle of incidence, ϵ. This calculation assumes that the incidence has a natural polarization state. The values at $\epsilon = 0°$ are given in Eq. (4.4) and corresponds to a case where $n = 1$ and $n' = 1.5$

$$R = \left(\frac{n-n'}{n+n'}\right)^2, \qquad T = \frac{4nn'}{(n+n')^2}, \quad (4.4)$$

where R and T are the reflectivity and transmissivity of the interface, respectively. If we calculate the numbers for an interface between air, $n_{air} = 1$, and the corneal tissue, $n_{cornea} = 1.376$, we find that $R = 0.975$ (97.5% of the energy enters the cornea) and $T = 0.025$ (2.5% of the incident light is reflected).

We cannot finish this description of the index of refraction without paying spatial attention to non-homogeneous materials. This is the case of the lens of the human eye. It is well-known that the lens is better described as a graded index of a refraction element [14–16]. The index of refraction at the core of the lens is the largest and decreases when moving toward the surface. This change is smooth over a limited range, but it bends the light trajectory in quite an efficient way. Therefore, when replacing the human lens by a single-material intra-ocular lens, we are also replacing a biologically graded index material by a polymer having a constant index of refraction over its whole volume. In the case of gradient media, the light trajectories do not follow a straight line, as it happens with homogeneous media. The actual propagation of light, within the geometrical model that only considers the trajectory of light, is given as the solution of a mathematical variational problem where a quantity defined as the optical path reaches an extremal point (a maximum or a minimum) [17]. The optical path, L, is defined as the product of the geometrical trajectory, the propagated distance (d), times the index of refraction (n) of the material where light travels, $L = nd$. This is the same as saying that, for going from point A to point B, light follows a trajectory that requires the minimum possible time. This can be easily understood by remembering that the index of refraction is inversely proportional to the speed of light within the media, so the larger the index of refraction is, the slower the light propagates. Then, a continuous variation of the index of refraction also changes the speed of light continuously as it travels to different portions of the non-homogeneous material, and the time of arrival to

a given point would change depending on the trajectory. This is where nature works and makes the light to spend the shortest time to arrive. All these previous concepts can be mathematically explained and derived in quite a safe way. Actually, there are some academic solutions, as the Luneburg lens, that is a sphere of an homogeneous material where the index of refraction increases when moving towards the center [18, 19]. In any case, graded index materials add a new parameter, the variation of the index of refraction, that can be used to improve the image-forming capabilities of an optical system.

Beyond Paraxial Optics

Why is paraxial optics so important? The reason is that it is robust, simple, and useful. Ray tracing, as a consequence of paraxial optics, makes it possible to understand how light travels from objects to images and how the objects and images can be real or virtual, larger or smaller, directed or inverted. Therefore, the location and size of the image can be easily obtained from quite a simple calculation or as back-of-the-envelope ray tracing [20, 21].

Besides, paraxial optics assures that optical system behaves perfectly. The conditions for an image-forming system to be perfect are defined as the three Maxwell's conditions representing quite common sense capabilities for such systems. The first Maxwell's condition states that the image of a point is a point, the second condition states that the image of a plane perpendicular to the optical axis of an optical system is also a plane, and the third condition states that the images are proportional to the objects.

Mathematically, the paraxial regime is based on an approximation for the trigonometric functions involved in the propagation of light: $\sin \epsilon \simeq \tan \epsilon \simeq \epsilon$, and $\cos \epsilon \simeq 1$ (where ϵ is given in radians, not in degrees). This means that Snell's law has a paraxial counterpart as $n\epsilon = n'\epsilon'$. Therefore, paraxiality is lost when the involved angles (e.g., the incidence and refraction angles) are large enough to surpass the previous approximation and Snell's law (Eq. 4.3) is strictly applied beyond its paraxial version.

Another useful simplification in the paraxial analysis of optical systems is to consider them as rotationally symmetric. This means that every plane containing the optical axis is equivalent, and any of them is valid to study the system. These planes are named as meridional planes. But this condition is broken easily and rays may have different behaviors for different meridional planes (e.g., astigmatic or toric lenses are not rotationally symmetric), or even more, they may travel as skew rays through the system. Although some paraxial calculations can be made for astigmatic lenses or systems, if we really need an accurate picture of how light travels through them, we have to use a three-dimensional representation of Snell's law. In this general and more realistic case, Snell's law becomes a slightly more complex relation (see Fig. 4.1a) that involves unitary vectors describing the incoming and outgoing rays (i and o, respectively) and another vector (k), the normal vector, that represents the orientation of the interface and points toward the media where the light is coming from [22]:

$$n\left|\vec{i} \times \vec{k}\right| = n'\left|\vec{o} \times \vec{k}\right|, \qquad (4.5)$$

where n and n^0 are the index of refraction of the two materials separated by the interface, and $\times$ means a cross product. The modulus of these cross products are $|i \times k| = \sin\theta$, and $|o \times k| = \sin\theta'$, that retrieves Eq. (4.3) from Eq. (4.5). The geometrical layout of the involved vectors is shown in Fig. 4.1a. Fortunately, computers deal very well with these calculations and evaluate the propagation of millions of optical rays through an optical system in a reasonable time. These computational capabilities make possible the analysis, and the optimization, of image-forming systems, including the human eye.

Some characteristic optical parameters of optical systems, such as refracting power, power, or focal distance, are well-defined within the paraxial approach, and their meaning remains after surpassing the paraxial domain. Also, the paraxial formalism predicts the location and size of the optical image for a given object provided by an optical system. This is described through the main paraxial image-forming equations exemplified for a thin lens of focal f immersed in air as:

$$-\frac{1}{a} + \frac{1}{a'} = \frac{1}{f'}, \qquad (4.6)$$

$$M = \frac{a'}{a}, \qquad (4.7)$$

where a and a' are the object and image distances, respectively, and M is the lateral magnification defined as the ratio between the lateral size of the image, y', and the object, y. These two paraxial equations serve as the first-order approximation to know where and how the image of an object is reproduced by an optical system. Equations (4.6) and (4.7) can be written in terms of vergences (V, V') and refracting power (P) as $-V + V' = P$ and $M = V/V'$, respectively. The convention's sign used here defines the distance of a real object as having a negative frontal distance, $a < 0$; meanwhile, the image of a real image has a positive sign. Vergences follow the same convention and are defined as $V = n/a$ and $V = n$ "/a," where n and n' are the index of refraction of the object and image spaces, respectively.

As we have seen, paraxial optics helps to grasp the main properties of an optical system. However, it fails when describing subtle details related to the quality of the image that is well beyond the paraxial approach. These discrepancies are also known as optical aberrations.

However, the paraxial approach is still valid when analyzing some aberrations related to the dependence of the index of refraction with wavelength, $n = n(\lambda)$, in the so-called chromatic aberrations. To show this, we present the value of the focal length of a thin lens in air in terms of its material and geometrical parameters:

$$\frac{1}{f'} = (n-1)\left(\frac{1}{r_1} - \frac{1}{r_2}\right), \qquad (4.8)$$

where r_1 and r_2 are the radii of curvature of the front and back surfaces, respectively, and n is the index of refraction of the material of the lens. Now, it is clear that if n varies with λ, then the focal distance, f', changes too. This behavior is split into two: a variation in the location of the focal length (longitudinal chromatic aberration) and a variation in the intersection of rays corresponding to different wavelengths with the paraxial image plane defined for a given wavelength of reference (transversal optical aberration). Given its treatment, we could think of these chromatic aberrations as paraxial aberrations.

Seidel Aberrations

Once we know that optical aberrations describe the discrepancies in paraxial performance, they can be classified and described using several categories [23, 24]. The Seidell classification of aberrations is based on their geometrical meaning (see Fig. 4.2).

When applying the ray tracing rules to the case of real optical systems, it is possible to classify aberrations depending on the location of the object point (on axis or off axis), the aperture of the system, and the geometry of the optical system with respect to the incoming radiation. Seidel aberrations (spherical, coma, astigmatism, field curvature, and distortion) are depicted in Fig. 4.2 and described below.

To analyze these aberrations, we rely on their relation with the three Maxwell's conditions of a perfect optical system. The first condition is related to the point-like property of the image for an object point source. This means that the optical rays departing from a point source, after propagating through the system, do not intersect at a single point but are distributed on the image plane as a finite size distribution of impacts. The aberrations violating the first Maxwell's condition are spherical aberration, coma, and astigmatism. Actually, spherical aberration and coma can be seen as two different flavors of the same phenomena. They appear when considering every ray impinging on the entrance pupil of an optical system. The difference between them is that spherical aberrations consider the object point source located at the optical axis, meanwhile coma happens for objects placed at a given distance, or angular deviation, from the optical axis. The third aberration, astigmatism, has a deeper

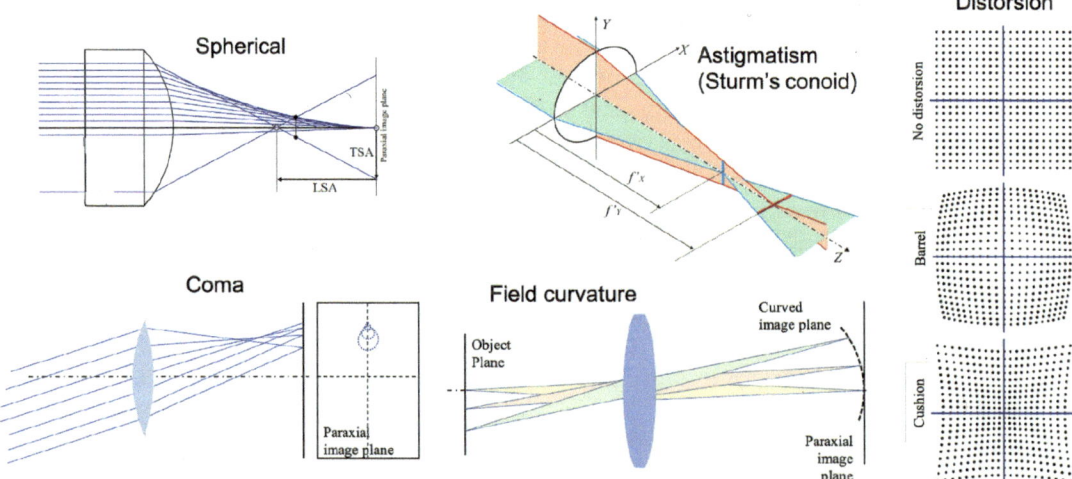

Fig. 4.2 The five primary Seidel aberrations are presented in this figure. Spherical aberration considers all the rays passing through the aperture of the system. It is sometimes characterized by the longitudinal spherical aberration (LSA) and the transversal spherical aberration (TSA) that compares the impact of the marginal rays with the paraxial ones. Coma is produced when the rays enter the full aperture of the system for an off-axis object. Astigmatism generates the so-called Sturm's conoid that contains two focal lines with a round spot in between them. Field curvature represents how the location of the image is no longer on a plane but it appears on a curved surface, also known as the Petzval surface. Both astigmatism and field curvature consider a narrow pencil of ray. Finally, the effect of distortion causes deformation of the location of the image point depending on its distance to the optical axis. In a real optical system, all these aberrations are mixed together

geometrical meaning. It occurs when a narrow pencil of rays strikes on a surface that shows two values of its radius of curvature along different planes. To better understand astigmatism, we first need to picture how a given surface may show two different radii of curvature, even for a spherical surface. A toric surface is quite a simple example. Let us consider the three-dimensional case of a donut. Every point on its surface has two curvatures aligned along the plane that we would use to split the donut in half. If the donut is sliced as a bagel sandwich, the radius of curvature is larger and the two sections have an "O" shape. When the donut is split to produce two "C" portions, the corresponding curvature at the cutting point has a smaller radius. Both radii of curvature are perpendicular to each other and can generate optical surfaces with different focusing characteristics. This fact is behind every toric lens prescribed to compensate the astigmatism ametropy. Moreover, this geometrical behavior also happens for oblique incidence on a spherical surface and generates oblique astigmatism. In any case, the two radii of curvature generate quite a unique three-dimensional structure known as Sturm's conoid. This behavior produces two focalization planes where the image of the point source collapses as a segment, and an intermediate plane where the light spot takes the form of a circle (this spot is also known as the circle of confusion).

The second Maxwell's condition establishes that the image of a plane perpendicular to the optical axis is another plane also perpendicular to the optical axis. The departure from this condition is explained as an aberration that is called field curvature. It describes how the image plane bends and departs from the paraxial image plane. The first approach to this aberration assumes that the image plane becomes a spherical surface that is tangent to the paraxial image plane at the optical axis. This surface where the image appears is known as the Petzval surface. This is quite disturbing for a lot of image-forming optical systems where the recording media is arranged on a flat surface (e.g., as a CMOS or CCD focal plane array). However, some optical systems, such as dome cinema projectors or the human eye, can

locate the image on a curved surface. Therefore, in the case of the human eye, field curvature should be taken into account when considering the role of optical aberrations for extra-foveal perception. Also, ophthalmic lenses make use of field curvature when optimizing their performance taking into account the eye movement behind the lens [25, 26].

Finally, the third Maxwell's condition assures that the image is similar to the object. This similarity should be taken in its strictest geometrical sense: the lateral dimensions are proportional, but the angular values are preserved. Distortion is the Seidel optical aberration that describes how the image is deformed with respect to the object, breaking the similarity condition between the object and the image. Mathematically, it means that the lateral magnification is not constant across the image plane, and the effect can be seen as a deformation of a rectangular grid that becomes closer to a pincushion or a barrel shape.

These previous descriptions have been developed to better understand the math behind the geometrical problem of image-forming system. Actually, they can provide simple geometrical relations applicable to the optimization of optical systems. However, Seidel aberrations never appear isolated and they are mixed together in real systems. Even more, when considering the chromatic behavior of optical systems, Seidel aberrations mix with chromatic aberrations to describe the behavior of optical systems working with white light [27].

Wavefront Aberrations

We have also explained how geometrical optics may help to understand the actual behavior of an optical system beyond the paraxial approach. Now, to complete the picture, we begin to move toward the electromagnetic model where light is a wave characterized by its wavelength, λ.

The propagation of light as a wave is better understood if we define and describe the optical wavefront. From an electromagnetic point of view, the wavefront is defined by those points sharing the same value of the phase of the propagating wave. This definition can be visualized by the evolution of the wavefronts when emitted from a point source (see Fig. 4.3). In the same way that the ripples of a pond surface caused by the impact of a stone propagate from the impact locations in circles, when moving to the three-dimensional domain, these circles become spheres, and the wavefront caused by a point source of electromagnetic waves travels at the speed of light in the medium, generating spherical wavefronts if the medium is homogeneous. This picture can be reinforced by assuming that upon departure from the point source, the light trajectories are accompanied by a time counter (a clock) that measures the travel time. Then, every point at the same wavefront shares the same time or the same optical path defined previously. The temporal period between ticks of this clock, T, is related to the frequency of the light, $\nu = 1/T$, that is larger for the blue portion than for the red part of the visible spectrum. These spherical wavefronts are deformed after propagating through an interface, and this deformation depends on the change in the index of refraction and also on the geometry of the interface. From this explanation, we can see that a point-like object emits spherical wavefronts. If the optical system were perfect and a point object produced a point image, then the outgoing wavefront exiting the optical system would also be spherical with its center at the point image (see Fig. 4.3a). Unfortunately, this is not the case for real sys-

tems, and the wavefront after the optical system shows deformations with respect to the ideal spherical wavefront with its center at the paraxial image point. These discrepancies are described by the wavefront aberration (see Fig. 4.3b). As far as these discrepancies are defined after the optical system, it is customary to evaluate them the plane of its exit pupil.

Graphically, the wavefront aberration is a map that shows the local differences between the actual wavefront and the reference spherical wavefront at the exit pupil. If the system were perfect, the wavefront aberration would be constant and null across the exit pupil [28, 29]. In most of the cases, the wavefront aberration is a smooth and continuous function defined within a circle having a radius equal to the radius of the exit pupil. Fortunately, some basic mathematical functions, known as Zernike polynomials, Z_j, come to the rescue of finding how simple contributions combine to produce any arbitrary wavefront aberration function. By doing this, the general wavefront aberration $W(\rho, \theta)$ is decomposed as a superposition of Zernike polynomials. Some of the basic Zernike polynomials are easily linked with the Seidel aberrations, and their coefficients in the expansion, c_j, are related to the importance of the corresponding term, Z_j. Mathematically, this can be written as:

$$W(\rho,\theta) = \sum_{j=1}^{N} c_j Z_j(\rho,\theta), \qquad (4.9)$$

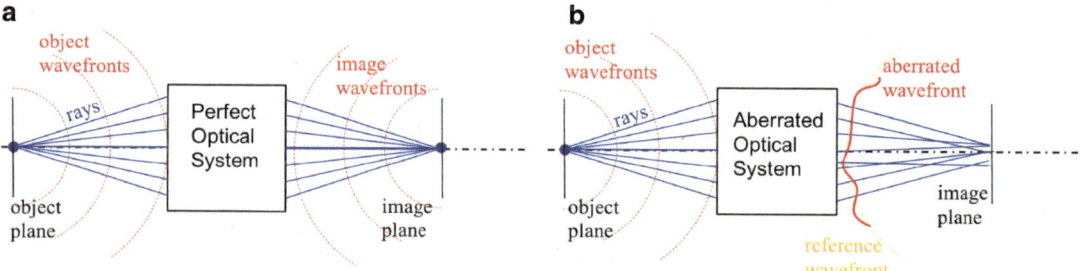

a

b

Fig. 4.3 A point source generates a collection of rays originated at the point-like object that, and collection of spherical concentric wavefronts. Rays and wavefronts are perpendicular to each other. In (**a**) we represent a perfect system, which transforms spherical wavefronts into spherical wavefronts that collapse at the image point.

When the system is aberrated, as represented in (**b**), the output wavefront is distorted and the rays departing the system do not intersect at a single point on the image plane. The difference between the aberrated wavefront and the ideal, spherical, wavefront is the wavefront aberration

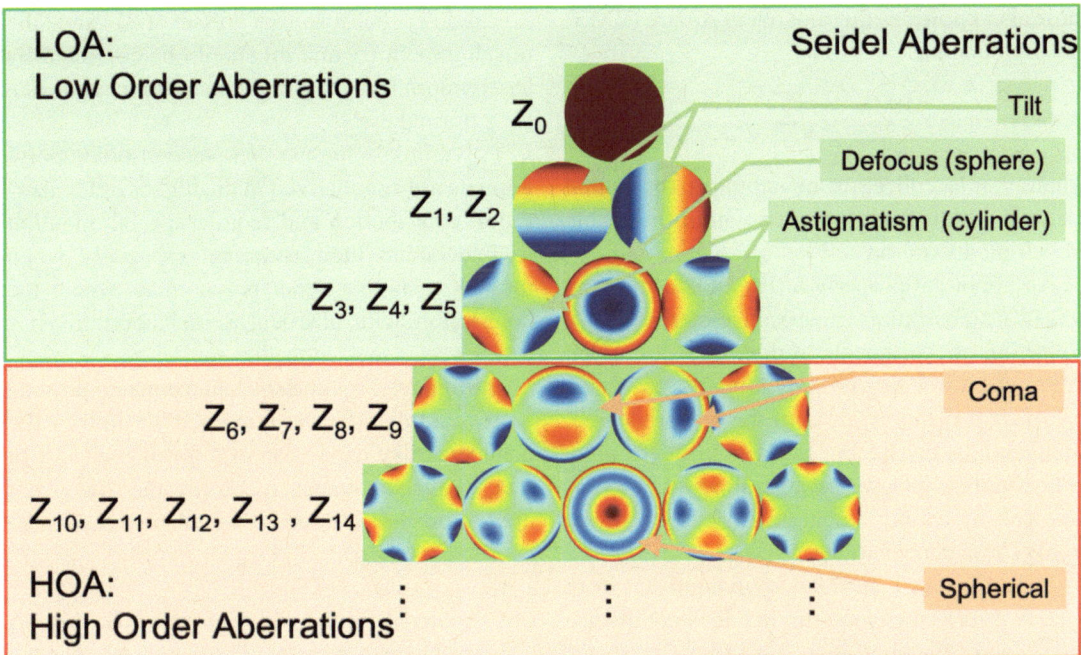

Fig. 4.4 An arrangement of the Zernike polynomials represented as phase maps. The order of the polynomial increases downward. The upper portion of the figure corresponds to the low-order aberrations (LOA), and the bottom portion, which can be extended toward higher order polynomials, is denoted as high-order aberrations (HOA). We have also identified the classical aberrations, Seidel aberrations, with the corresponding Zernike

where we have used polar coordinates (ρ, θ) with the origin at the center of the exit pupil. The mathematical form of the Zernike polynomials can be found elsewhere. In this contribution, we follow the notation presented by the Optical Society of America, where a single index j is used to denote a given polynomial [30]. An arbitrary Zernike polynomial can be seen as the product of a polynomial in ρ, times a sine or cosine function with an argument related to an integer multiple of θ. Then, the radial dependence is described by the polynomial in ρ, and the azimuthal dependence takes the form $\cos(m\theta)$ or $\sin(m\theta)$ (for some polynomials, the azimuthal dependence does not exist, and the Zernike polynomial shows a rotational symmetry around the center of the exit pupil). In Fig. 4.4, we show the maps of the first 15 Zernike polynomials organized in increasing order as we move downward and related to the classical Seidel aberration when possible. Each row contains polynomials of the same order (e.g., the fourth row includes four polynomials of third degree, i.e., involving ρ^3 and lower powers).

At this point, we want to pay attention to the units used in the previous expansion. This discussion is important to fully understand the optical meaning of the Zernike decomposition. These polynomials are defined on the unit circle (a circle having a radius equal to 1). To apply them to an actual circular aperture having an arbitrary value of its radius, the radial coordinate used with the Zernike polynomials is normalized as $\rho = r/R$, where R is the radius of the aperture, and r is the radial coordinate within the aperture. Then, ρ becomes a dimensionless variable, which also appears when defining the wavefront aberration, $W(\rho, \theta)$. However, W represents the distance between the reference sphere and the actual wavefront. Therefore, the coefficients c_j in Eq. (4.9) are also given as distances. In some applications, c_j are expressed in terms of a fraction of the wavelength. Using these coefficients, it is possible to define a global parameter that informs about the discrepancy with respect to the ideal wavefront due to a collection of Zernike aberrations. This parameter is also known as the root mean square (RMS) and is defined as

$$\mathrm{RMS}_J = \sqrt{\sum_{j \in J} c_j}, \qquad (4.10)$$

where J is a collection of subindex for c_j that identifies the terms of interest within the whole wavefront aberration.

An important property of Eq. (4.9) is that the wavefront aberration can be characterized by a collection of coefficients of the expansion. Even more, the lower degree polynomials, i.e., those involving ρ polynomials until the second degree, should not be considered as aberrations (from an optical point of view) because it could be compensated by adding a spherical (or toric) wavefront. These contributions.

correspond to Zernike polynomials from $j = 0.5$. Z_0 is a constant term that does not disturb the shape of the aberration function (it works as an offset). The combination of Z_1 and Z_2 represents a tilt that could cause a misalignment of the system with respect to the axis of reference. Zernike polynomials Z_3, Z_4, and Z_5 describe classical ametropies such as myopia, hypermetropia, and astigmatism. There exists a simple relation between the polynomial coefficients and the spherical (sphere + cylinder) ametropia of the eye:

$$S = -\frac{r\sqrt{3c_4}}{R^2} - C / 2, \qquad (4.11)$$

$$C = \frac{4\sqrt{6}\sqrt{c_3^2 + c_5^2}}{R^2}, \qquad (4.12)$$

$$\theta = \frac{1}{2}\tan^{-1}\left(\frac{c_3}{c_5}\right), \qquad (4.13)$$

where S, C, and θ are the sphere, cylinder, and angle of the conventional prescription notation (S, $C \times \theta$), respectively, c_3, c_4, and c_5 are the coefficients of the Zernike expansion related to the spherical (or cylindrical) deviation of the wavefront, and R is the radius of the exit pupil of the system (for the human eye, it is related to the size of the pupil). When applied to the human eye, all these polynomials, from Z_0 to Z_5, are also referred to as lower order aberrations (LOA), where the main contribution comes from the coefficients c_3,

c_4, and c_5 because the offset (c_0) and the misalignment (c_1 and c_2) should be corrected by an appropriate setting of the measurement device for a normal eye.

Polynomials higher than second-order polynomials are summarized in the higher order aberration contribution and require special attention to understand their meaning, especially when moving to higher order polynomials where the connection with classical Seidel aberrations is lost.

Fortunately, ophthalmic aberrometers provide quite a straightforward method to obtain the actual Zernike expansion of a given eye [31]. In fact, the aberrometer measures the wavefront aberration that is used to calculate the Zernike coefficients, c_j, as:

$$c_j = \int_0^{2\pi} d\theta \int_0^1 W(\rho,\theta) Z_j(\rho,\theta) \rho d\rho. \qquad (4.14)$$

These coefficients are the typical output of the measurement system. For a given Zernike decomposition until $j = N$ (where N is typically given by the resolution and accuracy of the aberrometer), Eq. (4.16) with $J = 0, \ldots, N$, provides an overall value of the wavefront aberration. This quantity can be split into two main components, LOA and HOA, just by selecting the appropriate subindex j, as $J_{\mathrm{LOA}} = 0, \ldots, 0.5$ and $J_{\mathrm{HOA}} = 6, \ldots, N$, when calculating $\mathrm{RMS}_{\mathrm{LOA}}$ and $\mathrm{RMS}_{\mathrm{HOA}}$, respectively. Even more, the amount of wavefront aberration that could be corrected using classical prescriptions (sphere + cylinder) would be represented by $\mathrm{RMS}_{j=3,4,5}$.

Wave Optics for Image-Forming Optical Systems

In the previous description of the index of refraction, we have briefly used the concept of wavelength, λ, to define the wavefront aberration. This parameter is directly linked to the electromagnetic nature of light. In this framework, light is seen as a propagating electromagnetic wave. The description of these waves was given by Maxwell through four fundamental equations that couple together electric and magnetic phenomena. Actually, one of the key points to accept this model was the prediction of electromagnetic waves, having a velocity related to both electric and magnetic parameters (the electric permittivity, ε, and the magnetic permeability, μ) that were already part of the description of electricity and magnetism. Then, it could be proved that $c = 1/\sqrt{\varepsilon_0 \mu_0}$ (where the subindex denotes that we are in vacuum). If light is a wave, it can generate interferences and diffraction when superposing light with light. This actually induces significant departures with respect to the geometrical model prediction. Now, shadows are not sharp any more (even for a single-point light source) and light can, slightly, bend around corners. This is diffraction, and this phenomenon explains very well the limit of resolution, the capability of distinguishing two separate objects in the image, of optical systems.

To understand this, we only need to think of light as a wave that travels across space. When this wave reaches an aperture (or an obstacle), a part of the light is blocked by the opaque portion of the aperture and only the open part is active for further propagation (see Fig. 4.5). From a geometrical optics point of view, the propagation of light would define a sharp transition between light and shadow after the aperture. But now, light is a wave, and when it reaches the aperture,

each portion of the wave passing through it acts a new emitter of waves propagating again from the aperture. The consequence of this is that light bends the edge and propagates beyond the geometrical shadow. If the aperture is circular, the distribution of light intensity can be described as

$$I(\theta) = I_0 \frac{2J_1\left(\frac{2\pi}{\lambda} a \sin\theta\right)}{\frac{2\pi}{\lambda} a \sin\theta}, \quad (4.15)$$

where λ is the wavelength, a is the radius of the circular aperture, and θ is the departure angle with respect to the propagation of the center of the light beam. This situation is depicted in Fig. 4.6, where we have represented the Airy spot that could be seen on a screen. When considering the case of the image point given by an optical system, even though the system can be perfect from a geometrical point of view, diffraction would cause the image of point-like source to be a finite spot (if the aperture is circular, it is described by Eq. (4.15) and plotted in Fig. 4.5). Moreover, if we have two-point sources, their images will be distinguished if their respective Airy spots do not overlap. The Airy disk has a characteristic pattern with a strong maximum at the center and several dark and bright rings

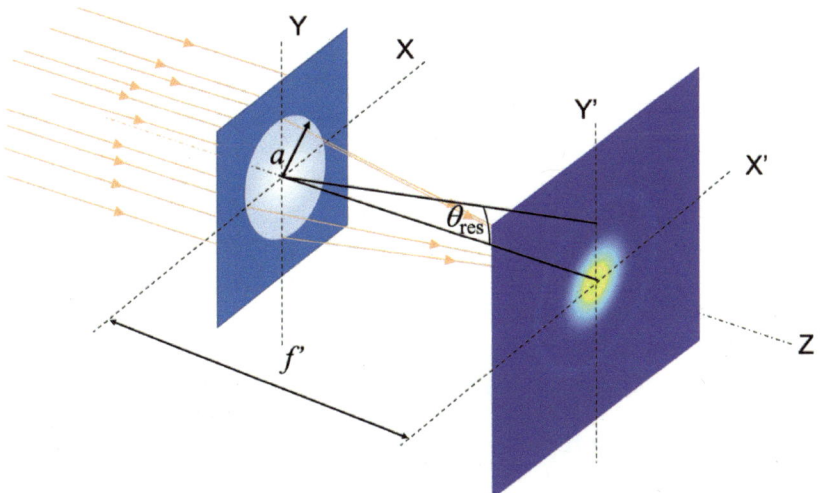

Fig. 4.5 A collection of parallel rays coming from an object located at infinity is also represented as a plane wave. This wave diffracts when passing through a lens located at the plane XY having a circular aperture with radius, a, and generates a distribution of light at its focal plane (located at the plane X^0Y^0). This spot is also known as the Airy disk (Eq. 4.15). The angle θ_{res} describes the angular location of the first dark ring of the Airy spot. This diffraction happens even for an unaberrated lens

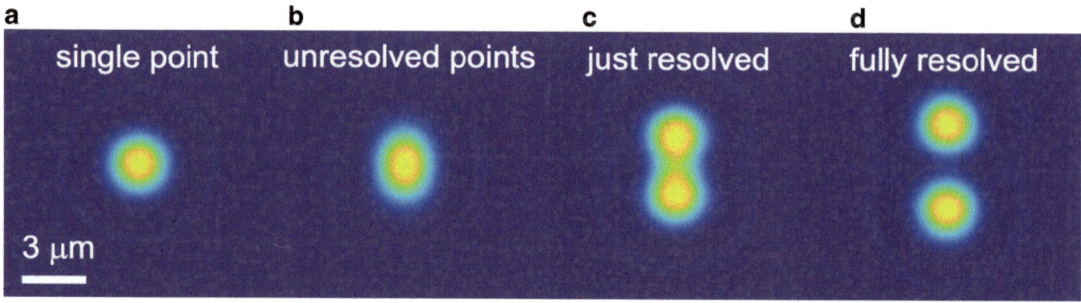

a single point **b** unresolved points **c** just resolved **d** fully resolved

3 μm

Fig. 4.6 A graphical representation of the image plane of an optical system having the same focal as the human eye, $f_{eye}^0 = 16$ mm, with a pupil diameter $D = 2a = 4$ mm, for a wavelength at the center of the visible spectrum, $\lambda = 555$ nm. (**a**) Each point-like source is imaged as a spatial light distribution (Airy spot) on the image plane of an optical system. (**b**) Two point sources are not resolved if they are located very close. (**c**) Light distribution for two point sources that are separated angularly $\theta_{res} = 1.22\lambda/D$. (**d**) Two points separated above the angle of resolution, θ_{res}, can be clearly distinguished

around it. The first ring is used to define the resolving power of the system through the well-known expression.

$$\theta_{res} = \frac{1.22\lambda}{D}, \qquad (4.16)$$

where D is the diameter of the aperture of the optical system, λ is the wavelength, and θ_{res} represents the angular separation of two point sources. If the angular separation is larger than θ_{res}, then they are resolved; if smaller, the optical instrument is unable to distinguish them as two separated point sources (see Fig. 4.6). This condition is also known as the Rayleigh criterion. Therefore, not only geometrical optics (or ray tracing) limits the quality of optical systems but also diffraction, as a consequence of the wave nature of light, constrains the capabilities of image-forming systems. As a simple application of the Rayleigh diffraction limit, the human eye, having a usable entrance pupil diameter of about $D = 6$ mm, generates a resolution angle of $\theta_{R,retina}' \; 0.4^0$, which fits very well with the angular separation between photodetectors at the retinal mosaic [32].

The Quality of an Optical System

In this section, we introduce a further refinement of the description of an optical system that is fully based on the electromagnetic model of the light. Then, optical rays and light trajectories will be replaced by wavefronts and the spatial distribution of irradiance (power per area unit) of the light. At the same time, when possible, we will look back to relate these new concepts to geometrical parameters and reasoning.

As the first step, let us recall the first Maxwell's condition for a perfect optical system: the image of a point source has also to be a point. However, we have seen that aberrations disrupt this ideal behavior and the generation of the point-like image is not achieved. From the wave optics point of view, a point object is a source of perfect spherical wavefronts, and a point image is attained when a perfect spherical wavefront collapses at it. This is why the wavefront aberration is defined as the departure between the ideal spherical wavefront and the actual one generated by the optical system. We have already seen how this wavefront aberration can be described in terms of Zernike polynomials and how the coefficients in this expansion (see Eqs. (4.9) and (4.14)) can be related to low- and high-order aberrations. Until here, we would have a mere mathematical description of the wavefront, but we need more: we have to know how aberrations impact the distribution of light at the image plane. Then, we define quite a simple but powerful concept that describes the actual distribution of light on the image plane when the object is a point-like source. This distribution is known as the point spread function, $PSF(x_i, y_i)$, where x_i and y_i are spatial coordinates at the image plane. Knowing that the PSF is applicable to a point source, if we have an extended source that can be seen as a collection of point sources, the resulting image is the superposition of the PSF at the location of the

images of every single point in the object. We can mathematically write this as follows:

$$I\left(x_i, y_i\right) = \iint O\left(x_o, y_o\right) \text{PSF}\left(x_i - Mx_o, y_i - My_o\right) dx_o dy_o, \tag{4.17}$$

where $O(x_o, y_o)$ represents the light distribution at the object plane (using spatial coordinates x_o and y_o), M is the lateral magnification of the system (describing the scale factor between the image and the object), and $I(x_i, y_i)$ is the light distribution at the image plane. Using a technical language, the previous integration is also known as a convolution product [33, 34].

Before going further, let us take a look at the PSF of an optical system. The behavior of waves is governed by a different set of rules when compared to geometrical ray tracing. One of the first consequences of a wave model is that optical wavefronts are distorted when passing through apertures. This phenomena is also known as diffraction, and it occurs even for perfect spherical wavefronts associated with point-like objects or images. The consequence is that, for any practical system, the image of a point will never be a point, which is a serious violation of the first Maxwell's condition for a perfect optical system. Then, we can conclude that perfect optical systems only happen within the paraxial approach. As a typical example, if we consider an optical system free of aberrations (a perfect optical system within the geometrical model), but having a finite transversal size realized as a circular aperture, the image of a point source (its PSF) has a distribution quite well-known as the Airy disk (see Figs. 4.5 and 4.6). When this happens, we have the best possible optical instrument that is qualified as a diffraction-limited optical system.

A dedicated discussion on how to overlap the images coming from two point-like sources

helped to define the Rayleigh criterium for the resolving power of an optical system (see Eq. 4.16 and Fig. 4.6). The same situation happens when trying to distinguish the bright and dark stripes of a periodic grating: if they are not resolved, the contrast between dark and bright is lower and they tend to look as a uniformly illuminated object. These objects are very useful in optics when describing the quality of an optical system. In fact, their use relies on a mathematical transformation known as Fourier transform. The concept is quite simple: a periodic distribution of light can be associated with a given spatial frequency, where this spatial frequency is just the inverse of the spatial period of the object. For example, if a periodic variation repeats itself only once over an angular extent of $1°$, then its spatial frequency is 1 cycle/deg., and if the spatial period repeats two times, then the spatial frequency will be 2 cycles/deg. The same could be said if the periodicity is repeated over a given length, providing spatial frequencies expressed as cycles/mm. The key advantage of this treatment is that any arbitrary light distribution can be expanded as the superposition of pure periodic light distributions, each one having its characteristic spatial frequency and a weight in this superposition calculated through a very sound mathematical relation. In optics, as far as the distribution of light is usually projected on a plane (meaning two dimensions), the applicable Fourier transform also needs to be 2D. From a mathematical point of view, this transformation is given as:

$$\Phi\left(\xi, \eta\right) = \int_{-\infty}^{\infty} \int_{-\infty}^{\infty} I\left(x, y\right) \exp\left[-i2\pi\left(x\xi + y\eta\right)\right] dx dy, \tag{4.18}$$

$$I\left(x, y\right) = \int_{-\infty}^{\infty} \int_{-\infty}^{\infty} \Phi\left(\xi, \eta\right) \exp\left[+i2\pi\left(x\xi + y\eta\right)\right] d\xi d\eta, \tag{4.19}$$

where $I(x, y)$ is the light distribution on a given plane with coordinates (x, y), and $\Phi(\xi, \eta)$ is the

so-called spatial frequency spectrum (or Fourier transform of I), where the coordinates ξ and η

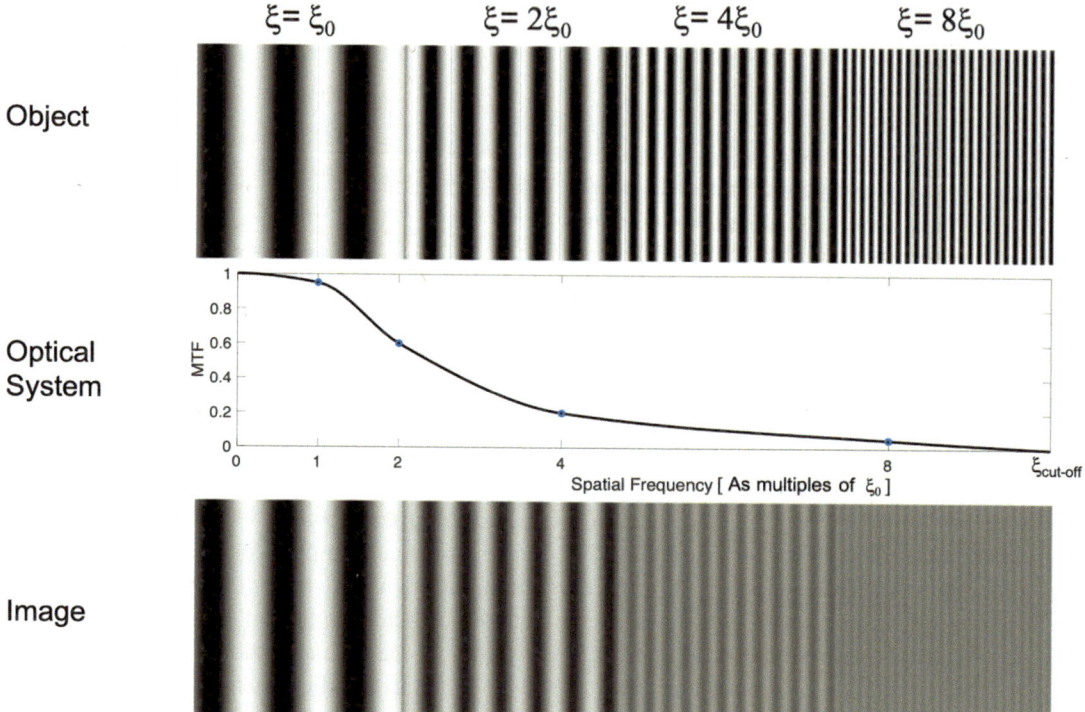

Fig. 4.7 An object having a sine wave distribution of light is imaged into another sine wave distribution that has a lower contrast than that of the object. The relation between the two contrasts is the value of the MTF at the spatial frequency of the object, $\xi = 1/p$, where p is the spatial period of the targets. In the upper row is a collection of four objects having a spatial frequency that increases when moving from the first to the fourth object (the spatial frequency is doubled in every step). We have considered an optical system that is represented by its MTF. The row at the bottom shows the image for every object. We can see how the contrast diminishes as the spatial frequency increases. The spatial frequency, ξ, is given as a multiple of a reference frequency ξ_0. We have also represented the value of the cut-off frequency, $\xi_{cut-off}$, where the MTF cancels

represent the spatial frequencies along the X and Y directions, respectively (i is the imaginary unit, $i^2 = -1$).

The explanation of the capabilities of this methodology, using the Fourier transform, are beyond the scope of this chapter, and they range from image-processing algorithms to the optical design of optical systems. However, there are a couple of things worth mentioning here: Fourier transforms provide a framework where the image-forming mechanism can be seen as the application of a filter in spatial frequencies; also, this formalism makes defining important figures of merit of optical systems, such as the modulation transfer function possible. Following this first point, we can rewrite Eq. (4.17) as.

$$\Phi_i(\xi,\eta) = \Phi_o(\xi,\eta)\text{OTF}(\xi,\eta), \quad (4.20)$$

where Φ_i and Φ_o are the Fourier transforms of the image and object, respectively, ($I(x_i, y_i)$ and $O(x_o, y_o)$ in Eq. (4.17)), and OTF is the Fourier transform of the optical transfer function (PSF). Eq. (4.20) has very important consequences, once we fully understand the meaning of the Fourier transform. The transformation from a distribution of light, $I(x, y)$, to its spatial frequency spectrum $\Phi(\xi, \eta)$ provides the same information but arranged in a different way. For example, the fine details in the object $O(x, y)$, i.e., those portions requiring higher resolution of the optical system, are represented by the value of Φ at larger values of the spatial frequencies ξ and/or η. If the OTF has a zero value at those spatial frequencies related to those details, the image will not contain such information and those high spatial frequency features will be lost.

The optical transfer function is a complex valued function that can be written in terms of its modulus, MTF, and phase, PTF: OTF = MTFexp(iPTF) (where $i = -1$, and the complex exponential can be written as a real part and an imaginary part as exp(iPTF) = cos(PTF) + $i$sin(PTF)). Here, we find the modulation transfer function (MTF) as the modulus of the optical transfer function. So, we have a mathematically sound way of describing the image-forming procedure within the electromagnetic model.

Another way of understanding how the MTF quantifies the quality of an optical system is by exemplifying its effect using quite a simple object: a collection of sine wave targets having different spatial periods (the spatial period, p, is related to the spatial frequency, $\xi = 1/p$) as those depicted in Fig. 4.7 that present as pure white at its maximum and as pure black at its minimum. Then, the contrast of these targets, defined as $M_o(\xi) = (I_{max} - I_{min})/(I_{max} + I_{min})$, is equal to 1. These light distributions are imaged by an optical system having an MTF, that is, typically, a decreasing function of ξ (see Fig. 4.7). The result is a collection of images, one for each target, where the maximum and the minimum are not pure white and black anymore and the images show a different contrast. Then, the ratio between the contrast of the image and the object is also the MTF at the given spatial frequency, ξ:

$$\text{MTF}(\xi) = \frac{M_i(\xi)}{M_o(\xi)}. \quad (4.21)$$

In every MTF plot, we find a value of the spatial frequency where the MTF reaches the value of zero. This maximum frequency is known as the cut-off frequency and strongly depends on the applicable diffractive effects. For example, for a diffraction-limited optical system, the cut-off frequency is $\xi_{cut-off} = D/\lambda$ if measured in cycles/rad and is $\xi_{cut-off} = Df'/\lambda$ if expressed in cycles/mm, where f'' is the focal length of the optical system [35]. We can see that this cut-off frequency is strongly related to the angular resolutions, θ_{res} (see Eq. (4.16)) (Fig. 4.8).

Therefore, the MTF becomes a figure of merit of the optical system that clearly describes how good an instrument is when reproducing a given

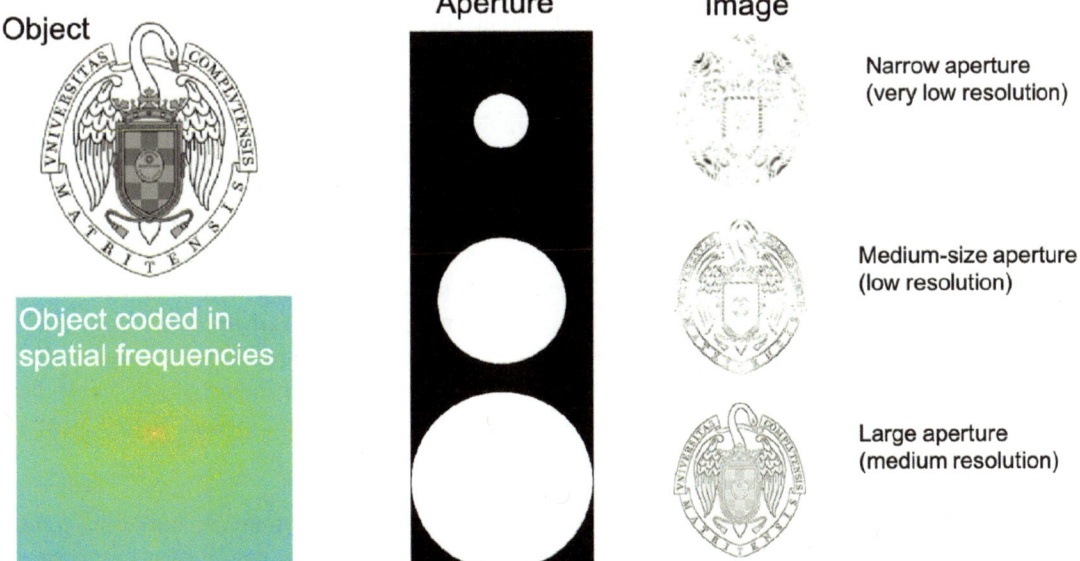

Fig. 4.8 The object at the top left can be coded in spatial frequencies through the application of the Fourier transformation (represented in logarithmic scale at the bottom left). Both representations to the left of this figure contain the same information. At the right, we have simulated how the object is reproduced when the system is not able to represent high frequency components (fine details). This filtering is strongly dependent on the aperture size of the optical system

object. As a matter of fact, by using this concept it is possible to understand that, even in the absence of aberrations, an optical instrument is not able to reproduce well all the details of the object because the value of MTF is only 1 at $\xi = 0$ ($\xi = 0$ means that the object has a constant distribution of light, and it is a uniform background) and the contrast for spatial frequencies larger than 0 will be diminished. This situation, where only diffraction is considered, established the attainable goal for the quality of an optical system, when all the aberrations are removed and the system reaches the diffraction-limited behavior.

When analyzing the actual behavior of the eye, there is a more psychophysical function known as the contrast sensitivity function, CSF, that measures the perceived contrast of sinusoidal patterns. The CSF contains contribution from the optical system of the eye plus the response of the processing unit, the visual cortex of the brain. Therefore, the information provided by the MTF has to be weighted with the neural response that is characterized by the neural contrast sensitivity function, CSF_N, to provide the actual value of the contrast sensitivity function in the form $CSF = MTF \times CSF_N$ [36].

Conclusions

These ideas and formalism are part of the tools necessary for the full understanding of the fitting of intra-ocular lenses. The optical behavior of the human eye can be outlined using the paraxial formalism. However, the results of the first-order approximation fall short with the new advances in science and technology: better tools for diagnosis, improved morphological characterization, and high-precision surgical procedures. Ophthalmic aberrometers and corneal topography systems provide sufficient information about the contribution of the optical elements of the eye: cornea and lens. Pachymetry and some optical coherence tomographic techniques measure the longitudinal dimensions of the eye, cornea, and lens. All these tools, along with the data obtained for the optical constant of the ocular media (corneal stroma, aqueous humor, lens, and vitreous body), can provide an estimate of the human's eye optical performance. Vision research laboratories are at the forefront in obtaining values of the wavefront aberration, $W(\rho,\varphi)$, the PSF and MTF of the eye, and analyzing the psychophysical response of the visual system to a wide variety of stimuli and conditions: monochromatic and polychromatic tests, photopic and scotopic illuminations, etc. Soon enough, the advances in research will be applied to ophthalmology's daily practices. As a practical example, the contribution to the total aberration coming from the corneal topography—external and internal surface—can be detached from the total aberration and the lens contribution can be extracted. Therefore, an advanced design of an intra-ocular lens that compensates both contributions, located at the lens position, could improve the quality of the eye toward the diffraction-limited situation. However, the neural adaptation of the visual system to the native aberration may temporarily jeopardize the improvements made: the brain must readapt itself to the new optical performance of the eye.

In this chapter, we have revisited the basic concepts of image-forming systems from two points of view: the geometrical realm and the physical optics model. We have seen that beyond paraxiality, it is still possible to understand how light propagates from the object to the image. Light trajectories can be calculated with quite a simple set of rules. These rules are efficiently applied by computers to provide an accurate evaluation of the system's performance. This performance is affected by aberrations, which disturb the ideal conditions, and by diffraction, which intrinsically limits the performance of an optical system. Although aberrations can be controlled in an efficient way, diffraction will ultimately limit the quality of the image.

Both diffractions and aberrations limit the optical performance of the human eye. A full understanding of these limitations may help us find efficient solutions when vision quality is compromised, and its recovery requires surgical treatments or the replacement of bio-elements by artificial ones. Modern intra-ocular lens designs are key in today's ophthalmological treatments. They offer controlled aberration, multiple foci, and improved biocompatibility and biostability. Moreover, advanced medical skills and procedures are now continuously challenging the limits of technology and science to provide better and more flexible solutions for the well-being of patients.

References

1. Padilla MLC. El pionero de la luz: Alhacén y su Libro de la Óptica. Universidad Complutense de Marid; 2019.
2. González-Cano A. Ibn al-haytham: an optical revolution. ARBOR Ciencia, Pensamiento y Cultura. 2015;191(775):a262.
3. Herzberger M. Optics from Euclid to Huygens. Appl Opt. 1966;5(9):1383–93.
4. Vazquez D, Gonzalez-Cano A, Diaz-Herrera N, Llombart N, Alda J. History of optics: a modern teaching tool. In: Groot Gregory G, editor. Optics education and outreach II, vol. 8481. International Society for Optics and Photonics, SPIE; 2012. p. 195–201.
5. de Valdés BD. Uso de los antojos para todo genero de vistas (1613). Editorial Maxtor; 2021.
6. González-Cano A. Eye gimnastics and a negative opinion on eyeglasses in the "libro del exercicio" by the spanish renaissance physician Cristóbal Méndez. Atti della Fondazione Giorgio Ronchi. 2004;49:559–63.
7. King HC. The history of the telescope. Dover Publcations; 2011.
8. Born M, Wolf E. Principles of optics. 7th ed. Cambridge University Press; 1999.
9. Casas J. Óptica. Librería General; 1994.
10. Hecht E. Optics. 5th ed. Pearson; 2016.
11. Pedrotti FL, Pedrotti LM, Pedrotti LS. Introduction to optics. 3rd ed. Cambridge University Press; 2017.
12. Slaleh BEA, Teich MC. Fundamentalas of photonics. Wiley; 2007.
13. Atchison DA, Smith G. Chromatic dispersions of the ocular media of human eyes. J Opt Soc Am A. 2005;22(1):29–37.
14. Cuadrado A, Sanchez-Brea LM, Torcal-Milla FJ, Quiroga JA, Gomez-Pedrero JA. Numerical model of the inhomogeneous scattering by the human lens. Biomed Opt Express. 2019;10(5):2161–76.
15. Navarro R, Palos F, Gonz'alez L. Adaptive model of the gradient index of the human lens. I. Formulation and model of aging ex vivo lenses. J Opt Soc Am A. 2007;24(8):2175–85.
16. Pierscionek BK, Regini JW. The gradient index lens of the eye: an opto-biological synchrony. Prog Retin Eye Res. 2012;31(4):332–49.
17. Janaswamy R. Geometrical optics and Fermat's principle. In: Engineering electrodynamics, 2053–2563. IOP Publishing; 2020. p. 9-1–9-26.
18. Luneburg RK. Mathematical theory of optics. University of California Press; 1944.
19. Morgan SP. General solution of the luneberg lens problem. J Appl Phys. 1958;29:1358–68.
20. Alda J, Arasa J. Encycolpedia of optical and photonic engineering, chapter ray tracing: paraxial. Routledge Handbooks Online (CRC); 2015.
21. Alda J. Encyclopedia of optical and photonic engineering, chapter paraxial optics. Routledge Handbooks Online (CRC); 2015.
22. Arasa J, Alda J. Encyclopedia of optical and photonic engineering, chapter ray tracing: real. Routledge Handbooks Online (CRC); 2015.
23. Barry Johnson R. Historical perspective on understanding optical aberrations. In: Smith WJ, editor. Lens design: a critical review, vol. 10263. International Society for Optics and Photonics, SPIE; 1992. p. 21–32.
24. Lin PD. Seidel primary ray aberration coefficients for objects placed at finite and infinite distances. Opt Express. 2020;28(9):12740–54.
25. Alda J, Alonso J. Encyclopedia of optical and photonic engineering, chapter ophthalmic optics. Routledge Handbooks Online (CRC); 2015.
26. Juan A, Alonso QJ, Gómez-Pedrero JA. Modern ophthalmic optics. Cambridge University Press; 2019.
27. Mahajan VN. Aberration theory made simple. SPIE Press; 2011.
28. Lakshminarayanan V, Fleck A. Zernike polynomials: a guide. J Mod Opt. 2011;58(7):545–61.
29. Mahajan VN. Zernike circle polynomials and optical aberrations of systems with circular pupils. Appl Opt. 1994;33(34):8121–4.
30. Thibos LN, Applegate RA, Schwiegerling JT, Webb R. Standards for reporting the optical aberrations of eyes. In: Vision science and its applications. Optical Society of America; 2000. p. SuC1.
31. Marcos S. Aberrometry: basic science and clinical applications. Bull Soc Belg Ophthalmol. 2006;306:197–213.
32. Miller DT, Williams DR, Michael Morris G, Liang J. Images of cone photoreceptors in the living human eye. Vis Res. 1996;36(8):1067–79.
33. Gaskill JD. Linear systems, Fourier transforms, and optics. Wiley-Interscience; 1978.
34. Goodman JW. Introduction to Fourier optics. 4th ed. W. H. Freeman; 2017.
35. Boreman GD. Modulation transfer function in optical and electro-optical systems. SPIE Press; 2001.
36. Michael R, Guevara O, de la Paz M, de Toledo JA, Barraquer RI. Neural contrast sensitivity calculated from measured total contrast sensitivity and modulation transfer function. Acta Ophthalmol. 2011;89(3):278–83.

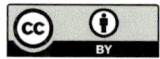

Pseudophakic Eye Models

5

Filomena Ribeiro, Pedro Ceia, and Leonor Jud

Introduction

Vision has always been a subject of interest for humans. Since the times of ancient Greece, with Democritus and Galenus being the most notable ones, to the Arabic scholars and Renaissance Europe through the work of Descartes, or more recently Snell's law and Gauss' paraxial theories, studies were conducted and theories were formulated to explain such a phenomenon and its properties [1, 2]. From the description of the detailed eye anatomy to the explanation of the optical system, step by step and aided by many developed instruments, human knowledge of vision has increased to an extent where one can expect to fully understand its functioning.

Eye models are necessary to study the optical characteristics of the human eye and to assess its diagnostic and therapeutic implications. The evolution of lens surgery and the development of different optical principles in intraocular lenses demand methods to select the most suitable intraocular lens (IOL) and predict the optical quality outcomes.

Pseudophakic eye models, with a realistic assessment of anatomy and visual performance in real life, when compared to the assessment using an optical bench or through interferometry, have been developed with several applications in ophthalmic implants. Possible clinical applications include IOL power calculation for cataract surgery, aspherical IOL power calculation, and the future development of customized lenses for full correction of optical aberrations.

Generic models have been successfully used for a variety of applications and have been very helpful for both diagnostic and therapeutic developments. However, only the emergence of personalized models and their subsequent clinical applications will pave the way for future customization.

F. Ribeiro (✉)
Hospital da Luz Lisboa, Lisbon, Portugal

Faculdade de Medicina da Universidade de Lisboa, Lisbon, Portugal

Visual Sciences Research Centre, Lisbon, Portugal

P. Ceia
Faculdade de Medicina da Universidade de Lisboa, Lisbon, Portugal
e-mail: pedro.ceia@campus.ul.pt

L. Jud
Instituto Superior Técnico, Universidade de Lisboa, Lisbon, Portugal

Schematic Eye Models

The first schematic eye model dates back to the nineteenth century, even though previous attempts had already been made [2, 3]. Since then, many others were formulated, each pretending to approach and solve particular questions.

© The Author(s) 2024
J. Aramberri et al. (eds.), *Intraocular Lens Calculations*, Essentials in Ophthalmology,
https://doi.org/10.1007/978-3-031-50666-6_5

In order to summarize and organize our ever-growing understanding of the eye as an optical system and to study particular properties of human optics and retinal image formation, various authors have dedicated their work to the development of schematic eye models [3]. Their purposes range from the study of retinal image sizing to light levels, refractive errors, aberrations and retinal image quality, design of spectacles, lenses, and individual customization, or even development and calibration of optical instruments [1]. In order to account for different populations, they can even be stratified by age, gender, ethnicity, refractive error, and accommodation and allow total customization [1]. As much as each model is different, the same applies to their intended purposes and focus.

As complex as theoretical eye models may be, they can essentially be grouped into two types: Paraxial models and finite models.

Paraxial Models

Paraxial models are simpler ones. They mechanistically summarize what we know about the optics of the eye [1] while describing refractive surfaces as spherical and centered on a common optical axis. Refractive indices are constant within each medium too [2]. Such models are only accurate within the paraxial region and are not capable of predicting aberrations and retinal image formation for large pupils or angles that are far from the optical axis. Since structures are centered and refractive surfaces are spherical while the lens is generally of a constant refractive index, paraxial models are poor predictors of monocular aberrations such as spherical aberrations and sagittal/tangential power errors and lack the ability to predict light distribution with larger field angles [2]. Nonetheless, they are sufficient for calculation of the entrance and exit pupil positions and diameters as well as retinal image sizes and effects of on-axis low-order aberrations. For this reason, they are commonly used as a learning tool for the theory of visual optics [1].

At last, paraxial models may be further divided into three groups as follows, according to the number of refractive surfaces that each offers [1, 3, 4].

Reduced Paraxial Models

Reduced eyes have a single refractive surface—the cornea–along with a shorter axial length and corneal radius of curvature. In these models, principal points (P and P′) and nodal points (N and N′) coincide since there is only one refractive surface. As a consequence of the absence of the crystalline lens, they cannot be used to examine the optical consequences of accommodation nor the changes in lens property changes in refractive errors, including aphakia [2]. Some examples are Emsley's and Bennett and Rabbetts' reduced eyes.

Simplified Paraxial Models

Simplified models have a total of three refractive surfaces—one for the cornea and two for the lens. For paraxial calculations, these models are now considered to be more adequate than many exact eyes, which are more complex than is required.

- Gullstrand's number 2 eye (1909): Although close to its exact counterpart, its lens (even though two-surfaced) has zero thickness, which limits its usefulness.
- Le Grand's simplified eye (1945): This is similar to Gullstrand's number 2 eye in terms of features.
- Gullstrand–Emsley eye (1952): This is modified from Gullstrand's number 2 eye to simplify calculations, including the same lens thickness as in Gullstrand's number 1 eye, while also changing the aqueous, vitreous, and lens refractive indices. This model offers two accommodation levels as does Gullstrand's number 2 eye, but the lens' refractive index is constant.
- Bennett and Rabbetts' simplified eye: This is a modification from the Gullstrand–Emsley eye in its relaxed form with different parameter values obtained through data from a larger study, with a mean power closer to 60 D. It also includes four levels of accommodation, an "elderly" version of the eye, and a refractive error of 1-D hypermetropia.

Exact Paraxial Models

Exact models represent the optical structure most accurately as possible, and, so, they must include at least four refractive surfaces: two for the cornea and two for the crystalline lens.

– Tscherning (1900): This is allegedly the first model to include a posterior corneal surface.
– Gullstrand's number 1 eye (1909): This is built with six refractive surfaces, of which the lens is composed of four, divided into a higher refractive power nucleus and a lower power cortex, accounting for refractive index variation within the medium. Therefore, it has a gradient index lens. It also offers adaptation to two levels of accommodation, being one of the few paraxial models that have this particularity. Despite that, Gullstrand's model presents an exaggerated spherical aberration, much higher than that of real eyes.
– Le Grand's full theoretical eye (1945): As a modification of Tscherning's, this is presented in both relaxed and accommodated forms.
– Blaker's eye (1980): Modified from Gullstrand's number 1 eye, this is the only paraxial model to feature a continuous gradient index for the lens. This is also called an adaptive model since parameters such as lens gradient index, lens surface curvature, thickness, and the anterior chamber depth (ACD) vary as linear functions of accommodation. This model was posteriorly revised to include aging effects.

Finite Eye Models

Finite models are more complex than paraxial models, and their primary interest is a reliable representation of the eye's functional capabilities instead of its constitution. They may be used for simulating human optics more accurately, and different models may be designed for different purposes. Their aim is to represent optical aberrations and retinal quality as closely as possible as they occur in vivo, incorporating aspheric surfaces [5–8], chromatic dispersion [5, 8], and a refractive index gradient lens [5], and may even include accommodation [5], age-dependent changes [9], or refractive error dependency [10, 11]. These models are called finite models, or wide-angle models, and have greatly contributed to improve the knowledge of the human eye's real optical performance and to the development of better technologies.

Applications of such models are various, including calculations of retinal image sizes, magnification, retinal illumination, entrance and exit pupil positions, and diameters for objects imaged with wide pupils or away from the optical axis. Finite eye models can also be used for a range of research and development purposes, including ophthalmic lens design, refractive surgery or IOL implantation, and studying the features of optical component systems [12].

– Lotmar (1971): This model was modified from Le Grand's full theoretical eye with anterior corneal asph.erization and a paraboloid posterior crystalline surface, to provide clinical levels of spherical aberration. However, it was shown that an ellipsoid shape for the anterior corneal surface would be a better fit and that the model is based on an anatomically inaccurate shape for the anterior lens surface.
– Drasdo and Fowler (1974): Based on a schematic eye attributed by Stine to Cowan, the purpose of this model was to determine retinal projection from the visual field using spherical lens surfaces since data supported the insignificance of such alteration.
– Kooijman (1983): Based on Le Grand's full theoretical eye, this predicts retinal illumination and adds aspheres to all four surfaces of the model. Corneal surfaces are aspherical, and the anterior lens surface is hyperbolic, whereas the posterior surface is parabolic. This model has two versions with retinal shape variations: spherical and elliptical.
– Liou and Brennan (1997): This model includes conicoid corneal and lenticular surfaces and a parabolic gradient index lens and is based on the average anatomical values of 45-year-old eyes if the parameter used is age-dependent. Its primary purpose was to model the spherical aberration of real eyes while also intending

to mimic normal levels of chromatic aberration—which was not successful. Additionally, it features a displacement of the aperture stop 0.5 mm to the nasal side and an angle of 5° between the line of sight and the optical axis regarding real eyes.

- Navarro and Escudero-Sanz (1999): This is a variable-accommodating model in which the lens parameters and anterior chamber depth are expressed as functions of accommodation in a logarithmic manner, based on Le Grand's full theoretical eye slightly modified for different anterior corneal radii and corneal indexes. Anterior corneal and lenticular surfaces are conicoids, whereas the retina is spherical.
- Atchison (2006): Based on Liou and Brennan's, a model was proposed to account for the displacement of the retina from the visual axis. The most distinctive features are the inclusion of a toric retina and its variation with refractive errors [4, 12].

Comparison of Finite Model Eyes

The abilities of different finite model eyes to evaluate the quality of vision have been discussed. Liou–Brennan and Atchison's models show the most similarities to in vivo eyes [12]. Lotmar's, Kooijman's, and Navarro and Escudero-Sanz' attempts were as accurate as Liou–Brennan's and Atchinson's at mimicking the real eye's performance reasonably well for on-axis and small-pupil diameters. For large-pupil diameters, however, the first ones were very inaccurate. Oppositely, Liou and Brennan and Atchison created schematic eyes that presented close-to-experimental in vivo values among spherical and higher order aberrations, even eccentrically, and peripheral refraction profiles for larger pupil diameters. Their corneal and lens spherical aberration and coma were similar but opposite in sign, which results in a good real eye representation [13]. Of the two models, Liou–Brennan's was considered the most reliable both anatomically and practically, even without considering the characteristic pupil nasal decentration [12, 14]. If lens and retina tilt and retinal decentration are taken into account, then Atchison's model has a peripheral refraction pro-

file that does not match real eye data well. Eccentric variation of coma-like aberration was much higher than expected in every model as well as retinal image quality probably due to the lack of scattering among the optical media [12].

Computational Eye Models

Computational eye models hold the promise of becoming a primary tool to optimize the selection of the IOL to be implanted in a cataract procedure, for they are excellent predictive tools for the optical quality in pseudophakic eyes, allowing for a better understanding of contributory factors.

Physics and mathematical models require an optical design software such as Zemax (Zemax Development Corporation, Bellevue, WA), Code V (Optical Research Associates, Pasadena, CA), OSLO (Lambda Research Corporation, Littleton, MA), or ASAP (Breault Research Organization, Inc., Tucson, AZ), for both the construction of models and optical analysis and optimization based on ray tracing technology.

The increasing performance of computers has consequently boosted the area of computer simulation. Ray tracing is a very promising technology which, along with wavefront technology, better describes the optics of the human eye and allows for exact calculations.

Previously, in order to use Gullstrand and Emsley models, it was necessary to reduce the number of surfaces represented for simplicity and ray tracing speed. However, nowadays computers can quickly ray trace eye models and more complexity can be added.

Even though paraxial ray tracing has been used in several studies, real ray tracing use has increased recently. This is due to increasing computational capacity and awareness of the importance of higher order aberrations and their current ability to be clinically measured.

It has also been used to go further in the study of optical phenomena and to allow the evaluation of the entrance pupil and optical properties of the eye [15], night vision [16], and extremely aberrated eyes as in keratoconus eye modeling [16].

	Surf:Type	Comment	Radius	Thickness	Glass	Semi-Diameter		Conic
OBJ*	Standard	OBJECT	Infinity	1.000000E+009		8.748867E+007		0.000000
1	Standard	INPUT BEAM	Infinity	50.000000		1.977588	U	0.000000
2*	Standard	CORNEA	7.770000	0.500000	CORNEA_L&B	5.000000	U	-0.180000
3*	Standard	AQUEOUS	6.400000	3.160000	AQUOSO/VITREO_L&B	5.000000	U	-0.600000
STO*	Standard	PUPIL	Infinity	0.000000	AQUOSO/VITREO_L&B	1.250000	U	0.000000
5*	Gradient 3	LENS-FRONT	12.400000	1.590000		5.000000	U	-0.940000
6*	Gradient 3	LENS-BACK	Infinity	2.430000		5.000000	U	0.000000
7*	Standard	VITREOUS	-8.100000	16.270000	AQUOSO/VITREO_L&B	5.000000	U	0.960000
IMA	Standard	RETINA	-12.000000	-		5.000000	U	0.000000

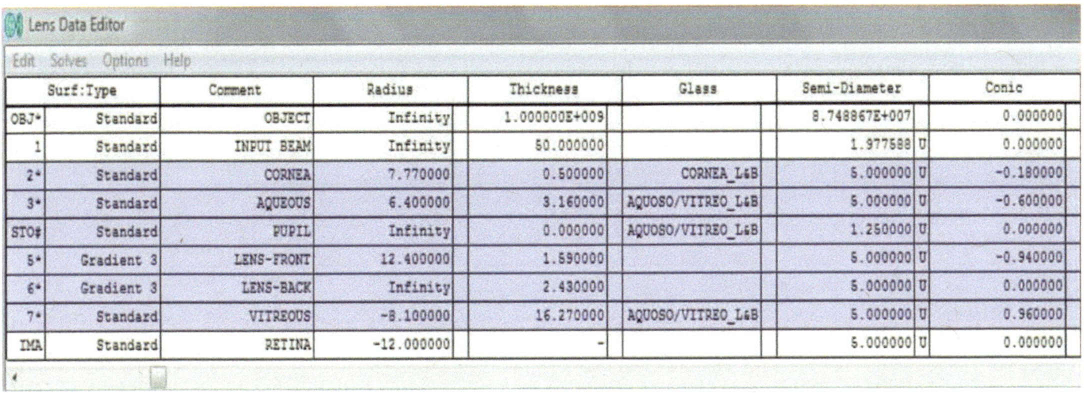

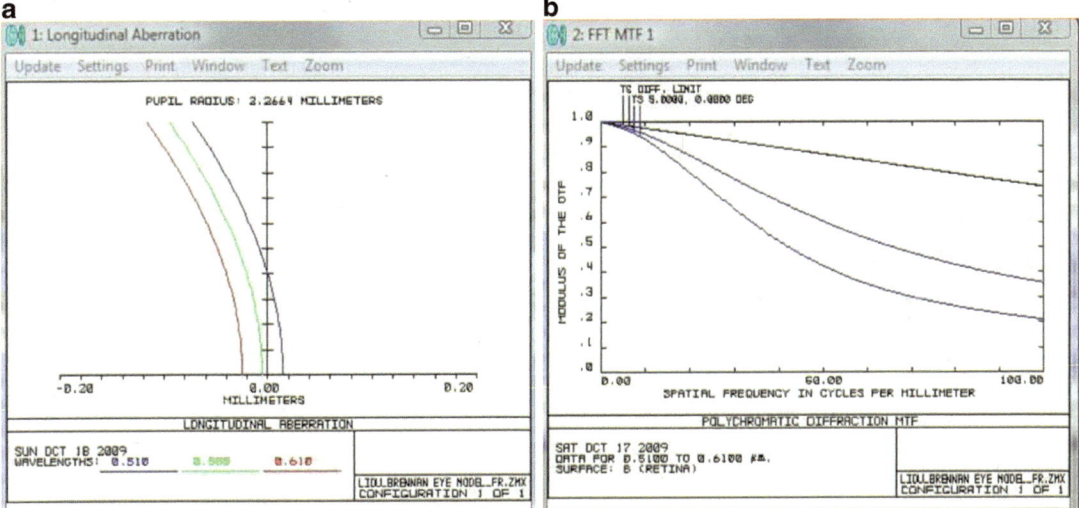

Fig. 5.1 Zemax lens data editor with data from the Liou–Brennan model. The rows describe the object (OBJ), the surfaces of cornea (surfaces 2 and 3), pupil (STO; aperture stop), crystalline lens (surfaces 5 and 6), and the surface of retina (IMA). All surfaces are characterized by the radius of curvature (anterior and posterior), thickness, refractive index, chromatic dispersion, and asphericity. With this setup, light rays can be traced from the OBJ sequentially through the system to the IMA

Fig. 5.2 Examples of optical performance evaluation using eye models. (**a**) Longitudinal chromatic aberration as a function of pupil height at each wavelength. (**b**) Polychromatic diffraction MTF (spatial frequency can be related to visual acuity measured by the Snellen chart, (considering that this chart has dark and bright bands subentending 1 minarc between them). For a visual acuity of 1.0, and considering a 100% contrast target, its correspondence to 100 cycles/mm may be established

Our research team published results [17] that identified the relative contribution of different optical elements to refractive error, using Zemax to model and evaluate the Liou–Brennan model (Figs. 5.1 and 5.2).

We used the Liou–Brennan eye model as a starting point, and its parameters were varied individually within a physiological range. The contribution of each parameter to the refractive error was assessed using linear regression curve fits. Formulas were obtained for each clinically measurable parameter, which represent the dioptric variation that each unit change on the optical element will cause (Table 5.1).

Table 5.1 Formulas for an easy and quick assessment of the effect of changes in each optical parameter on the refractive status of an eye, obtained by incorporating all of the aberrations of the eye. It should be noted that for the elements that did not show a good linear fit (corneal anterior radius, corneal posterior radius, and vitreous chamber depth), a variation around the nominal value or far from it will lead to different refractive errors. For instance, a small measurement error of corneal anterior radius below the nominal value may have more relevant repercussions on the refractive outcome than the same error above the nominal value

Optical element	Linear	Quadratic or inverse
Corneal elements		
Anterior radius (Ra)		$\Delta R_e(D) = [-2.588(Ra) + 26.720]\,(\Delta Ra)\,(mm)$
Posterior radius (Rp)		$\Delta R_e(D) = [-37.384/Rp^2]\,(\Delta Rp)\,(mm)$
Anterior asphericity (Qa)	$\Delta Re\,(D) = -1.120\Delta Qa$	
Posterior asphericity (Qp)	$\Delta Re\,(D) = 0.309\Delta Qp$	
Thickness (CT)	$\Delta Re\,(D) = -2.009\Delta CT\,(mm)$	
Axial length elements		
Anterior chamber depth (ACD)	$\Delta R_e\,(D) = -1.394\Delta ACD\,(mm)$	
Lens thickness (LT)	$\Delta R_e\,(D) = -2.414\Delta LT\,(mm)$	
Vitreous chamber depth (VCD)		$\Delta R_e(D) = [0.100(VCD) - 4.312]\,(\Delta VCD)\,(mm)$
Pseudophakie eye		
Postoperative ACD (ACD$_{post}$)	$\Delta R_e\,(D) = -1.334\Delta ACD_{post}\,(mm)$	

R_e refractive error; D diopter

Criteria for best-fit were r^2, F values, adjusted χ^2, and clinical significance. When values were similar, or when the difference between the linear fit and a more complex one was <10.251 diopters within a physiological range of the parameter variation, the linear fit was chosen. When all values were better for one of the models, that model was chosen. According to selection criteria, best fit was: linear for Qa, Qp, CT, ACD, and LT; quadratic for Ra and VCD; and inverse for Rp. A Δ preceding a parameter represents the variation of that parameter

Pseudophakic Eye Models

The growing developments in IOLs with new optical designs and corrective capabilities have not been on par with the methods that allow us to predict optical results. The previously mentioned models can be used for the evaluation of the pseudophakic eye, in which the lens is replaced by an IOL. In this new model, the complexity of the gradient refractive index of the crystalline lens is replaced by the IOL refractive index, the shape of the surfaces and optical design is made available by the manufacturer. All optical components of a pseudophakic eye are modeled by means of scientific computer methods so that physics and mathematical models can simulate and predict pseudophakic eye models' optics. With this methodology, the geometric optical properties, such as the wavefront aberration, can be simulated using Snell's refraction with ray tracing. The optical design process involves defining a conceptual optical design and giving an initial configuration input of the optical elements of the eye. The optical design software can be used to optimize an IOL by an iterative user-defined process to improve performance.

Real ray tracing has been used in several fields of ophthalmology to evaluate IOL performance on spherical aberration correction [18–22], interaction between monochromatic and chromatic aberrations [23], and aspheric intraocular lenses' optical performance in relation to tilt and decenter errors [24].

Personalized Pseudophakic Eye Models

The construction of personalized model and its subsequent clinical application will pave the way for future customization. The goal of eye modeling is to include the optical properties of one's entire eye into a complete custom virtual eye model. The modeling procedure of individual eyes is a complex task since it requires accurate biometric eye data such as the shape and thickness of the ocular elements.

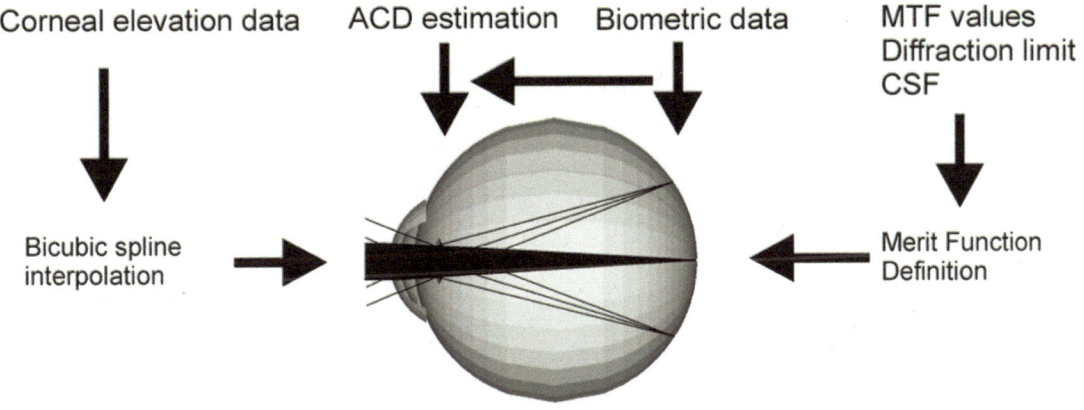

Corneal elevation data   ACD estimation   Biometric data   MTF values
                                                                       Diffraction limit
                                                                       CSF

Bicubic spline   Merit Function
interpolation   Definition

Personalized model

Fig. 5.3 An overview of the developed personalized pseudophakic model. The Liou–Brennan eye model was used as a starting point, and biometric values were replaced by individual measurements. Detailed corneal surface data were obtained from topography, and a grid of elevation values was used to define corneal surfaces in an optical ray tracing software (Zemax). Optimization criteria based on values of the modulation transfer function (MTF), weighted according to contrast sensitivity function (CSF), were applied

With the development of biometric measuring devices, we can accurately characterize the anterior and posterior surfaces of the cornea, intraocular distances, and aberrations of the ocular wavefront. All of these measurements can be incorporated into the construction of a customized model for functional optic nerve assessment.

The real ray tracing method may allow the highest degree of customization. Based on the principle that no single measurement of an eye can provide all the data required to achieve utmost individualization of therapeutic solutions, information from several sources, for example, corneal topography, corneal thickness, anterior chamber depth, lens thickness, and axial length, is considered. Some of its limitations are the current unavailability of measurements such as the shape of the lens, the retinal radius, the refractive indices of the ocular media and their relative distribution, and the lack of definition of the best optimization procedure.

Personalized models that can readily incorporate all these parameters as soon as our knowledge of them improves, or when measurement techniques become more accurate or available, will allow an easy progression toward customized refractive assessment. At last only the numerous stochastic errors associated with subjective examination will remain, along with IOL mislabeling errors and the uncertainty of how the interaction between higher order aberrations and neuroadaptation may influence refractive outcome.

Our research team has described the construction of personalized eye models, as seen in Fig. 5.3, which are based on the clinical measurement of individual human eyes [25], where computer-based technical implementation of the optical components and methods for calculations and optimizations in Zemax were implemented (Figs. 5.4 and 5.5). Optical optimization is the iteration algorithm that takes a starting optical design layout and changes the parameters in steps in order to achieve the specified targets.

IOL Power Calculation

One possible application is the calculation of intraocular lens power, with the potential to overcome the limitations of generic and population-related methods. This procedure can also be applied in the case of aspherical lenses and new optical designs.

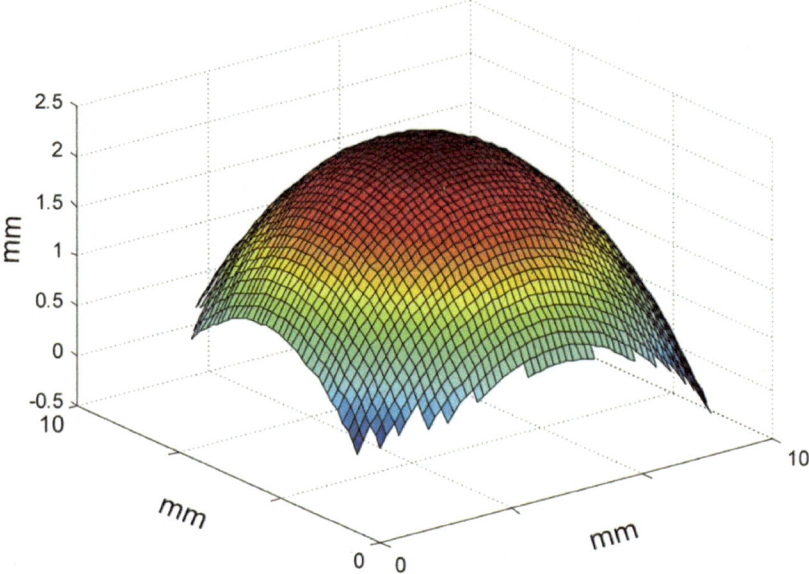

Fig. 5.4 Interpolated corneal elevation data for tridimensional corneal representation. Corneal elevation data generated from topography was re-formatted and imported to Zemax. Afterwards, a full definition of the surface shape was obtained through a bicubic spline interpolation of the imported data

Oper #	Freq			Target	Weight	Value	% Contrib
1 MTFA	3.000000			0.990000	29.760000	0.000000	7.552573
2 MTFA	10.000000			0.950000	70.430000	0.000000	16.458738
3 MTFA	17.000000			0.920000	91.790000	0.000000	20.116974
4 MTFA	27.000000			0.870000	99.970000	0.000000	19.592950
5 MTFA	34.000000			0.840000	96.240000	0.000000	17.583520
6 MTFA	50.000000			0.770000	75.450000	0.000000	11.583301
7 MTFA	70.000000			0.680000	46.930000	0.000000	5.619013
8 MTFA	100.000000			0.550000	19.060000	0.000000	1.492932

Merit Function Editor: 9.000000E+009

Edit Tools Help

Fig. 5.5 Merit function in which the used operands are the average MTF for different frequencies between 3 and 100 cycles/mm and the target is individually the system values by diffraction and the weights attributed depending on the CSF

Wavefront technology and ray tracing are very promising technologies that have been used to improve IOL power calculation errors [26–29], since they better describe the optics of the pseudophakic eye. Ray tracing allows for exact calculations, being simultaneously a better competitor when compared with paraxial optical methods, as long as the studied eye is properly modulated.

Since the calculation in the individual virtual eye is based on its complete geometry and is not limited to paraxial optics, it has the potential to overcome the limitations of current IOL calculation formulae and provide significant benefits to the eyes where current formulae are known to fail. This includes eyes that do not meet the population average such as eyes with irregular corneal surfaces as a result of refractive surgery (Fig. 5.6).

Possible clinical applications of this personalized model include the future development of customized lenses for full correction of optical aberrations (Fig. 5.7).

The results presented by our research group [25] suggest that the development of these eye models, considering individual aberrations, using wavefront technology and exact ray tracing, enhanced by the image metric based on MTF and CSF [30], allow for the prompt incorporation of parameters that are currently not measurable in clinical practice. This can be done in a personalized manner, if and when more clinical measurements become available, and can be incorporated,

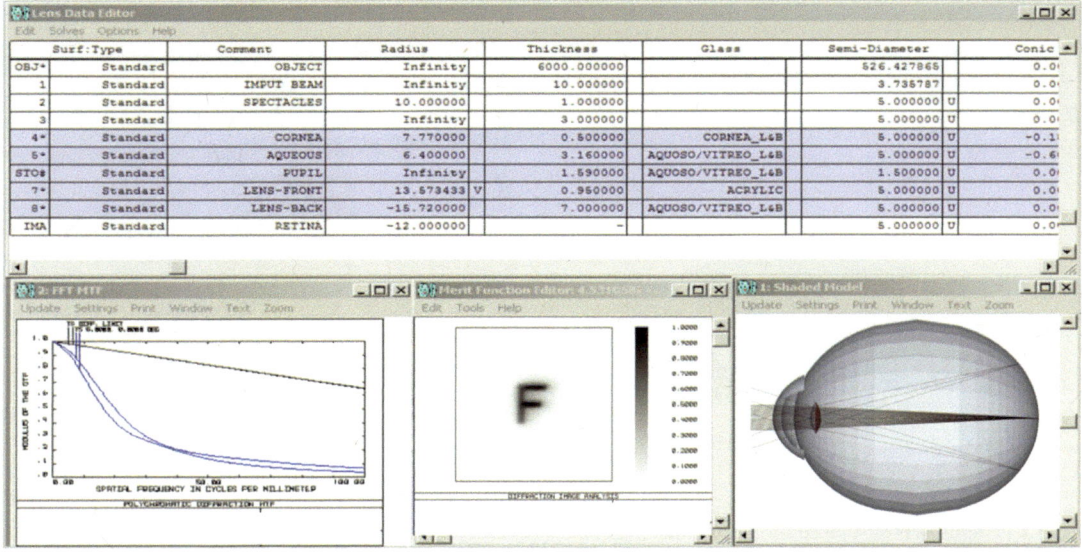

Fig. 5.6 Conversion in a pseudophakic model and its customization. Our model is prepared to incorporate all parameters in a personalized manner, as data becomes available in the clinical practice

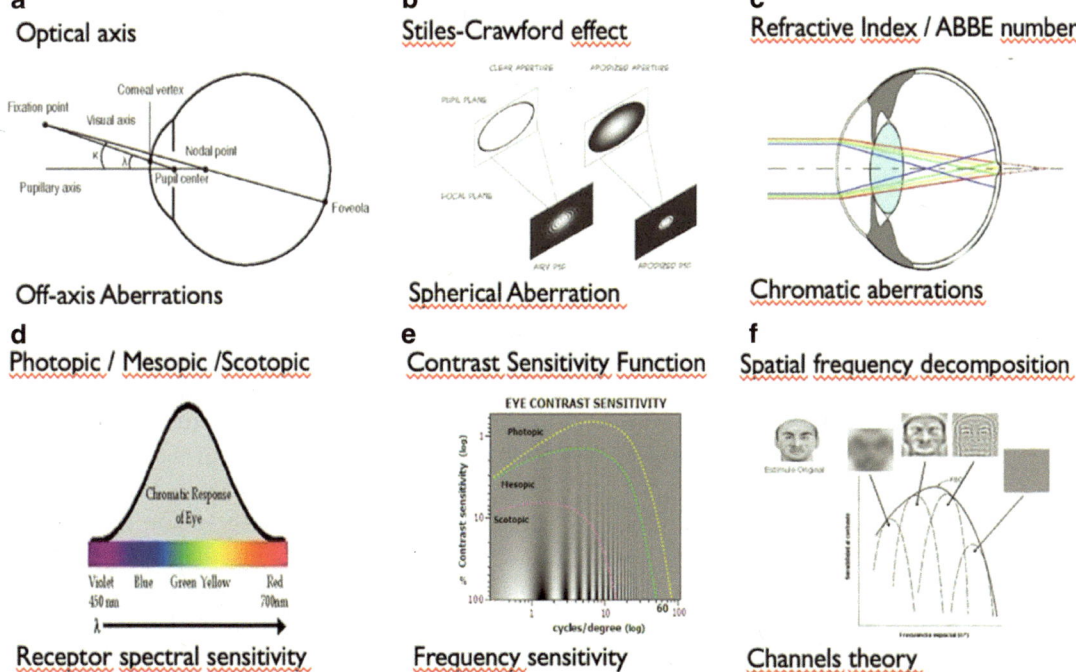

Fig. 5.7 Our optical phenomena simulation model for quality of vision evaluation. (**a**) Pupil decentration was set at 0.5 mm from the optical axis with a 5° angle between the visual and optical axis. (**b**) The Stiles–Crawford effect was incorporated as a Gaussian pupil apodization due to its relevance to eye aberrations. (**c**) In order to take chromatic dispersion into account, refractive indexes are calculated according to wavelength. (**d**) Receptor photopic spectral sensitivity was simulated using 510-, 555-, and 610-nm wavelengths, with relative weights of 1, 2, and 1, respectively. (**e**) The human CSF with a typical band-pass filter shape peaking at the spatial frequency at which the human eye is more sensitive in detecting contrast differences. The metric optimization defined different weights to each frequency (up to 100 cycles/mm, which corresponds to Snellen's 10/10 visual acuity) (**f**) in accordance with channel theory, which establishes that the visual pathway decomposes light in frequencies

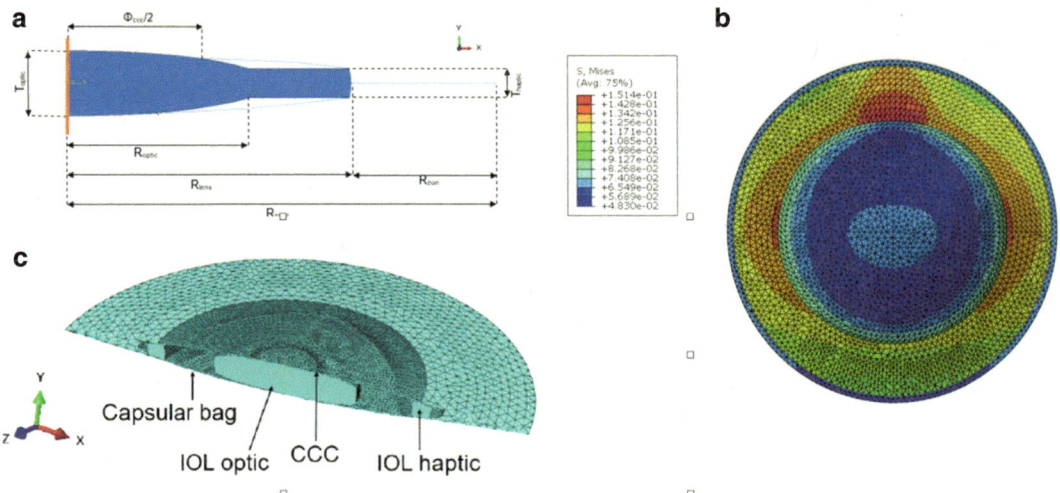

Fig. 5.8 Our models developed for the capsular bag–IOL complex: (**a**) axisymmetric geometry of the capsular bag–IOL complex [39]; (**b**) a finite element model of a three-dimensional pseudophakic [40]; and (**c**) von Mises stress (MPa) in the crystalline lens complex due to weakened zonular fibers

without the need for redefining population correction factors.

Pseudophakic Finite Element Models

The construction of biomechanical computational models of the human eye aims to understand its behavior in mechanical and optical terms. Finite element (FE) numerical simulation is an effective tool for analyzing phenomena that cannot be clarified by experimental methods, like most of the biomechanical processes.

This procedure has been applied in different anatomical features of the eye, such as the cornea [31] and the crystalline lens [32].

These simulations, however, depend heavily on the existence of experimental and clinical measurements, in order to provide the necessary data and validate the computational models' accuracy.

In order to portray the biomechanical behavior of the cornea, several in silico studies have been conducted. The condition of corneal ectasia and its response to cross-linking treatment [31] as well as the impact of laser ablative surgery on the long-term weakening of the corneal structure [33] and the implantation of intra-corneal ring segments have been assessed [34]. Other studies aimed to understand the biomechanics of the optical nerve head [35] and how it is influenced by scleral thickness [36].

Concerning the crystalline lens, initial studies compared the two main theories of accommodation: Helmoltz's and Schachar's [37]. Recent studies aim to understand the change of properties of the lens with age and their influence on presbyopia [38].

Computational models of the complete crystalline complex were already built but none for the pseudophakic eye. Our research group [39, 40] aimed to validate the previous knowledge of a healthy crystalline lens and to understand the biomechanical performance of the capsular bag and the effects of the implantation of an intraocular lens in cataract surgery (Fig. 5.8). With the objectives of modeling the new lens complex after surgery for removal of the cataractous lens, different configurations of IOL and capsular tension rings (CTR) can be considered as well as their position in the eye complex. This procedure can be applied to healthy and weakened zonular fibers in order to determine which mechanical factors contribute to capsular bag dislocation.

Furthermore, modeling of a pseudophakic eye can be relevant to understand behaviors that cannot be simulated experimentally, such as the

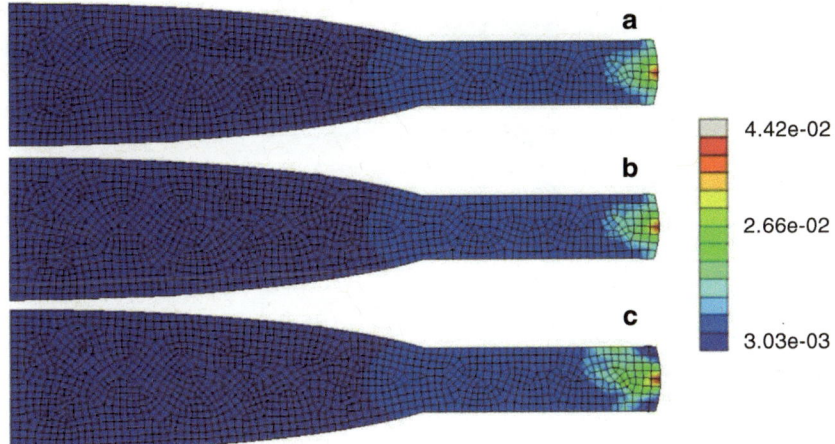

Fig. 5.9 von Mises stresses (in MPa) in the IOL for three different materials: (**a**) acrylic hydrophilic; (**b**) acrylic hydrophobic; (**c**) PMMA, after cataract surgery. All simu- lations were modeled with a 4-mm circular continuous capsulorrhexis [39]

assessment of the force acting on the IOL–capsular bag complex (Fig. 5.9).

The use of finite element analysis allows the search for solutions with great complexity that can support the experimental knowledge obtained so far. The underlying know-how for in silico experimentation is the subdivision of the modeled system into a number of small elements. For each of these elements, several equations are defined and solved, in order to understand the behavior of the structures both locally and globally, in terms of their geometric and mechanical alterations throughout the simulation.

However, these simulations require essential experimental knowledge in order to be accurately defined. Material properties of each of the system's components, geometric data, and boundary conditions are of utmost importance when defining the system's input data. Nonetheless, due to the computational effort that a simulation can require and lack of experimental data, some simplifications can be sometimes applied to the developed system.

Physical Eye Models

Wet-cell models with artificial cornea and IOL offer an alternative to schematic models, and they are often used in in vitro experiments. Although they perform well in evaluating ISO standards [41], they must keep up with the complexity of developing IOL designs and optics. New efforts are being developed to create physical models that better reproduce the anatomical and optical properties of a human eye.

Optomechanical eye models have been proposed to allow simulated in vivo testing of IOLs [42–44]. Also, due to the precision of three-dimensional printers and their flexibility at low cost, 3D physical models have been enhanced with the development in three-dimensional printing, with sliced images obtained with computed tomography [45] or defined with a 3D computer-aided design (CAD) [46]. Together with the main printed structure, poly(methyl methacrylate) (PMMA) aspherical corneas, variable iris, and IOLs can be assembled to a physical eye model.

Our research group has created a physical model of a custom-built pseudophakic eye to assess the accuracy of two commercially available measuring procedures of the pseudophakic anterior chamber (ACDpost) (Fig. 5.10). Knowing that OCT-based devices perform accurate measurements of anterior chamber depth (ACD), this technique will certainly contribute to improve intraocular lens position estimation methodologies and continue to push forward ray tracing-based methodologies, which make a direct use of the physical position of the IOL and

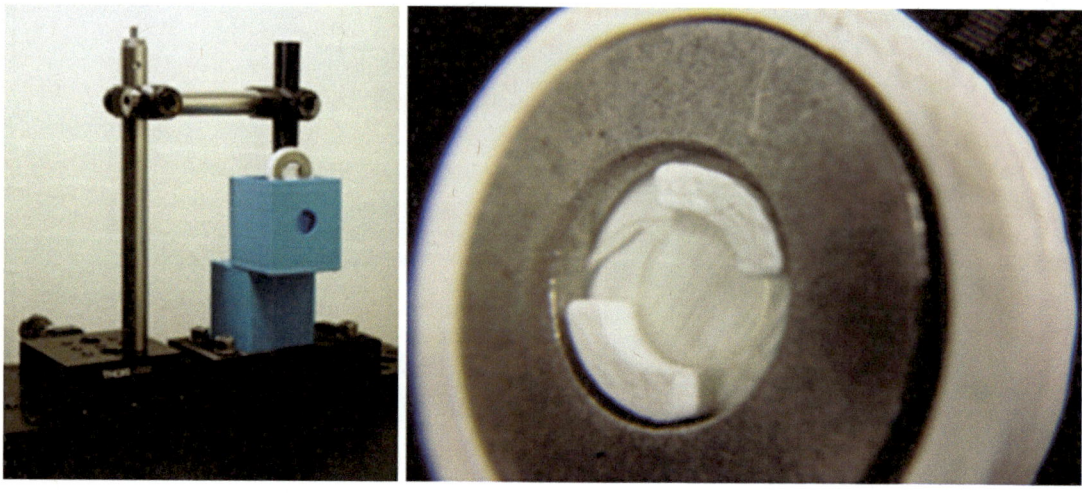

Fig. 5.10 A pseudophakic eye phantom and a custom IOL holder for micrometric axial displacements.

Fig. 5.11 Relation between Visante™ OCT and IOL's Phantom Eye relative displacement measurements in water with very good correlation

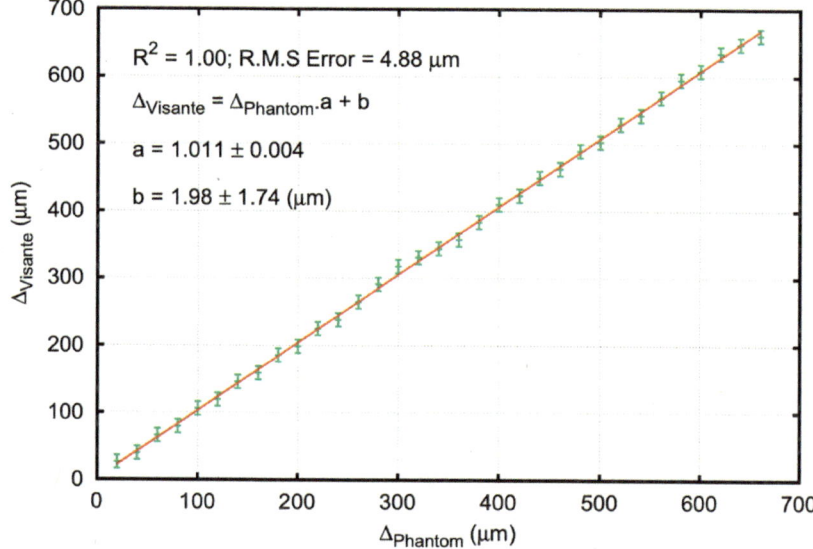

$R^2 = 1.00$; R.M.S Error = 4.88 μm

$\Delta_{Visante} = \Delta_{Phantom} \cdot a + b$

$a = 1.011 \pm 0.004$

$b = 1.98 \pm 1.74$ (μm)

not the effective lens position (ELP). The phantom was built using laboratory-grade optomechanical components, custom-designed components, and a 22D SA60AT Alcon AcrySof single-piece IOL. The IOL was installed in a custom IOL holder, allowing for precise axial displacements relative to the front surface. Calibrations were performed, and the span shift error was found to be virtually nonexistent.

With this physical model we concluded that measurements obtained with the Haag-Streit Lenstar are interchangeable with those of the Zeiss Visante. Moreover, this device had issues regarding accurate measurement of the IOL thickness in vivo, which is probably due to the difficulty in detecting the reflection from its posterior surface combined with an eventual mismatch of the refractive index of the IOL (Fig. 5.11). It is important to be aware that an inaccurate IOL thickness measurement will propagate its error to posterior eye structures which impacts the accuracy of axial length measurements. As such, performing biometry with this device in pseudophakic eyes will likely result in incorrect axial length measurements. Using the eye phantom, the performance of Visante device was also found to be superior with higher precision.

Conclusions

The modeling of anatomy, biomechanical properties, and optical phenomena are essential tools for the development of knowledge about the physiology of the pseudophakic eye and allow the development and validation of new therapeutic solutions for the final goal of customization for individual treatment.

References

1. Atchison DA, Thibos LN. Optical models of the human eye. Clin Exp Optom. 2016;99:99–106.
2. Smith G. Invited review schematic eyes: history, description and applications. Clin Exp Optom. 1995;78:176–89.
3. Atchison DA, Smith G. Optics of the human eye. 1st ed. Edinburgh: Butterworth-Heinemann; 2000.
4. Esteve-Taboada JJ, Montés-Micó R, Ferrer-Blasco T. Schematic eye models to mimic the behavior of the accommodating human eye. J Cataract Refract Surg. 2018;44:627–41.
5. Liou H-L, Brennan NA. Anatomically accurate, finite model eye for optical modeling. J Opt Soc Am A. 1997;14:1684.
6. Escudero-Sanz I, Navarro R. Off-axis aberrations of a wide-angle schematic eye model. J Opt Soc Am A. 1999;16:1881.
7. Kooijman AC. Light distribution on the retina of a wide-angle theoretical eye. J Opt Soc Am. 1983;73:1544–50.
8. Navarro R, Santamaría J, Bescós J. Accommodation-dependent model of the human eye with aspherics. J Opt Soc Am A. 1985;2:1273.
9. Norrby S. The Dubbelman eye model analysed by ray tracing through aspheric surfaces. Ophthalmic Physiol Opt. 2005;25:153–61.
10. Atchison DA. Optical models for human myopic eyes. Vis Res. 2006;46:2236–50.
11. Llorente L, Barbero S, Cano D, et al. Myopic versus hyperopic eyes: axial length, corneal shape and optical aberrations. J Vis. 2004;4:5.
12. Bakaraju RC, Ehrmann K, Papas E, et al. Finite schematic eye models and their accuracy to in-vivo data. Vis Res. 2008;48:1681–94.
13. Smith G, Bedggood P, Ashman R, et al. Exploring ocular aberrations with a schematic human eye model. Optom Vis Sci. 2008;85:330–40.

14. De Almeida MS, Carvalho LA. Different schematic eyes and their accuracy to the in vivo eye: a quantitative comparison study. Brazilian J Phys. 2007;37:378–87.
15. Aguirre GK. A model of the entrance pupil of the human eye. Sci Rep. 2019;9:9360.
16. Chen Y-L, Tan B, Baker K, et al. Simulation of keratoconus observation in photorefraction. Opt Express. 2006;14:11477.
17. Ribeiro F, Castanheira-Dinis A, Dias JM. Refractive error assessment: influence of different optical elements and current limits of biometric techniques. J Refract Surg. 2013;29:206–12.
18. Smith G, Pierscionek BK, Atchison DA. The optical modelling of the human lens. Ophthalmic Physiol Opt J Br Coll Ophthalmic Opt. 1991;11:359–69.
19. Werner W, Roth EH. [Image properties of spherical as aspheric intraocular lenses]. Klin Monatsbl Augenheilkd. 1999;214:246–50.
20. Altmann GE, Nichamin LD, Lane SS, et al. Optical performance of 3 intraocular lens designs in the presence of decentration. J Cataract Refract Surg. 2005;31:574–85.
21. Marcos S, Barbero S, Jiménez-Alfaro I. Optical quality and depth-of-field of eyes implanted with spherical and aspheric intraocular lenses. J Refract Surg. 2005;21:223–35.
22. Tabernero J, Piers P, Benito A, et al. Predicting the optical performance of eyes implanted with IOLs to correct spherical aberration. Investig Ophthalmol Vis Sci. 2006;47:4651–8.
23. Marcos S, Romero M, Benedí-García C, et al. Interaction of monochromatic and chromatic aberrations in pseudophakic patients. J Refract Surg. 2020;36:230–8.
24. Pérez-Gracia J, Varea A, Ares J, et al. Evaluation of the optical performance for aspheric intraocular lenses in relation with tilt and decenter errors. PLoS One. 2020;15:1–14.
25. Ribeiro FJ, Castanheira-Dinis A, Dias JM. Personalized pseudophakic model for refractive assessment. PLoS One. 2012;7:1–8.
26. Sun M, Pérez-Merino P, Martinez-Enriquez E, et al. Full 3-D OCT-based pseudophakic custom computer eye model. Biomed Opt Express. 2016;7:1074–88.
27. Olsen T, Hoffmann P. C constant: new concept for ray tracing–assisted intraocular lens power calculation. J Cataract Refract Surg. 2014;40:764–73.
28. Saiki M, Negishi K, Kato N, et al. Ray tracing software for intraocular lens power calculation after corneal excimer laser surgery. Jpn J Ophthalmol. 2014;58:276–81.
29. Rosales P, Marcos S. Customized computer models of eyes with intraocular lenses. Opt Express. 2007;15:2204–18.
30. Ribeiro F, Castanheira-Dinis A, Sanches JM, et al. Assessment of image quality using a pseudophakic eye model for refractive evaluation. Lecture Notes in Computer Science (Including Subseries Lecture Notes in Artificial Intelligence and Lecture Notes in Bioinformatics), vol. 7887. LNCS; 2013. p. 543–50.

31. Sinha Roy A, Rocha KM, Randleman JB, et al. Inverse computational analysis of in vivo corneal elastic modulus change after collagen crosslinking for keratoconus. Exp Eye Res. 2013;113:92–104.
32. Lanchares E, Navarro R, Calvo B. Hyperelastic modelling of the crystalline lens: accommodation and presbyopia. J Optom. 2012;5:110–20.
33. Sinha Roy A, Dupps WJJ. Patient-specific modeling of corneal refractive surgery outcomes and inverse estimation of elastic property changes. J Biomech Eng. 2011;133:11002.
34. Kling S, Marcos S. Finite-element modeling of intrastromal ring segment implantation into a hyperelastic cornea. Investig Opthalmology Vis Sci. 2013;54:881–9.
35. Sigal IA, Flanagan JG, Tertinegg I, et al. Finite element modeling of optic nerve head biomechanics. Investig Ophthalmol Vis Sci. 2004;45:4378–87.
36. Norman RE, Flanagan JG, Sigal IA, et al. Finite element modeling of the human sclera: influence on optic nerve head biomechanics and connections with glaucoma. Exp Eye Res. 2011;93:4–12.
37. Burd HJ, Judge SJ, Flavell MJ. Mechanics of accommodation of the human eye. Vis Res. 1999;39:1591–5.
38. Wang K, Venetsanos DT, Hoshino M, et al. A modeling approach for investigating opto-mechanical relationships in the human eye lens. IEEE Trans Biomed Eng. 2020;67:999–1006.
39. Cardoso MT, Feijó B, Castro APG et al. Axisymmetric finite element modelling of the crystalline under cataract surgery. 2019.
40. Paulino JS, Feijó B, Ribeiro FJ et al. 3D finite element modelling of the pseudophakic eye. 2020.
41. Alba-Bueno F, Vega F, Millán MS. Design of a test bench for intraocular lens optical characterization. J Phys Conf Ser. 2011;274:12105.
42. Gobbi PG, Fasce F, Bozza S, et al. Optomechanical eye model with imaging capabilities for objective evaluation of intraocular lenses. J Cataract Refract Surg. 2006;32:643–51.
43. Inoue M, Noda T, Mihashi T, et al. Quality of image of grating target placed in model of human eye with corneal aberrations as observed through multifocal intraocular lenses. Am J Ophthalmol. 2011;151:644–652. e1.
44. Inoue M, Noda T, Ohnuma K, et al. Quality of image of grating target placed in model eye and observed through Toric intraocular lenses. Am J Ophthalmol. 2013;155:243–252.e1.
45. Dobler B, Bendl R. Precise modelling of the eye for proton therapy of intra-ocular tumours. Phys Med Biol. 2002;47:593–613.
46. Xie P, Hu Z, Zhang X, et al. Application of 3-dimensional printing technology to construct an eye model for fundus viewing study. PLoS One. 2014;9:e109373.

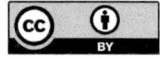

Data Analysis in IOL Power Calculations

6

Giacomo Savini and Kenneth J. Hoffer

When the results of intraocular lens (IOL) power calculation by one or more formulas are reported, different parameters should be provided and a proper statistical analysis should be performed. In recent years, specific guidelines on this subject have been published and updated, and it is likely that further recommendations will be given in the future, as the interest of researchers in this field is increasing [1–4].

Designing the Sample to be Analyzed

The first step of any study on IOL power calculation is the enrollment of an appropriate sample. The following guidelines should be followed:

- For patients who underwent bilateral cataract surgery, only one eye for each patient should be analyzed [1, 4]. Ocular measurements are more alike between fellow eyes than between eyes of different subjects, and measurements

G. Savini
G.B. Bietti Eye Foundation, Rome, Italy

Studio Oculistico d'Azeglio, Bologna, Italy
e-mail: giacomo.savini@startmail.com

K. J. Hoffer (✉)
St. Mary's Eye Center, Santa Monica, CA, USA

Stein Eye Institute, UCLA, Los Angeles, CA, USA
e-mail: KHofferMD@startmail.com

from fellow eyes cannot be treated as if they were independent [5]. If the correlation between the right and left eyes of each subject is not accounted for in statistical analysis, there may be errors in the results obtained [6]. It would be preferable to consider only one eye of each individual. In this case, several approaches can be followed such as random selection of one eye (right or left), arbitrary selection of all right eyes, or a clinically based selection (e.g., the eye with the best visual acuity). Alternatively, if both eyes of the same patient are included, appropriate statistical methods (generalized estimating equations), which estimate the correlation and adjust for it in the analysis, may be used [7]. However, in general, the fewer statistical adjustments performed, the better.

- Patients with preoperative and/or postoperative pathologies should be excluded, as well as those with a postoperative corrected distance visual acuity worse than 20/40, because poor acuity lessens the accuracy of the crucial postoperative refractive error [1, 4].
- A uniform sample is preferable. This means that we suggest enrolling eyes that underwent preoperative measurements with the same optical biometer, were operated with the same technique (standard phacoemulsification vs. femtosecond laser-assisted cataract surgery), received the same IOL model, and were refracted using the same method. Exceptions

J. Aramberri et al. (eds.), *Intraocular Lens Calculations*, Essentials in Ophthalmology,
https://doi.org/10.1007/978-3-031-50666-6_6

to this recommendation may be acceptable for studies where it is more difficult to enroll a large sample, such as eyes with keratoconus or eyes with previous corneal refractive surgery.

- The sample size should be sufficient to allow constant optimization. According to Langenbucher et al., at least 100 eyes should be enrolled in order to achieve a stable mean refractive error, at least with formulas with a single constant [8]. The same number was suggested in 2010 by Haigis (personal communication). We agree that such a sample size can be considered sufficient for most studies. Of course, larger samples may be more powerful to disclose statistically significant differences and for this reason we recently suggested a minimum sample size of 200 eyes [4], whereas Holladay et al. suggested a minimum sample size between 300 and 700 eyes [3]. The uncertainty on this issue depends on the fact that a universally accepted parameter to be selected and investigated does not yet exist: the calculated minimum sample size changes if we look at the standard deviation (SD) of the prediction error (PE), the median absolute error (MedAE), or the percentage of eyes with a PE within ±0.50 diopters (D). Although the SD has been recently advocated as the best parameter [3], there is not yet a global consensus on it. Moreover, the sample size calculation depends on the clinically significant difference that is looked for. Therefore, the help of a statistician is important when designing these studies.
- Also, depending on what is being studied, it is important to be sure that the AL and K ranges of the sample are not skewed toward longer eyes, shorter eyes, or only those with "normal values."
- Postoperative refraction should be measured when stable. With small-incision surgery and one-piece IOLs, the refraction can be considered to be stable at 1 week from surgery [9–11], but we suggest waiting at least 1 month. Three months may be even better, but no evidence exists for this. Waiting 6–12 months, as recently suggested [3], is quite impractical and leads to an unremarkable advantage. The highest accuracy should be used when assess-

ing the postoperative spherical equivalent: if the patient can read 20/20 for distance without any correction, the examiner should not simply report 0 (plano) as the postoperative refraction but should assess whether adding or subtracting 0.25 D can improve visual acuity further. The testing distance for visual acuity should be standardized. A 6-m (approximately 20-foot) distance, rather than 4 m (approximately 13 feet) or infinity, may be the preferred choice [12]. Refractions at 4 m can be converted to 6 m by adding a value of −0.08 D to the spherical equivalent (e.g., a refraction of 0.00 D at 4 m corresponds to a refraction of −0.08 D at 6 m).

Selecting the Data to be Reported

In addition to the demographics of the study population (age, gender, and ethnicity), the following values should be reported:

- Prediction error (PE): This is defined as the difference between the postoperative spherical equivalent refraction and the predicted refraction (not the target refraction!). It is calculated as the postoperative refraction minus the predicted refraction so that the PE is negative for myopic errors and positive for hyperopic errors. The mean PE with any formula should be zeroed out by means of constant optimization. The latter is a relatively easy task with published formulas [13–16], since it can be carried out on Excel (Microsoft, Redmond, VA), as previously explained [1, 4], or using the internal software of different optical biometers. For the Haigis formula, it is mandatory to optimize all three constants. Constant optimization is more complicated with the latest generation formulas, which are all unpublished and for which it is better to ask for the help of the formula's authors. Alternatively, it is possible to use specific computer programming languages able to extract data automatically from any database (e.g., Python Software Foundation, Wilmington, DE), enter them into the formula website, and generate a new database containing the predicted refraction for each eye. Regarding the Holladay 2 formula, which is also unpublished, it is possible to perform optimization using the Holladay IOL Consultant Software & Surgical Outcomes Assessment (www.hicsoap.com).

- There are also some situations where constant optimization should not be carried out or should be carried out with caution. The first scenario is the analysis of specific samples, such as long or short eyes. When evaluating only short eyes, it would be more appropriate to rely on the optimized constants of the whole population (which have to be separately calculated) rather than on the optimized constants specifically calculated for the short eye sample. In the clinical setting, in fact, no one uses separate constants for short and medium eyes. The same approach can be followed for unusual eyes (e.g., those with keratoconus), where it might be more appropriate to use optimized constants obtained from larger samples of healthy eyes rather than from keratoconic eyes. The second scenario is the analysis of eyes with previous corneal refractive surgery: here, constant optimization would be preferable, but the lack of large samples with the same IOL model often precludes it. When more IOL models have to be analyzed simultaneously, it can be acceptable to use (for each IOL) optimized constants from large databases such as those available on the User Group for Laser Interference Biometry (ULIB, http://ocusoft.de/ulib/c1.htm, accessed on February 27, 2021) or on the IOLcon website (https://iolcon.org, accessed on February 27, 2021).

- Standard deviation (SD) and variance of the PE: SD is the square root of the variance, which is the average of the squared differences from the mean. These values are extremely important as they provides us with the information about how spread out the individual PEs are. Accurate formulas have lower SDs (and variances), whereas higher SDs (and variances) are the consequence of many outliers. SD deviation has been recently indicated as the best parameter to compare the refractive outcomes of different formulas [3].

- Distribution of the PE: The PE has always been considered to be normally distributed [2], but recently this assumption has been negated by Holladay et al. [3] Actually, in previous studies with relatively small sample size our group found a normal distribution of the PE [17, 18], whereas the observation by Holladay and coauthors derives from the largest study ever published [19]. We recommend reporting whether the PE distribution is normal or not because the choice between parametric and nonparametric statistical methods (to be used when comparing the PEs of different formulas) depends on this issue. Additional values that should be provided with the distribution are skewness and kurtosis [3]. The former is related to the symmetry of the PE distribution: the tail may be longer to the left or the right. If skewness ranges between −0.5 and +0.5, the distribution is approximately symmetric. The latter describes the tailedness of the sample (and not its peak).

- Median absolute error (MedAE): The absolute prediction error has been considered the most important outcome for many years. Earlier studies reported the mean absolute error (MAE); we then switched our recommendation to the MedAE since Haigis and Norrby showed us that the distribution of the absolute prediction error cannot be normal. The absolute prediction error is still a mandatory outcome measure, especially once constant optimization leads to a mean arithmetic PE of zero.

- Interquantile range: This is the best way to show the spread of the absolute prediction error.

- Percentage of eyes with a PE within a given interval (e.g., ±0.50 D): This is probably the easiest way to report and remember the accuracy of any IOL power formula. The percentage of eyes with a PE within ±0.25 D is quite useful to predict the refractive outcomes and expectations for patients receiving multifocal IOLs, where the tolerance to refractive errors is minimal. The percentage of eyes with a PE within ±0.50 D is the most commonly reported value and can be used as a method to rank formulas.

Analyzing the Data

Once data are collected, they have to be analyzed. As previously stated, the first statistical analysis should investigate whether the PE is normally distributed. For this purpose, Shapiro-Wilk test and Kolmogorov-Smirnov test are probably the two most commonly used tests and are available with the majority of statistical software. Unfortunately, formal normality tests are notoriously affected by large samples in which small deviations from normality yield significant results. In other words, they display a higher probability of rejecting the null hypothesis of normality as sample size increases: for large samples ($n > 300$), these formal normality tests may be unreliable [20]. In this context, it is wise to refer to the central limit theorem [21], according to which in large samples ($n > 30$) the sampling distribution tends to be normal anyway, and to probability-probability plots (P-P plot): these graphs plot the cumulative probability of a variable (the PE) against the cumulative probability of a normal distribution. If values fall on the diagonal of the plot, then the variable is normally distributed [22].

The following questions should then be answered:

- Is the mean PE statistically significant from zero? If data are normally distributed, then one sample t-test is recommended; if the distribution is not normal, Wilcoxon rank sum test should be used.
- Is the SD of the PE statistically significant among formulas? Under the assumption that the values for each formula are matched (paired), if data are normally distributed, repeated-measures ANOVA with post-test is recommended; otherwise, the Friedman test with post-test should be used. Recently, the heteroscedastic method has been recommended [3]. This test can be used to compare the SD of different formulas when the PE distribution is not normal and is able to detect statistically significant differences that are missed by the Friedman test. Its main limitation is that it is difficult to use.

- Does the absolute error generated by the formulas under investigation show any statistically significant difference? Since the absolute error never has a normal distribution, nonparametric tests such as the Friedman test should be used.
- Does the percentage of eyes with a PE within ±0.50 D (or ±0.25) D show any statistically significant difference among formulas? Cochran's Q test is recommended for this purpose.

References

1. Hoffer KJ, Aramberri J, Haigis W, Olsen T, Savini G, Shammas HJ, Bentow S. Protocols for studies of intraocular lens formula accuracy. Am J Ophthalmol. 2015;160:403–5.
2. Wang L, Koch DD, Hill W, Abulafia A. Pursuing perfection in intraocular lens calculations: III. Criteria for analyzing outcomes. J Cataract Refract Surg. 2017;43:999–1002.
3. Holladay JT, Wilcox RR, Koch DD, Wang L. Review and recommendations for univariate statistical analysis of spherical equivalent prediction error for IOL power calculations. J Cataract Refract Surg. 2021;47:65–77.
4. Hoffer KJ, Savini G. Update on intraocular lens power calculation study protocols: the better way to design and report clinical trials. Ophthalmology. 2021;128(11):e115–20.
5. Katz J, Zeger S, Liang KY. Appropriate statistical methods to account for similarities in binary outcomes between fellow eyes. Invest Ophthalmol Vis Sci. 1994;35:2461–5.
6. Murdoch IE, Morris SS, Cousens SN. People and eyes: statistical approaches in ophthalmology. Br J Ophthalmol. 1998;82:971–3.
7. Hardin JW, Hilbe M. Generalized estimating equations. 2nd ed. New York: Chapman & Hall; 2012.
8. Langenbucher A, Schwemm M, Eppig T, Schröder S, Cayless A, Szentmáry N. Optimal dataset sizes for constant optimization in published theoretical optical formulae. Curr Eye Res. 2021;46(10):1589–96.
9. Lyle WA, Jin GJC. Prospective evaluation of early visual and refractive effects with small clear corneal incision for cataract surgery. J Cataract Refract Surg. 1996;22:1456–60.
10. Masket S, Tennen DG. Astigmatic stabilization of 3.0 mm temporal clear corneal cataract incisions. J Cataract Refract Surg. 1996;22:1451–5.
11. Nejima R, Miyai T, Kataoka Y, Miyata K, Honbou M, Tokunaga T, et al. Prospective intrapatient comparison of 6.0-millimeter optic single-piece and 3-piece

hydrophobic acrylic foldable intraocular lenses. Ophthalmology. 2006;113:585–90.

12. Simpson MJ, Chairman WN. The effect of testing distance on intraocular lens power calculation. J Refract Surg. 2014;30:726.

13. Haigis W, Lege B, Miller N, Schneider B. Comparison of immersion ultrasound biometry and partial coherence interferometry for intraocular lens calculation according to Haigis. Graefes Arch Clin Exp Ophthalmol. 2000;238:765–73.

14. Hoffer KJ. The Hoffer Q formula: a comparison of theoretic and regression formulas. J Cataract Refract Surg. 1993;19(11):700–12. Errata: 1994;20(6):677 and 2007;33(1):2–3

15. Holladay JT, Prager TC, Chandler TY, et al. A three-part system for refining intraocular lens power calculations. J Cataract Refract Surg. 1988;14:17–24.

16. Retzlaff JA, Sanders DR, Kraff MC. Development of the SRK/T intraocular lens implant power calculation formula. J Cataract Refract Surg. 1990;16:333–40. Errata: 1990;16:528 and 1993;19(5):444–446

17. Savini G, Hoffer KJ, Balducci N, Barboni P, Schiano LD. Comparison of formula accuracy for intraocular lens power calculation based on measurements by a swept-source optical coherence tomography optical biometer. J Cataract Refract Surg. 2020;46:27–33.

18. Taroni L, Hoffer KJ, Barboni P, Schiano-Lomoriello D, Savini G. Outcomes of IOL power calculation using measurements by a rotating Scheimpflug camera combined with partial coherence interferometry. J Cataract Refract Surg. 2020;46:1618–23.

19. Melles RB, Holladay JT, Chang WJ. Accuracy of intraocular lens calculation formulas. Ophthalmology. 2018;125:169–78.

20. Kim HY. Statistical notes for clinical researchers: assessing normal distribution. Restor Dent Endod. 2012;37:245–8.

21. Kwak SG, Kim JH. Central limit theorem: the cornerstone of modern statistics. Korean J Anesthesiol. 2017;70:144–56.

22. Hoffer KJ, Savini G. Reply. Ophthalmol. 2020;128(4):e21–22.

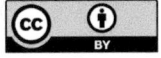

Demographics of Biometry

Ronald B. Melles

Introduction

The accurate prediction of refraction after cataract surgery refraction depends on the quality of the biometric measurements of the eye obtained preoperatively. These critical measurements typically include anterior chamber depth, lens thickness, axial length, and corneal curvature (expressed as radius of curvature or keratometry values) although recent biometry devices have introduced the use of additional values such as central corneal thickness and horizontal corneal diameter (aka white-to-white dimension). As several reports have shown, these parameters often are correlated and may vary by patient sex, race, and age [1–14]. To further explore these relationships, we analyzed a large dataset of biometry values obtained with modern biometry equipment and compared these measurements to those obtained in prior studies.

Methods

Kaiser Permanente Northern California (KPNC) is a large medical system providing comprehensive health care services to a diverse population of over 4.4 million patients. KPNC standardized biometry measurements using an optical low coherence reflectometry device (Lenstar 900, Haig-Streit, Köniz, Switzerland) platform across 25 eye care clinics in 2014. The export function of the biometry device was used to obtain and collate biometry values for 85,404 patients measured during the period from 2014 to 2019. An illustrative tracing of the biometry signals with component labels is shown in Fig. 7.1. The KPNC electronic medical record (Epic Systems, Verona, USA) was queried to capture race, sex, age, and diagnoses for these patients. Those with a prior history of keratorefractive surgery ($N = 4360$, 5.4%) or a diagnosis of keratoconus ($N = 295$, 0.3%) were excluded, leaving a study population of 80,479 eyes. Statistical analyses were performed only on right eye data using Stata 15.1 (StataCorp, College Station, TX). Because of the large sample size, even clinically small differences between average values were statistically significant, and thus percentage differences between means were typically calculated.

R. B. Melles (✉)
Department of Ophthalmology, The Permanente Medical Group, Kaiser Permanente Northern California, Oakland, CA, USA
e-mail: Ronald.Melles@va.gov

© The Author(s) 2024
J. Aramberri et al. (eds.), *Intraocular Lens Calculations*, Essentials in Ophthalmology,
https://doi.org/10.1007/978-3-031-50666-6_7

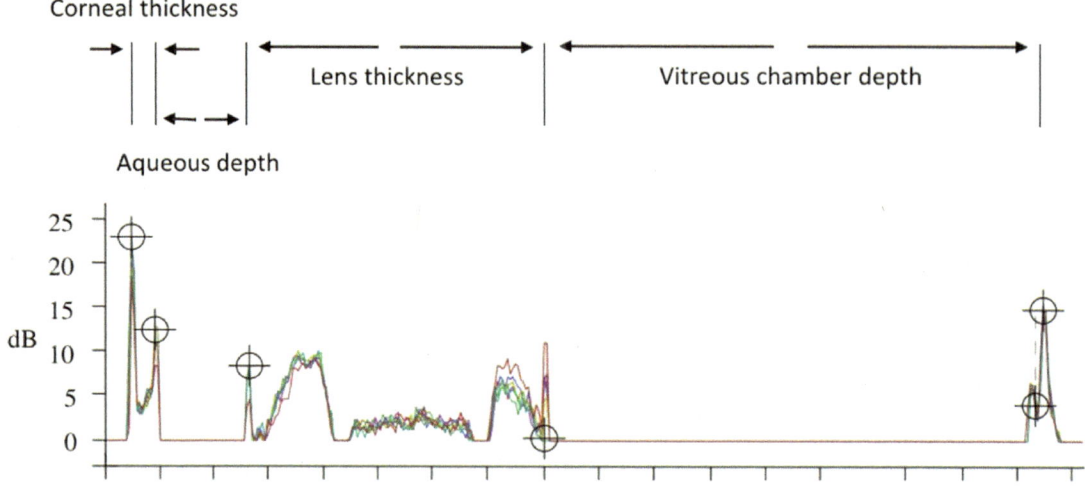

Fig. 7.1 An example optical low coherence reflectometry tracing of key biometric values

Results

Patients included in the study ranged in age from 21 to 102 (mean of 69.9, SD of 9.6). A diverse mix of racial/ethnic groups was represented including 14,768 Asian (18.4%), 5406 Black (6.7%), 7187 Hispanic (8.9%), 50,957 White (63.3%), and 2161 other race (2.7%) patients. As in many cataract-related studies, women ($N = 47,309$, 58.8%) outnumbered men ($N = 33,170$, 41.2%). Summary statistics of the biometry values are presented in Table 7.1. Using the Shapiro-Wilk test of normality on a random subcohort of 1000 patients, a normal distribution of values was found for aqueous depth and lens thickness but not for central corneal thickness, anterior corneal curvature, horizontal corneal diameter, or vitreous chamber depth. Skew and kurtosis values are also displayed in Table 7.1.

Sex-Related Differences

Differences in biometry values by sex are summarized in Table 7.2. In general, all values were larger in male patients, though in the case of central corneal thickness and lens thickness the differences were less than 1%. The most dramatic difference between the sexes is found in aqueous depth, where males had on average a 4.7% deeper

dimension than females (mean ± SD: 2.69 ± 0.41 vs. 2.57 ± 0.40, respectively).

Racial Differences

There are modest differences among the biometric measurements by race. Table 7.3 summarizes the key values for Asian, Black, Hispanic, White, and Others categories of race. Corneas are thinnest in Black patients and thickest in Whites. In general, Whites had the largest values in each measurement category, except for vitreous chamber depth and axial length, which were greatest in Asian patients, and radius of the anterior cornea, which was greatest in Blacks and Hispanics.

Age-Related Trends

The aqueous depth (Fig. 7.2) decreases with age due to thickening of the lens (Fig. 7.3). The vitreous chamber depth also decreases with age due to thickening of the lens, but the magnitude of this effect is difficult to ascertain in the current study population as myopic patients with deeper vitreous chamber depths tended to present at an earlier age for cataract surgery. The measured horizontal corneal diameter (aka White-to-White)

Table 7.1 Demographics and biometry measure summary statistics ($N = 80,479$). (All numbers represent millimeters unless otherwise indicated and are from right eye measurements only)

Measure	Mean	Median	SD	Minimum	Maximum	Skew	Kurtosis
Central corneal thickness	544.3 µ	543.9 µ	35.4 µ	356 µ	750 µ	0.10	0.35
Radius anterior cornea	7.69	7.69	0.27	6.31	9.47	0.14	3.30
Aqueous depth	2.62	2.61	0.41	1.25	4.83	0.14	0.01
Anterior chamber depth	3.17	3.16	0.41	1.76	5.40	0.14	0.01
Lens thickness	4.57	4.57	0.45	2.53	6.35	0.11	−0.12
Vitreous chamber depth	16.27	16.08	1.31	11.25	25.16	1.08	2.58
Axial length	24.00	23.80	1.38	18.60	33.25	1.05	2.39
Horizontal corneal diameter[a]	11.98	11.99	0.49	7.09	14.66	−0.83	4.41

[a]Also known as White-to-White (WTW)

Table 7.2 Sex differences in key biometry measures (all numbers represent millimeters unless otherwise indicated and are from right eye measurements only)

Measure	Female N (%)	Male N (%)	Difference of means	Percentage difference of means
Sex	47,309 (58.8%)	33,170 (41.2%)	–	–
	Mean ± SD	**Mean ± SD**		
Age at measurement (years)	70.0	69.8	0.2	0.2%
Central corneal thickness	543.1 µ ± 34.7	546.2 µ ± 36.3	3.1 µ	0.6%
Radius anterior cornea	7.65 ± 0.26	7.76 ± 0.27	0.11	1.5%
Aqueous depth	2.57 ± 0.40	2.69 ± 0.41	0.12	4.7%
Anterior chamber depth	3.11 ± 0.40	3.24 ± 0.41	0.13	4.0%
Lens thickness	4.56 ± 0.44	4.58 ± 0.47	0.02	0.6%
Vitreous chamber depth	16.11 ± 1.30	16.49 ± 1.29	0.38	2.4%
Axial length	23.78 ± 1.36	24.32 ± 1.38	0.54	2.2%
Horizontal corneal diameter[a]	11.90 ± 0.47	12.07 ± 0.51	0.17	1.4%

[a]Also known as White-to-White (WTW)

Table 7.3 Racial differences in the mean values of key biometry measures. The race with the minimum values for a given measure are shown in *italics* and maximum values in **bold** (all numbers represent millimeters unless otherwise indicated and are from right eye measurements only)

Measure	Asian	Black	Hispanic	White	Others	Difference[a]	Percentage difference
N (%)	14,768 (18.4%)	5406 (6.7%)	7187 (8.9%)	50,957 (63.3%)	2161 (2.7%)	–	–
Age at measurement (years)	67.4	68.9	67.9	**71.1**	*67.4*	3.7	5.5%
Central corneal thickness	540 µ	*524 µ*	539 µ	**549 µ**	540 µ	24.5	4.7%
Radius anterior cornea	7.68	**7.73**	**7.73**	7.69	7.71	0.05	0.6%
Aqueous depth	*2.57*	2.63	*2.57*	**2.64**	2.63	0.07	2.9%
Anterior chamber depth	*3.11*	3.15	*3.11*	**3.19**	3.17	0.08	2.7%
Lens thickness	4.55	*4.47*	4.55	**4.59**	4.51	0.12	2.7%
Vitreous chamber depth	**16.60**	16.36	*16.09*	16.19	16.26	0.51	3.2%
Axial length	**24.26**	23.98	*23.75*	23.97	23.94	0.52	2.2%
Horizontal corneal diameter	*11.73*	11.97	11.87	**12.06**	11.94	0.33	2.8%

[a]Absolute difference between the minimum and maximum values for measure row

Fig. 7.2 Decrease in aqueous depth with age. The change is approximated by the linear regression equation: aqueous depth$_{mm}$ = (−0.011*age) + 3.36. The central line within the box represents the median value for that age group; the box edges represent the 25th and 75th percentiles (Q1 and Q3) and the whiskers show the lower and upper extremes as calculated by Q1 − (1.5*(Q3 − Q1)) and Q3 + (1.5*(Q3 − Q1)), respectively

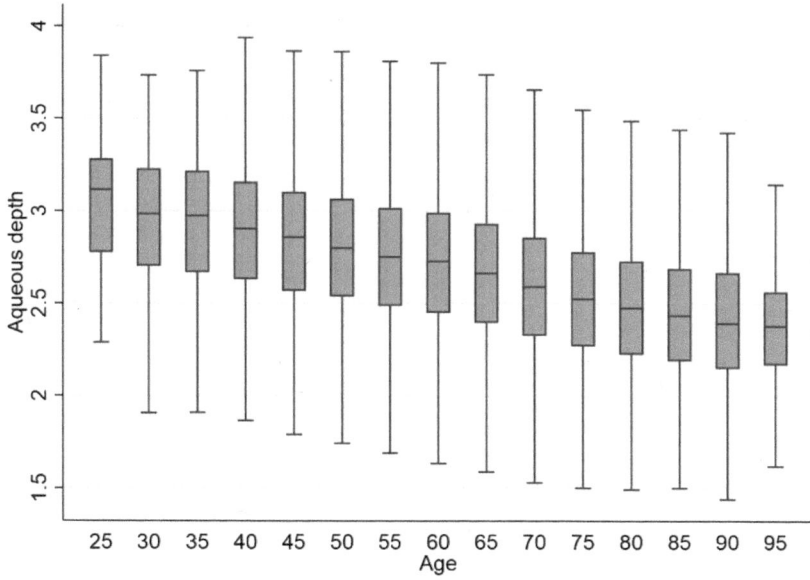

Fig. 7.3 Increase in lens thickness with age. The increase is approximated by the linear regression equation: lens thickness$_{mm}$ = (0.017*age) + 3.37

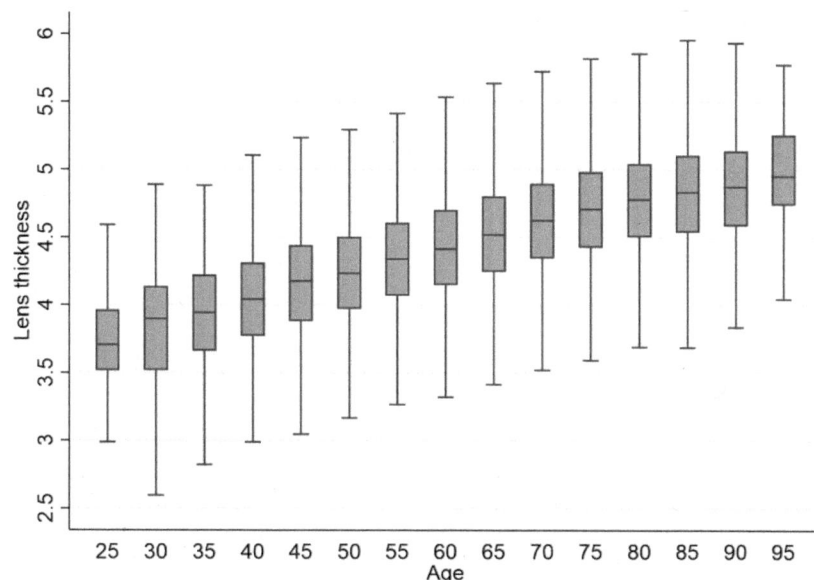

decreases slightly with age (Fig. 7.4), while central corneal thickness remains relatively stable (Fig. 7.5).

Corneal Astigmatism

Corneal astigmatism also varies with age, with younger patients on average having greater with-the-rule cylinder (Fig. 7.6), middle-aged patients having a decrease in overall astigmatism (Fig. 7.7), and older patients having an increase in against-the-rule cylinder (Fig. 7.8). The vertical astigmatism component was calculated as Vertical$_{astigmatism}$ = Sine (Axis) * Cylinder$_{diopters}$ and the horizontal astigmatism component as Horizontal$_{astigmatism}$ = Absolute (Cosine (Axis)) * Cylinder$_{diopters}$.

Fig. 7.4 Slight decrease in horizontal corneal diameter (aka White-to-White) with age

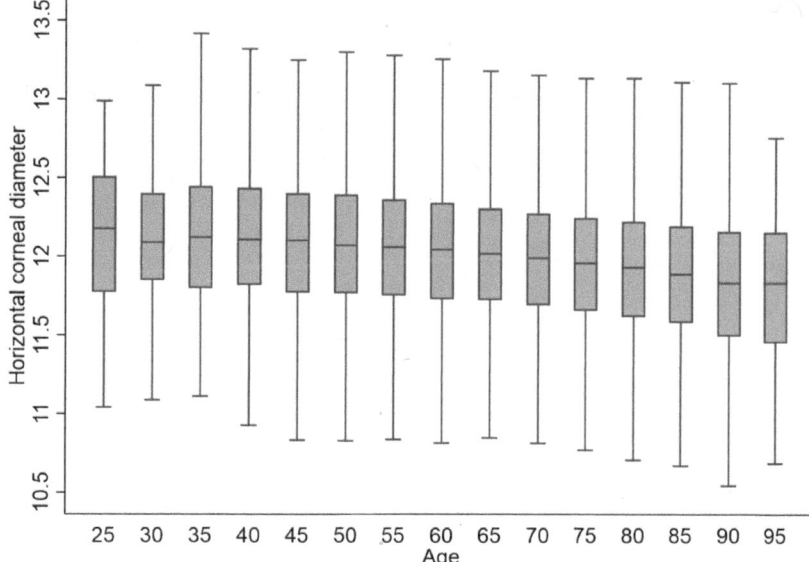

Fig. 7.5 Stable corneal thickness with age

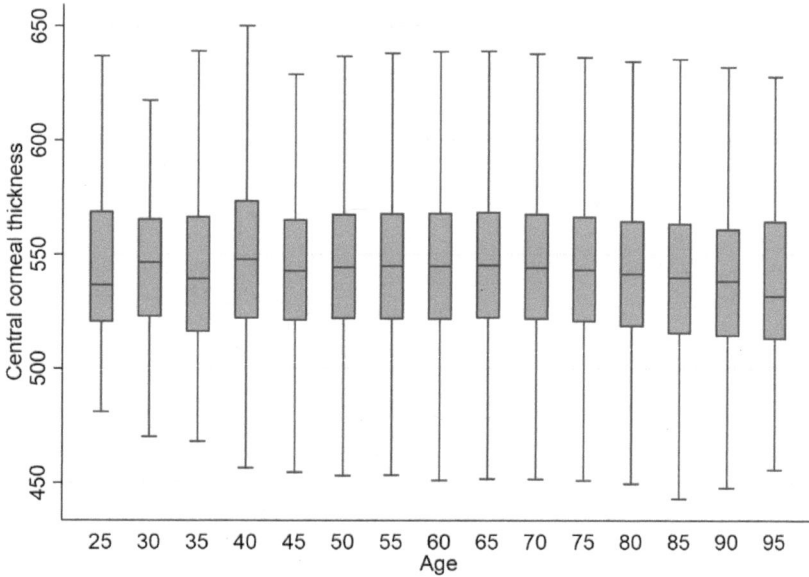

Correlation Among Biometry Variables

The highest correlation among the biometry measures are the aqueous depth-lens thickness, the anterior corneal radius-horizontal corneal diameter, the vitreous chamber depth-aqueous depth and vitreous chamber depth-anterior corneal radius, and the vitreous chamber depth-horizontal corneal diameter. Corneal measures are largely independent of the lens thickness (Table 7.4).

Inter-Eye Variation

All biometry values were very highly correlated between the right and left eyes (Table 7.5).

Fig. 7.6 Higher with-the-rule astigmatism in younger patients

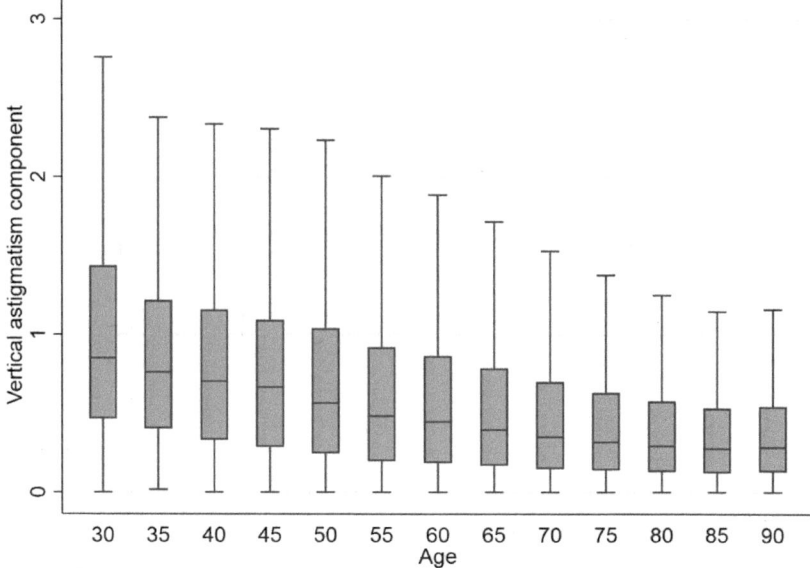

Fig. 7.7 Net astigmatism (cylinder) reaches a minimum near age 60

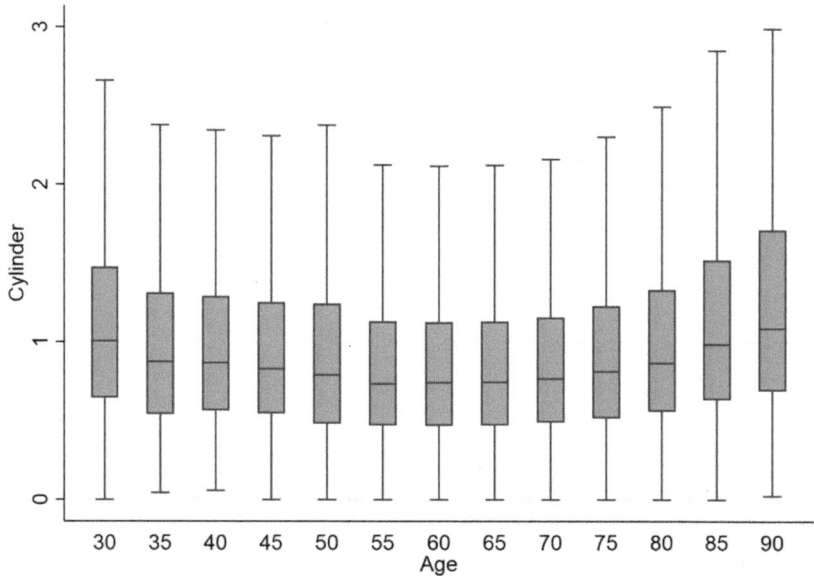

Conclusion

It is important for cataract surgeons to familiarize themselves with the normal ranges and correlations among biometry values in order to be able to quickly recognize outliers and possible measurement errors [15]. In addition, authors of intraocular lens calculation formulas should understand the variations in biometry values between the sexes [16, 17] and also how these measurements change with age. In particular, the continued increase in against-the-rule astigmatism late into life should be factored into toric intraocular implant selection. The decrease in horizontal corneal diameter seen with increased age may be an artifact of measurement as encroaching discoloration effects occur (such as from white limbal girdle of Vogt or arcus senilis).

Fig. 7.8 Against-the-rule astigmatism continues to increase with age in older patients

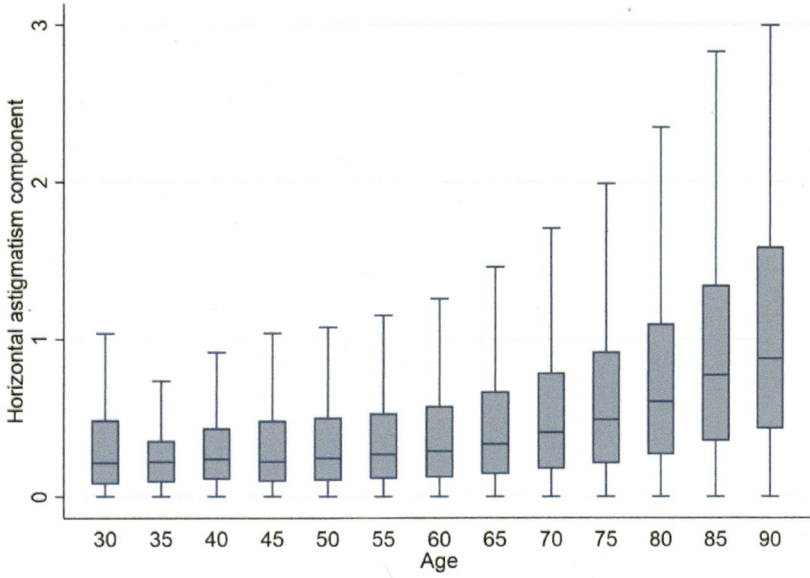

Table 7.4 Correlation matrix of key biometry variables

	R_{ac}	HCD	CCT	AD	LT	VCD
Radius anterior cornea (R_{ac})	–					
Horizontal corneal diameter (HCD)	0.387	–				
Central corneal thickness (CCT)	0.133	0.001	–			
Aqueous depth (AD)	−0.025	0.355	−0.048	–		
Lens thickness (LT)	0.001	−0.074	0.023	−0.625	–	
Vitreous chamber depth (VCD)	0.359	0.240	0.042	0.385	−0.326	–

Table 7.5 Inter-eye variation. All numbers represent values in millimeters, except where noted

Measure	Mean difference	Median difference	SD	Mean absolute difference	Median absolute difference	SD absolute difference
Central corneal thickness (microns)	−0.25 μ	−0.36 μ	9.85 μ	6.46 μ	4.82 μ	7.44 μ
Radius anterior cornea	0.01	0.01	0.09	0.06	0.05	0.06
Aqueous depth	−0.01	−0.01	0.19	0.12	0.07	0.15
Anterior chamber depth	−0.01	−0.01	0.19	0.12	0.07	0.15
Lens thickness	0.01	0.00	0.30	0.20	0.11	0.23
Vitreous chamber depth	0.02	0.03	0.44	0.27	0.17	0.35
Axial length	0.02	0.02	0.40	0.22	0.13	0.34
Horizontal corneal diameter	0.01	0.00	0.66	0.15	0.09	0.24

Table 7.6 Summary of biometry studies comparing race and sex differences. Percent differences calculated as: $(Value_{male} - Value_{female})/Value_{female}$. Values are expressed in millimeters. N/A = Not available

Study (year)	N	Method	Race	ACD female	ACD male	ACD percentage difference	AL female	AL male	AL percentage difference
Melles (2021)	80,479	Optical low coherence reflectometry (OLCR)	Multiple	3.11	3.24	4.2%	23.78	24.32	2.3%
Huang (2018)	6933	Partial coherence laser interferometry (PCLI)	Chinese	3.01	3.16	5.0%	23.88	24.79	3.8%
Hoffer (2017)	83,830	Various	Multiple	2.99	3.15	5.4%	23.23	23.75	2.2%
Hashemi (2012)	4869	OLCR	Iranian	2.58	2.66	3.1%	22.95	23.41	2.0%
Foster (2010)	2519	PCLI	White	3.08	3.15	2.3%	23.29	23.80	2.2%
Fotedar (2010)	1952	PCLI	White	3.06	3.16	3.3%	23.19	23.76	2.5%
Jivrajka (2008)	750	Immersion ultrasound	N/A	2.90	3.05	5.2%	23.27	23.76	2.1%
Warrier (2008)	1498	A-scan ultrasound	Burmese	2.79	2.86	2.5%	22.54	23.12	2.6%
Olsen (2007)	723	A-scan ultrasound	White	3.08	3.20	3.9%	23.20	23.74	2.3%

Table 7.6 summarizes the results from other large biometry studies. The results reported here closely aligned with those of previous reports, although the axial lengths were greater, possibly because the population studied included almost 20% Asian patients. In addition, values generated by different biometry methods may vary significantly. We have found in particular that optical low coherence reflectometry may overestimate anterior chamber depth and underestimate lens thickness compared to immersion ultrasound, a finding previously reported by Savini et al. [18]

References

1. Foster PJ, Broadway DC, Hayat S, Luben R, Dalzell N, Bingham S, Wareham JN, Khaw KT. Refractive error, axial length and anterior chamber depth of the eye in British adults: the EPIC-Norfolk Eye Study. Br J Ophthalmol. 2010;94:827–30.
2. Fotedar R, Wang JJ, Burlutsky G, Morgan IG, Rose K, Wong TY, Mitchell P. Distribution of axial length and ocular biometry measured using partial coherence laser interferometry (IOL Master) in an older white population. Ophthalmology. 2010;117:417–23.
3. Hashemi H, Khabazkhoob M, Miraftab M, Emanian MH, Shariati M, Abdolahinia T, Fotouhi A. The distribution of axial length, anterior chamber depth, lens thickness, and vitreous chamber depth in an adult population of Shahroud, Iran. BMC Ophthalmol. 2012;12:50.
4. He M, Huang W, Zheng Y, Alsbirk PH, Foster PJ. Anterior chamber depth in elderly Chinese: the Liwan eye study. Ophthalmology. 2008;115:1286–90.
5. Hoffer KJ. Biometry of 7,500 cataractous eyes. Am J Ophthalmol. 1980;90:360–8.
6. Hoffer KJ, Savini G. Effect of gender and race on ocular biometry. Int Ophthalmol Clin. 2017;57:137–42.
7. Huang Q, Huang Y, Luo Q, Fan W. Ocular biometric characteristics of cataract patients in western China. BMC Ophthalmol. 2018;18:1–9.
8. Jivrajka R, Shammas MC, Boenzi T, Swearingen M, Shammas HJ. Variability of axial length, anterior chamber depth, and lens thickness in the cataractous eye. J Cataract Refract Surg. 2008;34:289–94.
9. Lim LS, Saw S-M, Jeganathan VSE, Tay WT, Aung T, Tong L, Mitchell P, Wong TY. Distribution and determinants of ocular biometric parameters in an Asian population: the Singapore Malay Eye Study. Invest Ophthalmol Vis Sci. 2010;51:103–9.

10. Olsen T, Arnarsson A, Sasaki H, Sasaki K, Jonasson F. On the ocular refractive components: the Reykjavik Eye Study. Acta Ophthalmol Scand. 2007;85:361–6.

11. Pan CW, Wong TY, Chang L, Lin XY, Raghavan L, Zheng YF, Kok YO, Wu RY, Aung T, Saw SM. Ocular biometry in an urban Indian population: The Singapore Indian Eye Study (SINDI). Invest Ophthalmol Vis Sci. 2011;52:6636–42.

12. Warrier S, Wu HM, Newland HS, Muecke J, Selva D, Aung T, Casson RJ. Ocular biometry and determinants of refractive error in rural Myanmar: the Meiktila eye study. Br J Ophthalmol. 2008;92:1591–4.

13. Wickremasinghe S, Foster PJ, Uranchimeg D, Lee PS, Devereux JG, Alsbirk PH, Machin D, Johnson GJ, Baasanhu J. Ocular biometry and refraction in Mongolian adults. Invest Ophthalmol Vis Sci. 2004;45:776–83.

14. Yoon JJ, Misra SL, McGhee CH, Patel DV. Demographics and ocular biometric characteristics of patients undergoing cataract surgery in Auckland, New Zealand. Clin Exp Ophthalmol. 2016;44:106–13.

15. Kansal V, Schlendker M, Ahmed IK. Interocular axial length and corneal power differences as predictors of postoperative refractive outcomes after cataract surgery. Ophthalmology. 2018;125:972–81.

16. Zhang Y, Li T, Reddy A, Nallasamy N. Gender differences in refraction prediction error of five formulas for cataract surgery. BMC Ophthalmol. 2021;21:183.

17. Behndig A, Montan P, Lundstrom M, Zetterstrom C, Kugelberg M. Gender differences in biometry prediction error and intra-ocular lens power calculation formula. Acta Ophthalmol. 2014;92:759–63.

18. Savini G, Hoffer KJ, Schiano-Lomoriello D. Agreement between lens thickness measurements by ultrasound immersion biometry and optical biometry. J Cataract Refract Surg. 2018;44:1463–8.

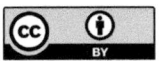

Part III

Measurements

Clinical Refraction

Sabong Srivannaboon

Postoperative refraction is one of the most important factors in determining the accuracy of intraocular lens (IOL) power calculation, as it plays a major role in the evaluation of each IOL formula and in the optimization of the IOL constant. Despite newer formulas, techniques, technologies, and IOL selections, patients still have postoperative refractive errors. This is where the method of back calculation using these postoperative refractions to evaluate and improve the accuracy of the next preoperative IOL power calculation can come into play. In addition, it has been reported that one of the three major sources contributing to the error of the IOL power calculation is the postoperative (PO) spectacle refraction [1]. Therefore, the most accurate PO refraction is essential to prevent future suboptimal refractive outcomes.

The accuracy of the IOL formula is usually evaluated by determining the prediction error (PE) [2] which is the difference between the predicted refraction from the IOL power implanted and the actual PO refraction. It is important to understand that this is not the same as the target refraction desired by the surgeon. For example, if the target refraction is −2.00 D and the IOL formula recommends a +22.0 D IOL with the prediction of the postoperative refraction of −2.15 D and the actual postoperative refraction is −2.25 D, then the prediction error (PE) is +0.10 D [(−2.15) − (−2.25) = (+0.10)]. The target refraction has nothing to do with the prediction error (PE).

Furthermore, optimization of the IOL constant also requires accurate postoperative refraction [3]. There are several methods for optimizing the IOL constant. For example, it can be calculated using the iterative method in which the IOL lens constant in each formula is varied in small steps (0.001) until the difference between the predicted postoperative refraction and the actual postoperative refraction is made equal to zero [3]. It can also be done automatically within some optical biometers by inputting the actual PO refraction or using an Excel spreadsheet (Microsoft, WA) Data Query function.

Basic Clinical Refraction

There are two types of clinical refractions: objective refraction and subjective refraction. The objective refraction includes the use of a retinoscope or an autorefractometer. The subjective refraction can be done using a trial lens set or a phoropter. The retinoscope is not commonly used in pseudophakic eyes, especially after the implantation of a multifocal IOL or an extended-depth-of-focus IOL. The luminous reflex from the retina can be ambiguous due to the aberration of the

S. Srivannaboon (✉)
Department of Ophthalmology, Siriraj Hospital, Mahidol University, Bangkok, Thailand

J. Aramberri et al. (eds.), *Intraocular Lens Calculations*, Essentials in Ophthalmology,
https://doi.org/10.1007/978-3-031-50666-6_8

Table 8.1 The mean ± standard deviation values of sphere, cylinder, axis, and spherical equivalent value derived from autorefractometer and subjective refraction. Note that both sphere and cylinder value as well as spherical equivalent show statistically significant differences between the groups but not the axis

	Auto-refractometer	Subjective refraction	p value
Sphere	−0.75 ±0.31	−0.33 ± 0.39	<0.05*
Cylinder	−0.60 ± 0.36	−0.35 ± 0.40	<0.05*
Axis	90.51	90.71	0.65
Spherical equivalent	−1.05 ± 0.26	−0.50 ± 0.41	<0.05*

IOL. Most of the time, the subjective refraction is the preferred method. There are some debates on whether to use the autorefractometer or subjective refraction. Bullimore et al. [4] found autorefraction to be more reproducible (SD ± 0.19 D) than subjective refraction. However, Zadnik et al. [5] reported differently. Srivannaboon et al. [6] also showed the difference between autorefractometer measurement and subjective manifest refraction in a group of monofocal pseudophakic patients as shown in Table 8.1. The spherical and cylindrical values as well as the spherical equivalent values show statistically significant differences between groups but not for the axis. Therefore, it is recommended to use subjective refraction for the evaluation of the accuracy of IOL power calculation and IOL constant optimization. If the autorefractometer is used, it must always be verified by the subjective refraction.

Key Points in Subjective Refraction

– Standardization

Since an accurate postoperative refraction is essential for optimal refractive outcomes in IOL calculation, a standardized refraction method must be carried out by anyone who performs refraction (surgeons and technicians). In the least, the network of co-management with any surgery center should apply a standardized method where all refractionists utilize the same methodology. This standardization leads to a better repeatability and reproducibility of manifest refraction for the evaluation of the refractive outcomes in IOL calculation. Taneri et al. [7] reported the intra-observer repeatability and inter-observer reproducibility of manifest refraction in a specialized refractive clinic with standardized protocol is better than the typical step used for manifest refraction (0.25 diopter). Reinstein et al. [8] also showed similar results. Therefore, it is imperative that a standardized protocol of refraction be achieved.

– Accurate Spherical and Cylindrical Values

Since the accurate PO refraction is very essential for the IOL power calculation, it is especially important to get the accurate spherical (Sph) and cylindrical (Cyl) values as well as the axis. Although the spherical equivalent (SE) refraction is mostly used for evaluation of the IOL formulas and optimization of the IOL constant, it is the combination of the spherical value and half of the cylindrical value [SE = Sph + (Cyl/2)]. Moreover, with the recent development of several toric IOL lens calculators, the toric evaluation also requires accurate cylindrical refractive measurement including the axis.

– Best-Corrected Visual Acuity

The best-corrected visual acuity must be the best visual acuity that can be achieved with refraction. Some technicians stop performing refraction when the patient reach 20/20 visual acuity, when in fact the patient can be better than that. Therefore, 20/20 visual acuity is not the end point of refraction.

– Testing Distance

The testing distance of the visual acuity chart must be set correctly. It is very important to understand that the measurement of the visual acuity at each refractive state of the eye is the measurement of minimal visual angle in which the patient resolves to see the letter (minimal resolvable acuity). It depends on the size of the letter and the testing distance. The required testing distance of each visual acuity chart must be checked. A 6-m distance (20 feet) is generally the preferred choice [9]. A 4-m chart test can be converted to a 6-m test chart by adding the value of −0.08 D to the spherical equivalent refraction derived by a 4-m chart [10].

– Timing

In general, postoperative refraction is recommended to be performed at least 1 month after the cataract surgery (preferably 3 months if a larger incision wound size is constructed) or when refraction is stable. With modern microincision cataract surgery (1.8–2.5-mm wound size) and foldable single-piece IOL, the refraction may seem stable at 2 weeks; however, it is still suggested to wait at least 1 month ideally.

– Correct Technique

The principle of subjective refraction in the pseudophakic eye is very similar to the phakic eye. The goal is to determine the strength of the corrective lens that will achieve the perfect focus of parallel rays of light from a distant object onto the retina as a single point. It is called the focal point of the eye. With the trial lens set or phoropter, the focal point of the eye can be identified by searching for the lens with the best-corrected visual acuity. Refining the power of the lens can be done using the same technique as in the phakic eye. The red-green duochrome test may be useful, but with some IOLs that filter a certain wavelength of the light, the red-green perception of the patient may be changed [11]. Thus, caution should be made with the red-green duochrome technique in these types of intraocular lenses. The fogging technique with a plus lens is recommended to get the most plus or the least minus focal point of pseudophakic eyes. Due to the modern technology of IOLs, the focal point of

the lens can be varied, such as monofocal IOLs, multifocal IOLs (bifocal or trifocal), and extended-depth-of-focus IOLs (an elongated focal point). The best way to understand the least minus end point is to understand the defocus curves of these pseudophakic eyes.

Defocus curves are plotted by presenting a series of negative and positive lenses (from +3.00 to −5.00 D in 0.50 D increments, or from +2.00 to −4.00 D in some studies) in front of the patient's eye and measuring the amount of "blur or defocus" that the lens induces. The amount of blur is determined by the visual acuity. The X-axis represents the power of the presenting lens, and the Y-axis represents the visual acuity. In general, the zero reference on the X-axis is set by the best-possible distance visual acuity. This is because the defocus curve is designed to evaluate the performance of the IOL without the bias of the error produced by the IOL power calculation. Therefore, defocus curves must be tested on the best-corrected visual acuity. Understanding defocus curves in each type of IOL will help to understand how the lens performs inside the eye and how the end point of refraction in these pseudophakic eyes is reached.

Refraction in the Presence of a Monofocal IOL

A monofocal IOL has only a single focal point. It is not difficult to identify the focal point of this lens because there is only one peak of the best-possible visual acuity. Therefore, subjective refraction is not difficult. Any refraction that achieves the best-possible visual acuity is the final subjective refraction.

Figure 8.1 shows the defocus curve of monofocal IOLs. There is only one peak of the best visual acuity.

The subjective refraction method is similar to that of phakic eyes. The sphere with the most plus or least minus power giving the best visual acuity is identified. The cross cylinder is then introduced

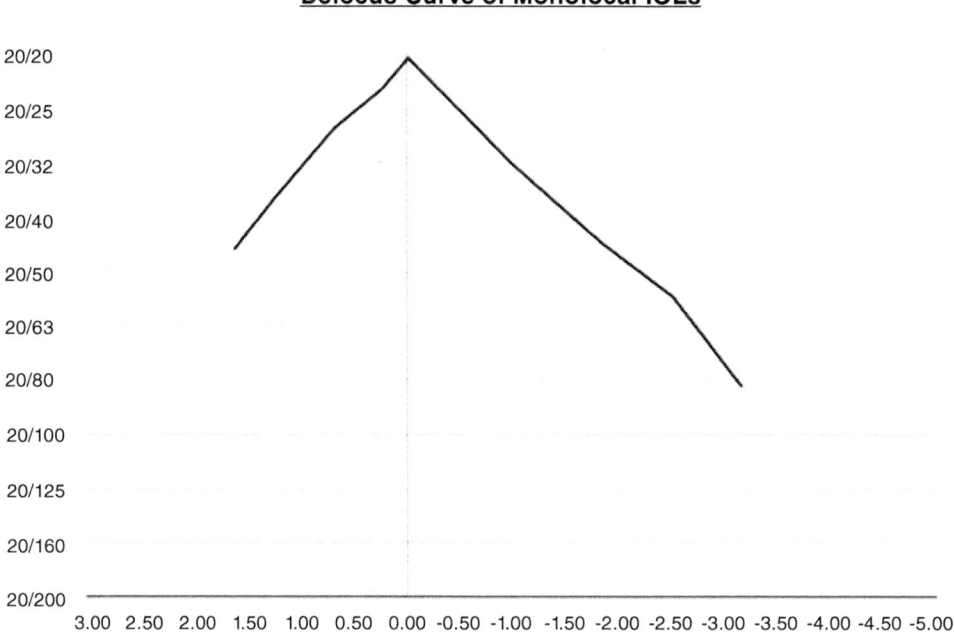

Fig. 8.1 A defocus curve of monofocal IOLs

to find the axis and amount of cylinder. Normally, the cylinder axis needs to be refined before the cylinder power, and it is recommended to use the ±0.25 D Jackson cross cylinder rather than the ±0.37 D or ±0.50 D for the evaluation of toric IOL outcomes. Refraction is measured with the natural pupil size in normal light conditions. Mydriasis can alter refraction outcome depending on the IOL design: certain aspheric and multifocal profiles are pupil dependent.

Generally, it is thought that there is no accommodation in pseudophakic eyes. Although this is true in most pseudophakic monofocal IOL patients, there are certain patients with monofocal IOLs who achieve good visual acuity for both distance and near. This phenomenon was previ-

ously known as apparent accommodation or pseudo-accommodation [12, 13]. In these cases, there is a range of refraction in which the patient can achieve best-possible visual acuity. This range is the amplitude of apparent accommodation. The final refraction should be on the most plus or least minus point of the best-possible visual acuity. Therefore, using the fogging technique with a plus lens is very useful in these cases.

Figure 8.2 shows a defocus curve of monofocal IOLs with pseudo-accommodation. There is a small range of refraction where patients can achieve the best-corrected visual acuity. The final refraction should be at point a (arrow).

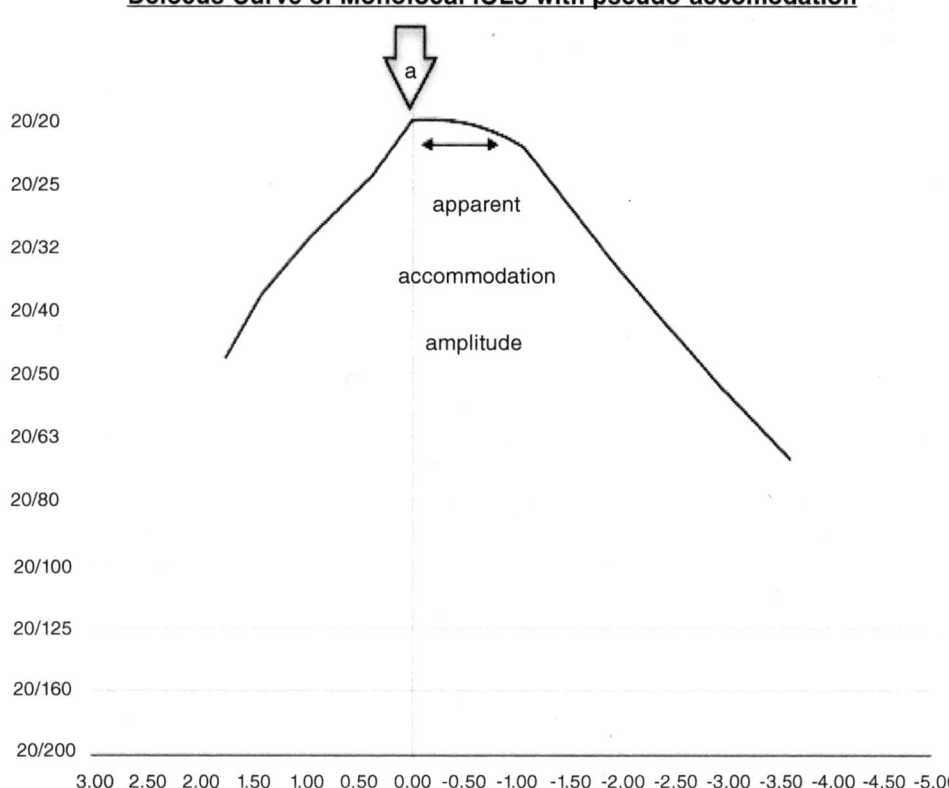

Fig. 8.2 A defocus curve of monofocal IOLs with pseudo-accommodation

Refraction in the Presence of Multifocal IOLs

A multifocal IOL has more than one focal point. It can be bifocal (two focal points) or trifocal (three focal points) depending on the design of the lens. There is only one "far" focal point, and this point should be the point of final refraction. In low-add power bifocal IOLs, the "near" focal point can be close to the "far" focal point. In trifocal IOLs, the "intermediate" focal point can also be very close to the "far" focal point. The proximity of these focal points can lead to an incorrect refraction. It is very crucial to locate the "far" focal point. In some eyes, identifying all focal points is very helpful to know which focal point is being measured. Because there are two or three points of the best-possi-

ble visual acuity in these lenses, the one with the most plus or least minus is the final refraction.

Figure 8.3 shows a defocus curve of bifocal IOLs . There are two points of the best-possible visual acuity in this lens: the far focal point (a) and the near focal point (b). There is a significant drop in visual acuity between both points. The final refraction should be at point a. Identify the existing point (b) should be identified to ensure that point (a) is the correct far focal point.

For example, if the refraction of −0.75 D achieves the best vision of 20/20 in a bifocal pseudophakic eye, searching for the other focal point is necessary to ensure that the far focal point is measured, not the near focal point (Fig. 8.4a, b).

Figure 8.4 shows a defocus curve of low-add bifocal IOLs. The second focal point (b) is moved

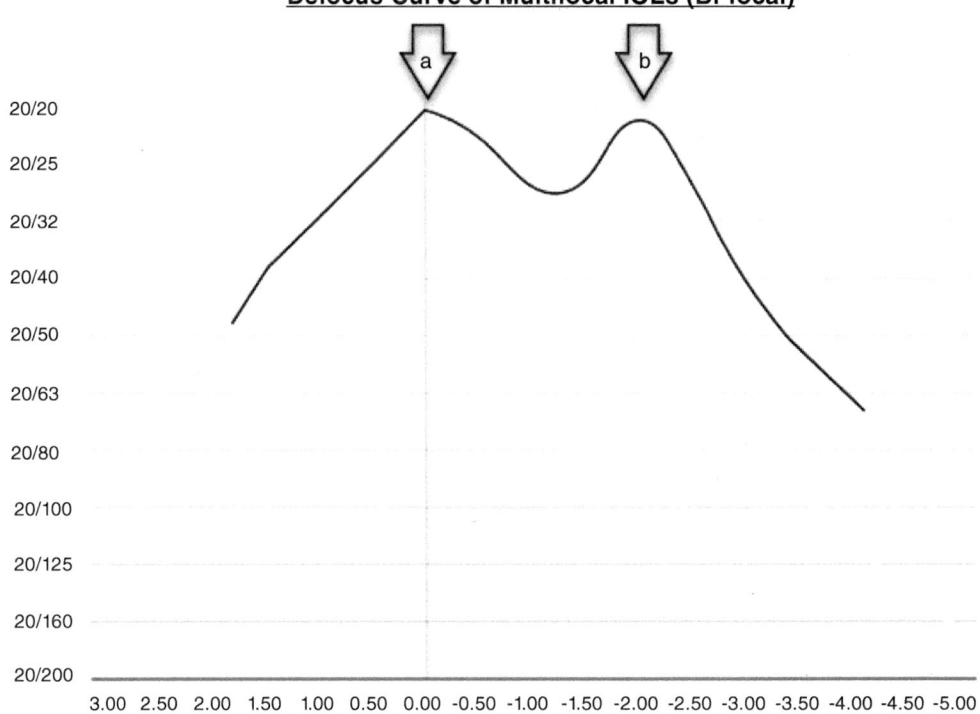

Fig. 8.3 A defocus curve of multifocal IOLs (bifocal)

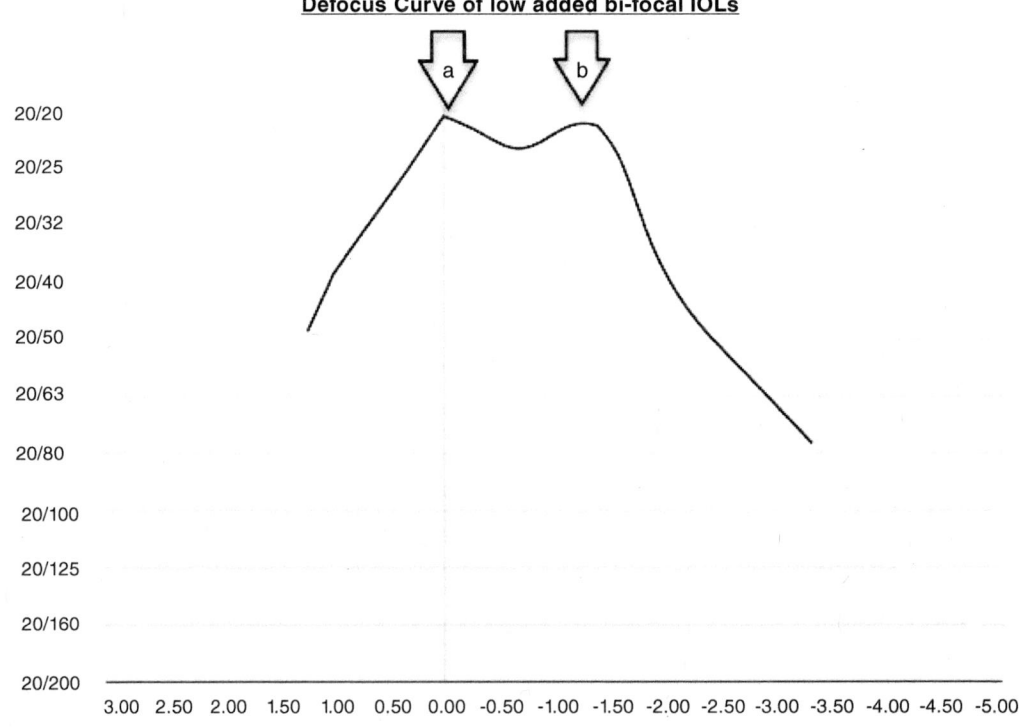

Fig. 8.4 A defocus curve of low-add bifocal IOLs

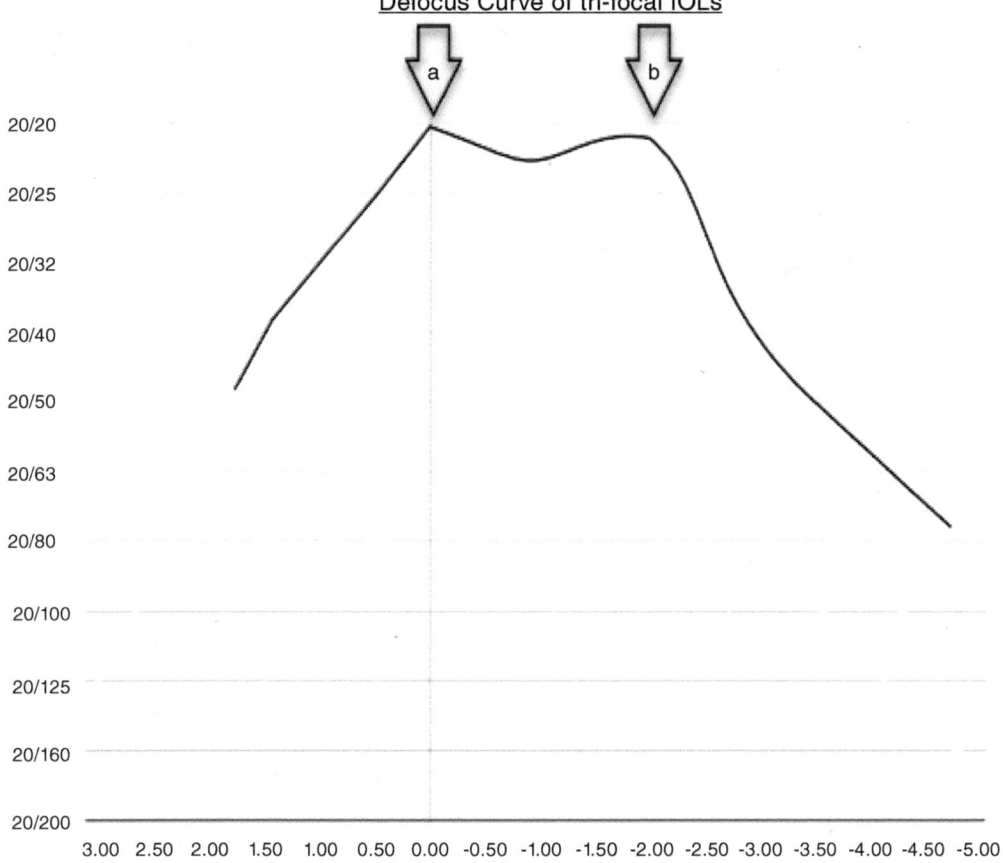

Fig. 8.5 A defocus curve of trifocal IOLs

close to the far focal point (a). The dropping of visual acuity between both points is less than high-add multifocal IOLs. Therefore, identifying the best-possible visual acuity is more difficult than high-add multifocal IOLs. The final refraction should be at point a.

Figure 8.5 shows a defocus curve of trifocal IOLs [14]. The intermediate focal point is not as distinct as the far (a) and near (b) focal points. Therefore, there are only two points of the best-possible acuity, but the dropping of visual acuity between these points is much less than bifocal IOLs. Again, identifying the best-possible visual acuity is more difficult than with bifocal IOLs. The final refraction should be at point a.

Refraction in the Presence of Extended-Depth-of-Focus (EdoF) IOL

Extended-depth-of-focus (EdoF) IOL technology has recently been introduced. It focuses incoming light into an extended longitudinal plane, rather than a focal point. Similar to phakic eyes with accommodation, there is a range of refraction that a patient can achieve their best-possible visual acuity. The final refraction should be on the most plus or least minus point of the best-possible visual acuity. Therefore, fogging technique with a plus lens is very useful in these cases.

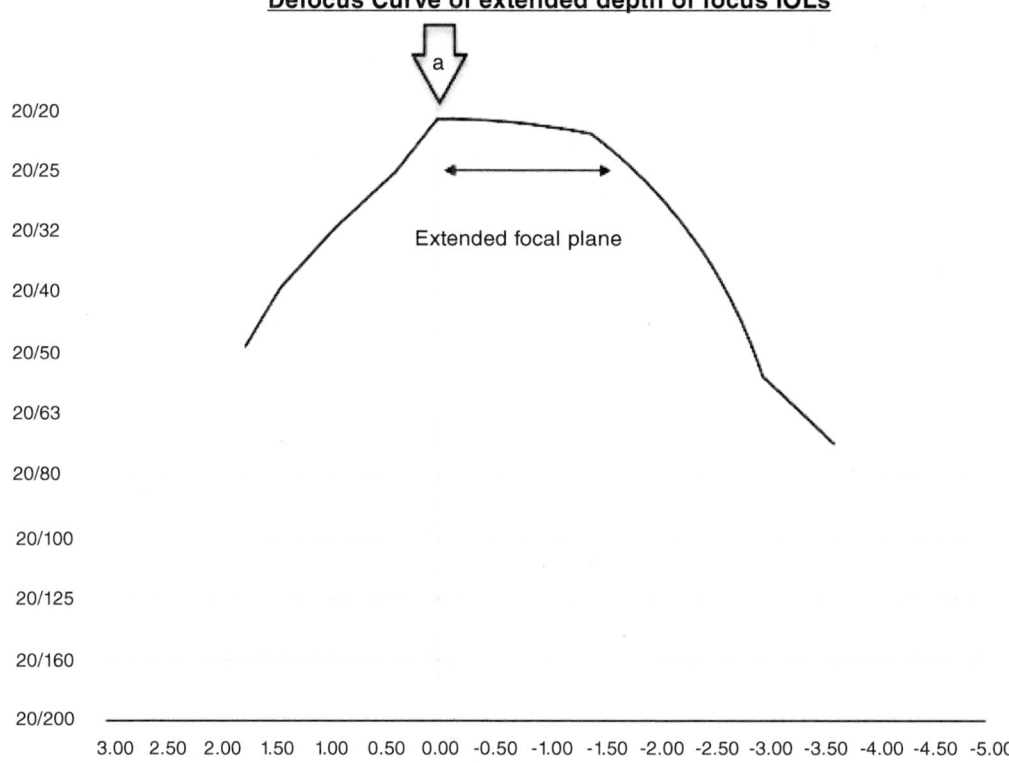

Fig. 8.6 A defocus curve of extended-depth-of-focus (EdoF) IOLs

Figure 8.6 shows a defocus curve of extended-depth-for focus (EdoF) IOLs. Note that there is a range of refraction that can achieve their best-corrected visual acuity. This is the extended longitudinal focal plane of the lens. The final refraction should be at point a.

end point is always on the most plus or least minus refraction that results in the best-possible visual acuity in that eye. The visual acuity of 20/20 is not always the end point of refraction. Using a pinhole occluder over subjective refraction might be useful to confirm the best-possible corrected visual acuity. Therefore, it is important to understand clinical refraction in the pseudophakic eye to achieve the most accurate postoperative refraction.

Summary

Identifying the end point of a subjective manifest refraction is an art. It requires proper technique to locate the correct far focal point. In pseudophakic eyes, the optic of the whole eye changes according to the type of IOL implanted in the eye. Various types of IOLs produce different ways of refracting light. Therefore, understanding the optics of the implanted IOL is very beneficial to performing the most accurate subjective manifest refraction in these patients. The defocus curve of the implanted IOL should be known before performing the subjective refraction. In general, the

Acknowledgment Thank you to Dr. Morakot Tanehsakdi, OD, for assistance in English language editing and writing input for this chapter.

References

1. Norrby S. Sources of error in intraocular lens power calculation. J Cataract Refract Surg. 2008;34(3):368–76.
2. Hoffer KJ, Aramberri J, Haigis W, Olsen T, Savini G, Shammas HJ, et al. Protocols for studies of

intraocular lens formula accuracy. Am J Ophthalmol. 2015;160(3):403–5.

3. Aristodemou P, Knox Cartwright NE, Sparrow JM, Johnston RL. Intraocular lens formula constant optimization and partial coherence interferometry biometry: refractive outcomes in 8108 eyes after cataract surgery. J Cataract Refract Surg. 2011;37(1):50–62.

4. Bullimore MA, Fusaro RE, Adams CW. The repeatability of automated and clinician refraction. Optom Vis Sci. 1998;75(8):617–22.

5. Zadnik K, Mutti DO, Adams AJ. The repeatability of measurement of the ocular components. Invest Ophthalmol Vis Sci. 1992;33(7):2325–33.

6. Srivannaboon S. Evaluation of the toric IOLs outcomes; expect the unexpected. In: Proceeding of the 34th meeting: the Royal College of Ophthalmologists of Thailand. Bangkok, Thailand: RCOPT;2014.

7. Taneri S, Arba-Mosquera S, Rost A, Kießler S, Dick HB. Repeatability and reproducibility of manifest refraction. J Cataract Refract Surg. 2020;46(12):1659–66.

8. Reinstein DZ, Yap TE, Carp GI, Archer TJ, Gobbe M. London Vision Clinic optometric group. Reproducibility of manifest refraction between surgeons and optometrists in a clinical refractive surgery practice. J Cataract Refract Surg. 2014;40(3):450–9.

9. Simpson MJ, Charman WN. The effect of testing distance on intraocular lens power calculation. J Refract Surg. 2014;30(11):726.

10. Hoffer KJ, Savini G. Update on intraocular lens power calculation study protocols: the better way to design and report clinical trials. Ophthalmology. 2020;S0161-6420(20):30638-2.

11. Friström B, Lundh BL. Color contrast sensitivity in cataract and pseudophakia. Acta Ophthalmol Scand. 2000;78(5):506–11.

12. Elder MJ, Murphy C, Sanderson GF. Apparent accommodation and depth of field in pseudophakia. J Cataract Refract Surg. 1996;22(5):615–9.

13. Niessen AGJE, de Jong LB, van der Heijde GL. Pseudo-accommodation in pseudophakia. Eur J Implant Refract Surg. 1992;4(2):91–4.

14. Böhm M, Petermann K, Hemkeppler E, Kohnen T. Defocus curves of 4 presbyopia-correcting IOL designs: diffractive panfocal, diffractive trifocal, segmental refractive, and extended-depth-of focus. J Cataract Refract Surg. 2019;45(11):1625–36.

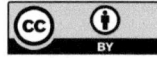

Ultrasound Biometry

9

Maya C. Shammas and H. John Shammas

Ultrasound biometry measures the axial length (AL) with an A-scan biometer. In the 1970s, 1980s, and 1990s, A-scan biometry was widely used to measure the AL [1–3]. Although modern biometry has evolved with the introduction of optical biometry in 1999 and swept-source optical coherence tomography in 2016, the acquisition rate never reached 100% of the cataractous eyes. In these eyes with advanced cataracts, A-scan biometry is still being used to acquire the AL.

During biometry, the ultrasound beam is aligned with the optical axis of the eye (Fig. 9.1). The emitted sound beam will meet multiple interfaces. At each interface, part of the sound beam is reflected toward the probe and the remainder of the sound beam keeps propagating deeper into the tissues. This process will generate echospikes from the different interfaces that have been intersected: the anterior surface of the cornea, posterior surface of the cornea, anterior surface of the lens, posterior surface of the lens, anterior surface of the retina, and the anterior surface of the sclera. When the ultrasound beam reaches the orbital tissues, it is attenuated until it loses all its energy. The reflected sound beam returns to the

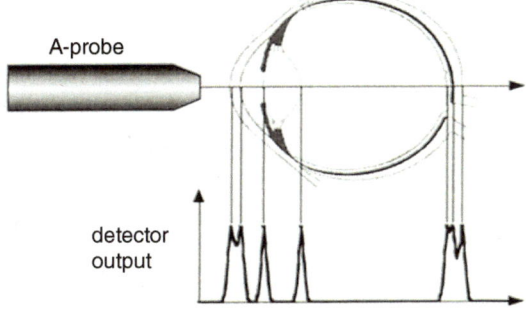

Fig. 9.1 The ultrasound beam is perpendicular to the cornea, the anterior and posterior lens surfaces, and to the retina. Please note the peaks generated when the beam intersects the anterior corneal surface, the posterior corneal surface, the anterior lens surface, the posterior lens surface, and the retina. Extra spikes are generated behind the retinal one by the sclera and the orbital tissues

transducer that also acts as a receiver. The pulses are then processed within the biometer to display "echo signals" on the screen.

Basic Principles of A-Scan Echography

In A-scan echography, an electro-acoustic device called a *transducer* is used as both a source and detector of sound. The transducer is typically mounted at the tip of a handheld probe. In an ideal world, the sound produced by the transducer would be an *impulse*. Each time this sound

M. C. Shammas
Shammas Eye Center, Lynwood, CA, USA

H. John Shammas (✉)
The Keck School of Medicine of USC,
Los Angeles, CA, USA

© The Author(s) 2024
J. Aramberri et al. (eds.), *Intraocular Lens Calculations*, Essentials in Ophthalmology,
https://doi.org/10.1007/978-3-031-50666-6_9

impulse crosses an interface, a similar "echo" impulse would be reflected back and detected by the transducer. For a variety of reasons, no real-world transducer can produce an ideal impulse. What we get instead is a sound pulse of finite duration, whose sound-pressure graph is like that shown in Fig. 9.2.

To turn these into a nice echo graph, something like that of Fig. 9.1, an electronic circuit called an *envelope detector* is used. Given the pulse shown in Fig. 9.3 as input, this circuit will output a voltage signal corresponding to the instantaneous intensity of the echo, as shown in Fig. 9.4.

The width or "thickness" of the detector output pulse determines how well the A-scan system can distinguish closely spaced interfaces—its *axial resolution*. Many factors combine to determine this pulse width, one of the most important being the *bandwidth* of the system electronics. An A-scan system with a large bandwidth will produce narrower echospikes—hence

higher resolution—than the one with a smaller bandwidth.

During A-scan biometry, alignment of the ultrasound beam is extremely important. To display the highest spikes possible, the ultrasound beam must stay perpendicular to the smooth and regular surfaces it intersects, whether it is the anterior and posterior corneal surfaces, the anterior and posterior lens surfaces, or most importantly the retinal surface, forming an incidence angle of 90° with each of these surfaces. If the ultrasound beam is aimed tangentially at any of the surfaces, the related echospike will be displayed much smaller or not at all (Fig. 9.4). Small echospikes can also be displayed if the surface in question is irregular due to scattering of the ultrasound beam when it intersects the irregular surface (Fig. 9.5).

In the displayed echograph (Fig. 9.1), the time axis of the graph indicates the "time-of-flight" of the impulse—the total time it takes for the impulse to travel from the transducer to a given

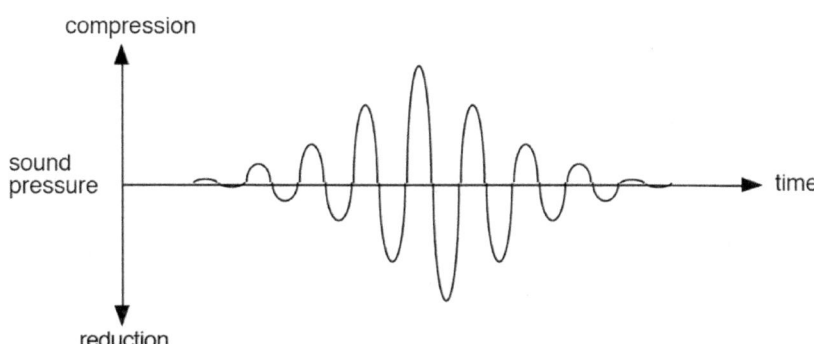

Fig. 9.2 A sound-pressure graph of a realistic A-scan pulse

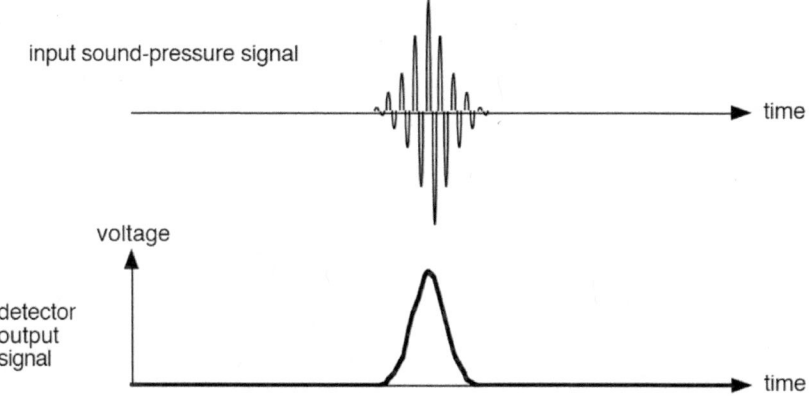

Fig. 9.3 An envelope-detector response to a realistic A-scan pulse

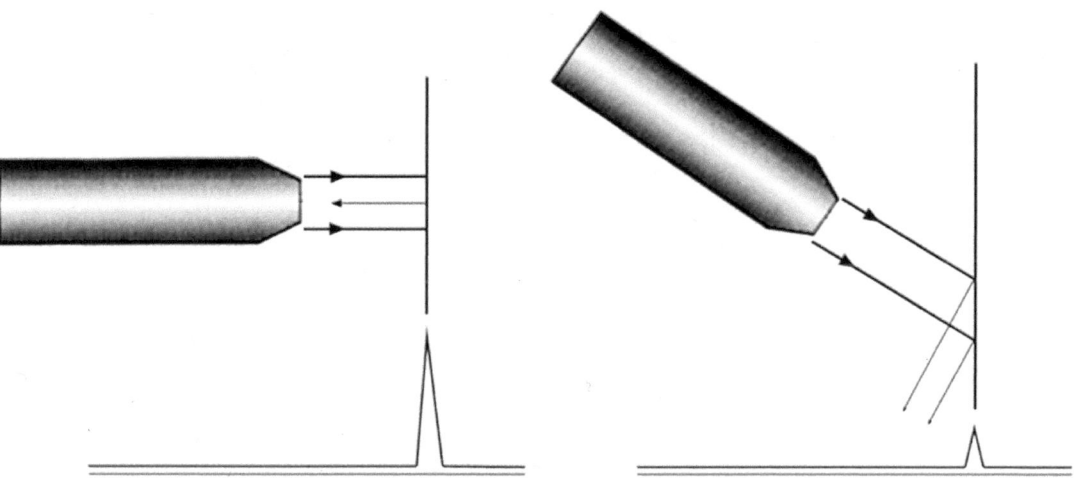

Fig. 9.4 A sharp and tall echospike is displayed when the ultrasound beam is kept perpendicular to the surface under study. A smaller echospike is displayed when the ultrasound beam is tangential to the same surface

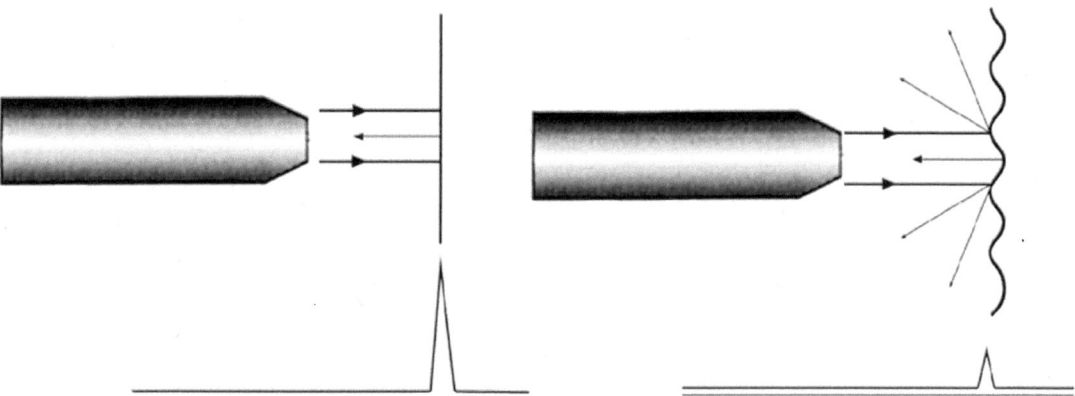

Fig. 9.5 A smaller echospike is displayed when the ultrasound beam encounters an irregular surface. Note the scattering of the beam when it intersects the irregular surface

interface and back to the transducer. The times at which echo impulses are received can be used to compute the distances between the corresponding interfaces, provided we know the sound velocity. The formula is:

$$d = tv / 2,$$

where d is distance, t is echospike time (taken from the horizontal axis of the echo graph in Fig. 9.1), and v is sound velocity. The factor of 2 occurs because the echospike time t is a time-of-flight measurement of the time required for the sound to travel the distance d twice (outward from the transducer, then back).

A little careful analysis reveals that this formula can be slightly modified to compute distances *between* adjacent interfaces, based on the time *difference* between the corresponding echospikes, using the specific velocity for the intervening medium. For example, the first two echospikes in the graph shown in Fig. 9.1 correspond, as shown, to the anterior and posterior surfaces of the cornea. The velocity of sound in the corneal tissue has been measured experimentally to be 1641 m/s. So, if the anterior and posterior corneal echospikes occur at points t_{C1} and t_{C2}, respectively, on the echo graph time axis, the corneal thickness, T_C can be computed as.

$$T_C = \left[(t_{C2} - t_{C1}) \times 1641\right] / 2.$$

Similarly, the anterior chamber depth can be computed from the time between the posterior cornea and anterior lens echospikes using the velocity 1532 m/s for aqueous; the lens depth can be computed from the time between the anterior and posterior lens spikes using the velocity 1641 m/s for the natural lens, and the vitreous cavity depth can be computed from the time between the posterior lens and retina spikes using the velocity 1532 m/s for vitreous. Moreover, we can correct for other media by using the proper velocities, for example, 980 m/s for silicone IOLs, 2718 m/s for PMMA IOLs, and so on. Modern A-scan biometers perform such calculations automatically.

Measurement Technique

Immersion Technique

The immersion technique is the preferred examination method [4] because it eliminates any corneal compression during the exam:

- The patient is placed in a supine position on a flat examination table or in a reclining examination chair, and a drop of local anesthetic is instilled in both eyes.
- A scleral shell is applied to the eye. The most used scleral shells are the Hansen shell, the Prager shell, and the Kohn shell (Fig. 9.6).

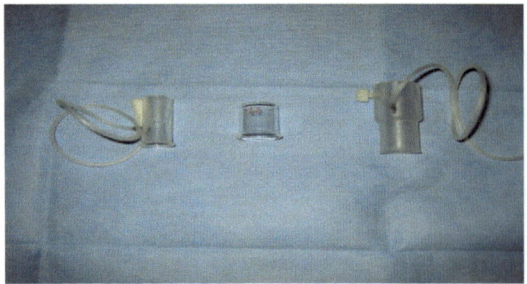

Fig. 9.6 Popular shells used for immersion biometry. From left to right, the Kohn shell, the Hansen shell, and the Praeger shell

The Hansen shells are available in 16-, 18-, 20-, 22-, and 24-mm diameter. Other types of scleral shells are also available from different manufacturers.

- The flared edges of the scleral shell are placed between the lids, making sure that the cup is stable on the eye (Fig. 9.7).
- The Hansen shell is filled with gonioscopic solution (Fig. 9.8). Methylcellulose 1% is preferred over the 2.5% concentration (too thick) and over saline solutions (too liquid). The solution should be free of air bubbles; the presence of bubbles causes variations in the speed of sound and is responsible for noise formation within the ultrasound pattern. The easiest way to avoid bubbles is to remove the bottle's nipple and pour the solution into the cup. If bubbles do form within the solution, they are removed with a syringe, and, if unsuccessful, the cup must be emptied, cleaned, repositioned, and refilled with gonioscopic solution.
- The ultrasound probe is immersed in the solution keeping it 5–10 mm away from the cornea (Fig. 9.9). The patient is asked to look, with the fellow eye, at a fixation point placed at the

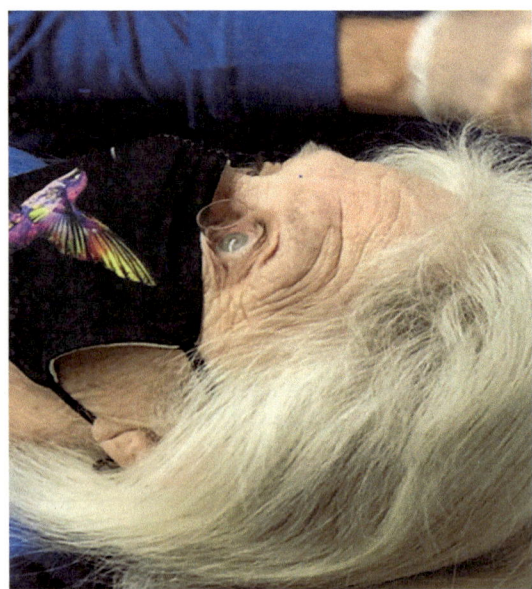

Fig. 9.7 Immersion A-scan biometry. The Hansen shell with its flared edges is placed between the lids

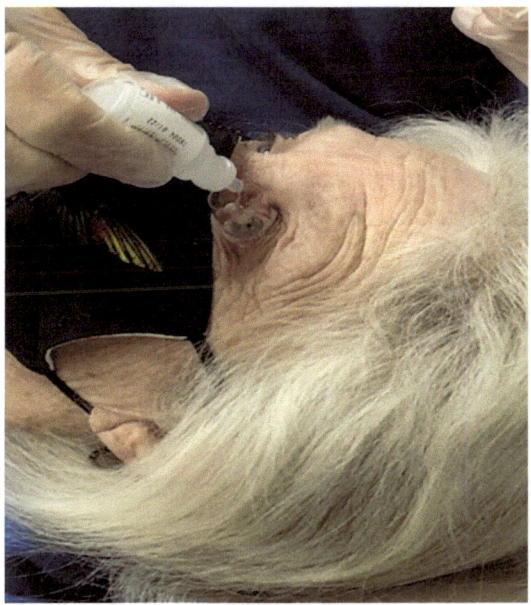

Fig. 9.8 Immersion A-scan biometry. The Hansen shell is filled with gonioscopic solution

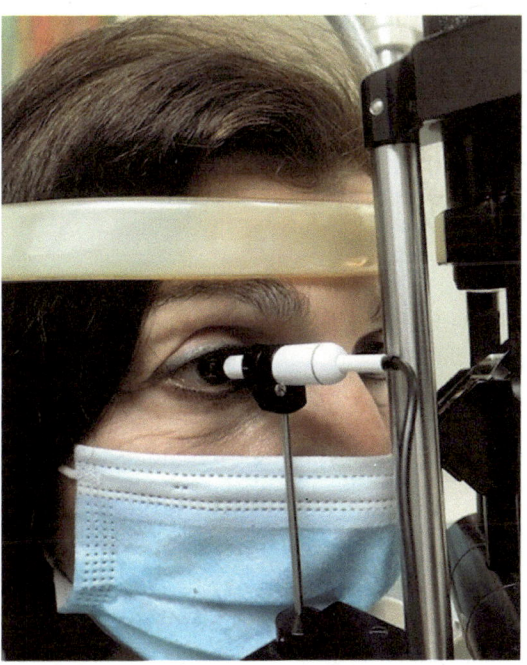

Fig. 9.10 Contact A-scan biometry. The patient is examined in the seated position. The technician uses the joystick to align the probe with the eye to be measured

Contact Technique

The contact technique was popularized in the 1980s [5–7]. The probe is brought forward to gently touch the cornea without indenting it (Fig. 9.10). In a prospective study on 180 eyes performed by the author [6], axial length measurements were obtained on each eye with both contact and immersion techniques. Axial length measurements obtained with the contact technique were shorter than those obtained with the immersion technique by an average of 0.24 mm.

The two methods of examination differ in the patient's position and the possible corneal applanation by the ultrasound probe. The patient is conventionally examined in the seated position with the contact technique, and the probe is brought forward to touch the cornea.

The patient is conventionally examined in the supine position with the immersion technique, and the solid probe is kept 5–10 mm away from the cornea. These differences in the methods of examination, mainly the corneal indentation and the subsequent shallowing of the anterior cham-

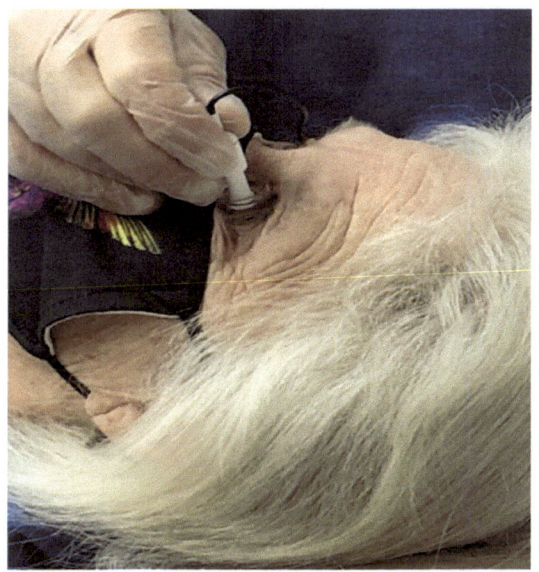

Fig. 9.9 Immersion A-scan biometry. The ultrasound probe is immersed in the solution, keeping it 5–10 mm away from the cornea

ceiling. Attention is then focused on the screen. The probe is gently moved until it is properly aligned with the optical axis of the eye and an acceptable A-scan echogram is displayed on the screen. A printout is obtained.

ber, are responsible for the shorter measurement obtained with the contact technique.

A-Scan Pattern of the Phakic Eye

Identifying the Echospikes

The A-scan pattern of a normal phakic eye examined with an immersion technique (Fig. 9.11) displays the following echospikes from left to right [8, 9]:

IS: The initial spike (IS) is produced at the tip of the probe. It has no clinical significance. Many units will allow the technician to move the whole A-scan pattern to the left and remove the IS from the picture.

C: The corneal spike (C) is double-peaked representing the anterior and posterior surfaces of the cornea.

L1: The anterior lens spike (L1) is generated from the anterior surface of the lens.

L2: The posterior lens spike (L2) is generated from the posterior surface of the lens and is usually smaller than L1.

R: The retinal spike (R) is generated from the anterior surface of the retina. This surface is highly reflective resulting in a straight, high-reflective, and tall echospike whenever the ultrasound beam is perpendicular to the retina, as it should be during axial length measurement. The scleral spike is another high-reflective spike generated from the scleral surface, right behind the retinal spike, and should not be confused with it. The orbital spikes are low reflective behind the scleral spike.

With a contact technique, the probe touches the cornea, and the initial spike merges with the anterior corneal echospike forming an overloaded first echospike that appears wider and truncated at the top (Fig. 9.12). The remainder of the echospikes are displayed the same as in the immersion technique.

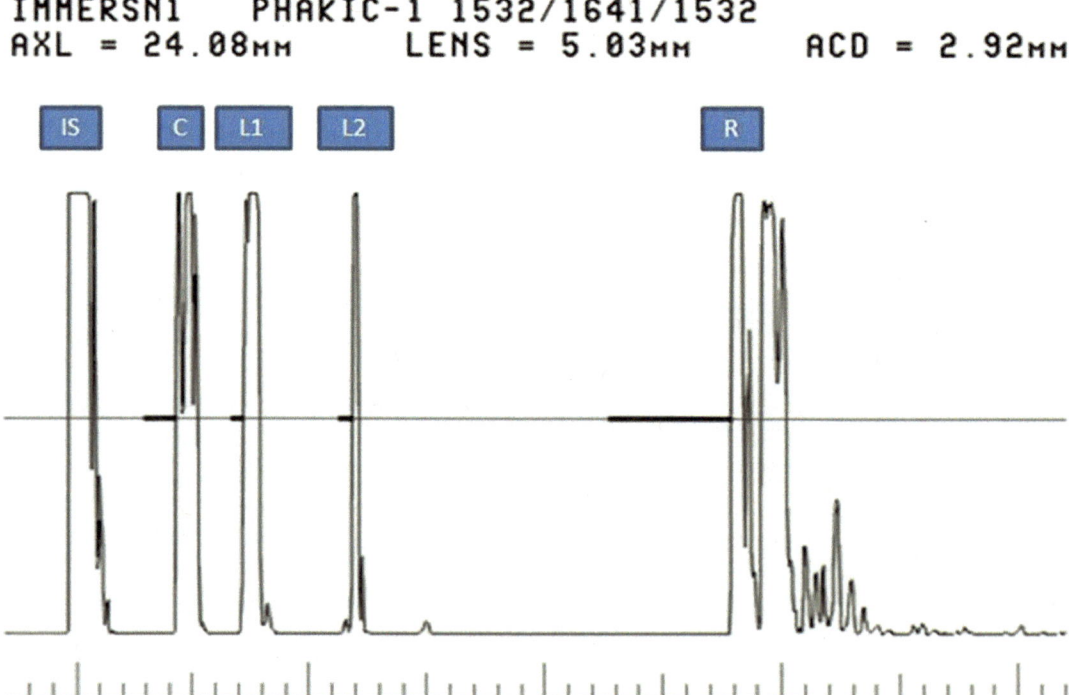

Fig. 9.11 An A-scan display of a phakic eye during immersion A-scan biometry, identifying the initial spike (IS), the cornea (C), the anterior lens surface (L1), the posterior lens surface (L2), and the retina (R)

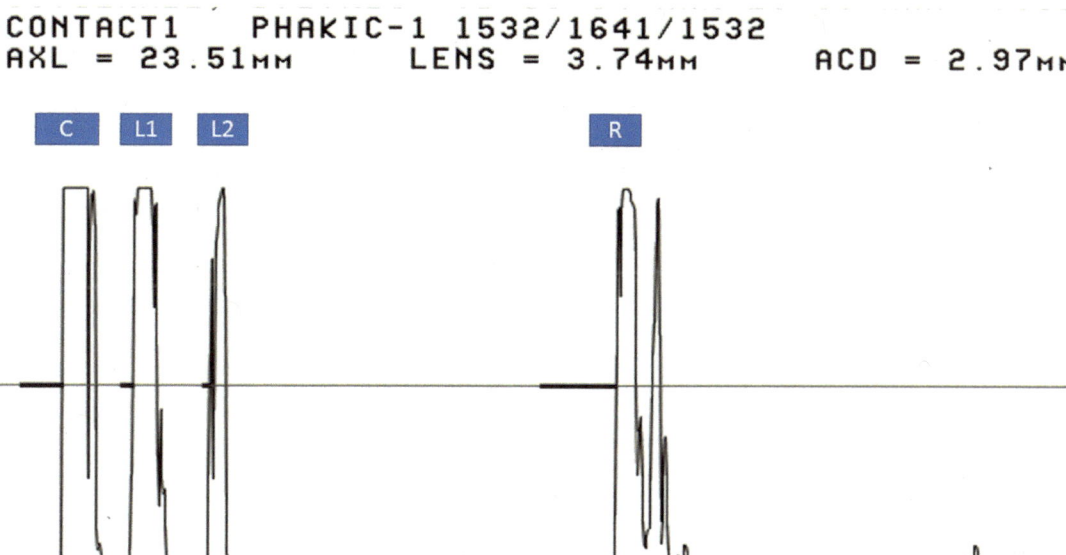

```
CONTACT1     PHAKIC-1 1532/1641/1532
AXL = 23.51mm        LENS = 3.74mm        ACD = 2.97mm
```

Fig. 9.12 An A-scan display of a phakic eye during contact A-scan biometry, identifying the cornea (C), the anterior lens surface (L1), the posterior lens surface (L2), and the retina (R)

Setting the Appropriate Velocities

Most modern biometers use separate sound velocities for the different eye components to obtain the total axial length [10–14]. The eye is divided ultrasonically into four compartments:

- The corneal thickness is measured between the anterior and posterior surfaces of the cornea using a velocity of 1620 m/s.
- The aqueous depth is measured between the posterior corneal surface and the anterior lens surface using a velocity of 1532 m/s. The anterior chamber depth, usually displayed on the screen, is the sum of the corneal thickness and aqueous depth.
- The lens thickness is measured between the anterior and the posterior lens surfaces, using a velocity of 1641 m/s. The sound velocity in cataractous eyes varies from 1588 to 1622 m/s with a slower velocity (average 1590 m/s) in the intumescent cataracts due to their high water content, and a higher velocity in the posterior capsular cataracts.

- The vitreous cavity's depth is measured between the posterior lens surface (L2) and the anterior surface of the retina (R) using a velocity of 1532 m/s.

Although it is best to measure the different ocular compartments at their specific sound velocities, the use of an average sound velocity of 1553 m/s yields clinically insignificant errors in the average 23.5-mm eye. However, it can yield around a 0.05-mm longer measurement in the long eye and around a 0.07-mm shorter measurement in the short eye.

In the presence of an intumescent cataract, the lens increases its water content and becomes thicker (over 5.0 mm). Concomitantly, the sound velocity decreases to around 1590 m/s from the usual 1641 m/s. Many biometers do an internal adjustment for an intumescent cataract; however, the erroneous use of a 1641-m/s sound lens velocity will yield a 0.10–0.15-mm longer measurement, calling for a weaker IOL and resulting in a slightly more hyperopic final refraction.

Errors in Axial Length Measurement and the Final Refraction

Variations in axial length measurement affect the final refraction differently in the average, long, and short eyes [4]. In an average 23.5-mm eye, a 0.1-mm difference in AL measurement affects the final postoperative refraction by 0.25 D. In a long 26.0-mm eye, a 0.1-mm difference in the AL measurement affects the final postoperative refraction by only 0.20 D. In the short 2 1.0-mm eye, a 0.1-mm difference in the AL measurement affects the final postoperative refraction by 0.31 D.

Axial Length Measurement of the Challenging Eye

Aphakic eyes, pseudophakic eyes, and eyes with a posterior pole staphyloma or filled with silicone-filled vitreous are best measured with optical biometry or swept-source optical coherence tomography. Measuring these eyes with ultrasound can be challenging.

The Aphakic Eye

In the aphakic eye, a medium reflective echospike from the anterior vitreous face replaces the two lens peaks of the phakic eye.

The axial length is measured between the anterior corneal surface and the anterior retinal surface using an average sound velocity of 1.532 mm/μs (1532 m/s), which is the velocity in aqueous and vitreous. Certain units use a slightly higher sound velocity of 1534 m/s to account for the faster speed of sound within the cornea. If the ultrasound unit uses only fixed 1550 m/s velocity and does not allow the use of 1534 m/s velocity, the axial length of the aphakic eye can then be calculated as follows:

$$\text{APHAKIC AL} = (1534/1550) \times \text{AL measured with } 1550 \, \text{m/s}.$$

The Pseudophakic Eye

In a pseudophakic eye (Fig. 9.13), a high reflective spike from the anterior surface of the pseudophakic lens is visualized following the corneal spikes. It is usually followed by multiple smaller echospikes (arrows) that represent reverberations of the ultrasound beam between the anterior and posterior surfaces of the implant. The operator must remember to lower the beam's amplification to better differentiate the different peaks and to reduce artifacts.

In pseudophakic eyes, most biometers make an internal adjustment and the operator can choose the "pseudophakic mode" and the IOL material. The average sound velocity (V_L) and central thickness (T_L) of each IOL vary according to the IOL material (Table 9.1).

It is best to measure the AL at the velocity of 1532 m/s as if it is an aphakic eye and then add or subtract a corrected axial length factor (F):

$$PAL = AL_{1532} + F$$

$$\text{and } F = T_L \times (1 - 1532/V_L)$$

where

- PAL is the true axial length of the pseudophakic eye.
- F is the corrected axial length factor.
- AL_{1532} is the axial length measured at the velocity of 1532 m/s.
- T_L is the central IOL thickness.
- V_L is the average sound velocity within the IOL.

If the measurement of the AL is taken at a velocity of 1550 m/s (AL_{1550}) like measuring a phakic eye with an average velocity of 1550 m/s, the measurement can be converted to an aphakic measurement (AL_{1532}) where:

$$AL_{1532} = (1532/1550) \times AL_{1550}.$$

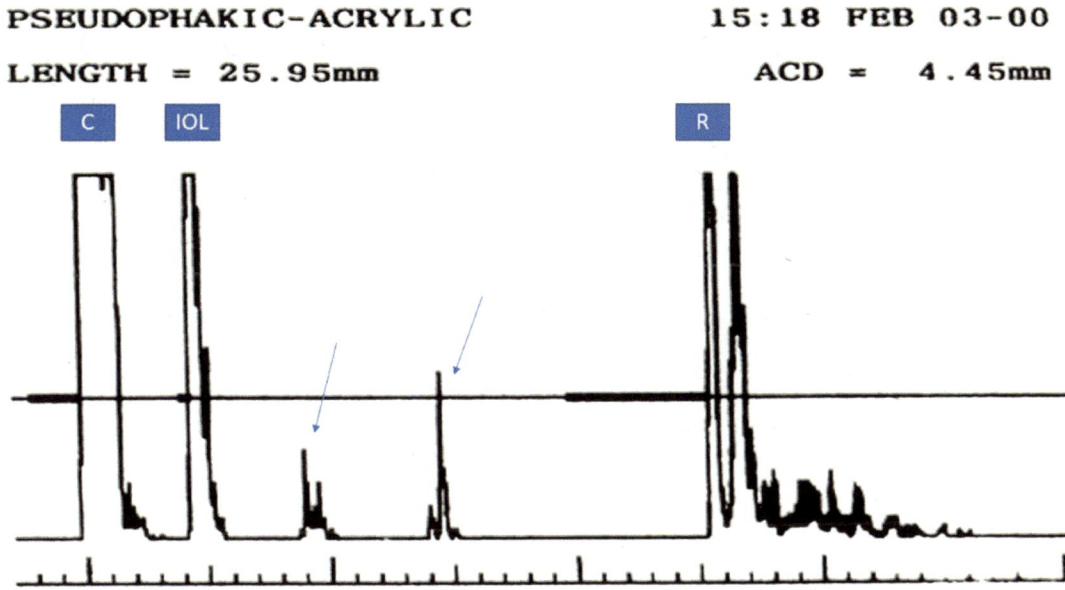

PSEUDOPHAKIC–ACRYLIC   **15:18 FEB 03-00**

LENGTH = 25.95mm   **ACD = 4.45mm**

C   IOL   R

Fig. 9.13 An A-scan display of a pseudophakic eye. Note the presence of reverberation spikes (arrows) behind the intraocular lens (IOL)

Table 9.1 Average sound velocity and central thickness of different intraocular lens materials

Implant	Sound velocity (m/s)	Central thickness (mm)
PMMA	2660	0.6–0.8
Silicone	980	1.2–1.5
Glass	6040	0.3–0.4
Acrylic	2200	0.7–0.9

Table 9.2 IOL correction factors

IOL power	Acrylic IOL	Silicone IOL	PMMA IOL
+10.0 D	+0.18	−0.50	+0.23
+12.0 D	+0.18	−0.52	+0.25
+14.0 D	+0.18	−0.54	+0.28
+16.0 D	+0.22	−0.55	+0.30
+18.0 D	+0.23	−0.56	+0.33
+20.0 D	+0.25	−0.59	+0.36
+22.0 D	+0.26	−0.60	+0.39
+24.0 D	+0.27	−0.62	+0.41
+26.0 D	+0.29	−0.64	+0.44
+28.0 D	+0.30	−0.65	+0.46
+30.0 D	+0.31	−0.67	+0.50

- The average correction factor (F) is "+0.4 mm" for the PMMA IOL, "+0.2 mm" for the acrylic IOL, and "−0.6 mm" for the silicone IOL.

The following table details the correction factors according to the IOL power (Table 9.2):

If the eye is to be measured with an average sound velocity instead of using preceding formulas, the following velocities are recommended:

- 1555 m/s for an eye with PMMA IOL
- 1476 m/s for an eye with a silicone IOL
- 1549 m/s for an eye with a glass IOL
- 1554 m/s for an eye with an acrylic IOL

If a pseudophakic eye is measured at the phakic average velocity of 1550 m/s, the error is <0.1 mm for the eye with a PMMA, glass, or acrylic IOL. However, this error exceeds 1.0 mm for the eye with a silicone IOL.

The Eye with Silicone-Filled Vitreous

Silicone oil is used to fill the vitreous cavity to prevent recurrent retinal detachments in high-risk cases. Silicone oil can have varying viscosity, measured in centistokes (cSt). The commonly used 1000 centistoke oil has a velocity of 980 m/s, whereas the 5000 centistoke oil's velocity is 1040 m/s. The low velocity within the silicone oil will cause an erroneous measurement of the vitreous cavity depth (VCD). Some biometers provide an option to measure the axial length in the presence of silicone oil. If this option is not available, the eye is measured as usual. The vitreous cavity depth measurement will need to be corrected.

The formula to correct the axial length in any silicone oil-filled vitreous is:

1. The vitreous cavity depth as measured by the biometer is calculated:

$$VCD_{1532} = AL - (ACD + LENS).$$

2. The vitreous cavity depth measurement is corrected using the correct velocity of 980 instead of 1532 m/s: $VCD_{corrected} = VCD_{1532} \times (1/1532) \times 980$ m/s *

   * or 1040 m/s (depending on the oil placed in the patient's eye).

3. $AL_{CORRECTED} = VCD_{corrected} + ACD + LENS$

In some cases, silicone oil must remain in the vitreous cavity for a long period. In this case, we must consider some IOL power adjustments. The additional IOL power for a silicone oil-filled vitreous is +3.0 to 3.5 D to obtain emmetropia.

In cases of eyes filled with gas or Perfluorocarbon liquid, ultrasound echoes are blocked. Measuring the AL with ultrasound becomes almost impossible.

Avoiding Errors in Axial Length Measurement

During AL measurement, the technician aligns the ultrasound beam with the optical axis of the eye by being perpendicular to the four major surfaces of the eye: the anterior surface of the cornea, the anterior surface of the lens, the posterior surface of the lens, and the anterior surface of the retina. Errors in AL measurement are due to an improper technique yielding shorter or longer measurements [1–3]. Often, manufacturers recommend using the average value of multiple measurements to improve precision and avoid errors. Although this is a good practice, one should remember that multiple readings of an erroneous measurement will still yield an erroneous average measurement.

Avoiding Shorter Axial Length Measurement

Shorter AL measurement might occur with corneal compression, off-axis measurement, and sometimes in the presence of asteroid hyalosis. Entering a shorter measurement of the AL in IOL power calculations will call for the use of a stronger IOL than is required, resulting in an induced myopia in the final postoperative refraction.

Corneal compression is the most common cause of shorter AL measurements with the "contact technique." An unskilled technician can indent the cornea with the A-scan probe more than needed, resulting in a shallower anterior chamber depth and a shorter axial length, even though an acceptable A-scan echogram has been displayed on the screen. Using an "immersion technique" will keep the probe away from the cornea and will avoid any corneal compression.

Off-axis measurement occurs when the ultrasound beam is not perpendicular to the surfaces of the eye components. A minimal off-axis scan is characterized by the absence of a posterior lens spike or the presence of an exceedingly small one (Fig. 9.14). The remainder echospikes from the cornea, the anterior surface of the lens, and the retina usually appear normal. A larger off-axis measurement occurs when the patient is not looking at the fixation light due to the presence of a dense cataract or the inability of the patient to hold the eye in a steady position. A larger off-axis scan is characterized by the absence of the poste-

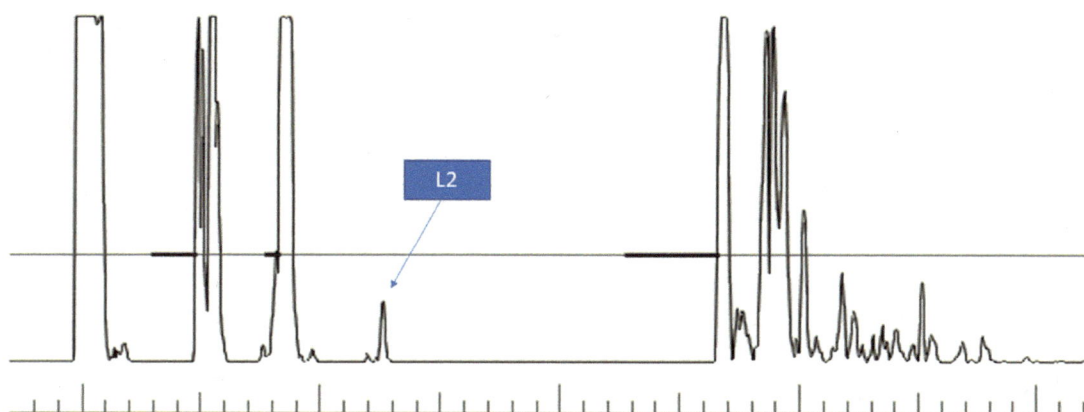

```
IMMERSN1    PHAKIC-1 1532/1641/1532
AXL =   0.00mm       LENS = 0.00mm        ACD = 0.00mm
```

Fig. 9.14 An A-scan display of a phakic eye that is not acceptable. The unit recognizes the absence of the posterior lens spike (L2) and does not give any measurement

rior lens spike and the presence of a jagged retinal spike.

The presence of asteroid hyalosis will create echospikes within the vitreous cavity that can be confused by the biometer as the retinal surface. By decreasing the biometer's system sensitivity, the amplitude of all the echospikes will decrease to a point where the weaker vitreous spikes almost disappear. Also, when in doubt as to the nature of the vitreous pathology, a B-scan ultrasound can be helpful.

Avoiding Longer Axial Length Measurement

Longer measurements of the axial length might occur in the presence of a pre-corneal echospike, a poor retinal echospike, or the use of an inaccurate velocity. Entering a longer measurement of the AL in IOL power calculations will call for the use of a weaker IOL than is required, resulting in an induced hyperopia in the final postoperative refraction.

A pre-corneal echospike is usually generated by an air bubble within the scleral shell during an immersion technique.

A poor retinal echospike is the result of an off-axis measurement. The biometer will miss the retinal spike and read a longer measurement between the corneal and the scleral spike (Fig. 9.15).

An inaccurate velocity can be inadvertently used when measuring an aphakic eye.

Detecting Significant Intraocular Pathology

There are cases where the ultrasound pattern is difficult to interpret. In most cases, this is due to posterior pathology that cannot be visualized due to an advanced cataract. The most common cause is the presence of a staphyloma in a highly myopic eye. Other causes include a retinal detachment, macular changes, or an intraocular mass. In such cases, a B-scan will determine the correct diagnosis.

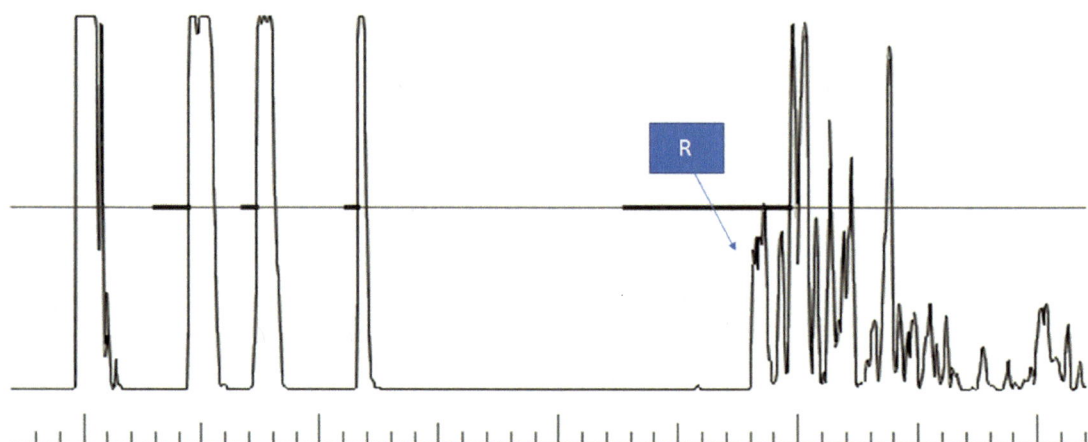

IMMERSN1   PHAKIC-1 1532/1641/1532
AXL = 25.73ᴍᴍ   LENS = 4.62ᴍᴍ   ACD = 2.92ᴍᴍ

Fig. 9.15 An A-scan display of a phakic eye with a poorly defined retinal spike (R). The erroneous long measurement is taken between the cornea and the sclera (instead of the retina)

References

1. Byrne SF. Standardized echography, Part I: a-scan examination procedures. Int Ophthalmol Clin. 1979;19:267–81.
2. Ossoinig KC. Standardized echography: basic principles, clinical applications and results. Int Ophthalmol Clin. 1979;19:127–285.
3. Kendall CJ. Ophthalmic echography, The ophthalmic technical series. Thorofare, NJ: Springer; 1990. p. 57–106.
4. Shammas HJ. Axial length measurement and its relation to intraocular lens power calculations. Am Intraocular Implant Soc J. 1982;8:346–9.
5. Shammas HJ, Swearingen M. Clinical evaluation of the Bio-Pen for axial length measurement. J Cataract Refract Surg. 1990;16:120–2.
6. Shammas HJ. A comparison of immersion and contact techniques for axial length measurement. Am Intraocul Implant Soc J. 1984;10:444–7.
7. Olsen T, Nielsen PJ. Immersion versus contact technique in the measurement of axial length by ultrasound. Acta Ophthalmol (Copenh). 1989;67:101–2.
8. Shammas HJ. Manual versus electronic measurement of the axial length. In: Hillman JS, LeMay MM, editors. Ultrasonography in ophthalmology, Proceedings of the 1982 Ninth SIDUO Congress. The Hague: Dr. W. Junk Publishers; 1983. p. 225–9.
9. Shammas HJ. A-Scan biometry of 1000 cataractous eyes. In: Ossoining KC, editor. Ophthalmic echography. Proceedings of the 10th SIDUO Congress, Documenta Ophthalmologica Proceedings Series, vol. 48. The Hague: Dr. W. Junk Publisher; 1987. p. 57–63.
10. Oksala A, Lehtinen A. Measurement of the velocity of sound in some parts of the eye. Acta Ophthalmol. 1958;36:633–9.
11. Jansson F, Kock E. Determination of the velocity of ultrasound in the human lens and vitreous. Acta Ophthalmol. 1962;40:420–33.
12. Coleman DJ, Lizzi FL, Franzen LA, Abramson DH. A determination of the velocity of ultrasound in cataractous lenses. Bibl Ophthalmol. 1975;83:246–51.
13. Pallikaris I, Gruber H. Determination of sound velocity in different forms of cataracts. Doc Ophthalmol. 1981;29:165–9.
14. Massin M, Lambrinakis I. In vivo determination of the speed of ultrasound in cataractous lenses. In: Ultrasonography in ophthalmology, vol. 12. Springer; 1990. p. 131–4.

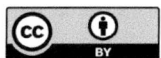

Optical Biometry

10

Magdalena Nenning, Nino Hirnschall, and Oliver Findl

Cataract surgery has greatly improved by innovative techniques and advanced technology. Patients' expectations and demands for an optimal outcome have increased and have contributed to the fact that, besides obtaining visual rehabilitation, it has also become a refractive procedure.

An accurate calculation of intraocular lens (IOL) power is crucial for satisfactory refractive outcomes. Several factors, including keratometry (K) readings, axial length (AL), postoperative IOL position, and IOL power formulae, affect the IOL power calculation, with preoperative biometry, primarily the assessment of the axial eye length, being its most essential component. Postoperative refractive errors are the main cause for dissatisfaction or lens exchange, and studies have shown that 54% of those errors arise from imprecise AL measurements. Historically, measurements of AL, ACD, and crystalline lens thickness have been commonly performed by ultrasound biometry.

The introduction of optical biometry was a major development in cataract surgery and has led to more precise biometry systems that are now considered as the gold standard in ocular biometry [1–3].

History of Optical Biometry

Ultrasound Biometry

Since its introduction in 1956, ultrasound biometry has steadily improved and has been the gold standard for AL measurement before the introduction of partial coherence interferometry [2, 4]. Two types of A-scan ultrasound biometry are available.

In contact applanation biometry, an ultrasound probe is directly placed on the central cornea and a high frequency sound wave travels into the eye, with part of it reflecting back toward the probe when encountering a media interface, allowing to calculate the distance between the probe and various intraocular structures. A limitation to this method is the inadvertent indentation of the cornea and the resulting shallowing of the anterior chamber which arises from the compression of the probe. This results in a shortening of the eye and an overestimation of the IOL power. Since

M. Nenning · O. Findl (✉)
Vienna Institute for Research in Ocular Surgery (VIROS), A Karl Landsteiner Institute, Hanusch Hospital, Vienna, Austria
e-mail: oliver@findl.at

N. Hirnschall
Department for Ophthalmology and Optometry, Kepler University Hospital GmbH, Linz, Austria
e-mail: nino@hirnschall.at

© The Author(s) 2024
J. Aramberri et al. (eds.), *Intraocular Lens Calculations*, Essentials in Ophthalmology,
https://doi.org/10.1007/978-3-031-50666-6_10

this error is variable, it cannot be compensated for by a constant.

In immersion ultrasound biometry, a saline immersion bath is placed between the probe and the eye. While avoiding the indentation of the cornea, this method was shown to be more accurate compared to contact ultrasound. A mean difference of 0.25–0.33 mm has been reported between the two methods, which translates to an error of approximately 1 diopter (D) [1, 5, 6].

In A-scan ultrasound biometry in general, relatively long, low-resolution wavelengths (10 MHz) are used. This has the advantage of excellent penetration through dense media, but the disadvantage of low resolution. An accuracy of AL measurement of approximately 100–200 μm has been reported, whereas an error of 100 μm results in a corresponding postoperative refractive error of 0.28 D. Also, inconsistent measurements may occur due to discrepancies of retinal thickness in the central retina and off-axis measurements [1, 5, 6].

Partial Coherence Interferometry (PCI)

Although the birthplace of optical biometry is Vienna, Austria, the concept of coherence interferometry was introduced before as a new method for high-range resolution measurement of light scattering in optically dense inhomogeneous media in the 1970s [7].

However, it was not until 1986, when Fercher and coworkers introduced this method for the purpose of ocular biometry [8]. They used a long-coherence Helium-Neon laser beam to illuminate the patient's eye, which represented an interferometer with the cornea and the retina forming the interferometer mirrors. The reflections from the cornea and the retina created an interferogram consisting of concentric interference fringes (Fig. 10.1), which pulsated with the patient's heartbeat. An interferometer in the illuminating beam enabled the determination of the optical path length between those two mirrors. This technique offered the advantages of high transversal

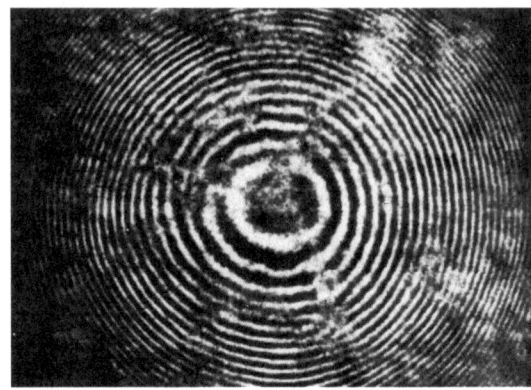

Fig. 10.1 Interference pattern caused by the light remitted by the fundus and the light reflected at the cornea [9]

resolution at the fundus and no need for anesthesia or mechanical contact with the eye [9].

The use of a low temporal coherence allowed accurate measurement of intraocular distances, especially the axial eye length. On the contrary, high temporal coherence was used to measure distance variations resulting from blood pulse-induced dilatation of ocular tissues, which contributed to clinical applications in vascular diseases or glaucoma [8].

Concerning the axial eye length measurement, however, it was difficult to meet the requirements such as a high spatial coherence and a very low temporal coherence in those early times. Until 1985, dye lasers, which suffered from problems like beam instabilities, were used and later replaced with multimode semiconductor lasers, which, on the other hand, offered only low spectral bandwidth [8].

In early experiments with a Michelson interferometer, an optical dual-beam illumination scheme was used. A short coherence length beam was split into a direct and a delayed beam, and the eye was illuminated along a coaxial pathway. An overlapping of the two exit beams, reflected at fundus and cornea, indicated an identical total path length, and an interferogram was created at the observation plane.

Figure 10.2 shows an A-scan of a myopic eye, measured by PCI as described above. The peak position indicates the optical distance to the anterior corneal surface, which, in this case, yields an

Fig. 10.2 A-scan of a myopic eye, measured with the first dual-beam heterodyne PCI instrument. The signal peak indicates the optical length of the eye (33.56 mm). Divided by the refractive index of the ocular media in sum, the geometrical length of the eye can be obtained (24.78 mm) [10]

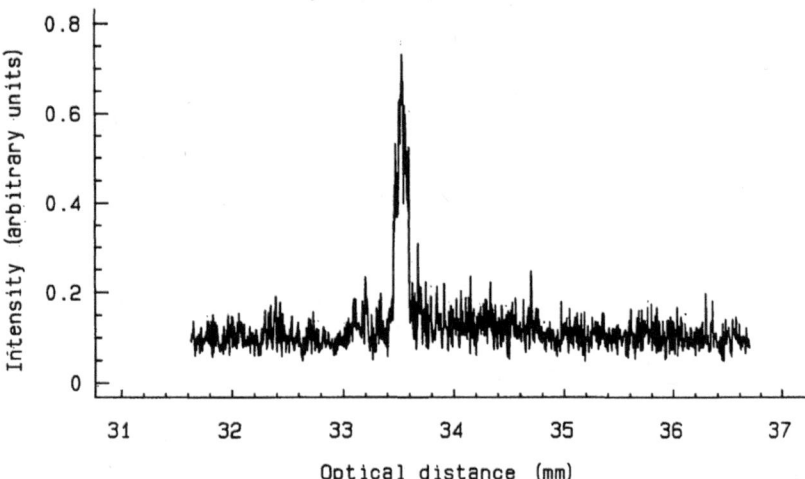

optical length of 33.56 mm. This value has to be divided by the group refractive index of the traversed ocular media to convert to a geometric length of 24.78 mm [10]. Later, the resolution was further refined by replacing the multimode laser diode by a broadband superluminescent diode, which allowed measurements of the cornea and anterior segment [8].

In the meantime, the PCI method has almost completely replaced ultrasound-based biometry.

Its commercial launch took place in 1999 by Zeiss with the introduction of the IOL Master (Carl Zeiss Meditec AG, Germany), while several other devices of various manufacturers have been developed later (Lenstar LS900, Haag-Streit; Aladdin, Topcon; OA-2000, Tomey; AL-Scan, Nidek; Galilei G6, Ziemer, etc.). All optical biometry devices are somewhat based on the concept of PCI [11].

Ultrasound Biometry vs. PCI

A direct comparison between ultrasound and optical biometry cannot be drawn, as ultrasound biometry measures the distance from the cornea to the inner limiting membrane, while optical biometry measures the distance from the cornea to the retinal pigment epithelium, which explains a discrepancy in axial length values obtained

from these two methods. Therefore, the optical biometry measurements were "adjusted" to be interchangeable with immersion ultrasound measurements (with a correction factor of 0.18 mm) [5].

Optical biometry is superior to ultrasound biometry in several aspects. Orientation is easier for optical biometry because the patient fixates the laser beam, whereas orientation of the scan is more of an estimation for ultrasound measurements. Other advantages of optical biometry are that it is examiner independent, easy to be performed, and there is no risk of infection [5].

Regarding the prediction of IOL power, it was shown that PCI can improve the refractive outcome by about 30% when using the SRK II formula [1]. In a study that compared PCI with ultrasound biometry by applying both methods to four commonly used IOL power formulae (SRK II, Olsen, SRK/T, Holladay I), the refractive outcome was significantly improved with all four IOL power formulae when using PCI instead of ultrasound [12].

One limitation of optical biometry is the absorption and reflection of light in dense media resulting in unsuccessful scans in the case of very dense cataracts or corneal scars.

Optical biometry has replaced ultrasound biometry worldwide, with an exception in cases of very dense cataracts [13].

Concept of PCI

Figure 10.3 shows a diagram of the principal setup of a dual-beam partial coherence interferometer. A superluminescent diode (SLD) emits an infrared light beam ($\lambda \sim 780$ nm) of high spatial coherence but very short coherence length (l_c). Long, red wavelengths are chosen because they are scattered less than blue light. This results in a better penetration in dense cataracts. The SLD emits a broader spectrum of color than does a laser, so the measurement is more sensitive than it would be with only one frequency of light. An external Michelson interferometer splits the beam into two parts by means of a fixed reference mirror (1) and a moveable measurement mirror (2), resulting in a reference beam and a measurement beam. Those two beam components are parallel and coaxial and due to being reflected once at both interferometer plates, they have a mutual time delay of twice the interferometer arm length difference (d). At the interferometer exit, they are combined again, forming a coaxial dual beam [1, 10, 14, 15, p. 261]

The laser beam appears as a weak red spot (the wavelength is just visible), which acts as a fixation target for the patient [16]. The eye is illuminated, and reflected beams are generated at every intraocular interface, splitting both beam components into further subcomponents. Hence, two coaxial beams that are both reflected at the cornea (C) and the retina (R) result in four reflected beams, yielding an additional path difference of twice the optical length (OL) between each of the two pairs of beams [10]. The total of the reflected beams is detected by and superimposed on a photodetector.

The axial eye length, in this method, extends from the anterior corneal surface to the retinal pigment epithelium, so the reflections of those two interfaces are measured. If the coherence length of the laser is shorter than two times the optical length, no interference will be observed. If, however, the delay of these two beam components produced by the interferometer (the interferometer arm length difference) equals the optical distance between the two interfaces, there are two subcomponents that traverse the same total path length and will consequently interfere. That means, two arm length differences equal twice the optical length within a difference of the coherence length. For AL measurement, the subcomponent of the reference beam that is reflected at the retinal pigment epithelium (R_1) will interfere with the subcomponent of the measurement beam that is reflected at the cornea (C_2) [14]. The photodetector senses the intensity distribution (the interference pattern consists of concentric fringes) and records the corresponding displacement of the measurement mirror and the interferometer arm length difference, respectively. As the mirror position can be determined precisely, this method yields very accurate results [17, p. 129].

Each interferometer arm length difference for which an interference pattern is observed equals an intraocular optical distance within the coherence length of the light source. The interference pattern is called a partial coherence interferometry signal, similar to that of ultrasound A-scans, but with a much higher resolution (approximately 12 m) and precision (0.3–10 m). The anterior corneal surface acts as the reference surface, for all intraocular distances are measured from this point. Hence, any influence of longitudinal eye movement during measurement can be neglected [1, 14].

In order to accelerate the process, a dynamic approach based on the heterodyne detection principle has been established. In this technique, the measurement mirror is shifted with constant speed by a stepper motor. This causes a Doppler shift of the light frequency of the measurement beam, where

$$f_D = 2v / \lambda$$

v is the speed with which the mirror is moved (plate speed), and λ is the wavelength of light.

Interference patterns will occur in case of path length coincidence, as described above, but in this case, intensity is modulated by the Doppler frequency. A photodetector measures and amplifies the intensity of the reflected beams and a band pass filter is interposed, which digitally filters the signals in a manner that it only transmits signals with the Doppler frequency f_D. A personal

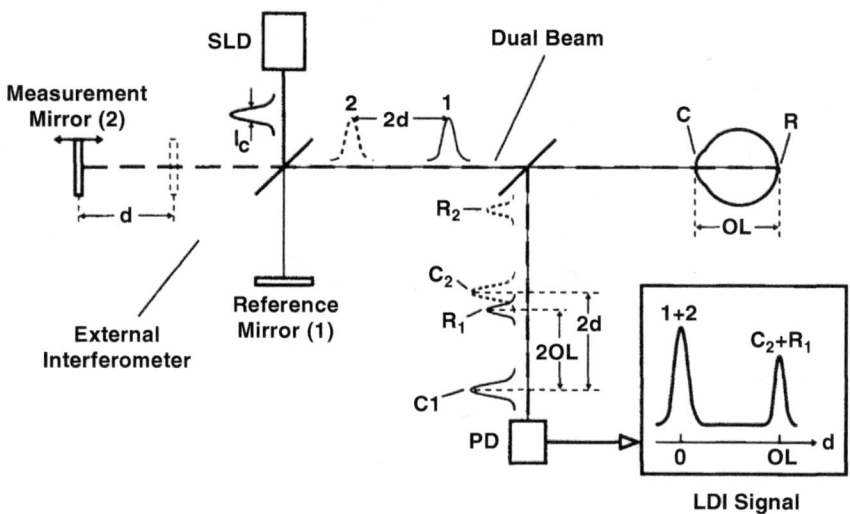

Fig. 10.3 Principle of the dual-beam PCI. An external Michelson interferometer illuminates the eye with a coaxial dual beam. The reflections are detected by and super-imposed on a photodetector. A partial coherence interferometry signal of the optical distance is imaged, which equals the optical axial eye length [14]

computer records the intensity of the measured signal as a function of d and displays it as an LDI scan as shown in Fig. 10.3. At $d = 0$, the two beam components (1 + 2) interfere, which is shown as a peak in the scan that can be considered as a calibration point. At $d = OL$, the two beam components R_1 and C_2 interfere and the resulting peak corresponds with the optical distance between C and R [10, 14].

Calibration of the instrument can be performed by measuring the optical length of a plane glass pate of known thickness and refractive index. Once the instrument is calibrated, d doesn't have to be measured along the total eye length, but instead, $d = OL$ is located and a surrounding range of up to 3 mm is scanned to register the field in which retinal peaks are expected. The LDI scans therefore only contain the peak at $d = OL$, whereas the peak at $d = 0$ is waived. The information gathered this way suffices to measure the AL and the retinal thickness and helps to decrease the measuring time as well as the computer storage space needed [10, 14].

.An additional helium neon (HeNe) laser and a single-mode laser diode (SMLD) serve for alignment purposes. The latter has the same wavelength as the measurement beam, but an l_c larger than twice the OL. Hence, regardless the interferometer arm length difference, permanent interference happens for the reflected beams and since λ is the same, no difference is visible in the interference pattern. This procedure helps to align the photodetector with the center of the interference fringes before starting the measurement. Once finished, the laser input can simply be switched from SMLD to SLD [10].

The coherence length of the light source correlates directly with the precision of the measurement: the shorter the l_c, the higher the accuracy. A signal with f_D is usually recorded in the range $d = OL \pm l_c/2$, while the amplitude of the signal varies within this range and its maximum is obtained at $d = OL$. Therefore, if the signal peak is located, the precision is higher than $l_c/2$. Hence, an SLD that emits a light beam with an l_c of 15 μm achieves a precision <7.5 μm [10, 14].

Since the concept of dual-beam PCI is to match an unknown intraocular distance with a known distance within the Michelson interferometer and the cornea is used as a reference surface, the location of the eye relative to the instrument is insignificant for the measurement and longitudinal eye movement doesn't impair the procedure. Lateral eye movements, on the other hand, are capable of influencing the measurement [14].

PCI yields optical distances, so the values obtained need to be divided by the group refractive index of the traversed ocular media (cornea, aqueous humor, lens, vitreous) to convert to geometrical distances [1].

The IOL Master uses PCI for AL measurement, while the ACD is measured by optical principles using not a PCI method but rather a photographic technique. The first commercially available PCI instrument for anterior segment biometry was the AC Master (Carl Zeiss Meditec AG). Measurements of the anterior segment using PCI have to be performed along the optical axis, so the device includes a display to steer the direction of fixation of the eye. This mechanism also enables to present a defocus in order to induce accommodation; thus, the AC Master can also be used during accommodation [18, 19]. The technique of PCI for anterior segment biometry measures central corneal thickness, ACD, and lens thickness with high precision and reproducibility [20, 21].

The PCI technique as described above has been extended to a fully computerized scanning instrument. It is not only capable of measuring intraocular distances parallel to the visual axis but also at arbitrary angles. The performance of scans in horizontal and vertical directions facilitates to maintain topographic and tomographic images as well as cross-sectional images and thickness maps of different fundus structures [14].

As measurements are carried out in vivo, the laser safety regulations have to be met. The intensity of about 190 μW (or 490 μW/cm²) of the SLD is allowed to be applied to the eye for approximately 47 min. Maximum illumination time of one point of the eye in this procedure is about 2–4 s, which is far below the safety limit. The HeNe alignment laser delivers a power of approximately 5 μW (or 13 μW/cm²), which is below the limit of permanent illumination of 18 μW/cm² [14].

Optical Low-Coherence Reflectometry (OLCR)

Related to PCI technology, OLCR was introduced in the form of Lenstar LS900 (Haag-Streit AG, Switzerland), followed by the Aladdin (Topcon, Japan). Those devices use a laser diode infrared light with a wavelength of 820 nm. Similar to PCI, the concept is based on a Michelson interferometer and an A-scan is obtained as a result. While the devices differ in AL measurement, the same technology is used to measure keratometry readings and corneal diameter distance. OLCR-based devices are capable of acquiring central corneal thickness and lens thickness, and all measurements are obtained simultaneously, without the need for realignment. The difference of the results from both methods has found to be clinically irrelevant [22–24].

Advancements of PCI

Although optical biometry is preferred over ultrasound biometry due to higher accuracy and comfort of the method, one relevant drawback of this technique is its inability to be performed in cases with dense opacities of the cornea or the lens [25].

The accuracy of PCI is strongly related to the signal-to-noise ratio (SNR), which is the ratio of the interference signal amplitude relative to the background noise amplitude. A high SNR reflects higher quality of the AL readings and for a measurement to be reliable, a ratio above 2.0 has been determined. Values between 1.6 and 1.9 are classified as borderline and should entail additional measurements for verification [26, 27].

Main reason for a low SNR and the failure to perform a PCI measurement is the presence of very dense media, such as dense corneal scars, dense cataracts, or a vitreous hemorrhage. Other reasons include patients with poor fixation and macular pathologies [25]. These opacities are capable of causing different optical phenomena, such as absorption, reflection, and light scattering (particularly Rayleigh scattering). Any opacity in media traversed by the laser can interfere with the result, but above all, mature cataracts and particularly posterior subcapsular cataracts were responsible for the first generations of PCI measurement failures. In such cases, the SNR may amount to less than 2.0, which requires ultrasound biometry to be performed subsequently in order to gain AL readings [25].

To overcome this problem, software and hardware upgrades of the commonly used biometers have been developed [24]. In the first approach, the averaging of consecutive scans was used to increase the SNR by dampening all noise variance, including shot noise. As a result of this method, structural elements, that have been hidden under the noise floor, became visible. However, one remaining problem was that actual signals were low in amplitude [28].

In the second approach to enhance image quality, the so-called composite scan was introduced in a software upgrade (version 5.0) of the IOL Master 500. The composite scan allows averaging of consecutive optical scans by digital processing of signals of multiple measurements. As true peaks, although low in amplitude, are present in multiple scans, their signal enhances as more scans are performed. Background noise, on the other hand, is a random signal, so by superimposing multiple scans, those peaks cancel each other out. This technique helps to improve the SNR and therefore allows to successfully gain biometry readings in part of the eyes that previously failed the measurement. A clinical evaluation of the composite scan showed that the rate of acquisition failure could be reduced from 10.6% to 4.7%. The new algorithm was successful in 30% of the eyes that could not be measured with version 4.0 of the IOL Master 500 and was particularly advantageous in eyes with posterior subcapsular cataract [25].

Introduction of OCT-Based Biometry

In 1991, Huang and coworkers adapted the technique of low-coherence reflectometry with the aim of generating not only one-dimensional (A-Scan), but two-dimensional (B-Scan) images of biological tissues. Although its predecessor and basic ranging technology was applied since the 1970s, as mentioned earlier in this chapter, it was with this development that the term optical coherence tomography was first introduced [1, 8, 29].

The process of creating a one-dimensional, longitudinal scan is repeated at incremental steps across the tissue sample, and the reflection sites in those individual scans are brought together to provide a two-dimensional map [30].

The operating mode is therefore analogous to ultrasonic pulse-echo imaging (ultrasound B-mode), and the device utilized is an extension to previously used low-coherence reflectometers. An incorporated transverse scanning mechanism enables two-dimensional imaging, and higher-speed longitudinal scanning increases the data collection rate. The amplitudes and delays of tissue reflections are measured similarly to the PCI method, and the lateral resolution of the image is limited by the beam diameter. The resulting image can be viewed directly as a gray scale or false-color image. The optical sectioning capability of OCT is similar to confocal microscopic systems. However, it bears the advantage of not being limited by the available numerical aperture but only by the coherence length of the light source. Thus, high-resolution, transpupillary imaging of the posterior eye can be achieved [29].

The change from A-scan to B-scan was a major development in ophthalmic imaging. By generating cross-sectional slices of tissue, peaks can directly be assigned to their corresponding tissue structures and boundaries can be verified, which prevents from potential errors. Furthermore, OCT-based biometry is able to image a longitudinal cross section through the entire length of the eye including the anterior segment, which makes it a useful imaging tool particularly in irregular cataracts or eyes with phakic IOLs, but also in pseudophakic eyes in order to measure postoperative ACD.

A direct comparison between an A-scan from the IOL Master 500 (Fig. 10.4) and a B-scan from the IOL Master 700 (Fig. 10.5) demonstrates that the added information B-scans provide on ocular tissues.

Time-Domain OCT

Traditional OCT imaging, as introduced in 1991, uses time-domain detection. A low-coherence light source is coupled into the interferometer

Fig. 10.4 A-scan (IOL Master 500)

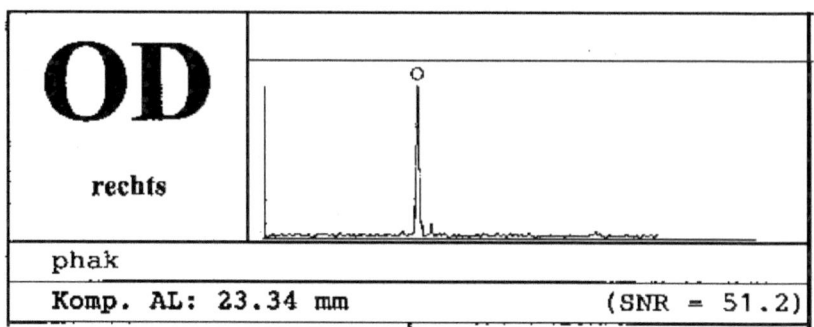

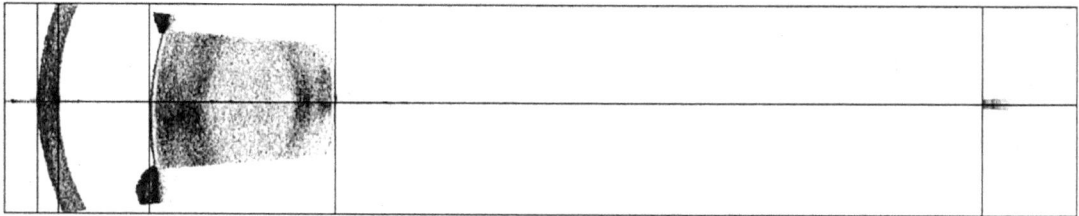

Fig. 10.5 B-scan (IOL Master 700)

and split into two components by a beam splitter. One arm of the interferometer aims a beam to the sample being investigated while the other arm directs a beam to a reference mirror. The signals from both arms are then reflected and scattered back and recombined by the beam splitter, which lies in the path from the light source to the sample, before being sensed by a photodetector [30].

In time-domain OCT (TD-OCT), the position of the reference mirror is displaced by a stepper motor. The photodetector detects interferometric signals only when the reflections from both interferometer arms are nearly matched in group delay (time-of-flight) and the amplitude of the interferometric signal is highest, when the reference arm length is matched to the backscattering interface's distance, or, in other words, when the two arms are matched in distance so that the reflections reach the detector at the same time [29]. The photodetector records the amplitude of the signal and simultaneously, the corresponding position of the reference mirror is scanned in order to measure amplitudes and delays of tissue reflections. Usually, a piezoelectric transducer in the sample arm is used to measure the length of the optical delay line. The detector output gener-

ates the interferometric signals, which are collected by a computer and, after sophisticated processing, produce a cross-sectional image. Multiple of those parallel images can be used to gather a three-dimensional data set.

The broadness of the interference signal is given by the coherence length; the short coherence length and broad spectral bandwidth of the light source cause the signal to fall off rapidly with delay mismatch and by observing the interference peaks during the scan, the location of the reflections from the sample can be determined with high resolution [29–31, p. 12ff].

Eye motion during measurement is capable of decreasing the resolution and the SNR in OCT imaging. In TD-OCT, movement only affects the image pixel for which the signal is captured at that time, so those artefacts are usually insignificant. TD-OCT B-scans have an axial resolution of approximately 10 μm and a transverse resolution of 20–25 μm. To increase the resolution and scan density, the scan time can be prolonged in order to achieve more A-scans that contribute to the final image. However, as the scan time increases, so does the likelihood of eye motion-induced artefacts [30, 32].

Spectral-Domain OCT

In 2006, the first Spectral-Domain OCT (SD-OCT) device became available on the market. The principle of SD-OCT, also known as Fourier-Domain OCT (FD-OCT) or Frequency-Domain OCT, is similar to that of TD-OCT. However, instead of changing and scanning the position of the reference mirror, it is fixed and stationary at one position; hence, no mechanical scanning of its location is required. The interference pattern is recorded as a function of optical frequency with a spectrometer, instead of a photodetector and Fourier transformation is applied to convert the interferogram to a frequency-domain spectrum [33]. The spectrometer is a charge-coupled device (CCD) with an array of photodetectors that are each sensitive to a certain range of frequencies. The CCD senses all frequency components of the interference pattern, and all components of the spectral variation of the detected signal correspond to a specific depth within the tissue. Fringe patterns from closer tissue planes are spaced farther apart than those arising from deep tissue interfaces, and higher reflective tissues result in higher amplitude interferograms. Thus, the information needed to produce an A-scan is obtained from the spacing and amplitude of the fringe pattern. Similar to TD-OCT, multiple A-scans are acquired along a transverse plane and assembled into B-scans [15, p. 261, 30, 32, 33].

SD-OCT is principally more prone to motion-induced signal fading, since the signal is detected over time from various interfaces of different depths inside the tissue, but as imaging speed is easy to increase in SD-OCT systems, those motion artefacts can be reduced to a minimum. A lower illumination time achieved by a pulse instead of a broadband light source further helps to alleviate this problem. Moreover, motion-induced artefacts can be compensated for by image registration, which is a technique that aligns multiple B-scans based on structural features of the tissue examined, such as blood vessels [30, 32].

The introduction of FD-OCT not only depicted the foundation of all modern OCT systems today but also for functional extensions such as OCT angiography [8].

Swept-Source SD-OCT

The swept-source version of SD-OCT became available in clinical practice in 2012, with the IOL Master 700 (Carl Zeiss Meditec AG) being the first Swept-Source OCT (SS-OCT)-based biometry device.

SS-OCT is a variation of FD-OCT, in which a Fourier transformation is applied to the interference pattern to convert measurements of interfered light into physical delays or distances to allow simultaneous measurements of all light echoes.

In SS-OCT, the SLD's band of frequencies is replaced with a rapidly tunable narrowband laser. Instead of separating the broad wavelength light into single wavelength components by a spectrometer, the tunable swept laser emits different wavelengths, but only one single wavelength at a time; thus, the light is divided into a spectrum from the very beginning without the need of a spectrometer [34]. Each laser frequency labels a different time delay, which is detected by interference and whenever the wavelength of the laser is swept, a single photodetector records the interference spectrum of the light waves returning to the device. The A-scan rate is determined by the frequency at which the light source is swept. Although the light source is more complex in the SS-OCT setting, compared to SD-OCT, the mechanism of the device is simplified, which contributes to data acquisition rates that are twice as fast [33]. The modulation of the reference arm length in the TD-OCT setting limits the speed of the scan, so the primary advantage of SD-OCT is its much higher acquisition speed. With its reference mirror remaining stationary, SD-OCT attains data quickly and renders images 40–110 times faster than TD-OCT devices. While the scan speed in TD-OCT is approximately 400 A-scans/s, it varies between 16,000 and 55,000 A-scans/s in SD-OCT, which means that a B-scan containing 2048 A-scans can be acquired in 0.04–0.13 s. This allows for three-dimensional data sets to be achieved, which consists of a series of rapidly acquired B-scans. In the swept-source version of SD-OCT, up to a million A-scans can be obtained per second [30, 32].

Apart from highly increased scanning speeds, the fact that SS-OCT detects one single wavelength at a time avoids signal roll off, which occurs at the fringes of the imaging spectrum in FD-OCT, as the whole spectrum of wavelengths is detected at the same time. This results in enhanced depth range and enables for simultaneous imaging of different ocular structures without changing the focus of the device [30].

The overall resolution of the OCT image is determined by both axial and transverse resolution. As described above, transverse resolution depends on the beam diameter, while axial resolution depends on the properties of the optical light source. High spectral bandwidth leads to a short coherence length and high axial resolution [30, 32].

In TD-OCT, however, increasing the spectral bandwidth of the light source also involves higher electronic detection bandwidth, which results in a poor SNR. To overcome this problem, either the A-scan rate or depth scan range has to be decreased, or the incident optical power has to be increased, which is limited by the maximum permissible incident power on the eye, as stated by the American National Standards Institute (ANSI).

Both spectrometer- and swept-source-based SD-OCT systems benefit from higher speed and scan depth, enabling the acquisition of higher numbers of depth scans and resulting in high transverse resolution, which is not possible to achieve to the same extent in TD-OCT systems.

This sensitivity advantage over TD-OCT and the much shorter illumination time required allows for high-resolution imaging with illumination intensities well below the legal requirements [30, 32].

Another feature of SS-OCT is its capability of heterodyne detection, which means that the interferometric signal frequency spectrum is shifted away from the zero frequency. Hence, positive as well as negative displacements are taken into account [30].

The depth of tissue penetration depends on the wavelength of the light source. While SD-OCT usually employs an SLD with a wavelength of 800–900 nm, SS-OCT devices use wavelengths above 1000 nm. Shorter wavelengths involve higher degrees of scattering and attenuation, particularly from the retinal pigment epithelium (RPE), as it contains melanin. Consequently, SS-OCT is superior to SD-OCT in tissue penetration when it comes to increased tissue depth, dense retinal hemorrhage, exudates and imaging of structures beyond the RPE, such as the choroid or sclera. In SD-OCT, enhanced depth imaging (EDI), an averaging technique, has been employed to overcome this problem.

However, the longer wavelengths used in SS-OCTs result in a lower image resolution [30, 33–35].

OCT and Dense Cataracts

As described in previous sections of this chapter, the introduction of PCI has significantly improved the accuracy of AL measurement, due to its higher precision compared to applanation ultrasound as well as its excellent intra- and interobserver reliability. The most important drawback of conventional PCI technology in contrast to ultrasound is its failure of measurement when it comes to dense posterior subcapsular (PSC), mature or brunescent cataracts, owing to a reduced SNR (<2.0) [36, 37]. Freeman et al. assessed cataract gradings (LOCS III) related to unsuccessful measurements using the IOL Master 500 and reported that AL values could not be obtained in either of the eyes with mature cataract. Additionally, they provided a clinical cut-off value for PSC cataracts (P-scale) of 3.5, as 100% of PSC cataracts exceeding a P-scale value of 3.5 failed to be measured using the PCI method. As the LOCS III grading system doesn't specify the location of the opacity, measurement failure may sometimes occur at lower levels (P-scale value >2.5). No significant relation could be detected for nuclear opalescence (NO) or cortical (C) cataracts. As visual acuity (VA) decreases with the development of cataract, one could suggest VA to be related to measurement failure rates. While most of the data supports this conclusion, some patients with severe PSC cataracts can still retain good VA. Hence, the relationship is not strong enough to define a convenient cut-off value that defines whether IOL Master measurements will be obtainable [38].

The overall rate of acquisition failure for conventional PCI technology varies from 8% to 20% [36, 39–41], and could be reduced to 4.7% owing to the introduction of the composite scan method [25].

A newer approach to be used in optical biometry is SS-OCT, as employed in the IOL Master 700. The detailed differences between PCI and SS-OCT have been described in previous sections, but in general, the two technologies differ in terms of measurement setup and wavelength used (PCI: 780 nm; SS-OCT: 1055 nm) [37, 38].

Hirnschall et al. conducted a study to assess whether cases of measurement failure using the PCI method could be resolved by the SS-OCT technology. 1226 scans were evaluated, and measurement failure was defined as an SNR <2.0 in the IOL Master 500 acquisition. As the IOL Master 700 does not provide an SNR or a composite scan, each scan was analyzed separately and classified as successful if an AL value could be obtained and no warning was given by the device. Figure 10.6 shows a comparison of a successful and an unsuccessful SS-OCT scan. Twenty-one out of 23 (91.3%) of the unsuccessful scans using the PCI method were measurable with SS-OCT, yielding an estimated failure rate

of 0.5%, when considering the total amount of participants (6/1226). Thus, SS-OCT was shown to significantly improve the rate of attainable AL measurements. While AL values of 80% of dense nuclear or white cataracts that failed to be measured by the IOL Master 500 could be attained by the IOL Master 700, all eyes with PSC cataract were measurable by the latter [37]. Similar results were reported by Srivannaboon et al. [42] and Akman et al. [43]

The main cause for the better outcomes of SS-OCT is that it operates with higher wavelengths compared to PCI. As higher wavelengths undergo lower amounts of light scattering, they result in a deeper penetration of tissue. The phenomenon which describes the correlation between wavelength and scattering is called Rayleigh scattering. It states that the amount of scattering is inversely proportional to the fourth power of the wavelength; thus, longer wavelengths are significantly less affected by Rayleigh scattering. Perhaps, the number of successful measurements could be further increased by using an even higher wavelength; however, it would happen at the cost of the scan resolution [37].

In general, the technology of SS-OCT significantly increases the number of successful AL measurements, but as in rare cases the scan acquisition is not feasible, optical biometry still cannot fully supersede ultrasonic biometry. In order to benefit from the higher accuracy of optical biometry, both techniques should be available in the presurgical setting, with ultrasound biometry being reserved for cases of measurement failure [38].

Fig. 10.6 Comparison of a successful and an unsuccessful SS-OCT scan. The scan on top has successfully recognized the macula, while the scan at the bottom failed [37]

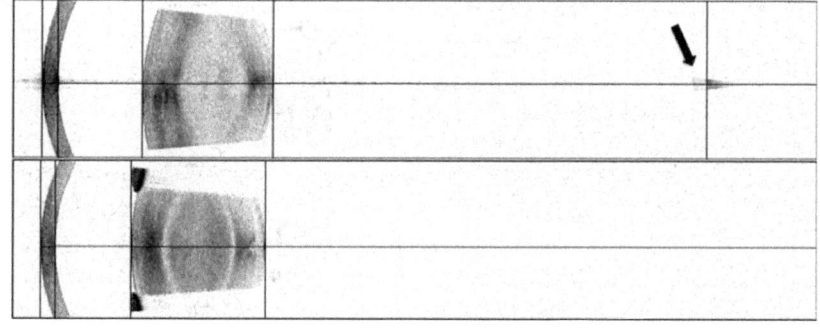

Optical Biometry: Cornea

Besides accurate determination of ocular distances, such as AL or ACD, measurement of the corneal power is also critical for precise IOL power calculation [44].

Keratometry readings can be achieved using keratometers and topography devices. In manual keratometry, the measurement is limited to the central 3.0 mm of the anterior cornea. The curvature is determined at two axes; the first meridian measured is the steep meridian where the radius of curvature is smallest. This meridian yields the maximum keratometry reading (Max K). The second meridian determined is the axis that is 90° apart from the steep meridian, which equals the flat meridian with the minimum keratometry reading (Min K). Thus, besides the assessment of the corneal radius of curvature, the presence of corneal astigmatism as well as its degree and orientation can be determined [45].

One of the first devices developed for this purpose was the Javal-Schiøtz keratometer, a manual keratometer which utilizes the principals of reflection as well as fixed image size and variable object size. Its rotating mechanism enables measurements in multiple meridians. The cornea and tear film act as a reflecting surface in the shape of a convex mirror. The image of an object of known size and distance is reflected and analyzed to determine the curvature of the cornea over a 3.0–4.0 mm diameter area, depending on the dioptric power of the cornea [44–46]. As a result, the device generates the anterior corneal radius of curvature in millimeters [47]. To estimate the total corneal power, a theoretical calculation based on the anterior corneal curvature and a standard refractive index is applied [48]. Although the actual refractive index of the cornea is 1.376, a slightly lower index of 1.3375 is used to account for the shorter radius of curvature of the posterior corneal surface [49]. The measurement is performed at two paraxial corneal radii, and the assumption is made that the shape of the cornea between these two points is spherical. Hence, due to the aspheric corneal surface because of the flattening toward its periphery, measurements obtained by manual keratometry are only accurate for the central, spherical part of the cornea and moreover, those devices are of limited value in cases of irregularly shaped corneas [45, 49].

With developments in electronic systems, automated keratometers, which mostly use television monitors instead of an eyepiece system to view the reflected image, were introduced. A popular device is the Topcon automated keratorefractometer (Topcon, Tokyo, Japan), which simultaneously determines refraction and keratometry. For the purpose of keratometry, infrared light is used to illuminate the target mires and an infrared photodetector measures the image size to translate to radius of curvature [45, 49].

Although the Javal-Schiøtz keratometer and similar devices developed over time obtained useful measurements of regular spherocylindrical corneas, they were mainly replaced by optical biometry devices which simultaneously offer integrated keratometry measurement [47]. As refractive indices used in different devices may vary, it is more accurate to describe the cornea in terms of radius of curvature than power [49].

The IOL Master, as described above, relies on PCI for the measurement of AL, while an integrated automated keratometer similarly performs telecentric keratometry by implementing five measurements at six spots on a 2.5 mm diameter to obtain the average keratometry values at the two major perpendicular meridians [45]. Another optical biometry device to offer integrated keratometry is the Lenstar LS900. While the device differs from the IOL Master in measuring optical distances, as it uses OLCR instead of PCI, the same technology is used to measure keratometry readings [50].

Many of the subsequently introduced devices are based on the Placido disk principle. The patient fixates at the center of a disc painted with alternating black and white rings, which are reflected from the anterior cornea and the reflections are analyzed to gain information about the surface shape of the cornea and to calculate its radius of curvature. A schematic diagram of a Placido disk topographer is shown in Fig. 10.7.

While keratoscopy using a Placido disk was initially complicated and time-consuming, as a

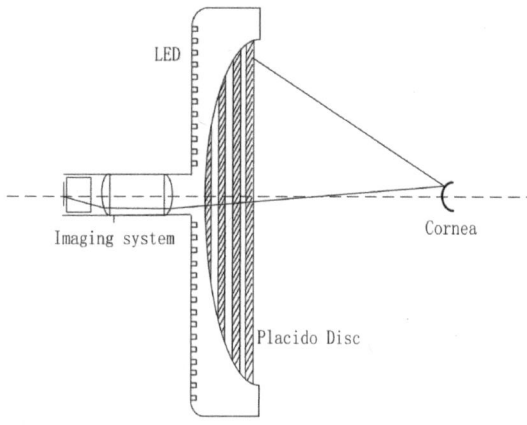

Fig. 10.7 Schematic diagram of a Placido disk topographer [51]

handheld device was used, following photography of the reflections and comparison of the photographs to images reflected by spheres of known radius, computer technology enabled the development of an automated use of the Placido disk. Many modern devices, such as some videokeratography devices, rely on the Placido disk principle. In computer-assisted videokeratography, computer programs are used to derive topographic information from a high-resolution cylindrical photokeratoscope. The images are digitized and, at the same time, displayed as color-coded maps of corneal power, photokeratoscopic images, wire mesh models, or solid models. Examples of commercially available systems are the EyeSys 3000 (EyeSys Laboratories, Houston, USA) and the TMS-I (Computer Anatomy Inc., New York, USA). A disadvantage of those devices is that they only take into account the anterior corneal surface and various assumptions must still be made regarding the relationship between the anterior and posterior corneal surface, in order to calculate the total corneal power [46, 49].

The primary advantage of modern technologies, which include slit-scanning Scheimpflug photography, very high-frequency ultrasound and optical coherence tomography, are increased accuracy, an extended area of measurement and the ability to directly measure the posterior corneal surface [46]. Those devices offer simulated keratometry readings (Sim K), based on the central 3.0 mm of the anterior corneal curvature alone, to allow for comparison with other instruments [44].

The first device to offer the possibility of measuring the posterior corneal surface was the Orbscan (Orbtek Inc., New York, USA), which uses optical slit-scanning. The cornea is scanned by multiple slit light beams to obtain two-dimensional, cross-sectional images which are then translated to a topographical map. The newer Orbscan II (Bausch & Lomb, New York, USA) and the TMS 5 (Tomey GmbH, Nürnberg, Germany) combine the slit-scanning method with a Placido disk to take advantage of both technologies [46]. Ring topography and slit-scan images are taken separately, and after the assessment of both, the data is merged [50].

Another keratometric method is Scheimpflug photography, whose technique is employed in the Pentacam (Oculus Inc., Wetzlar, Germany), the GALILEI (Zeimer Group, Port, Switzerland), and the SIRIUS (CSO, Scandicci, Italy). The Scheimpflug principle describes a condition that allows documentation of an obliquely tilted object (i.e., the planes of image, lens, and object are not parallel to each other) with maximum depth of focus and minimum image distortion. The principle allows for a specific arrangement of the three planes in order to increase the focal depth. In Scheimpflug photography, a rotating camera captures images of the anterior eye segment at different meridians around the optical axis, including anterior corneal surface, posterior corneal surface, and lens. In approximately 2 s, between 25 and 50 slit images are taken, with 500 elevation points incorporated in every one of them. A three-dimensional model of the anterior eye segment is created, and the software incorporated in the device calculates and displays topographical maps as well as power maps of the cornea (Fig. 10.8) [46, 50, 52].

Another method for corneal imaging is very high-frequency ultrasound. This technique is used in the Artemis (ArcScan Inc., Golden, USA) to allow for a direct visualization and measurement of the posterior corneal surface. Furthermore, three-dimensional maps of individual corneal layers can be obtained, which makes

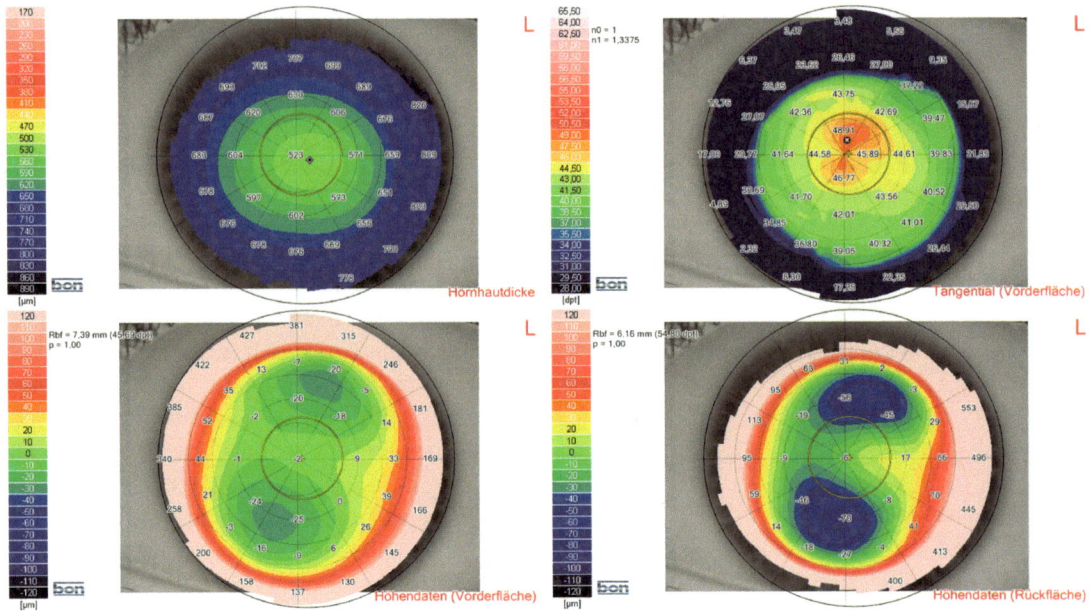

Fig. 10.8 Topographical maps and power maps of the cornea, generated by Scheimpflug photography

it an important tool in the field of keratorefractive surgery [46].

SS-OCT devices, such as the Casia 2 (Tomey, Nagoya, Japan), which is designed specifically for imaging the anterior segment, can be used for keratometric purposes. It is indicated for cross-sectional imaging of the anterior segment components such as anterior chamber or cornea, as well as for their dimension measurements such as curvature, length, area, or volume. To generate corneal maps, the shape of the cornea is analyzed similar to a topographer [53].

For all those devices, attention has to be paid to patients who underwent keratorefractive surgery prior to the measurement procedure, as their K readings need correction concerning the refractive power of the cornea and the predicted post-operative IOL position [47].

Although all these techniques provide reasonable results to be used in IOL power calculation, discrepancies concerning the mean spherical equivalent were found when comparing the devices. Those discrepancies may arise due to differences in the optical or mathematical methods used to calculate the total corneal power. Hamer et al. compared the results of different keratometers and found the corneal curvature to be measured steepest with the manual keratometer, followed by automated keratometry and Scheimpflug imaging. The flattest measurements were obtained with instruments that calculated Sim K from Placido disc topography. The corneal curvature was steeper when measured with the IOL Master compared to Placido disc topographers, which can be attributed to the small area that is used to simulate the K readings [44]. Reuland et al. compared the IOL Master and the Pentacam and showed that the results of the two devices are comparable [54].

The assessment of the mean spherical equivalent does not depend on the orientation of the power meridians and is therefore affected to a lower extent by erroneous readings at one meridian than the determination of astigmatic orientation and power. The latter is more prone to variable outcomes, which can be evaluated by intra-observer, interobserver, and between-session repeatability. In the study conducted by Hamer et al., repeatability was weaker for topographic devices and manual keratometers when compared to the Pentacam and the IOL Master.

The tear film has a significant influence on the repeatability of corneal topographers due to the likelihood of localized disturbances in an unstable tear film that may affect readings along a specific meridian and hence distort the measurement of astigmatism. This limitation, from which devices based on the Placido principle suffer more than those based on Scheimpflug imaging or automated keratometry, can be counteracted by administrating ocular lubricants prior to the measurement in order to stabilize the tear film [44]. However, instruments working with Placido discs deliver a higher level of spatial resolution compared to Scheimpflug devices and SS-OCT [50]. Instruments such as the IOL Master are more resistant to tear film-induced errors, owing to the small measurement zone. Furthermore, the integrated software provides numerous quality checks that may improve the measurement's reliability [44].

Concerning the Pentacam, total corneal power, which includes both the anterior and posterior corneal curvature, is a better representative for subjective cylinder than Sim K.

Devices that combine two methods, such as hybrid topographers, in which the anterior corneal surface is measured by the Placido disk principle, while Scheimpflug imaging is used for both the anterior and posterior surface, can potentially achieve more accurate results than one of the two techniques alone. Therefore, the results obtained by the TMS 5 are superior to Placido or Scheimpflug measurements alone [50]. Keratometric data can also be merged with topographic output to improve the results [55].

Hoffmann et al. compared multiple keratometry devices to the newer anterior segment OCT Casia SS-1000 and reported that SS-OCT measurements offer not only a good reproducibility in normal eyes but also in post-LASIK eyes and eyes with keratoconus. In their series, Casia SS-1000 delivered the best predictive power concerning astigmatism, compared to the Lenstar LS900 and the Pentacam. This may be due to the fact that it renders images much faster than the Pentacam and therefore minimizes motion artefacts. The results of the TMS 5 were comparable to the Casia SS-1000 [50].

In general, when calculating toric IOLs, not only the anterior but also the posterior corneal surface should be taken into account, as it plays a sig-

nificant role when evaluating the total amount of corneal astigmatism. While keratometric data is more stable than tomographic data, corneal tomography is more precise, as it includes the measurement of the posterior corneal curvature. For most patients, the best results may be obtained by combined keratometry, topography of the anterior corneal curvature, and tomography of the anterior and posterior curvature. Anterior segment OCT may be a useful tool for corneal tomography [5].

Intraoperative OCT

As discussed in previous sections of this chapter, modern techniques such as optical biometry have significantly improved IOL power calculation during the last decades. Although the latest generation of IOL power calculation formulae has further enhanced the postoperative refractive outcome, a relevant unpredictability still remains. When aiming for emmetropia, approximately 8.5% of all patients need a refractive correction of more than 1.0 D after cataract surgery, as stated by the data collected by the EUREQUO system for the purpose of quality control [56]. The incidence of unsatisfactory refractive outcomes depends on the length of the eye and is particularly apparent in shorter eyes (~30%) [57]. As shown by Olsen [6] and Norrby [58], the main source of postoperative refractive errors is an imprecise prediction of the final postoperative IOL position or postoperative ACD. In modern IOL power formulae, the so-called effective lens position (ELP), which is a virtual position predicted by preoperative measurements such as corneal radii, AL, or ACD, was developed to optimize the formulae for empirical data [59, 60]. However, the ELP does not directly correlate with the anatomical IOL position and is not capable of predicting the IOL position after surgery or the ACD shift within the first postoperative months with certainty [59]. It was shown that a better prediction factor for the final postoperative IOL position, compared to preoperative methods, is the real-time assessment of the intraoperative distance between the endothelium and the anterior lens capsule of the aphakic eye [57, 61].

The field of intraoperative OCT (iOCT) has advanced in several ways in recent years. The first iOCT system, which was a handheld probe that employed time-domain detection, was reported in 2001 by Radhakrishnan [62]. With the advent of Fourier-domain techniques, iOCT systems have further developed, using both spectrometer and swept-source systems to increase measurement speed and to allow for larger field-of-views and higher sampling densities [63]. Handheld probes had the advantage that the patient's head did not need to be positioned at a chin-rest, thus allowing image acquisition in supine position as well as in sterile settings for the first time, which was the major shift that initiated the evolution of OCT into the operating room. However, the images were affected by motion artefacts, they had a challenging reproducibility and frequent pauses were required during surgery for image acquisition. To address these issues, in a first attempt, the devices were mounted on conventional operating microscopes and later permanently integrated into the microscope optics to combine the two optical paths, allowing for visualization of two-dimensional OCT sections through the microscope's oculars or on an external display, thus providing the opportunity of real-time OCT during surgery [64]. Current-generation microscope-integrated iOCT systems can be combined either with direct or with indirect ophthalmic viewing systems and enable both anterior and posterior segment imaging intraoperatively [63].

In cataract surgery, microscope-integrated OCT is used extensively in training novel surgeons to improve surgical precision [64, 65]. It can be used to visualize corneal incisions, to evaluate the adequacy of stroma hydration at the end of the procedure to prevent postoperative wound leak or to assess trenching depth during phacoemulsification in order to prevent iatrogenic capsular rupture. Senior surgeons may also benefit from microscope-integrated OCT when facing clinically suspected complicated cases, such as identifying a true posterior polar cataract or capsular defects in traumatic cataracts [64].

In patients with mature cataracts in whom preoperative AL acquisition failed, iOCT can be used to assess AL values prior to IOL implanta-tion. Moreover, it can be helpful in patients with very low compliance.

The idea behind using iOCT for biometrical purposes, particularly for ACD measurement, stems from the lens haptic plane concept. The lens haptic plane can be considered the plane through the vertices of the IOL haptics, which is associated with the anatomical position of the IOL to be implanted, hence its fixation plane, when the site of fixation equals the equator of the capsular bag. The lens haptic plane is reasonably independent of the IOL model used [66, 67]. Measuring the anterior lens capsule of the aphakic eye intraoperatively allows to depict a position close to the theoretical lens haptic plane [57].

To evaluate the benefit of iOCT for ocular biometry, Hirnschall et al. performed intraoperative ACD measurements to predict the postoperative IOL position. They used a prototype of a continuous iOCT that was directly connected to the surgical microscope. In the surgical setting, intraoperative measurements of the aphakic eye were obtained following phacoemulsification and implantation of a capsular tension ring to tauten the lens capsule. A partial least-square regression model for ACD was created that proved the distance between corneal endothelium and anterior lens capsule to be a significantly better predictor for postoperative ACD compared to preoperative measurements. Intraoperatively measured ACD had the highest predictive power, and AL had the second highest predictive power, followed by preoperatively measured ACD. Improvement could further be achieved by using regression models combining preoperative and intraoperative ACD measurements [57, 59].

In the second step, Hirnschall et al. evaluated whether the implication of intraoperatively measured ACD into IOL power calculation formulae improves the postoperative refractive outcome. A partial least-regression model was generated to compare conventional optimized formulae with a formula including the ACD measured intraoperatively. As a result, it was shown that the latter was useful to better predict postoperative refraction and AL dependency could be significantly lowered. Future steps may be an automation of iOCT as well as its implementation into fourth-generation power formulae or ray tracing using the anatomical lens position instead of the currently used virtual ELP [60].

Optical biometry has evolved significantly in the last decades. Accuracy in preoperative measurements is vital for satisfactory postoperative refractive outcomes, so the latest biometry technologies combined with newer IOL power calculation formulae and lens designs have become necessary tools in the field of cataract surgery. With all the developments discussed in the chapter, refractive outcomes in a range of ±0.5 D have become achievable in a majority of the patients. However, as the attainment of the target postoperative refraction is not achieved in all cases, further research is still required [68].

References

1. Drexler W, Findl O, Menapace R, Rainer G, Vass C, Hitzenberger CK, Fercher AF. Partial coherence interferometry: a novel approach to biometry in cataract surgery. Am J Ophthalmol. 1998;126(4):524–34. https://doi.org/10.1016/S0002-9394(98)00113-5.
2. Fontes BM, Fontes BM, Castro E. Intraocular lens power calculation by measuring axial length with partial optical coherence and ultrasonic biometry. Arq Bras Oftalmol. 2011;74(3):166–70. https://doi.org/10.1590/S0004-27492011000300004.
3. Goto S, Maeda N, Noda T, Ohnuma K, Koh S, Iehisa I, Nishida K. Comparison of composite and segmental methods for acquiring optical axial length with swept-source optical coherence tomography. Sci Rep. 2020;10(1):4474. https://doi.org/10.1038/s41598-020-61391-7.
4. Hitzenberger CK, Fercher AF, Juchem M. Measurement of the axial eye length and retinal thickness by laser Doppler interferometry. In: Puliafito CA, editor. Optics, electro-optics, and laser applications in science and engineering. SPIE; 1991. p. 46–50. https://doi.org/10.1117/12.43956.
5. Lee AC, Qazi MA, Pepose JS. Biometry and intraocular lens power calculation. Curr Opin Ophthalmol. 2008;19(1):13–7. https://doi.org/10.1097/ICU.0b013e3282f1c5ad.
6. Olsen T. Sources of error in intraocular lens power calculation. J Cataract Refract Surg. 1992;18(2):125–9. https://doi.org/10.1016/S0886-3350(13)80917-0.
7. Ivanov AP, Chaikovskii AP, Kumeisha AA. New method for high-range resolution measurements of light scattering in optically dense inhomogeneous media. Opt Lett. 1977;1(6):226. https://doi.org/10.1364/OL.1.000226.
8. Hitzenberger CK, Drexler W, Leitgeb RA, Findl O, Fercher AF. Key developments for partial coherence biometry and optical coherence tomography in the human eye made in Vienna. Invest Opthalmol Vis Sci. 2016;57(9):OCT460. https://doi.org/10.1167/iovs.16-19362.
9. Fercher AF, Roth E. Ophthalmic laser interferometry. In: Mueller GJ, editor. Optical instrumentation for biomedical laser applications, vol. 658. SPIE; 1986. p. 48. https://doi.org/10.1117/12.938523.
10. Hitzenberger CK. Optical measurement of the axial eye length by laser Doppler interferometry. Invest Ophthalmol Vis Sci. 1991;32(3):616–24.
11. Kunert KS, Peter M, Blum M, Haigis W, Sekundo W, Schütze J, Büehren T. Repeatability and agreement in optical biometry of a new swept-source optical coherence tomography–based biometer versus partial coherence interferometry and optical low-coherence reflectometry. J Cataract Refract Surg. 2016;42(1):76–83. https://doi.org/10.1016/j.jcrs.2015.07.039.
12. Findl O, Drexler W, Menapace R, Heinzl H, Hitzenberger CK, Fercher AF. Improved prediction of intraocular lens power using partial coherence interferometry. J Cataract Refract Surg. 2001;27(6):861–7. https://doi.org/10.1016/S0886-3350(00)00699-4.
13. Cech R, Utíkal T, Juhászová J. [Comparison of optical and ultrasound biometry and assessment of using both methods in practice]. Ceska Slov Oftalmol Cas Ceske Oftalmol Spolecnosti Slov Oftalmol Spolecnosti. 2014;70(1):3–9.
14. Drexler W. Measurement of the thickness of fundus layers by partial coherence tomography. Opt Eng. 1995;34(3):701. https://doi.org/10.1117/12.191809.
15. Cantor LB, Rapuano CJ, Cioffi GA. Basic and clinical science course (BCSC), section 03: clinical optics. American Academy of Ophthalmology; 2014.
16. Hitzenberger C, Mengedoht K, Fercher AF. [Laser optic measurements of the axial length of the eye]. Fortschritte Ophthalmol Z Dtsch Ophthalmol Ges. 1989;86(2):159–61.
17. Kohnen T, editor. Modern cataract surgery. Karger; 2002.
18. Sacu S, Findl O, Buehl W, Kiss B, Gleiss A, Drexler W. Optical biometry of the anterior eye segment: interexaminer and intraexaminer reliability of ACMaster. J Cataract Refract Surg. 2005;31(12):2334–9. https://doi.org/10.1016/j.jcrs.2005.04.035.
19. Lavanya R, Teo L, Friedman DS, Aung HT, Baskaran M, Gao H, Alfred T, Seah SK, Kashiwagi K, Foster PJ, Aung T. Comparison of anterior chamber depth measurements using the IOLMaster, scanning peripheral anterior chamber depth analyser, and anterior segment optical coherence tomography. Br J Ophthalmol. 2007;91(8):1023–6. https://doi.org/10.1136/bjo.2006.113761.
20. Buehl W, Stojanac D, Sacu S, Drexler W, Findl O. Comparison of three methods of measuring corneal thickness and anterior chamber depth. Am J Ophthalmol. 2006;141(1):7–12.e1. https://doi.org/10.1016/j.ajo.2005.08.048.

21. Kriechbaum K, Leydolt C, Findl O, Bolz M, Drexler W. Comparison of partial coherence interferometers: Acmaster versus laboratory prototype. J Refract Surg (Thorofare, NJ, 1995). 2006;22(8):811–6.

22. Huang J, McAlinden C, Huang Y, Wen D, Savini G, Tu R, Wang Q. Meta-analysis of optical low-coherence reflectometry versus partial coherence interferometry biometry. Sci Rep. 2017;7(1):43414. https://doi.org/10.1038/srep43414.

23. Hoffer KJ, Shammas JH, Savini G. Comparison of 2 laser instruments for measuring axial length. J Cataract Refract Surg. 2010;36(4):644–8. https://doi.org/10.1016/j.jcrs.2009.11.007.

24. Epitropoulos A. Axial length measurement acquisition rates of two optical biometers in cataractous eyes. Clin Ophthalmol. 2014;8:1369. Published online Jul 2014. https://doi.org/10.2147/OPTH.S62653.

25. Hirnschall N, Murphy S, Pimenides D, Maurino V, Findl O. Assessment of a new averaging algorithm to increase the sensitivity of axial eye length measurement with optical biometry in eyes with dense cataract. J Cataract Refract Surg. 2011;37(1):45–9. https://doi.org/10.1016/j.jcrs.2010.07.023.

26. Dietlein TS, Roessler G, Lüke C, Dinslage S, Roters S, Jacobi PC, Walter P, Krieglstein GK. Signal quality of biometry in silicone oil–filled eyes using partial coherence laser interferometry. J Cataract Refract Surg. 2005;31(5):1006–10. https://doi.org/10.1016/j.jcrs.2004.09.049.

27. Suto C, Sato C, Shimamura E, Toshida H, Ichikawa K, Hori S. Influence of the signal-to-noise ratio on the accuracy of IOLMaster measurements. J Cataract Refract Surg. 2007;33(12):2062–6. https://doi.org/10.1016/j.jcrs.2007.07.031.

28. Szkulmowski M, Wojtkowski M. Averaging techniques for OCT imaging. Opt Express. 2013;21(8):9757. https://doi.org/10.1364/OE.21.009757.

29. Huang D, Swanson E, Lin C, Schuman J, Stinson W, Chang W, Hee M, Flotte T, Gregory K, Puliafito C, et al. Optical coherence tomography. Science. 1991;254(5035):1178–81. https://doi.org/10.1126/science.1957169.

30. Yaqoob Z, Wu J, Yang C. Spectral domain optical coherence tomography: a better OCT imaging strategy. BioTechniques. 2005;39(6S):S6–S13. https://doi.org/10.2144/000112090.

31. Drexler W, Fujimoto JG, editors. Optical coherence tomography. Springer International Publishing; 2015. https://doi.org/10.1007/978-3-319-06419-2.

32. Schuman JS. Spectral domain optical coherence tomography for glaucoma (an AOS thesis). Trans Am Ophthalmol Soc. 2008;106:426–58.

33. Alibhai YA, Or C, Witkin AJ. Swept source optical coherence tomography: a review. Curr Ophthalmol Rep. 2018;6(1):7–16. https://doi.org/10.1007/s40135-018-0158-3.

34. Kishi S. Impact of swept source optical coherence tomography on ophthalmology. Taiwan J Ophthalmol. 2016;6(2):58–68. https://doi.org/10.1016/j.tjo.2015.09.002.

35. Cole ED, Duker JS. OCT technology: will we be "swept" away? Rev Ophthalmol. Published online Apr 2017. https://www.reviewofophthalmology.com/article/oct-technology-will-we-be-swept-away.

36. Kiss B, Findl O, Menapace R, Wirtitsch M, Drexler W, Hitzenberger CK, Fercher AF. Biometry of cataractous eyes using partial coherence interferometry: clinical feasibility study of a commercial prototype I. J Cataract Refract Surg. 2002;28(2):224–9. https://doi.org/10.1016/s0886-3350(01)01272-x.

37. Hirnschall N, Varsits R, Doeller B, Findl O. Enhanced penetration for axial length measurement of eyes with dense cataracts using swept source optical coherence tomography: a consecutive observational study. Ophthalmol Ther. 2018;7(1):119–24. https://doi.org/10.1007/s40123-018-0122-1.

38. Freeman G, Pesudovs K. The impact of cataract severity on measurement acquisition with the IOLMaster. Acta Ophthalmol Scand. 2005;83(4):439–42. https://doi.org/10.1111/j.1600-0420.2005.00473.x.

39. Rajan MS, Keilhorn I, Bell JA. Partial coherence laser interferometry vs conventional ultrasound biometry in intraocular lens power calculations. Eye. 2002;16(5):552–6. https://doi.org/10.1038/sj.eye.6700157.

40. Findl O, Drexler W, Menapace R, Hitzenberger CK, Fercher AF. High precision biometry of pseudophakic eyes using partial coherence interferometry. J Cataract Refract Surg. 1998;24(8):1087–93. https://doi.org/10.1016/S0886-3350(98)80102-8.

41. Haigis W, Lege B, Miller N, Schneider B. Comparison of immersion ultrasound biometry and partial coherence interferometry for intraocular lens calculation according to Haigis. Graefes Arch Clin Exp Ophthalmol. 2000;238(9):765–73. https://doi.org/10.1007/s004170000188.

42. Srivannaboon S, Chirapapaisan C, Chonpimai P, Loket S. Clinical comparison of a new swept-source optical coherence tomography–based optical biometer and a time-domain optical coherence tomography–based optical biometer. J Cataract Refract Surg. 2015;41(10):2224–32. https://doi.org/10.1016/j.jcrs.2015.03.019.

43. Akman A, Asena L, Güngör SG. Evaluation and comparison of the new swept source OCT-based IOLMaster 700 with the IOLMaster 500. Br J Ophthalmol. 2016;100(9):1201–5. https://doi.org/10.1136/bjophthalmol-2015-307779.

44. Hamer CA, Buckhurst H, Purslow C, Shum GL, Habib NE, Buckhurst PJ. Comparison of reliability and repeatability of corneal curvature assessment with six keratometers: comparison of six keratometers. Clin Exp Optom. 2016;99(6):583–9. https://doi.org/10.1111/cxo.12329.

45. Mehravaran S, Asgari S, Bigdeli S, Shahnazi A, Hashemi H. Keratometry with five different techniques: a study of device repeatability and inter-device agreement. Int Ophthalmol. 2014;34(4):869–75. https://doi.org/10.1007/s10792-013-9895-3.

46. Gutmark R, Guyton DL. Origins of the keratometer and its evolving role in ophthalmology. Surv

Ophthalmol. 2010;55(5):481–97. https://doi.org/10.1016/j.survophthal.2010.03.001.

47. Hirnschall N, Findl O. Patient-assessment techniques for cataract surgery. Expert Rev Ophthalmol. 2011;6(2):211–9. https://doi.org/10.1586/eop.11.4.

48. Hoshikawa R, Kamiya K, Fujimura F, Shoji N. Comparison of conventional keratometry and total keratometry in normal eyes. Biomed Res Int. 2020;2020:1–6. https://doi.org/10.1155/2020/8075924.

49. Fowler CW, Dave TN. Review of past and present techniques of measuring corneal topography. Ophthalmic Physiol Opt. 1994;14(1):49–58. https://doi.org/10.1111/j.1475-1313.1994.tb00556.x.

50. Hoffmann PC, Abraham M, Hirnschall N, Findl O. Prediction of residual astigmatism after cataract surgery using swept source Fourier domain optical coherence tomography. Curr Eye Res. 2014;39(12):1178–86. https://doi.org/10.3109/02713683.2014.898376.

51. Sui C, Wo S, Cai P, Gao N, Xu D, Han Y, Du C. Design and implementation of optical system for Placido-disc topography. J Mod Opt. 2017;64(21):2413–9. https://doi.org/10.1080/09500340.2017.1366567.

52. Wegener A, Laser-Junga H. Photography of the anterior eye segment according to Scheimpflug's principle: options and limitations—a review. Clin Exp Ophthalmol. 2009;37(1):144–54. https://doi.org/10.1111/j.1442-9071.2009.02018.x.

53. Angmo D, Nongpiur M, Sharma R, Sidhu T, Sihota R, Dada T. Clinical utility of anterior segment swept-source optical coherence tomography in glaucoma. Oman J Ophthalmol. 2016;9(1):3. https://doi.org/10.4103/0974-620X.176093.

54. Reuland MS, Reuland AJ, Nishi Y, Auffarth GU. Corneal radii and anterior chamber depth measurements using the IOLmaster versus the Pentacam. J Refract Surg (Thorofare, NJ, 1995). 2007;23(4):368–73.

55. Hoffmann PC, Wahl J, Hütz WW, Preußner P-R. A ray tracing approach to calculate toric intraocular lenses. J Refract Surg. 2013;29(6):402–8. https://doi.org/10.3928/1081597X-20130515-04.

56. Lundström M, Barry P, Henry Y, Rosen P, Stenevi U. Evidence-based guidelines for cataract surgery: guidelines based on data in the European registry of quality outcomes for cataract and refractive surgery database. J Cataract Refract Surg. 2012;38(6):1086–93. https://doi.org/10.1016/j.jcrs.2012.03.006.

57. Hirnschall N, Farrokhi S, Amir-Asgari S, Hienert J, Findl O. Intraoperative optical coherence tomography measurements of aphakic eyes to predict postoperative position of 2 intraocular lens designs. J Cataract Refract Surg. 2018;44(11):1310–6. https://doi.org/10.1016/j.jcrs.2018.07.044.

58. Norrby S. Sources of error in intraocular lens power calculation. J Cataract Refract Surg. 2008;34(3):368–76. https://doi.org/10.1016/j.jcrs.2007.10.031.

59. Hirnschall N, Amir-Asgari S, Maedel S, Findl O. Predicting the postoperative intraocular lens position using continuous intraoperative optical coherence tomography measurements. Invest Opthalmol Vis Sci. 2013;54(8):5196. https://doi.org/10.1167/iovs.13-11991.

60. Hirnschall N, Norrby S, Weber M, Maedel S, Amir-Asgari S, Findl O. Using continuous intraoperative optical coherence tomography measurements of the aphakic eye for intraocular lens power calculation. Br J Ophthalmol. 2015;99(1):7–10. https://doi.org/10.1136/bjophthalmol-2013-304731.

61. Pujari A, Agarwal D, Chawla R, Kumar A, Sharma N. Intraoperative optical coherence tomography guided ocular surgeries: critical analysis of clinical role and future perspectives. Clin Ophthalmol. 2020;14:2427–40. https://doi.org/10.2147/OPTH.S270708.

62. Radhakrishnan S. Real-time optical coherence tomography of the anterior segment at 1310 nm. Arch Ophthalmol. 2001;119(8):1179. https://doi.org/10.1001/archopht.119.8.1179.

63. El-Haddad MT, Tao YK. Advances in intraoperative optical coherence tomography for surgical guidance. Curr Opin Biomed Eng. 2017;3:37–48. https://doi.org/10.1016/j.cobme.2017.09.007.

64. Posarelli C, Sartini F, Casini G, Passani A, Toro MD, Vella G, Figus M. What is the impact of intraoperative microscope-integrated OCT in ophthalmic surgery? Relevant applications and outcomes. A systematic review. J Clin Med. 2020;9(6):1682. https://doi.org/10.3390/jcm9061682.

65. Carrasco-Zevallos OM, Viehland C, Keller B, Draelos M, Kuo AN, Toth CA, Izatt JA. Review of intraoperative optical coherence tomography: technology and applications [Invited]. Biomed Opt Express. 2017;8(3):1607. https://doi.org/10.1364/BOE.8.001607.

66. Norrby SNE, Koranyi G. Prediction of intraocular lens power using the lens haptic plane concept. J Cataract Refract Surg. 1997;23(2):254–9. https://doi.org/10.1016/S0886-3350(97)80350-1.

67. Norrby NES. The lens haptic plane (LHP) a fixed reference for IOL implant power calculation. Eur J Implant Refract Surg. 1995;7(4):202–9. https://doi.org/10.1016/S0955-3681(13)80035-4.

68. Nazm N, Chakrabarti A. Update on optical biometry and intraocular lens power calculation. TNOA J Ophthal Sci Res. 2017;55(3):196. https://doi.org/10.4103/tjosr.tjosr_44_17.

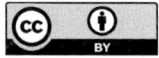

Axial Length Measurement

11

David L. Cooke

Introduction

Optical biometry has markedly improved postoperative predictions after cataract surgery. Prior to this time, ultrasound (US) was the standard. The IOLMaster (Carl Zeiss, Jena, Germany) was markedly less user-dependent, and its axial length (AL) measurements were shown to be more repeatable than those by US biometry; it became the gold standard shortly after its release in 1999.

For nearly 20 years, there has been only one way to optically measure the AL—the way Haigis set up in late 1990s and published in 2000. It is used in the IOLMaster (version 500 and earlier), and most competitors have tuned their machine to that method. It has been unclear what to label this AL. It has been called "Axial Length Measurements Based on Single Refractive Index" [1], "Composite method for acquiring optical axial length" [2], "Axial Length Using a Single Group Refractive Index" [3], and "Displayed AL" [3]. There are some problems with each of these labels. In this chapter, it will be called "Traditional AL."

Recently, another method has arisen, where the segment lengths are added together and a theoretical retinal thickness (fudge factor) is sub-

tracted from all values until the average AL for the dataset is equal to the average IOLMaster AL. It has correctly been called by at least all these labels, "Segmented AL," "Segmental AL," "Segment-wise AL," "Axial Length Measurements Based on Multiple Refractive Indices," "Segmental method for acquiring optical axial length," and "Axial Length Using different Refractive Indices for Each Ocular Segment." In this chapter, it will be called sum-of-segments AL.

The goal of this chapter is to explain and explore these two AL methods. Topics will be presented in this order, with these headings: basic science, definitions of commonly used terms, history, ocular segments, and areas for potential improvement.

Basic Science

Axial Length Measurements

Since the geometric length of the eye or its segments cannot be measured directly (such as using a ruler or caliper), technologies had to be developed to measure them *indirectly*. Two of them which provide adequate resolution for ophthalmic purposes are US and optical biometry.

D. L. Cooke (✉)
Department of Neurology and Ophthalmology, Michigan State University, College of Osteopathic Medicine, East Lansing, MI, USA

Great Lakes Eye Care, St. Joseph, Michigan, USA

© The Author(s) 2024
J. Aramberri et al. (eds.), *Intraocular Lens Calculations*, Essentials in Ophthalmology,
https://doi.org/10.1007/978-3-031-50666-6_11

Ultrasound (US) Biometry

US biometry measures the time (*T*) that sound takes to reflect off the interfaces in the eye. These times are converted to geometrical lengths by multiplying the time by the sound velocities *V*.

$$\text{Length} = T_{\text{measured}} * V_{\text{Media}} \qquad (11.1)$$

Early US machines only measured reliable signals from the retina internal limiting membrane (ILM). Later, high-precision immersion US systems, like those used today, detected signals from the ocular segments as well. Besides providing the individual segmental lengths (aqueous, lens, vitreous), these systems provided the initial sum-of-segments axial length measurements of the eye. Widely used sound velocities are $V_{\text{aqueous}} = 1532\,\text{m/s}$, $V_{\text{lens}} = 1641\,\text{m/s}$, and $V_{\text{vitreous}} = 1532\,\text{m/s}$.

Carefully performed, segmental immersion ultrasound measurements provide the most accurate US sum-of-segments ALs. There are some drawbacks compared to optical biometry, however. Because US reflects off the ILM, retinal pathologies such as an epiretinal membrane, may adversely affect US ALs. In addition, its resolution and reproducibility are less than those of optical biometry.

Optical Biometry (Interferometry)

All optical biometers and OCTs (Optical Coherence Tomography) are interferometers. The original, time-domain biometers work in this fashion (see Fig. 11.1): a beam of light is emitted from the machine toward the eye, passing through a beam splitter. Beam 1 travels to the eye, and beam 2 travels through air to a moveable mirror. After reflections, these beams travel to a photosensor which detects the intensity of light formed by the constructive and destructive interference of the two beams.

Reflections of beam 1 occur where there are sharp changes in refractive index such as at media boundaries. Spikes from constructive interference occur when the optical time for beam 1 to travel from the light source to the eye and back to the photodetector is identical to the optical time for beam 2 to travel from the light source to the beam splitter, to the moveable mirror, and back to the photodetector.

The mirror may move either backward or forward. For this example, it will move backward. As it does, an initial photodetector spike is generated due to beam 1 reflection from the anterior cornea. This is typically the reference point for the rest of the measurements. As the mirror moves further, the next spike occurs at the posterior corneal surface. The distance moved by the mirror between the first and the second spikes is the "air distance" or "optical path length" (OPL) of the cornea. The distance the mirror moves between the second and third spikes is the OPL of the aqueous and so on through the eye.

If we knew the speed of light through the cornea (mm/s), and we knew the time (s) it took to travel through the cornea, we could multiply the speed of light by that time to get the true geomet-

Fig. 11.1 Interferometer

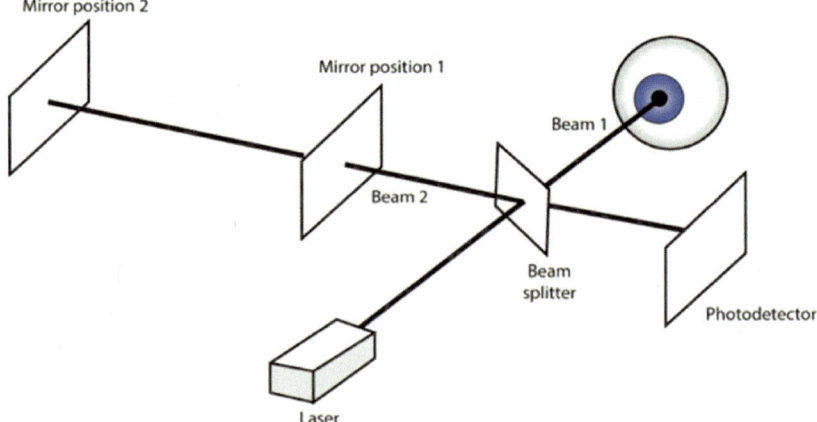

ric thickness of the cornea in mm. Unfortunately, we cannot directly measure the speed of light in the cornea. However, because the refractive index (RI) is the ratio of the speed of light in the cornea to the speed of light in air, we can set up the following ratios:

$$\frac{\text{Speed of light in air}}{\text{Speed of light in cornea}} = RI = \frac{\text{Air length of cornea}\,(\text{OPL})}{\text{Geometric corneal length}} \quad (11.2)$$

Rearranging this equation, we can determine the geometric length of the cornea

$$\text{Geometric length} = \frac{\text{OPL}}{\text{RI}} \quad (11.3)$$

where OPL is the optical path of the cornea and RI is the refractive index of the cornea.

Newer instruments use more efficient methods of interferometry than time-domain interferometry, such as swept-source interferometry. The concepts of air distance, optical path length, and refractive indices all still apply to every optical biometer as well as to every OCT machine.

An optical biometer produces a picture that is very similar to an ultrasound A-scan (Fig. 11.2). The OCT lines up several optical "A-scans" to create a two-dimensional image in the same way an ultrasound B-scan lines up several A-scans to create a two-dimensional image. The OCT is an "optical B-scan" while a simple optical biometer is an "optical A-scan."

Refractive Indices (RIs)

Refractive indices are typically measured with a refractometer that is temperature-controlled between 20 and 25 °C because temperature has a large effect on refractive index. It is customary for a single wavelength to be used, such as the sodium D line at 589 nm. Refractive indices in literature typically refer to this D line. The refractive index of a single wavelength is called a phase RI. A group RI results when more than one wavelength is used, as is the case with partial or low-coherent light.

Scaling Formulas

A prism-induced "rainbow" is a good demonstration of the speed of light varying by wavelength. If all wavelengths traveled at the same speed, white light would exit a prism the same way it entered, as white light. Obviously this isn't the case. The shorter, violet wavelengths are bent most. That is the same as saying the RI of violet waves is higher than for longer red waves.

The rule to remember is that as a light wavelength changes, one must use a different refractive index for the same substance. An example might be the aqueous. Gullstrand found a phase refractive index of 1.336. It is a bit unclear whether this was at green light (555 nm) or yel-

Fig. 11.2 Typical "A-scan" produced by an optical biometer. The first spike is the reflection produced by the air–corneal interface of the anterior cornea. The first "×" is above the spike produced at the posterior cornea. The second "×" is above the spike of the anterior capsule of the crystalline lens. The third "×" is above the spike of posterior capsule; the fourth "×" is above the junction of the anterior retina and the vitreous. This spike is not visible in some eyes. The final "×" is above the spike of the retinal pigment epithelium

low light (593 nm). However, it is clear that for a light wave of 1050 nm—the light wave of the ARGOS biometer (Movu, Santa Clara, California) [4]—the RI should be a different value than 1.336, the value ARGOS uses.

Because the change in RI by wavelength is not linear, scaling formulas are necessary. These formulas attempt to predict what the RI of a substance (e.g., the cornea) will be at different wavelengths.

The key points from the basic science section

- All OCTs and optical biometers measure an "air distance" which must be divided by a group refractive index to determine the actual length of an ocular segment, such as the cornea.
- Gullstrand RIs apply to green or yellow light, but likely not to the invisible wavelength used in optical biometers.
- Because the actual group RIs for the measuring wavelengths of biometers at body temperatures aren't known, we don't know the actual thicknesses of the ocular segments. Instead, the axial length was calibrated to ultrasound AL of the eye (discussed further in the "History" section).
- Though current measurements may not be physiologically accurate, both US AL and optical AL could be physically correct if either correct sound velocities (V) or group refractive indices (RIs) were known.

Definitions of Commonly Used Terms.

Coherence

The term "coherence" is used in the label of many ocular machines: OCT (optical coherence tomography), OLCR (optical low-coherence reflectometry), OLCI (optical low-coherence interferometry), and PCI (partial coherence interferometry). The ARGOS has been called a "large-coherence length" swept-source OCT.

The difference between coherent and non-coherent light is in the capability of generating interference. Generally speaking, if incoherent light arrives from two sources, its intensity just adds up from the two sources and you see the illuminated spot brighter. For example, by shin-

ing two flashlights at the same spot at night, you get twice the intensity.

From our interferometry example, beams 1 and 2 both go to separate mirrors and instead of having the beams converge on a photosensor, they project onto a screen. When both beams travel the same distance in air (OPL), the optical path difference (OPD) between the two paths is zero.

For each tiny part of the final image, the two waves either amplify or weaken each other, depending on the OPD between the two beams at that exact point. If the OPD = 0, constructive interference happens and the intensity increases to 4 times that of a single beam. If the OPD = half a wavelength, then the peak of one wave meets the trough from the other wave, and they cancel each other out leading to an intensity of zero at that spot. This often causes adjacent bright and dark lines referred to as interference fringes (see Fig. 11.3). The pattern of lines on the screen looks like fingerprint lines. The main difference between coherent and incoherent light is that the former interferes causing fringes while the latter just makes the spot brighter.

If a beam of white light is used in our interference example, you will see fringes when the OPD between the two paths is zero. When OPD is increased very slightly, the fringes "wash out" and you just see a spot of light. For a Helium–Neon (HeNe) laser, you can move one mirror by 25 m and still get interference fringes. Coherence

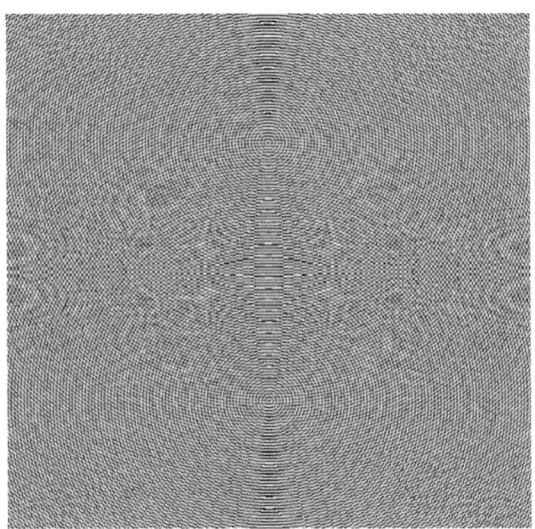

Fig. 11.3 Interference fringe

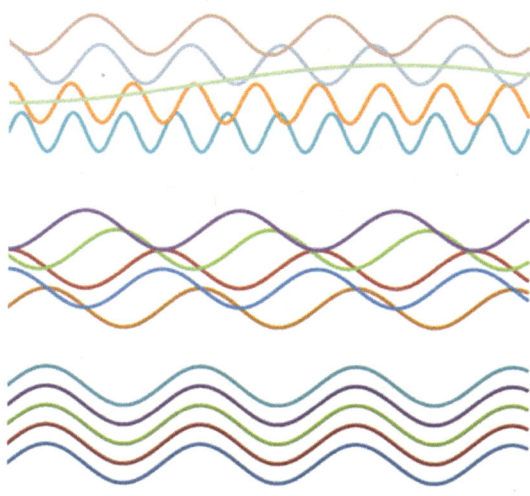

Fig. 11.4 Coherence diagram. Waves align for highly coherent light (bottom row); they partially align for partial coherence light (middle row). Incoherent waves do not align (top row)

length is the OPD between the two beams over which you still get interference fringes. In other words, the coherence length is the maximum OPD between the two paths of an interferometer over which the light wave maintains a harmonic shape such that you can still see interference fringes (before the fringes wash out).

White light has a very short coherence length of a few nm. Low coherence length is approximately 160 μm [5], and large coherence length is in the range of 15–30 mm [6]. "Partial coherence," "low coherence," and "short coherence length" are equivalent terms (Fig. 11.4). Reflectometer is another name for interferometer (in an ophthalmology setting).

Group RI

Group RI and *phase RI* are often discussed together because they are related. The refractive index of a single wavelength, such as a HeNe laser, is called a *phase RI*. Biometers use laser diodes or super-luminescent diodes which emit a bandwidth centered about a single wavelength. The bandwidth reduces the coherence length. This group of wavelengths is treated as if it were one wavelength. It is called a *group RI*, and it has a slightly different RI than the *phase RI*.

History

Haigis calibrated optical biometry to segmental immersion US AL measurements. He calculated a weighted-average of the segment group refractive indices (RIs). Note that he didn't use segment phase RIs, and note that the weighted average RI is not called a group RI.

In the English literature, he measured only 98 eyes with both immersion US biometry and optical biometry optical path lengths (OPLs) [7]. However, he actually measured more than 600 eyes [8], and he later confirmed this with 320 eyes, obtaining 5 measurements for each eye [9]; he then correlated optical biometry OPL with immersion sum-of-segments US AL. He couldn't calculate optical biometry sum-of-segments AL because the IOLMaster could only measure two spikes: one at the anterior cornea and one at the retinal pigment epithelium (RPE).

He initially used a weighted-average group refractive index RI ("composite RI") approximated from the Gullstrand eye (1.3549). However, a regression formula worked better than using the average RI. He kept 1.3549 in the formula, and this decision has caused some confusion. When a regression includes a formula, the regression often undoes it, creating a new formula instead. Haigis showed this in a German-language article [10]. Haigis stated that the original formula (containing the composite RI of 1.3549) used in the IOLMaster algorithm:

$$AL_{GBS} = \left(OPL_{IOLMaster} / 1.3549 - 1.3033 \right) / 0.9571 \tag{11.4}$$

was identical to this new formula, which he labeled "calibration function":

$$AL_{Zeiss} = 0.7711 \times OPL_{IOLMaster} - 1.3617 \tag{11.5}$$

AL$_{GBS}$ was the measured segmental immersion US AL. Haigis replaced this with AL$_{Zeiss}$ which is the algorithm used in the IOLMaster (version 500 and earlier). Haigis emphasized, "Consequently, the calibration function (Eq. 11.5) also contains no group refractive indices as a variable." Simply-put, he had the OPL and found a regression which converted that OPL to an ultrasound-equivalent AL. When he regressed to US, it negated the average group RI of 1.3549. Any RI could have been included in that original formula, and the regression coefficients would have changed accordingly, ending up with Eq. (11.5).

Shortly after the IOLMaster was introduced, debate arose as to whether Haigis had properly calibrated it. At least two groups which use ray-tracing [11, 12] used a different calibration algorithm. Fam [13] and later Wang [14] adjusted the biometric parameters for eyes of certain ALs, to compensate for observed refractive errors.

Haigis's calibrated AL (Eqs. 11.4 or 11.5) has become the traditional AL to which other biometers have been calibrated [10]. It is important to note that this distance is not the physiological AL, from the anterior cornea to the RPE (where the photoreceptors lie), but rather from the anterior cornea to the internal limiting membrane of the retina.

Lenstar

When Haag-Streit initially developed the Lenstar, its plan was to use sum-of-segments AL instead of traditional AL. However, in order to release the Lenstar with the FDA's 510K-approval [15], the Lenstar had to be made substantially equivalent to the IOLMaster. Because of this, Haag-Streit disabled the sum-of-segments capability. It would only be available as a research option.

Sum-of-Segments AL

Sum-of-segments AL is quite different from traditional AL at the extremes. Compared to sum-of-segments AL, traditional AL is shorter for short eyes and longer for long eyes. Figure 11.5 illustrates the difference between these two methods of calculating optical AL. Trend lines are plotted instead of the actual data from the 1442 eyes which were used to develop these trend lines. Figure 11.5a is a Bland-Altman plot which shows that sum-of-segments AL is the same length as traditional AL in the normal AL range of 24 mm, but not at the extremes.

The effect of sum-of-segments AL on prediction errors is illustrated in Fig. 11.5b. Prediction errors are about the same for both methods of calculating AL, when ALs are in the typical range of approximately 24 mm. At extreme ALs, sum-of-segments AL (dashed line in Fig. 11.5b) gave a

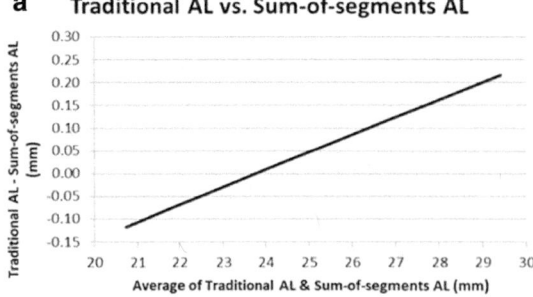

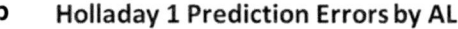

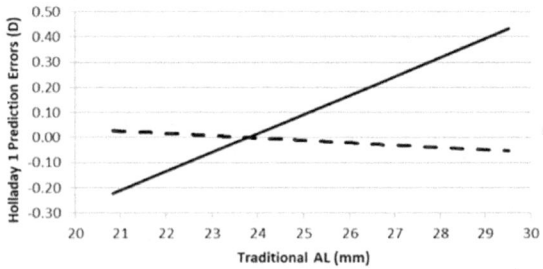

Fig. 11.5 (**a**) (Left) Bland-Altman graph of traditional AL vs. sum-of-segments AL, using the trend line of 1442 ALs measured with Lenstar. Axial length was calculated by two methods: traditional AL and sum-of-segments AL (modified from Cooke and Cooke [16]). (**b**) (Right) shows the trend lines of 1442 Holladay 1 prediction errors by traditional AL and sum-of-segments AL (modified from Cooke and Cooke [16]). The solid line represents the prediction error when using traditional AL. Sum-of-segments AL was used in calculating the dashed line. All other formula inputs were identical, including lens constants

notable improvement over using Holladay 1 with traditional AL (solid line) and it nearly optimized the Holladay 1 prediction error trend line.

The dashed line in Fig. 11.5b illustrates the findings of at least two studies [3, 16], which have shown that original vergence formulas (such as Holladay 1) are improved when sum-of-segments AL is used instead of traditional AL. The Olsen formula is known to have an internal AL recalibration. As expected, it was shown to be worse with sum-of-segments AL in both studies. Presumably, newer formulas have internal AL adjustments for long and short eyes such that they would perform worse when using sum-of-segments AL than when using traditional AL.

For most biometers, segment OPLs are only available in a research mode, if they are available at all. Because sum-of-segments AL requires these segment OPLs, we developed a way to closely approximate sum-of-segments AL using CMAL (Cooke-modified AL). CMAL does not require OPLs, but rather, uses displayed biometer values:

$$\text{CMAL} = 1.23853 + 0.95855 \times \text{traditional AL} - 0.05467 \times \text{lens thickness} \qquad (11.6)$$

where all measurements are in millimeters. CMAL seems to work well on the Lenstar, but it still needs to be validated with other machines. Theoretically, it should work for all biometers, assuming that the displayed lens thickness (LT) and AL are equivalent between that biometer and the Lenstar machine. However, this does not mean CMAL represents the true axial length because it is based on the Lenstar group refractive indices. Also, there is not necessarily industry-wide agreement as to where on a spike to place the cursors. Referring to Fig. 11.2, the second "×" is above the spike of the anterior capsule of the crystalline lens. Perhaps this is incorrect. Perhaps it should be placed at the initiation (i.e., bottom) of the spike.

Not all segments are equivalent between biometers. For example, the ARGOS LT has been shown to be greater than the Lenstar's LT by 0.22 mm [4] and the OA-2000 central corneal thickness (CCT) has been shown to be 30 μm less than the IOLMaster 700's CCT [17].

Key points of the history section

- Haigis calibrated optical biometry to immersion segmental ultrasound biometry.
- He used sum-of-segments AL for ultrasound, but couldn't for optical biometry because optical LT was not available.
- Sum-of-segments AL can be well-approximated by using only LT and AL (CMAL formula). Note, this has currently only been shown on the Lenstar biometer.

- "Single Refractive Index" and "composite" are technically incorrect terms for traditional AL.
- It is not yet finalized as to which formulas sum-of-segments AL makes better or worse. Simple vergence formulas have been shown to be better at the extremes when sum-of-segments AL is used instead of traditional AL. Newer formulas, designed with only optical biometry, seem to adjust to optical AL, and in fact, may be made worse with sum-of-segments AL.
- It is comparably easy to empirically standardize traditional AL across biometers because it only requires that the corneal and retinal interfaces (RPE) are measured. It is complex to standardize sum-of-segments AL because it requires consistent industry-wide agreement for:
  - Group RI values for the four eye segments.
  - A scaling formula because biometers measuring wavelengths range from 780 to 1300 nm.
  - The definition of segment interface locations (where on a spike to place the cursor).

Segments

There is a general uniformity of axial length measurements [10]. Each biometer tends to give the same traditional axial length (AL). For there to be uniformity of sum-of-segments AL between biometers, however, there needs to be uniformity of the segment lengths. This has not been the case so far. Segment lengths are not as standardized as traditional AL. This could create a scenario where IOL power formulas need to vary based on measuring device, which is not ideal.

This section will evaluate the magnitude of the differences in segment lengths as well as why these differences exist. Some generalizations about measured ocular segments will be presented.

The geometric lengths of segments are calculated according to Eq. (11.3). A machine measures the optical path length (OPL) in air of the segment and divides it by that segment's refractive index (RI), given the wavelength used by the machine.

Recently, 1695 eyes were measured with a Lenstar [18]; OPLs were obtained for all ocular segments. Thirteen RI models were used to find segment RIs for a measuring wavelength of 820 nm. A fourteenth RI model was added for this chapter. The calculated geometric lengths of the segments varied, depending on the model used. The article described how to standardize sum-of-segments axial length for various RI models. For this study, the vitreous OPL started at the posterior lens surface and ended at the RPE. So the vitreous actually should probably have been called the vitreo-retinal complex because it always included the retinal thickness.

Table 11.1 is modified from that article [18]. Each model gives a different unadjusted sum-of-segments axial length (sixth column in Table 11.1). This is the total sum-of-segments AL from anterior cornea to retinal pigment epithelium (RPE) using the Lenstar measurements with RI values from the RI model listed in column 1. Note the large disparity of average ALs in column 6, depending on the RI method used. The

Table 11.1 Mean segment and unadjusted sums-of segments length for the different refractive index models using 1695 eyes originally measured with Lenstar biometer. Each value represents the average for all 1695 values (mean axial length from Lenstar printout = 23.76 mm; table is modified from Cooke et al. [18])

Refractive index model	Cornea (mm)	Aqueous (mm)	Lens (mm)	Vitreous (mm)	Unadjusted sum-of-segments AL (mm)	Theoretical retinal thickness (mm)
Navarro	0.536	2.70	4.60	16.03	23.86	0.106
D&M Le Grand (589)	0.536	2.70	4.60	16.04	23.89	0.127
D&M Le Grand (555)	0.537	2.70	4.61	16.06	23.91	0.147
A&S Le Grand (589)	0.537	2.70	4.61	16.06	23.91	0.153
Cornu Le Grand	0.537	2.71	4.60	16.07	23.91	0.155
A&S Le Grand (555)	0.537	2.71	4.61	16.08	23.94	0.177
D&M-Gullstrand (589)	0.537	2.70	4.67	16.04	23.96	0.198
Lenstar RIs	0.553	2.70	4.64	16.07	23.96	0.201
D&M-Gullstrand (555)	0.537	2.71	4.68	16.06	23.98	0.219
A&S Gullstrand (589)	0.537	2.71	4.67	16.06	23.98	0.224
A&S Cauchy (HL)	0.538	2.71	4.66	16.08	23.98	0.226
A&S Gullstrand (555)	0.538	2.71	4.68	16.08	24.01	0.248
A&S Cauchy (LL)	0.538	2.71	4.73	16.08	24.05	0.293
Liou & Brennan	0.546	2.75	4.77	16.33	24.40	0.636

average sum-of-segments AL for the 1695 eyes varied between 23.86 and 24.40 mm.

The last, seventh, column shows the adjustment to subtract from every AL to make the mean of that RI model equal to the mean traditional AL displayed by the Lenstar. Theoretically, if the values of an RI model were correct, the sum-of-segments AL would be the actual distance from the anterior cornea to the RPE. The Lenstar machine printout intentionally reports AL distance to the internal limiting membrane of the retina. The difference between the average Lenstar-displayed AL (23.76 mm) and the value in column 6 is listed in column 7. This is theoretically the difference between the RPE and the ILM. This would be the retinal thickness. That is why the last column is labeled "Theoretical Retinal Thickness."

The study found that "when the shortest *adjusted* sum-of-segments AL was subtracted from the longest one for each eye, mean difference was only 0.01 ± 0.01 mm and the maximum difference for any eye was only 0.04 mm." This adjustment method standardizes sum-of-segments AL well, even at extreme ALs. The Liou and Brennan unadjusted length was not included in that analysis. When adjusted, it varied only slightly more than the other methods.

Some items are notable about this table. The first is that several of the theoretical retinal thicknesses in column 7 are outside the physiological range for retina. This is particularly true for the Navarro schematic eye with a retinal thickness of only 106 μm and for the Liou and Brennan model which has a retinal thickness of 636 μm.

The sum-of-segments method is used by the ARGOS as well. The ARGOS was not included in this study, but it would have been near the bottom of the list because its theoretical retinal thickness is 300 μm.

There is one other commercial machine which measures sum-of-segments AL, the Galilei G6.

It actually displays both traditional and sum-of-segments AL. It uses the label "tAL (total axial length)" for sum-of-segments axial length. It defines this as "the distance from the anterior cornea to the posterior retina; optical axial length is converted to geometrical axial length using segment-specific, wavelength-adjusted, group refractive indices; for use with specifically designed formulas such as Okulix, etc." It is important to note that this axial length is different from all other sum-of-segments AL in that it is the *unadjusted* sum-of-segments AL, equivalent to column 6 in Table 11.1. Two cautions are in order:

1. It is the only commercially available sum-of-segments AL which is calculated to the retinal pigment epithelium. This has the potential to be the most accurate AL, but all other biometers adjust their AL to the anterior retina. Caution: Using tAL with standard formula lens constants could give wildly unexpected results.
2. Ziemer has not released the refractive index model (segmental refractive indices) used in developing tAL. So it is uncertain what theoretical retinal thickness to subtract in order to standardize the Galilei G6 AL to the standard IOL power formulas and lens constants.

It is worth noting that sum-of-segments isn't really the sum of all the segments; retinal thickness is subtracted to standardize it to the traditional AL. So the sum-of-segments AL, as used clinically, is only the sum of the cornea, aqueous, lens, and vitreous. Ideally, the retinal thickness would be included because the photoreceptors are located at the posterior retinal surface, not the anterior retinal surface.

Though the sum-of-segments AL can be standardized between machines, Table 11.1 shows that the segments can vary wildly; this is particularly true for the vitreous (because it is the longest) and for the lens (because it is the least understood). Haag-Streit and Movu are to be commended because other than for the Lenstar and ARGOS, companies don't list the segment RIs or OPLs that their biometers use.

To gain a better understanding of how the machine segments compare, several generalizations or "rules of thumb" are presented in Table 11.2. These derive from Table 11.3, which contains all the summaries for the comparative studies presented in Tables 11.4, 11.5, 11.6, 11.7,

Table 11.2 Generalizations from Tables 11.3, 11.4, 11.5, 11.6, and 11.7

Central corneal thickness	Anterior chamber depth	Lens thickness	Axial length
Lenstar ≈ IOLM 700 Pentacam ≈ US	Anterion ≈ OA-2000 OA-2000 ≈ Argos	OA-2000 ≈ Argos Argos ≈ Anterion	*All axial lengths are similar except for ARGOS, which is shorter in long eyes and longer in short eyes.*
US > (7μ) Lenstar; almost all others are smaller than Lenstar	Aladdin ≈ Lenstar Lenstar ≈ IOLM 700	Argos > (0.04 mm) IOLM 700 IOLM 700 > (0.04 mm) Lenstar	
IOLMaster 00 > (18μ) Argos Argos > (10μ) OA-2000	Argos > (0.06 mm) Lenstar Lenstar > (0.05 mm) IOLMaster 500	*Almost all are >LS Pent AXL did not measure LT*	

IOLM IOLMaster, *Pent AXL* Pentacam AXL. Pentacam axial length values were not listed in table because there were less than 300 such eyes available

Table 11.3 Summary (with weighted averages from Tables 11.4, 11.5, 11.6, 11.7, and 11.8)

Comparisons	N	CCT (μm)	ACD (mm)	LT (mm)	AL (mm)
Aladdin minus IOLMaster 500	422		0.08		0.02
OA-2000 minus IOLMaster 500	994		0.03		−0.01
IOLM-700 minus IOLMaster 500	742		−0.01		0.00
Lenstar minus IOLMaster 500	2696		0.05		0.02
Aladdin minus Lenstar	434	−10	0.00	0.16	0.00
Argos minus Lenstar	356	−9	0.06	0.22	−0.01
IOLM-700 minus Lenstar	1168	1	−0.01	0.04	0.01
OA-2000 minus Lenstar	377	−13	0.05	0.06	−0.02
Pent (AXL) minus Lenstar	815	4	N/A		N/A
US minus Lenstar	1432	7			
Argos minus IOLMaster 700	1143	−18	0.09	0.04	−0.05
Anterion minus IOLMaster 700	708	−5	0.07	0.07	−0.02
OA-2000 minus IOLMaster 700	793	−28	0.06	0.04	−0.02
OA-2000 minus Argos	690	−10	−0.03	0.00	0.04

US ultrasound, *IOLM* IOLMaster, *Pent (AXL)* Pentacam combined with Pentacam AXL. Sample size (*N*) is not necessarily the value for all segments in a given row (e.g., in the "ARGOS minus Lenstar" row, 356 eyes were evaluated, but only 62 eyes measured ACD)

Table 11.4 Machine CCT minus Lenstar CCT

Machine	Sample size	μm
Ultrasound [22]	80	10
Ultrasound [23]	256	3
Ultrasound [24]	55	1.2
Ultrasound [24]	50	−1.7
Ultrasound [25]	65	5.6
Ultrasound [26]	530	13.2
Ultrasound [27]	50	13
Ultrasound [28]	76	7
Ultrasound [29]	184	−3.5
Ultrasound [30]	86	8
Galilei [22]	80	28
Galilei [31]	100	17
Galilei [32]	47	15
Galilei [33]	120	−1
Pentacam [29]	184	7
Pentacam [28]	76	22
Pentacam [34]	108	5
Pentacam [35]	37	3
Pentacam [36]	27	−9
Pentacam [32]	47	6
Pentacam [33]	120	2
Sirius [37]	40	4
Sirius [23]	256	−7
Sirius [27]	50	−4
RTVue OCT [23]	256	−7
RTVue-OCT [27]	50	−4

CCT central corneal thickness

and 11.8. These were drawn from comparisons found in the literature. They are almost all English-language articles from peer-reviewed journals. This is not meant to be an exhaustive list. It is hoped that these tables will highlight the

Table 11.5 Machine minus IOLMaster 500

Machine	N	CCT (μm)	ACD (mm)	LT (mm)	AL (mm)
Aladdin [38]	231		0.10		0.04
Aladdin [39]	60		0.16		0.01
Aladdin [39]	56		0.05		−0.01
Aladdin [40]	75		0.00		0.01
ARGOS [41]	129		−0.06		−0.03
ARGOS [4]	42		0.17		0.01
OA-2000 [42]	119		N/A		0.00
OA-2000 [43]	65		0.01		0.01
OA-2000 [44]	58		0.01		0.11
OA-2000 [45]	108		0.01		−0.06
OA-2000 [46]	138		0.18		−0.05
OA-2000 [47]	102		−0.09		−0.06
OA-2000 [42]	119		N/A		0.00
OA-2000 [48]	140		0.05		0.00
OA-2000 [49]	99		−0.01		−0.01
OA-2000 [50]	46		−0.06		0.02
IOLM700 [41]	129		−0.07		0.00
IOLM700 [42]	119		N/A		0.00
IOLM700 [51]	111		0.02		0.00
IOLM700 [52]	171		−0.08		−0.01
IOLM700 [53]	100		0.04		0.02
IOLM700 [54]	112		0.11		0.00
Lenstar [54]	112		0.12		0.01
Lenstar [55]	51		0.06		0.01
Lenstar [4]	42		0.24		0.02
Lenstar [38]	231		0.10		0.04
Lenstar [56]	112		0.10		0.01
Lenstar [57]	100		0.14		0.02
Lenstar [58]	105		0.10		0.02
Lenstar [46]	138		0.01		0.02
Lenstar [59]	200		0.17		0.01
Lenstar [60]	76		0.05		0.03
Lenstar [61]	125		0.02		0.00
Lenstar [62]	109		N/A		0.01
Lenstar [63]	76		N/A		0.01
Lenstar [64]	1079		0.01[a]		0.00
Lenstar [48]	140		0.00		0.03

N sample size, *CCT* central corneal thickness, *ACD* anterior chamber depth, *LT* lens thickness, *AL* axial length
[a] ACD is unpublished data obtained from Cooke and Cooke [64]

Table 11.6 Machine minus Lenstar

Machine	N	CCT (μm)	ACD (mm)	LT (mm)	AL (mm)
Aladdin [38]	231	N/A	0.00	N/A	0.00
Aladdin [65]	101	−10	−0.01	0.16	−0.01
Aladdin [66]	102	N/A	0.00	N/A	0.01
ARGOS [4]	62	N/A	−0.07	0.22	−0.01
ARGOS [67]	294	−9	0.09	N/A	−0.01
IOLM700 [68]	64	N/A	−0.02	0.14	0.00
IOLM700 [69]	183	−5	0.03	−0.03	0.01
IOLM700 [70]	129	−1	−0.02	−0.03	0.00
IOLM700 [71]	127	−2	0.01	−0.02	0.13
IOLM700 [72]	80	3	−0.02	0.04	0.00
IOLM700 [73]	100	6	−0.03	0.06	−0.01
IOLM700 [74]	48	6	N/A	0.04	N/A
IOLM700 [74]	50	5	N/A	0.08	N/A
IOLM700 [75]	164	5	−0.07	0.17	−0.01
IOLM700 [54]	112	N/A	−0.01	N/A	−0.01
IOLM700 [51]	111	0	N/A	0.02	0.00
OA-2000 [46]	138	N/A	0.08	N/A	−0.03
OA-2000 [76]	99	−13	0.00	0.08	0.01
OA-2000 [48]	140	N/A	0.06	0.04	−0.03
Pent-AXL [77]	136	−10	0.00	N/A[a]	−0.02
Pent-AXL [78]	40	4	0.03	N/A[a]	−0.08
Pent-AXL [78]	40	6	−0.04	N/A[a]	0.02

N sample size, *CCT* central corneal thickness, *ACD* anterior chamber depth, *LT* lens thickness, *AL* axial length
[a] Currently, the Pentacam AXL or "AXL Wave" has a PCI system like the IOL Master 500. As such it does not include a lens thickness

wide variation present in measuring segments and to provide some of the supporting data for the generalizations presented in Table 11.2. The most-notable findings were italicized. Any such generalizations are likely to change as more studies become available.

Table 11.7 Machine minus IOLMaster 700

Machine	N	CCT (µm)	ACD (mm)	LT (mm)	AL (mm)
ARGOS [41]	129	−24	0.00	0.07	−0.03
ARGOS [79]	106	−26	0.10	0.01	−0.08
ARGOS [42]	119	N/A	N/A	N/A	0.00
ARGOS [80]	218	−5	0.12	0.08	−0.01
ARGOS [17]	571	−20	0.10	0.03	−0.07
Anterion [81]	389	−6	0.07	0.06	−0.01
Anterion [82]	49	−7	0.06	−0.06	0.00
Anterion [71]	127	2	0.04	0.07	−0.08
Anterion [83]	41	1	0.08	0.09	0.01
Anterion [84]	102	−7	0.07	0.06	–
Anterion [85]	125	−9	0.07	0.07	−0.01
Anterion [86]	78	–	0.07	0.07	−0.01
OA-2000 [42]	119	N/A	N/A	N/A	−0.01
OA-2000 [17]	571	−30	0.07	0.03	−0.02
OA-2000 [87]	103	−17	0.00	0.08	0.00

N sample size, *CCT* central corneal thickness, *ACD* anterior chamber depth, *LT* lens thickness, *AL* axial length

Table 11.8 Machine minus ARGOS

Machine	N	CCT (µm)	ACD (mm)	LT (mm)	AL (mm)
OA-2000 [42]	119	N/A	N/A	N/A	0.00
OA-2000 [17]	571	−10	−0.03	0.00	0.05

N sample size, *CCT* central corneal thickness, *ACD* anterior chamber depth, *LT* lens thickness, *AL* axial length

Comparative studies were included in Tables 11.3, 11.4, 11.5, 11.6, and 11.7 only if there were at least two papers making the same analysis. In addition, at least 300 eyes total were required. Instead of showing the absolute differences between machines, the values in Tables 11.3, 11.4, 11.5, 11.6, and 11.7 show the direction of the difference. This should identify if one machine consistently measures shorter or longer than another. Hopefully, adjustments can be made to equalize segment distances.

Summary of Segments

- Other than for the Argos biometer, AL between biometers is similar. Machines have been calibrated to the original IOLMaster.
- Argos has been adjusted so that normal ALs are fairly similar to the original IOLMaster.
- Galilei G6 has two AL options. One of them has been calibrated to the IOLMaster; the other (tAL) has not been calibrated to the IOLMaster and might give markedly different predictions in "unsuspecting" IOL power formulas.
- Segmental thicknesses, especially LTs, differ between biometers. This means that the CMAL formula might only work on the Lenstar machine.
- Though the AL can be made to be equivalent to the sum-of-segments AL of other machines, segments are likely to vary wildly. This is particularly true of the vitreous (because it is the longest) and the lens (because it is the least understood).
- Other than for the Lenstar and ARGOS, companies don't list either the RIs or the OPLs their biometers use. Haag-Streit and MOVU are to be commended.
- Sum-of-segments AL appears to help original vergence formulas, assuming that it is adjusted to original IOLMaster AL by subtracting a theoretical retinal thickness.

Areas for Potential Improvement

Some questions remain, such as, "Why does the AL measurement decrease after cataract extraction?" Many studies have shown the AL measures about 0.07 mm shorter after cataract extraction. There seem to be three possible answers: (1) RIs are incorrect; (2) segmental AL is needed, instead of traditional AL; or (3) the eye shortens after cataract extraction. The answer is currently unknown.

If ALs were all correct, then merely adding 200 μm to the adjusted sum-of-segments AL would give the distance to the RPE. But we don't know that all measurements (traditional AL and all of the ocular segments) are correct. Hopefully, work will be done to try to determine the physiological RIs for the various measuring wavelengths used.

Ueda [19], Prinz [20], and Cooke [21] have shown that increasing cataract density causes eyes to measure longer. Presumably, this is due to the lenticular RI increasing more than the machine predicts, thereby measuring the eye as too long. Could biometers auto-adjust RIs based on the density of the cataract?

Probably, the biggest future improvement would be for companies to publicize their OPLs. If not, they could publicize their RIs; OPLs could be back-calculated from Eq. (11.3). To date, only Haag-Streit (Lenstar) and Movu (ARGOS) have released their RIs.

Chapter Summary

- The traditional ALs we measure may not be physiologically accurate.
  - Optical biometry approximately equals immersion US AL, and immersion US AL might not be physiologically correct, particularly since the standard sound velocities have not been challenged in decades.
  - Current techniques tend to make displayed ALs equivalent between machines.
- Sum-of-segments ALs are different from traditional AL, especially at extremes.
  - Traditional AL reports measurements to the ILM, optical sum-of-segments AL measures to the RPE; they can be made similar by subtracting retinal thickness from each sum-of-segments AL.
  - RIs are not currently known.
  - Different sum-of-segments ALs can be made equivalent to each other in their

means, even with widely varied RIs. This can limit differences between RI models.
  - Individual segment lengths of the eye (e.g., the lens) can vary widely, with varied RIs. There is not currently an acceptable standard for these thicknesses, but knowing the OPLs for the segments would enable others to help standardize segment lengths.
  - Unadjusted optical sum-of-segments AL, measuring to the RPE, likely more closely approximates physiologically correct (accurate) values if accurate RIs can be obtained.
- Creating AL measurements with improved physiologic accuracy holds promise for further improvement of IOL power calculations.

Acknowledgment Special thanks to Marwan Suheimat for the explanation of coherence and to Michael Trost of Zeiss for the translation of Haigis's German article as well as extensive proof-reading of this chapter.

References

1. Shammas HJ, Shammas MC, Jivrajka RV, Cooke DL, Potvin R. Effects on IOL power calculation and expected clinical outcomes of axial length measurements based on multiple vs single refractive indices. Clin Ophthalmol. 2020;14:1511–9. https://doi.org/10.2147/OPTH.S256851.
2. Goto S, Maeda N, Noda T, Ohnuma K, Koh S, Iehisa I, Nishida K. Comparison of composite and segmental methods for acquiring optical axial length with swept-source optical coherence tomography. Sci Rep. 2020;10(1):4474. https://doi.org/10.1038/s41598-020-61391-7.
3. Wang L, Cao D, Weikert MP, Koch DD. Calculation of axial length using a single group refractive index versus using different refractive indices for each ocular segment: theoretical study and refractive outcomes. Ophthalmology. 2019;126(5):663–70. https://doi.org/10.1016/j.ophtha.2018.12.046. Epub 2018 Dec 31.
4. Shammas HJ, Ortiz S, Shammas MC, Kim SH, Chong C. Biometry measurements using a new large-coherence-length swept-source optical coherence tomographer. J Cataract Refract Surg. 2016;42(1):50–61. https://doi.org/10.1016/j.jcrs.2015.07.042.
5. Vogel A, Dick HB, Krummenauer F. Reproducibility of optical biometry using partial coherence interferometry: intraobserver and interobserver reliability. J Cataract Refract Surg. 2001;27(12):1961–8. https://doi.org/10.1016/s0886-3350(01)01214-7.

6. Chong C, Suzuki T, Morosawa A, Sakai T. Spectral narrowing effect by quasi-phase continuous tuning in high-speed wavelength-swept light source. Opt Express. 2008;16(25):21105–18. https://doi.org/10.1364/oe.16.021105.

7. Haigis W, Lege B, Miller N, Schneider B. Comparison of immersion ultrasound biometry and partial coherence interferometry for intraocular lens calculation according to Haigis. Graefes Arch Clin Exp Ophthalmol. 2000;238(9):765–73. https://doi.org/10.1007/s004170000188.

8. Haigis W, Kohnen T, editors. Modern cataract surgery, Dev ophthalmol, vol. 34. Basel: Karger; 2002. p. 119–30. https://doi.org/10.1159/000060791.

9. Haigis W, Mlynski J. Comparative axial length measurements using optical and acoustic biometry in normal persons and in patients with retinal lesions. In: White Paper, Carl Zeiss Meditec. 2009.

10. Optische und geometrische Weglänge in der Laserinterferenzbiometrie. http://www.dgii.org/uploads/jahresband/2013/025_Haigis.pdf. Accessed 14 Jan 2021.

11. Preussner PR, Olsen T, Hoffmann P, Findl O. Intraocular lens calculation accuracy limits in normal eyes. J Cataract Refract Surg. 2008;34(5):802–8. https://doi.org/10.1016/j.jcrs.2008.01.015.

12. Olsen T. Calculation of intraocular lens power: a review. Acta Ophthalmol Scand. 2007;85(5):472–85. https://doi.org/10.1111/j.1600-0420.2007.00879.x. Epub 2007 Apr 2.

13. Fam HB, Lim KL. Improving refractive outcomes at extreme axial lengths with the IOLMaster: the optical axial length and keratometric transformation. Br J Ophthalmol. 2009;93(5):678–83. https://doi.org/10.1136/bjo.2008.148452. Epub 2009 Jan 23.

14. Wang L, Shirayama M, Ma XJ, Kohnen T, Koch DD. Optimizing intraocular lens power calculations in eyes with axial lengths above 25.0 mm. J Cataract Refract Surg. 2011;37(11):2018–27. https://doi.org/10.1016/j.jcrs.2011.05.042.

15. U.S. Food and Drug Administration. 510(K) summary. Available at: https://www.accessdata.fda.gov/cdrh_docs/pdf8/K082891.pdf. Accessed 14 Jan 2021.

16. Cooke DL, Cooke TL. A comparison of two methods to calculate axial length. J Cataract Refract Surg. 2019;45(3):284–92. https://doi.org/10.1016/j.jcrs.2018.10.039.

17. Tamaoki A, Kojima T, Hasegawa A, Yamamoto M, Kaga T, Tanaka K, Ichikawa K. Clinical evaluation of a new swept-source optical coherence biometer that uses individual refractive indices to measure axial length in cataract patients. Ophthalmic Res. 2019;62(1):11–23. https://doi.org/10.1159/000496690. Epub 2019 Mar 19.

18. Cooke DL, Cooke TL, Suheimat M, Atchison DA. Standardizing sum-of-segments axial length using refractive index models. Biomed Opt Express. 2020;11(10):5860–70. https://doi.org/10.1364/BOE.400471.

19. Ueda T, Ikeda H, Ota T, Matsuura T, Hara Y. Relationship between postoperative refractive outcomes and cataract density: multiple regression analysis. J Cataract Refract Surg. 2010;36(5):806–9. https://doi.org/10.1016/j.jcrs.2009.12.024.

20. Prinz A, Neumayer T, Buehl W, Kiss B, Sacu S, Drexler W, Findl O. Influence of severity of nuclear cataract on optical biometry. J Cataract Refract Surg. 2006;32(7):1161–5. https://doi.org/10.1016/j.jcrs.2006.01.101.

21. Cooke DL, Cooke TL, Atchison DA. Effect of cataract-induced refractive change on intraocular lens power formula predictions. Biomed Opt Express. 2021;12(5):2550–6. https://doi.org/10.1364/BOE.422190.

22. Can E, Eser-Ozturk H, Duran M, Cetinkaya T, Arıturk N. Comparison of central corneal thickness measurements using different imaging devices and ultrasound pachymetry. Indian J Ophthalmol. 2019;67(4):496–9. https://doi.org/10.4103/ijo.IJO_960_18.

23. Şimşek A, Bilak Ş, Güler M, Çapkin M, Bilgin B, Reyhan AH. Comparison of central corneal thickness measurements obtained by rtvue oct, lenstar, sirius topography, and ultrasound pachymetry in healthy subjects. Semin Ophthalmol. 2016;31(5):467–72. https://doi.org/10.3109/08820538.2014.962173. Epub 2014 Nov 20.

24. Huang J, Liao N, Savini G, Li Y, Bao F, Yu Y, Yu A, Wang Q. Measurement of central corneal thickness with optical low-coherence reflectometry and ultrasound pachymetry in normal and post-femtosecond laser in situ keratomileusis eyes. Cornea. 2015;34(2):204–8. https://doi.org/10.1097/ICO.0000000000000329.

25. Koktekir BE, Gedik S, Bakbak B. Comparison of central corneal thickness measurements with optical low-coherence reflectometry and ultrasound pachymetry and reproducibility of both devices. Cornea. 2012;31(11):1278–81. https://doi.org/10.1097/ICO.0b013e31823f7701.

26. Gursoy H, Sahin A, Basmak H, et al. Lenstar versus ultrasound for ocular biometry in a pediatric population. Optom Vis Sci. 2011;88:912–9.

27. Bayhan HA, Aslan Bayhan S, Can I. Comparison of central corneal thickness measurements with three new optical devices and a standard ultrasonic pachymeter. Int J Ophthalmol. 2014;7(2):302–8. https://doi.org/10.3980/j.issn.2222-3959.2014.02.19.

28. Borrego-Sanz L, Sáenz-Francés F, Bermudez-Vallecilla M, Morales-Fernández L, Martínez-de-la-Casa JM, Santos-Bueso E, Jañez L, García-Feijoo J. Agreement between central corneal thickness measured using Pentacam, ultrasound pachymetry, specular microscopy and optic biometer Lenstar LS 900 and the influence of intraocular pressure. Ophthalmologica. 2014;231(4):226–35. https://doi.org/10.1159/000356724. Epub 2014 Mar 13.

29. Tai LY, Khaw KW, Ng CM, Subrayan V. Central corneal thickness measurements with differ-

ent imaging devices and ultrasound pachymetry. Cornea. 2013;32(6):766–71. https://doi.org/10.1097/ICO.0b013e318269938d.

30. El Chehab H, Giraud JM, Le Corre A, Chave N, Durand F, Kuter S, Ract-Madoux G, Swalduz B, Mourgues G, Dot C. Comparaison de la biométrie sans contact cornéen par LENSTAR LS 900 et de la biométrie contact par OCUSCAN RXP dans le cadre de la délégation de tâches [Comparison between Lenstar LS 900 non-contact biometry and OcuScan RXP contact biometry for task delegation]. J Fr Ophtalmol. 2011;34(3):175–80. French. https://doi.org/10.1016/j.jfo.2010.09.026. Epub 2011 Jan 22.

31. Huerva V, Ascaso FJ, Soldevila J, Lavilla L. Comparison of anterior segment measurements with optical low-coherence reflectometry and rotating dual Scheimpflug analysis. J Cataract Refract Surg. 2014;40(7):1170–6. https://doi.org/10.1016/j.jcrs.2013.10.045. Epub 2014 May 20.

32. Han SH, Hwang HS, Shin MC, Han KE. Comparison of central corneal thickness and anterior chamber depth measured using three different devices. J Korean Ophthalmol Soc. 2015;56:694–701.

33. Miranda I. Comparación de los valores del espesor corneal central según los equipos Lenstar, Galilei y Pentacam. Rev Cubana Oftalmol. 2012;25(1):65–71.

34. Huang J, Pesudovs K, Wen D, Chen S, Wright T, Wang X, Li Y, Wang Q. Comparison of anterior segment measurements with rotating Scheimpflug photography and partial coherence reflectometry. J Cataract Refract Surg. 2011;37(2):341–8. https://doi.org/10.1016/j.jcrs.2010.08.044.

35. Sen E, Inanc M, Elgin U, Yilmazbas P. Comparison of anterior segment measurements with LenStar and Pentacam in patients with newly diagnosed glaucoma. Int Ophthalmol. 2018;38(1):171–4. https://doi.org/10.1007/s10792-016-0440-z. Epub 2017 Jan 21.

36. O'Donnell C, Hartwig A, Radhakrishnan H. Comparison of central corneal thickness and anterior chamber depth measured using LenStar LS900, Pentacam, and Visante AS-OCT. Cornea. 2012;31(9):983–8. https://doi.org/10.1097/ICO.0b013e31823f8e2f.

37. Chen W, McAlinden C, Pesudovs K, Wang Q, Lu F, Feng Y, Chen J, Huang J. Scheimpflug-Placido topographer and optical low-coherence reflectometry biometer: repeatability and agreement. J Cataract Refract Surg. 2012;38(9):1626–32. https://doi.org/10.1016/j.jcrs.2012.04.031. Epub 2012 Jul 3.

38. Ortiz A, Galvis V, Tello A, Viaña V, Corrales MI, Ochoa M, Rodriguez CJ. Comparison of three optical biometers: IOLMaster 500, Lenstar LS 900 and Aladdin. Int Ophthalmol. 2019;39(8):1809–18. https://doi.org/10.1007/s10792-018-1006-z. Epub 2018 Aug 22.

39. Hoffer KJ, Shammas HJ, Savini G, Huang J. Multicenter study of optical low-coherence interferometry and partial-coherence interferometry optical biometers with patients from the United States

and China. J Cataract Refract Surg. 2016;42(1):62–7. https://doi.org/10.1016/j.jcrs.2015.07.041.

40. Mandal P, Berrow EJ, Naroo SA, Wolffsohn JS, Uthoff D, Holland D, Shah S. Validity and repeatability of the Aladdin ocular biometer. Br J Ophthalmol. 2014;98(2):256–8. https://doi.org/10.1136/bjophthalmol-2013-304002. Epub 2013 Nov 13. Erratum in: Br J Ophthalmol. 2015 Dec;99(12):1746.

41. Yang CM, Lim DH, Kim HJ, Chung TY. Comparison of two swept-source optical coherence tomography biometers and a partial coherence interferometer. PLoS One. 2019;14(10):e0223114. https://doi.org/10.1371/journal.pone.0223114.

42. Huang J, Chen H, Li Y, Chen Z, Gao R, Yu J, Zhao Y, Lu W, McAlinden C, Wang Q. Comprehensive comparison of axial length measurement with three swept-source OCT-based biometers and partial coherence interferometry. J Refract Surg. 2019;35(2):115–20. https://doi.org/10.3928/1081597X-20190109-01.

43. Huang J, Savini G, Hoffer KJ, Chen H, Lu W, Hu Q, Bao F, Wang Q. Repeatability and interobserver reproducibility of a new optical biometer based on swept-source optical coherence tomography and comparison with IOLMaster. Br J Ophthalmol. 2017;101(4):493–8. https://doi.org/10.1136/bjophthalmol-2016-308352. Epub 2016 Aug 8.

44. Ghaffari R, Mahmoudzadeh R, Mohammadi SS, Salabati M, Latifi G, Ghassemi H. Assessing the validity of measurements of swept-source and partial coherence interferometry devices in cataract patients. Optom Vis Sci. 2019;96(10):745–50. https://doi.org/10.1097/OPX.0000000000001433.

45. Hua Y, Qiu W, Xiao Q, Wu Q. Precision (repeatability and reproducibility) of ocular parameters obtained by the Tomey OA-2000 biometer compared to the IOLMaster in healthy eyes. PLoS One. 2018;13(2):e0193023. https://doi.org/10.1371/journal.pone.0193023.

46. Goebels S, Pattmöller M, Eppig T, Cayless A, Seitz B, Langenbucher A. Comparison of 3 biometry devices in cataract patients. J Cataract Refract Surg. 2015;41(11):2387–93. https://doi.org/10.1016/j.jcrs.2015.05.028.

47. Kongsap P. Comparison of a new optical biometer and a standard biometer in cataract patients. Eye Vis (Lond). 2016;3:27. https://doi.org/10.1186/s40662-016-0059-1.

48. Reitblat O, Levy A, Kleinmann G, Assia EI. Accuracy of intraocular lens power calculation using three optical biometry measurement devices: the OA-2000, Lenstar-LS900 and IOLMaster-500. Eye (Lond). 2018;32(7):1244–52. https://doi.org/10.1038/s41433-018-0063-x. Epub 2018 Mar 12.

49. Guo XX, You R, Li SS, Yang XF, Zhao L, Zhang F, Wang YL, Chen X. Comparison of ocular parameters of two biometric measurement devices in highly myopic eyes. Int J Ophthalmol. 2019;12(10):1548–54. https://doi.org/10.18240/ijo.2019.10.05.

50. Du YL, Wang G, Huang HC, Lin LY, Jin C, Liu LF, Liu XR, Zhang MZ. Comparison of OA-2000 and

IOL Master 500 using in cataract patients with high myopia. Int J Ophthalmol. 2019;12(5):844–7. https://doi.org/10.18240/ijo.2019.05.23.

51. Kunert KS, Peter M, Blum M, Haigis W, Sekundo W, Schütze J, Büehren T. Repeatability and agreement in optical biometry of a new swept-source optical coherence tomography-based biometer versus partial coherence interferometry and optical low-coherence reflectometry. J Cataract Refract Surg. 2016;42(1):76–83. https://doi.org/10.1016/j.jcrs.2015.07.039.

52. Akman A, Asena L, Güngör SG. Evaluation and comparison of the new swept source OCT-based IOLMaster 700 with the IOLMaster 500. Br J Ophthalmol. 2016;100(9):1201–5. https://doi.org/10.1136/bjophthalmol-2015-307779. Epub 2015 Dec 16.

53. Srivannaboon S, Chirapapaisan C, Chonpimai P, Loket S. Clinical comparison of a new swept-source optical coherence tomography-based optical biometer and a time-domain optical coherence tomography-based optical biometer. J Cataract Refract Surg. 2015;41(10):2224–32. https://doi.org/10.1016/j.jcrs.2015.03.019.

54. Song JS, Yoon DY, Hyon JY, Jeon HS. Comparison of ocular biometry and refractive outcomes using IOL Master 500, IOL Master 700, and Lenstar LS900. Korean J Ophthalmol. 2020;34(2):126–32. https://doi.org/10.3341/kjo.2019.0102.

55. Mylonas G, Sacu S, Buehl W, Ritter M, Georgopoulos M, Schmidt-Erfurth U. Performance of three biometry devices in patients with different grades of age-related cataract. Acta Ophthalmol. 2011;89(3):e237–41. https://doi.org/10.1111/j.1755-3768.2010.02042.x. Epub 2011 Feb 11.

56. Buckhurst PJ, Wolffsohn JS, Shah S, Naroo SA, Davies LN, Berrow EJ. A new optical low coherence reflectometry device for ocular biometry in cataract patients. Br J Ophthalmol. 2009;93(7):949–53. https://doi.org/10.1136/bjo.2008.156554. Epub 2009 Apr 19.

57. Hoffer KJ, Shammas HJ, Savini G. Comparison of 2 laser instruments for measuring axial length. J Cataract Refract Surg. 2010;36(4):644–8. https://doi.org/10.1016/j.jcrs.2009.11.007. Erratum in: J Cataract Refract Surg. 2010 Jun;36(6):1066.

58. Epitropoulos A. Axial length measurement acquisition rates of two optical biometers in cataractous eyes. Clin Ophthalmol. 2014;8:1369–76. https://doi.org/10.2147/OPTH.S62653.

59. Holzer MP, Mamusa M, Auffarth GU. Accuracy of a new partial coherence interferometry analyser for biometric measurements. Br J Ophthalmol. 2009;93(6):807–10. https://doi.org/10.1136/bjo.2008.152736. Epub 2009 Mar 15.

60. Cruysberg LP, Doors M, Verbakel F, Berendschot TT, De Brabander J, Nuijts RM. Evaluation of the Lenstar LS 900 non-contact biometer. Br J Ophthalmol. 2010;94(1):106–10. https://doi.org/10.1136/bjo.2009.161729. Epub 2009 Aug 18.

61. Rohrer K, Frueh BE, Wälti R, Clemetson IA, Tappeiner C, Goldblum D. Comparison and evaluation of ocular biometry using a new noncontact optical low-coherence reflectometer. Ophthalmology. 2009;116(11):2087–92. https://doi.org/10.1016/j.ophtha.2009.04.019. Epub 2009 Sep 10.

62. Chen YA, Hirnschall N, Findl O. Evaluation of 2 new optical biometry devices and comparison with the current gold standard biometer. J Cataract Refract Surg. 2011;37(3):513–7. https://doi.org/10.1016/j.jcrs.2010.10.041. Epub 2011 Jan 17.

63. Jasvinder S, Khang TF, Sarinder KK, Loo VP, Subrayan V. Agreement analysis of LENSTAR with other techniques of biometry. Eye (Lond). 2011;25(6):717–24. https://doi.org/10.1038/eye.2011.28. Epub 2011 Mar 11.

64. Cooke DL, Cooke TL. Comparison of 9 intraocular lens power calculation formulas. J Cataract Refract Surg. 2016;42(8):1157–64. https://doi.org/10.1016/j.jcrs.2016.06.029.

65. Yeu E. Agreement of ocular biometry measurements between 2 biometers. J Cataract Refract Surg. 2019;45(8):1130–4. https://doi.org/10.1016/j.jcrs.2019.03.016. Epub 2019 Jul 3.

66. McAlinden C, Gao R, Yu A, Wang X, Yang J, Yu Y, Chen H, Wang Q, Huang J. Repeatability and agreement of ocular biometry measurements: Aladdin versus Lenstar. Br J Ophthalmol. 2017;101(9):1223–9. https://doi.org/10.1136/bjophthalmol-2016-309365. Epub 2017 Jan 27.

67. Cummings AB, Naughton S, Coen AM, Brennan E, Kelly GE. Comparative analysis of swept-source optical coherence tomography and partial coherence interferometry biometers in the prediction of cataract surgery refractive outcomes. Clin Ophthalmol. 2020;14:4209–20. https://doi.org/10.2147/OPTH.S278589.

68. Passi SF, Thompson AC, Gupta PK. Comparison of agreement and efficiency of a swept source-optical coherence tomography device and an optical low-coherence reflectometry device for biometry measurements during cataract evaluation. Clin Ophthalmol. 2018;12:2245–51. https://doi.org/10.2147/OPTH.S182898.

69. Hoffer KJ, Hoffmann PC, Savini G. Comparison of a new optical biometer using swept-source optical coherence tomography and a biometer using optical low-coherence reflectometry. J Cataract Refract Surg. 2016;42(8):1165–72. https://doi.org/10.1016/j.jcrs.2016.07.013.

70. El Chehab H, Agard E, Dot C. Comparison of two biometers: a swept-source optical coherence tomography and an optical low-coherence reflectometry biometer. Eur J Ophthalmol. 2019;29(5):547–54. https://doi.org/10.1177/1120672118802918. Epub 2018 Oct 7.

71. Shetty N, Kaweri L, Koshy A, Shetty R, Nuijts RMMA, Roy AS. Repeatability of biometry measured by IOLMaster 700, Lenstar LS 900 and Anterion,

and its impact on predicted intraocular lens power. J Cataract Refract Surg. 2020;47:585. https://doi.org/10.1097/j.jcrs.0000000000000494. Epub ahead of print.

72. Arriola-Villalobos P, Almendral-Gómez J, Garzón N, Ruiz-Medrano J, Fernández-Pérez C, Martínez-de-la-Casa JM, Díaz-Valle D. Agreement and clinical comparison between a new swept-source optical coherence tomography-based optical biometer and an optical low-coherence reflectometry biometer. Eye (Lond). 2017;31(3):437–42. https://doi.org/10.1038/eye.2016.241. Epub 2016 Nov 11.

73. Kurian M, Negalur N, Das S, Puttaiah NK, Haria D, Tejal SJ, Thakkar MM. Biometry with a new swept-source optical coherence tomography biometer: repeatability and agreement with an optical low-coherence reflectometry device. J Cataract Refract Surg. 2016;42(4):577–81. https://doi.org/10.1016/j.jcrs.2016.01.038.

74. Bullimore MA, Slade S, Yoo P, Otani T. An evaluation of the IOLMaster 700. Eye Contact Lens. 2019;45(2):117–23. https://doi.org/10.1097/ICL.0000000000000552.

75. Cheng H, Li J, Cheng B, Wu M. Refractive predictability using two optical biometers and refraction types for intraocular lens power calculation in cataract surgery. Int Ophthalmol. 2020;40(7):1849–56. https://doi.org/10.1007/s10792-020-01355-y. Epub 2020 Apr 15.

76. Gao R, Chen H, Savini G, Miao Y, Wang X, Yang J, Zhao W, Wang Q, Huang J. Comparison of ocular biometric measurements between a new swept-source optical coherence tomography and a common optical low coherence reflectometry. Sci Rep. 2017;7(1):2484. https://doi.org/10.1038/s41598-017-02463-z.

77. Pereira JMM, Neves A, Alfaiate P, Santos M, Aragão H, Sousa JC. Lenstar® LS 900 vs Pentacam®-AXL: comparative study of ocular biometric measurements and intraocular lens power calculation. Eur J Ophthalmol. 2018;28(6):645–51. https://doi.org/10.1177/1120672118771844. Epub 2018 May 22.

78. Ruiz-Mesa R, Abengózar-Vela A, Ruiz-Santos M. Comparison of a new Scheimpflug imaging combined with partial coherence interferometry biometer and a low-coherence reflectometry biometer. J Cataract Refract Surg. 2017;43(11):1406–12. https://doi.org/10.1016/j.jcrs.2017.08.016.

79. Omoto MK, Torii H, Masui S, Ayaki M, Tsubota K, Negishi K. Ocular biometry and refractive outcomes using two swept-source optical coherence tomography-based biometers with segmental or equivalent refractive indices. Sci Rep. 2019;9(1):6557. https://doi.org/10.1038/s41598-019-42968-3. Erratum in: Sci Rep. 2020 Jul 31;10(1):13181.

80. Sabatino F, Matarazzo F, Findl O, Maurino V. Comparative analysis of 2 swept-source optical coherence tomography biometers. J Cataract Refract Surg. 2019;45(8):1124–9. https://doi.org/10.1016/j.jcrs.2019.03.020. Epub 2019 Jun 4.

81. Fişuş AD, Hirnschall ND, Findl O. Comparison of two swept-source optical coherence tomography-based biometry devices. J Cataract Refract Surg. 2021;47(1):87–92. https://doi.org/10.1097/j.jcrs.0000000000000373.

82. Tañá-Rivero P, Aguilar-Córcoles S, Tello-Elordi C, Pastor-Pascual F, Montés-Micó R. Agreement between two swept-source OCT biometers and a Scheimpflug partial coherence interferometer. J Cataract Refract Surg. 2020;47:488. https://doi.org/10.1097/j.jcrs.0000000000000483. Epub ahead of print.

83. Oh R, Oh JY, Choi HJ, Kim MK, Yoon CH. Comparison of ocular biometric measurements in patients with cataract using three swept-source optical coherence tomography devices. BMC Ophthalmol. 2021;21(1):62. https://doi.org/10.1186/s12886-021-01826-5.

84. Tañá-Sanz P, Ruiz-Santos M, Rodríguez-Carrillo MD, Aguilar-Córcoles S, Montés-Micó R, Tañá-Rivero P. Agreement between intraoperative anterior segment spectral-domain OCT and 2 swept-source OCT biometers. Expert Rev Med Devices. 2021;18(4):387–93. https://doi.org/10.1080/17434440.2021.1905518. Epub 2021 Mar 30.

85. Panthier C, Rouger H, Gozlan Y, Moran S, Gatinel D. Comparative analysis of 2 biometers using swept-source optical coherence tomography technology. J Cataract Refract Surg. 2021;48:26. https://doi.org/10.1097/j.jcrs.0000000000000704. Epub ahead of print.

86. Pfaeffli OA, Weber A, Hoffer KJ, Savini G, Baenninger PB, Thiel MA, Taroni L, Müller L. Agreement of IOL power calculation between IOLMaster 700 and Anterion swept source optical coherence tomography-based biometers. J Cataract Refract Surg. 2021;48:535. https://doi.org/10.1097/j.jcrs.0000000000000788. Epub ahead of print.

87. Liao X, Peng Y, Liu B, Tan QQ, Lan CJ. Agreement of ocular biometric measurements in young healthy eyes between IOLMaster 700 and OA-2000. Sci Rep. 2020;10(1):3134. https://doi.org/10.1038/s41598-020-59919-y.

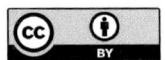

Technology of SS-OCT Biometer: Argos Biometer

Changho Chong

Background

Optical coherence tomography was developed by two groups, D. Hwang and J. Fujimoto in MIT in 1990 [1], Japanese researcher, Tanno in 1989, almost simultaneously but independently. Since it was commercialized for retinal imaging in 1994, it has been indispensable diagnostic modality for early diagnosis of retinal diseases in ophthalmic practice. Some years later, Swept Source-Optical Coherence Tomography was first proposed by A. Fercher in 1995 as a variation of Fourier-Domain OCT [2] (Fig. 12.1). Technologies advocated and demonstrated at the time were in lack of robustness so as to be developed into viable and prac-

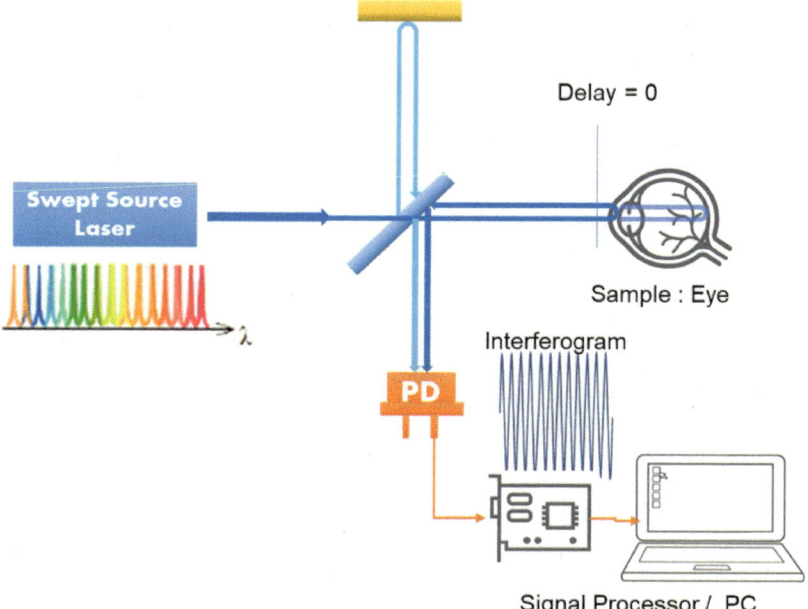

Fig. 12.1 Principle of swept-source OCT

C. Chong (✉)
Santec Holdings Corporation, Komaki, Japan
e-mail: changho.chong@santec.com

J. Aramberri et al. (eds.), *Intraocular Lens Calculations*, Essentials in Ophthalmology,
https://doi.org/10.1007/978-3-031-50666-6_12

tical applications. J. Fujimoto started to re-examine this approach in 2001 and thereafter many researchers followed and demonstrated faster imaging and higher sensitivity system over the course of years [3–7]. First commercial SS-OCT system was a 3D Anterior segment imaging system in 2008, Casia (Tomey, Nagoya, Japan) with a 30 kHz A-line rate which used high-speed-scanning laser (HSL-200, Santec Corporation).

Challenges

SS-OCT system boasts incomparable fast imaging speed due to fast swept rate of the laser wavelength change and high sensitivity due to intrinsically high signal efficiency based on Fourier transform in signal processing. Fast swept rate is an essential feature when imaging the large area with short acquisition time as well

as overcoming the motion blur during the image acquisition. However, in order to realize the continuous wavelength sweep at the rate of 10 kHz to several hundred kHz, the other performance comes at a cost. Narrow spectral width which is conversely defined as "coherence length" of laser cannot be sustained as "long" enough as the laser that oscillates at stationary wavelength. As a result, imaging depth is limited to the order of a few millimeters because of its short coherence length. Researchers attempted many different approaches [3–7] to overcome this trade-off to achieve (1) continuous sweep with (2) large coherence length (narrow spectral width) during (3) faster swept rate, all simultaneously. For most of the applications, point of interest resides in subsurface of biological tissues such as in retinal imaging, or cancer assessment, two to five millimeters of coherence length was sufficient to serve as diagnostic modality as seen in Fig. 12.2.

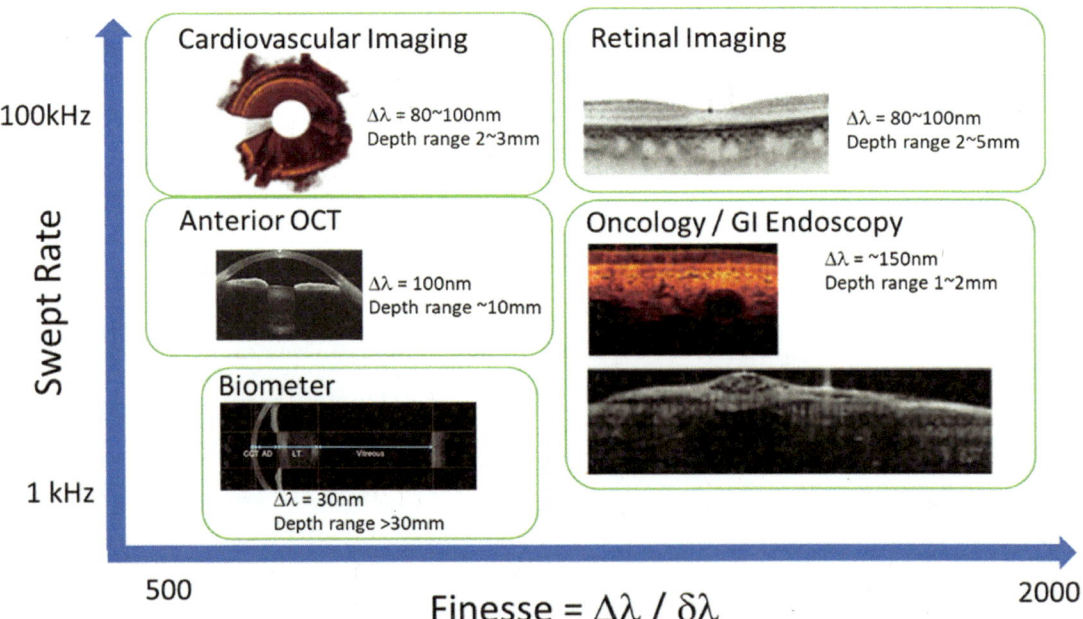

Fig. 12.2 Swept rate requirement in different clinical applications

Large Coherence Length

Coherence length of an SS-OCT system is defined by the optical path length difference between interferometer's sample path and reference path (see Fig. 12.1) where signal decays 6-dB (one-fourth) compared to nominal signal at zero path length or optical delay. And in the conventional definition, a half of coherence length corresponds to physical imaging depth in the system where signal amplitude, in the other words, image contrast is worsened by 6-dB. This doesn't necessarily mean image is cropped at this depth. Image is still visible as long as contrast is sufficient to reveal the lesion of interest.

$$\text{Coherence length} = \frac{2\ln 2\lambda_0^2}{\pi\delta\lambda}$$

Swept-Source Biometer

Early Work and Breakthrough

As advocated by Lexer et al. [8], the first demonstration of swept-source-based interferometer was indeed for the biometer application (see Fig. 12.3) in one-dimensional measurement. This was realized by the setup using a single longitudinal mode laser which has intrinsically narrow spectral width despite its slow wavelength tunability.

In order to overcome the increased output linewidth at higher scan rates, several ideas have been introduced such as the phase matching technique using an acousto-optic filter that matches the wavelength shift over a round trip to the phase shift generated by the filter itself [6]. Another technique is Fourier domain mode locking (FDML), whereby the tunable filter scan frequency is matched to the optical round-trip time resulting in a higher Q factor of the cavity in frequency domain [7, 9]. These two approaches, however, require both to operate at a preset resonant condition, i.e., at fixed swept rate, and the latter case needs long fiber length to accommodate several tens of kHz swept rate or slower. Other than using these techniques, adding the ambiguity or complex conjugate removal by adding external phase shifter in the OCT system is known as an alternative way [10], but it is not preferable when the system design is cost-sensitive.

After a decade later since the Lexer's demonstration in one-dimensional biometer at very slow speed, author's group demonstrated 28 mm coherence length at 2.5 kHz swept rate [12] using the method called Quasi-Phase Continuous Tuning technique [11] (Fig. 12.4) and achieved successful two-dimensional OCT of whole eye.

To our knowledge, this was the first demonstration of imaging whole eye of porcine with SS-OCT (Fig. 12.5).

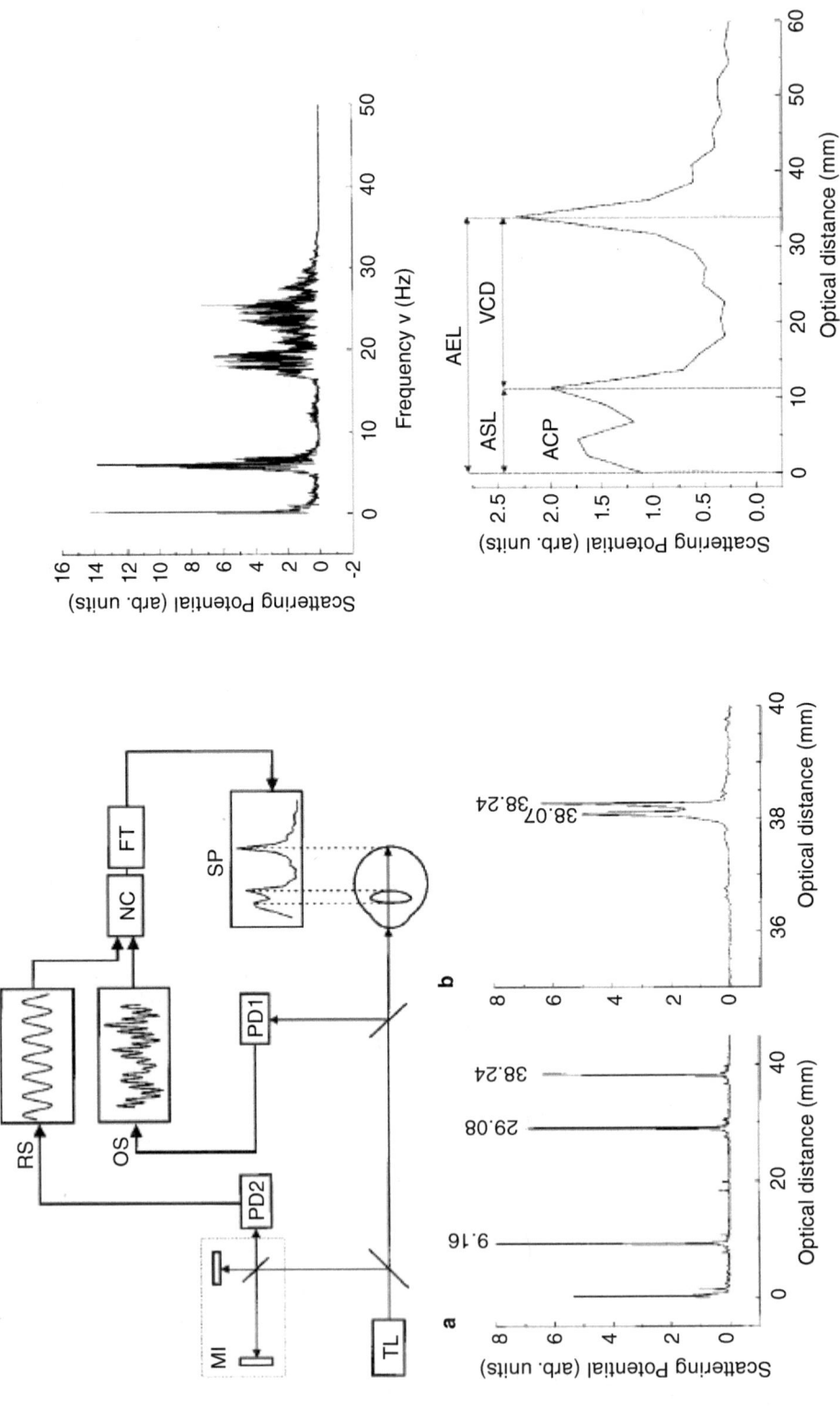

Fig. 12.3 First demonstration of axial length measurement (Lexer et al. [8]). Top left: Scheme of the WTI: wavelength tuning interferometer. *TL* tunable laser, *NC* numerical correction, *FT* Fourier transform. Top right: WTI scan of an eye model with 9 nm tun-ing. Bottom left: WTI scan of an eye model after numerical correction. Bottom right: WTI scan of a human eye in vivo obtained by high-speed piezotuning over 0.15 nm.

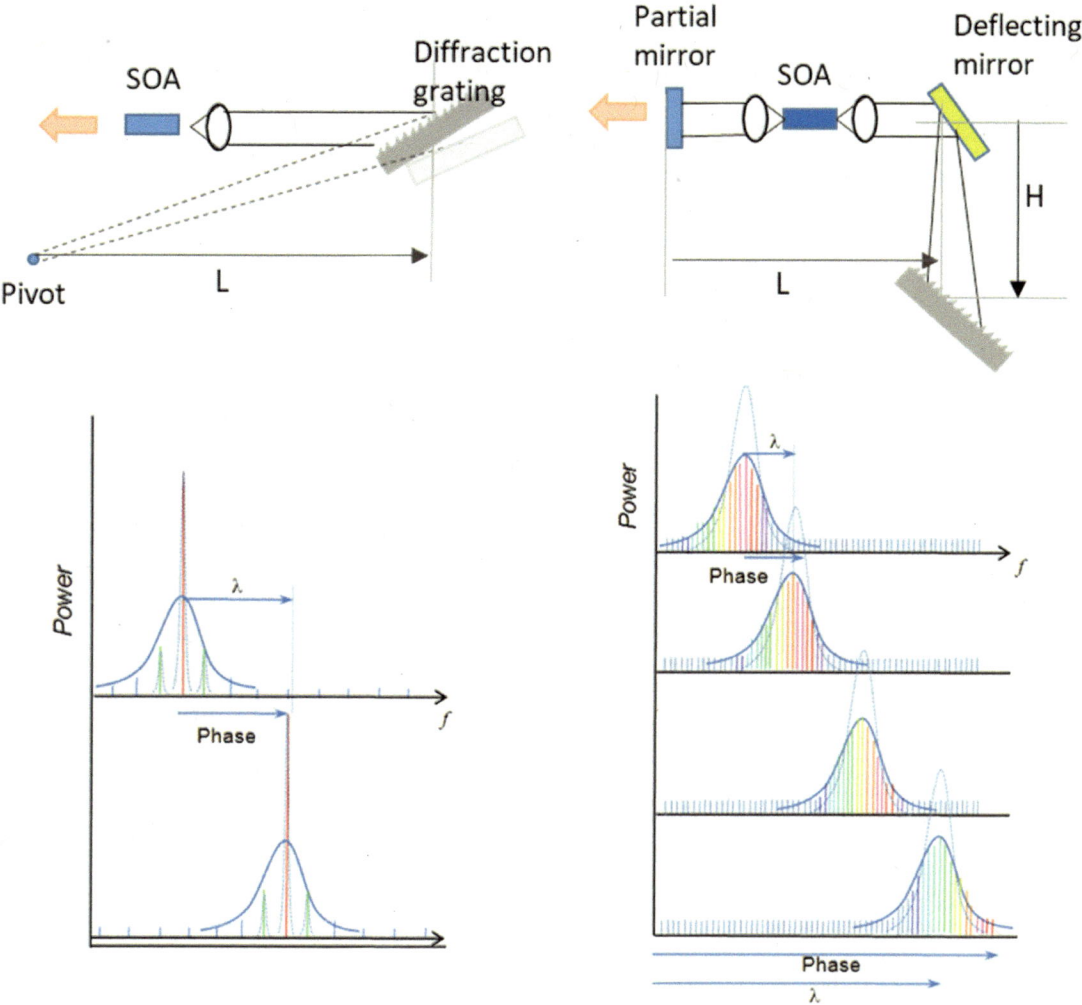

Fig. 12.4 Conceptual diagram for Quasi-Phase Continuous Tuning [11]

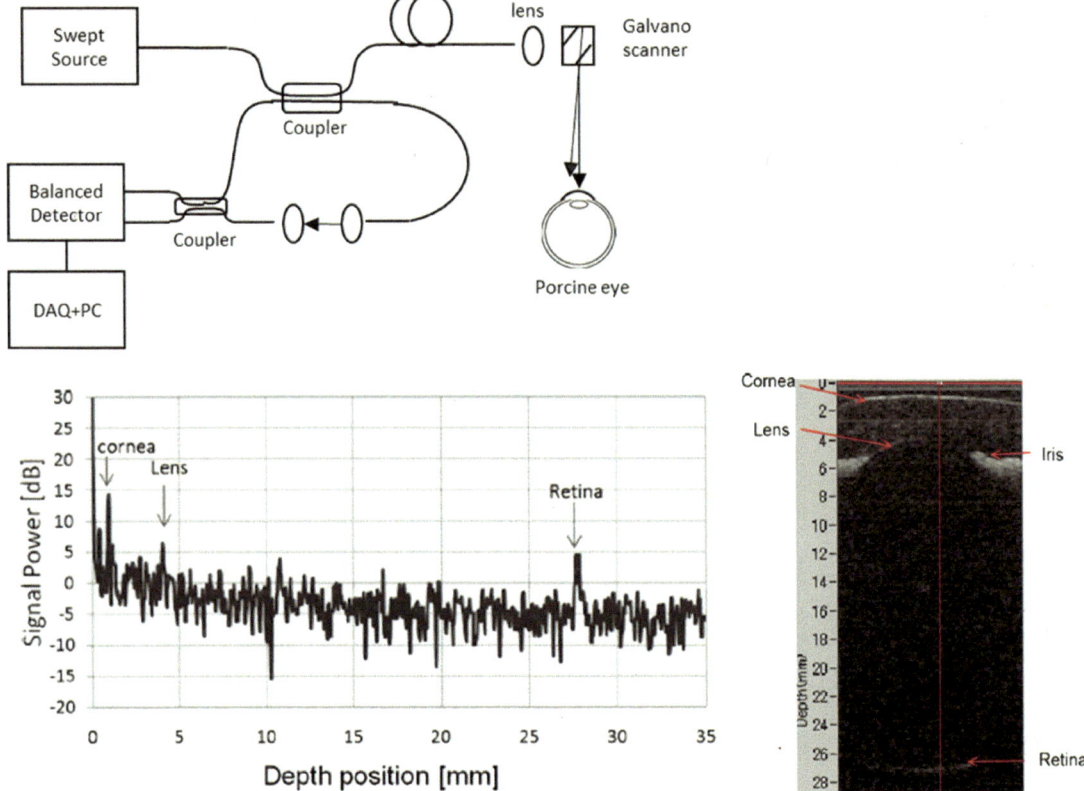

Fig. 12.5 First demonstration of whole eye imaging [12]

Argos SS-OCT Biometer

Basic Performance

Argos was first introduced to the market in 2014 in annual conference of ESCRS (European Society of Cataract & Refractive Surgeons) in London. ARGOS uses a proprietary swept-laser source (Santec Corp., Komaki, Japan) designed for deep (>50 mm) imaging at a fast 3000 lines/s A-line rate. Argos's performance specifications are listed in Fig. 12.6.

ARGOS is a swept-source OCT that captures an image of the whole eye from the cornea to the retina prior to cataract surgery. The measured image is used to calculate the biometric parameters necessary for IOL power calculation.

High Success Rate

The swept-source OCT technique for biometry delivers various advantages over traditional optical biometer as well as other non-contact techniques. First, the 1050 nm light used experiences less scatter than shorter wavelengths leading to more photons being available to make the measurement as seen in Fig. 12.7. Second, this technique has an inherent sensitivity advantage over other interferometric techniques. In addition, for ARGOS, the measurement beam scans across the eye capturing a full 2D image of the anterior chamber. For dense localized cataracts, this scanning helps ensures light travels past the cataract to reach the retina so that axial length can be measured. ARGOS even measures the densest

Parameter	Symbol	Range	Repeatability(s)
Central Corneal thickness	CCT	300-800 μm	< 10 μm
Anterior Chamber Depth	ACD	1.5-5.0 mm	10 μm
Lens Thickness	LT	0.5 – 6.5 mm	20 μm
Axial Length	AL	15 – 30 mm	10 μm
Corneal curvature	R_1, R_2(K_1, K_2)	5.5 – 10 mm (60-34D)	20 μm (0.13D)
Corneal Diameter	CD	7 – 15 mm	60 μm
Pupil Size	PS	2 – 13 mm	90 μm
Astigmatism angle	AST	0 – 180 deg	5deg (Cyl >1D)

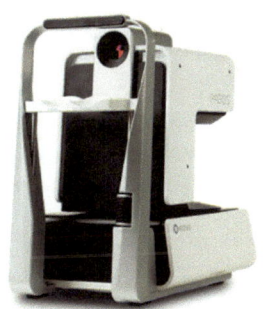

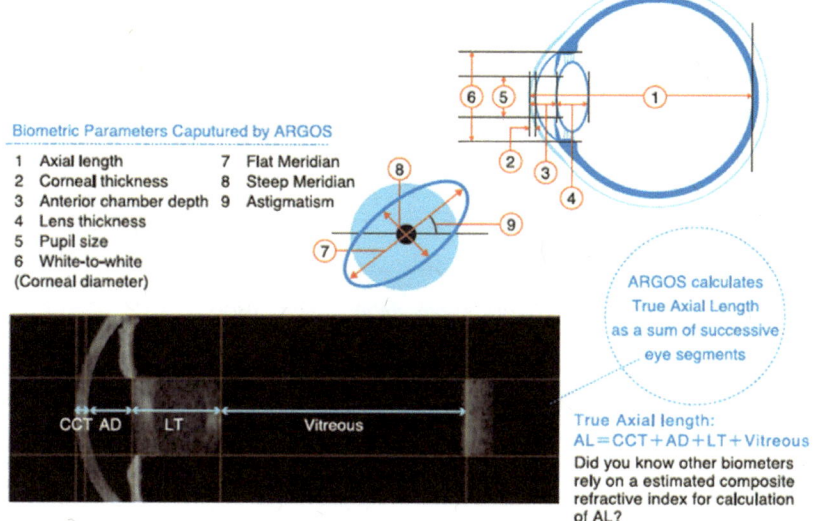

Biometric Parameters Caputured by ARGOS

1 Axial length
2 Corneal thickness
3 Anterior chamber depth
4 Lens thickness
5 Pupil size
6 White-to-white
(Corneal diameter)

7 Flat Meridian
8 Steep Meridian
9 Astigmatism

CCT AD LT Vitreous

ARGOS calculates True Axial Length as a sum of successive eye segments

True Axial length:
AL = CCT + AD + LT + Vitreous
Did you know other biometers rely on a estimated composite refractive index for calculation of AL?

Fig. 12.6 SS-OCT biometer ARGOS

cataracts that usually require the use of ultrasound A-scan. Furthermore, faster real-time OCT imaging during alignment ensures the confidence of fixation and provides assurance of accurate measurement with instant validation.

ERV Mode

The Fourier domain techniques as applied to optical coherence tomography (OCT), such as spectral domain OCT (SD-OCT) and swept-source OCT (SS-OCT), rely on the basis of an immovable mirror that creates a window where interference is possible, thereby also defining the OCT image. The information contained in this window is encoded in spatial or temporal frequencies, depending on if the technique is spectral domain (SD-OCT) or swept-source

(SS-OCT). It is only after performing the Fourier transform that it is possible to transform the frequencies (spatial or temporal) into spatial information. The window position depends on the position of the mirror, while the axial range of information depends on the bandwidth of the light source (coherence function). The amount of information, encoded in frequencies, depends on the ability to collect them: in SD-OCT, the separation power of the diffraction grating and the pixel size of the camera; in SS-OCT, the sampling of the signal. In the "normal mode," the coherence function is centered before the cornea, while in the "Enhanced Retinal Visualization" (ERV) it is centered closer to the retinal region. The intensity of the obtained image depends on the intensity of the backscattered light from the

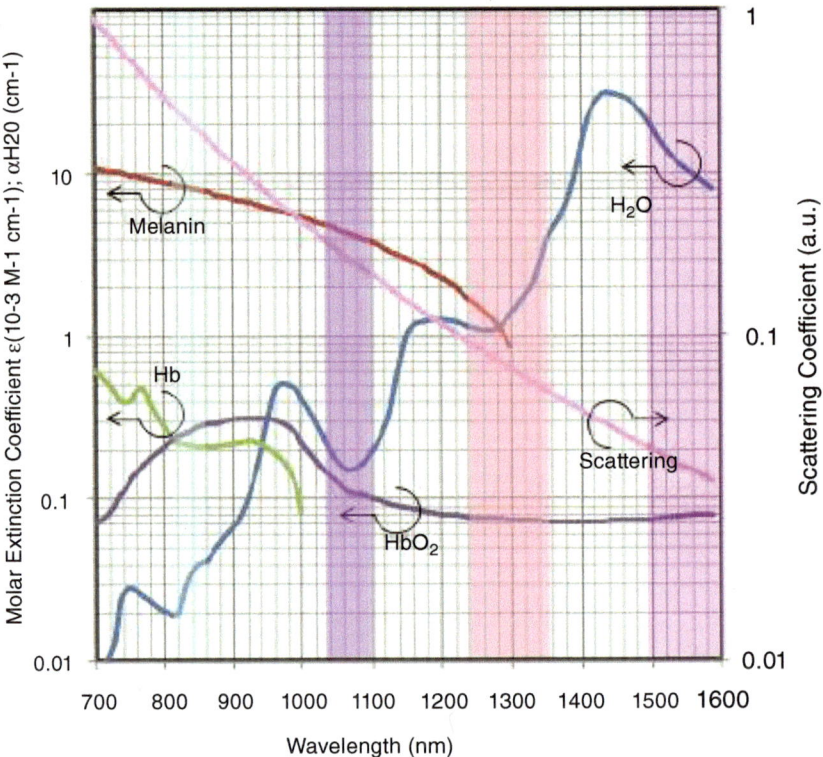

Fig. 12.7 Absorption and scattering coefficient of water

eye structures and their positions such that the acquired signal is the result of the convolution of the backscattered signal and the coherence function. When a dense cataract is present, the backscattered signal from the lens can partially or completely block the light coming back from the retina. In the normal mode, when the signal is convolved with the coherence function to produce the acquired signal, the retina can be hardly or not visible at all. However, in the ERV mode, the use of a shifted coherence function (due to the movement of the mirror) provides an additional opportunity to visualize the retina and therefore on evaluating the axial length (AL). In Fig. 12.8a–d, a conceptual image of the acquired signal of the system is shown. The backscattered signal from a cataract patient (one A-scan, i.e., columns of the image) is depicted in red. The coherence function is represented in blue and the acquired signal in black. (a) Simulated backscattered signal and normal coherence function (blue solid line). (b) Normal mode acquired signal (black solid line). (c) Simulated backscattered signal and ERV coherence function (blue dashed line). (d) ERV acquired signal (black dashed line). While this feature has been denominated as "Enhanced Retinal Visualization," it is not restricted to only dense cataracts or is it suggested to be used on all dense cataracts that may be encountered by the operator. Figure 12.8e–h present two cases from two different patients where the use of the ERV mode can be recommended. Top case: Retina not visible. (e) Normal mode where retina is not visible. (f) ERV mode where the retina is visible and AL can be evaluated. Bottom case: Retina appears fragmented. (g) Normal mode where retina appears fragmented and retinal signal is faint. (h) ERV mode where the retina is clearly visible and retinal signal is stronger. ERV boosts about 8–10 dB sensitivity to detect the retinal segment that compensates the signal decay by coherence length in normal mode so that it could make successful measurement in the densest cataract.

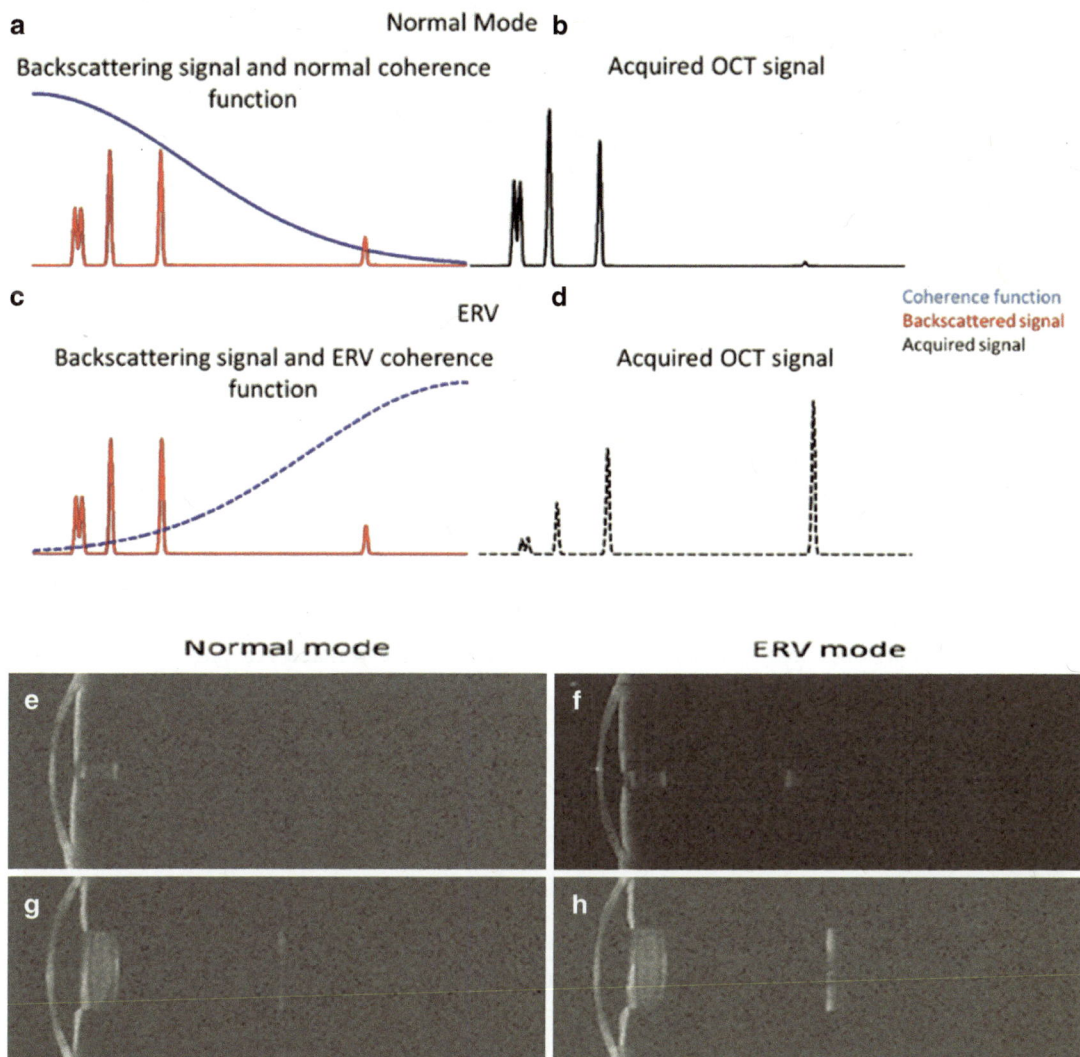

Fig. 12.8 ERV mode measurement

True Axial Length

In many of early clinical studies showing comparison of Argos, the conventional optical biometers tend to overestimate axial length at larger end, underestimate at shorter end, which is primarily the reason for not being able to predict short/long eyes with good precision in the past. Additional adjustment to the AL value calculated by tradition biometers is required to take into account the offset from true AL value before substituting to IOL power formula.

Argos calculates axial length as the sum of physical distances of four segments: central corneal thickness, aqueous depth, lens thickness, thickness of vitreous humor to the retina each calculated by dividing optical distance by corresponding refractive indices (1.375, 1.336, 1.41, 1.336) at infra-red wavelength range which implies the true physical scale of AL (Fig. 12.9). On the other hand, the conventional biometer uses composite refractive index where a statistically average proportion of axial length to lens thickness is assumed [13]. This approach does

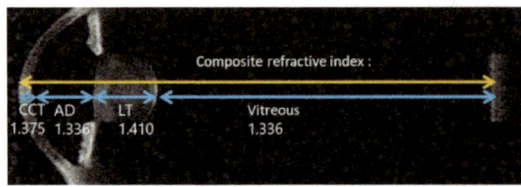

Fig. 12.9 True axial length—sum of segmented optical length

not take into account the actual lens thickness that could be out-of-proportion from normal distribution.

Composite refractive index used in traditional optical biometers was calibrated against ultrasound A-scan biometer's measurement. However, it is important to note that ultrasound and light have completely different behavior. Ultrasound travels faster in dense material while light travels slower in denser medium. The average composition or ratio of lens thickness to axial length is believed to be around 20%, and it decreases as the axial length is larger than average AL of 23.5 mm, which means total density gets lowered; thus, ultrasound travels slower and light travel faster. If a biometer is calibrated against ultrasound-based biometer and taken with average axial length demography, composite refrac-

tive index and formula for adjustment will reflect this effect in a linear extrapolated manner. That means it assumes the ratio of lens to AL is linear proportional to AL. So, what if lens thickness is disproportionate when axial length is large? The most Asian adults have a larger axial length compared to people in western country. And quite a few people have larger than "average" lens thickness which doesn't follow the linearly extrapolated distribution. If one applies formula based on composite refractive index, or IOLMaster (Zeiss Meditec, Germany) based value, it overestimates AL in the case of larger lens thickness because the device assumes it is measuring the eye with lens with smaller ratio while it is not. Wang and Koch did the studies on population with the eye with longer AL to account for this discrepancy and proposed adjustment which is also linear extrapolation. However, the distinction between overestimated AL and apparently true AL is difficult for users to judge according to intended use of the device. It is confusing for users whether AL output is actually true or overestimate and whether device is correcting for either of cases. Without knowing it, additional adjustment is simply a bet based on statistics.

$$AL_{ARGOS} = \frac{CCT}{1.375} + \frac{AD}{1.336} + \frac{LT}{1.41} + \frac{Vitreous}{1.336} - \text{Retinal thickness offset} \tag{12.1}$$

$$AL_{IOLMaster} = \frac{\left(\dfrac{OPL*}{1.3549} - 1.3033\right)}{0.9571} \tag{12.2}$$

Figure 12.10 shows the distribution of the ratio of lens thickness to true axial length measured by ARGOS. Linear approximation in red represents interpretation of proportion that traditional optical biometer is considering.

Assuming this linear approximation of LT/AL found, $y = -0.0149x + 0.5513$, whereas y is LT/AL and x is AL, is ground-truth data of proportion, let's mathematically estimate both the composite refractive index of whole eye and composite ultrasound velocity by weighing the refractive indices of crystalline lens (1.410) and vitreous (1.336), respectively, as well as sound velocity, 1641 m/s for lens and 1532 m/s for vitreous in the same way.

$$\text{Composite Refractive Index}: n(y) = 1.41y + 1.336(1-y) \tag{12.3}$$

$$\text{Composite Sound Velocity}: v(y) = 1641y + 1532(1-y) \tag{12.4}$$

If the weight, $y = -0.0149x + 0.5513$, is substituted, they become as following forms:

$$\text{Composite Refractive Index}: n(x) = -0.0011x + 1.3767 \tag{12.5}$$

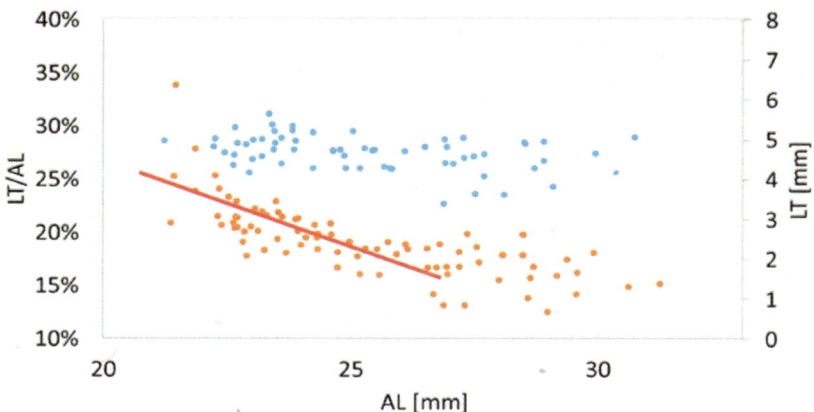

Fig. 12.10 The ratio of lens thickness to axial length of the eye (conceptual image of actual data)

$$\text{Composite Ultrasound Velocity}: v(x) = -1.6241x + 1592 \tag{12.6}$$

"True" AL should be adjusted by multiplying a factor of $n(x)/n(23.5)$ which is the difference of refractive index at AL = x with respect to the refractive index at nominal of 23.5 mm. In the same way, ultrasound velocity can be adjusted by multiplying $v(23.5)/v(x)$ in relative to those in average axial length, 23.5 mm. Total adjustment is the sum of these two factors:

$$\text{AL}_{\text{optical biometer}} = \text{AL}_{\text{measured}} + \left(\frac{v_0}{v(x)} + \frac{n(x)}{n_0} \right) \text{AL}_{\text{measured}} \tag{12.7}$$

whereas $v_0 = v(x = 23.5)$, $n_0 = n(x = 23.5)$, $\text{AL}_{\text{measured}}$ is the value of optical length measured divided by nominal refractive index (e.g., 1.3549 in Eq. 12.2).

When Eqs. (12.3) and (12.4) are substituted into Eq. (12.4) and approximated in the first order around $x = 23.5$ mm, equation is deduced to the following form:

$$\text{AL}_{\text{optical biometer}} = 1.043\text{AL}_{\text{measured}} - 1.005 \tag{12.8}$$

$$\text{AL}_{\text{IOLMaster}} = \frac{\left(\frac{\text{OPL}*}{1.3549} - 1.3033 \right)}{0.9571} = 1.045 \left(\frac{\text{OPL}*}{1.3549} - 1.303 \right) = 1.045 \left(\frac{\text{OPL}*}{1.3549} \right) - 1.36 \tag{12.9}$$

Coefficient of first term 1.043 is close to reciprocal of 0.9571 (1.045) in Eq. (12.2) suggesting the agreement of this assumption. This proves our assumption that the conventional optical biometers suffer the inherent issue with contradictory nature of speed of light and ultrasound velocity. The difference in the second term of Eqs. (12.8) and (12.9) is simply the offset of retinal thickness to account for IOL formula based on ultrasound.

Those eyes in the larger axial length over 25 mm as seen in the graph of Fig. 12.9, distribution spreads wider and becomes no longer correlated well with linear approximation; thus, it increases the ambiguity when the linear approximation is still used. This is not something resolved by machine learning techniques on top to cover it up if the measurement itself contains ambiguity. That is why it is important to measure true axial length.

A number of clinical studies were reported to prove clinical and statistical significance on the use of true axial length applied to IOL power determination [14].

Future of SS-OCT with Tunable VCSEL

VCSEL (Vertical Cavity Surface Emitting Laser) becomes now popular even in consumer electronics such as smartphones that use VCSEL for 3D

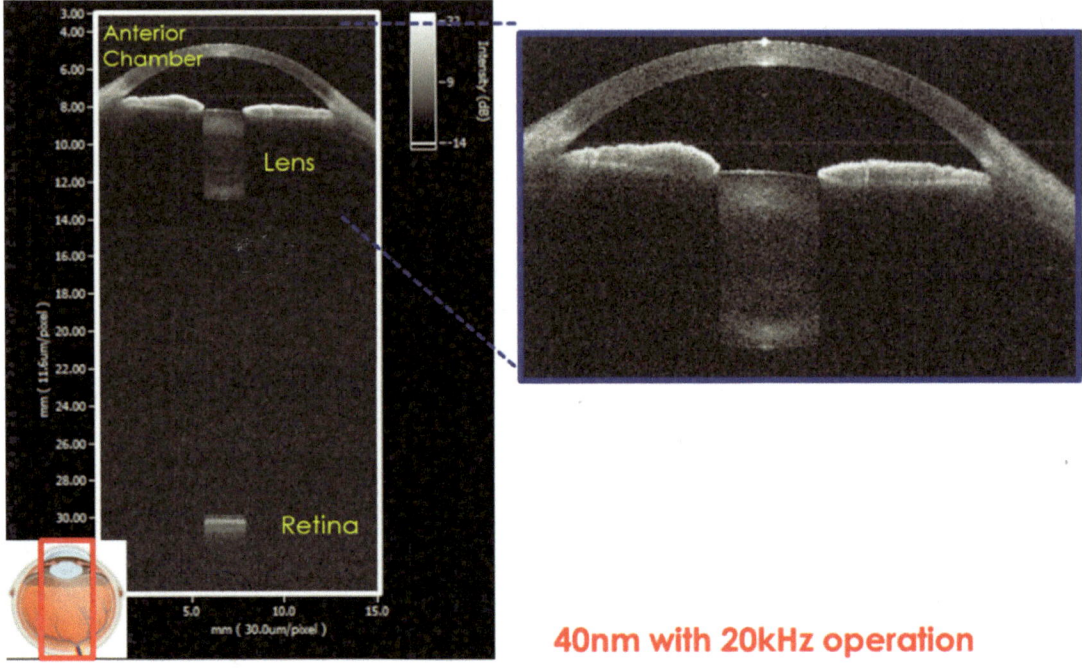

Fig. 12.11 SS-OCT whole eye image measured with tunable VCSEL

sensing for face recognition or lidar applications. Wavelength tunable version of this is the most coveted ultimate solution for the next generation SS-OCT [15, 16]. It boasts wide wavelength swept range of over 80 nm at 1050 nm band and intrinsically single-mode laser oscillation, thus very long coherence length. That means the depth range trade-off is no longer trade-off at faster swept rate. In fact, with integrated MEMS (Micro-Electro-Mechanical System) mirror enables several hundred kHz swept rate while maintaining large coherence length. One another advantage of tunable VCSEL that differentiate from the other swept-source is the reconfigurability of performance specifications. In the other words, one can software-define the swept range, swept rate in various required settings. Tunable VCSEL has a potential to bring multiple OCT functions in one device, for example, anterior OCT, optical biometer, and retinal OCT. Figure 12.11 shows the example image of in vivo human eye measured with a prototype that used a tunable VCSEL having the performance shown in Fig. 12.12.

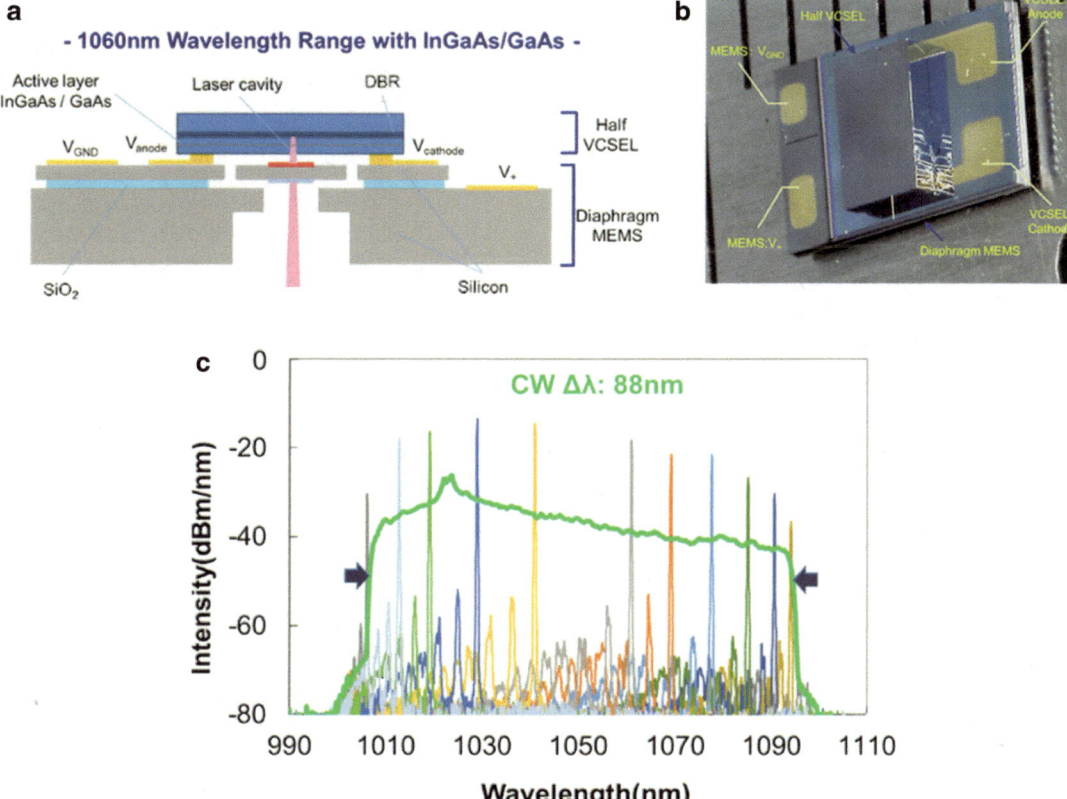

Fig. 12.12 Tunable VCSEL swept-source [15]. (**a**) Cross-sectional image of device structure, (**b**) an image of device, and (**c**) wavelength swept performance

References

1. Huang D, Swanson EA, Lin CP, Schuman JS, Stinson WG, Chang W, Hee MR, Flotte T, Gregory K, Puliafito CA, Fujimoto JG. Optical coherence tomography. Science. 1991;254:1178–81.
2. Fercher AF, Hitzenberger CK, Kamp G, Elzaiat SY. Measurement of intraocular distances by backscattering spectral interferometry. Opt Commun. 1995;117:43–8.
3. Chinn SR, Swanson EA, Fujimoto JG. Optical coherence tomography using a frequency-tunable optical source. Opt Lett. 1997;22:340–2.
4. Yun SH, Tearney GJ, de Boer JF, Iftimia N, Bouma BE. High-speed optical frequency-domain imaging. Opt Express. 2003;11:2953–63.
5. Yun SH, Tearney GJ, de Boer JF, Bouma BE. Motion artifacts in optical coherence tomography with frequency domain ranging. Opt Express. 2004;12:2977–98.
6. Yun SH, Richardson DJ, Culverhouse DO, Kim BY. Wavelength-swept fiber laser with frequency shifted feedback and resonantly swept intra-cavity acoustooptic tunable filter. IEEE J Sel Top Quant Electron. 1997;3(4):1087.
7. Huber R, Adler DC, Srinivasan VJ, Fujimoto JG. Fourier domain mode locking at 1050 nm for ultra-high-speed optical coherence tomography of the human retina at 236,000 axial scans per second. Opt Lett. 2007;32:2049–51.
8. Lexer F, Hitzenberger CK, Fercher AF, Kulhavy M. Wavelength-tuning interferometry of intraocular distances. Appl Opt. 1997;36(25):6548.
9. Srinivasan V, Huber R, Gorczynska I, Fujimoto J, Jiang J, Reisen P, Cable A. High-speed, high resolution optical coherence tomography retinal imaging with a frequency-swept laser at 850 nm. Opt Lett. 2007;32:361–3.
10. Yun SH, Tearney GJ, de Boer JF, Bouma BE. Removing the depth-degeneracy in optical frequency domain imaging with frequency shifting. Opt Express. 2004;12(20):4822–8.
11. Chong C, Suzuki T, Morosawa A, Sakai T. Spectral narrowing effect by quasi-phase continuous tuning

in high-speed wavelength-swept light source. Opt Express. 2008;16:21105–2118.

12. Chong C, Takuya S, Totsuka K, Morosawa A, Sakai T. Large coherence length swept source for axial length measurement of eye. Appl Opt. 2009;48(10):D144.

13. Haigis W, Lege B, Miller N, Schneider B. Comparison of immersion ultrasound biometry and partial coherence interferometry for intraocular lens calculation according to Haigis. Graefes Arch Clin Exp Ophthalmol. 2000;238(9):765–73.

14. John Shammas H, Ortiz S, Shammas MC, Kim SH, Chong C. Biometry measurements using a new large-coherence–length swept-source optical coherence tomographer. J Cataract Refract Surg. 2016;42(1):P50.

15. Okano M, Chong C. Swept source lidar: simultaneous FMCW ranging and nonmechanical beam steering with a wideband swept source. Opt Express. 2020;28(16):23898–915.

16. Khan MS, Keum C-D, Isamoto K, Sakai T, Doi T, Kawasugi M, Totsuka K, Chong C, Nishiyama N, Toshiyoshi H. High reliability electrically pump MEMS based widely tunable VCSEL for SS-OCT. In: SPIE photonics west, MOEMS and miniaturized systems XVIII; 2019. p. 10931–44.

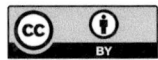

Influence of Anterior Chamber Depth, Lens Thickness, and Corneal Diameter on Intraocular Lens Power Calculation

Tiago Bravo Ferreira and Nuno Campos

In this chapter, we will summarize the different intraocular lens (IOL) power calculation formulas, especially those that consider the variables anterior chamber depth (ACD), lens thickness (LT), and/or horizontal corneal diameter (CD), also known as corneal diameter (CD). We will describe the preoperative evaluation of these biometric parameters and their normal values. We will review the influence of each of these three parameters in different IOL power calculation formulas. Finally, highlighting the need for further improvement of refractive results in cataract surgery, we will enumerate future directions for research in this area.

Introduction

In the past decade, cataract surgery transitioned from a replacement of the opacified crystalline lens to a refractive procedure. Residual refractive errors became less frequent, with an increased precision of optical biometry and new IOL power calculation formulas [1].

For spherical IOL power calculation, the combination of optical biometry with last generation formulas such as the Barrett Universal II (BU II) or the Hill-Radial Basis Function (RBF) formulas results in a postoperative refractive result

within ±0.50 D of the target in at least 72–84% of the eyes [2, 3], results that still reflect the need for increased precision in IOL power calculation. This is further supported by the knowledge that implantation of new aspheric, multifocal, or toric IOL designs is ineffective unless minimal residual refractive error is achieved [4].

Intraocular Lens Power Calculation Formulas

A number of different mathematical formulas have been proposed to improve postoperative refractive prediction.

These formulas have been subject to several improvements since the first analytical formulas proposed by Fedorov [5], Fyodorov [6], and Colenbrander [7], and the first empirical formula, the SRK, proposed by Sanders, Retzlaff, and Kraff [8, 9]. Analytical formulas rely on a thin lens system to calculate the IOL power, and they all use approximately the same vergence formula.

Given most presently available formulas use non-realistic models for the optics of the eye, they require a number of retrospective corrective factors from observed data in order to work accurately. Therefore, empirical formulas are based on large retrospective populational studies.

The most commonly used empirical formula, the SRK, has been improved with corrective

T. B. Ferreira (✉) · N. Campos
CUF Tejo Hospital, Lisbon, Portugal

J. Aramberri et al. (eds.), *Intraocular Lens Calculations*, Essentials in Ophthalmology,
https://doi.org/10.1007/978-3-031-50666-6_13

factors for extreme eyes and an enhanced algorithm for effective lens position (ELP) estimation, evolving to the SRK II, SRK-T, and, more recently, the SRK-T2 [10]. The effect of these factors is to correct for any off-set errors arising in the formula by applying an average corrective term, making the predictions accurate in the average eye.

In fact, formulas do not account for the actual physical lens position in the pseudophakic eye, but instead use a theoretical position defined as the effective distance from the anterior surface of the cornea to the lens plane as if the lens was of negligible thickness (ELP). This value is provided by the manufacturer as the A-constant is formula-dependent and does not reflect the true ACD in the anatomical sense, which hampers the comparison with postoperative measurements of the pseudophakic ACD, i.e., the postoperative anterior chamber depth (ACD_{post}).

Estimates of postoperative ELP were initially a constant (4 mm). In second-generation formulas, axial length (AL) was introduced as a predictor, and on third-generation formulas, corneal power and AL were used as predictors of postoperative ELP. Given these limitations, and given that the actual postoperative lens position is correlated with AL, ACD, anterior segment depth, and CD [11], new formulas that integrate some or all of the parameters subject of this chapter (ACD, LT, and CD) to predict ELP emerged (Fig. 13.1).

More recent formulas, Holladay 2 (unpublished formula) and Olsen 2 [12], introduce new correlation parameters to compensate for the above-mentioned flaws of third generation formulas. The introduction of more parameters improves the predictive ability of the formulas, decreasing or even removing (Haigis formula) the contribution of the error associated with corneal dioptric power. However, care should be taken with the reproducibility of measuring more parameters and also the fact that regressive factors depend on the measurement technique.

Eyes considered to be average comprise the majority of cases, with the results generally degrading in non-average eyes, due to the statistical nature of the formulas.

Nowadays, multiple formulas exist [13], casting some confusion in clinical practice.

The processing capability of computers no longer requires the simplifications of paraxial optics used nor lengthy population studies. Computerized methods such as artificial intelligence (AI) or ray-tracing emerged as alternatives.

Other new formulas further improved IOL power calculation results by merging the thin lens framework with statistical regression techniques. The main difference between formulas of this type is the variables used and weighting attributed to each one when performing the regression for the ELP value.

New IOL power calculation formulas (Fig. 13.2) include:

- Barrett Universal II (BU II) [14, 15] is a multiple-parameter vergence-based thick-lens formula (although reported to use paraxial ray tracing by Barrett in several personal communications), which has been modified by the author over the years. The formula is unpublished and freely accessible online at calc.apacrs.org/barrett_universal2105/ (accessed March 18, 2021). It uses AL, keratometry (K), and ACD to predict the ELP. Two additional optional parameters may be used, namely LT and CD.
- Emmetropia Verifying Optical (EVO) formula (version 2.0) is a thick-lens formula based on the theory of emmetropization. The formula is unpublished. Version 2.0 of the formula freely accessible online at www.evoiolcalculator.com (accessed March 18, 2021). Predictors of ELP are AL, K, and ACD, with LT and central corneal thickness (CCT) being optional.
- Hill-RBF formula uses AI through a pattern recognition algorithm that considers a form of data interpolation for calculating the IOL power. The Hill-RBF calculator is freely accessible online at www.rbfcalculator.com (accessed March 18, 2021) and also available

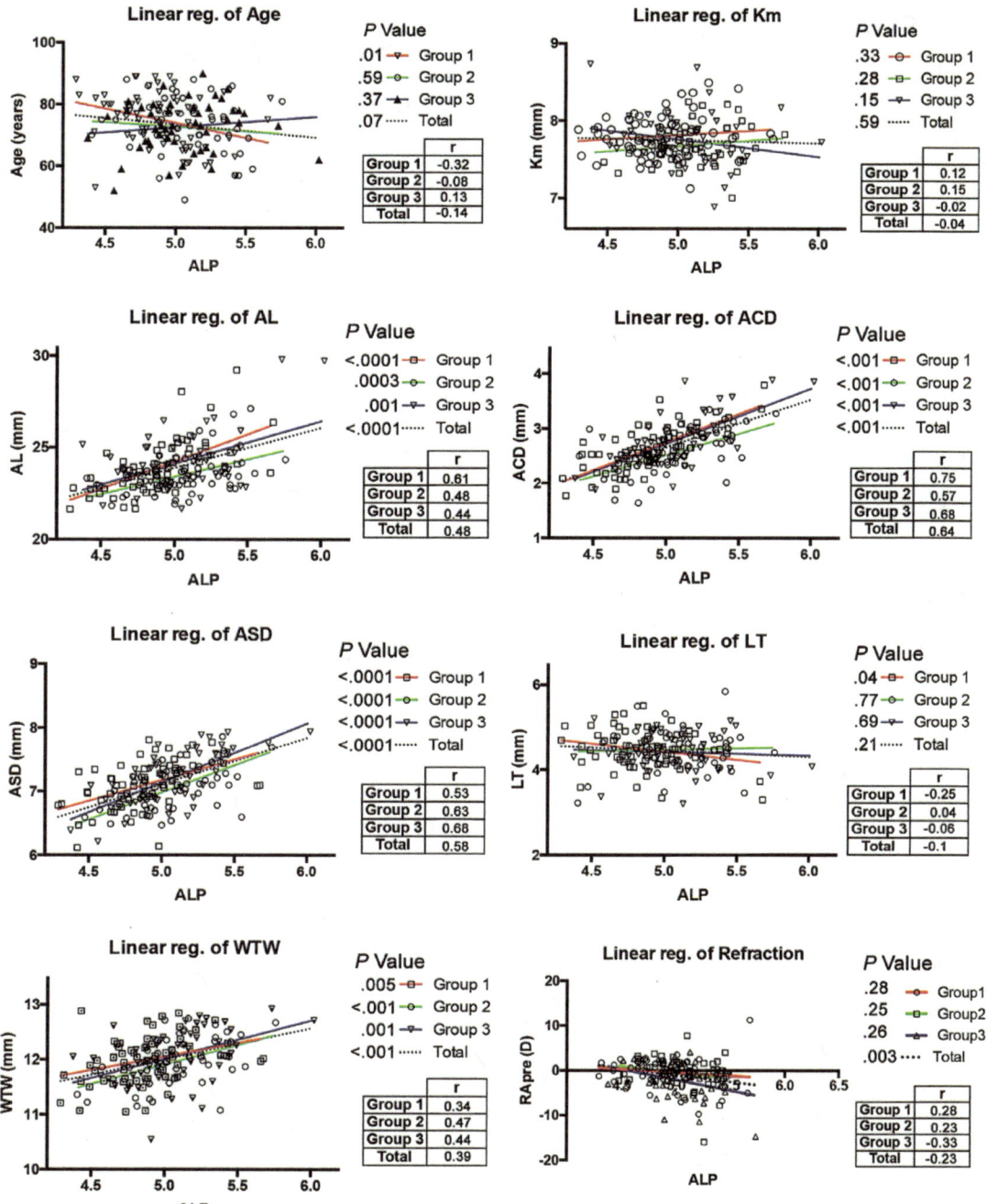

Fig. 13.1 Correlations of actual lens position with age, mean K data, AL, ACD, anterior segment depth, lens thickness, CD distance, and refraction. *ACD* anterior chamber depth, *AL* axial length, *ALP* actual lens position, *ASD* anterior segment depth, *Km* mean keratometry, *LT* lens thickness, *RApre* preoperative refraction assessment, *reg.* regression, *CD* corneal diameter. (Reproduced with permission from J Cataract Refract Surg. 2017 Feb;43(2):195–200)

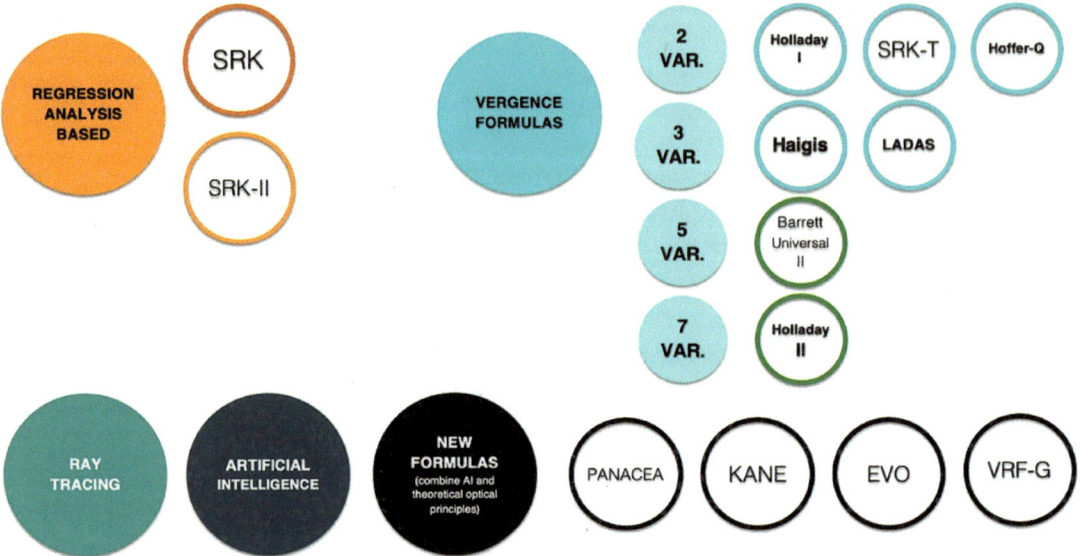

Fig. 13.2 Classification of new intraocular lens power calculation formulas. (Reproduced with permission from Ophthalmology. 2019 Sep;126(9):1334–1335)

on the Lenstar biometer. It is now in version 3.0. AL, K, and ACD are the mandatory data for IOL calculation. LT, CCT, and CD are optional.

- Kane formula is based on a combination of theoretical optics and AI. It is unpublished and freely accessible online at www.iolformula.com (accessed March 18, 2021). The predictors of ELP are AL, K, ACD, and gender. LT and CCT are optional.

- Ladas Super Formula is a combination of the Holladay 1, Holladay 2 (with Wang-Koch adjustment), Hoffer Q, and SRK/T formulas. It is based on a three-dimensional model, adjusting the best formula for a specific eye. The current version of the formula (Ladas Super Formula AI) was developed in 2019. This new version is based on AI and is freely available at www.iolcalc.com (accessed March 18, 2021).

- Næser 2 is a thick-lens formula [16]. It predicts the geometric ACD and not the ELP. The Næser 2 formula, and improvement over the Næser 1 formula, uses calculated data of the IOL architecture and optimized AL measurements to achieve equal results on small, aver-

age, and large eyes. The formula is available from its author in Excel (Microsoft Corporation, Redmond, WA, USA).

- Olsen formula was first developed in 1987, undergoing several modifications in the following years [17–19]. The current version is based on ray-tracing [20]. The C constant estimates IOL position based on ACD and LT. The formula can be downloaded at www.phacooptics.net (accessed March 18, 2021). Besides ACD and LT, PhacoOptics software uses four determinants for ELP prediction: AL, K, ACD, and LT. Two versions of Olsen formula are then described: the 4-factor version, also known as Olsen$_{Standalone}$ and the 2-factor version, which is installed on optical biometers.

- VRF formula is a vergence based thin-lens formula. The formula is published and uses four variables to predict the ELP (AL, K, ACD, and CD) [21]. The formula is available in its proprietary software (ViOL Commander software v. 2.0.0.0 (V/B/C Systems, Kiev, Ukraine)).

- VRF-G formula is a modification of the VRF formula. The new formula is based on theoretical optics, including regression and ray-tracing components. It uses eight variables for ELP prediction (AL, K, ACD, CD, LT, preoperative refraction, CCT, and gender).

- The Prediction Enhanced by ARtificial Intelligence and output Linearization-Debellemanière, Gatinel, and Saad (PEARL-DGS) formula uses machine learning (ML) and output linearization for estimating ELP and calculation the IOL power. It uses adjustments for the biometric values and is unpublished. It is available online at www.iolsolver.com (accessed March 18, 2021).

- T2 formula is an improvement of the SRK/T to circumvent its nonphysiological behavior [10]. It enhances the corneal height calculation of the original formula.

A summary of the constants and metrics used by each formula is presented in Table 13.1.

Performance of Different Formulas

Of all the available formulas, the best performing formulas use more than two parameters for ELP prediction and therefore should be preferred clinically [22].

In two landmark clinical studies [2, 23], Melles et al. investigated the performance of different IOL power calculation formulas. In their second study [23], the authors found Kane formula to be the most accurate, with 84% of the eyes within ±0.50 D of the target. Olsen, BU II, and EVO 2.0 formulas showed the next best results (Fig. 13.3). This was true when both SS-OCT and PCI-based biometers were used to acquire preoperative data.

In a 2016 study [24], Kane et al. reported the BU II to be similarly accurate for both small and long eyes, a finding confirmed in a subsequent study. The formula was superior to Haigis, SRK/T, and T2 formulas for all ALs (Fig. 13.4).

Similar findings were reported by Cooke and Cooke [25] when using the IOLMaster biometer,

Table 13.1 Summary of each intraocular lens formula constants and metrics (adapted from Clinical Ophthalmology 2020;14:4395–4402—open access)

Formula	Constants		Metrics
BARRETT UII	LF	2.035	AL, K, ACD, LT, HCD
EVO 2.0	A constant	119.20	AL, K, ACD, LT, CCT
HAIGIS	a0; a1; a2	−0.66; 0.234; 0.217	AL, K, ACD
HILL-RBF 2.0	A constant	119.23	AL, K, ACD
HOFFER Q	pACD	5.75	AL, K
HOLLADAY 1	SF	1.97	AL, K
KANE	A constant	119.18	AL, K, ACD, gender, LT, CCT
NÆESER 2	Korr AL constants	1.43; 0.94	AL, K, ACD
PEARL-DGS	A constant	119.03	AL, K, ACD, LT, HCD, CCT
SRK/T	A constant	119.22	AL, K
T2 FORMULA	A constant	119.22	AL, K
VRF	CACD	5.66	AL, K, ACD, HCD
VRF-G	A constant	119.19	AL, K, ACD, gender, LT, CCT, HCD, preoperative SE

SF surgeon factor, *pACD* personalized anterior chamber depth, *LF* lens factor, *CACD* optical constant of the anterior chamber depth, *AL* axial length, *K* keratometry, *ACD* anterior chamber depth, *LT* lens thickness, *HCD* horizontal cornea diameter, *CCT* central corneal thickness, *SE* refractive spherical equivalent

while the Olsen$_{Standalone}$ version was superior to BU II when using the Lenstar biometer. Figure 13.5 depicts two tables with the main study findings.

Shajari et al. [22] also found BU II to be the most precise formula. However, in contrast to the study by Kane et al., the authors found no significant differences between BU II, SRK/T, and T2 formulas. Also, in the study by Shajari et al. [22], differences in mean absolute error (MAE) between Hoffer Q, Holladay 1, and SRK/T formulas were not statistically significant.

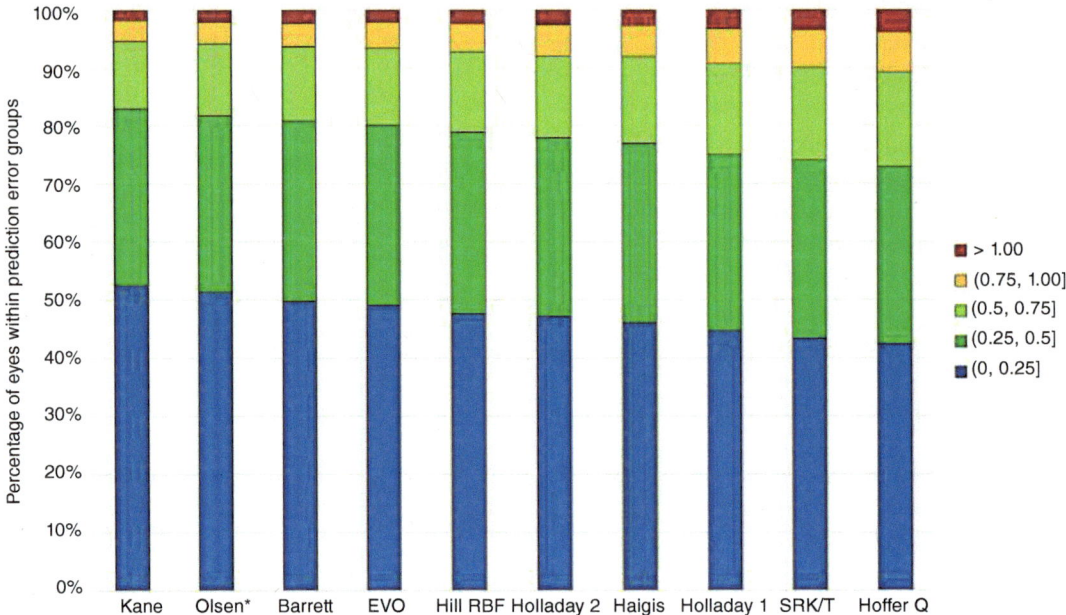

Fig. 13.3 Stacked histogram comparing the percentage of cases within a given diopter range of predicted spherical equivalent refraction outcome for the SN60WF (Alcon Laboratories, Inc., Forth Worth, TX) model intraocular lens. *H1* Holladay 1, *H2* Holladay 2, *HS* Haag-Streit, *WK* Wang-Koch. (Reproduced with permission from Ophthalmology. 2019 Sep;126(9):1334–1335)

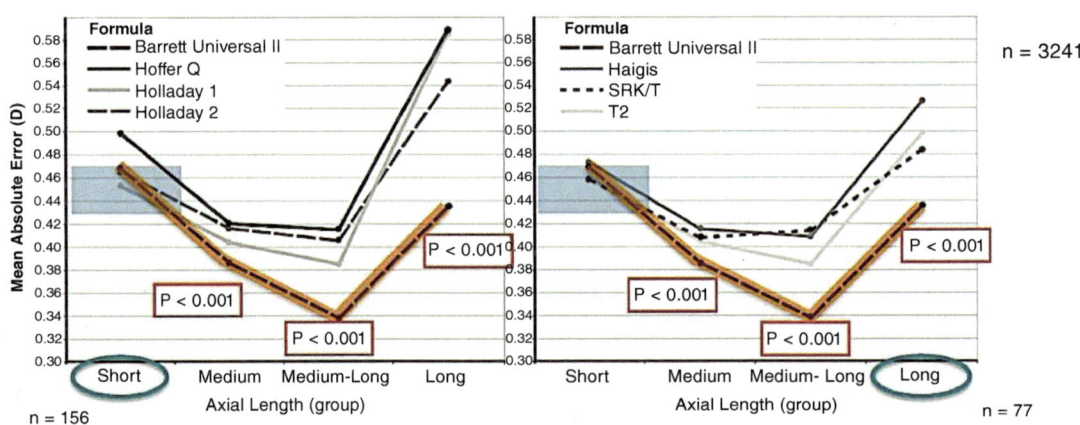

Fig. 13.4 Mean absolute error plotted against AL groups for the Barrett Universal II, Hoffer Q, Holladay 1, Holladay 2, Haigis, SRK/T, and T2 formulas. The formulas are grouped to allow easier visualization. (Adapted with permission from J Cataract Refract Surg. 2016 Oct;42(10):1490–1500)

Table 1. Formula performance for all eyes using optimized lens constants with PCI measurements (mean AL = 23.81 mm; range = 20.87 to 29.44 mm; N = 1079).

Formula	ME (D)	MAE (D)	Med AE(D)	SD	MAX Err	±0.5 D	±1.0D
Barrett	0.00	0.306	0.255	0.387	1.35	80.6	99.3
Haigis*	0.00	0.319	0.271	0.401	1.71	79.8	98.7
T2	0.00	0.319	0.265	0.404	1.70	79.0	98.7
Super Formula	−0.06	0.326	0.275	0.410	1.72	79.9	98.3
Holladay 1*	0.00	0.326	0.270	0.414	1.54	79.5	98.4
Holladay 2$_{NoRef}$	0.00	0.331	0.287	0.417	1.52	79.3	97.7
Holladay 2$_{PreSurgRef}$	0.00	0.346	0.297	0.432	1.47	75.2	98.1
Hoffer Q*	0.00	0.341	0.281	0.432	1.81	77.0	97.4
SRK/T*	0.00	0.346	0.290	0.440	1.89	75.1	98.1
Olsen$_{Standalone}$	0.01	0.348	0.285	0.446	1.59	75.1	97.1

Barrett = Barrett Universal II formula; Holladay 2$_{NoRef}$ = Holladay 2 formula that used all preoperative variables except preoperative refraction; Holladay 2$_{PreSurgRef}$ = Holladay 2 formula that used the refraction from the preoperative examination; MAE = mean absolute error; Max Err = maximum prediction error; ME = mean prediction error; Med AE = median absolute error, Olsen$_{Standalone}$ = purchased Olsen formula
*Formulas that were evaluated in a previous study[1]
[†]Percentage of refractions within ±0.5 D of prediction
[‡]Percentage of refractions within ±1.0 D of prediction

Table 2. Formula performance for all eyes using optimized lens constants with OLCR measurements (mean AL = 23.81 mm; range = 20.84 to 29.51 mm; N = 1079).

Formula	ME (D)	MAE (D)	Med AE(D)	SD	MAX Err	±0.5 D	±1.0D
Olsen$_{Standalone}$	0.00	0.284	0.225	0.361	1.51	83.7	99.1
Barrett	0.00	0.285	0.230	0.365	1.25	82.9	99.2
Olsen$_{OLCR}$	0.00	0.296	0.245	0.378	1.53	82.0	98.6
Haigis*	0.00	0.314	0.268	0.393	1.78	80.4	98.7
T2	0.00	0.313	0.262	0.397	1.62	79.6	98.8
Super Formula	−0.06	0.321	0.269	0.403	1.54	79.1	98.4
Holladay 2$_{NoRef}$	0.00	0.318	0.261	0.404	1.39	79.0	98.1
Holladay 1*	0.00	0.320	0.268	0.408	1.69	79.1	98.6
Holladay 2$_{PreSurgRef}$	0.00	0.336	0.288	0.423	1.48	76.6	98.4
Hoffer Q*	0.00	0.340	0.285	0.428	1.66	77.8	97.4
SRK/T*	0.00	0.342	0.289	0.433	1.79	75.7	98.1

Barrett Universal II formula; Holladay 2$_{NoRef}$ = Holladay 2 formula that used all preoperative variables except preoperative refraction; Holladay 2$_{PresurgRef}$ = Holladay 2 formula that used the refraction from the preoperative examination; MAE = mean absolute error; Max Err = maximum prediction error; ME = mean prediction error; Med AE median absolute error; Olsen$_{OLCR}$ = preloaded Olsen formula; Olsen$_{Standalone}$ = purchased Olsen formula
*Formulas that were evaluated in a previous study[1]
[†]Percentage of refractions within ±0.5 D of prediction
[‡]Percentage of refractions within ± 1.0 D of prediction

Fig. 13.5 Formula performance for all eyes using optimized lens constants with partial coherence interferometry (PCI) measurements (Table 13.1) and optical low coherence reflectometry (OLCR) measurements (Table 13.2). (Reproduced with permission from *J Cataract Refract Surg.* 2016;42:1157–1164)

BU II, EVO 2.0, Kane, and Olsen formulas superiority was confirmed in different studies [26, 27]. A study suggested Kane may be superior in ALs >22 mm [26]. Another study [27] reported similar results for the VRF-G formula when compared with the three other formulas, for eyes of all ALs.

Refractive Prediction Errors after Cataract Surgery

Even if the current formulas offer excellent results, the potential for postoperative ametropia still exists due to pre-, intra-, or postoperative causes. Preoperatively, the current

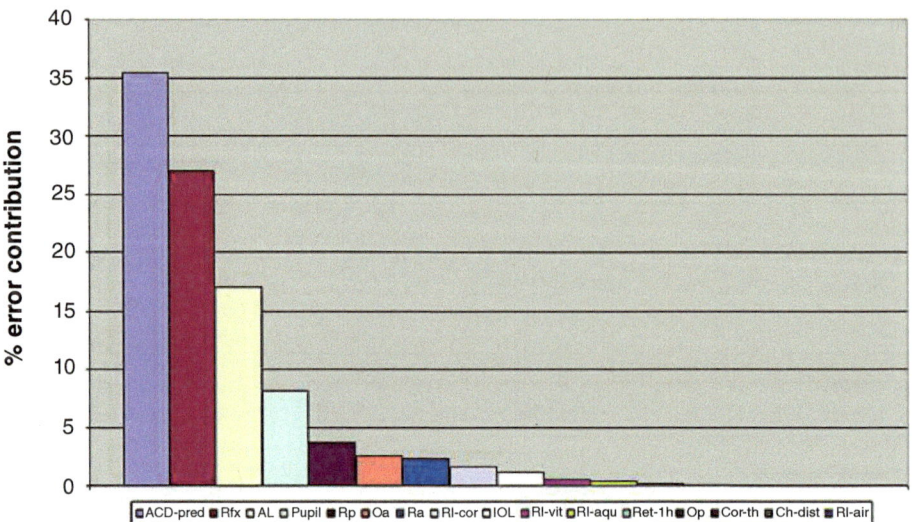

Fig. 13.6 Relative (percentage) error contribution of all factors influencing the refractive outcome of cataract surgery, arranged in order of decreasing magnitude. Eye of average dimensions and properties implanted with a 21.5 D IOL with spherical surfaces. *ACD-pred* prediction of postoperative IOL position, *AL* axial length, *Ch-dist* chart distance, *Cor-th* corneal thickness, *IOL* IOL power, *Pupil* pupil size, *Qa* corneal anterior asphericity, *Qp* corneal posterior asphericity, *Ra* corneal anterior radius, *Ret-th* retinal thickness, *Rfx* postoperative spectacle refraction, *RIair* air refractive index, *RI-aqu* aqueous refractive index, *RIcor* corneal refractive index, *RI-vit* vitreous refractive index, *Rp* corneal posterior radius. (Reproduced with permission from J Cataract Refract Surg 2008;34:368–376)

limitations of biometric data acquisition accuracy and repeatability [28], ocular surface disease [29–31], previous refractive surgery, and ELP prediction limitations should be considered. Our study group showed [32] that, in the phakic eye, AL measurements taken by ultrasound (vitreous chamber depth, LT, and ACD were the most sensitive to biometric errors, with a contribution to the refractive error of 62.7%, 14.2%, and 10.7%, respectively). When optical biometry measurements were considered, postoperative ACD was the most important contributor, followed by the anterior corneal surface and corneal asphericity. A Monte Carlo simulation showed that current limit of refractive assessment is 0.26 D for the phakic eye [32].

It is known that the error in ELP prediction is of major importance to the refractive outcome [33], having a 42% relative contribution to the total refractive error, contrasting with a 36% relative contribution of AL measurement errors and 22% relative contribution of corneal power measurement errors.

Similar values were found by Norrby [28], with the largest contributors of error being estimation of ELP (35%), postoperative refraction determination (27%), and AL measurement errors (17%) (Fig. 13.6).

During surgery, a decentration of the capsulorrhexis of more than 0.4 mm is associated with a 0.25 D change in spherical equivalent (SE) [34]. As our study group showed [35], the surgically induced astigmatism varies significantly, even with fixed incision size and meridian, also contributing to residual refractive error.

Postoperatively, the variability on subjective refraction and shift in IOL position are potential sources of refractive error.

We can conclude that estimation of postoperative IOL position is a major determinant of residual refractive error, hence the importance of considering elements that may improve this estimation in IOL calculation.

Preoperative Evaluation

Accurate biometric measurements are paramount for the correct evaluation of the eye.

Although there are several techniques to measure AL, optically based systems, such as PCI or OLCR, have gained increased popularity in recent years. These systems are more accurate and less dependent on the operator than ultrasound biometry [36–39]. Furthermore, most optical biometers evaluate additional parameters, including corneal curvature, ACD, LT, and CD.

Anterior Chamber Depth

The ACD is an important parameter for IOL power calculation, being used as a variable for ELP prediction in several formulas. ACD can be measured by various techniques:

- A-Scan ultrasound (US)
- Ultrasound biomicroscopy (UBM)
- Optical biometry
- Slit-beam photography
- Scheimpflug imaging
- Anterior segment optical coherence tomography (AS-OCT)

Measurement devices based on these techniques were developed for measuring the ACD. Using them to measure ACD_{post} results in significant discrepancies between measurements obtained with different techniques, being unclear which one is more adequate to accurately measure ACD_{post}. Figure 13.7 demonstrates the concept of ACD measurement pre- and postoperatively.

It is important to note that different measurement techniques have variable agreements between them when evaluating ACD. Thus, their interchangeability should be studied (see topic "Agreement Between Measurement Techniques").

Lens Thickness

US, optical biometry, Scheimpflug photography, and OCT may be used to evaluate LT.

US techniques are more reliable in measuring posterior lens shape in the cataractous eye, whilst OCT [40], or Scheimpflug photography may both be used for analyzing the anterior lens shape. Scheimpflug photography [41] should not be used for posterior lens imaging since the required geometrical distortion induced by the acute angles leads to a significant loss of resolution.

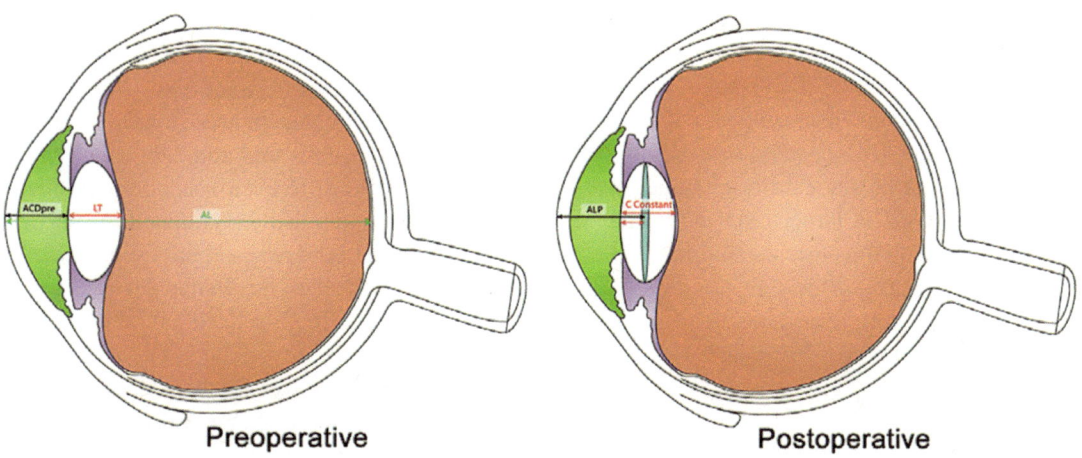

Preoperative   **Postoperative**

Fig. 13.7 Description of the anterior lens position. *ACDpre* preoperative anterior chamber depth, *AL* axial length, *ALP* actual lens position, *LT* lens thickness. (Reproduced with permission from J Cataract Refract Surg 2017; 43:195–200)

Another technique capable of imaging the cataractous lens shape with high resolution is magnetic resonance imaging (MRI), but the associated costs are still considered too high.

Corneal Diameter

CD can be evaluated using:

- Manual calipers
- UBM
- Digital photography
- Optical biometry
- Corneal topography
- AS-OCT

Definitions of normal CD, as determined by the horizontal CD, are controversial. The generally accepted values of normal horizontal CD of 11.0–13.0 mm are not established by any evidence-based studies, with definitions of microcornea ranging from 10.0 [42–45] to 11.0 mm [46, 47] and of macrocornea from 12.5 [43–46] to 13 mm [48]. It is important to remember that most of these ranges are based on measurements with manual calipers, as automated devices are relatively new.

With any technique, it must be noted that CD measurements are not equivalent to angle-to-angle (ATA) measurements and no accurate prediction of ATA may be derived from CD [48]. When comparing AS-OCT (Visante) with automated CD measurements using the IOLMaster and the Orbscan IIz, a study showed that the internal diameter of the anterior chamber evaluated with AS-OCT is larger than the horizontal CD measured with the other techniques [49].

Agreement Between Measurement Techniques

Repeatability and reproducibility of the above-mentioned techniques are high for most measured parameters. However, agreement is variable. Numerous studies evaluated the agreement between different techniques in the mea-

surement of the biometric parameters topic of this chapter (ACD, LT, and CD).

ACD measurements with the IOLMaster are generally shallower than those of other optical biometers, probably because the slit source that measures ACD is projected from the temporal side, with ACD measured slightly off-center. Sabatino et al. [50] compared two biometers, the IOLMaster and a biometer based on optical low-coherence interferometry (OLCI) in ACD measurement, finding statistically significant differences (3.13 ± 0.36 mm vs. 3.16 ± 0.30 mm, respectively). Repeatability was high for both instruments. On the contrary, Hoffer et al. [51] showed PCI to measure a deeper ACD than OLCR (3.11 ± 0.47 mm vs. 2.98 ± 0.49 mm, respectively; $P < 0.0001$).

When assessing the agreement and comparing ACD measurements between two optical devices (Orbscan II and IOLMaster) and contact US A-Scan, Reddy et al. [52] showed the mean ACD was 3.32 ± 0.60 mm, 3.33 ± 0.61 mm, and 2.87 ± 0.55 mm, respectively ($P < 0.01$). A high agreement between Orbscan II and IOLMaster was noted.

Lee et al. [53] compared ACD measurements (endothelium to anterior capsule of the lens) using the Orbscan IIz and UBM. The authors found a deeper ACD with UBM (2.91 ± 0.43 mm vs. 2.82 ± 0.46 mm, respectively; $P < 0.001$).

Even when using the same technique, differences may still exist. Savini et al. [54] investigated the differences between two Scheimpflug camera devices (Pentacam and Sirius). The mean ACD was 2.90 ± 0.48 mm and 2.94 ± 0.47 mm, respectively. The difference was considered statistically but not clinically significant. Aramberri et al. [55] studied the repeatability, reproducibility, and agreement of the Pentacam HR and a dual-camera Scheimpflug device (Galilei G2) in analyzing the anterior segment. The ACD measurement precision was high, with a within-subject standard deviation (Sw) value of 0.02 mm, and intraclass correlation coefficient (ICC) values higher than 0.993. Other authors [56] showed that the Galilei G4 yielded a significantly shallower ($P < 0.05$) ACD measurement than the Pentacam HR.

One study [57] compared the ACD and CD using the Zeiss Meditec Atlas, IOLMaster 500, Orbscan II, and Pentacam and found the largest agreement to exist between the IOLMaster and the Pentacam.

Baikoff et al. [58] compared a PCI device (IOLMaster 500) with an AS-OCT prototype (Carl Zeiss Meditec). The mean ACD was 3.53 ±0.35 mm with the IOLMaster and 3.64 ±0.33 mm with the AS-OCT. OCT measurements were more reproducible.

When studying OCT biometers, Hoffer et al. [59] showed small differences exist between OLCR and swept-source (SS)-OCT (IOLMaster 700) in ACD measurement (-0.03 mm; $P < 0.001$). Comparing a new SS-OCT biometer (Argos) with the IOLMaster 500 and the Lenstar LS900, Shammas et al. [60] found a difference in ACD of -0.17 ± 0.20 mm for the PCI device, and 0.08 ± 0.15 mm for the OLCR device.

Recently, Tañá-Rivero et al. [61] compared a Scheimpflug-PCI device (Pentacam AXL) with two SS-OCT biometers (IOLMaster 700 and ANTERION). The authors found a statistically significant difference in ACD, LT, and CD between the biometers ($P < 0.001$), with the IOLMaster showing the shallowest and ANTERION the deepest ACD.

In another recent study [62], intraoperative OCT yielded a significantly deeper ACD value than PCI. However, this difference did not reflect a significant difference in IOL calculation using the BU II formula.

Differences between measurement devices should be remembered when using formulas that consider ACD in IOL power calculation.

Savini et al. [63] investigated the differences in LT between immersion US and three optical biometers (OA-2000, Alladin and Galilei G6). Differences were small but statistically significant and influenced IOL selection, resulting, when using the optical biometry measurements, in a selection of a lower power IOL in between 43.2% and 62.5% of eyes, depending on the optical biometer.

In the study by Kurian et al. [64] there were significant differences between OLCR and SS-OCT biometry when evaluating LT (-0.06 mm; $P < 0.001$).

Fisus et al. [65] compared the IOLMaster 700 with a new SS-OCT biometer (ANTERION), finding a difference of and 0.07 ± 0.04 mm in both LT and ACD between both biometers. Although the differences were small, the authors suggested the devices are not interchangeable.

Domínguez-Vicent et al. [66] reported that CD depends not only on image quality but also on the algorithms chosen for limbus detection. Differences in formulas that use CD as a variable, such as Holladay 2 or BU II, may be found. The authors [56] also found that the mean CD was 11.84 ± 0.31 mm and 11.90 ± 0.43 mm when measured with the Galilei G4 and the Pentacam HR, respectively.

It is also known that measurements of CD with the Pentacam HR and the Orbscan IIz are similar [67].

In the study by Tañá-Rivero et al. [61], the IOLMaster showed the largest CD and the Pentacam the shortest (12.00 ± 0.51 mm vs. 11.67 ± 0.51 mm, respectively; $P < 0.001$). The LT measured with IOLMaster was thicker than that measured with ANTERION (4.23 ± 0.57 mm vs. 4.20 ± 0.58 mm, respectively; $P < 0.001$).

A recent metanalysis [68] demonstrated a high agreement between measurements of AL, ACD, and corneal power with the Lenstar and IOLMaster. However, significant differences in CD between the two devices were found (mean difference OLCR to PCI -0.14 mm; 95% CI -0.25 to -0.02 mm; $P = 0.02$).

Thus, significant differences in CD should be considered in the case of formulas that use this parameter for IOL power calculation, the same being true for ACD and LT.

When evaluating these biometric parameters, it is important to remember that pupil dilation causes a significant variation of their values [69–73], with some studies also showing differences in IOL power when using some formulas, particularly BU II [55]. Hence, biometry should always be acquired in the same standard conditions, preferably through an undilated pupil and by the same experienced operator.

Population Means

Given the paucity of published studies of ocular biometric parameters using optical biometry, we recently characterized the ocular biometric parameters and their associations in a population of cataract surgery candidates in Portugal, using the Lenstar LS900 optical biometer [74].

The mean values of ACD, LT, and CD are shown in Table 13.2.

The histograms of the distribution of the ACD, LT, and CD values are shown in Figs. 13.8, 13.9, and 13.10, respectively.

The AL, ACD, LT, and CD were all significantly correlated between each other ($P < 0.001$).

Table 13.2 Demographic data and mean ocular biometric parameters in a Portuguese population

Parameter	Mean ± SD (range)		
Eyes (*n*)	6506		
Patients (*n*)	6506		
Anterior chamber depth (mm) ± SD	3.25 ± 0.44	3.30 ± 0.40	3.14 ± 0.43
Range	(2.04–5.28)	(2.06–5.42)	(2.04–4.99)
Lens thickness (mm) ± SD	4.32 ± 0.49	4.35 ± 0.49	4.38 ± 0.41
Range	(2.73–5.77)	(2.75–5.77)	(2.73–5.42)
Corneal diameter (mm) ± SD	12.02 ± 0.46	12.03 ± 0.43	11.98 ± 0.49
Range	(10.50–14.15)	(10.51–14.15)	(10.50–14.09)

Fig. 13.8 Histogram of anterior chamber depth (ACD) of the study population

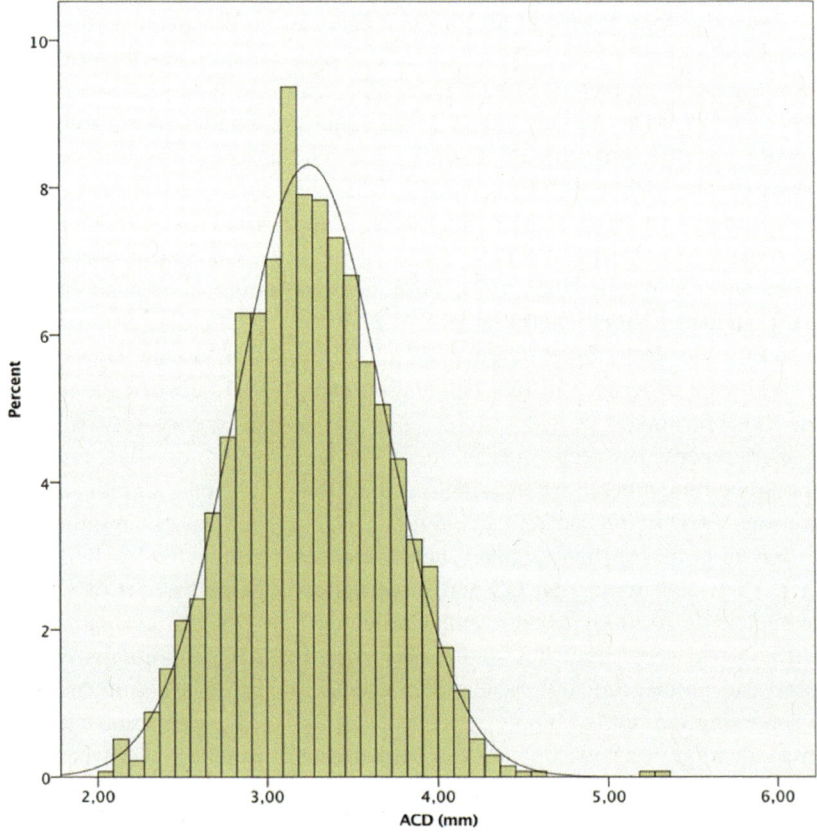

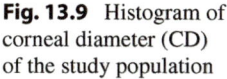

Fig. 13.9 Histogram of corneal diameter (CD) of the study population

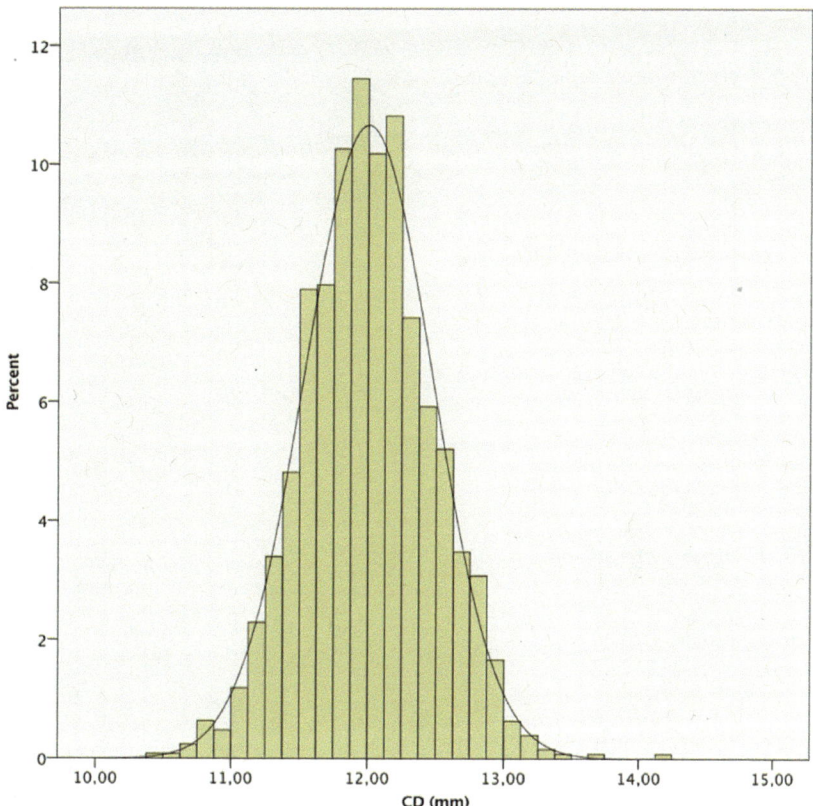

The mean ACD in our population (3.25 ± 0.44 mm) was higher than that reported in most studies in Eastern [75–78] and Western populations, and it is comparable with that reported by Hoffer in the USA [79].

The mean LT was 4.32 ± 0.49 mm, and it was directly proportional to age and inversely proportional to AL. These findings confirm those of the studies by Jivrajka et al. [64] and Hoffer [65, 80], although LT in our study was thinner than those studies reported. The mean CD in our study (12.02 ± 0.46 mm) was similar to that reported in other series in the literature [64, 81].

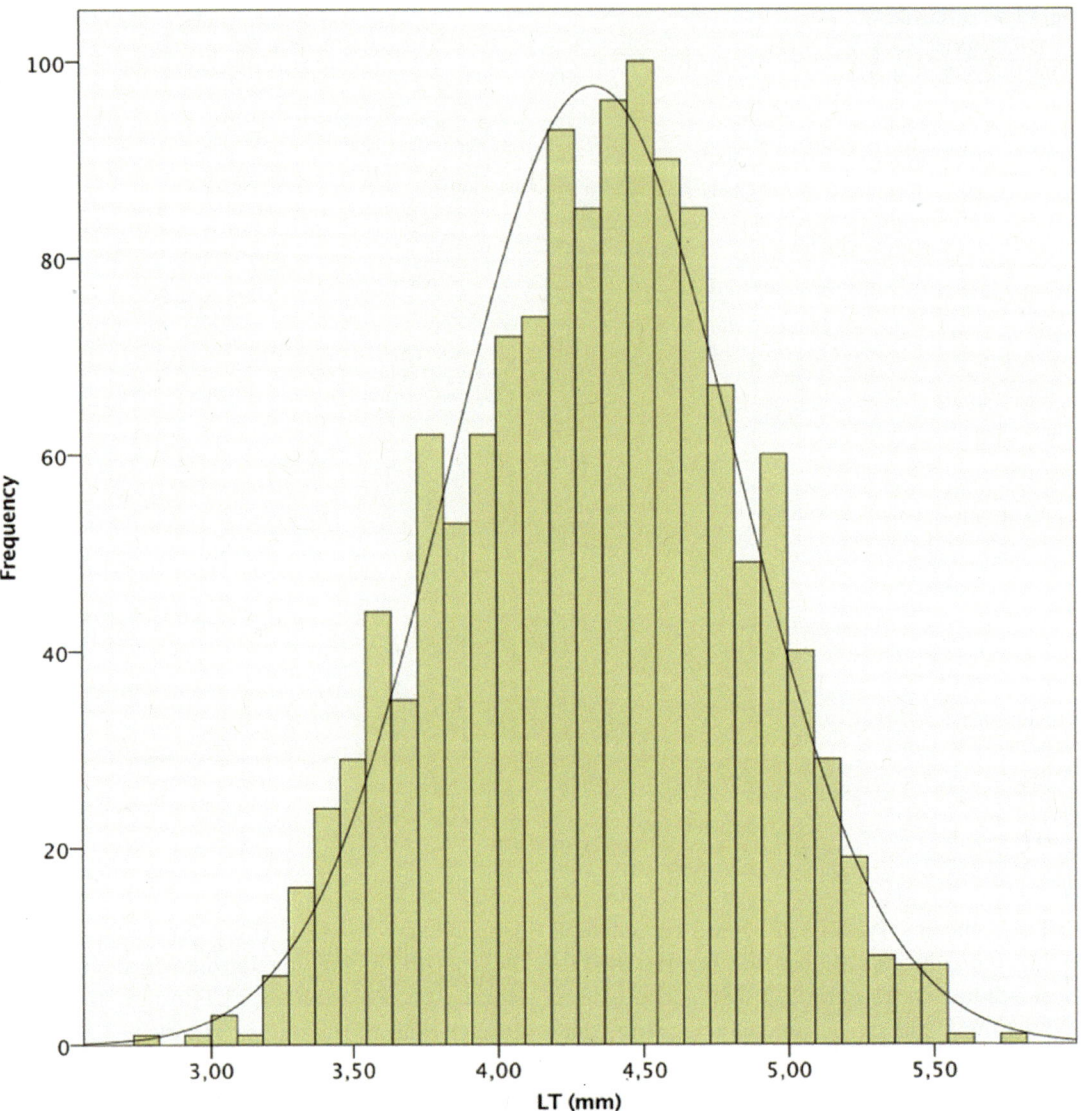

Fig. 13.10 Histogram of lens thickness (LT) of the study population

Influence of Anterior Chamber Depth on Intraocular Lens Power Calculation

It is known that the change in ACD after cataract surgery has an impact on postoperative refractive error (a hyperopic shift will small changes and a myopic shift with larger changes) [82].

Formulas may fail in short eyes and shallow ACDs. Also, there is no agreement on the accu-

racy of different formulas in long eyes with deep ACDs [2, 83–85].

In a 2013 study, our group evaluated the effect of changes in each optical parameter on the refractive status of the eye [32]. We found that, for each 1% increase in ACD, refractive error changes −0.044 D. Thus, a change of 0.179 mm in ACD is required for a 0.25 D variation in refractive error. If we also consider AL, a change of 0.25 mm in ACD measurement corresponds to an error of 0.10 D in an eye with an AL of 30.0 mm. This error increases 5 times (to 0.50 D) in an eye with an AL of 20.0 mm. This is the reason because precisely estimating ACD is much more important in short than in long eyes.

It is interesting to note that Savini et al. [13] studied two formulas—(BU II) and EVO 2.0—where ACD is an optional parameter, and results of each of these formulas were better when no ACD was entered. However, the authors point out that errors in ACD measurement may explain the results.

When using the BU II formula [86], the optional variables (ACD, LT, and CD) seem to have the least effect in long eyes (AL ≥26.0 mm) and the greatest effect in short eyes (AL ≤22.0 mm), where clinically significant differences are found, further stressing the importance of the optional parameters in these eyes.

In the study by Melles et al. [2], the relationship between ACD and refractive prediction error was investigated. For Hoffer Q, Holladay 1, and Olsen formulas, there was a significant bias in prediction error with variations in ACD (Fig. 13.11).

In a study of third-generation and Haigis formulas [87], Jeong et al. showed ACD was the key factor for the difference between third-generation formulas and Haigis. Of the third-generation for-

mulas, larger errors with ACD variations were observed with the Hoffer Q than with the SRK-T formula.

Hipólito-Fernandes et al. [88] studied the influence of ACD and LT in the accuracy of five vergence based and four new generation formulas. The authors divided the eyes in three groups, according to ACD. The Vergence-based two-variable formulas (SRK/T, Holladay 1, and Hoffer Q) revealed a significant myopic shift in group 1 (ACD ≤3.00 mm) and a significant hyperopic shift in group 3 (ACD ≥3.50 mm). In group 1, Kane and Hill-RBF v2.0 were better than the other formulas. The same formulas outperformed others in group 2, while in group 3 Hill-RBF performed the best (Fig. 13.12). Kane, PEARL-DGS, EVO 2.0, and BU II had lower MAE, median absolute errors (MedAE), and a higher percentage of eyes within ±0.25 D than the other formulas.

Gökce et al. [70] studied the influence of ACD on nine formulas in eyes with normal ALs. In eyes with ACD ≤3.0 mm or ≥3.5 mm, ACD was an important variable in the accuracy of IOL calculation. In eyes with normal ALs and ACD ≤3.0 mm or ≥3.5 mm, the BU II, Haigis, Holladay 2, and the Olsen$_{Standalone}$ formulas performed better than two variable formulas (Hoffer Q and Holladay 1) and the Olsen$_{OLCR}$ formula.

Fig. 13.11 Correlations between anterior chamber depth and postoperative prediction error for different formulas. (Reproduced with permission from Ophthalmology 2018 Feb;125(2):169–178)

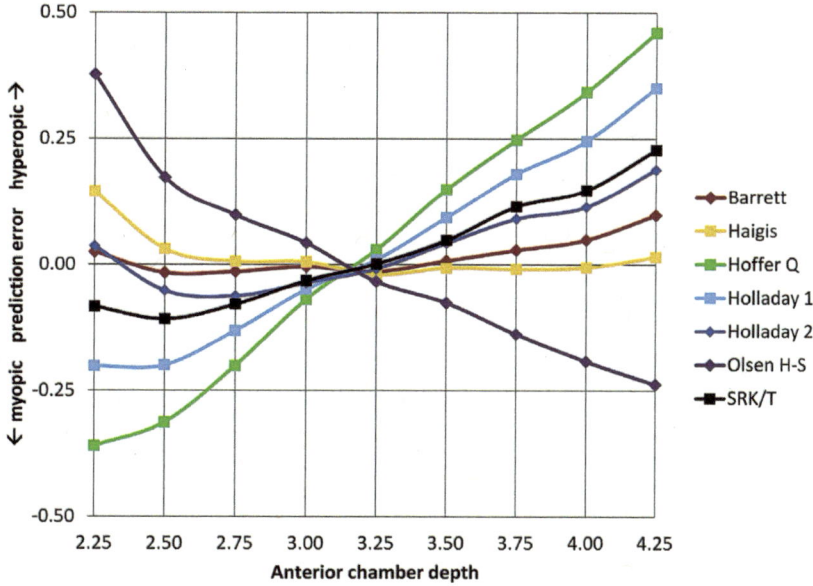

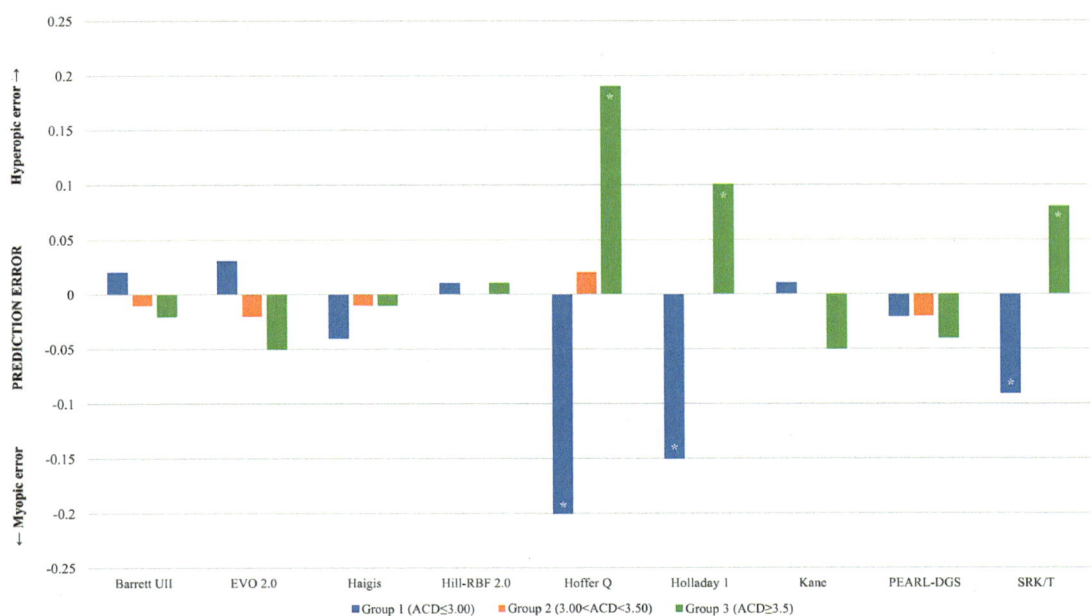

Fig. 13.12 Mean prediction error (in diopters) of each formula, distributed by anterior chamber depth (ACD) group, listed by alphabetic order. *$P < 0.05$—one sample *t*-test. *EVO* emmetropia verifying optical. (Reproduced with permission from Br J Ophthalmol. 2020 Nov 23:bjophthalmol-2020-317822)

The effect of ACD in eyes with different ALs was studied by Yang et al. [85] The Hoffer Q formula was preferred over other formulas in eyes with AL <22.0 mm and ACD <2.5 mm. In eyes with AL <24.5 mm and ACD <2.5 mm, the Haigis formula resulted in myopic refractive prediction errors, while in eyes with AL ≥25.0 mm and ACD ≥3.5 mm it was the preferred formula.

Similarly, Fernandez et al. [89] showed that predictability of different formulas was reduced in eyes with very shallow ACD (ACD ≤2.46 mm). However, in contrast with other studies, and probably due to the low number of eyes in these groups in the study by Fernandez et al., a decrease in accuracy was not found in short eyes or shallow ACD (>2.46 mm).

The accuracy of formulas in short eyes (AL <22 mm) was studied by Shrivastava et al. [90] The performance of seven formulas (BU II, Haigis, Hill-RBF, Hoffer Q, Holladay 1, Holladay 2, and SRK/T) on these eyes was evaluated. In eyes with ACD ≥2.4 mm, Haigis was the best performing formula, with SRK/T being the worst, while in eyes with ACD <2.4 mm, although the differences were not significant, Haigis performed the worst.

Influence of Lens Thickness on Intraocular Lens Power Calculation

Lenticular growth, mainly sagittal, occurs throughout life, and it has been estimated that the equatorial diameter increases about 0.02 mm/year [91]. This thickening occurs predominantly in the anterior direction [92], with the consequent anterior movement of the center of the lens and shallowing of the anterior chamber [93]. This has clear implications on ACD_{post} estimation, given in a younger population a higher lens thickness should correspond to a greater IOL depth, while in an older population, such as a cataract population, a greater lens thickness and smaller IOL depth should be found.

In a study where our group evaluated the effect of changes in each optical parameter on the refractive status of the eye [73], we found that for each 1% increase in LT refractive error changes −0.097, with a change of 0.104 mm in LT required for a 0.25 D variation in refractive error.

The relationship between different ocular biometric parameters and prediction error of different formulas was studied by Melles et al. [2] When considering LT, Haigis and Holladay 2 were the formulas most affected by its variation (Fig. 13.13).

Similarly, Hipolito-Fernandes et al. [76] found a tendency for a myopic shift with thinner lenses and a hyperopic shift with thicker lenses. This effect was particularly evident for the Haigis and Hill-RBF v2.0 formulas. According

to what was shown by Melles et al., BU II had higher prediction errors (hyperopic shifts) with thicker lenses, when compared with the Hoffer Q and Holladay 1 formulas. For the Kane and PEARL-DGS formulas, the MAE was never significantly different from zero across all the LT range (Fig. 13.14).

In another study supporting these findings, Kim et al. [94] showed BU II formula to have the least bias in prediction error according to variations in LT. Refractive errors predicted by the Haigis and Holladay 2 formulas were correlated with LT ($P < 0.001$).

Fig. 13.13 Correlations between lens thickness and postoperative prediction error for different formulas. (Reproduced with permission from Ophthalmology 2018 Feb;125(2):169–178)

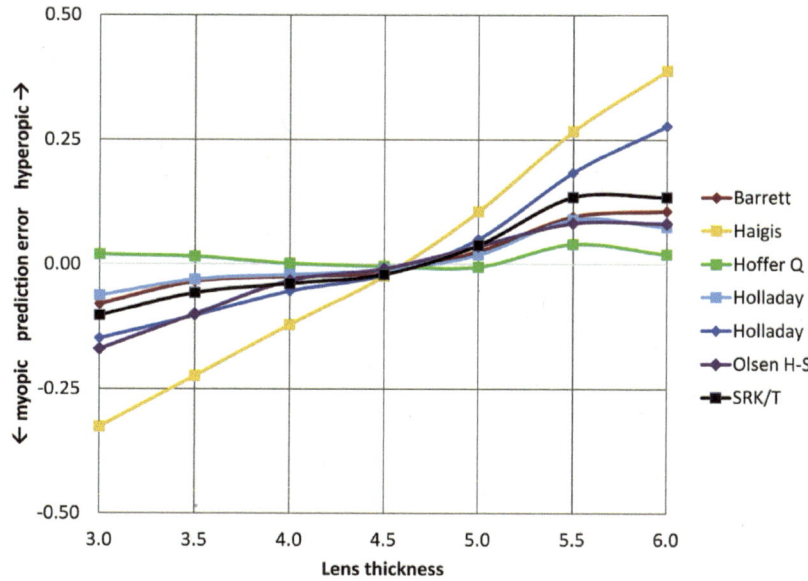

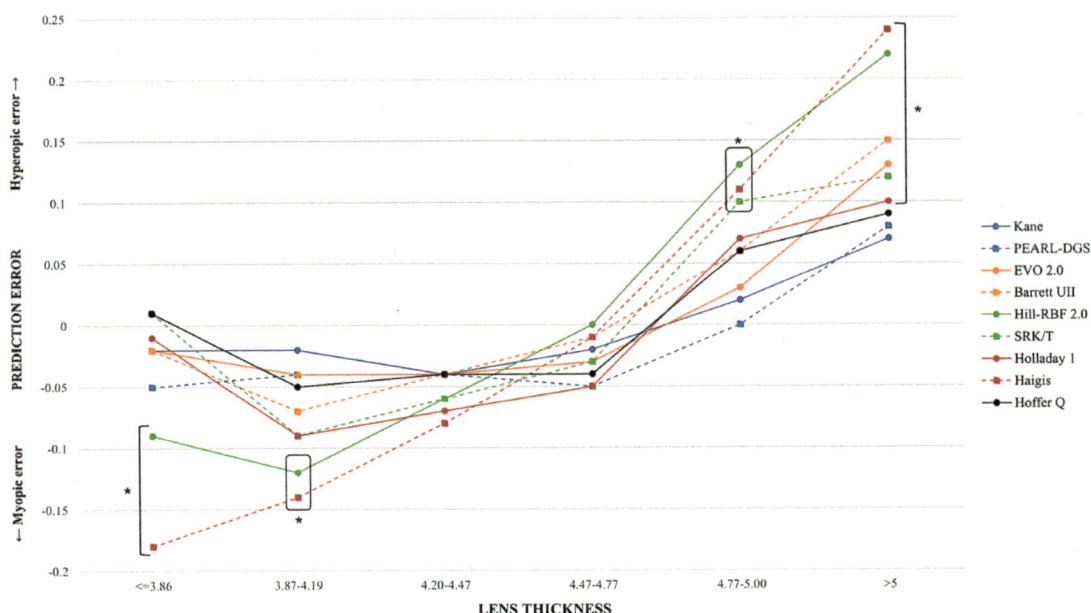

Fig. 13.14 Mean prediction error (in diopters) of each formula, from lens thickness percentile tenth until 90th (in millimeters). *P < 0.05—one sample t-test. *EVO* emmetropia verifying optical. (Reproduced with permission from Br J Ophthalmol. 2020 Nov 23:bjophthalmol-2020-317822)

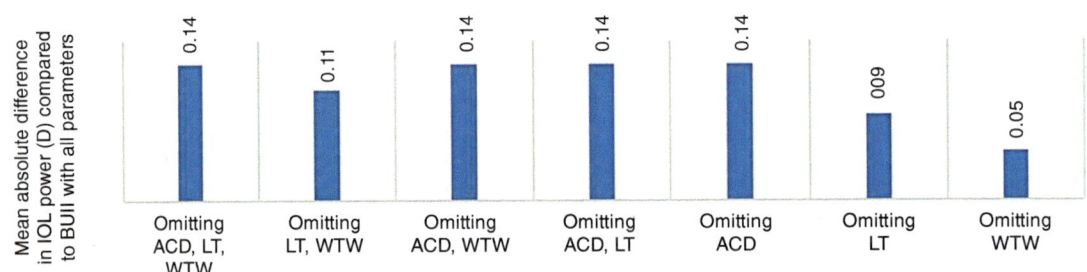

Fig. 13.15 The mean absolute difference in IOL power calculation between partial biometry data and all Barrett Universal II (BUII) parameters in the whole cohort. *ACD* anterior chamber depth, *D* diopters, *IOL* intraocular, *LT* lens thickness, *CD* corneal diameter. (Reproduced with permission from J Clin Med. 2021;10(3):542—open access)

Influence of Corneal Diameter on Intraocular Lens Power Calculation

When studying the influence of optional parameters in BU II, Vega et al. [74] showed that the effect of omitting CD was less than that of omitting ACD or LT (Fig. 13.15), which have more profound and similar effects across all ALs.

The Case of Toric Intraocular Lenses

With the increasing importance of a precise refractive outcome in cataract surgery, accuracy in planning of astigmatic correction also became critical. The classical toric calculators had several limitations in the calculation of the cylindrical power of toric IOLs. Besides not considering the IOL's spherical power or the posterior corneal surface, it is known that, for each cylindrical power at the IOL plane, a corresponding magnitude of astigmatism is corrected at the corneal plane. This variability depends on the distance between the cornea and the IOL [95, 96]. Most classical toric IOL calculators (e.g., the original toric calculator from Alcon (Alcon Laboratories Inc., Fort Worth, TX, USA)) [97] assumed a fixed ratio (in Alcon's case, 1.46) between the cylindrical power at the corneal and IOL plane. This results in undercorrections in long eyes and overcorrections in short eyes (e.g., in an eye with an axial length of 20.0 mm the real ratio is 1.29 and in an eye with an axial length of 30.0 mm the real ratio is 1.86) [98, 99].

Recently, strategies to overcome this limitation, such as including the ACD and CCT in toric IOL power calculation, were described [100–102].

Future Perspectives

Several paths of investigation aim to improve the main source of error we have identified in this chapter, ELP. These include the use of new imaging techniques or AI strategies.

The use of OCT imaging for improving ELP estimation has been approached by different authors [103]. Goto et al. [104] developed and validated a formula for predicting ACD_{post} from preoperative ATA depth measured by AS-OCT. ATA depth proved to be the most effective parameter for predicting ACD_{post}. Results seem to improve the accuracy of IOL power calculation, with postoperative ACDs of the new formula, the SRK/T formula, and Haigis formulas being predicted with R^2 of 0.71, 0.36, and 0.55, respectively, and the MedAEs being 0.10 mm, 0.65 mm, and 0.30 mm, respectively.

Martinez-Henriques et al. developed an OCT model to improve ELP estimation [105]. The authors obtained a three-dimensional full image of the crystalline lens with quantitative AS-OCT eye imaging. The IOL position after surgery was used to calculate refraction estimation errors. The authors showed that considering the full lens shape is valuable for calculating the ELP.

Satou et al. [106] developed and validated a new method of IOL power calculation based on paraxial ray tracing of the postoperative IOL position captured with AS-OCT. The percentage of eyes within ±0.50 D of the newly developed formula was 84.3% and results showed no correlation with AL or keratometry, which may improve the outcomes in eyes with abnormal proportions.

Different AI strategies for predicting ELP are also being used, namely ML processes. Li et al. [107] showed ACD was the most important input in an ML model, followed by LT, AL, and CD. Subsequently [108], the authors integrated an ML-based method for predicting ELP into existing formulas (Haigis, Hoffer Q, Holladay, and SRK/T) and showed that replacing each of the formulas ELP estimation with the new model improved the performance of all the formulas.

In conclusion, ACD, LT, and CD are important parameters for IOL power calculation and should, in the future, play a primordial role in improving ELP prediction.

Financial Disclosure The author has no proprietary or financial interests in any of the subjects described in this chapter.

References

1. Koch DD, Hill W, Abulafia A, Wang L. Pursuing perfection in intraocular lens calculations: I. Logical approach for classifying IOL calculation formulas. J Cataract Refract Surg. 2017;43(6):717–8.
2. Melles RB, Holladay JT, Chang WJ. Accuracy of intraocular lens calculation formulas. Ophthalmology. 2018;125(2):169–78.
3. Kane JX, Van Heerden A, Atik A, Petsoglou C. Accuracy of 3 new methods for intraocular lens power selection. J Cataract Refract Surg. 2017;43(3):333–9.
4. Hayashi K, Hayashi H, Nakao F, Hayashi F. Influence of astigmatism on multifocal and monofocal intraocular lenses. Am J Ophthalmol. 2000;130:477–82.
5. Fedorov SN, Kolinko AI. A method of calculating the optical power of the intraocular lens. Vestn Oftalmol. 1967;80(4):27–31.

6. Fyodorov SN, Galin MA, Linksz A. Calculation of the optical power of intraocular lenses. Investig Ophthalmol. 1975;14(8):625–8.

7. Colenbrander MC. Calculation of the power of an iris clip lens for distant vision. Br J Ophthalmol. 1973;57(10):735–40.

8. Retzlaff J. Posterior chamber implant power calculation: regression formulas. J Am Intra Ocular Implant Soc. 1980;6(3):268–70.

9. Sanders DR, Kraff MC. Improvement of intraocular lens power calculation using empirical data. J Am Intra-Ocular Implant Soc. 1980;6(3):263–7.

10. Sheard RM, Smith GT, Cooke DL. Improving the prediction accuracy of the SRK/T formula: the T2 formula. J Cataract Refract Surg. 2010;36(11):1829–34.

11. Plat J, Hoa D, Mura F, Busetto T, Schneider C, Payerols A, Villain M, Daien V. Clinical and biometric determinants of actual lens position after cataract surgery. J Cataract Refract Surg. 2017;43(2):195–200.

12. Jin H, Rabsilber T, Ehmer A, Borkenstein AF, Limberger IJ, Guo H, et al. Comparison of ray-tracing method and thin-lens formula in intraocular lens power calculations. J Cataract Refract Surg. 2009;35(4):650–62.

13. Savini G, Di Maita M, Hoffer KJ, Næser K, Schiano-Lomoriello D, Vagge A, Di Cello L, Traverso CE. Comparison of 13 formulas for IOL power calculation with measurements from partial coherence interferometry. Br J Ophthalmol. 2020;105:484. Epub ahead of print.

14. Barrett GD. Intraocular lens calculation formulas for new intraocular lens implants. J Cataract Refract Surg. 1987;13:389–96.

15. Barrett GD. An improved universal theoretical formula for intraocular lens powerprediction. J Cataract Refract Surg. 1993;19:713–20.

16. Næser K, Savini G. Accuracy of thick-lens intraocular lens power calculation based on cutting-card or calculated data for lens architecture. J Cataract Refract Surg. 2019;45(10):1422–9.

17. Olsen T. Theoretical approach to intraocular lens calculation using Gaussian optics. J Cataract Refract Surg. 1987;13:141–5.

18. Olsen T, Corydon L, Gimbel H. Intraocular lens power calculation with an improved anterior chamber depth prediction algorithm. J Cataract Refract Surg. 1995;21:313–9.

19. Olsen T. Prediction of the effective postoperative (intraocular lens) anterior chamber depth. J Cataract Refract Surg. 2006;32:419–24.

20. Olsen T, Hoffmann P. C constant: new concept for ray tracing-assisted intraocular lens power calculation. J Cataract Refract Surg. 2014;40:764–73.

21. Voytsekhivskyy OV. Development and clinical accuracy of a new intraocular lens power formula (VRF) compared to other formulas. Am J Ophthalmol. 2018;185:56–67.

22. Shajari M, Kolb CM, Petermann K, Böhm M, Herzog M, de'Lorenzo N, Schönbrunn S, Kohnen T. Comparison of 9 modern intraocular lens power calculation formulas for a quadrifocal intraocular lens. J Cataract Refract Surg. 2018;44(8):942–8. Erratum in: J Cataract Refract Surg. 2018 Nov;44(11):1409.

23. Melles RB, Kane JX, Olsen T, Chang WJ. Update on intraocular lens calculation formulas. Ophthalmology. 2019;126(9):1334–5. Epub 2019 Apr 11.

24. Kane JX, Van Heerden A, Atik A, Petsoglou C. Intraocular lens power formula accuracy: comparison of 7 formulas. J Cataract Refract Surg. 2016;42:1490–500.

25. Cooke DL, Cooke TL. Comparison of 9 intraocular lens power calculation formulas. J Cataract Refract Surg. 2016;42:1157–64.

26. Cheng H, Kane JX, Liu L, Li J, Cheng B, Wu M. Refractive predictability using the IOLMaster 700 and artificial intelligence-based IOL power formulas compared to standard formulas. J Refract Surg. 2020;36(7):466–72.

27. Hipólito-Fernandes D, Elisa Luís M, Gil P, Maduro V, Feijão J, Yeo TK, Voytsekhivskyy O, Alves N. VRF-G, a new intraocular lens power calculation formula: a 13-formulas comparison study. Clin Ophthalmol. 2020;14:4395–402.

28. Norrby S. Sources of error in intraocular lens power calculation. J Cataract Refract Surg. 2008;34:368–76.

29. Chuang J, Shih KC, Chan TC, Wan KH, Jhanji V, Tong L. Preoperative optimization of ocular surface disease before cataract surgery. J Cataract Refract Surg. 2017;43:1596–607.

30. Holladay JT, Hill WE, Steinmueller A. Corneal power measurements using Scheimpflug imaging in eyes with prior corneal refractive surgery. J Refract Surg. 2009;25:862–8. Erratum in: J Refract Surg 2010;26(6):387.

31. Latkany RA, Chokshi AR, Speaker MG, Abramson J, Soloway BD, Yu G. Intraocular lens calculations after refractive surgery. J Cataract Refract Surg. 2005;31:562–70.

32. Ribeiro F, Castanheira-Dinis A, Dias JM. Refractive error assessment: influence of different optical elements and current limits of biometric techniques. J Refract Surg. 2013;29(3):206–12.

33. Olsen T. Sources of error in intraocular lens power calculation. J Cataract Refract Surg. 1992;18(2):125–9.

34. Okada M, Hersh D, Paul E, van der Straaten D. Effect of centration and circularity of manual capsulorrhexis on cataract surgery refractive outcomes. Ophthalmology. 2014;121:763–70.

35. Ferreira TB, Ribeiro FJ, Pinheiro J, Ribeiro P, O'Neill JG. Comparison of surgically induced astigmatism and morphologic features resulting from femtosec-

ond laser and manual clear corneal incisions for cataract surgery. J Refract Surg. 2018;34(5):322–9.

36. Binkhorst RD. The accuracy of ultrasonic measurement of the axial length of the eye. Ophthalmic Surg. 1981;12:363–5.

37. Seres A, Németh J, Süveges I. Unexpected ametropia after intraocular lens implantation: the role of different factors of ultrasound biometry and surgery. Doc Ophthalmol Proc Ser. 1997;61:415–20.

38. Drexler W, Findl O, Menapace R, et al. Partial coherence interferometry: a novel approach to biometry in cataract surgery [letter]. Am J Ophthalmol. 1998;126:524–34.

39. Kiss B, Findl O, Menapace R, et al. Refractive outcome of cataract surgery using partial coherence interferometry and ultrasound biometry. Clinical feasibility study of a commercial prototype II. J Cataract Refract Surg. 2002;28:230–4.

40. Zeng Y, Liu Y, Liu X, Chen C, Xia Y, Lu M, He M. Comparison of lens thickness measurements using the anterior segment optical coherence tomography and A-scan ultrasonography. Invest Ophthalmol Vis Sci. 2009;50(1):290–4.

41. Wegener A, Laser-Junga H. Photography of the anterior eye segment according to Scheimpflug's principle: options and limitations—a review. Clin Exp Ophthalmol. 2009;37:144–54.

42. Leibowitz HM, et al. Corneal disorders: clinical diagnosis and management. 2nd ed. Philadelphia: Saunders; 1998. p. 204–6.

43. Rapuano C, et al. Anterior Segment. St. Louis: Mosby, Inc.; 2000. p. 47–9.

44. Smolin G, et al. The cornea. 3rd ed. Little, Brown; 1994. p. 538–9.

45. Khng C, Osher RH. Evaluation of the relationship between corneal diameter and lens diameter. J Cataract Refract Surg. 2008;34:475–9.

46. Albert DM. Albert & Jakobiec's principles & practice of ophthalmology. 3rd ed. Philadelphia: Elsevier Inc.; 2008.

47. Arffa RC. Diseases of the cornea. 4th ed. St Louis: Mosby; 1997. p. 86.

48. Piñero DP, Plaza Puche AB, Alió JL. Corneal diameter measurements by corneal topography and angle-to-angle measurements by optical coherence tomography: evaluation of equivalence. J Cataract Refract Surg. 2008;34(1):126–31.

49. Kohnen T, Thomala MC, Cichocki M, Strenger A. Internal anterior chamber diameter using optical coherence tomography compared with white-to-white distances using automated measurements. J Cataract Refract Surg. 2006;32(11):1809–13.

50. Sabatino F, Findl O, Maurino V. Comparative analysis of optical biometers. J Cataract Refract Surg. 2016;42(5):685–93.

51. Hoffer KJ, Shammas HJ, Savini G. Comparison of 2 laser instruments for measuring axial length. J Cataract Refract Surg. 2010;36(4):644–8. https://doi.org/10.1016/j.jcrs.2009.11.007. Erratum in: J Cataract Refract Surg. 2010 Jun;36(6):1066.

52. Reddy AR, Pande MV, Finn P, El-Gogary H. Comparative estimation of anterior chamber depth by ultrasonography, Orbscan II, and IOLMaster. J Cataract Refract Surg. 2004;30(6):1268–71.

53. Lee JY, Kim JH, Kim HM, Song JS. Comparison of anterior chamber depth measurement between Orbscan IIz and ultrasound biomicroscopy. J Refract Surg. 2007;23(5):487–91.

54. Savini G, Carbonelli M, Sbreglia A, Barboni P, Deluigi G, Hoffer KJ. Comparison of anterior segment measurements by 3 Scheimpflug tomographers and 1 Placido corneal topographer. J Cataract Refract Surg. 2011;37(9):1679–85.

55. Aramberri J, Araiz L, Garcia A, Illarramendi I, Olmos J, Oyanarte I, Romay A, Vigara I. Dual versus single Scheimpflug camera for anterior segment analysis: precision and agreement. J Cataract Refract Surg. 2012;38(11):1934–49.

56. Domínguez-Vicent A, Monsálvez-Romín D, Aguila-Carrasco AJ, García-Lázaro S, Montés-Micó R. Measurements of anterior chamber depth, white-to-white distance, anterior chamber angle, and pupil diameter using two Scheimpflug imaging devices. Arq Bras Oftalmol. 2014;77(4):233–7.

57. Hsu M, Christiansen SM, Moshirfar M. Comparison of white-to-white horizontal corneal diameter and anterior chamber depth using the atlas, IOLMaster, Orbscan II, and Pentacam instruments. ARVO annual meeting abstract, Mar 2012.

58. Baikoff G, Jitsuo Jodai H, Bourgeon G. Measurement of the internal diameter and depth of the anterior chamber: IOLMaster versus anterior chamber optical coherence tomographer. J Cataract Refract Surg. 2005;31(9):1722–8.

59. Hoffer KJ, Hoffmann PC, Savini G. Comparison of a new optical biometer using swept-source optical coherence tomography and a biometer using optical low-coherence reflectometry. J Cataract Refract Surg. 2016;42(8):1165–72.

60. Shammas HJ, Ortiz S, Shammas MC, Kim SH, Chong C. Biometry measurements using a new large-coherence-length swept-source optical coherence tomographer. J Cataract Refract Surg. 2016;42(1):50–61.

61. Tañá-Rivero P, Aguilar-Córcoles S, Tello-Elordi C, Pastor-Pascual F, Montés-Micó R. Agreement between two swept-source OCT biometers and a Scheimpflug partial coherence interferometer. J Cataract Refract Surg. 2020;47:488.

62. Muniz Castro H, Tai AX, Sampson SJ, Wade M, Farid M, Garg S. Accuracy of intraocular lens power calculation using anterior chamber depth from two devices with Barrett universal II formula. J Ophthalmol. 2019;2019:8172615.

63. Savini G, Hoffer KJ, Schiano-Lomoriello D. Agreement between lens thickness measurements by ultrasound immersion biometry and optical biometry. J Cataract Refract Surg. 2018;44(12):1463–8.

64. Kurian M, Negalur N, Das S, Puttaiah NK, Haria D, Tejal SJ, Thakkar MM. Biometry with a new swept-source optical coherence tomography biometer: repeatability and agreement with an optical low-coherence reflectometry device. J Cataract Refract Surg. 2016;42(4):577–81.

65. Fişuş AD, Hirnschall ND, Findl O. Comparison of two swept-source optical coherence tomography-based biometry devices. J Cataract Refract Surg. 2021;47:87.

66. Dominguez-Vicent A, Pérez-Vives C, Ferrer-Blasco T, et al. Device interchangeability on anterior chamber depth and white-to-white measurements: a thorough literature review. Int J Ophthalmol. 2016;9:1057–65.

67. Salouti R, Nowroozzadeh MH, Zamani M, Ghoreyshi M, Khodaman AR. Comparison of horizontal corneal diameter measurements using the Orbscan IIz and Pentacam HR systems. Cornea. 2013;32(11):1460–4.

68. Huang J, McAlinden C, Huang Y, Wen D, Savini G, Tu R, Wang Q. Metaanalysis of optical low-coherence reflectometry versus partial coherence interferometry biometry. Sci Rep. 2017;7:43414. Available at: https://www.ncbi.nlm.nih.gov/pmc/articles/PMC5324074/pdf/srep43414.pdf. Accessed 18 Mar 2021.

69. Teshigawara T, Meguro A, Mizuki N. Influence of pupil dilation on the Barrett universal II (new generation), Haigis (4th generation), and SRK/T (3rd generation) intraocular lens calculation formulas: a retrospective study. BMC Ophthalmol. 2020;20:299.

70. Arriola-Villalobos P, et al. Effect of pharmacological pupil dilation on measurements and IOL power calculation made using the new swept-source optical coherence tomography-based optical biometer. J Fr Ophtalmol. 2016;39:859.

71. Wang X, Dong J, Tang M. Effect of pupil dilation on measurements and intraocular lens power calculations in schoolchildren. PLoS One. 2018;13(9):e0203677.

72. Bakbak B, Koktekir BE, Gedik S. The effect of pupil dilation on biometric parameters of the Lenstar 900. Cornea. 2013;32:e21–4.

73. Huang J, McAlinden C, Su B. The effect of cycloplegia on the Lenstar and the IOLMaster biometry. Optom Vis Sci. 2012;89:1691–6.

74. Ferreira TB, Hoffer KJ, Ribeiro F, Ribeiro P, O'Neill JG. Ocular biometric measurements in cataract surgery candidates in Portugal. PLoS One. 2017;12(10):e0184837.

75. Wong TY, Foster PJ, Ng TP, Tielsch JM, Johnson GJ, Seah SK. Variations in ocular biometry in an adult Chinese population in Singapore: the Tanjong Pagar survey. Invest Ophthalmol Vis Sci. 2001;42:73–80.

76. Lege BA, Haigis W. Laser interference biometry versus ultrasound biometry in certain clinical conditions. Graefes Arch Clin Exp Ophthalmol. 2004;242:8–12.

77. Cao X, Hou X, Bao Y. The ocular biometry of adult cataract patients on lifeline express hospital eye train in rural China. J Ophthalmol. 2015;2015(5):171564.

78. Jivrajka R, Shammas MC, Boenzi T, Swearingen M, Shammas HJ. Variability of axial length, anterior chamber depth, and lens thickness in the cataractous eye. J Cataract Refract Surg. 2008;34:289–94.

79. Lee KE, Klein BK, Klein R, Quandt Z, Wong TY. Age, stature, and education associations with ocular dimensions in an older white population. Arch Ophthalmol. 2009;127:88–93.

80. Hoffer KJ. Axial dimension of the human cataractous lens. Arch Ophthalmol. 1993;111(7):914–8. Erratum 1993;111(12):1626.

81. Hoffmann PC, Hutz WW. Analysis of biometry and prevalence data for corneal astigmatism in 23,239 eyes. J Cataract Refract Surg. 2010;36(9):1479–85.

82. Ning X, Yang Y, Yan H, et al. Anterior chamber depth—a predictor of refractive outcomes after age-related cataract surgery. BMC Ophthalmol. 2019;19:134.

83. Gökce SE, Montes De Oca I, Cooke DL, Wang L, Koch DD, Al-Mohtaseb Z. Accuracy of 8 intraocular lens calculation formulas in relation to anterior chamber depth in patients with normal axial lengths. J Cataract Refract Surg. 2018;44:362–8.

84. Jeong J, Song H, Lee JK, Chuck RS, Kwon JW. The effect of ocular biometric factors on the accuracy of various IOL power calculation formulas. BMC Ophthalmol. 2017;17:62.

85. Yang S, Whang WJ, Joo CK. Effect of anterior chamber depth on the choice of intraocular lens calculation formula. PLoS One. 2017;12:e0189868.

86. Vega Y, Gershoni A, Achiron A, et al. High agreement between Barrett universal II calculations with and without utilization of optional biometry parameters. J Clin Med. 2021;10(3):542.

87. Jeong J, Song H, Lee JK, et al. The effect of ocular biometric factors on the accuracy of various IOL power calculation formulas. BMC Ophthalmol. 2017;17:62.

88. Hipólito-Fernandes D, Luís ME, Serras-Pereira R, Gil P, Maduro V, Feijão J, Alves N. Anterior chamber depth, lens thickness and intraocular lens calculation formula accuracy: nine formulas comparison. Br J Ophthalmol. 2020;106:349.

89. Fernández J, Rodríguez-Vallejo M, Poyales F, Burguera N, Garzón N. New method to assess the accuracy of intraocular lens power calculation formulas according to ocular biometric parameters. J Cataract Refract Surg. 2020;46(6):849–56.

90. Shrivastava AK, Behera P, Kacher R, Kumar B. Effect of anterior chamber depth on predictive accuracy of seven intraocular lens formulas in eyes with axial length less than 22 mm. Clin Ophthalmol. 2019;13:1579–86.

91. Weekers R, Delmarcelle Y, Luyckx J. Biometrics of the crystalline lens. In: Bellows JG, editor. Cataract and abnormalities of the lens. New York: Grune & Stratton; 1975. p. 134–47.

92. Farnsworth PN, Shyne SE. Anterior zonular shifts with age. Exp Eye Res. 1979;28(3):291–7.

93. Cook CA, Koretz JF, Pfahnl A, Hyun J, Kaufman PL. Aging of the human crystalline lens and anterior segment. Vis Res. 1994;34(22):2945–54.

94. Kim SY, Lee SH, Kim NR, Chin HS, Jung JW. Accuracy of intraocular lens power calculation formulas using a swept-source optical biometer. PLoS One. 2020;15(1):e0227638.

95. Eom Y, Song JS, Kim YY, Kim HM. Comparison of SRK/T and Haigis formulas for predicting corneal astigmatism correction with toric intraocular lenses. J Cataract Refract Surg. 2015;41:1650–7.

96. Symes RJ, Ursell PG. Automated keratometry in routine cataract surgery: comparison of Scheimpflug and conventional values. J Cataract Refract Surg. 2011;37(2):295–301.

97. http://acrysoftoriccalculator.com. Accessed 12 Jul 2018.

98. Savini G, Hoffer KJ, Ducoli P. A new slant on toric intraocular lens power calculation. J Refract Surg. 2013;29(5):348–54.

99. Savini G, Hoffer KJ, Carbonelli M, Ducoli P, Barboni P. Influence of axial length and corneal power on the astigmatic power of toric intraocular lenses. J Cataract Refract Surg. 2013;39:1900–3.

100. Savini G, Naeser K. An analysis of the factors influencing the residual refractive astigmatism after cataract surgery with toric intraocular lenses. Invest Ophthalmol Vis Sci. 2015;56:827–35.

101. Goggin M, Moore S, Easterman A. Outcome of toric intraocular lens implantation after adjusting for anterior chamber depth and intraocular lens sphere equivalent power effects. Arch Ophthalmol. 2011;129:998–1003; correction, 1494.

102. Fam HB, Lim KL. Meridional analysis for calculating the expected spherocylindrical refraction in eyes with toric intraocular lenses. J Cataract Refract Surg. 2007;33:2072–6.

103. Ribeiro F, Prata M, Mendanha DJ. Position measurement to improve refractive outcomes in cataract surgery. Adv Ophthalmol Vis Syst. 2016;4(3):84–5.

104. Goto S, Maeda N, Koh S, Ohnuma K, Hayashi K, Iehisa I, Noda T, Nishida K. Prediction of postoperative intraocular lens position with angle-to-angle depth using anterior segment optical coherence tomography. Ophthalmology. 2016;123(11):2474–80.

105. Martinez-Enriquez E, Pérez-Merino P, Durán-Poveda S, et al. Estimation of intraocular lens position from full crystalline lens geometry: toward a new generation of intraocular lens power calculation formulas. Sci Rep. 2018;8:9829.

106. Satou T, Shimizu K, Tsunehiro S, et al. Development of a new intraocular lens power calculation method based on lens position estimated with optical coherence tomography. Sci Rep. 2020;10:6501.

107. Li T, Yang K, Stein JD, Nallasamy N. Gradient boosting decision tree algorithm for the prediction of postoperative intraocular lens position in cataract surgery. Transl Vis Sci Technol. 2020;9(13):38.

108. Li T, Stein JD, Nallasamy N. AI-powered effective lens position prediction improves the accuracy of existing lens formulas. medRxiv. 2020; https://doi.org/10.1101/2020.10.29.20222539.

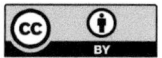

Keratometry

14

Thomas Olsen

Keratometry

What is the corneal power? Most clinicians will ask for the "K-reading" neglecting the fact that the keratometer does not measure the power directly. What is measured is the size of the Purkinje I image reflected from the front surface of the cornea in a para-central ring of 3 mm or so and from this the radius of curvature is calculated [1].

The measurement of corneal curvature is among the oldest disciplines in ocular biometry. Since the front corneal surface acts as a convex mirror, it is a straightforward task to measure the curvature by measuring the magnification of that mirror. This is the principle of all Placido-based keratometers and topographers. We will have a detailed look at the conditions for this measurement.

The dioptric power of a reflecting convex mirror is given by

$$F_m = -\frac{2n}{r} \qquad (14.1)$$

where F_m is reflective power of mirror (corneal surface) in diopters and r is radius of curvature in meters. For example, if $r = 7.8$ mm and $n = 1$ (air), then F_m becomes −260 D. This corresponds to a focal length of about −3.9 mm (=1/−260). In

other words, a distant object (e.g., the mires of the keratometer) will be focused 3.9 mm behind the cornea. Since the magnification is inversely related to power (or directly proportional to curvature), one can get a curvature measurement from the magnification of the mires observed in the reflection by the corneal surface.

The size of the object reflected by the cornea determines the effective area of the cornea to be measured. A large object means a larger zone to be examined and vice versa. There is a trade-off here as decreasing the diameter will increase the measurement error. Standard keratometers often use bright ring objects to be reflected in a 3 mm dimeter ring on the cornea. It is important to note that in this way keratometry does not measure the very central power of the cornea. To get the full picture of the cornea, it is often better to use Placido keratoscopy or topography by which the entire area of optical interest can be examined (Fig. 14.1).

One may ask why we do not use topography as the standard rather than keratometry which only gives the radius in a small area? The reading of the keratometer is however often more accurate than the topographer because of automated alignment control and other measures to ensure a consistent reading. It is also a good idea regularly to check the reading against calibrated steel balls or other spheres with a known curvature.

T. Olsen (✉)
Aros Private Hospital, Aarhus N, Denmark

© The Author(s) 2024
J. Aramberri et al. (eds.), *Intraocular Lens Calculations*, Essentials in Ophthalmology,
https://doi.org/10.1007/978-3-031-50666-6_14

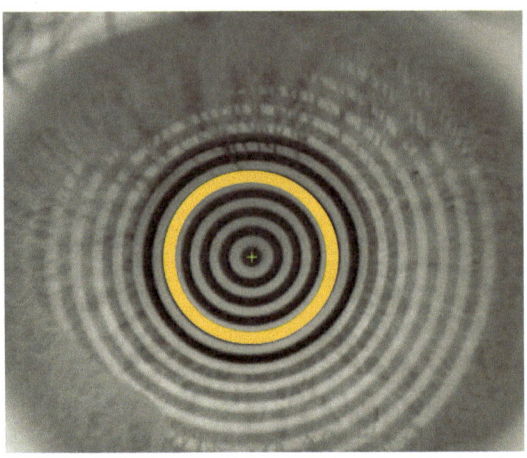

Fig. 14.1 Photokeratoscopy of the normal cornea. The standard keratometer measures the image size in the standard 3 mm ring zone (ring insert)

Instrumentation

The world's first keratometer was built by Herman Helmholtz in 1854, just a couple of years after he invented the ophthalmoscope. The optical principle of the Helmholtz keratometer was very advanced and allowed high precision measurements to be taken that was independent of the distance between the patient's eye and that of the observer. The optical principle was later implemented in the "ophthalmometer" manufactured by the Zeiss company in 1950—about 100 years after Helmholtz disclosed his principle. A clever arrangement was the use of image doubling through plane-parallel plates (compensating for eye movements) so that the observer would have to superimpose two images projected to infinity by adjusting a beam splitter that would eventually translate into radius of curvature.

Later in the eighteenth century, Émile Javal and Hjalmar Schiötz designed a keratometer that gained widespread use because of its simplicity. Rather than doubling the image, the Javal instrument doubles the object and the task of the observer is to move the distance between the two mire objects so that they will align through the eyepiece. The Bausch & Lomb keratometer produced from 1932 onwards was also based on this concept. The Javal type instrument was mainly meant to measure astigmatism and was less accurate that the Helmholtz model because the measuring result depends on the distance between the patient's eye and the instrument.

Modern keratometers have shifted from manual to automated principles using LED (mostly infrared) as test mires and CCD to capture the image. The sensitivity of modern CCDs is so high that the exposure time can be kept sufficiently low so that the effect of eye movements is minimized. For the same reason, there is no need for image doubling and many mechanical features have been replaced by electronic processing and image analysis.

At the time of development of the early keratometers, the clinical interest was focused on astigmatism measurement and contact lens fitting. Little interest was given to the exact translation of radius into dioptric power. Of course, this is the most important subject of IOL power calculation for which accuracy is the top priority.

A detailed description of modern instrumentation is beyond the scope of this chapter.

The Calculation of Power from Curvature

The refractive power of a single spherical surface is given by

$$F = \frac{n_2 - n_1}{r} \qquad (14.2)$$

where F is refractive power of the surface, n_1 and n_2 are the refractive indices of the first and second medium, respectively, and r is radius of curvature in meters. For example (front surface of the cornea), if $r = 7.7$ mm, $n_1 = 1$ (air), $n_2 = 1.376$ (cornea), then F becomes +48.83 D. For example (back surface of the cornea), if $r = 6.8$ mm, $n_1 = 1.336$ (aqueous), $n_2 = 1.376$ (cornea), then F becomes −5.88 D.

Now, the cornea is not a single surface but rather two surfaces that combine to produce the total refraction (Fig. 14.2). The paraxial, refractive power of two spherical surfaces in combination is given by

Fig. 14.2 The refraction of the cornea occurs at the front and back surface

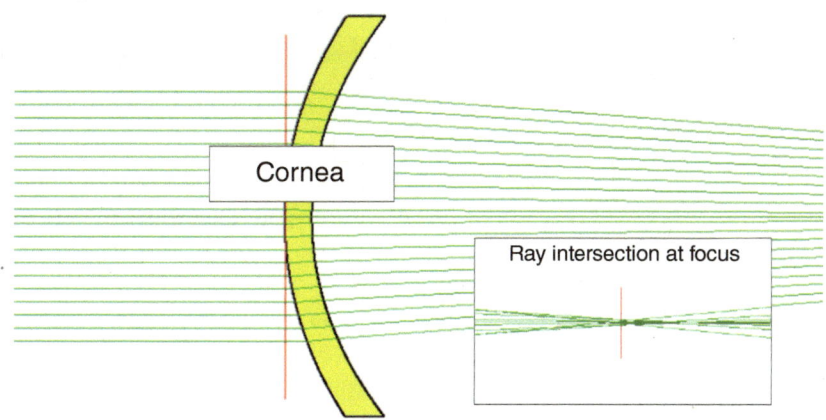

Cornea

Ray intersection at focus

$$F_{12} = F_1 + F_2 - \frac{D}{n} * F_1 * F_2 \qquad (14.3)$$

where F_{12} is total refractive power of the two surfaces, F_1 and F_2 are refractive power of the first and second surface, respectively, D is distance between the two surfaces, and n is refractive index between the two surfaces. Equation (14.3) is also called the paraxial formula for the combination of two surfaces or the "thick-lens equation."

The dark horse is the curvature of the posterior surface of the cornea, which is not directly visible from the outside. So, for anterior keratometry to give a meaningful diopter reading for the whole cornea, certain assumptions need to be made.

One such assumption might be to use a schematic eye as a model for the ratio between the front and back surface of the cornea. The front and back corneal curvature of the Gullstrand exact schematic eye are 7.7 and 6.8 mm, respectively, giving a "Gullstrand ratio" between front and back curvature of 6.8/7.7 = 0.883. (Modern Scheimpflug and OCT techniques tend to give a slightly lower values—typically 0.83 or 0.84—but we will come back to that later.) If we assume a Gullstrand ratio of 0.883, then it is a straightforward calculation to calculate the total refractive power of the standard cornea (0.5 mm thick) as

$$F_{12} = 48.83 - 5.88 + \frac{0.0005}{1.376} * 48.8 * 5.9 = 43.05\,\text{D} \qquad (14.4)$$

Now, if we want this value to be read directly from the anterior curvature, we can try and simulate what the assumed index of refraction should be using the single surface model (Eq. 14.2). Thus, if we substitute the power and curvature and solve for the assumed refractive index of the cornea, we get:

$$43.05 = \frac{n-1}{7.7} \geq n = 43.05 * 7.7 + 1 = 1.3315$$
$$(14.5)$$

Note that this value is lower from the value of 1.3375 used by standard keratometry. The difference amounts to about 0.8 D higher reading of the standard keratometer as compared to the Gullstrand cornea!

Why has index 1.3375 become the standard? The reason seems to be from early days of instrument making where the exact corneal power was of less clinical interest than the astigmatism which can be found as the difference between the flat and the steep meridian. For practical purposes, the value of 1.3375 means that a corneal curvature of 7.5 mm would give a reading of 45 D so it was easy to check the calibration of the instrument. In 1909, Gullstrand wrote *Diese Zahl wurde aus technischen Gründe gewählt, damit 45 Dptr einem Radius von 7.5 mm entsprechen zollte* [2]. ("This number was chosen for technical reasons, so that 45 D corresponded to a radius of 7.5 mm.")

For realistic IOL power calculation, it is very important that the power of the cornea is correct. If we start the process by making an error of 1.0 D, we will have to correct it at the end to avoid off-set errors.

Asphericity and Ray Tracing

The above considerations are valid in the paraxial domain with the fundamental assumption that all angles "i" are so small that $\sin(i) = i$. As we move away from the central axis, this assumption is no longer valid; therefore, paraxial imagery cannot be used to describe the effective refraction that includes higher order aberrations like spherical aberrations.

The cornea is not a spherical surface but rather an ellipsoid that tends to flatten at the periphery thereby decreasing the spherical aberration, but not all of it. Many studies have been published on the spherical aberration of the cornea, and many modern clinical Scheimpflug or OCT instruments offer comprehensive analysis of the higher order aberrations, including the spherical aberrations. To demonstrate the effect of the corneal asphericity, the author uses the values obtained by Dubbelman [3] for the normal cornea (Table 14.1).

The asphericity has some implications for the measurements of corneal curvature. As mentioned above, the standard keratometer is actually blind to the very center of the cornea—which is the steepest—but uses a ring zone of about 3 mm (often called the SimK) depending on the device. The 3 mm diameter of the cornea corresponds to about 11–12° of the cornea, assuming a normal curvature of 7.7 mm.

A relevant question is how much error the 3 mm zone reading deviates from the central zone? For this study, we can model the corneal shape as a conic section and use the abundance of

Table 14.1 Dubbelman model for corneal asphericity

Dubbelman cornea model	Apical radius (mm)	Q-value
Cornea front	7.70	−0.18
Cornea back	6.48	−0.38

mathematical methods to describe conical sections. Baker (1943) [4] described a simple formula that is useful for ray tracing:

$$y^2 = 2rx - px^2 \quad (14.6)$$

where x and y are the coordinates of the conic surface with origin in (0, 0), r = apical radius and p is a constant describing the shape. For $0 < p < 1$, the shape is a prolate. Another term commonly used is the Q-value defined as $Q = p - 1$. Typical values for the front corneal surface range from −0.2 to −0.4 which means the shape of the cornea is a prolate.

Now, assuming an apical radius of 7.7 mm and a Q-value of −0.18, we can calculate what the sagittal radius of the cornea—the one that is measured by the keratometer—will be as a function of displacement from the axis (Fig. 14.3). From this graph, the keratometer reading of a standard 3 mm diameter (green rectangle) would give a 7.72 mm radius as compared to 7.70 at the apex. This corresponds to a 0.12 D difference. Of course, this difference may be higher when the cornea is abnormal, i.e., with a post-LASIK or a keratoconus cornea.

This asphericity reduces the spherical aberration, but not all of it. Depending on the contribution from the lens, the total optics of the eye typically shows some spherical aberration which is dependent on the pupil size. This is responsible for the night myopia found in many individuals.

What does the asphericity of the cornea mean for the effective power of the cornea? This can be studied by exact ray tracing that does not have the limitations of paraxial imagery. The only assumption of exact ray tracing is Snell's law:

$$\frac{\sin\theta_1}{\sin\theta_2} = \frac{n_2}{n_1} \quad (14.7)$$

where n_1 and n_2 are the refractive indices of medium 1 and 2, respectively, and θ_1 and θ_2 are the incident angles in medium 1 and the outgoing angle in medium 2, respectively.

In the following ray tracing experiments, we again assume the cornea model of Dubbelman with a conic coefficient of the cornea of −0.18 and −0.38 for the anterior and posterior surface, respectively (Table 14.1). Assuming an

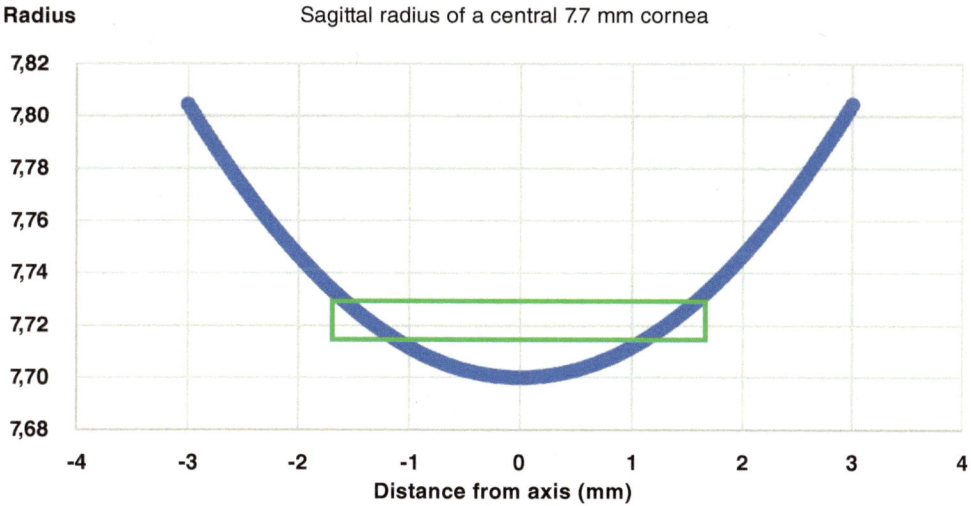

Fig. 14.3 Sagittal radius of cornea as a function of distance from axis. The rectangle insert illustrates the keratometer area of measurement

anterior apical radius of 7.70 mm and a posterior radius of 6.47 mm (Dubbelman's mean value) and a thickness of 0.5 mm, we trace a high number of rays through the cornea (Fig. 14.4) and look for the focus, which may be defined as the point on the axis having the least spread or the highest point spread function (PSF) (Fig. 14.5). Once the focal distance "d" has been found, we can then calculate the corresponding power as $F = n/d$ where n is the refractive index of aqueous (1.336).

To study the effect of pupil size, experiments were made with pupil sizes varying between 0 and 6 mm. As expected, the effective power of the cornea was found to increase with larger pupil diameter. The spherical aberration can be found as the difference between the central power and the power at the larger pupil. For normal pupil size (3 mm), the spherical aberration is within 0.25 D. To reach more than 0.5 D, the pupil size should be more than 5 mm.

All of the above concerns the normal cornea and ways to predict the effective corneal power. To study the effect of varying degrees of asphericity, we may conduct experiments varying the Q-values of the cornea around the normal value (Fig. 14.6). As can be seen in the figure, the spherical aberration is linearly correlated with the Q-value of both surfaces. However, the posterior cornea has a much lower influence.

As can be seen, the effective corneal power is very much influenced by the shape of the cornea. Simply taking a K-reading is only part of the story. We must consider the total area of refraction and most preferably use ray tracing, nomograms or other techniques to get the effective corneal power to be used in the IOL power calculation.

According to the author's own experience using Scheimpflug photography (Oculus Pentacam HR), the normal Q-values range from −0.80 to +0.65 (mean value −0.05 with a standard deviation of 0.23) and from −0.90 to +0.85 (mean value −0.34 with a standard deviation of 0.21) of the front and back corneal surfaces, respectively. For comparison, post-myopic LASIK corneas may have higher Q-values (higher spherical aberration) of the front surface, ranging from −1.00 to +3.1 (mean value of 0.60 with a standard deviation of 0.80, illustrating the larger spread) and mean value −0.24 ranging from −0.90 to +0.40 (mean value −0.24 with a standard deviation of 0.22) of the back corneal surface.

An advantage of exact ray tracing is that it is possible to study the image quality by means of

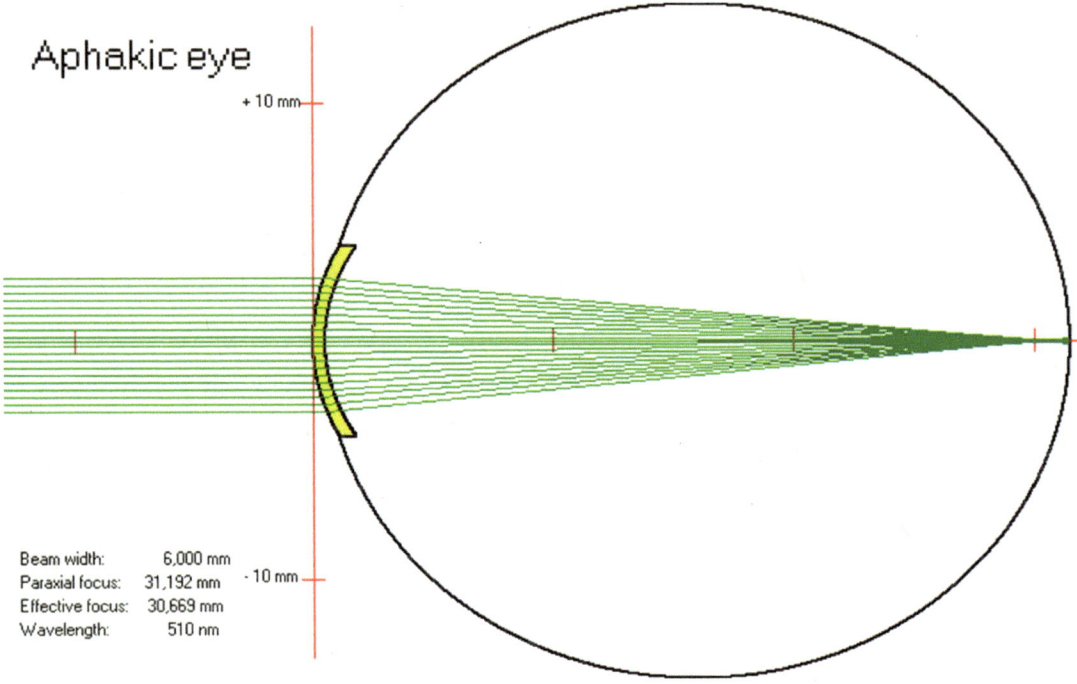

Fig. 14.4 Exact ray tracing of the cornea, simulated by a long, aphakic eye

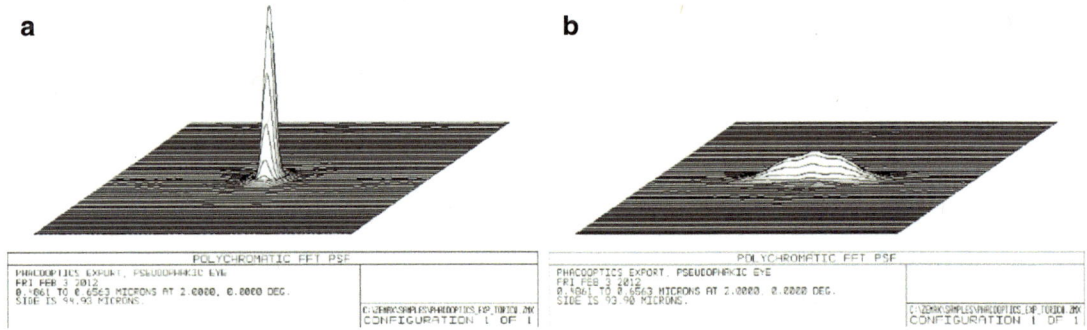

Fig. 14.5 Point spread function showing a good (**a**) and a bad (**b**) focus

the blur or point spread function observed at the focus. The blurring can be quantitated as the root-mean-square (RMS) of the ray intersections with the image plane around the axis. Figure 14.7 shows the RMS as a function of varying the front and back Q-values around the mean.

As can be seen from Fig. 14.7, the best image is found at zero spherical aberration which is found for a front corneal Q-value around −0.5.

As the value for the normal cornea is around −0.18, we see that there is room for improvement. The clinical tools to reduce spherical aberration of the IOL eye include: (1) altering the cornea profile toward more asphericity and (2) implant an aspheric IOL with a proper wavefront correction of the spherical aberration. It should be remembered; however, that an ultra-sharp, aberration-free focus comes at the expense of depth of focus.

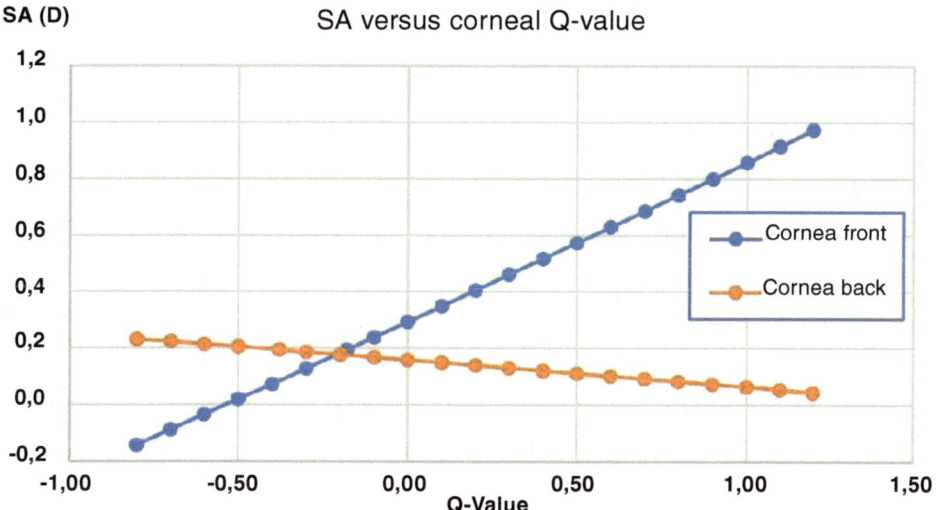

Fig. 14.6 The spherical aberration of the cornea is directly proportional to the Q-value of the front cornea. The posterior cornea has a much lower influence

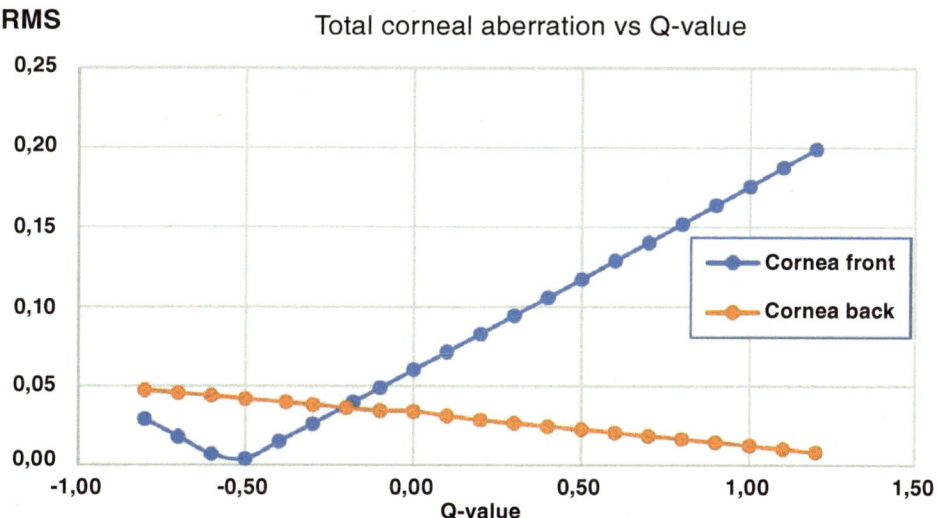

Fig. 14.7 Total corneal aberration as a function of front and back Q-value of the cornea

Clinical Studies Using Scheimpflug Data

As mentioned, exact ray tracing is an established technique often used in optical engineering to examine optical properties of any physical object. The advantage of the technique is that it does not use any assumptions on the shape of the surface if the surface is completely described in physical terms.

With the advent of modern scanning techniques (Scheimpflug, OCT) that measure both surfaces of the cornea in multiple points, we have an opportunity to study the optics of the cornea by exact ray tracing, which has obvious advantages over more assumptive methods. In the following, an example is shown of the steps involved in the calculation of the corneal power by ray tracing from raw matrix elevation data and how this compares with conventional methods [5].

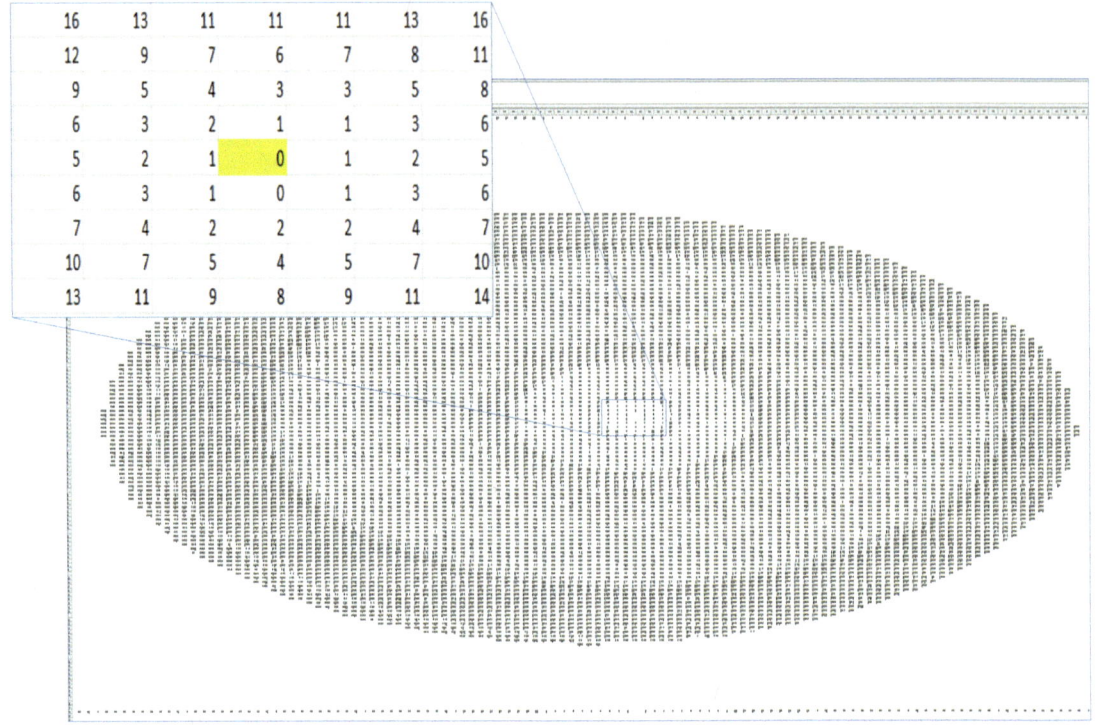

16	13	11	11	11	13	16
12	9	7	6	7	8	11
9	5	4	3	3	5	8
6	3	2	1	1	3	6
5	2	1	0	1	2	5
6	3	1	0	1	3	6
7	4	2	2	2	4	7
10	7	5	4	5	7	10
13	11	9	8	9	11	14

Fig. 14.8 A 3D matrix of mapped corneal data exported by the Oculus Pentacam HR ©. The Pentacam captures the height data in a (*xy*) matrix of a maximum of 140 × 140 points of 0.1 mm interval. The insert shows the height (elevation) of the individual points in μm. The apex has an elevation of 0 μm (yellow point)

An example of the dataset exported by the Oculus Pentacam HR is shown in Fig. 14.8. The elevation data can be used to create a physical meshwork of individual points by a process called triangulation (Figs. 14.9 and 14.10). In this way, the cornea surface is represented by a continuous surface of minute triangles, which can be used by the ray tracing software.

An example of optical engineering software is the Zemax® program which has been used by the author to import the 3D triangulated dataset and analyze for refraction by ray tracing. A pupil can be inserted, and the effective focal length can be analyzed from a high number of rays refracted through the system. The focal distance is found as the point where the rays form the least blur and the highest point spread function (PSF) (Fig. 14.11). The effective power of the cornea is then found as the reciprocal of the effective focal distance.

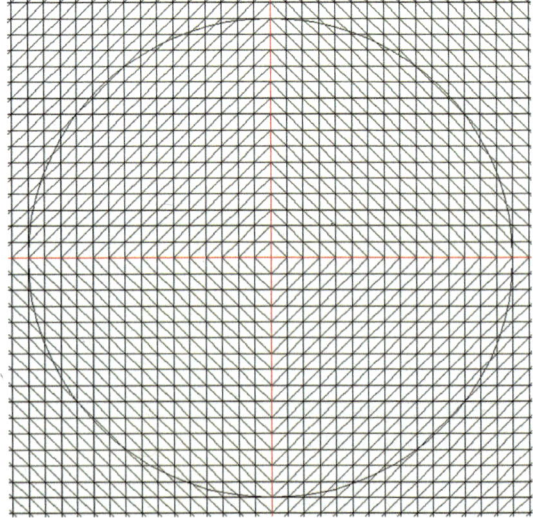

Fig. 14.9 This diagram is a front view of the triangulation around the vertex (0, 0). Each grid intersection represents a measurement point of a certain elevation in the Z-axis. The circle represents the pupil at a width of 3 mm

Fig. 14.10 Ray tracing through anterior and posterior cornea based on 3D elevation data exported by the Pentacam

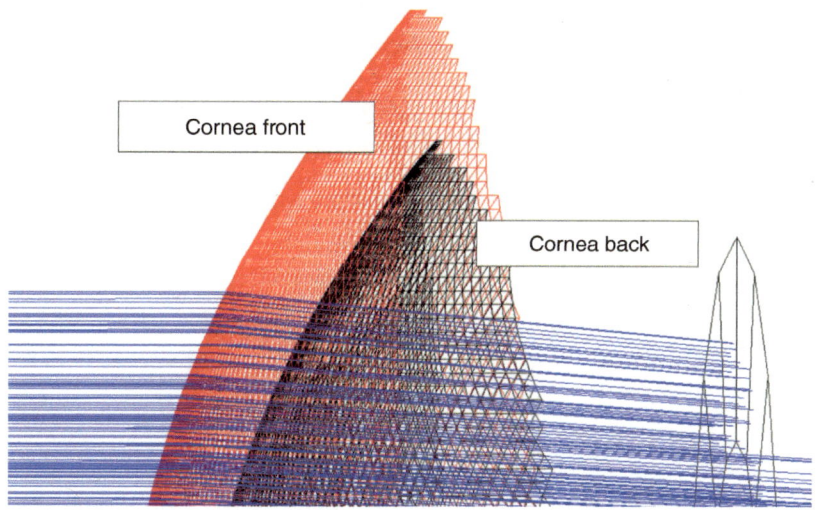

Fig. 14.11 The focal distance is found as the point where the rays form the least blur and the highest point spread function (PSF)

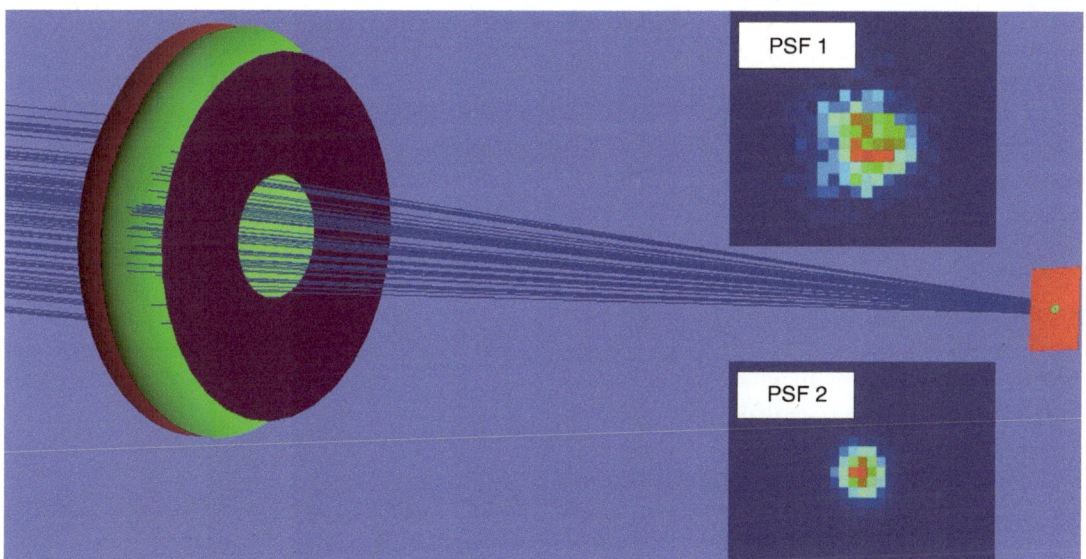

Table 14.2 shows the ray traced corneal power at different pupil sizes as compared to the Pentacam-derived True Net Power (TNP) and Total Corneal Refractive Power (TCRP) as well as the standard reading of the keratometer. The ray-traced corneal power is seen to increase as the pupil increases because of spherical aberration. The TNP gives the lowest value as this

value is calculated from the apical curvatures of the front and back surfaces of the cornea (paraxial domain) without the effect of the corneal asphericity. The standard K-reading is about 1 D higher than the ray-traced corneal power at 3 mm pupil.

You may ask the question: If keratometer index 1.3375 is bad, what is the best index

Table 14.2 Results of varying the pupil size on the estimated corneal power from ray tracing analysis of 20 normal subjects. The Pentacam variables "TNP" ("True Net Power," based on thick-lens calculation of the corneal power by the Pentacam software) and "TCRP" ("Total Corneal Refractive Power" based on an exact ray tracing algorithm)

	Zemax-derived corneal power (D)/pupil size			Pentacam variables (D)		Keratometer (D)
$N = 20$	3 mm	4 mm	5 mm	TNP	TCRP	"K-reading"
Mean (± SD)	42.34 (±1.33)	42.52 (±1.38)	42.64 (±1.41)	41.91 (±1.29)	42.38 (±1.28)	43.36 (±1.53)
Range	39.79–44.69	39.86–45.19	39.96–46.46	39.50–43.65	39.90–44.05	40.74–45.95

Table 14.3 Equivalent keratometer index that gives the same corneal power as the ray-traced value

Keratometric index (single surface equivalent)	Pupil 3 mm	Pupil 4 mm	Pupil 5 mm
Mean (±SD)	1.3207 (±0.0037)	1.3310 (±0.0041)	1.3320 (±0.0043)
Range	1.3165–1.3329	1.3165–1.3378	1.3170–1.3403

based on the ray tracing experiments? This value can be back-calculated in each case solving for the single-surface index giving the observed ray-traced corneal power. The results are shown in Table 14.3. As can be seen, the fictitious index for a 3 mm pupil was 1.3207 on average with a range from 1.3165 to 1.3329. The range actually includes the Gullstrand-derived value of 1.3315 as proposed by Olsen many years ago (see section "The Refractive Power of the Cornea" above). In other words, if one uses the Gullstrand ratio of 0.88 rather than the Scheimpflug-derived value of 0.83–0.84, then the corneal power includes the spherical aberration and may be regarded as the effective corneal power.

Figure 14.12 shows the comparison of K-reading, Pentacam Total Net Power (TNP) and Total Corneal Refractive Power (TCRP) versus the ray-traced corneal power assuming a 3 mm pupil in a large series of normal cataractous case ($n = 443$). The conventional K-reading gives the highest and the TNP the lowest value. There is remarkable good agreement between the TCRP and the ray-traced corneal power (regression coefficient 1.00 with no significant off-set and correlation coefficient $r = 0.99$).

Notes on the Stiles–Crawford Effect

These ray tracing calculations are valid from a purely optical point of view. However, the retina does not act like a simple screen. For many years, it has been known that the sensitivity of the retina is dependent on the incident angle of light on the retina. This directional sensitivity of the retina was discovered by Stiles and Crawford in 1933 [6] as a discrepancy between the objective and the effective area of the pupil in terms of luminous effectivity. The phenomenon predicts rays off axis to be less effective than central (paraxial) rays as a perceptive stimulus. The Stiles–Crawford equation is:

$$I = I_0 * e^{-0.108*y^2} \tag{14.8}$$

where I is stimulus efficacy of peripheral ray, I_0 efficacy of axial ray, y is distance of peripheral ray from axis. To correct for the Stiles–Crawford effect, we therefore put a weight on each ray according to this formula and solve for the best focus as described by Olsen in 1993 [7]. The result appears as the lower curve in Fig. 14.13. The Stiles–Crawford effect is insignificant in the normal area (pupil less than 4 mm). For a large pupil (8 mm), the effect amount to about 0.3 D less corneal power than predicted by optics alone.

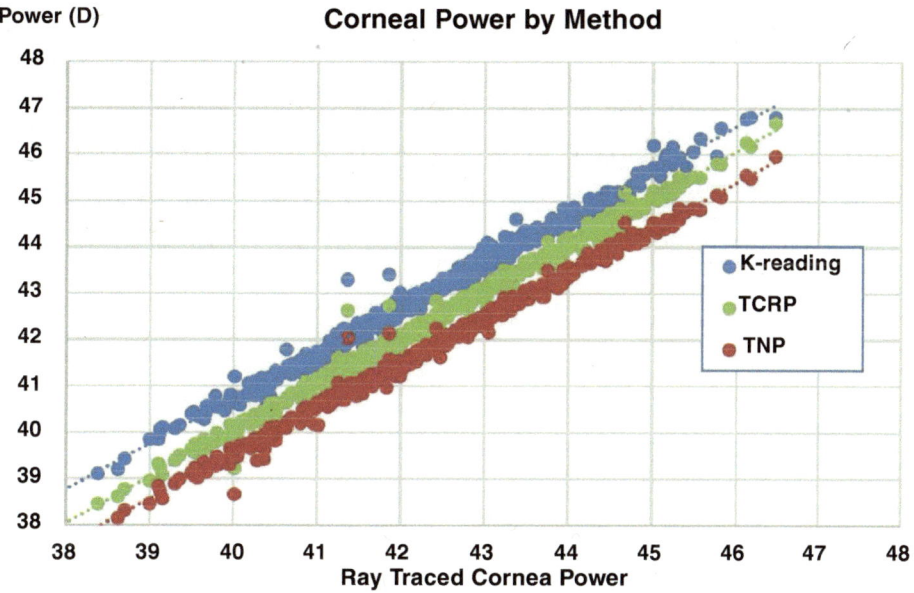

Fig. 14.12 The corneal power found by K-reading, Pentacam TNP, and TCRP versus the ray-traced power based on mapped elevation data assuming a 3 mm pupil ($n = 443$ normal cases)

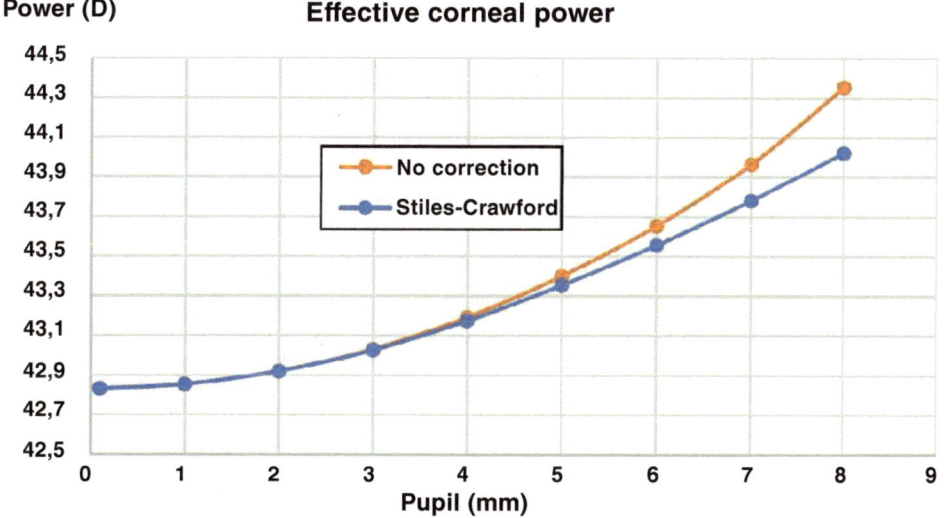

Fig. 14.13 The effective corneal power as a function of pupil size

References

1. Bennett AG, Rabbetts RB. What radius does the conventional keratometer measure? Ophthal Physiol Opt. 1991;11(3):239–47.
2. Gullstrand A. Einführung in die Methoden der Dioptrik des Auges des Menschen. In: Helmholtz H, editor. Handbuch der physiologischen Optik des Auges. Leipzig: Verlag von S. Hirzel; 1911. p. 152.
3. Dubbelman M, Weeber HA, van der Heijde RG, Volker-Dieben HJ. Radius and asphericity of the posterior corneal surface determined by corrected Scheimpflug photography. Acta Ophthalmol Scand. 2002;80:379–83.
4. Baker TY. Ray tracing through non-spherical surfaces. Proc Phys Soc. 1943;55:361–4.
5. Olsen T, Jeppesen P. Ray-tracing analysis of the corneal power from Scheimpflug data. J Refract Surg. 2018;34(1):45–50.
6. Stiles WS, Crawford BH. The luminous effectivity of rays entering the eye pupil at different points. Proc R Soc Lond. 1933;112:428–50.
7. Olsen T. On the Stiles-Crawford effect on ocular imagery. Acta Ophthalmol Scand. 1993;71:85–8.

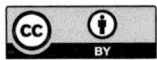

Corneal Topography and Tomography

15

Jaime Aramberri

Introduction

Corneal optics determines the optical performance of the eye. The present day intraocular lens (IOL) technologies and the high expectations of cataract and refractive lensectomy patients demand an exhaustive preoperative analysis of corneal shape and optics with latest generation tomographers. In this way, corneal optics can be evaluated further beyond simple keratometry; any irregularity described in terms of aberrometry, the possibility of later laser refractive treatments ascertained, and other subtle problems that could affect visual function can be detected. This diagnostic method has become by its own right the cornerstone of IOL selection in lens surgery.

There has been a significant evolution from Placido topographers, where only the anterior corneal surface is analyzed, to elevation tomographers that can also measure corneal thickness and the posterior surface rendering a total corneal assessment. The early devices were based on scanning-slit technology, then on Scheimpflug imaging, and more recently on optical coherence tomography (OCT). At present, corneal tomography is a powerful tool that provides essential information about the cornea in order to help select the type of IOL, calculate its power and toricity accurately, and estimate the final visual quality. This helps the surgeon to maintain a tight control of the process.

Technologies

Reflection Topography

This method studies the shape of the anterior corneal surface from the analysis of the size of the image of a test mire pattern projected from a known distance. Nearly all commercial devices use a pattern composed of alternating black and white rings called a Placido disk [1] (Fig. 15.1a). Some instruments use color rings to improve the identification of boundaries which can be useful in case of irregular corneas where there might be edge overlapping. The Cassini®, Ioptics, topographer uses a multiple dot color pattern instead of concentric rings [2] (Fig. 15.1b).

Placido mires are normally non-planarly arranged, inside a rotationally symmetric aspherical surface to achieve a wide-angle ring projection and to obtain an image reflected onto one plane so that the central CCD camera gets a sharp image. Instruments can be classified as small-target (cone topographer) and large-tar-

J. Aramberri (✉)
Clínica Miranza BEGITEK, San Sebastián, Spain

Clínica ÓKULAR, Vitoria, Spain

J. Aramberri et al. (eds.), *Intraocular Lens Calculations*, Essentials in Ophthalmology,
https://doi.org/10.1007/978-3-031-50666-6_15

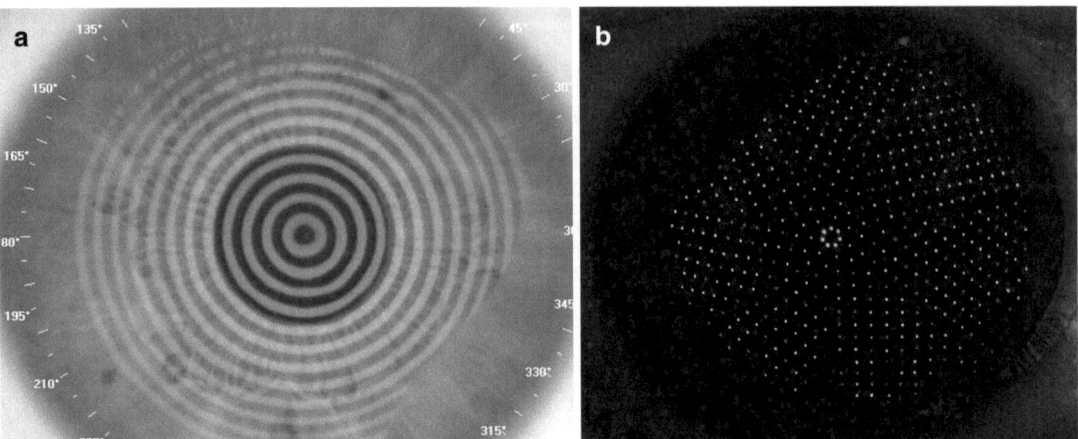

Fig. 15.1 Reflection topography test mires. (**a**) Placido rings and (**b**) Cassini color dot pattern

get (disk topographer). In the former, the ring pattern is arranged in a small highly curved surface and the projecting distance is small, while in the latter the projecting surface has smaller curvature and the working distance is longer [3]. These configurations allow covering a wide field of cornea, 8–10 mm, and measuring around 6000–15,000 points depending on the instrument. In IOL power calculation, the area of interest is the central, so-called optical cornea.

The image is captured by a digital camera in a short period of time and first processed by ring boundaries identification. The software reconstructs the corneal shape with a proprietary algorithm. The accuracy and precision of each device will depend on this hardware–software combination. Most topographers use arc-step algorithms that trace arcs sequentially, dot by dot, from the corneal vertex to the periphery. They have been proven to be more accurate in height and instantaneous curvature calculation than old algorithms that assumed a spherical geometry, with less than 0.25 μ error in the central 3 mm [4].

In reflection topography, a small distance between rings (or dots) means a steep curvature and vice versa. Any corneal surface or tear film irregularity will translate into ring irregularity. A visual check of the Placido ring image provides some qualitative information about the corneal surface and/or tear film (Fig. 15.2).

Cassini is a unique reflection topographer in that it uses a multiple dot color pattern (679 LEDs) that facilitates a true object-image correspondence decreasing reconstruction errors in case of skew rays [5]. This is especially important when the cornea is not rotationally symmetric, for example, astigmatism, especially if it is irregular. This device can also measure posterior corneal keratometry from the reflection of a ring of dots produced by seven infrared LEDs.

Elevation Topography

The advent of technologies that can obtain cross-sectional images of the cornea allowing simultaneous anterior and posterior corneal topography represented a quantum leap in corneal diagnostics. These instruments project some light on the cornea and record corneal sections in different meridians from the backscattered light (Rayleigh scattering) (Table 15.1).

– *Scanning slit*: In 1995, the Orbscan® topographer, Orbtek, was the first to use a slit of light that scanned horizontally the cornea assessing both corneal surfaces. In 1999, it evolved to Orbscan II®, Bausch & Lomb, incorporating a Placido disk to increase its accuracy in anterior corneal measurement [6].
– *Scheimpflug*: In 2003, Pentacam®, Oculus, was the first corneal tomographer that used the

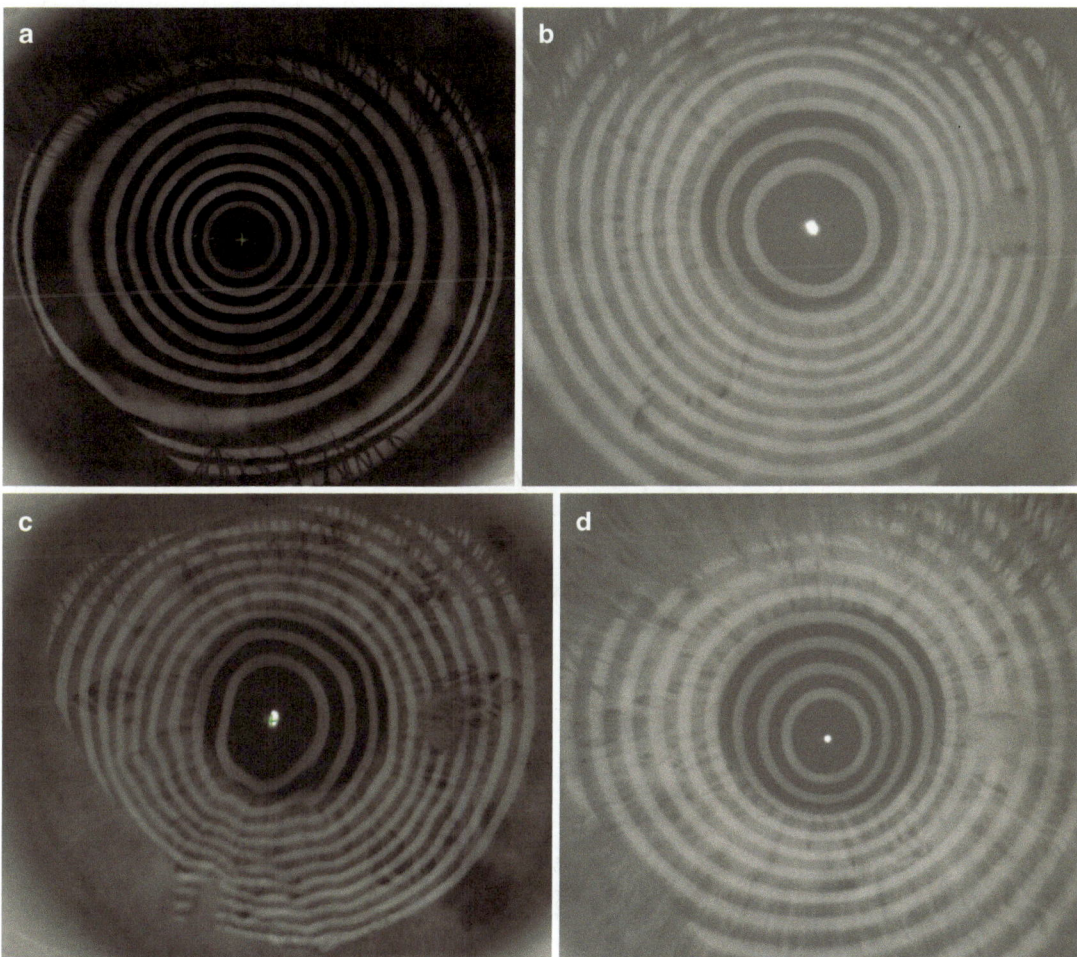

Fig. 15.2 (**a**) Central thin rings in a steep cornea ($K = 48$ D). (**b**) Central thick rings in a flat cornea ($K = 34$ D). (**c**) Irregular rings in a case of corneal scar. (**d**) Paracentral inferior steepening in a case of keratoconus

Table 15.1 Scheimpflug and OCT corneal tomographers

Technology	Model	Hardware	Wavelength (nm)	Scan time (s)	Meridians	AL
Scheimpflug	PENTACAM HR/AXL	1 camera	475	2	25	Yes
	GALILEI G4/G6	2 cameras Placido	470	1	60	Yes
	SIRIUS	1 camera Placido	475	1	25	No
	TMS 5	1 camera Placido	475	1	64	No
OCT	ANTERION	Swept source	1300	0.5	65	Yes
	MS39	Spectral Placido	845	1	25	No
	CASIA 2	Swept source	1310	0.3	16	No
	REVO NX	Spectral	830	0.17	16	No

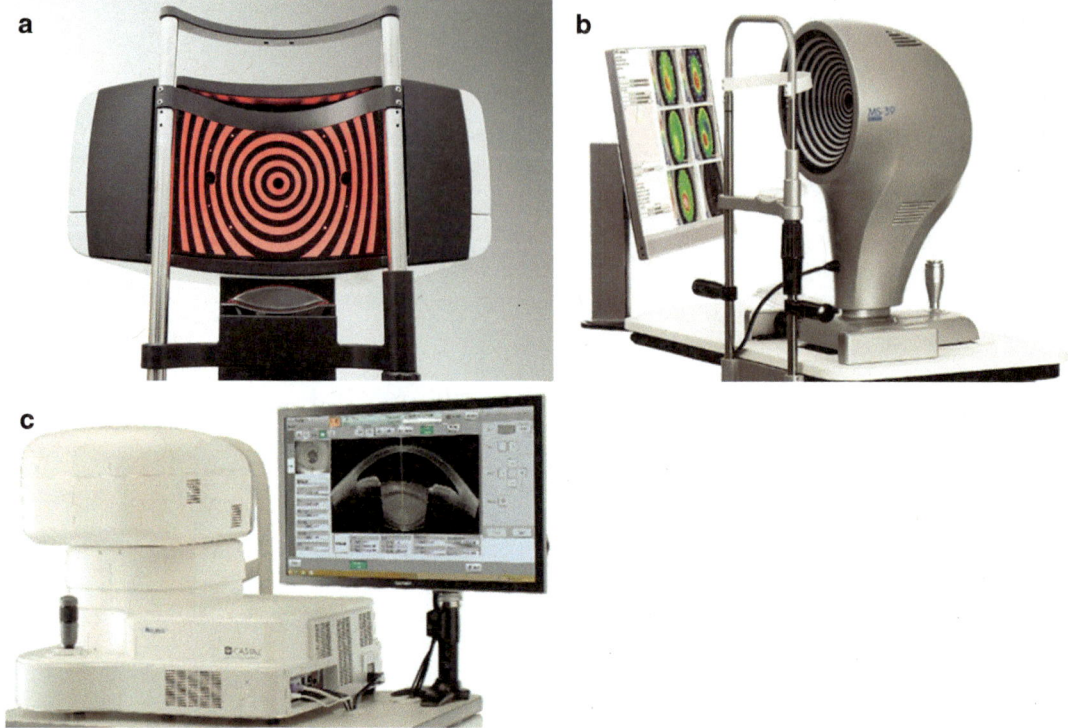

Fig. 15.3 From left to right: (**a**) Orbscan scanning-slit, (**b**) MS 39 Placido/FD-OCT, and (**c**) Casia 2 FD-OCT

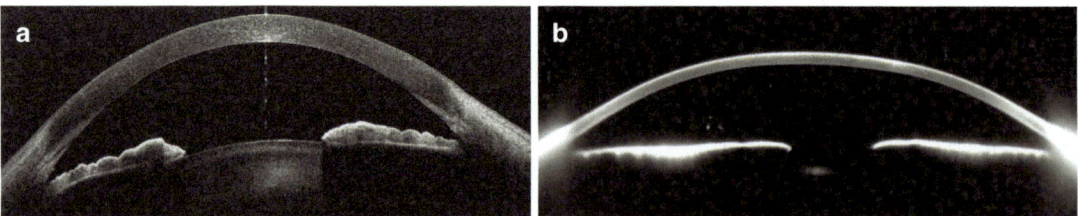

Fig. 15.4 Corneal image by OCT (**a**) has higher resolution and presents less light scatter with sharper boundaries than Sheimpflug image (**b**)

Scheimpflug photography principle to analyze the cornea by means of a rotating camera. Later, other instruments using the same principle were marketed: Galilei®, Ziemer, TMS®, Tomey, Sirius®, CSO, etc.

– *Optical Coherence Tomography (OCT)* (Fig. 15.3): This technology has boosted corneal tomography due to a significant improvement in image quality. In 2009, Zeiss commercialized the Visante-Omni® that used Time-Domain (TD)-OCT to measure the posterior corneal surface. The anterior topography was measured with a Placido system. The evolution to Frequency-Domain (FD)-OCT technology has decreased the image acquisition time allowing anterior surface topography from OCT data. At present time, there are three devices that measure both anterior and posterior corneal topography just from OCT data: Casia 2® (Tomey), Anterion® (Heidelberg), and Copernicus/Revo NX® (Optopol). The MS39® (CSO) still combines Placido disk for anterior cornea and spectral FD-OCT for the posterior topography.

Compared to other technologies, OCT has increased posterior corneal analysis accuracy due to a significant image quality improvement (Fig. 15.4). OCT has higher axial resolution in tissue: 5 µm in the case of spectral FD-OCT and 10 µm in the case of Swept Source FD-OCT [7].

Measurements

All devices will describe both corneal surfaces in terms of elevation, curvature, and optical function. Reflection topographers can obtain elevation and curvature information by an arc step calculation method applied to the obtained reflected image, while elevation tomographers will directly get the elevation fitting a curve to the cross-sectional image of the cornea (Fig. 15.5). Afterwards, curvature will be calculated by differentiation.

The relationship between curvature and elevation is a function of the distance to the optical axis. Using a conic function formula, it can be found that the difference in elevation for two curves of 7.85 mm (43 D) and 7.67 mm (44 D) is around 1.5 µm at a distance of 1 mm to the center. This value is under the resolution of any current elevation tomographer, and this is why many instruments, Scheimpflug and OCT, still use a Placido disk to measure the anterior cornea. However, there are other models that rely exclusively on elevation to calculate corneal curvature having shown excellent repeatability and good agreement with other devices [8, 9].

Axial and Tangential Radii

The curvature radius of each surface point can be calculated in two ways [10]:

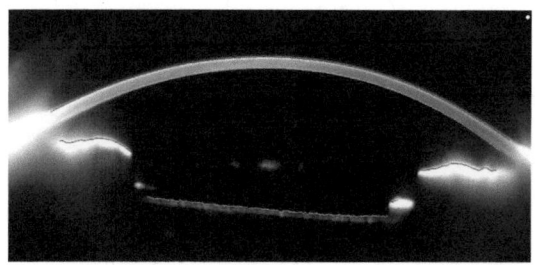

Fig. 15.5 Boundaries identified in a Scheimpflug image (Pentacam). Initial step before best fitting function is calculated

– Axial (sagittal) radius: The distance from the optical axis to the surface normal at that point.
– Tangential (instantaneous, meridional) radius: The distance from the center of curvature of the best fit sphere of each point to the surface normal at that point.

The axial radius only describes adequately symmetrical profiles like the central cornea where the radius of curvature can be assumed to be in the optical axis. Tangential radius will better describe asymmetrical features and the corneal periphery.

Metrics

Three types of metrics are available to the user:

Curvature Metrics
– Radii of curvature: Both axial and tangential radii (in mm) are available in color-coded maps and in indices for different areas of analysis, for example, Sim K, 5 mm semi-meridians.
– Keratometric curvature: Applying the paraxial formula for spheres with the standard keratometric index of refraction (SKIR = 1.3375), the axial and tangential powers are calculated.

$$P = \frac{n_2 - n_1}{r} = \frac{1.3375 - 1}{r} = \frac{0.3375}{r} \quad (15.1)$$

where P is power, n_2 is index of refraction of cornea, n_1 is index of refraction of air, and r is radius of curvature.

This convention has been followed by all manufacturers accepting the heritage of keratometry. The mean value for an annular region of an approximate diameter of 3 mm is known as Sim K (simulated keratometry). There can be small systematic differences among instruments because each one calculates this value in a particular way, for example, Sirius and MS-39 define this value as the mean of the sagittal power from the fourth to the eighth Placido ring (Phoenix 4.0 manual) and Pentacam defines it as the mean value of a ring 15° around the vertex normal (software 6.10r53). Powers are also calculated for other diameters as well as it has been mentioned above for radii.

Color-coded maps are also displayed where steep areas are represented by long wavelengths (*hot* colors) and flat areas represented by short wavelengths (*cold* colors).

It should be emphasized that keratometric diopters do not represent actual optical power but only curvature: A perfectly spherical cornea with a 7.5 mm curvature radius will be 45 diopters all over the surface. Spherical aberration, higher power in the periphery, is not taken into account.

- Keratometric astigmatism is the difference between the steepest and flattest meridian. It can be expressed as Sim K astigmatism, where both axes are 90° apart, or for other areas of analysis.
- Asphericity index (shape factor): This parameter expresses the rate of change of curvature from the center to the periphery of the cornea for a certain analyzed diameter. It determines the spherical aberration of the aphakic eye. The mean value is available for the anterior and posterior corneal surfaces. Four different coefficients are usually provided: Q, p, e, and E [11].

Elevation Metrics

Measured elevation data are displayed in color-coded maps that express the difference with respect to a certain reference plane. As the cornea is best fitted with an asphero-toric curve, this will be the reference body that will disclosure more accurately the tiniest irregularities. Some topographers also describe the surface elevation with a Zernike polynomial expansion.

Refractive Power Metrics

Ray-tracing methodology is used to calculate the actual optical properties of the cornea. An incoming collimated bundle of rays is traced through the anterior and posterior (if measured) corneal surface applying Snell's law. Some devices use Gullstrand's refractive indices for cornea (1.376) and aqueous (1.336), while others use proprietary values.

- Refractive power map: the distribution of power is displayed in a color-coded map.
- Refractive power indices: There is no standardization on the name of a central mean total power parameter, and thus each instrument uses a different name for it. The total corneal refractive astigmatism is the difference in total refractive power between the steepest and flattest meridians.
- Wavefront analysis: The anterior, posterior, and total wavefront aberration maps and Zernike coefficients are calculated by all topo-tomographers. The latter are expressed in RMS values. The wavefront error map represents the difference in height between the corneal wavefront and an ideal wavefront within the analysis diameter.

Precision and Agreement

Central curvature measurement is similar to automated keratometers: the within-subject standard deviation value of repeated measurements around 0.10 D (Sim K) [12]. Placido topographers are usually slightly more imprecise than elevation ones probably due to their tear film quality dependence. Table 15.2 shows different values obtained by our group in different precision studies in healthy eyes presented at IOL Power Club meetings over the past 10 years. The impact of this error level in IOL power calculation is small and can be calculated by Gaussian error propagation analysis: a two-fold increase of Sim K imprecision will barely affect final refraction prediction

Table 15.2 Precision of 3 repeated measurements on healthy eyes in different studies with different topo-tomographers. S_w within-subject standard deviation from ANOVA. *CV* coefficient of variation

Device	Year	N	Sim K	S_w	CV
Pentacam HR	2011	35	43.22 ± 1.43	0.06	0.14
MS 39	2019	29	43.88 ± 1.19	0.08	0.17
Casia 2	2017	41	44.05 ± 1.34	0.08	0.17
Galilei G2	2011	35	43.19 ± 1.39	0.10	0.23
IOL master 700	2015	34	43.85 ± 1.79	0.10	0.23
Anterion	2019	29	43.43 ± 1.19	0.12	0.27
Sirius	2017	41	43.94 ± 1.41	0.16	0.37

error and the distribution of cases within ±0.50 and ±1.00 D of the prediction (Table 15.3).

Measurement precision will be worse under any circumstance that affects corneal regularity and/or tear film quality: previous corneal surgery, aging, dry eye, etc. [13].

Curvature measurement agreement is fairly good among different technologies and instruments. Most studies report differences between 0.05 and 0.4 D in Sim K. This value can be sig-

Table 15.3 Contribution of Sim K standard deviation, $\sigma(K)$, to the final refraction standard deviation, $\sigma(R_x)$. Calculations performed for three different axial lengths. The last two columns display the proportion of eyes within certain refraction ranges. These standard deviation values have been set constants in the model: AXL = 0.02 mm; ELP = 0.2 mm; IOL = 0.13 D; $n = 0.002$

AXL (mm)	$\sigma(K)$	$\sigma(R_x)$	±0.50 D	±1.00 D
23.50	0.1	0.33	87.03%	99.76%
	0.2	0.37	82.34%	99.31%
21.50	0.1	0.42	76.61%	98.27%
	0.2	0.46	72.29%	97.03%
27.00	0.1	0.19	99.15%	100%
	0.2	0.26	94.55%	99.99%

nificant if the parameter is used to calculate IOL power; therefore, it should be measured and compensated for this task. IOL constant optimization for a new device will take this bias into account.

Software

In addition to the regular topographic software, all topo-tomographers integrate specific modules oriented for IOL power calculations, where corneal measurements are combined with biometry values. Four modules can be distinguished:

Surgical Planning Information (Fig. 15.6)

The important metrics are keratometry based data like Sim K and keratometric astigmatism; ray-tracing based refractive power values like total power and total astigmatism; shape factor; Zernike aberrometry coefficients; pupil position

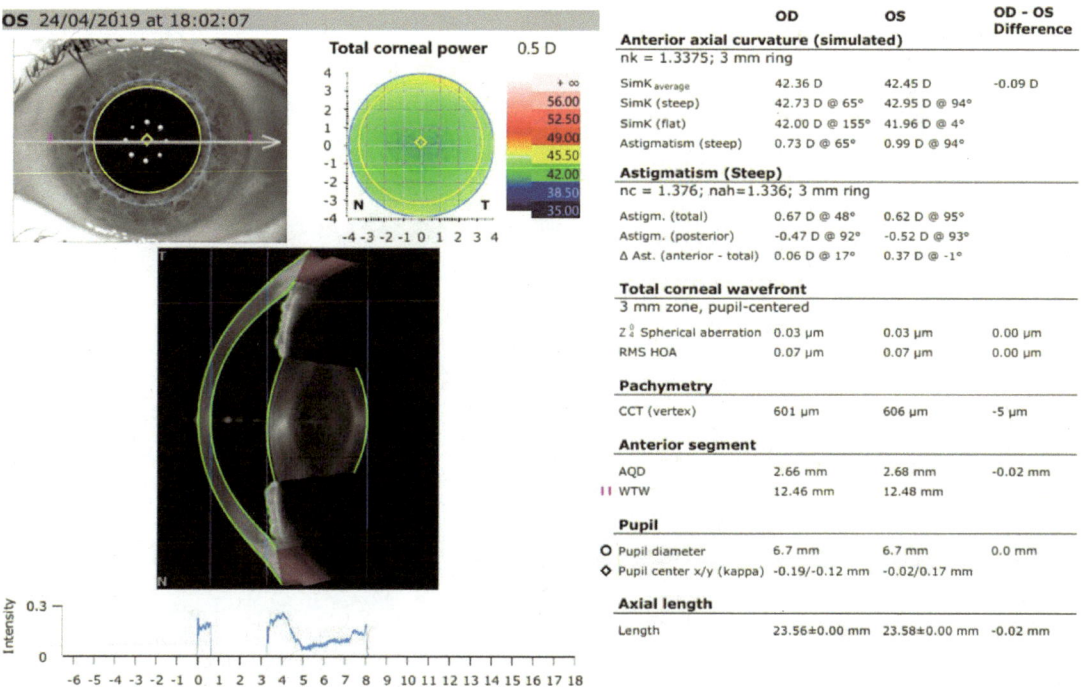

Fig. 15.6 IOL surgery planning module of Anterion tomographer

and diameter; lens thickness (only some devices with PCI and SS-OCT technologies); other biometric parameters like axial length, corneal diameter, corneal thickness, ACD, etc.

IOL Calculation

IOL calculation formulas are programmed in order to perform these calculations. Third-generation formulas like Hoffer Q, Holladay 1, and SRK/T are present in all of them. Newer formulas like Barrett Universal II, Hoffer QST, Kane, RBF, specific post-LASIK formulas like Shammas-PL, and ray-tracing software like Okulix and Phaco-Optics are available only in certain platforms. CSO devices, Sirius®, and MS39® incorporate a proprietary ray-tracing module adequate for odd corneas (post-LASIK, etc.) [14].

Toric IOL Calculations

Tomographers can base their calculations both in keratometric astigmatism and in total corneal astigmatism measured by ray-tracing of anterior and posterior cornea. One of the best-known toric calculators is normally available: Abulafia-Koch, Barrett toric, Holladay 2 toric, Naeser-Savini, etc.

Post-surgical Analysis

Refractive data can be entered to keep track of results and optimize the IOL constant. Some devices can image the rotational position of the toric IOL and calculate the rotation necessary to improve the refractive astigmatism. The Casia 2® has an IOL position analysis module that can measure centration and tilt of the IOL (Fig. 15.7).

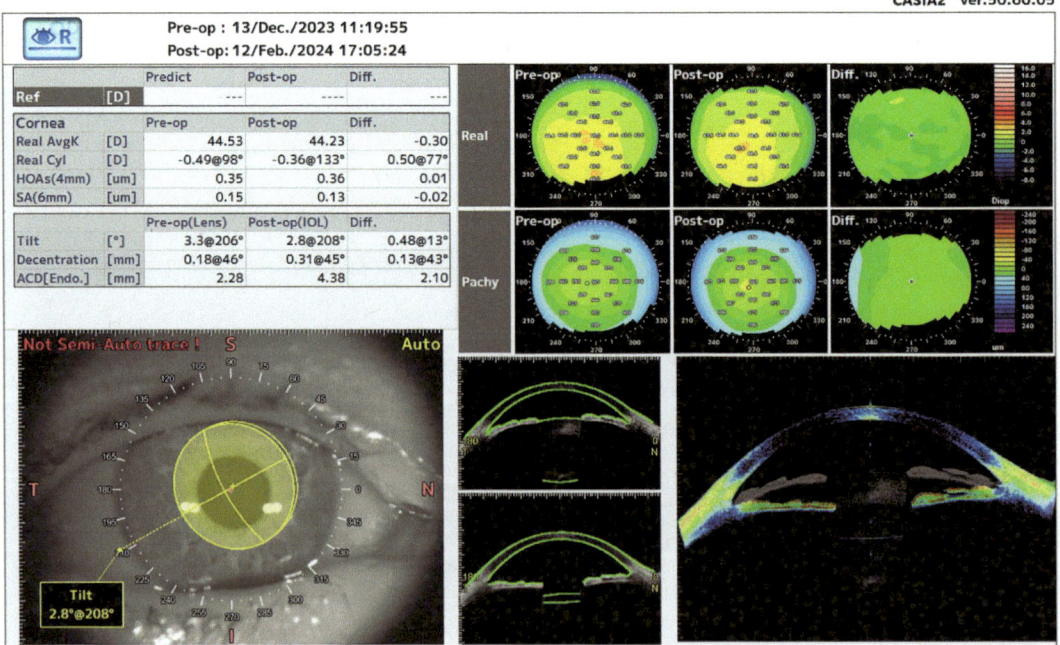

Fig. 15.7 Postoperative analysis module of CASIA 2®

IOL Selection

The IOL selection process implies choosing among different levels of optical performance and compromise, where one design can fit one type of eye but can be contraindicated in another, i.e., a multifocal diffractive IOL can provide good visual quality combined with a regular cornea but not with one that presents a post-LASIK decentered topographical optical zone. The toricity and shape of the IOL are also a matter of consideration in this context. All these decisions are primarily based on corneal topo-tomographic information.

Corneal Optical Quality

Corneal optical quality measurement allows determining if the eye is suitable for the implantation of an IOL design that entails some functional compromise that occurs with many multifocal models. It is also useful to estimate the visual performance after surgery allowing the surgeon to provide the correct information to the patient and define reasonable expectations. This will undoubtedly affect the perceived result and improve the quality of the surgery.

Corneal optical quality is usually assessed by wavefront error aberration analysis. All tomographers present such a software module where Zernike polynomial expansion of the wavefront error is calculated, and some metrics are displayed: Zernike coefficients for several orders, RMS of different combinations of terms (higher and lower order aberrations, HOA and LOA, coma, trefoil, etc.), point spread function, PSF, modulation transfer function (MTF), Strehl ratio, etc. (Fig. 15.8).

Zernike polynomials contribute differently to the overall visual quality. The lower the order and the more central in the pyramid the greater the effect on visual quality. Fourth-order spherical aberration and third-order coma are usually the most relevant HOA values. In aberrated corneas, it is interesting to check the image simulation because the final effect on visual quality will depend on how these terms combine.

There are not universally accepted normality cut-off values. It has been suggested that a relative contraindication for multifocal IOLs is a value over 0.3 μm of corneal HOA in 4 mm diameter, due to equivalency with 0.50 D blur [15]. But there is lack of empirical evidence to support any precise threshold value. Another related issue

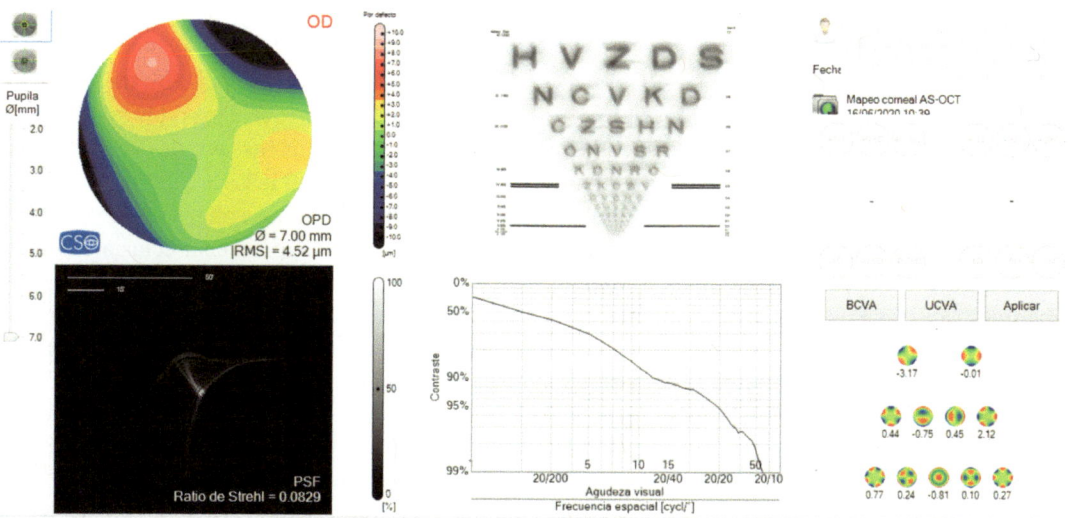

Fig. 15.8 Optical quality display: in the upper row, the wavefront error map (OPD) with some indices and the image simulation. In the lower row, the PSF figure and the Strehl ratio, the MTF curve and the Zernike coefficients pyramid are displayed

Table 15.4 Corneal aberrations. Diameter analysis is not the same and this affects the RMS values [17–20]

	Vinciguerra $n = 1000$; diameter = 5 mm; EyeTop	Wang $n = 228$; diameter = 6 mm Atlas	Zheleznyak $n = 40$; diameter = 5 mm Orbscan	Nur Colak $n = 81$; diameter = 6 mm; Sirius
HOA (µm)	0.16 ± 0.06	0.48 ± 0.12	0.29 ± 0.1	0.36 ± 0.1
Spherical (µm)	0.15 ± 0.05	0.28 ± 0.08	0.15 ± 0.09	0.22 ± 0.05
Coma (µm)	0.14 ± 0.08	0.25 ± 0.13	0.15 ± 0.08	0.48 ± 0.09
Trifoil (µm)	n.d.	n.d.	0.14 ± 0.09	0.13 ± 0.04

is that there is not very good agreement in corneal HOA measurements among devices [16]. It is important to know the normal range of the tomographer in use. Table 15.4 shows some references in normal eye samples. In our practice, we refrain from implanting multifocal IOLs when the HOA RMS value is three standard deviations away from the mean value.

Corneal Anatomical Quality

Corneal topography can detect surface pathology that can affect the optical performance of the pseudophakic eye and is a valuable tool for evolutionary follow up. A frequent situation is epithelial basement membrane dystrophy (EBMD) where corneal epithelial irregularities can alter central corneal power over time and lead to biometric error [21]. Surgery and post-surgical treatments can trigger epithelial changes that finally disturb the corneal surface. Corneal topography can detect and quantify central irregularity. The epithelial map available in some OCT tomographers is a powerful tool to diagnose this sort of pathology. A focal thickening is a characteristic feature in this map with values over 60 µm. In the cross-sectional OCT image sometimes, an intraepithelial white nodule can be seen (Fig. 15.9).

Surface irregularity is a habitual feature of dry eye disease that also affects both optical performance of the pseudophakic eye and keratometry precision and accuracy [13]. It is a recognized source of dissatisfaction in patients with multifocal IOLs; therefore, it should always be taken into consideration in candidates for this type of

lens [22]. In addition to curvature and epithelial maps, some topographers can perform the NIBUT test (non-invasive break-up time), dynamic tear study and non-contact meibography. This can be completed by tear meniscus measurement with OCT which has shown to be a reliable diagnostic test [23].

Topographies of contact lens users must be examined carefully looking for any irregularity that can yield a keratometric and, consequently, an IOL power error. If this is the case, biometry should be repeated after the situation has cleared. Figure 15.10 shows a case with mild asymmetric keratometric astigmatism. The patient had stopped wearing soft contact lenses 10 days before. One month later the steepening of the superior semi-meridian had disappeared, the Sim K had flattened 1.05 D and keratometric astigmatism had reduced by 1.30 D.

In modern IOL surgery, patient expectations are very high and the final goal is to achieve a refractive status of emmetropia with the best possible uncorrected vision. The odds of needing some excimer treatments are around 5–10%, especially if multifocal IOLs are implanted where tolerance to any residual ametropia is very low. Any sign of subclinical corneal ectasia can lead to the contraindication of excimer laser surgery, and this can alter the surgical plan. Corneal tomography has boosted the detection of subclinical keratoconus by epithelium and pachymetry and analysis. The earliest morphological feature in keratoconus is a focal stromal thinning, usually in the inferior-temporal quadrant, with epithelium thinning, which is thought to be a compensating phenomenon that decreases the optical impact of the anterior protrusion [24].

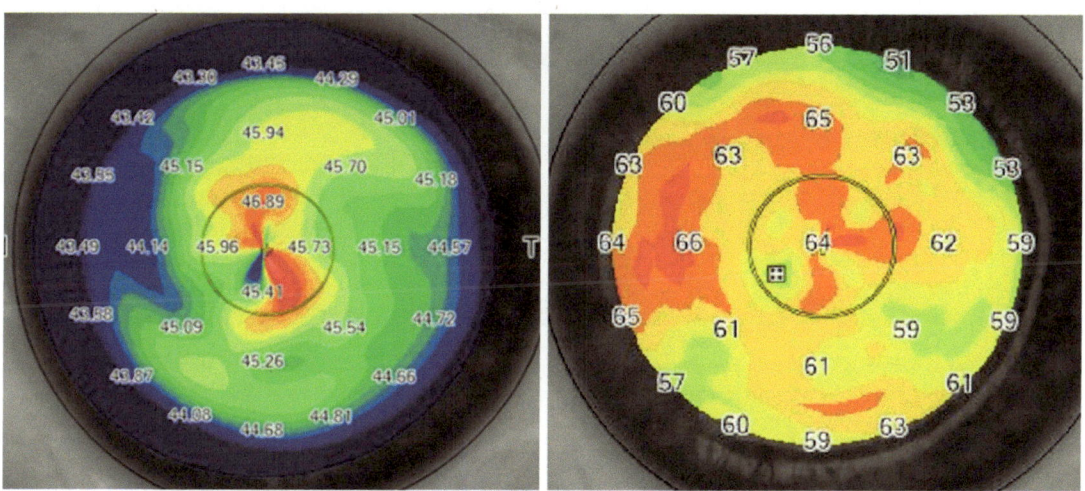

Fig. 15.9 Central corneal topographic irregularity in a case of epithelial basement membrane dystrophy. The epithelial map shows central irregular thickening

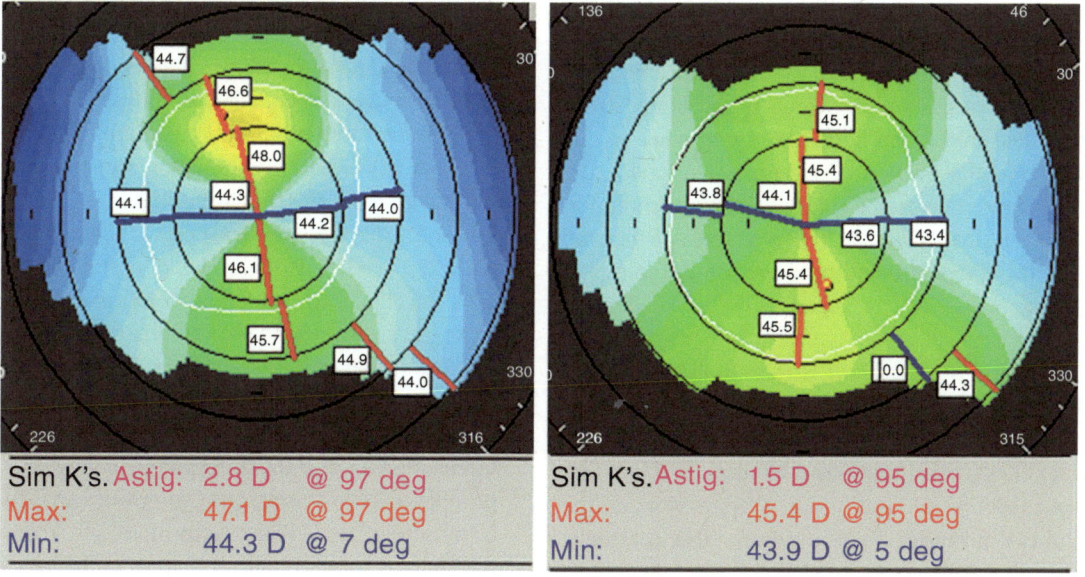

Fig. 15.10 Topographic and keratometric changes after discontinuing soft contact lenses. On the left, 10 days without contact lenses and on the right 1 month later

This is why the posterior elevation value is always higher than anterior. The epithelial map provided by some OCT tomographers can detect this pattern distinguishing it from other clinical entities, for example, epithelium focal hyperplasia rendering a pseudokeratoconic topographic pattern (Fig. 15.11).

The rate of corneal thickening from the thinnest point to the periphery is higher in the kera-toconic cornea. This relevant feature was found by Ambrosio who developed two graphs in order to detect it: CTSP (corneal thickness spatial profile) and PTI (percentage thickness increase) [25].

Most topo-tomographers incorporate software modules dedicated to keratoconus diagnosis that help the clinician in the detection of this condition.

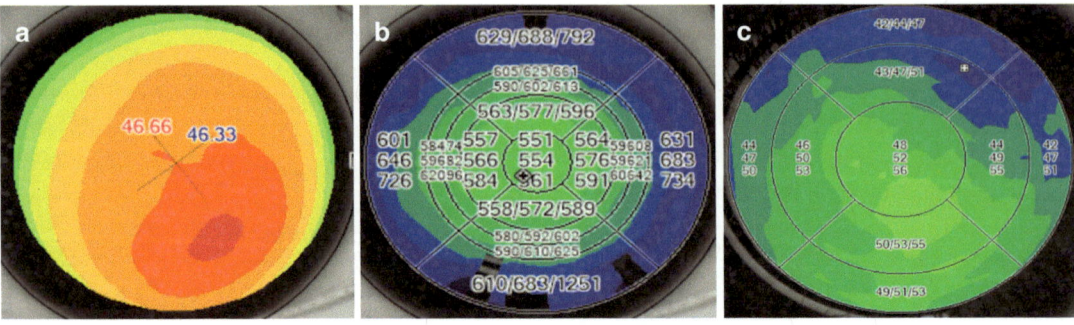

Fig. 15.11 (**a**) Possible keratoconus pattern in the axial keratometric map (left). (**b**) Pachymetry map looks normal (center). (**c**) There is epithelium thickening in the epi- thelial map coincident with the steepened area: pseudoectasia produced by surface pathology

IOL Power Calculation

IOL power has been calculated for many years using optical vergence thin lens formulas. The corneal power parameter, essential in this calculation, has been provided by the keratometer in the form of a K value, which is calculated from the measured mean paracentral curvature radius applying the SKIR (1.3375) to account for the unmeasured posterior corneal power (see section "Measurements" above in this chapter). Since the first topographers, and now the tomographers, a similar value is calculated from an equivalent central corneal area, around 3 mm in diameter. This value is called Sim K (simulated keratometry) and can be used in the IOL calculation formulas as the agreement with K is fairly good. K does not correspond to any classic Gaussian optics definition. Although it approximates the corneal posterior vertex power, the reference plane is a little posterior to this [26].

Since corneal topographers can measure many points of the anterior surface and tomographers can measure the posterior surface curvature and power new options arise to parameterize corneal optics in order to calculate the IOL.

Important Concepts

- The actually measured area depends on curvature radius and asphericity. The steeper the cor-

nea, the smaller the measured area and vice versa. Corneal asphericity will finally determine if K is over or underestimated. In a very flat physiologically prolate cornea, K will be underestimated because the more peripheral curvature is smaller. On the contrary, in a very flat post-LASIK oblate cornea, K will be overestimated because the more peripheral curvature is higher (Fig. 15.12). This overestimation can be very significant if the shape factor is high.

- The accuracy of corneal power calculated with the SKIR depends on a certain ratio between the anterior and posterior corneal curvatures. The so-called Gullstrand ratio, whose normal value is: anterior radius/posterior radius = 1.21 ± 0.02 [9]. If it is expressed inversely: posterior radius/anterior radius = 0.82 ± 0.02. In corneas, where this proportion is different, corneal power (K) will be miscalculated. If the ratio increases, there will be an overestimation of K value because the calculation will miss the relative anterior flattening effect. This happens after myopic LASIK/PRK [27], keratoconus [28], and DSAEK [29], to mention some frequently found conditions. If the ratio decreases, there will be an underestimation of K value because the calculation will miss the relative steepening effect. This happens after hyperopic LASIK/PRK, some presby-LASIK profiles and radial keratotomy (RK) [30] (Fig. 15.13). K values changes approximately five times the

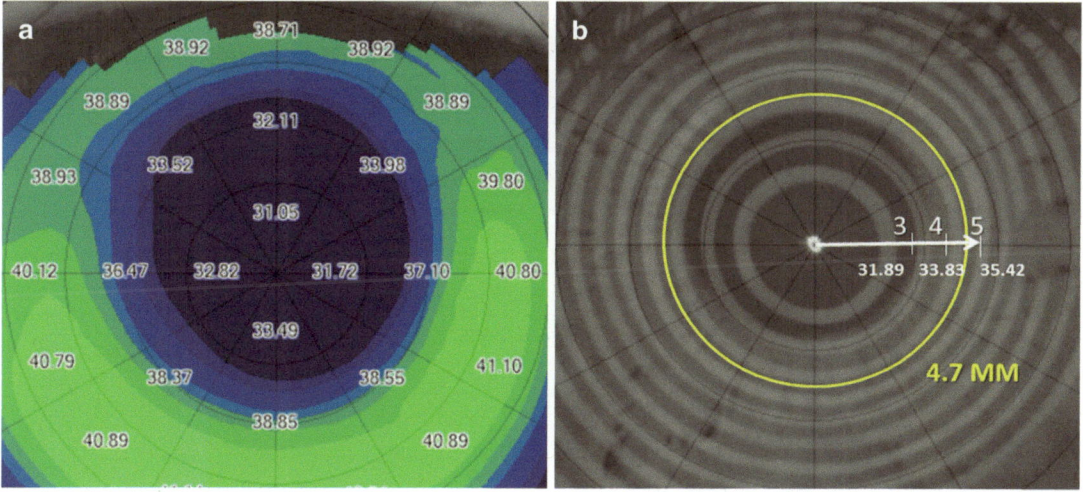

Fig. 15.12 Placido topography after LASIK-M. (**a**) The actually measured area diameter is 4.7 mm due to corneal curvature and shape. (**b**) Curvature gradient is very high as it can be seen in three reference positions: 3, 4, and 5 mm

Fig. 15.13 Anterior/posterior corneal ratio. Normality range is within red dotted lines. Central line scale is not proportional

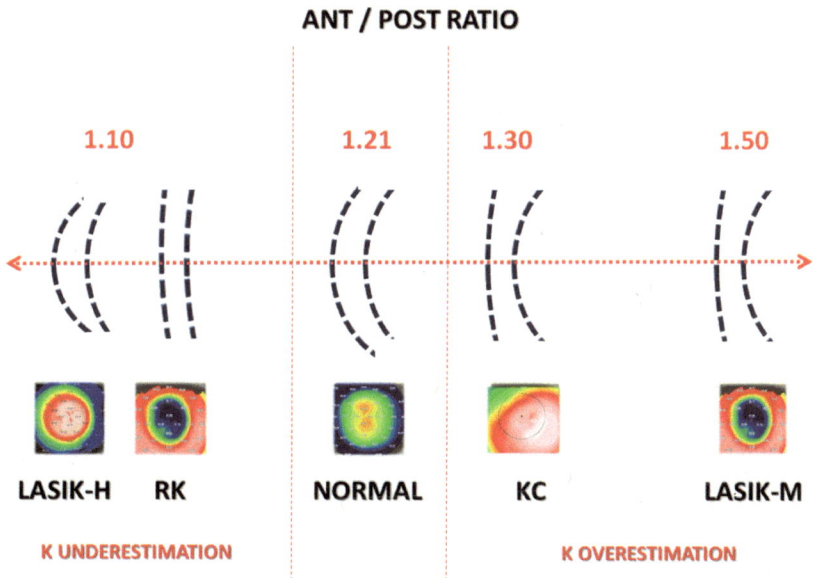

corneal ratio change, for example, 0.3 corneal ratio converts to 1.5 in *K*.

Ant/post ratio change is proportional to the anterior curvature change produced by the laser in excimer surgery. This explains why a function can be fit to predict the effect (e.g., Haigis-L and Barrett true K formulas). While there is no such proportionality after RK and similar surgeries, the same number of cuts can produce different effects on this ratio [30]. The accuracy of any predicting function will be worse by definition.

Parameters for IOL Calculations

Sim K

It can be used in any formula that requires a keratometric *K* value. In our practice, we use it as a double check of the keratometer measurement.

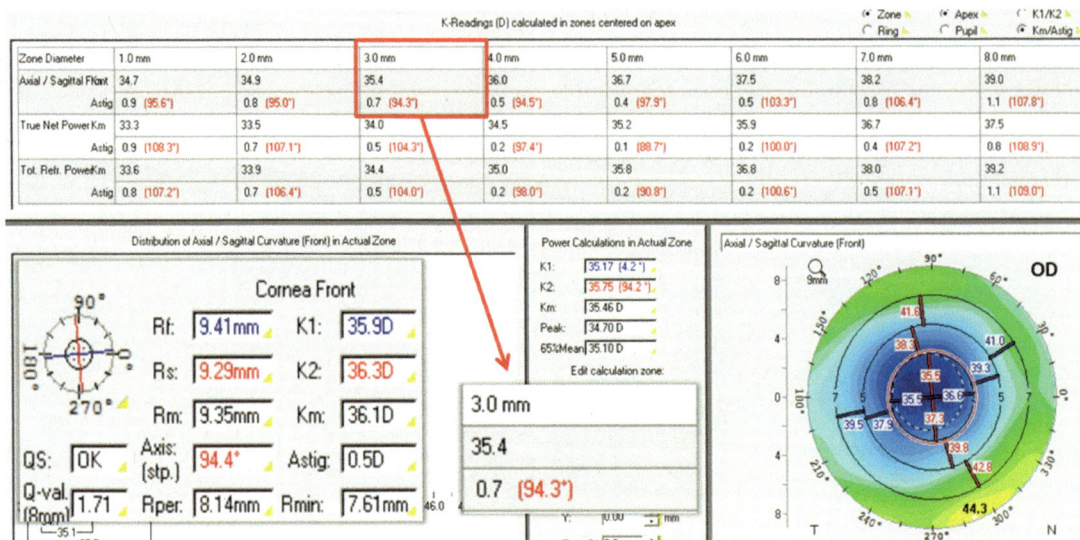

Fig. 15.14 Power distribution map in Pentacam. Post LASIK-M case. 36.1 D Sim K value becomes 35.40 D once adjusted to the 3 mm area in the Axial/sagittal front option

We know the bias between both devices from previous home-made agreement study.

In case of curvature and shape extreme values, the measurement area should be adjusted. This is particularly important in very flat and oblate corneas after LASIK/PRK and RK. The way to proceed depends on the topographer model. For example, with the Pentacam it can be done in the power distribution map module, adjusting the area of analysis to 3 mm of the parameter axial/sagittal curvature front (Fig. 15.14). In the Sirius and MS39, the Sim K option is changed by Meridians in the Indices table. The mean value for 3 mm will be the adjusted new K.

Equivalent K Reading (EKR)

Described first by Holladay for the Pentacam®, it can be defined as the total central power calculated from both measured anterior and posterior surfaces and adjusted to a reference plane similar to the keratometric K value [31]. Therefore, it can be used in any IOL power calculation formula designed to input K as the corneal parameter avoiding the ant/post ratio induced error. In a normal eye, this value should be very similar to Sim K, with just some difference from the variance of this ratio in the normal eye (SD = 0.02). In the

Pentacam®, the recommended value is EKR 4.5 mm which shows a 95% agreement range with keratometer measured K of 1.48 D [32]. However, there is some controversy on the results obtained with the EKR, both in normal and previously operated eyes [31–33]. In cases of DSAEK, Xu reported the lowest predictive error with EKR: -0.05 ± 1.02 D, achieving a good compensation for the altered ant/post ratio [29].

EKR is also available in the Cassini® software. We obtained good results using it with the Haigis formula in a series of 26 eyes after myopic LASIK with a mean ant/post ratio of 1.31 ± 0.06. The predictive error was -0.16 ± 0.73 D, which is comparable to other published series (presented at the IOL Power Club meeting in Athens in 2017).

The Galilei® has a conceptually similar index called TCPIOL calculated by ray-tracing and referenced to the posterior corneal surface in order to equal Sim K, but it does not seem to improve the results in normal eyes [34].

Total Corneal Power

All tomographers calculate a central corneal power parameter by ray tracing through the anterior and posterior surfaces normally using the

Gullstrand values for the index of refraction of cornea (≈ 1.376) and aqueous (≈ 1.336). This measurement has been given different names: It is called total corneal refractive power (TCRP) in the Pentacam®, total corneal power (TCP) in the Galilei® and Anterion®, real power in the Casia® and Revo NX®, and mean pupilar power (MPP) in the Sirius® and MS39®. It should be pointed out that the Galilei® presents three different values: TCP1, TCP2, and TCP-IOL, depending on the index of refraction used and the corneal reference plane (see the Galilei® chapter in this book).

Some tomographers offer alternatively a K value calculated using the Gaussian equivalent power formula:

$$P = K_{ant} + K_{post} - \left(\frac{d}{n}\right) * K_{ant} * K_{post} \quad (15.2)$$

where P is power, K_{ant} is the anterior corneal power, K_{post} is the posterior corneal power calculated using Eq. (15.1), d is corneal thickness, and n is corneal refractive index. In the Pentacam®, this value is called true net power (TNP).

All these powers have reference planes anterior to the Sim K and thus have lower dioptric values. Although they all share the interesting feature of taking into account the posterior measured curvature and avoiding the proportion assumption of the Sim K, they cannot be directly input into regular IOL formulas as these are designed for the Sim K. Internally, the formula converts the K to a more accurate value using another corneal refractive index that will be between 1.3215 and 1.3333 depending on the formula [35]. However if a new IOL constant is calculated specifically for any of these values results can be correct both in normal eyes and post-corneal refractive surgery IOL power calculations [34, 36]. This new IOL constant will correct the bias between the total corneal power and the Sim K.

Radii of Curvature

A simple way of avoiding this K confusion is using the radii of curvature values in mm that all formulas allow as input. It also prevents from any error in the adjustment of the keratometry index of refraction.

Central Corneal Elevation Data

The cornea can be represented by a topographic data matrix which will be implemented in an exact ray-tracing eye model in order to calculate the optical performance of the pseudophakic eye. It can be done just using the anterior corneal surface but accuracy will certainly be better if the posterior cornea is represented in the same way by a tomographer. This will take account of HOAs and the best IOL power, both in terms of spherical equivalent and toricity and can be selected regarding different visual optical metrics beyond spectacle refraction as optimization factor. This methodology should provide better outcomes than paraxial methods whenever the amount of HOA is high.

Okulix software works in this way and is available in different biometry and topography devices (Fig. 15.15). It can also perform paraxial calculations based on indices (Sim K). The exact ray-tracing mode does not seem to offer any advantage in normal eyes over regular formulas or over the paraxial calculation by the same software. However, it has been shown to be a very good option after corneal refractive surgery: Savini reported 63.6% of cases within ±0.50 D of the target [36]. Results might be even better if measurements are obtained with a SS-OCT device: Gjerdrum et al. have found excellent outcomes with Anterion® and Okulix: PE within ±0.5 D in 88% of eyes [37].

The tomographers Sirius® and MS39® have a software module that performs IOL calculations by exact ray-tracing. The IOL position is estimated with a proprietary algorithm using several anterior segment parameters as predictors. Savini et al. reported 71% of eyes within ±0.50 D of prediction with Sirius [14] and 75% of eyes in a non-published series with the MS 39 instrument using optical-segmented AL.

Our group calculates the irregular cornea cases, mainly post-refractive and keratoconus, exporting the corneal elevations from the tomographer to Zemax® optical design software, first performing a 3D model with an algorithm programmed in Matlab®, and selecting the IOL power based on an optimizing function with the through-focus visual Strehl metrics which has a

Fig. 15.15 Simulation of Landolt C image with different IOL powers. The effect of HOA is considered and the IOL that produces the best quality image should be the best option

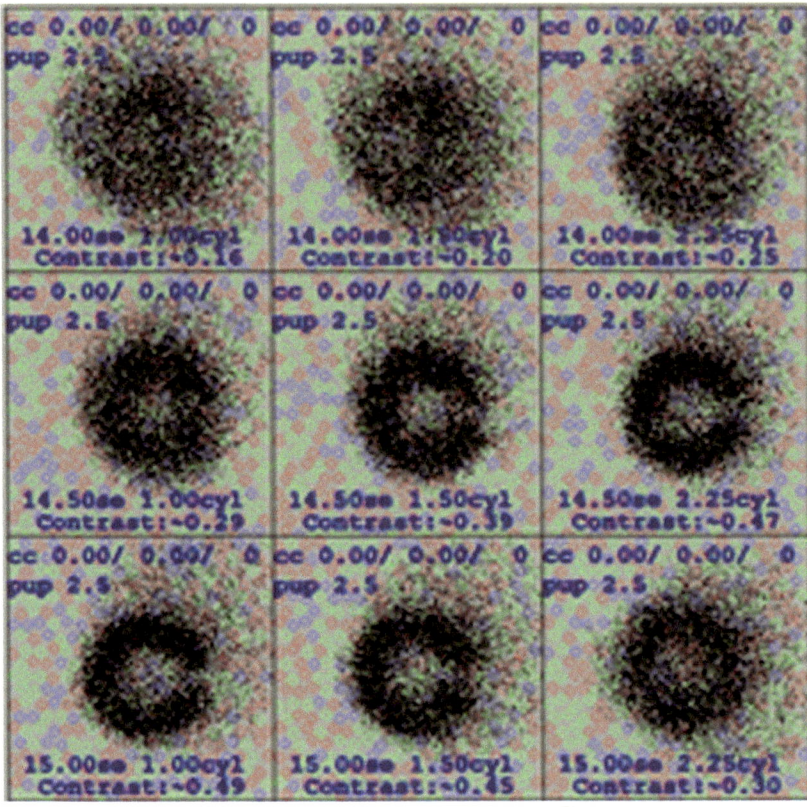

good correlation with the subjective refraction [38] (Fig. 15.16). At the 2021 IOL Power Club meeting, we presented a series of 75 eyes post-LASIK where 78.4% of eyes were ±0.50 D of predicted refraction (SE), and these values were 84% and 83% for J0 and J45 vectors, respectively.

Corneal Asphericity and Spherical Aberration

IOL designs have different shape factors to compensate the spherical aberration of the cornea. Hence, it is useful to know this value in the cornea to aim for a certain target, either zero or not. This can be particularly relevant in situations like keratoconus or after corneal refractive surgery where spherical aberration can be very high and impair visual quality.

All topo-tomographers measure corneal asphericity expressing this value in any of the well-defined coefficients: Q, p, e, and E. More useful is the spherical aberration measurement, in

μm, obtained from the wavefront error Zernike polynomial expansion, that can be found in the IOL calculation menu and in the Wavefront analysis menu. The spherical aberration Zernike coefficient is the C12 or Z(4, 0). It is a general consensus in refractive surgery to measure this value for 6 mm analysis diameter.

It should be remarked that the objective is the spherical aberration (anterior + posterior) and not the asphericity. This will yield a different spherical aberration depending on the radius of curvature: The higher the curvature, the higher the induced spherical aberration for a constant asphericity value [39].

Axis of Reference

All topographers measure the distance between two cardinal references: pupil center and corneal vertex. Although there is some terminology confusion about these axes, they are usually named angle kappa (in degrees) and distance chord μ (in mm). Several reports have found a relationship

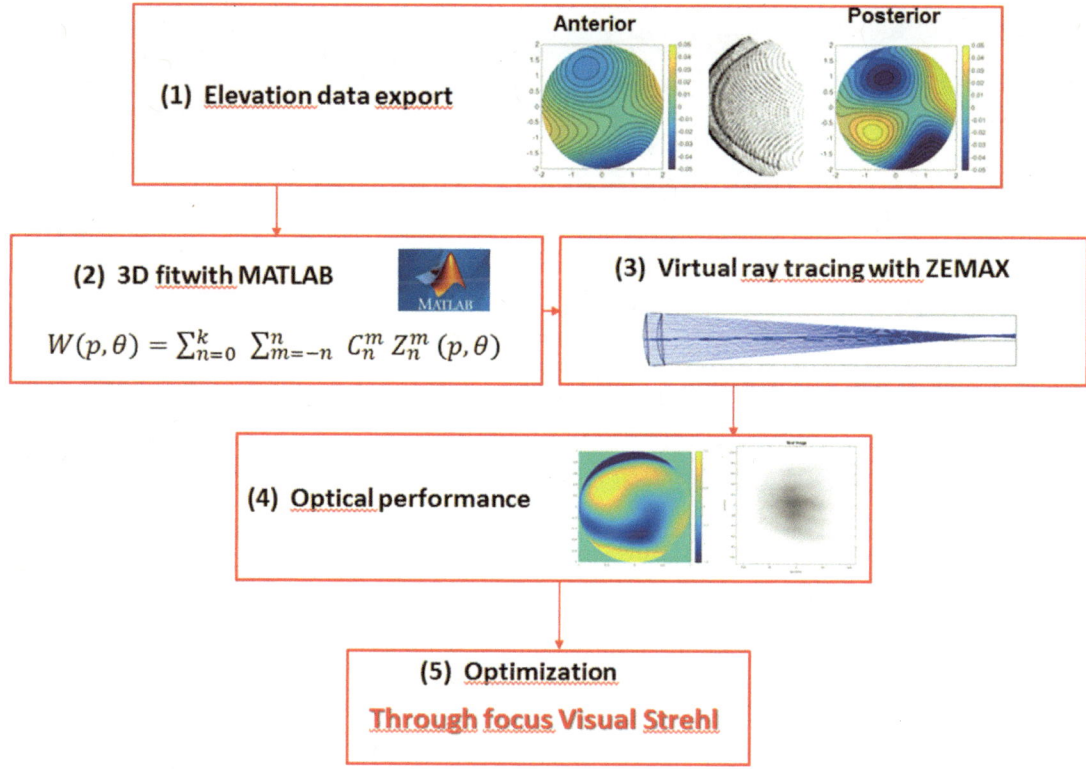

Fig. 15.16 IOL calculation from corneal elevations. Flow chart

between these values and the optical quality and patient satisfaction with different types of IOLs. Large angle kappa is related to higher risk of unwanted photic phenomena with multifocal IOLs [40, 41]. Therefore, measuring these values can be useful to select the type of IOL and properly center the capsulorrhexis and the IOL.

Toric IOL Calculation

Many studies show that the prevalence of significant corneal astigmatism is high with 30–43% of corneas presenting more than 1 D of keratometric astigmatism. Vision degradation is relevant over this value and can be a practical threshold to indicate the implantation of a toric IOL [42]. Corneal topo-tomography is the cornerstone in corneal astigmatism quantitative and qualitative analysis and, therefore, the essential tool in toric IOL selection.

Regular and Irregular Astigmatism

Regular astigmatism occurs if the refracting toric surface has two orthogonal meridians with geometrically identical semi-meridians. The curvature topographic feature will be a symmetric bowtie. The size and the color distribution of this bowtie will depend on corneal shape and curvature. As the shape gets more prolate, the bowtie becomes smaller and the steep axis stands out (Fig. 15.17).

Irregular astigmatism can also be defined as the presence of HOA. With regular toric IOLs, only regular astigmatism can be fully corrected. However, with advanced optic calculations there is room for IOL selection in order to achieve some compensation of the HOA. Frequent cases of irregular astigmatism are: post-LASIK/PRK/RK corneas, keratoconus, scars, etc. In very aberrated corneas paraxial calculations are non-sense and topography data-based calculations should

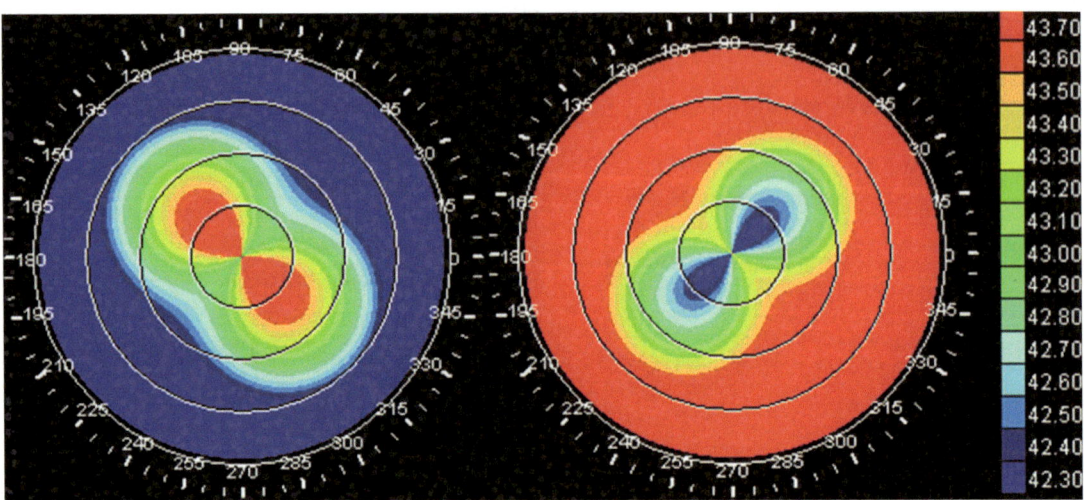

Fig. 15.17 Axial map simulation: Same astigmatism in both cases with apical radii 8.00 and 7.8 mm. The only difference is the shape factor. Left image is prolate ($p = 0.75$), and right image is oblate ($p = 1.25$). The prominent meridian is the steep one in the first case and the flat one in the second

be done using a ray-tracing method on a thick lens model. In Fig. 15.18, a very aberrated cornea that had undergone RK years before was calculated with a ray-tracing software obtaining an accurate refractive prediction.

Measured and Estimated Total Astigmatism

Keratometric astigmatism (K and Sim K) estimates total corneal astigmatism using the SKIR, 1.3375, value, which assumes a normal anterior/posterior corneal ratio and symmetry between steep-flat meridians in both surfaces. Since corneal tomographers can measure the posterior cornea, it has become evident that this is not always true. Koch et al. measured 715 corneas with the Galilei® and found that the steep meridian was vertical in 51.9% of anterior surfaces and 86.6% of posterior ones. This discrepancy means that keratometric astigmatism tends to overestimate with-the-rule (WTR) astigmatism and underestimate against-the-rule (ATR) astigmatism. The mean error vector was 0.22 D a 180°. In 5% of cases, the error was higher than 0.50 D [43]. Savini et al. reported similar findings with the Sirius® in 157 eyes. Sim K astigmatism overesti-

mated WTR astigmatism, 0.22 ± 0.32 D, underestimated ATR, 0.21 ± 0.26 D, and overestimated the oblique, 0.13 ± 0.37 D. In this study, there was a difference higher than 0.50 D between keratometric astigmatism and total astigmatism in 16% of cases [44]. Therefore, corneal total astigmatism, as measured from both the anterior and posterior corneal surfaces with a tomographer, is better than keratometric astigmatism as a toric IOL target. All tomographers display this value in the total corneal power analysis. This value can also be found in the total cornea wavefront error analysis, where the common vector for $Z(2, 2)$ and $Z(2, -2)$ in an area of 3 mm should be a very similar value (Fig. 15.19).

However, published evidence shows that empirical formulas that estimate the target total astigmatism from the keratometric astigmatism yield more accurate toric IOL calculations than the total corneal astigmatism mentioned in the previous paragraphs. Some of the most used formulas are: Barrett Toric, Abulafia-Koch, Holladay 2 Toric Naeser-Savini, Kane Toric, etc. [45, 46].

It has been proposed that IOL tilt can be the source for that residual astigmatism than cannot be predicted from the corneal measurements. It seems that IOL tilt can be estimated from preoperative lens tilt. If this is so, the incorporation of

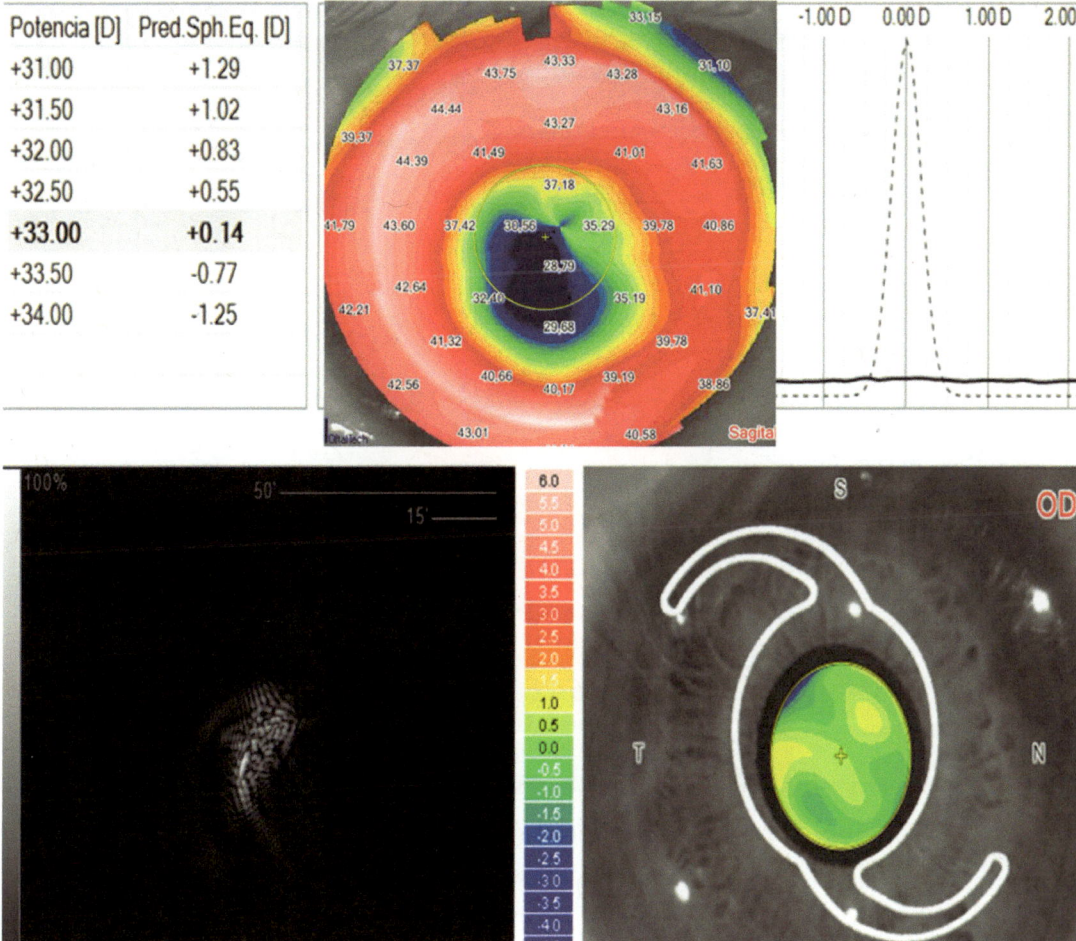

Potencia [D]	Pred.Sph.Eq. [D]
+31.00	+1.29
+31.50	+1.02
+32.00	+0.83
+32.50	+0.55
+33.00	**+0.14**
+33.50	-0.77
+34.00	-1.25

Fig. 15.18 Decentered and small optical zone after RK. AL = 24.63 mm; *K* (Lenstar): 31.87/33.53 D. Ray-tracing calculation (MS39) predicts +0.14 D refraction with +33.00 IOL power. After surgery subjective residual refraction was plano. PSF and wavefront error graphics display the bad visual quality of this eye

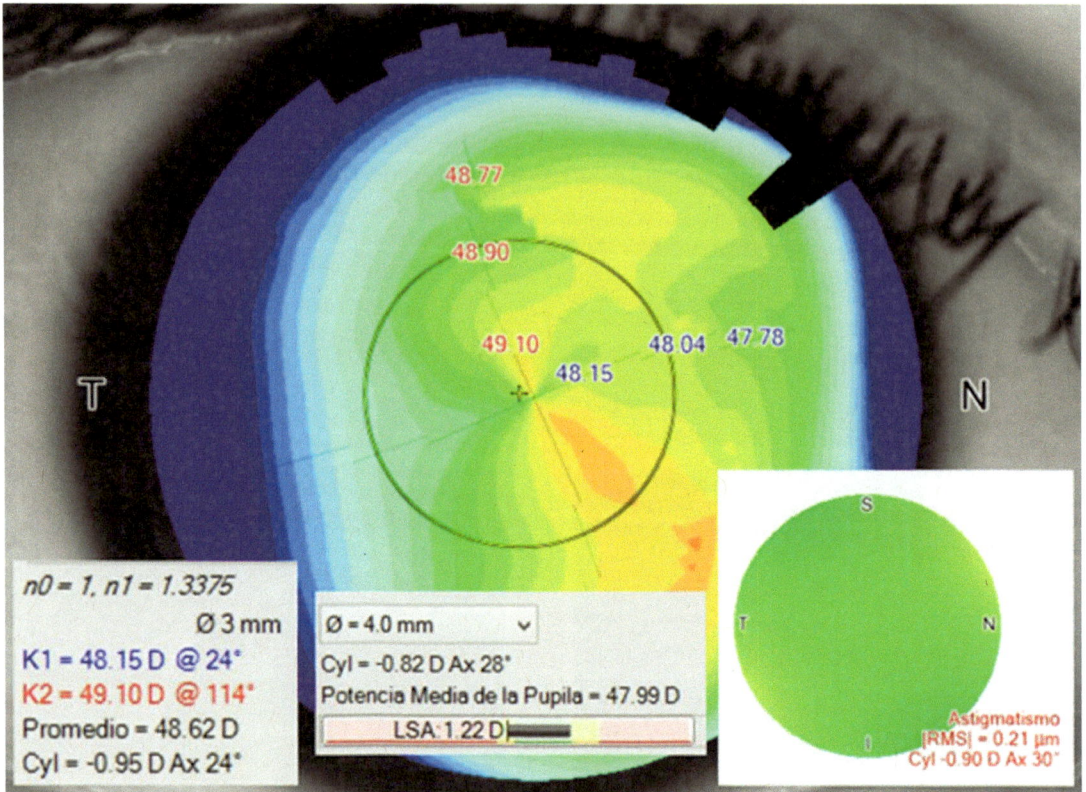

Fig. 15.19 Corneal tomography. Keratometric astigmatism is −0.95 D a 24°, total astigmatism is −0.82 D a 28° and total aberrometric astigmatism (3 mm) is −0.90 D a 30°

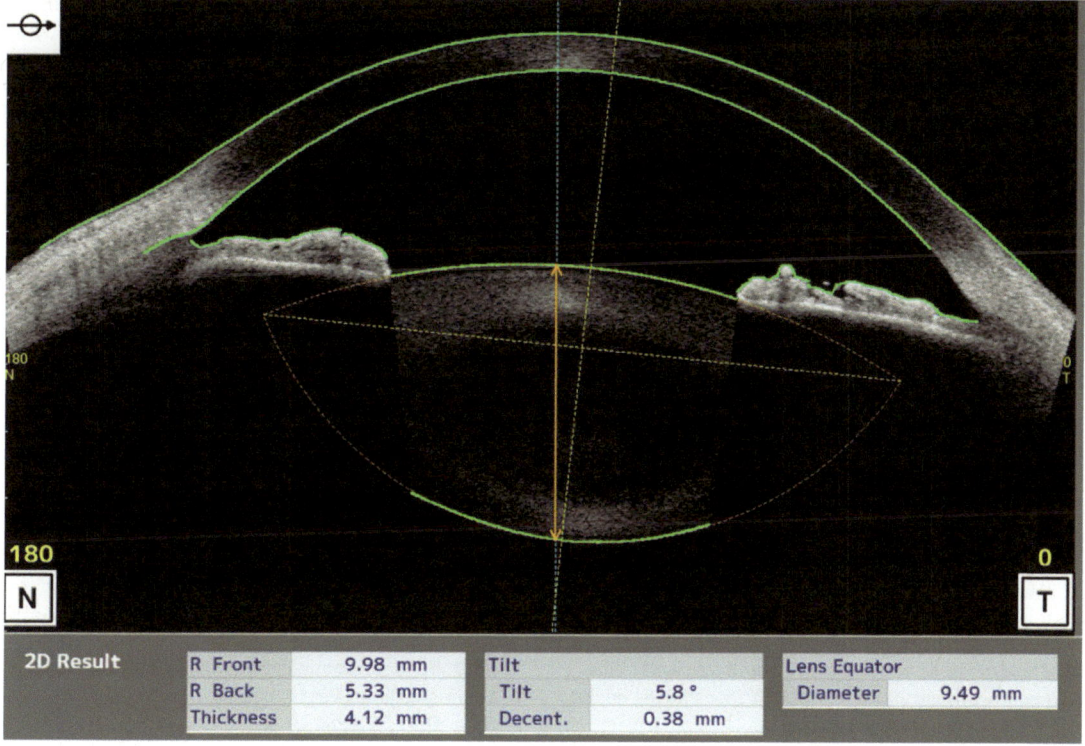

2D Result

			Tilt		Lens Equator	
R Front	9.98 mm		Tilt	5.8 °	Diameter	9.49 mm
R Back	5.33 mm					
Thickness	4.12 mm		Decent.	0.38 mm		

Fig. 15.20 Natural lens analysis with CASIA 2: curvatures, thickness, and tilt are measured

this variable in a theoretical model might improve results in the near future. SS-OCT tomographers can measure the tilt of the natural lens (Fig. 15.20) [47, 48].

References

1. Gills JP, et al. Corneal topography: the state of the art. Thorofare, NJ: Slack Incorporated; 1995. p. 1–328.
2. Ventura BV, Al-Mohtaseb Z, Wang L, Koch DD, Weikert MP. Repeatability and comparability of corneal power and corneal astigmatism obtained from a point-source color light-emitting diode topographer, a Placido-based corneal topographer, and a low-coherence reflectometer. J Cataract Refract Surg. 2015;41(10):2242–50.
3. Kaschke M, Donnerhacke K-H, Rill MS. Optical visualization, imaging, and structural analysis. In: Optical devices in ophthalmology and optometry. 1st ed. Weinheim: Wiley-VCH; 2014.
4. Mattioli R, Carones F, Cantera E. New algorithms to improve the reconstruction of corneal geometry on the keratron videokeratographer. Invest Ophthalmol Vis Sci. 1995;36(Suppl):1400.
5. Klein SA. Axial curvature and the skew ray error in corneal topography. Optom Vis Sci. 1997;74(11):931–44.
6. Cairns G, McGhee CN. Orbscan computerized topography: attributes, applications, and limitations. J Cataract Refract Surg. 2005;31(1):205–20.
7. Wang SB, Cornish EE, Grigg JR, McCluskey PJ. Anterior segment optical coherence tomography and its clinical applications. Clin Exp Optom. 2019;102(3):195–207.
8. Szalai E, Berta A, Hassan Z, et al. Reliability and repeatability of swept-source Fourier-domain optical coherence tomography and Scheimpflug imaging in keratoconus. J Cataract Refract Surg. 2012;38(3):485–94.
9. Aramberri J, Araiz L, Garcia A, Illarramendi I, Olmos J, Oyanarte I, Romay VI. Dual versus single Scheimpflug camera for anterior segment analysis: precision and agreement. J Cataract Refract Surg. 2012;38:19341949.
10. Corbett MC, Rosen ES, O'Brart DPS. Assessment of corneal shape. In: Corneal topography. Principles and applications. 1st ed. London: BMJ Books; 1999.
11. Calossi A. Corneal asphericity and spherical aberration. J Refract Surg. 2007;23(5):505–14.
12. Savini G, Schiano-Lomoriello D, Hoffer KJ. Repeatability of automatic measurements by a new anterior segment optical coherence tomographer combined with Placido topography and agreement

with 2 Scheimpflug cameras. J Cataract Refract Surg. 2018;44(4):471–8.

13. Epitropoulos AT, Matossian C, Berdy GJ, Malhotra RP, Potvin R. Effect of tear osmolarity on repeatability of keratometry for cataract surgery planning. J Cataract Refract Surg. 2015;41:1672–7.

14. Savini G, Bedei A, Barboni P, Ducoli P, Hoffer KJ. Intraocular lens power calculation by ray-tracing after myopic excimer laser surgery. Am J Ophthalmol. 2014;157:150–3.

15. Goto S, Maeda N. Corneal topography for intraocular lens selection in refractive cataract surgery. Ophthalmology. 2020;19. pii: S0161-6420(20)31108-8.

16. Piccinini AL, Golan O, Hafezi F, Randleman JB. Higher-order aberration measurements: comparison between Scheimpflug and dual Scheimpflug-Placido technology in normal eyes. J Cataract Refract Surg. 2019;45(4):490–4.

17. Vinciguerra P, Camesasca FI, Calossi A. Statistical analysis of physiological aberrations of cornea. J Refract Surg. 2003;19:S265–9.

18. Wang L, Dai E, Koch DD, Nathoo A. Optical aberrations of the human anterior cornea. J Cataract Refract Surg. 2003;29:1514–21.

19. Zheleznyak L, Kim MJ, MacRae S, Yoon G. Impact of corneal aberrations on through-focus image quality of presbyopia-correcting intraocular lenses using an adaptive optics bench system. J Cataract Refract Surg. 2012;38(10):1724–33.

20. Colak HN, Kantarci FA, Yildirim A, et al. Comparison of corneal topographic measurements and high order aberrations in keratoconus and normal eyes. Cont Lens Anterior Eye. 2016;39:380–4.

21. Ho WM, Stanojcic N, O'Brart N, O'Brart D. Refractive surprise after routine cataract surgery with multifocal IOLs attributable to corneal epithelial basement membrane dystrophy. J Cataract Refract Surg. 2019;45:685–9.

22. Gibbons A, Ali TK, Waren DP, Donaldson KE. Causes and correction of dissatisfaction after implantation of presbyopia-correcting intraocular lenses. Clin Ophthalmol. 2016;10:1965–70.

23. Chan HH, Zhao Y, Tun TA, Tong L. Repeatability of tear meniscus evaluation using spectral-domain Cirrus® HD-OCT and time-domain Visante® OCT. Cont Lens Anterior Eye. 2015;38(5):368–72.

24. Reinstein DZ, Archer TJ, Gobbe M. Corneal epithelial thickness profile in the diagnosis of keratoconus. J Refract Surg. 2009;25(7):604–10.

25. Ambrosio R Jr, Caiado AL, Guerra FP, et al. Novel pachymetric parameters based on corneal tomography for diagnosing keratoconus. J Refract Surg. 2011;27:753–8.

26. Wang L, Mahmoud AM, Anderson BL, Koch DD, Roberts CJ. Total corneal power estimation: ray tracing method versus gaussian optics formula. Invest Ophthalmol Vis Sci. 2011;52(3):1716–22.

27. Seitz B, Torres F, Langenbucher A, et al. Posterior corneal curvature changes after myopic laser in situ keratomileusis. Ophthalmology. 2001;108:666–73.

28. Tomidokoro A, Oshika T, Amano S, Higaki S, Maeda N, Miyata K. Changes in anterior and posterior corneal curvatures in keratoconus. Ophthalmology. 2000;107:1328–32.

29. Xu K, Qi H, Peng R, Xiao G, Hong J, Hao Y, Ma B. Keratometric measurements and IOL calculations in pseudophakic post-DSAEK patients. BMC Ophthalmol. 2018;18:268.

30. Camellin M, Savini G, Hoffer K, et al. Scheimpflug camera measurement of anterior and posterior corneal curvature in eyes with previous radial keratotomy. J Refract Surg. 2012;28:275–9.

31. Holladay JT, Hill WE, Steinmuller A. Corneal power measurements using Scheimpflug imaging in eyes with prior corneal refractive surgery. J Refract Surg. 2009;25:862–8.

32. Karunaratne N. Comparison of the Pentacam equivalent keratometry reading and IOL Master keratometry measurement in intraocular lens power calculations. Clin Exp Ophthalmol. 2013;41(9):825–34.

33. Lam S, Gupta BK, Hahn JM, Manastersky NA. Refractive outcomes after cataract surgery: Scheimpflug keratometry versus standard automated keratometry in virgin corneas. J Cataract Refract Surg. 2011;37:1984–7.

34. Savini G, Negishi K, Hoffer KJ, Lomoriello DS. Refractive outcomes of intraocular lens power calculation using different corneal power measurements with a new optical biometer. J Cataract Refract Surg. 2018;44:701–8.

35. Holladay JT. Standardizing constants for ultrasonic biometry, keratometry, and intraocular lens power calculations. J Cataract Refract Surg. 1997;23:1356–70.

36. Savini G, Hoffer KJ, Schiano-Lomoriello D, Barboni P. Intraocular lens power calculation using a Placido disk-Scheimpflug tomographer in eyes that had previous myopic corneal excimer laser surgery. J Cataract Refract Surg. 2018;44(8):935–41.

37. Gjerdrum B, Gundersen KG, Lundmark PO, Aakre BM. Refractive precision of ray tracing IOL calculations based on OCT data versus traditional IOL calculation formulas based on reflectometry in patients with a history of laser vision correction for myopia. Clin Ophthalmol. 2021;15:845–57.

38. Young LK, Love GD, Smithson HE. Accounting for the phase, spatial frequency and orientation demands of the task improves metrics based on the visual Strehl ratio. Vis Res. 2013;90:57–6.

39. Holladay JT. Effect of corneal asphericity and spherical aberration on intraocular lens power calculations. J Cataract Refract Surg. 2015;41:1553–4.

40. Fu Y, Kou J, Chen D, Wang D, Zhao Y, Hu M, Lin X, Dai Q, Li J, Zhao YE. Influence of angle kappa and angle alpha on visual quality after implantation of multifocal intraocular lenses. J Cataract Refract Surg. 2019;45(9):1258–64.

41. Karhanová M, Pluháček F, Mlčák P, Vláčil O, Šín M, Marešová K. The importance of angle kappa evaluation for implantation of diffractive multifocal intraocular lenses using pseudophakic eye model. Acta Ophthalmol. 2015;93(2):e123–8.

42. Kessel L, Andresen J, Tendal B, et al. Toric intraocular lenses in the correction of astigmatism during cataract surgery: a systematic review and meta-analysis. Ophthalmology. 2016;123(2):275–86.

43. Koch DD, Ali SF, Weikert MP, et al. Contribution of posterior corneal astigmatism to total corneal astigmatism. J Cataract Refract Surg. 2012;38(12):2080–7.

44. Savini G, Versaci F, Vestri G, et al. Influence of posterior corneal astigmatism on total corneal astigmatism in eyes with moderate to high astigmatism. J Cataract Refract Surg. 2014;40(10):1645–53.

45. Ferreira TB, Ribeiro P, Ribeiro FJ, O'Neill JG. Comparison of methodologies using estimated or measured values of total corneal astigmatism for toric intraocular lens power calculation. J Refract Surg. 2017;33(12):794–800.

46. Kane JX, Connell B. A comparison of the accuracy of 6 modern toric intraocular lens formulas. Ophthalmology. 2020;127(11):1472–86.

47. Hirnschall N, Buehren T, Bajramovic F, Trost M, Teuber T, Findl O. Prediction of postoperative intraocular lens tilt using swept-source optical coherence tomography. J Cataract Refract Surg. 2017;43(6):732–6.

48. Weikert MP, Golla A, Wang L. Astigmatism induced by intraocular lens tilt evaluated via ray tracing. J Cataract Refract Surg. 2018;44:745–9.

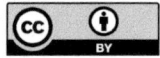

The A-Scan Biometer

16

Maya C. Shammas and H. John Shammas

A-scan ultrasonography has been used for diagnostic purposes since the 1960s. Biometry was then limited to measuring eyes with deformities affecting the axial length (AL), i.e., congenital glaucoma, axial myopia, and phthisis bulbi. Around the mid-1970s, the use of intraocular lenses during cataract surgery gained in popularity and many intraocular lens (IOL) theoretical formulas were published to determine the IOL power. All these formulas required an AL measurement, and A-scan biometry was the only way to accomplish the task. The original units required manual measurement of the ultrasound travel time with a caliper from a Polaroid picture of the A-scan and converting it to millimeters. The measurement was then entered into a calculator to obtain the IOL power needed for emmetropia. Through the years, the ultrasound biometer evolved with the introduction of electronic gates, automatic calibration, and computerized capabilities. Most available A-scan biometers are now compact, efficient, computerized, and complete with IOL power calculation capabilities.

Routine use of A-scan ultrasound biometry has been largely replaced by the more accurate, precise, and reproducible optical biometry. However, the use of optical biometry is limited when measuring eyes with a mature cataract or other vitreoretinal pathology. A-scan biometry is needed in these cases. A-scan biometry can be achieved by contact or immersion techniques. The contact technique applanates the probe against the cornea to obtain the measurements; errors can occur with axial length measurements from excessive indentation of the probe against the cornea. With the immersion technique, the probe is immersed in a gonioscopic solution or balanced salt solution (BSS) contained within a scleral shell; because it does not cause indentation of the cornea, the results are more reliable and therefore the preferred method whenever possible.

Basic Technology

An ultrasound unit is composed of four basic elements: *the pulser*, *the receiver*, and *the display screen* all contained within the same chassis and connected to *the transducer*, located at the tip of the probe by an electrically shielded cable (Fig. 16.1a). The pulser produces electrical pulses at a rate of 1000 pulses/s. Each pulse will excite the electrodes of the piezo-electric crystal of the transducer, generating sound waves. The returning echoes are received by the transducer and transformed into electrical signals. These signals are processed in the receiver and demodulator and then displayed on the screen.

M. C. Shammas
Shammas Eye Center, Lynwood, CA, USA

H. J. Shammas (✉)
Ophthalmology, The Keck School of Medicine of USC, Los Angeles, CA, USA

© The Author(s) 2024
J. Aramberri et al. (eds.), *Intraocular Lens Calculations*, Essentials in Ophthalmology,
https://doi.org/10.1007/978-3-031-50666-6_16

Fig. 16.1 (**a**) An ultrasound unit is composed of four basic elements: the pulser, the receiver, and the display screen all contained within the same chassis and connected to the transducer, located at the tip of the probe by an electrically shielded cable. (**b**) The piezo-electric principle: changes in the polarity of an electric current passing through a quartz crystal will cause changes in the shape and size of the crystal, and vice versa. This in turn will transform the electrical energy into mechanical energy in the form of sound waves. When the sound waves return to the probe, the mechanical energy will modify the thickness of the crystal and produce electrical energy. (**c**) A crystal with a flat surface emits a non-focused beam, essential for biometry. (**d**) A crystal with a concave surface emits a focused beam essential for B-scan echography

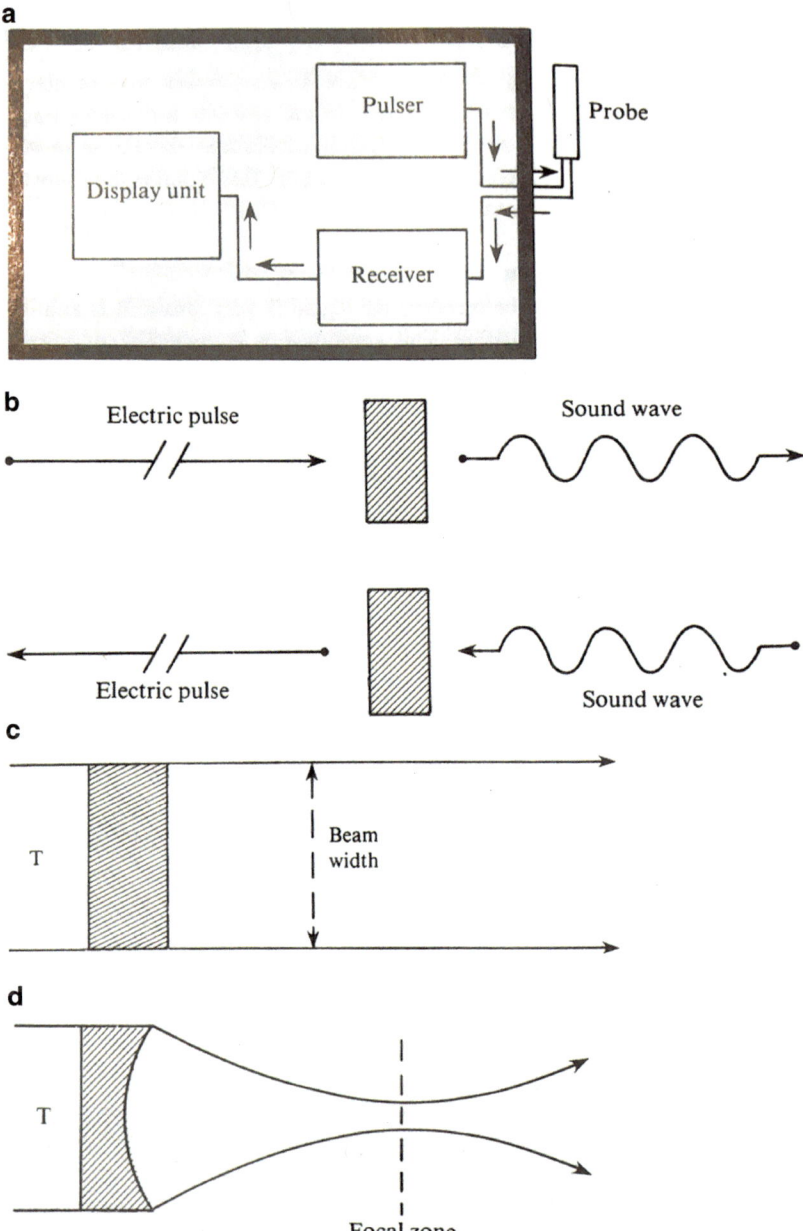

This process is based on the piezo-electric principle (Fig. 16.1b); changes in the polarity of an electric current passing through a quartz crystal will cause changes in the shape and size of the crystal, and vice versa. This in turn will transform the electrical energy into mechanical energy in the form of sound waves. When the sound waves return to the probe, the mechanical energy will modify the thickness of the crystal and produce electrical energy. The performance of the crystal depends mainly on its shape and thickness. A flat surface emits a non-focused beam (Fig. 16.1c) essential for biometry; a concave surface emits a focused beam essential for B-scan echography (Fig. 16.1d).

Physical Principles of A-Scan Ultrasound

Ultrasound refers to sound waves beyond the range of human hearing. In order to make this definition more precise and to explain the properties of ultrasound, we must first explain *sound*. Consider knocking on a door. When the knuckles of the hand strike the door's surface, the molecules of which the door is made are temporarily forced closer together. The compression or "mechanical disturbance" has thus *moved* or "propagated" deeper into the "medium" which is the material of the door. Disturbances which propagate in this way are generally called *waves*; hence, we speak of "sound waves."

A *point source* of sound creates a spherical wavefront, with sound propagating in all directions away from the source. A piston-like sound source creates a quasi-planar wavefront, with sound propagating mostly in a single direction, as shown in Fig. 16.2.

When the piston is moving repetitively back and forth at a constant *frequency,* we can plot a graph of the piston's position against time and we would obtain a curve as shown in Fig. 16.3. Such a curve is called *periodic* because it repeats itself continuously. The smallest repeated portion is called a *cycle*, and the length of time required for one cycle is called the *period*. The study of periodic sound provides the theoretical basis of ophthalmic ultrasound. Frequency is measured in cycles per second, also called *Hertz* (after Heinrich Hertz, a German physicist who studied wave phenomena at the end of the nineteenth century), which is abbreviated Hz. One *kilohertz*, abbreviated kHz, equals 1000 cycles/s. One *megahertz*, abbreviated MHz, equals 1,000,000 cycles/s. The healthy human ear can detect sound frequencies in a range of about 20 Hz to as much as 20 kHz. *Ultrasound* is sound at frequencies well above the 20 kHz.

Real-world ultrasound equipment generates sound pulses whose energy is confined to a lim-

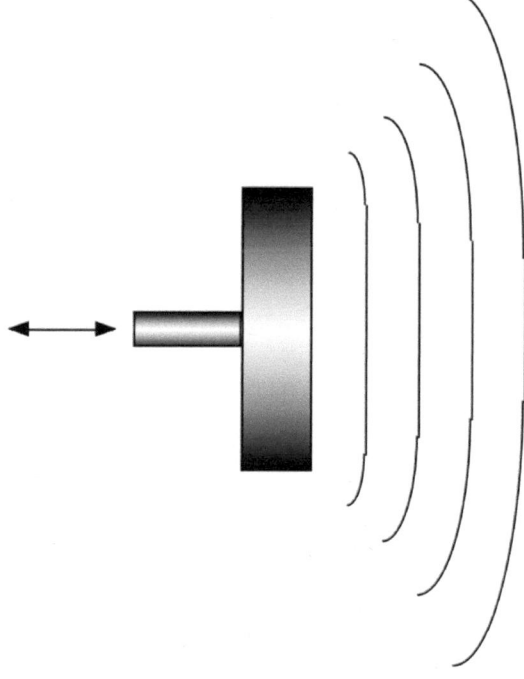

Fig. 16.2 Quasi-planar wavefronts created by a broad, flat sound source (piston)

ited range or *band* of frequencies. The size of the range is called the *bandwidth*. The midpoint of the range is called the *center frequency*. Both are typically measured in MHz. A typical A-scan biometry system, for example, might have a center frequency of 10 MHz and a bandwidth of 4–6 MHz.

The amount of distance corresponding to one cycle (Fig. 16.4) is called the *wavelength*, and it depends on both the *frequency* of the sound and the speed or *velocity* at which it propagates through the medium, according to the formula:

$$\lambda = v / f$$

where "λ" represents wavelength, "v" represents velocity, and "f" represents frequency. Most ocular ultrasound images work at frequencies of 8–10 MHz. The average velocity of sound in human tissue is about 1550 m/s. 10 MHz sound in human tissue has a wavelength of 155 µm (millionths of a meter).

Fig. 16.3 Piston's position plotted against time

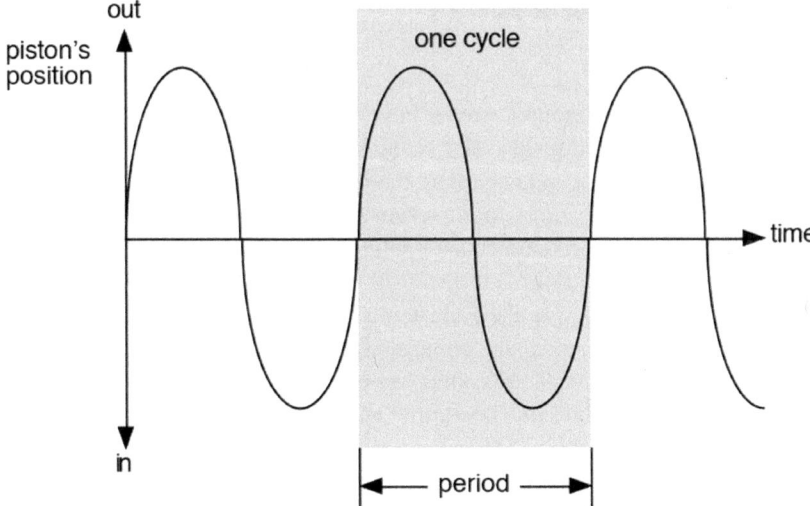

Fig. 16.4 Plot of sound pressure vs. distance along sound beam, at a single instant

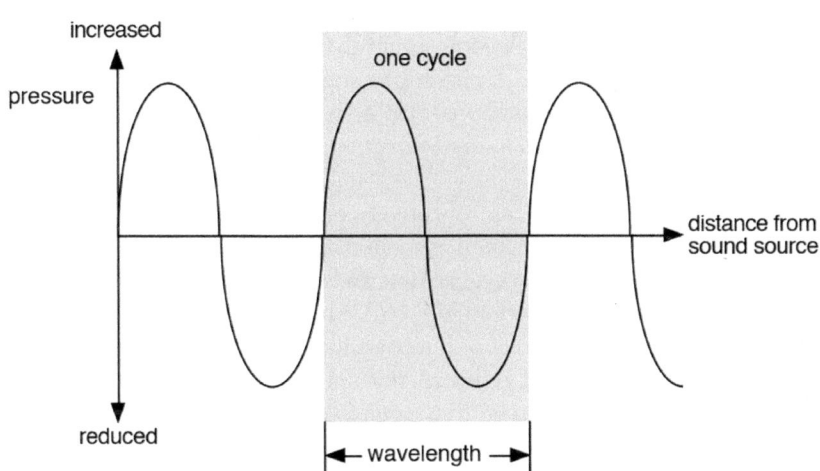

Major Components of a Biometer

Four different components are herein discussed including the probe and its transducer, the sensitivity setting, the velocity setting, and data analysis with IOL calculation.

The Probe and Its Transducer

The probe is connected to the main chassis of the biometry by an electronically shielded cable and contains a transducer at its tip [1–3]: The original solid probe (Fig. 16.5) has been designed for standardized A-scan echography using the Kretztechnik 7200 MA ultrasound unit. This probe can also be used to measure the axial length through an immersion technique. The newer probe (Fig. 16.6) is thinner and designed specifically for biometry.

The transducer emits the ultrasound beam. Ultrasound consists of high-frequency sound waves over 20,000 cycles/s, which is the highest frequency audible to the human ear [4]. The ultrasound beam is formed of ultrasound waves that display different characteristics depending on the ultrasound frequency, wavelength, velocity, and direction.

The *frequency* [5] is the number of hertz (Hz) or cycles per second. Higher frequencies provide

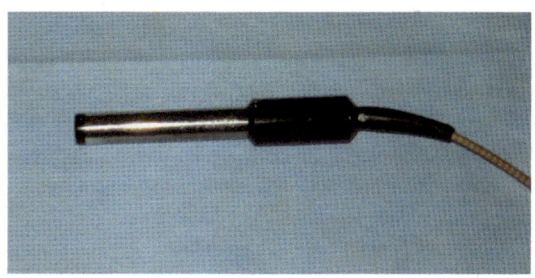

Fig. 16.5 The Kretztechnik 7200 solid probe is used for diagnostic standardized A-scanning and for biometry

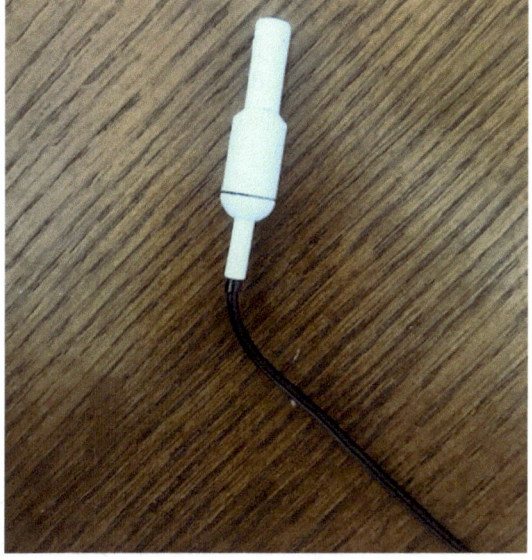

Fig. 16.6 Smaller solid probe designed for biometry

a higher resolution while lower frequencies provide better penetration but a reduction in the resolution. To obtain the high resolution needed for axial length measurement, biometry units use ultrasound frequencies ranging between 8 and 25 MHz (1 MHz = 1 megahertz = 1 million cycles/s).

The *wavelength* [6] is the distance between two particles in the same phase of oscillation. Within the ocular tissues, the wavelength is approximately 0.19 mm if an 8 MHz probe is used and 0.15 mm if a 10 MHz probe is used.

The *velocity* [7] is the speed of sound propagation and is expressed in meters per second (m/s). The velocity varies according to the medium through which sound propagates; within

the eye, the ultrasound velocity is 1532 m/s in aqueous and vitreous, 1640 m/s in a clear lens, and 1550 m/s in solid tissues. During an accurate measurement of the different eye components, the proper sound speed must be used for each of these entities.

The *direction* of the ultrasound beam [8, 9] affects the display of the tissues under examination. During biometry, the emitted sound beam will meet multiple interfaces. At each interface, part of the sound beam is reflected toward the probe and the remainder of the sound beam keeps propagating deeper into the tissues. This process will generate echo spikes from the different interfaces that have been intersected, i.e., anterior surface of the cornea, posterior surface of the cornea, anterior surface of the lens, posterior surface of the lens, anterior surface of the retina, and anterior surface of the sclera. When the ultrasound beam reaches the orbital tissues, it is attenuated until it loses all its energy. The sound beam returns to the transducer that also acts as a receiver. The pulses are then processed within the biometer to display "echo-signals" on the screen.

The Sensitivity Setting

The sensitivity setting controls the height of the echo spikes displayed on the screen.

The axial length is more accurately measured at a lower system sensitivity that allows a better pattern recognition of the anterior and posterior corneal surfaces, anterior and posterior lens surfaces, and anterior retinal surface.

The Velocity Setting

The velocity setting controls the speed of sound propagation. The velocity, measured in meters per second (m/s), varies according to the medium through which sound propagates. Most units use an average velocity of 1548–1556 m/s in a cataractous eye and 1532 m/s in an aphakic eye. Newer units measure each ocular compartment at its correct velocity; the anterior chamber depth is measured with a velocity of 1532 m/s; the cataractous lens is measured with an average velocity of 1640 m/s; the vitreous cavity's depth is measured with a velocity of 1532 m/s like the aqueous. These measurements are then computed within the instrument to display one axial length reading.

The Electronic Gates

Electronic gates allow ultrasound units to provide an electronic read-out of the axial length in millimeters. The gates will measure the travel time between the leading edges of the spikes (Fig. 16.7) or the peaks of the spikes (Fig. 16.8). Biometers are equipped with 2, 4, or 5 gates. The two main gates are the "corneal gate" placed in

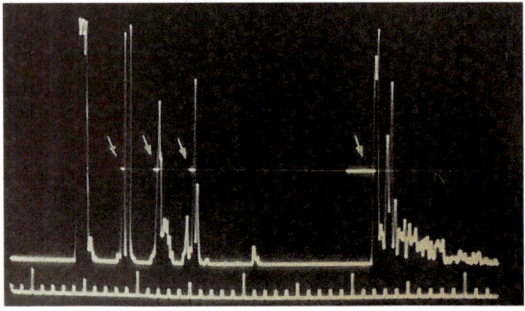

Fig. 16.7 The four gates of this horizontal caliper lights (arrows) measure the distances between the leading edges of the anterior corneal surface, anterior lens surface, posterior lens surface, and the retina

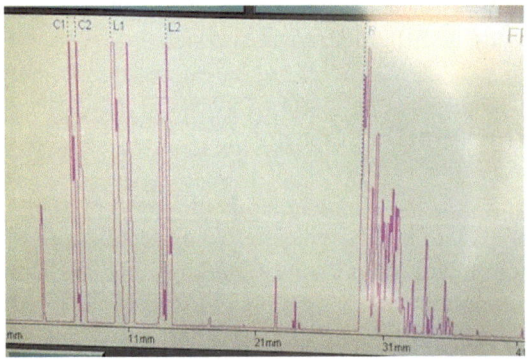

Fig. 16.8 Five vertical gates (dotted lines) measure the distances between the peaks of the anterior cornea (C_1), the posterior cornea (C_2), anterior lens surface (L_1), posterior lens surface (L_2), and retina (R)

the region of the anterior corneal spike and the "retinal gate" placed in the region of the retinal spike. Such instruments measure the travel time between the anterior surface of the cornea and the anterior surface of the retina and use an average sound velocity for the measurement of the axial length.

Instruments equipped with four gates (Fig. 16.7) allow the positioning of these gates over the leading edges or the peaks of the echoes generated from the anterior surface of the cornea, the anterior surface of the lens, posterior surface of the cornea, the anterior surface of the lens, the posterior surface of the lens, and the anterior surface of the retina. A measurement of the anterior chamber depth, lens thickness, and the total axial length is displayed on the screen.

Instruments equipped with five gates (Fig. 16.8) will additionally locate the posterior corneal surface and include a measurement of the corneal thickness.

Data Analysis and IOL Calculation

Most biometers will analyze the measurements and will display the axial length, anterior chamber depth, and lens thickness. IOL power calculations are provided using available modern formulas. Many will be able to provide a print out or connect directly to an imaging system or Electronic Medical Record. These programs are also able to store information, compare results, review data, and refine the ELP constants.

Choosing the Appropriate Ultrasound Biometer

Most biometers provide reproducible and accurate measurements and are programmed with popular formulas. However, each biometer is characterized by specific features and components that have been discussed in length in this chapter. Here are some essential features to look for in a biometer:

– A display screen that allows pattern recognition of the displayed echogram. Biometers shaped like a pen without a display unit are not advisable.
– Measurement capability of the anterior chamber depth and of the lens thickness, in addition to measuring the entire axial length. Newer formulas require these measurements.
– Measurement capability of aphakic and pseudophakic eyes.
– A freeze frame capability and a print out of the A-scan echogram for review.
– Visible electronic gates.
– IOL power calculation capability.

Some biometers are available with diagnostic B-scan, ultrasound biomicroscopy (UBM), and/or pachymetry within the same chassis. Practices that handle vitreoretinal pathology and/or perform corneal surgery will enjoy the added features in one compact unit.

Commonly Used Ultrasound Biometers

There are many excellent ultrasound machines available. Here is a list of some of the currently available machines. All the companies offer models that complete axial length measurements utilizing contact or immersion technique, measure anterior chamber depth and lens thickness, and have formulas pre-programmed in their system (Table 16.1).

Table 16.1 Commonly used ultrasound biometers

Company	Product	Additional features	Other models
Quantel Medical/Ellex	Aviso S	Pachymetry UBM B scan	Aviso Axis Nano Compact
MEDA	ODM-2200	B scan	MD-1000A
Suoer	SW-1000P	Pachymetry Tonometry	SW-1000
Keeler	Accutome A-Scan Plus Connect	Optional UBM Optional B scan	
Nidek	US-4000	Pachymetry B scan	US-500
Sonomed	MV4500 Master-Vu	Optional B scan	
DGH	Scanmate A Flex	Alignment ranking UBM B scan	Scanmate A
Ellex/Quantel	Eye Cubed	UBM B scan	
Tomey	AL-4000	Auto alignment	AL-100
SonoStar	SPA-100	Pachymetry	
Micromedical	PalmScan AP2000 Pro	Pachymetry Mobile	A2000T, AP2000T, A2000

References

1. Buschman W. Special transducer probes for diagnostic ultrasonography of the eyeball. In: Goldberg R, Sarin L, editors. Ultrasonics in ophthalmology. Philadelphia: W.B. Saunders Co.; 1967. p. 87–101.
2. Coleman DJ, Carlin B. Transducer alignment and electronic measurement of visual axis dimensions in the human eye using time amplitude ultrasound. In:

Oksala A, Gernet H, editors. Ultrasonics in ophthalmology. Basel: S. Karger; 1967. p. 207–13.

3. Gordon D. Transducer design for ultrasonic ophthalmology. In: Gitter K, et al., editors. Ophthalmic ultrasound. St. Louis: The C.V. Mosby Co.; 1969. p. 65–6.

4. Shammas HJ. Atlas of ophthalmic ultrasonography and biometry. St. Louis: The C.V. Mosby Co.; 1984. p. 273–308.

5. Herrman G, Buschmann W. Methods of measuring the HF oscillation frequency in ultrasound pulses of equipment for diagnostic ultrasonography. Ophthalmol Res. 1972;3:274–82.

6. Till P. Solid tissue model for the standardization of the echo-ophthalmograph 7200 MA (Kretztechnik). Doc Ophthalmol. 1976;41:205–40.

7. Ludwig GD. The velocity of sound through tissues and the acoustic impedence of tissue. J Acoust Soc Am. 1950;22:862–6.

8. Lizzi F, Burt W, Coleman DJ. Effects of ocular structures on the propagation of ultrasound in the eye. Arch Ophthalmol. 1970;84:635–40.

9. Lowe R. Time amplitude ultrasonography for ocular biometry. Am J Ophthalmol. 1968;66:913–8.

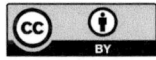

Oliver Klaproth

Introduction

The ZEISS IOLMaster 700 with SWEPT Source Biometry® is the latest optical biometer in the more than 20-year long history of biometry innovation from ZEISS (Fig. 17.1). It combines all measurements required for modern IOL power calculation formulas at very precise levels [1]. It combines those with innovative technologies to support the improvement of refractive outcomes such as Total Keratometry (TK®), which enables the use of posterior corneal curvature measurements in IOL power calculation [2–5], the cornea-to-retina scan, the unique fixation check [6], and central topography. The ZEISS IOLMaster 700 is an integral part of the ZEISS Cataract Workflow, which enables remote IOL power calculation and surgical planning, IOL ordering, and more, in combination ZEISS EQ Workplace® for ZEISS FORUM® and ZEISS Veracity® Surgical software. It also enables markerless toric IOL alignment in combination with ZEISS CALLISTO eye® for surgical microscopes OPMI LUMERA® or ARTEVO® 800. It adheres to applicable DICOM standards and can therefore be networked with EMR and PACS systems. Overall, the ZEISS IOLMaster 700 builds on more than 20 years of experience in optical biometry, delivers precise and reliable measurements, and helps optimizing clinical cataract workflows [2, 3, 7]. It is designed to increase patient throughput and for getting fewer refractive surprises.

O. Klaproth (✉)
ZEISS Ophthalmology, Berlin, Germany
e-mail: oliver.klaproth@zeiss.com

J. Aramberri et al. (eds.), *Intraocular Lens Calculations*, Essentials in Ophthalmology,
https://doi.org/10.1007/978-3-031-50666-6_17

Fig. 17.1 ZEISS
IOLMaster 700

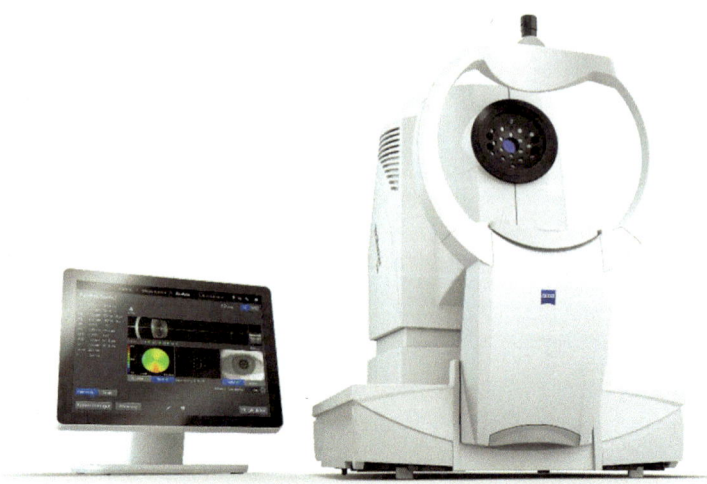

SWEPT Source Biometry®

OCT Technology

The ZEISS IOLMaster 700 is a SWEPT Source OCT Biometer that operates at a wavelength from 1035 to 1080 nm with a scanning rate of 2 kHz and 44 mm scan depth, to generate a 2D OCT cornea-to-retina cross-section scan of the eye in six meridians (0°, 30°, 60°, 90°, 120°, and 150°). Each meridional scan is averaged from three single scans. This technology is used to derive all axial biometry measurements, including **axial lengths**, **central corneal thickness**, **anterior chamber depths** from epithelium and endothelium, and **lens thickness**, at very precise levels (Table 17.1) [4, 5, 9–17].

The seamless cornea-to-retina cross-section scan furthermore aids surgeons in detecting unusual eye geometries. In contrast to A-Scan biometers, it furthermore enables to verify the correctness of measurements by displaying the anatomical structures and overlaying the seg-mentation used for axial measurements (Fig. 17.2).

The ZEISS IOLMaster 700 is designed to optimize workflow efficiency, even when handling dense cataracts.

The combination of SWEPT Source OCT 6-meridian scan pattern and the use of approx. 1055 nm wavelengths (rather than, for example, 1300 nm, which has a higher energy absorption rate in the vitreous) enables a cataract penetration rate of up to 99% [18].

Unique Fixation Check

The ZEISS IOLMaster 700 also utilizes the SWEPT Source OCT to take a horizontal cross section image of the central 1 mm of the macula, which is averaged from 4 scans (Fig. 17.2). This enables users to verify whether the axial lengths and keratometry measurement were taken during correct fixation, to reduce the risk of refractive surprises due to incorrect measurements caused by undetected poor fixation.

Table 17.1   ZEISS IOLMaster 700 technical data

Measurement range	• Axial length 14–38 mm
	• Corneal radii 5–11 mm
	• Anterior chamber depth 0.7–8 mm
	• Lens thickness
	  – 1–10 mm (phakic eye)
	  – 0.13–2.5 mm (pseudophakic eye)
	• Central corneal thickness 0.2–1.2 mm
	• Corneal diameter 8–16 mm

Display scaling	• Axial length 0.01 mm • Corneal radii 0.01 mm • Anterior chamber depth 0.01 mm • Lens thickness 0.01 mm • Central corneal thickness 1 µm • Corneal diameter 0.1 mm
SD of repeatability [8]	• Axial length 5 µm • Corneal radii 0.09 D • Cylinder >0.75 D, axis 3.8° • Anterior chamber depth 7 µm • Lens thickness 6 µm • Central corneal thickness 2.5 µm • Corneal diameter 111 µm
IOL calculation formulas	• See Table 17.2
Interfaces	• ZEISS VERACITY surgical • ZEISS EQ workplace • ZEISS EQ Mobile • ZEISS FORUM eye care data management system • ZEISS computer-assisted cataract surgery system CALLISTO eye (via USB, EQ workplace and EQ Mobile, and FORUM) • Data interface for electronic medical record (EMR)/patient management systems (PMS) • Holladay IOL consultant software and PhacoOptics® • Data export to USB storage media, including comprehensive CSV batch export. • Ethernet port for network connection and network printer • Import of IOL data from IOLCon.org
Line voltage	• 100–240 V ± 10%
Line frequency	• 50–60 Hz
Power consumptions	• Max. 150 VA
Laser class	• 1

Fig. 17.2 ZEISS
IOLMaster analysis
screen, showing
measurement values,
SS-OCT images, central
topography maps,
telecentric 3-kone
keratometry spots, and
CD/reference images,
and plausibility checks

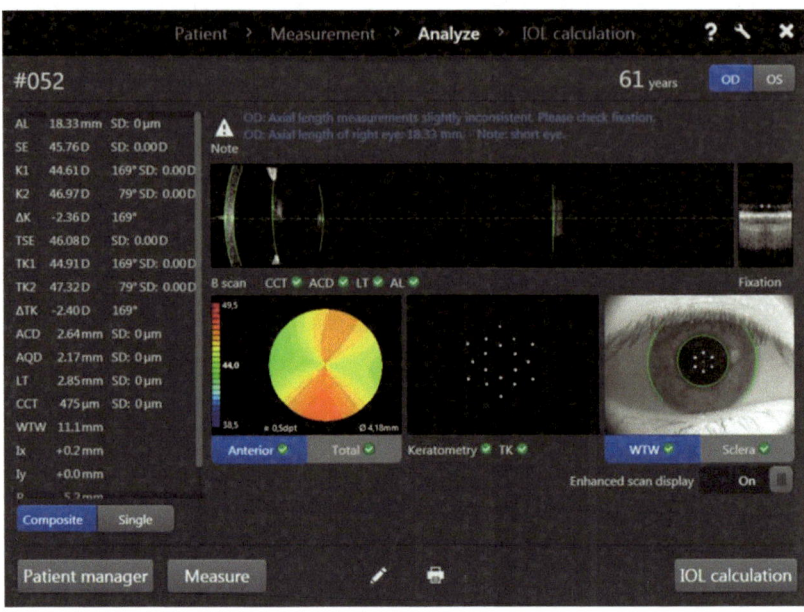

Distance Independent Telecentric 3-Zone Keratometry

Telecentric Keratometry utilizes projection of keratometry points on the cornea via a parallel ray system, rather than reflecting divergent light directly from LEDs, thus simulating an infinite light source incident on the precorneal tear film. The light spots are then diffusely reflected by the tear film. Due to an aperture stop placed in the focus of the objective lens in the observation beam path, only the rays parallel to the optical axis are detected by the sensor. A slight change of distance between the cornea and the objective thus has no effect on the measurement.

Keratometry values are generated in 3 zones out of 18 spots in an area of about 3.2 mm for an 8 mm radius cornea. The system is designed to sample local irregularities in the central zone of the cornea into the final keratometry, which would not be possible with a ring measurement only. This 3-zone approach also allows for measurement of the central topography (see below). The keratometry measurement is repeated 15 times, with an algorithm detecting and erasing outliers and providing warnings to users in case of inconsistencies between single measurements or the different measurement rings. This telecen-

tric approach to keratometry has proven to be precise and repeatable in many studies. [4, 5, 9–17]

The **keratometric index** on the IOLMaster 700 can be chosen by the user to match individual requirements. The choice of keratometric index has no effect on IOL power calculation though, as for the internal calculation algorithms, only directly measured radii are used, which are unaffected by the keratometric index.

Additional Measurements

Angle Alpha- and Kappa-Chords

The ZEISS IOLMaster 700 measures the Subject Fixated—Coaxially Sighted Corneal Light Reflex (SF-CSCLR) as described by Chang and Waring [19], or corneal vertex, which gives an approximation of the position of the corneal intercept of the visual axis. It then displays the **chord of angle alpha** and the **chord of angle kappa**, as the angles (in degrees) cannot be measured directly. The chords are defined as the distance between the corneal vertex and the limbus center (alpha)/ the pupil center (kappa). They are displayed either in cartesian (*Ix/Iy* and *Px*, *Py*, for alpha and kappa, respectively) or polar coordinates (alpha (chord) and kappa (chord)/CW-Chord, respectively).

Corneal and Pupil Diameter

The horizontal corneal diameter and pupil diameter are measured from the image of the eye taken at 860–880 nm.

Total Keratometry: Replacing Assumptions with Measurements

Principle of Total Keratometry

A known limitation of classic keratometry is that the posterior surface of the cornea is not measured but considered via a keratometric index only. However, several studies have confirmed that posterior corneal astigmatism magnitude and axis orientation cannot be adequately predicted by measuring the anterior corneal curvature alone [20–22]. Therefore, nomograms and mathematical models have been created in order to predict the posterior surface astigmatism and optimize toric IOL power calculation [23–25]. Yet, these methods are based on theoretical assumptions of posterior corneal astigmatism and, therefore, generally cannot fully account for outliers and irregularities.

This led ZEISS to the development of technology able to measure, not estimate, the posterior curvature: **Total Keratometry (TK®)** [22]. TK® considers measured corneal thickness and measured posterior corneal curvature in addition to the anterior corneal curvature measurements. It combines telecentric 3-Zone Keratometry of the ZEISS IOLMaster 700 with its SWEPT Source OCT cornea-to-retina scan [4, 11, 26].

TK® has been designed to match the Gullstrand ratio in normal eyes. However, it still can detect the impact of posterior astigmatism in individual eyes, such as eyes with post corneal laser vision correction. An additional significant advantage of this approach is that TK® can be directly incorporated in classic IOL power calculation

formulas, while using existing optimized IOL constants, such as ULIB and IOLCon [27, 28].

Precision of Total Keratometry Measurements

Goggin and LaHood first published data confirming that the ZEISS IOLMaster 700 is capable of measuring the posterior corneal surface [22]. Savini et al. [29] assessed the repeatability of TK® and standard keratometry measurements provided by ZEISS IOLMaster 700. They conclude that TK® measurements offer high repeatability in unoperated and post-excimer laser surgery eyes.

Clinical Results with Total Keratometry in Non-toric and Toric IOL Power Calculation

While TK® values are equivalent to K values in normal eyes, they will differ in eyes with an unusual ratio of anterior-to-posterior corneal curvature or in patients with an unusual posterior astigmatism. In these cases, the classic posterior corneal astigmatism nomograms cannot detect these outliers, while TK® can. Therefore, one can expect that TK® and K will overall perform relatively similar in terms of mean refractive outcomes after cataract surgery in normal eyes. However, TK® will be able to help surgeons avoid outliers or refractive surprises in the unusual cases mentioned above. Published studies by Fabian and Wehner or Srivannaboon and Chirapapaisan confirm this behavior with respect to spherical equivalent and cylinder prediction errors [27, 28].

Clinical Performance of Total Keratometry in Post-corneal Refractive Surgery Eyes

Eyes after refractive corneal laser surgery are the most prominent example of unusual anterior and posterior corneal curvature ratio, as the anterior surface has been altered. In these eyes,

TK® becomes very beneficial, as it does not rely on assumptions on the posterior surface but is a measurement of total corneal power taking actual posterior corneal curvatures into consideration.

Wang et al. have shown, for example, that TK® can be used in classic IOL power calculation formulas such as the Haigis formula, resulting in overall similar results like specifically designed post-LVC formulas as the Barrett True K without taking historical refraction data into account [30].

Lawless et al. have shown in their publication that when using the Barrett True K TK® formula,

which was specifically designed for TK®, it outperformed any other non-history formula in postmyopic LASIK eyes evaluated in this study [31] (Fig. 17.3). They also confirm, that Haigis with TK provides similar results as Barrett True K with K and no history.

Yeo et al. analyzed in this open-access paper 64 eyes with previous myopic laser refractive surgery by comparing the prediction error on different formulas [32]. In their analysis, EVO with TK® followed by Barrett True-K TK® and Haigis with TK® achieved the highest percentages of patients with absolute prediction error within 0.50 and 1.00 D (Fig. 17.4).

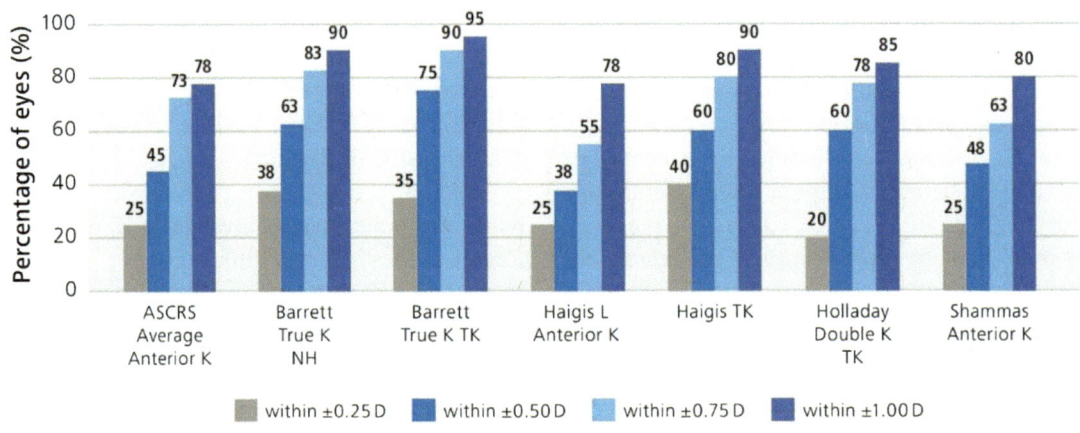

Fig. 17.3 Percentage of eyes within 0.25, 0.50, 0.75, and 1.00 D of absolute prediction error; no-history formulas followed by formulas using TK. (Taken from Lawless et al. 2020)

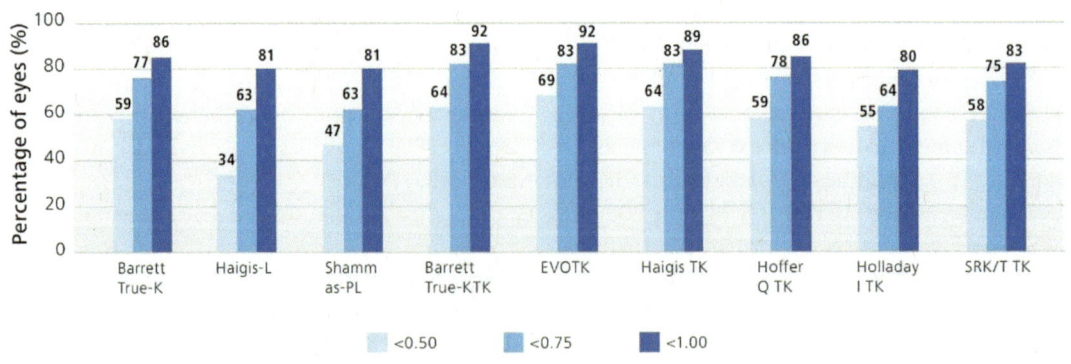

Fig. 17.4 Percentage of eyes within 0.50, 0.75, and 1.00 D of absolute prediction error. (Taken from Yeo et al. 2020)

Central Topography: Starting Your Workflow with More Insights

Central topography combines keratometry data from the 3-Zone Telecentric Keratometry with data of the corneal thickness measurement of the SWEPT Source OCT to create a **total axial power map** from the anterior and posterior corneal surface. This provides surgeons with more information on the central corneal shape right from the start without changing workflow or taking more time (Fig. 17.2).

Wang et al. compared central topography maps to topographic maps from a Placido-dual-Scheimpflug Topographer. This study included 105 eyes with various corneal conditions such as regular/irregular corneas, previous corneal refractive surgery, and keratoconus or pellucid marginal degeneration. In 68.6–89.5%, similar overall shape was observed which leads to the same decision for premium IOL selection in 75.2–97.1% of cases [33].

Markerless Toric IOL Alignment

The ZEISS IOLMaster 700 is able to acquire a red-free (520 nm) image of the limbal vessels and iris structures during the keratometry measurement.

Both reference image and keratometry data (Fig. 17.5) can be transferred to ZEISS CALLISTO® eye, e.g., together with your surgical planning from VERACITY® Surgical or EQ Workplace. During surgery, the image is then used for intraoperative matching with the live eye image. All data needed is displayed in the eyepiece or 3D screen of the surgical microscopes OPMI LUMERA® or ARTEVO® 800 from ZEISS. Preoperative corneal marking and additional measurements for Toric IOL alignment thus become obsolete. Solomon and Ladas conclude that within their study, the use of ZEISS CALLISTO® eye yields less remaining refractive cylinder than Toric IOL placement guided by intraoperative aberrometry [3].

Fig. 17.5 Example of IOLMaster 700 reference image with planned toric IOL, predicted refraction, formula information, and implantation axis information based on TK®

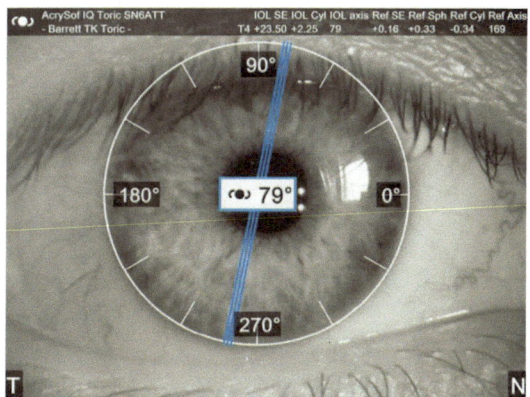

IOL Power Calculation

The ZEISS IOLMaster 700 offers a broad range of formula to calculate IOLs for a wide range of eyes, from long to short eyes, including toric IOL power calculation (Fig. 17.6) and post-corneal refractive surgery IOL power calculation, including post-RK cases (Table 17.2).

The ZEISS IOLMaster 700 supports import of IOL power steps and ranges as well as constants from the IOLCon.org website. Download of IOL data directly from IOLCon.org is recommended to always have access to the latest and best optimized IOL data directly from the respective IOL manufacturer.

Fig. 17.6 ZEISS IOLMaster 700 toric IOL power calculation report

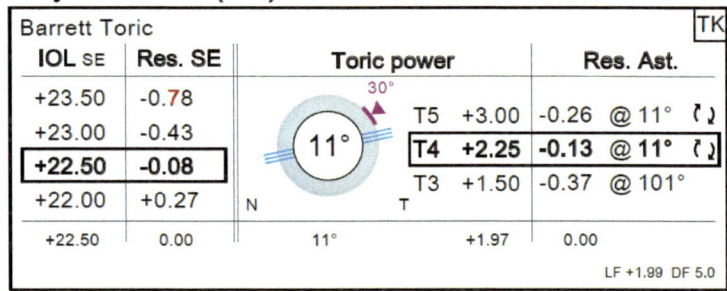

Table 17.2 IOL power calculation formulas available on ZEISS IOLMaster 700, ZEISS EQ Workplace, and ZEISS Veracity Surgical (June 2021)

Formula	K/TK	Non-toric	Toric	Post-refractive surgery	Post-refractive surgery toric	IOLMaster 700	EQ Workplace	Veracity Surgery Planner (US only)
Abulafia-Koch	K		•					•
SRK/T	K/TK®	•				•	•	•
Hoffer Q	K/TK®	•				•	•	•
Holladay Holladay 1 Holladay 2	K/TK®	•				•	•	•
Haigis suite						•	•	
Haigis	K/TK®	•		• TK® only				
Haigis-T	K/TK®		•		• TK® only			
Haigis-L	K			•				
Haigis-L toric	K				•			
Barrett suite	K/TK®					•	•	•
Barrett universal II		•						
Barrett toric calculator			•					
Barrett true K				•				
Barrett true K toric					•			
Kane suite	K/TK®						• (2024)	•
Kane		•						
Kane toric			•					
Z CALC (ZEISS IOL only)	K/TK®	•	•	•	•		•	

ZEISS Cataract Workflow

ZEISS offers a selection of software solutions to complement the ZEISS IOLMaster 700 and help cataract surgeons to streamline their cataract workflow. From a wider selection of formulas, remote IOL power calculation, remote surgery planning, constant optimization, IOL ordering to postop quality assessment. Those will be addressed in the following chapter: ZEISS Cataract Workflow.

References

1. Montés-Micó R, Pastor-Pascual F, Ruiz-Mesa R, Tañá-Rivero P. Ocular biometry with swept-source optical coherence tomography. J Cataract Refract Surg. 2021;47:802–14.
2. Mayer WJ, Kreutzer T, Dirisamer M, Kern C, Kortuem K, Vounotrypidis E, Priglinger S, Kook D. Comparison of visual outcomes, alignment accuracy, and surgical time between 2 methods of corneal marking for toric intraocular lens implantation. J Cataract Refract Surg. 2017;43:1281.
3. Solomon JD, Ladas J. Toric outcomes: computer-assisted registration versus intraoperative aberrometry. J Cataract Refract Surg. 2017;43:498.
4. Srivannaboon S, Chirapapaisan C, Chonpimai P, Loket S. Clinical comparison of a new swept-source optical coherence tomography-based optical biometer and a time-domain optical coherence tomography-based optical biometer. J Cataract Refract Surg. 2015;41:2224–32.
5. Sel S, Stange J, Kaiser D, Kiraly L. Repeatability and agreement of Scheimpflug-based and swept-source optical biometry measurements. Contact Lens Anterior Eye. 2017;40:318.
6. Yang JY, Kim HK, Kim SS. Axial length measurements: comparison of a new swept-source optical coherence tomography-based biometer and partial coherence interferometry in myopia. J Cataract Refract Surg. 2017;43:328.
7. Passi SF, Thompson AC, Gupta PK. Comparison of agreement and efficiency of a swept source-optical coherence tomography device and an optical low-coherence reflectometry device for biometry measurements during cataract evaluation. Clin Ophthalmol. 2018;12:2245.
8. Carl Zeiss Meditec, Clinical Trial, IOLMaster 700-2015-1.
9. Shetty N, Kaweri L, Koshy A, Shetty R, Nuijts RMMA, Sinha Roy A. Repeatability of biometry measured by three devices and its impact on predicted intraocular lens power. J Cataract Refract Surg. 2021;47:585–92.
10. Kurian M, Negalur N, Das S, Puttaiah NK, Haria D, Tejal SJ, Thakkar MM. Biometry with a new swept-source optical coherence tomography biometer: repeatability and agreement with an optical low-coherence reflectometry device. J Cataract Refract Surg. 2016;42:577–81.
11. Kunert KS, Peter M, Blum M, Haigis W, Sekundo W, Schütze J, Büehren T. Repeatability and agreement in optical biometry of a new swept-source optical coherence tomography-based biometer versus partial coherence interferometry and optical low-coherence reflectometry. J Cataract Refract Surg. 2016;42:76–83.
12. Martínez-Albert N, Esteve-Taboada JJ, Montés-Micó R, Fernández-Vega-Cueto L, Ferrer-Blasco T. Repeatability assessment of biometric measurements with different refractive states and age using a swept-source biometer. Expert Rev Med Devices. 2019;16:63–9.
13. Jung S, Chin HS, Kim NR, Lee KW, Jung JW. Comparison of repeatability and agreement between swept-source optical biometry and dual-Scheimpflug topography. J Ophthalmol. 2017;2017:1516395.
14. Garza-Leon M, La Fuentes-de Fuente HA, García-Treviño AV. Repeatability of ocular biometry with IOLMaster 700 in subjects with clear lens. Int Ophthalmol. 2017;37:1133–8.
15. Bullimore MA, Slade S, Yoo P, Otani T. An evaluation of the IOLMaster 700. Eye Contact Lens. 2019;45:117.
16. Huang J, Zhao Y, Savini G, Yu G, Yu J, Chen Z, Tu R, Zhao Y. Reliability of a new swept-source optical coherence tomography biometer in healthy children, adults, and cataract patients. J Ophthalmol. 2020;2020:8946364.
17. Chan TCY, Wan KH, Tang FY, Wang YM, Yu M, Cheung C. Repeatability and agreement of a swept-source optical coherence tomography-based biometer IOLMaster 700 versus a Scheimpflug imaging-based biometer AL-scan in cataract patients. Eye Contact Lens. 2020;46:35–45.
18. Hirnschall N, Varsits R, Doeller B, Findl O. Enhanced penetration for axial length measurement of eyes with dense cataracts using swept source optical coherence tomography: a consecutive observational study. Ophthalmol Therapy. 2018;7:119.
19. Chang DH, Waring GO. The subject-fixated coaxially sighted corneal light reflex: a clinical marker for centration of refractive treatments and devices. Am J Ophthalmol. 2014;158:863–874.e2.
20. Tonn B, Klaproth OK, Kohnen T. Anterior surface-based keratometry compared with scheimpflug tomography–based total corneal astigmatism. Investig Ophthalmol Vis Sci. 2014;56:291.
21. Koch DD, Ali SF, Weikert MP, Shirayama M, Jenkins R, Wang L. Contribution of posterior corneal astigmatism to total corneal astigmatism. J Cataract Refract Surg. 2012;38:2080.

22. LaHood BR, Goggin M. Measurement of posterior corneal astigmatism by the IOLmaster 700. J Refract Surg. 2018;34:331.

23. Koch DD, Jenkins RB, Weikert MP, Yeu E, Wang L. Correcting astigmatism with toric intraocular lenses: effect of posterior corneal astigmatism. J Cataract Refract Surg. 2013;39:1803–9.

24. Abulafia A, Koch DD, Wang L, Hill WE, Assia EI, Franchina M, Barrett GD. New regression formula for toric intraocular lens calculations. J Cataract Refract Surg. 2016;42:663–71.

25. Canovas C, Alarcon A, Rosén R, Kasthurirangan S, Ma JJK, Koch DD, Piers P. New algorithm for toric intraocular lens power calculation considering the posterior corneal astigmatism. J Cataract Refract Surg. 2018;44:168–74.

26. Akman A, Asena L, Güngör SG. Evaluation and comparison of the new swept source OCT-based IOLMaster 700 with the IOLMaster 500. Br J Ophthalmol. 2016;100:1201–5.

27. Fabian E, Wehner W. Prediction accuracy of total keratometry compared to standard keratometry using different intraocular lens power formulas. J Refract Surg. 2019;35:362.

28. Srivannaboon S, Chirapapaisan C. Comparison of refractive outcomes using conventional keratometry or total keratometry for IOL power calculation in cataract surgery. Graefe's archive for clinical and experimental ophthalmology. Albrecht Von Graefes Arch Klin Exp Ophthalmol. 2019;257:2677–82.

29. Savini G, Taroni L, Schiano-Lomoriello D, Hoffer KJ. Repeatability of total Keratometry and standard Keratometry by the IOLMaster 700 and comparison to total corneal astigmatism by Scheimpflug imaging. Eye (London, England). 2020;35:307.

30. Wang L, Spektor T, de Souza RG, Koch DD. Evaluation of total keratometry and its accuracy for intraocular lens power calculation in eyes after corneal refractive surgery. J Cataract Refract Surg. 2019;45:1416–21.

31. Lawless M, Jiang JY, Hodge C, Sutton G, Roberts TV, Barrett G. Total keratometry in intraocular lens power calculations in eyes with previous laser refractive surgery. Clin Exp Ophthalmol. 2020;48:749–56.

32. Yeo TK, Heng WJ, Pek D, Wong J, Fam HB. Accuracy of intraocular lens formulas using total keratometry in eyes with previous myopic laser refractive surgery. Eye. 2020;35:1705.

33. Wang L, Canedo ALC, Wang Y, Xie KC, Koch DD. Comparison of central topographic maps from a swept-source OCT biometer and a Placido disk-dual Scheimpflug tomographer. J Cataract Refract Surg. 2021;47:482–7.

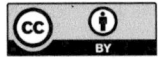

Digital Solutions in the Cataract Workflow from ZEISS

18

Melanie Schüle, Kyle Smith, Stephan Dreyer, and Jeremiah Elliott

Introduction

Cataract surgeons in today's competitive business environment demand solutions that enhance efficiency, cost-effectiveness, and clinical outcomes. Patients, at the same time, are demanding more from their surgeons. They want to maintain an active lifestyle into their later years, performing their everyday activities mostly without visual aids. Cataract surgeons must be thoughtful business people, striving for maximum efficiency in the clinic while taking the time to manage the concerns and expectations of every individual patient. Most patients expect a great deal more from their cataract surgery than they did 20 years ago, in part because modern technology has brought cataract surgery outcomes close to what corneal refractive surgery provides. With modern IOL calculation formulas, more sophisticated and accurate diagnostic devices, many high-quality toric and presbyopia-correcting IOLs on the market, and constantly improving surgical techniques, patients can expect excellent results from their surgery. This advanced technology creates more challenges for the busy surgeon, especially when patients are willing to pay extra for premium results. Surgeons understand that outstanding surgical results are directly related to the quality of the planning done prior to the surgery itself. The voluminous data available for every patient and the rapidly expanding treatment options make surgical planning a time-consuming prospect if the surgeon must process all that information with traditional manual methods.

For these reasons, cataract surgeons are focusing more intently on achieving excellent outcomes through meticulous surgical planning and more precise alignment of toric lenses during surgery. Thankfully, ZEISS has created several powerful digital solutions to support cataract surgeons and their teams by integrating the entire process of cataract surgery—from the office to the OR and back.

ZEISS FORUM

FORUM® from ZEISS is a scalable and flexible ophthalmic data management solution. It streamlines practice workflows by connecting involved devices and providing access to all patient examination data, allowing healthcare professionals to make confident decisions at a glance.

Streamline the Workflow

ZEISS FORUM enables a fully electronic workflow that automatically sends patient demograph-

M. Schüle (✉) · K. Smith · S. Dreyer · J. Elliott
ZEISS, Oberkochen, Baden-Württemberg, Germany
e-mail: melanie.schuele@zeiss.com;
kyle.smith.md@zeiss.com; stephan.dreyer@zeiss.com;
jeremiah.elliott@zeiss.com

© The Author(s) 2024

J. Aramberri et al. (eds.), *Intraocular Lens Calculations*, Essentials in Ophthalmology,
https://doi.org/10.1007/978-3-031-50666-6_18

ics to diagnostic devices. It facilitates a completely paperless workflow that saves storage space and reduces the cost of printing.

Decide with Confidence

ZEISS FORUM facilitates clinical case visualization by preparing ophthalmic data and images in a way that lets healthcare professionals make decisions with confidence. ZEISS FORUM effectively supports patient care with unique features and workplaces designed specifically for glaucoma, retina, and cataract surgery.

Simplify the Environment

ZEISS FORUM integrates conveniently with the healthcare providers' existing IT infrastructure using established standards as well as customized tools. Its centralized storage of all examination data ensures patient record consistency across the network, including EMR, HIS, DICOM, and non-DICOM instruments—those created by ZEISS as well as instruments from other manufacturers. FORUM's multi-site solution ensures that patient data is consistently available and shared across multiple sites.

ZEISS EQ Workplace

The EQ Workplace® software from ZEISS is a cataract surgery planning software based on ZEISS FORUM allowing cataract surgeons to streamline and automate processes in the cataract workflow. The software gives users the ability to access and review ZEISS IOLMaster and other diagnostic data in one place, calculate, select, and order IOLs remote of the measurement device, and prepare surgery for CALLISTO eye® from ZEISS. It also generates personalized IOL constants for future improvement of outcome prediction.

Preoperative Surgical Planning

Data Review

ZEISS EQ Workplace enables automatic data transfer and auto-population of data, saving cataract surgeons valuable time preoperatively. Biometry and diagnostic data can be accessed and reviewed remotely in the workplace or from any FORUM workstation, supporting the complex decision of selecting the right IOL for the patient.

IOL Calculation

With all relevant data for IOL calculation already pre-populated, ZEISS EQ Workplace allows a quick and easy calculation and selection of the IOL for surgery. It uses state-of-the-art IOL power estimation formulas to determine the proper IOL power and automatically uses the right calculator depending on the eye status and within the surgeon's preferred formulas. Available formulas include the Barrett Suite and Haigis Suite, Holladay I and II, Z CALC, and more. Users can compare multiple IOLs and formulas, can change and add IOL models, select a different formula or power, and see the results update immediately.

IOL Ordering

ZEISS EQ Workplace can send an e-mail order of the planned IOL directly from the workplace to pre-defined recipients. The essential data related to the IOL planned in EQ Workplace automatically transfers to the IOL in order to avoid error-prone manual transcription.

Surgery Preparation

ZEISS EQ Workplace allows users to set all relevant surgical assistance parameters in the workplace. It then automatically transfers these parameters, the planned IOL, and reference image to ZEISS CALLISTO eye.

Documentation

ZEISS EQ Workplace produces a planning PDF that can be printed, saved, forwarded, or archived as DICOM in ZEISS FORUM. Surgical teams may reference this document to be sure everyone is familiar with the plan.

Individual Constant Personalization

ZEISS EQ Workplace uses post-op refractions entered into the post-up screen of the workplace to personalize the surgeon's constants for each IOL model. Surgeons can use their own personalized optimized constants, or optimized constants imported from IOLCon (https://iol-con.org).

Intraoperative Assistance.

Surgery Preparation and Digital Toric Alignment

The surgical plans created in EQ Workplace can be imported by ZEISS CALLISTO eye in the operating room. This means that the OR team will have the details of every patient's surgical plan available in the device used for toric alignment without additional manual data entry.

During surgery and to further protect against never-events, the IOL at hand can be verified by comparing it with the IOL selected prior to surgery as displayed in ZEISS CALLISTO eye.

ZEISS VERACITY Surgery Planner

ZEISS VERACITY Surgery Planner is only available in the USA and Canada.

ZEISS created **VERACITY Surgery Planner** to address the challenge of time-consuming surgical planning for a variety of treatment options based on traditional manual methods. ZEISS VERACITY Surgery Planner represents an entirely new category of medical software, a tool that serves as the hub for all information related to ophthalmic surgery, a web-based digital assistant that brings the relevant data together in one location and automates much of the planning process, intraoperative documentation, and outcome analysis. The primary objective is to save time and prevent errors that could adversely affect outcomes.

Preoperative Surgical Planning

Configurability

Even though surgical teams can begin using ZEISS VERACITY Surgery Planner with minimal initial setup, the tool is highly configurable—flexible—so each team can continue working without disruption of its normal workflow.

Electronic Medical Record (EMR) Integration

Surgeons and their team members spend a great deal of time entering patient information into their EMR systems as part of the normal clinic workflow. ZEISS VERACITY Surgery Planner exploits that effort by importing that data directly from the EMR system, so team members are not duplicating effort. VERACITY Surgery Planner can import data from most EMR systems in the USA. This automated data transfer typically includes patient demographics, refractions, visual acuities, problem lists, medications, allergies, and prior surgical procedures.

Diagnostic Device Integration

ZEISS VERACITY Surgery Planner directly interfaces with most of the diagnostic devices commonly used in planning cataract surgery: optical biometry, corneal topography, and OCT. This includes devices made by ZEISS (IOLMaster 700, ATLAS topography, CIRRUS OCT) and many non-ZEISS devices: Lenstar (Haag-Streit), OPD-scan III (Nidek), Pentacam (Oculus), Cassini (Cassini), iTrace (Tracey Technologies), and more. VERACITY Surgery Planner imports the discrete data generated by these devices as well as the images they produce.

Patient Questionnaire

ZEISS VERACITY Surgery Planner incorporates answers from a configurable patient questionnaire that can be sent to patients in advance of their appointments via text message. This digital process automatically captures the patient's concerns, desires, and expectations for surgery. The text message can also include embedded patient education videos unique to each practice.

Data Validation and Alerts

ZEISS VERACITY Surgery Planner analyzes the imported data and alerts the surgical team to data inconsistencies, abnormal data, and other patient-related issues that could be of concern for the cataract surgeon.

Suggestions

ZEISS VERACITY Surgery Planner processes the available patient data acquired from the EMR, diagnostic devices, and the patient questionnaire and then generates a suggested treatment plan focused on the patient's desired outcome, and consistent with the surgeon's configured preferences.

IOL Calculations

ZEISS VERACITY Surgery Planner uses some of the most well-respected IOL power estimation formulas and toric calculators to determine the proper IOL power. These include the ZEISS AI IOL Calculator, Barrett Suite, Kane, Holladay II, the Abulafia-Koch toric calculator, and more. The system automatically uses the Barrett True-K calculator for eyes with prior corneal refractive surgery. ZEISS VERACITY Surgical displays the net astigmatism and the predicted final refraction for every surgical plan. When users change the IOL model or power, they see the results update immediately. ZEISS VERACITY Surgical also calculates the proper powers for a series of back-up lenses.

Automated Constant Optimization

ZEISS VERACITY Surgery Planner uses post-op refractions imported from the EMR system to optimize the constants automatically for each IOL model. Surgeons can use community-based optimized constants or their own personal optimized constants.

Arcuate Incisions

ZEISS VERACITY Surgery Planner also includes formulas for calculating the appropriate arcuate incisions for astigmatism reduction when a toric IOL is not possible.

Surgical Plan

The surgical plan ZEISS VERACITY Surgery Planner produces is much more than an IOL calculation. It includes documentation of the pre-ferred surgical method (standard phaco vs. femtosecond laser), supplemental procedures (i.e., MIGS), supplemental techniques (i.e., ZEISS miLOOP, capsular tension ring), anesthesia method, and many other details.

Surgery Scheduling

ZEISS VERACITY Surgery Planner assists with scheduling procedures, including non-cataract eye surgeries, so the entire surgical team can plan and work efficiently in the same digital environment.

Documentation

ZEISS VERACITY Surgery Planner generates a planning document for each case that can be sent to the ASC in advance of the surgery. Some surgical teams use it to be sure everyone is familiar with the plan.

Intraoperative Assistance

Digital Toric Alignment

The surgical plans created in ZEISS VERACITY Surgery Planner can be imported by ZEISS CALLISTO eye in the operating room. This means the OR team will have the details of every surgical plan available in the device used for toric alignment without additional manual data entry.

OR Display

ZEISS VERACITY Surgical generates a display of the surgical plan appropriate for use in the OR so every member of the surgical team is aware of the essential information for that case, including the proper IOL model and power, supplemental procedures or techniques planned, and any other patient-related concerns (Flomax, allergies, etc.).

Automated Operative Note

When the procedure has been completed, ZEISS VERACITY Surgical automatically generates a comprehensive operative note that includes the relevant details of the procedure. The system comes with preconfigured notes for virtually every type of cataract surgery and the most common supplemental procedures, but users can edit these templates as needed.

Postoperative Data Analytics

ZEISS VERACITY Surgery Planner imports post-op refractions from the EMR for use in its data analytics tool. Surgeons can view graphical displays of their surgical results in multiple formats depending on filter settings. Without any manual data entry in ZEISS VERACITY Surgery Planner, surgeons can see how often their patients' post-op refraction is within 0.5 D of target, or see which formula is providing the best results, or see how many premium lenses they are implanting each month.

ZEISS CALLISTO eye

Surgeons understand that toric IOLs are superior to arcuate incisions in the management of astigmatism. A correctly aligned toric IOL is the key to reduce postoperative astigmatism because a malrotation of only 3° will reduce the astigmatism correction by as much as 10% [1]. For these reasons, surgeons who desire excellent surgical outcomes require precise toric IOL alignment, which requires the appropriate adjustment for cyclotorsion. Historically, surgeons have turned to marker-based technologies, intraoperative aberrometry, and markerless computer-guided alignment to add precision to their toric alignment during surgery.

With ZEISS CALLISTO eye markerless alignment, manual marking steps can be skipped altogether for an efficient [2] and precise [3, 4] toric IOL alignment to reduce residual astigmatism. ZEISS CALLISTO eye imports surgical plans created in EQ Workplace or VERACITY Surgery Planner, or IOL selections made in ZEISS IOLMaster 700, and uses that information to generate intraoperative overlays for computer-guided cataract surgery. This efficient technology saves time for the OR team by eliminating the need for manual preoperative marking, manual data transfer, and manual intraoperative marking.

In a single-center study ($n = 57$ eyes), the mean overall surgical time for toric IOL patients treated with ZEISS CALLISTO markerless was significantly shorter than for patients using manual marking (727.2 ± 198.4 s versus 1110.0 ± 382.2 s; $P < 0.001$). The mean deviation from the target induced astigmatism was also significantly lower in the digital (CALLISTO eye) group (0.10 ± 0.08 D versus 0.22 ± 0.14 D; $P = 0.008$) [2]. The authors conclude that the "digital tracking approach for toric IOL alignment was efficient and safe to improve refractive outcomes [and] image-guided surgery helped streamline the workflow in refractive cataract surgery" [2]. A single center, randomized, contralateral, controlled study ($n = 104$ eyes) that compared the outcomes of markerless toric lens alignment (ZEISS CALLISTO eye) with intraoperative aberrometry (Alcon ORA system) demonstrated a residual astigmatism of 0.29 ± 0.22 D for CALLISTO eye group and 0.46 ± 0.25 D for ORA group ($P = 0.00039$). More than 25% of the patients in CALLISTO eye group had no postoperative astigmatism, whereas only four patients (8%) in ORA group showed no postoperative astigmatism. 92.2% of patients had <0.5 D in CALLISTO eye group and 76.5% in ORA group. 100% of patients were below 1.0 D in CALLISTO eye group and 96.1% in ORA group. The median absolute error in predicting cylindrical correction was reported to be similar for both groups: 0.35 D for CALLISTO eye group and 0.39 D for ORA group ($P = 0.91$). The authors concluded that "intraoperative markerless computer-assisted registration and biometric guidance summarily yielded less remaining refractive cylinder than toric IOL placement guided by intraoperative aberrometry" [5].

The assistance functions provided by ZEISS CALLISTO eye are surgeon-controlled via foot control panel or hand grips. CALLISTO eye's Z ALIGN® feature facilitates rotational alignment of toric IOLs and centration of IOLs on the visual axis (from data provided by IOLMaster 700). ZEISS CALLISTO eye's incision assistant helps to position incisions (optionally on the step axis and opposite clear cornea incisions when needed) and paracentesis. The device's rhexis assistant helps surgeons to size and shape the capsulorrhexis and center it on the visual axis provided by the ZEISS IOLMaster. And the LRI assistant guides surgeons in performing limbal relaxing incisions when a toric IOL is either insufficient or inappropriate for astigmatism management.

ZEISS CALLISTO eye helps surgeons address increasingly lofty patient expectations by projecting valuable information directly into the surgeon's view through the microscope.

Summary

ZEISS supports cataract surgeons with two cataract planning solutions, EQ Workplace and VERACITY Surgery Planner, and the intraoperative surgical guidance system, ZEISS CALLISTO eye, all created to improve efficiency and reduce errors while adapting to the surgeon's existing workflow.

ZEISS EQ Workplace supports cataract surgeons and their staff by streamlining the entire cataract surgery planning process. It saves valuable time during preoperative processes, reduces the risk of an IOL selection error, further protecting against never-events, and gives surgeons access to relevant data from anywhere in the clinic. By connecting ZEISS IOLMaster via FORUM to the ZEISS CALLISTO eye in the OR, EQ Workplace builds a secure data trail into the OR by remotely preparing all the surgical assistance functions for ZEISS CALLISTO eye. This digitization improves patient safety and efficiency in the clinical workflow.

ZEISS VERACITY Surgery Planner is a tool conceived by surgeons and perfected over the years by gathering feedback from surgeons using the product in actual clinical settings. It was designed to save time, and it does. In a recently published, prospective study, ZEISS VERACITY Surgical significantly reduced surgical planning time when compared with traditional paper-based methods ($P < 0.00001$) [6]. Improved efficiency is but one advantage. The automated data transfer and data validation ZEISS VERACITY Surgery Planner provides can help prevent errors that could result in poor patient outcomes. And the automated data analytics tool provides valuable insights that could lead to improvements in techniques and surgical decision-making.

References

1. Till JS, Yoder PR Jr, Wilcox TK, Spielman JL. Toric intraocular lens implantation: 100 consecutive cases. J Cataract Refract Surg. 2002;28:295–301.
2. Mayer WJ, Kreutzer T, Dirisamer M, Kern C, Kortuem K, Vounotrypidis E, Priglinger S, Kook D. Comparison of visual outcomes, alignment accuracy, and surgical time between 2 methods of corneal marking for toric intraocular lens implantation. J Cataract Refract Surg. 2017;43:1281–6.
3. Findl O, Hirnschall S, Weber M. Influence of rhexis size and shape on postoperative IOL tilt, decentration and anterior chamber depth. In: XXXI congress of the ESCRS; 2013.
4. Varsits RM, et al. Evaluation of an intraoperative toric intraocular lens alignment system using an image-guided system. J Cataract Refract Surg. 2019;45:1234–8.
5. Solomon LJ, Ladas J. Toric outcomes: computer-assisted registration versus intraoperative aberrometry. J Cataract Refract Surg. 2017;43(4):498–504.
6. Gujral T, Hovanesian J. Cataract surgical planning using online software vs traditional methods: a time/motion and quality of care study. Clin Ophthalmol. 2021;15:3197–203.

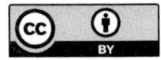

Biometry Measurements Using a New Large Coherence Length Swept-Source Optical Coherence Tomography

19

Clinical Experience with the Argos Biometer

H. John Shammas and Maya C. Shammas

Optical coherence tomography (OCT) presents several advantages over other techniques to evaluate biometry [1]. It is noninvasive and its high speed allows the collection of two- or three-dimensional data in hundreds of milliseconds with high lateral resolution and axial resolution. Most of the previously proposed swept-source OCTs have a depth range that is defined by a coherence length ranging around 2 mm, far below the measurement range required for the axial length of the eye. The coherence length was improved by using a swept-source technology that implements quasi-phase continuous tuning (QPCT) combined with multiple beam expanders at a swept rate of 2.5 kHz, which is about 5 to 10 times larger than what can be achieved in current systems. This swept-source OCT enables simple measurements of the axial length of the eye, where you need to only divide the obtained distance by the known refractive index. This technology has been the foundation of developing the Argos biometer [2], allowing a high-speed measurement (~30× faster than optical biometry), with two-dimensional

imaging of the eye and measuring all 9 parameters in a fraction of a second.

Recently presented systems with extended axial range allow the capturing of the anterior segment or even the full eye. OCT systems based on swept-source technology provide an extended imaging axial range without compromising the axial resolution. Furthermore, the use of OCT 2-D data should improve the success ratio in measuring the axial length, as well as improve the repeatability of its measurements.

The Argos uses a 1060 nm wavelength and 20 nm bandwidth swept-source technology to collect 2-D OCT data of the full eye [1]. The device provides 3 OCT images in every acquisition to measure not only the axial length (AL) and the anterior chamber depth (ACD) but also the central corneal thickness (CCT), aqueous depth (AD), lens thickness (LT), pupil size (PS), and the corneal diameter (CD). An automatic algorithm evaluates all the biometry parameters, and the optical distances are converted into geometric distances using the standard refractive indices of 1.376 for the cornea, 1.336 for the aqueous and vitreous, and 1.410 for the lens (Fig. 19.1); this is in contrast of other biometers that use different proprietary functions to convert the optical path length into millimeters (Fig. 19.2).

H. John Shammas (✉)
The Keck School of Medicine of USC,
Los Angeles, CA, USA

M. C. Shammas
Shammas Eye Center, Lynwood, CA, USA

© The Author(s) 2024
J. Aramberri et al. (eds.), *Intraocular Lens Calculations*, Essentials in Ophthalmology,
https://doi.org/10.1007/978-3-031-50666-6_19

Fig. 19.1 Argos uses a segmented method to measure the AL using multiple indices of refraction. A specific refractive index is used for each segment, where: AL = CCT/1.375 + AD/1.336 + LT/1.41 + VIT/1.336 − RT

Fig. 19.2 The Lenstar and IOLMaster 500 biometers use proprietary calibration functions to convert the optical path length into millimeters

To minimize measurement errors, manual adjustment of the parameters from the OCT images is possible and is recommended in the presence of outliers. Keratometry (flattest and steepest meridians and astigmatism) is obtained from OCT information in combination with a ring LED; the OCT information locates the eye in space, and this information is introduced to the equations that allow evaluating the curvature of the anterior cornea. The unit displays the anterior corneal radius of curvature (R) at the flattest and steepest meridians along with the average value (R_{AV}) and the K readings using a 1.3375 corneal index of refraction.

Argos also contains a double-checking system for those cases where the patient is not fixating correctly: the camera provides a panoramic view of the eye and allows alignment of the patient eye with respect to the pupil center, and a manual adjustment of the parameters provided by the OCT images is included to minimize the impact of possible errors in the distances provided by the automatic algorithm. While the former is used in the acquisition process, the latter is used to re-process (manually adjust) the eyes identified as outliers. An alert system is activated if any unsuc-cessful measurement or a higher-than-normal standard deviation is detected; it urges the user to check the plausibility in analysis mode, and it suggests manual adjustment if necessary.

We have been using the Argos biometer since 2014, and I would like to share my clinical experience with this biometer.

Repeatability and Reproducibility of the Argos Measurements

The repeatability and reproducibility of the Argos measurements have been tested by means of variation analysis study, and our study clearly demonstrated that the new OCT biometer produces precise and reproducible measurements [1].

The repeatability of the Argos measurements was analyzed as the average, standard deviation (SD), and range of the standard deviations of the biometric parameters (AL, ACD, CCT, AD, LT, PS, CD, and R_{AV}) obtained from the 3 images provided by the instrument in every acquisition. The repeatability analysis of the measurements was performed on the 3 OCT data images provided by Argos in a single acquisition. The intra-set average difference was 0.01 mm for AL, 0.01 mm for CCT, 0.01 mm for ACD, 0.01 mm for AD, 0.02 mm for LT, 0.05 mm for PS, 0.11 mm for CD, and 0.01 mm for R_{AV}.

The reproducibility of the Argos measurements was analyzed by means of variance analysis using the data provided from 3 sets of measurements and each set containing 3 images. Realignment was performed between measurements in all patients. To measure the reproducibility of the measurements, the average and standard deviation of the variation of the 9 images were calculated for every parameter. The obtained average of standard deviations of the 9 images were 0.01 mm for AL, 0.01 mm for the CCT, 0.01 mm for the AD, 0.01 mm for the ACD, 0.03 mm for LT, 0.10 mm for PS, 0.14 mm for CD, and 0.02 mm for R_{AV}. No statistically significant differences in paired t test ($p < 0.01$) were found in the data provided.

Comparing the Argos Measurements to the IOLMaster 500 and Lenstar Biometers

We compared the AL, ACD, and R_{AV} measurements to the results obtained with the IOLMaster 500 and the Lenstar LS900 biometers, while CCT, AD, LT, PS, and CD are also compared to those results provided by the Lenstar LS900 biometer. Three different examiners, one for each instrument, performed the measurements in a randomized manner, and without knowledge of the results of the other two instruments. Measurements were performed under natural conditions (no dilation drops were used) using the artificial ambient light in the clinic. For each measurement, the subjects were stabilized using the forehead and chin rests of each biometer and alignment was achieved with the subjects fixating on a light projected at optical infinity. For the IOLMaster and Lenstar measurements, the procedures from their respective manuals were followed and the result printouts were used for the study.

AL is defined as the measurement between the anterior corneal surface and the retinal surface; ACD is the measurement between the anterior corneal surface and the anterior lens surface; R_{AV} is the average anterior corneal radius of curvature; CCT is the measurement between the anterior and posterior corneal surfaces; AD is the measurement between the posterior corneal surface and the anterior lens surface; PS and CD measure the pupil size and the corneal diameter, respectively, taken from a horizontal section.

In one study [1], there was general agreement between the AL measurements taken by the OCT unit and those taken by the PCI unit and the ones taken the OLCR unit with a correlation coefficient of 1.00 compared to both instruments, with an average difference of −0.01 mm when compared to the IOLMaster and 0.01 mm when compared to the Lenstar.

The clinical relevance of these measurement differences is insignificant when performing IOL power calculation in an average eye. All commonly used third-generation formulas, including the Hoffer Q [3], Holladay I [4], and SRK/T [5],

base their calculations on AL and K measurements. A 0.01 mm longer AL decreases the calculated IOL power by less than 0.05 D depending on the AL and keratometry of the eye. We always recommend personalizing formula constants when any measurement or surgical technique is modified; however, initial calculations with the new OCT unit can be accurately performed using the same ACD constant for the Hoffer Q, surgeon factor for the Holladay 1, and A constant for the SRK/T formula used with the PCI unit. The Haigis formula [6] uses preoperative ACD measurements in addition to AL values. In our study, the OCT biometer measured on average a 0.17 mm deeper ACD. Clinically, the deeper ACD increased the IOL power by 0.1 D when the standard Haigis constants are used. We recommend a small decrease of approximately 0.02 in the a0 constant when the Haigis formula is first used with the OCT unit until all three constants in the Haigis formula are properly personalized.

Acquisition Rate

The patient group in this study [1] included many eyes with advanced cataracts. The AL could not be measured in 14 cases by one or more biometer; two patients had mature white cataracts and could not be measured by all three instruments. In the case of Argos, 54 out of the 56 eyes (96%) could be measured for all parameters and only the 2 cases with the mature cataracts were discarded due to no visibility of the retina. In the case of the IOLMaster, the success rate for AL measurement was 77% (43/56 eyes) and 13 eyes could not be successfully measured; these included the 2 mature cataracts, 2 cases with stage 5 nuclear sclerosis with posterior subcapsular changes, and 9 cases of stage 2 to stage 3 nuclear sclerosis with stage 3 posterior subcapsular changes. Finally, for the AL measurements by Lenstar, the success rate was 79% (44/56 eyes) and 14 eyes could not be successfully measured; these included the 2 mature cataracts, 3 cases with stage 4 cortical changes, and 7 cases with stage 3 posterior subcapsular changes.

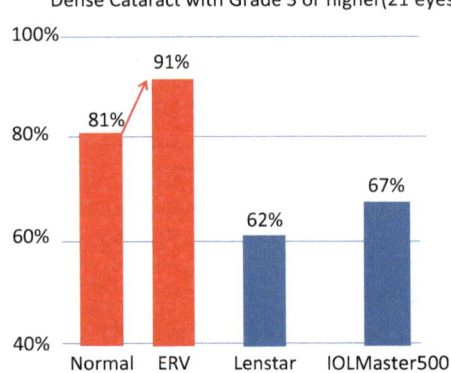

Fig. 19.3 In dense cataracts, the acquisition rate is much higher with the Argos biometer compared to the Lenstar and the IOLMaster 500. The acquisition rate increases with the use of the ERV mode

The high success rate of acquiring the axial length measurement in eyes with dense cataracts is due to two main differences between the Argos and other biometers: the wide scanning beam in OCT bypasses the cataract region allowing the light reaching the retina not to be blocked; furthermore, the OCT in the Argos unit uses a longer wavelength centered at 1060 nm which penetrates deeper in the cataract tissue compared to the PCI and OLCR units whose wavelengths are centered at 840 nm for the Lenstar LS900 unit and 780 nm for the IOLMaster 500 unit.

In very dense cataracts (Grade 3 or higher) (Fig. 19.3), the acquisition rate of the Lenstar biometer dropped to 62% and the IOLMaster 500 to 67%. The Argos biometer maintained a high 81% acquisition rate, which could even improve to 91% with the use of the ERV mode (Enhanced Retinal Visualization).

The Value of Using Multiple Indices of Refraction

The Argos® swept-source optical coherence tomographer measures the optical path length (OPL) of each segment of the eye and uses a specific refractive index (SRI) for each of these segments (cornea, anterior chamber, lens, and vitreous). As such, when there are variations in the relative lengths of these components, the

axial length calculation is appropriately adjusted. In this new study [7], we compared the AL measurements obtained with the Argos biometer with its multiple indices, one for each segment of the eye (ALmultiple) to a simulated axial length that uses a single index of refraction for the entire eye (ALsingle). We noticed that the use of a single index of refraction for the entire eye yielded longer measurements in the long eyes and shorter measurements in the short eyes (Fig. 19.4).

This is consistent with the notion that a single refractive index is developed based on a normative dataset, effectively presuming a fixed ratio of eye segments in the total axial length. In cases where this ratio is less likely to be observed (e.g., short eyes, long eyes), the use of different refractive indices for each ocular segment would be more reliable.

The difference in axial length measurements based on multiple specific refractive indices for each segment of the eye to those obtained using a single refractive index for the entire eye had subsequent effects on IOL power calculation.

We evaluated the results in 595 eyes undergoing cataract surgery where biometry and IOL power calculations were based on axial length calculated with multiple specific refractive indices (ALmultiple) versus those with a simulated axial length based on using a single refractive index (ALsingle). The expected residual refractions based on different IOL formulas were calculated for both single and multiple groups. Formulas were then optimized, and the mean prediction errors (MPE) and mean absolute prediction errors (MAE) were calculated, based on the difference between the (optimized) expected value and the actual refractive outcome. In nearly all cases, the average MPE in the ALmultiple group was lower than that for the ALsingle group across all axial lengths and formulas (Fig. 19.5). When larger differences in MAE were present, the multiple group results were more often lower (better).

Two other studies [8, 9], compared axial length measurements from an OLCR biometer using a single refractive index to calculate AL measurements using multiple refractive indices for each ocular segment, in reverse of the present study. Both studies found that the single

Fig. 19.4 Bland–Altman graph confirming that the use of a single index of refraction for the entire eye yielded longer measurements in the long eyes and shorter measurements in the short eyes

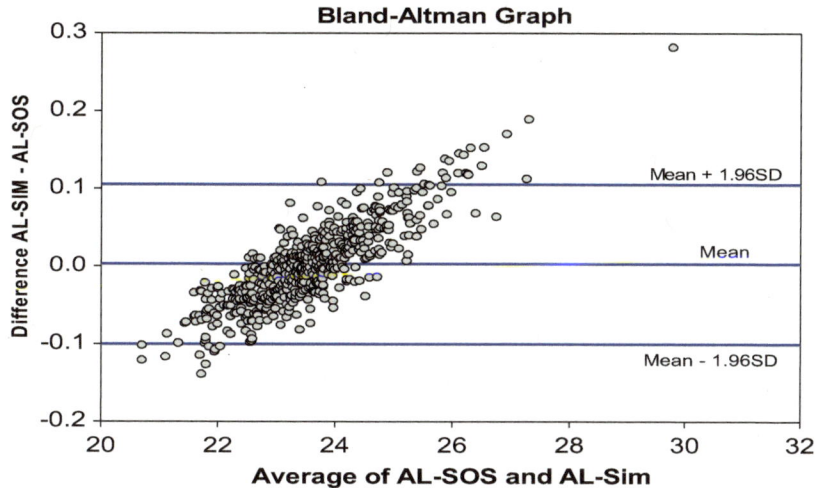

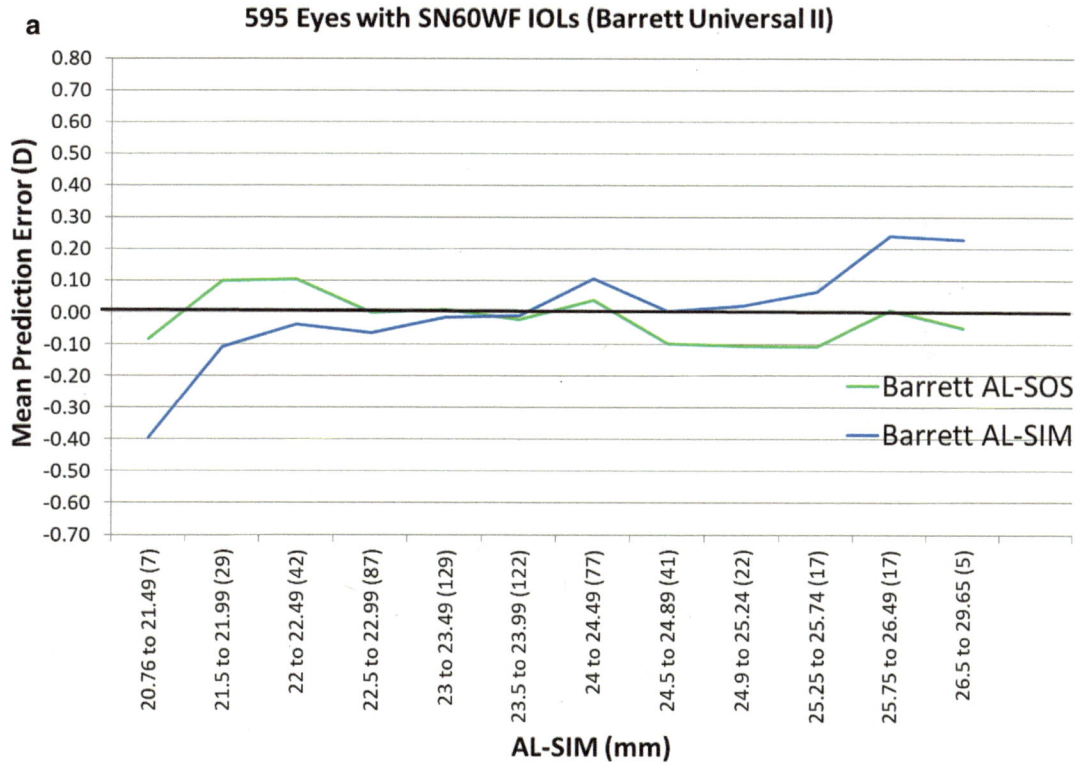

Fig. 19.5 The use of the sum-of-segments method (AL-SOS) using multiple indices improved the prediction results compared to the simulated method (AL-SIM) across the entire range of the axial length with the Barrett 2 formula (**a**), Haigis (**b**), Hoffer Q (**c**), Holladay1 (**d**), and SRK/T (**e**)

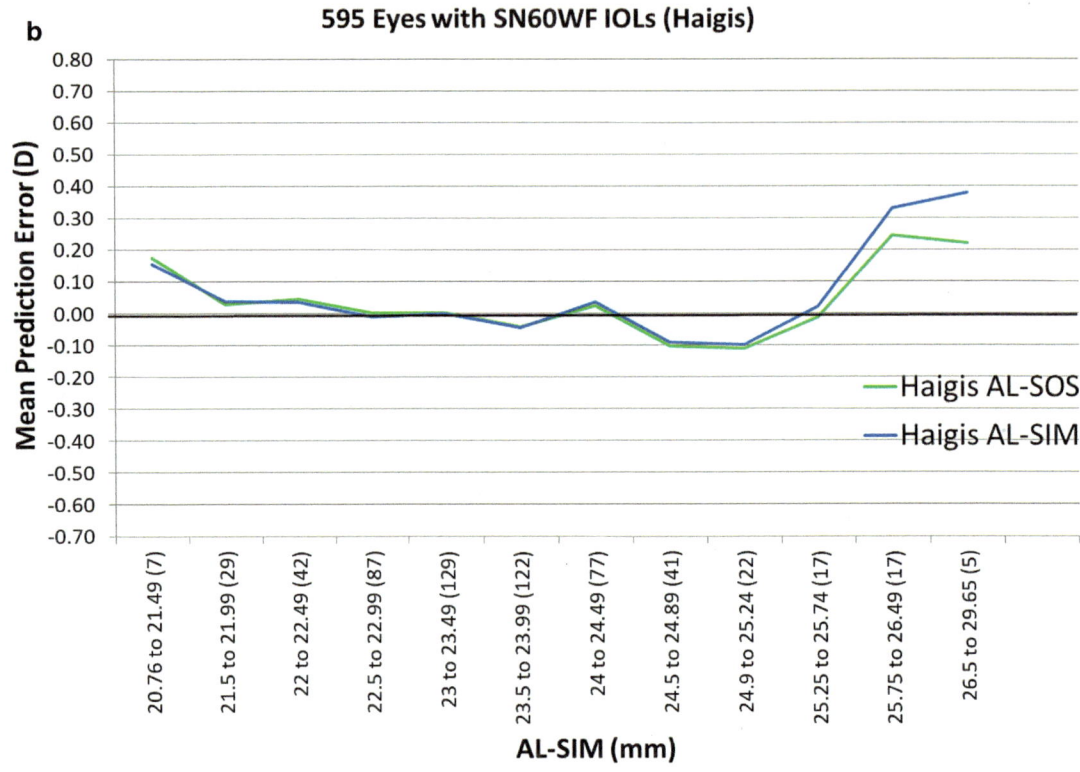

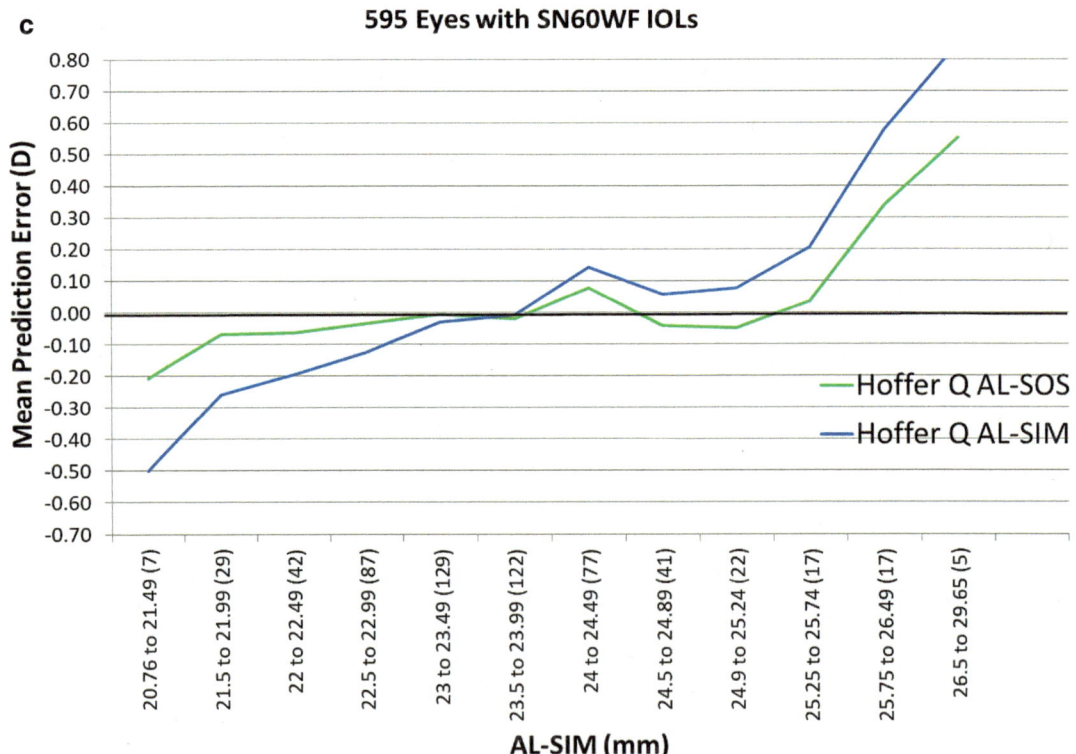

Fig. 19.5 (continued)

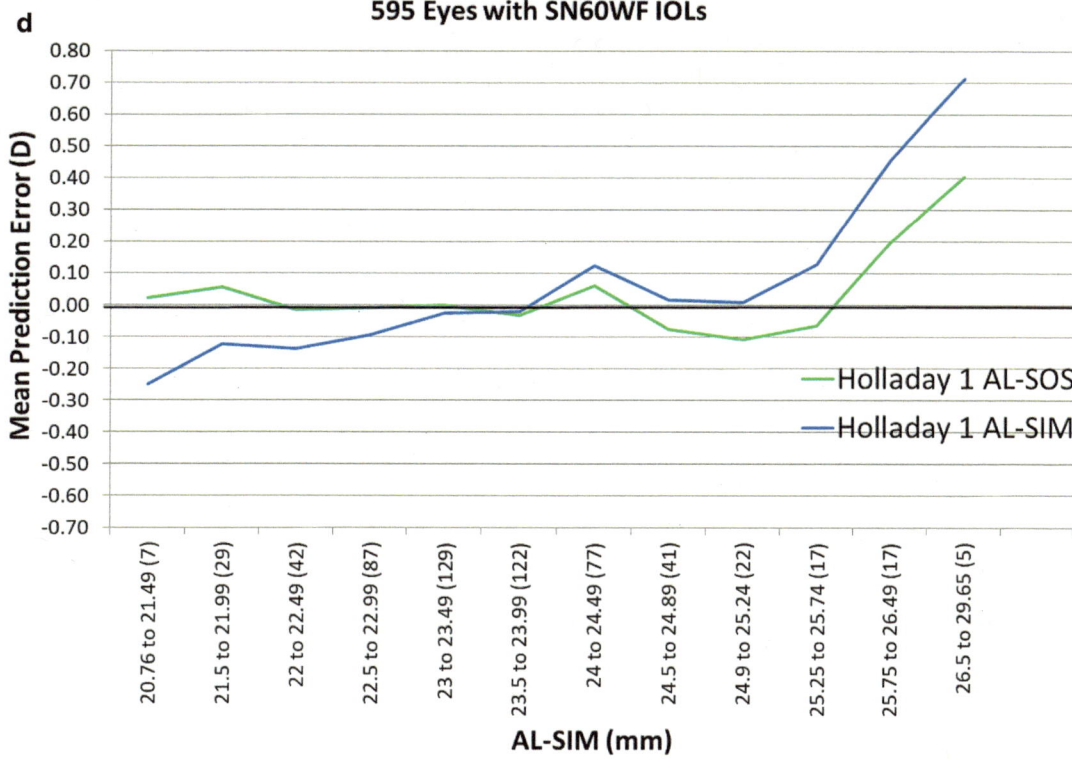

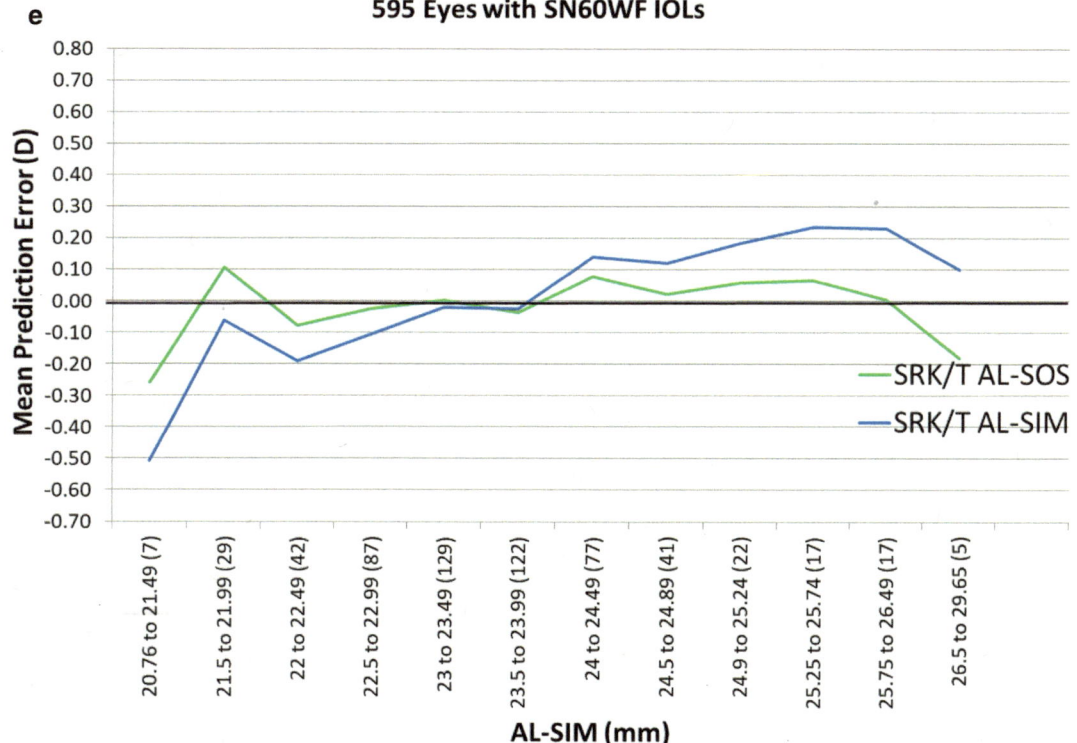

Fig. 19.5 (continued)

index AL measurements taken from the OLCR biometer were on average too short in short eyes and too long in long eyes, when compared to the calculated measurements based on multiple refractive indices. Wang et al. [8] found the refractive accuracy using multiple indices of refraction to calculate AL and IOL power in 4992 eyes to be improved in short eyes with Hoffer Q and Holladay 1 formulas and in long eyes with all formulas except the Olsen formula.

Using multiple indices instead of a single index to calculate AL in 1442 eyes, Cooke and Cooke [9] improved predictions for formulas designed on US data (SRK/T, Holladay 1, Holladay 2, Hoffer Q, and Haigis) although predictions were worse with the Barrett and Olsen formulas. Both studies agree with our study in that most of the accuracy improvements are noted in short and in long eyes.

References

1. Shammas HJ, Ortiz S, Shammas MC, Kim SH, Chong C. Biometry measurements using a new large-coherence-length swept-source optical coherence tomographer. J Cataract Refract Surg. 2016;42:50–61. https://doi.org/10.1016/j.jcrs.2015.07.042.

2. Chong C, Suzuki T, Totsuka K, Morosawa A, Sakai T. Large coherence length swept source for axial length measurement of the eye. Appl Opt. 2009;48:144–50.

3. Hoffer KJ. The Hoffer Q formula: a comparison of theoretic and regression formulas. J Cataract Refract Surg. 1993;19(11):700–12. Errata: 1994;20(6):677 and 2007;33(1):2–3

4. Holladay JT, Praeger TC, Chandler TY, Musgrove KH, Lewis JW, Ruiz RS. A three-part system for refining intraocular lens power calculations. J Cataract Refract Surg. 1988;14:17–24.

5. Retzlaff J, Sanders DR, Kraff MC. Development of the SRK/T intraocular lens implant power calculation formula. J Cataract Refract Surg. 1990;16:333–40. Errata: 1990;16:528 and 1993;19(5):444–446

6. Haigis W. The Haigis formula. In: Shammas HJ, editor. Intraocular lens power calculations. Thorofare, NJ: Slack; 2004. p. 41–57.

7. Shammas HJ, Shammas MC, Jivrajka RV, Cooke DL, Potvin R. Effects on IOL power calculation and expected clinical outcomes of axial length measurements based on multiple vs single refractive indices. Clin Ophthalmol. 2020;14:1511–9. https://doi.org/10.2147/OPTH.S256851.

8. Wang L, Cao D, Weikert MP, Koch DD. Calculation of axial length using a single group refractive index versus using different refractive indices for each ocular segment: theoretical study and refractive outcomes. Ophthalmology. 2019;126(5):663–70. https://doi.org/10.1016/j.ophtha.2018.12.046.

9. Cooke DL, Cooke TL. Approximating sum-of-segments axial length from a traditional optical low-coherence reflectometry measurement. J Cataract Refract Surg. 2019;45(3):351–4. https://doi.org/10.1016/j.jcrs.2018.12.026.

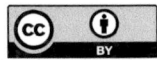

Argos Verion Image-Guided System

20

Raiju J. Babu and Jessica Voegtle

Cataract surgery has evolved with improved technologies, advanced biometers, and increasing patient expectations to achieving complete spectacle independence. The goal of the cataract surgeon is to implant an intraocular lens (IOL) with an appropriate IOL power to compensate for the refractive error and leave the patient emmetropic (plano target). Based on the patient need, the surgeon may chose a target refraction of emmetropia at distance or, in certain instances, target a myopic outcome to address spectacle independence at near. Occasionally, a mono vision or mini mono vision approach where one eye is targeted for distance and the other eye is targeted for myopic outcomes is also seen in practice [1].

The planning and execution of the process involve several steps:

- A preoperative diagnostic examination of the eye captures all parameters necessary for the selection of the optimal spherocylindrical power. In addition, for patients needing astigmatism correction, the pre-op evaluation also determines the ideal toric IOL orientation relative to reference landmarks that will be visible to the physician at the time of surgery.

- Alternatively, on the day of surgery the clinician may use a femtosecond laser as a first treatment step, to create surgical incisions and sometimes also to treat astigmatism via additional corneal shape-altering cuts.
- During the actual surgery, the clinician implants the IOL with the correct spherocylindrical power and aligns each toric implant correctly to minimize astigmatism, if applicable.

Astigmatism Correction

Accurately determining the power of an IOL can be done using online web-based calculators or those supplied by the IOL manufacturer. The post-surgical refractive error is dependent upon the parameters used in the IOL power calculation. New generation calculators account for posterior corneal astigmatism (PCA), anterior chamber depth (ACD), effective lens position (ELP), and surgically induced astigmatism (SIA), in addition to the usual biometry parameters of keratometry and axial length [2]. If the patient has preoperative astigmatism, the surgeon can correct it using a toric IOL or other methods such as Limbal relaxing incisions [3]. When aligning the axis of a toric IOL, it is essential to accurately determine the steep axis of the cornea. This should be done with the patient in the seated position, to account for cyclotorsion that would occur when the patient is supine. Manual corneal

R. J. Babu (✉) · J. Voegtle
Alcon Vision LLC, Fort Worth, TX, USA
e-mail: raiju.babu@alcon.com;
jessica.voegtle@alcon.com

J. Aramberri et al. (eds.), *Intraocular Lens Calculations*, Essentials in Ophthalmology,
https://doi.org/10.1007/978-3-031-50666-6_20

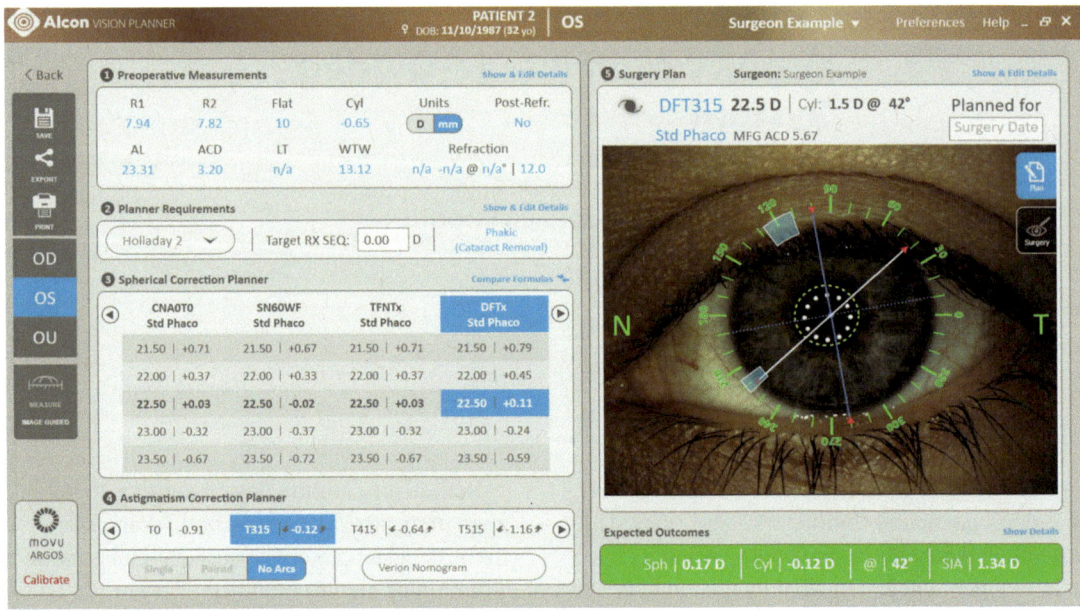

Fig. 20.1 Figure displays the reference image captured by the Argos Biometer and the Alcon Vision planner used to create the surgical plan including IOL power calculation

marking consists of preoperative marking of the horizontal axis, intraoperative alignment of the reference marks with the degree gauge of the fixation ring, and intraoperative marking of the target axis. The marking may be done with a skin-marking pen with a thin slit beam, a weighted thread, a pendulum marker, or a bubble marker [4]. Femtosecond laser-assisted corneal and capsulotomy marking provides more permanent markings for postoperative assessment of IOL position [5]. Image-guided systems capture preoperative digital photography of iris landmarks and conjunctival, scleral, or limbal blood vessels (Fig. 20.1). Based on the features of the eye, an intraoperative registration with the surgery image allows displaying the preoperative calculated toric implantation axis in the microscope.

Intraoperative wavefront aberrometry provides refinement of IOL selection and axis rotation by providing intraoperative aphakic refractive information to the surgeon to determine the correct IOL power and pseudophakic refractive data to correctly align the axis of a toric IOL [6]. With respect to toric IOL axis determination, risks associated with manual reference

marking include smudging or smearing, irregular or thick markings, parallax error, corneal abrasions, significant learning curve, intersurgeon variability, and anterior chamber bacterial contamination [4, 7, 8]. In one study, they showed that 30% of the ink markings were poorly visible due to washout [9]. Anterior stromal puncture offers the benefits of precise marking with no smudging [4].

Argos and Verion Digital Marking

The Argos Biometer with Image Guidance by Alcon is an integrated biometer that provides image guidance to the surgeons (Fig. 20.2). The image guidance is provided by having hardware (Verion Digital Marker) to provide overlays in the operating room and also at the Alcon LenSx Laser. The Verion Reference Unit is also an integrated keratometer with image guidance capability at Alcon LenSx system and Operating room. Verion Reference Unit is not capable of providing biometry; therefore, another biometer would be required to input the information into the Vision Planner.

The Digital Marker exists in 2 variants:

Digital Marker L (DML) and Digital Marker M (DMM)

The core of the Digital Markers is the Digital Marker Panel PC running software for image processing (registration and tracking) and displaying of tracking results during surgery. The Panel PC is placed at the LenSx Laser or next to the surgeon's microscope and receives the image signal of the microscope. Via established network connection or USB stick, preoperative data from

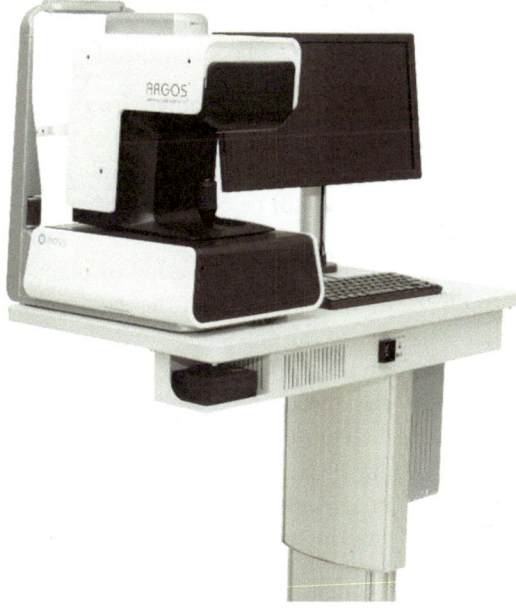

Fig. 20.2 The Argos Biometer with Image guidance by Alcon

the Argos Biometer or Verion Reference Unit is loaded into the planning screen of the system. If required, with user interaction, the planned surgery parameters can be modified.

The Digital Marker L imports patient information and provides this to the Alcon LenSx Laser. Additionally, the eye image from the Argos Biometer is provided to the Digital Marker L to determine the cyclotorsion angle between reference image and image from the digital laser microscope. Based on the determined cyclotorsion angle and planned centration options for arcuate incisions and capsulotomy, positions of treatment patterns are proposed to the operator.

The Digital Marker M consists of the Panel PC, Microscope Integrated Display (MID), foot pedal, and optionally the VERION Link (established connection to Alcon Centurion phaco system). The Microscope Integrated Display (MID) is mounted into the surgery microscope and connected via communication cable to the Digital Marker M. The MID acquires digitally a microscope image, passing this to the Panel PC for the image processing, and injects context information received by the Digital Marker M into the surgeons optical microscopes view (Fig. 20.3). After potential adjustment and confirmation of the registration angle, the tracker will be initialized. A live image with the planned tracking overlay is shown. If the eye is moving and/or rotating, the difference to the new position of the eye will be determined and the overlay adjusted. According to every surgery step on the Digital

Fig. 20.3 The final registration angle determined by the Digital Marker L and provided to the LenSx Laser for adjustment of the treatment parameters, i.e., incisions and centration of Capsulotomy and Lens fragmentation

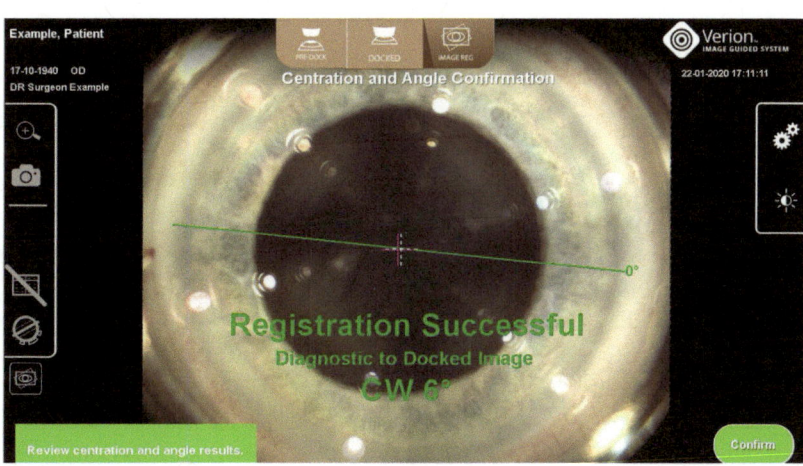

Fig. 20.4 Figure displays the toric overlay providing thereby image guidance with respect to IOL implantation axis based on the preoperative plan

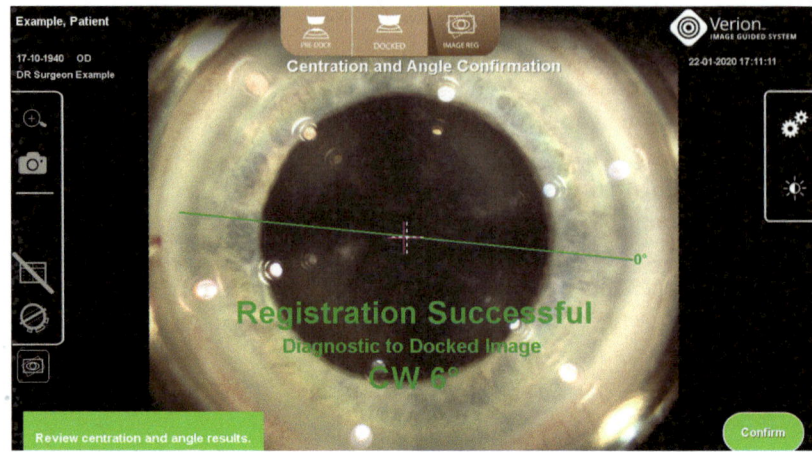

Marker M, an equivalent overlay will be displayed at the MID. With the footpedal (connected via USB) user interactions with the Digital Marker can be controlled, without physical touch of the computer screen (e.g., getting into live mode, start, and confirmation of registration, and to toggle through the different surgery steps). Overlays may show incision locations, capsulorrhexis size and location, IOL centration, toric alignment axis, or IOL centration + toric alignment axis (Fig. 20.4). During surgery, the displayed overlay can be adjusted with appropriate buttons on the screen. Optional Aphakic, Pseudophakic, and Lens Axis Marker phases are available to trigger measurements with the ORA VerifEye Lynk System (Intraoperative aberrometer) or display corresponding information (e.g., measurement data) on the screen or in the MID.

In detail, the Digital Marker provides:

- Patient Eye Confirmation: Automated consistency check of reference image from VERION Reference Unit or Argos Biometer with Alcon Image guidance and patient eye image under microscope at the beginning of the surgery at the Digital Marker. The doctor receives feedback, whether the reference image and the microscope image do or do not match.
- Incision Guide: Online overlay of planned incision areas on the microscope live image. Lateral and rotational movements of the eye will be compensated relative to the reference image.

- Capsulorrhexis Guide: Online overlay of planned capsulorrhexis position and radius on the microscope live image. Lateral movements of the eye will be compensated relative to the reference image.
- Centration Guide: Online overlay of planned (multifocal) IOL position on the microscope live image. Lateral movements will be compensated relative to the reference image.
- Toric Alignment Guide: Online overlay of preop planned implantation axis on the microscope live image. Lateral and rotational movements of the eye will be compensated relative to the reference image (Fig. 20.4).
- Finalization check: Combined overlay of the centration and toric alignment information on the microscope live image for a final IOL position check. Lateral and rotational movements of the eye will be compensated relative to the reference image.
- Documentation: Storage of reference and measurement data, surgery, and surgery image data on an external storage.

The benefits of image-guided systems include accurate alignment of the toric axis relative to anatomic landmarks in photographs of the iris and limbal vessels [4, 6–8, 10–13] and minimizing marking errors and improving postoperative alignment [11, 13]. In a randomized controlled trial [14], the IOL misalignment was significantly less with image-guided system compared to manual marking. This has implications with respect to astigmatic outcomes, as 1 degree of IOL misalignment can translate to 3.3% reduction in effectiveness of astigmatic correction [15] using one method. In another method where the vector difference between the target and achieved astigmatic outcomes, an error of 4.9 degree would result in remaining astigmatism magnitude of 17% of the preoperative astigmatism [16]. The randomized control trial did not find the difference in Uncorrected VA or residual astigmatism, although a statistically significant difference was seen in degree of IOL misalignment [14]. The key differentiation is that image-guided systems eliminates or accounts for the possible change in head position when keratometry and steep axis is determined impacts ability to account for cyclotorsion and thereby affecting precision [9, 17]. In addition, image-guided systems reduce the risk of anterior chamber bacterial contamination [7]. A risk of image-guided systems is that the eye tracker may disengage during surgery and a repeat registration may be required [4]. Additional risks include intraoperative changes in the appearance of the limbal vessels, including conjunctival chemosis, ballooning, and bleeding, which may interfere with intraoperative registration [4, 10]. Furthermore, registration may not be possible in extremely uncooperative patients or for difficult orbital anatomy, including extremely deep-set eyes or narrow palpebral apertures [4]. Image-guided technologies primarily help to reduce any source of error and variability from manual processes. It also helps in eliminating transcription errors as the data is integrated. An additional benefit is that the Vision Planner that is part of the image-guided system helps the surgeon to move away from additional tools and calculators for astigmatism correction for toric alignment axis and arcuate incision and Global IOL constants by providing personal optimization algorithms for constants and SIA which is intended to improve outcome.

Disclaimer Raiju Babu and Jessica Voegtle are employee's of Alcon Vision LLC.

References

1. Labiris G, Toli A, Perente A, Ntonti P, Kozobolis VP. A systematic review of pseudophakic monovision for presbyopia correction. Int J Ophthalmol. 2017;10(6):992–1000. https://doi.org/10.18240/ijo.2017.06.24.
2. Findl O, Hirnschall N. Principles of corneal measurement for intraocular lens power calculation. Exp Rev Ophthalmol. 2016;11(2):93–9.
3. Hirnschall N, Gangwani V, Crnej A, Koshy J, Maurino V, Findl O. Correction of moderate corneal astigmatism during cataract surgery: toric intraocular lens versus peripheral corneal relaxing incisions. J Cataract Refract Surg. 2014 Mar;40(3):354–61. https://doi.org/10.1016/j.jcrs.2013.08.049.
4. Kaur M, Shaikh F, Falera R, Titiyal JS. Optimizing outcomes with toric intraocular lenses. IJO. 2017;65(12):1301–13.
5. Diakonis VF, Swann BF, Weinstock RJ. Femtosecond laser–assisted capsulotomy markings for the alignment of toric IOLs: a new technique. J Refract Surg. 2018;34(10):711–2.
6. Donaldson K, Fernandez-Vega-Cueto L, Davidson R, Dhaliwal D, Hamilton R, Jackson M, et al. Perioperative assessment for refractive cataract surgery. J Cataract Refract Surg. 2018;44(5):642–53.
7. Panagiotopoulou EK, Ntonti P, Gkika M, Konstantinidis A, Perente I, Dardabounis D, et al. Image-guided lens extraction surgery: a systematic review. Int J Ophthalmol. 2019;12(1):135–51.
8. Sivagnanam S, Arunkumar GL, Srinivasan U, Kathirvel PSA, K, Gurubaran K. A new system of axis marking for toric intraocular lenses - the Toric max system. Del J Ophthalmol. 2016;27(1):62–3.
9. Lin H-Y, Fang Y-T, Chuang Y-J, et al. A comparison of three different corneal marking methods used to determine cyclotorsion in the horizontal meridian. Clin Ophthalmol. 2017;11:311–5.
10. Behshad S, Tucker J, Garg SS. Toric intraocular lens alignment: manual versus automated alignment techniques for toric IOLs. Int Ophthalmol Clin. 2016;56(3):71–84.
11. Coleman MJ, Stark WJ, Daoud YJ. A comprehensive guide to managing astigmatism in the cataract patient. Exp Rev Ophthalmol. 2014;9(6):539–44.
12. Thulasi P, Khandelwal SS, Randleman JB. Intraocular lens alignment methods. Curr Opin Ophthalmol. 2016;27(1):65–75.
13. Ventura BV, Wang L, Weikert MP, Robinson SB, Koch DD. Surgical management of astigmatism with toric intraocular lenses. Arq Bras Oftalmol. 2014;77(2):125–31.
14. Webers VSC, Bauer NJC, Visser N, Berendschot TTJM, van den Biggelaar FJHM, Nuijts

RMMA. Image-guided system versus manual marking for toric intraocular lens alignment in cataract surgery. J Cataract Refract Surg. 2017 Jun;43(6):781–8.

15. Lipsky L, Barrett G. Comparison of toric intraocular lens alignment error with different toric markers. J Cataract Refract Surg. 2019 Nov;45(11):1597–601.

16. Visser N, Berendschot TT, Bauer NJ, Jurich J, Kersting O, Nuijts RM. Accuracy of toric intraocular lens implantation in cataract and refractive surgery. J Cataract Refract Surg. 2011 Aug;37(8):1394–402. https://doi.org/10.1016/j.jcrs.2011.02.024.

17. Xiang W, Chen W, Liu R, et al. Ocular cyclorotation and corneal axial misalignment in femtosecond laser-assisted cataract surgery. Curr Eye Res. 2019;44(12):1313–8.

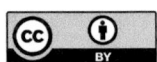

Optical Biometer OA-2000

21

Naoko Hara, Kathrin Benedikt,
and Hirofumi Owaki

Introduction

Optical biometer OA-2000 (Tomey Corporation, Nagoya Japan) can measure all biometric parameters needed for pre-cataract surgery: axial length, anterior chamber depth, lens thickness, corneal radius of curvature over a 2.5 mm and 3.0 mm diameter, corneal topography, central corneal thickness, pupil diameter, and Corneal Diameter (Fig. 21.1 and Table 21.1). It is done almost automatically by one measurement in short time. The touch screen enables intuitive operation, measurement, data checking, IOL calculation, and data output within one compact

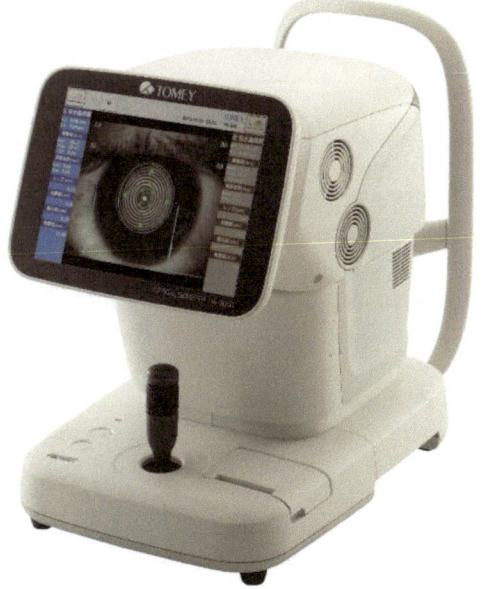

Fig. 21.1 Optical biometer OA-2000

N. Hara · K. Benedikt · H. Owaki (✉)
Tomey Corporation, Aichi, Japan
e-mail: kathrin@tomey.de; matsu@tomey.co.jp

© The Author(s) 2024
J. Aramberri et al. (eds.), *Intraocular Lens Calculations*, Essentials in Ophthalmology,
https://doi.org/10.1007/978-3-031-50666-6_21

Table 21.1 Specifications of OA-2000

Measurement method	Axial length Anterior chamber depth Lens thickness Central corneal thickness	Optical low-coherence interferometer using swept-source laser
	Corneal radii Topography	5.5 mm 9 rings Placido ring cone topography
Measurement range	Axial length	14.0–40.0 mm
	Corneal radii	5.0–11.0 mm
	Anterior chamber depth	1.5–7.0 mm
	Lens thickness	0.5–6.0 mm
	Central corneal thickness	0.2–1.2 mm
	Corneal Diameter	7.0–16.0 mm
Display resolution	Axial length	0.01 mm
	Corneal radii	0.01 mm
	Anterior chamber depth	0.01 mm
	Lens thickness	0.01 mm
	Central corneal thickness	1 μm
	Corneal Diameter	0.3 mm

IOL calculation formulae	Standard formulas
	  SRK/T, Holladay, Hoffer Q
	  Haigis optimized, Haigis standard, Olsen, OKULIX [a]
	  Barrett Universal II [b]
	For toric IOL
	  Olsen Toric Calculator, OKULIX [a]
	  Barrett Toric Calculator [b], Barrett True K Toric Calculator [b]
	For post-refractive surgery
	  Shammas-PL, Double K SRK/T, OKULIX [a], EASY IOL
	  Barrett True K [b]	

[a] Optional, depending on sales area
[b] Optional

unit. The OA-2000 supports doctors to reduce stress on patients and accurate and smooth preoperative examination and planning for high-quality cataract surgery by these features on daily practice [1].

Axial Length Measurement

The touch-alignment system is employed on OA-2000. It can provide a stable measurement and a high reproducibility between operators because OA-2000 aligns itself automatically to patient eye once an operator only touches the center of the pupil on the screen. Operators can measure all data easily without any special skills (Fig. 21.2) [2].

OA-2000 achieves a high signal–noise ratio (SNR) and high transmitting on opacity parts by using swept-source coherence tomography method. In addition, long coherence length allows high penetration and high success rate on long axial length myopic eyes (Fig. 21.3) [3]. Additionally, OA-2000 obtains not only A-scan wave form but also B-scan image of 1 mm width on retina by 2D scanning. On a measurement result of normal eye (Fig. 21.4), SNR is high and standard deviation (SD) is very low because the measurement light isn't reduced as the crystalline lens is clear. It means the measurement is very stable.

On the other hand, there are some cases where it is difficult to obtain the signal around the center of the retina as shown in Fig. 21.5a. In such case, OA-2000 measures the axial length by detecting a stronger signal from peripheral area automatically. When the retinal signal cannot be detected even with that way, V scan (Fig. 21.6) is performed instead of horizontal scan to find less opacity position so that the retinal signal can be

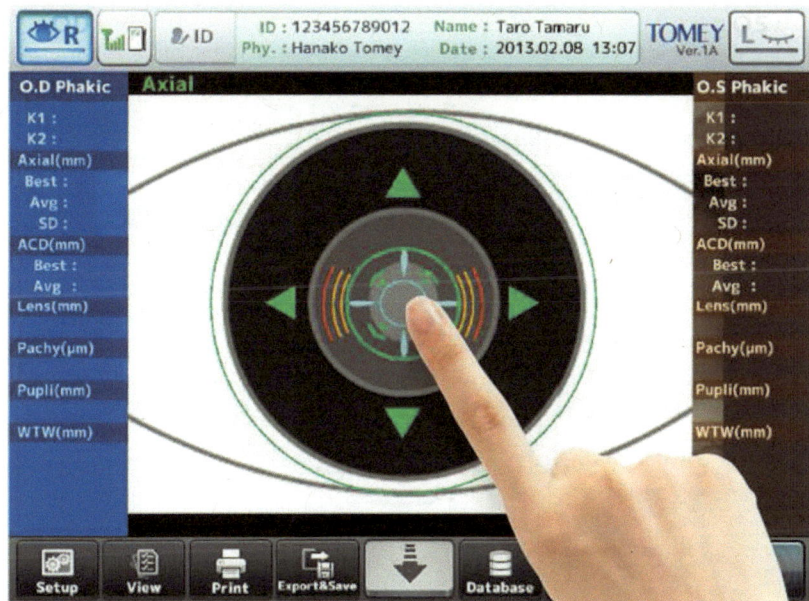

Fig. 21.2 Touch alignment, easy operation. http://vimeo.com/259629303?width=640&height=480

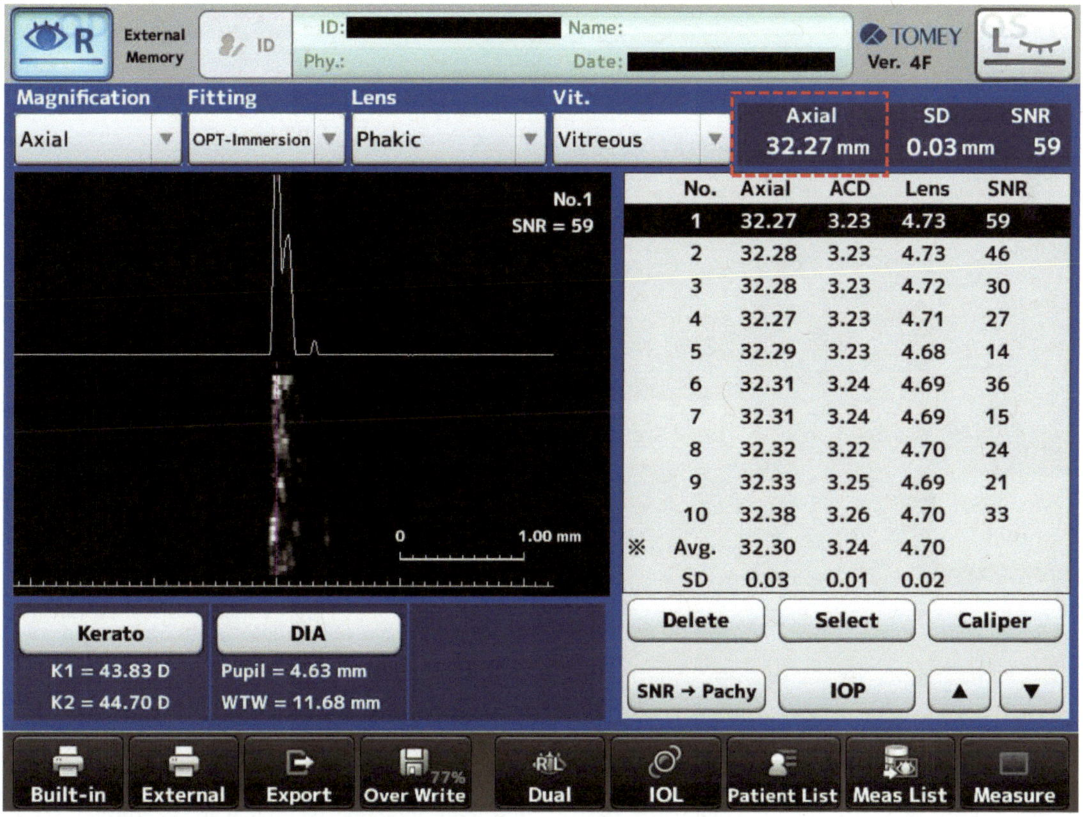

Fig. 21.3 Results of cataract eye with long axis length

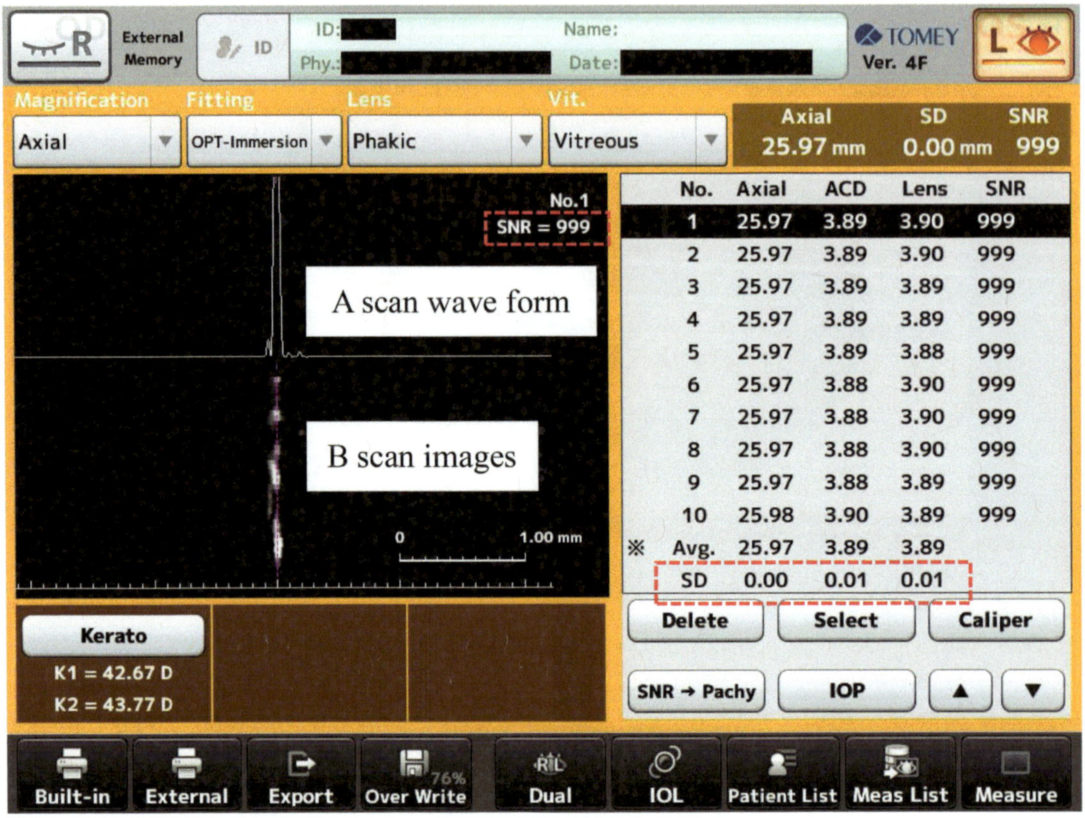

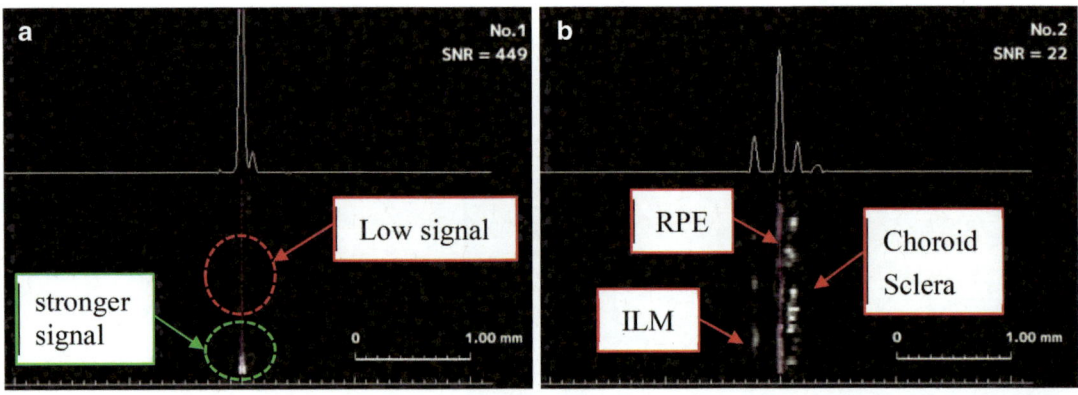

Fig. 21.4 Measurement result of normal eye

Fig. 21.5 Wave forms and B-scan images on retina of cataract eyes. (**a**) Lens central opacity. (**b**) Multi-peaks wave form

detected. High success rate is achieved by these techniques in combination.

In the case of dense cataract with low SNR, multi-peaks retinal waveforms may appear as Fig. 21.5b shows. OA-2000 detects retinal pig-ment epithelium (RPE) automatically by an orig-inal algorithm based on signal appearance ratio and peak analysis results. It is recommended to judge it comprehensively including the results of other examinations, when it is suspected if the

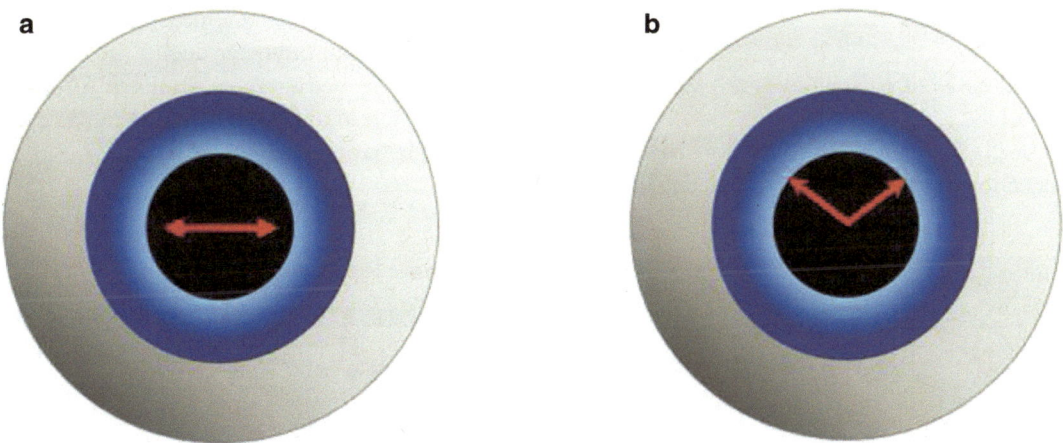

Fig. 21.6 Scanning methods on OA-2000. (**a**) Horizontal scan. (**b**) Vertical scan

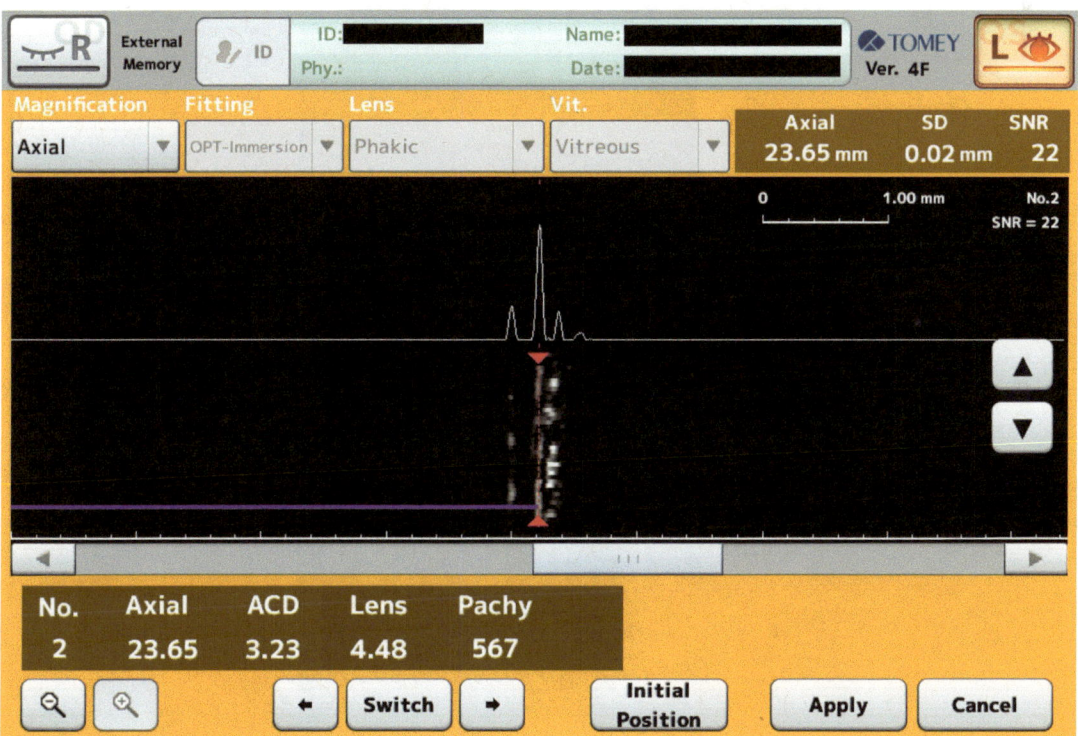

Fig. 21.7 Caliper function

detected retinal peak is correct or not, for example, miss-detecting epiretinal membrane as RPE. Caliper function (Fig. 21.7) allows operators to select RPE position manually if the auto-detected RPE is not correct.

For converting optical path lengths (OPLs) to geometrical distances, an original conversion formula was established by clinical dataset of ultrasound biometer and OA-1000, how to be performed based on the way by Haigis [4, 5]. OPLs of OA-2000 are in good agreement with OA-1000, which is the previous model; OA-2000 also uses the same conversion formula.

Clinical Cases

Clinical cases of cataract eyes are introduced in Fig. 21.8.

OA-2000 includes the function of wireless connection with ultrasound biometer AL-4000 (Fig. 21.9). It is useful when measurement is difficult by an optical biometer due to subject eyes conditions. The measurement results of AL-4000 can be transferred to OA-2000, and it can be used for IOL calculation on OA-2000.

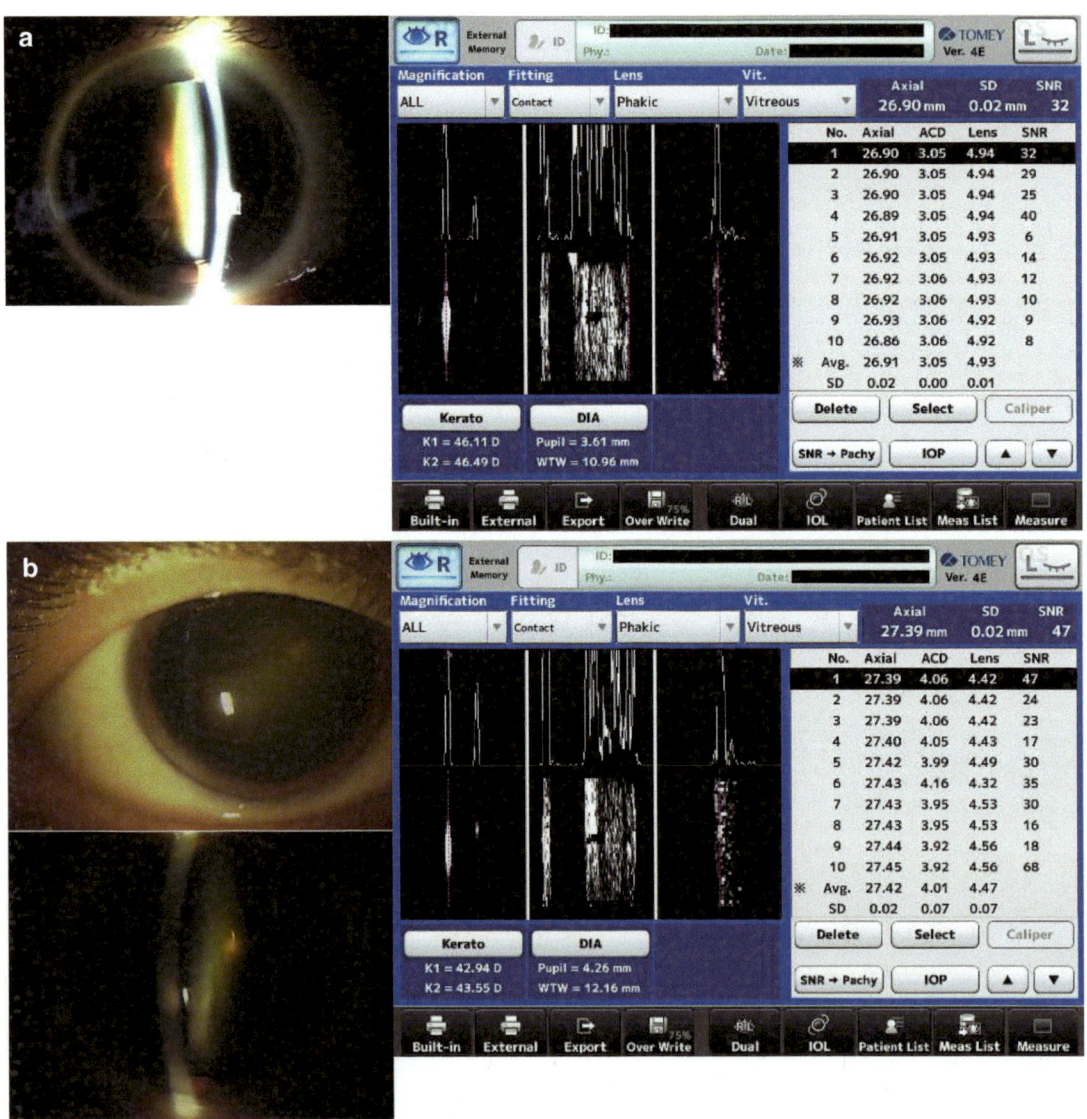

Fig. 21.8 Clinical cases of cataract eyes, Provided by Dr. Hitoshi Tabuchi, Chief director of Department of Ophthalmology, Tsukazaki Hospital. (**a**) Hypermature cataract eye. The nuclear sclerosis is Emery class V. SDs for axial length, ACD, and lens show small numbers even with relatively low SNRs; measurement result is stable. (**b**) Cortex and posterior subcapsular cataract eye. The nuclear sclerosis is Emery class III. SDs for axial length, ACD, and lens show small numbers even with relatively low SNRs; measurement result is stable.. (**c**) Cortex and posterior subcapsular cataract eye. The nuclear sclerosis is Emery class II-III. The retinal signal is very low because the opacity of the cortex and the posterior subcapsular is strong. However, SDs are small enough and the measurement result is stable

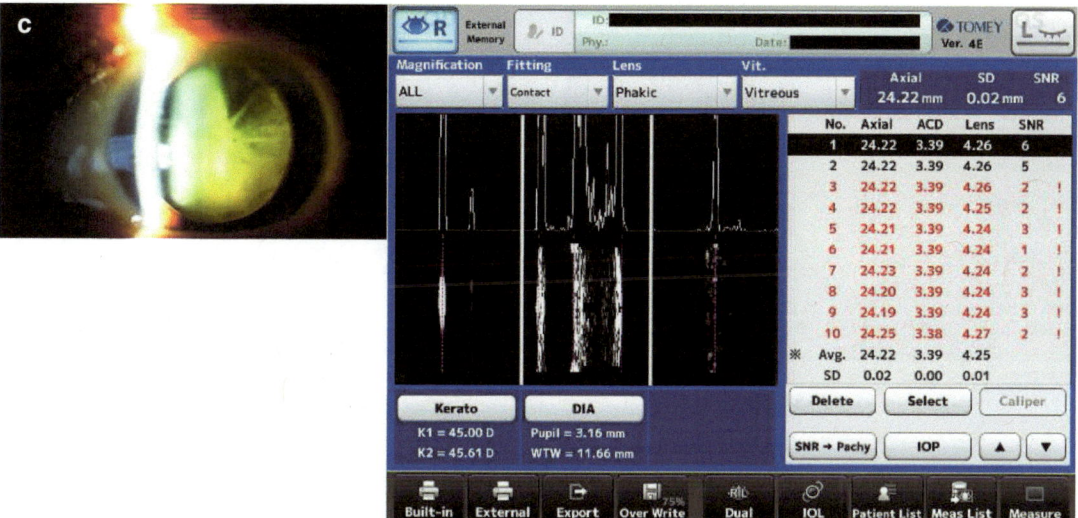

Fig. 21.8 (continued)

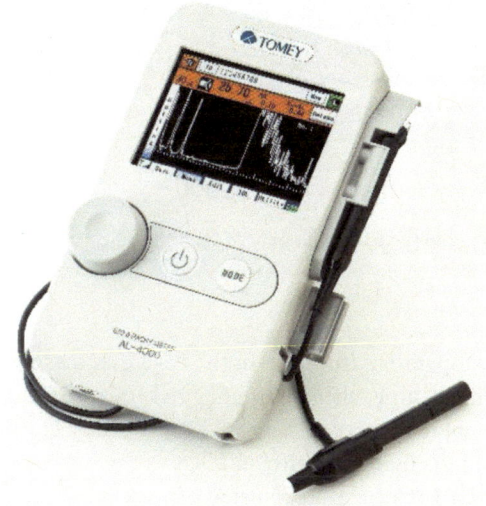

Fig. 21.9 Ultrasound biometer AL-4000

Measurement of Corneal Radius of Curvature and Topography

OA-2000 employs a Placido disc for measuring corneal radii and topography, which has been proven being an accurate measurement method and used for many years [6]. The Placido-based topography can capture image in a single shot; therefore, it is hard to be affected by eye motion, when performed at the same time as the axial length measurement. Figure 21.10 shows examples of comparison of topography map between TMS-4N and OA-2000 for same eyes. The measurement range of OA-2000 is 5.5 mm which is narrower than TMS-4N. However, it is enough for evaluating visual function, and they have good consistency in that range.

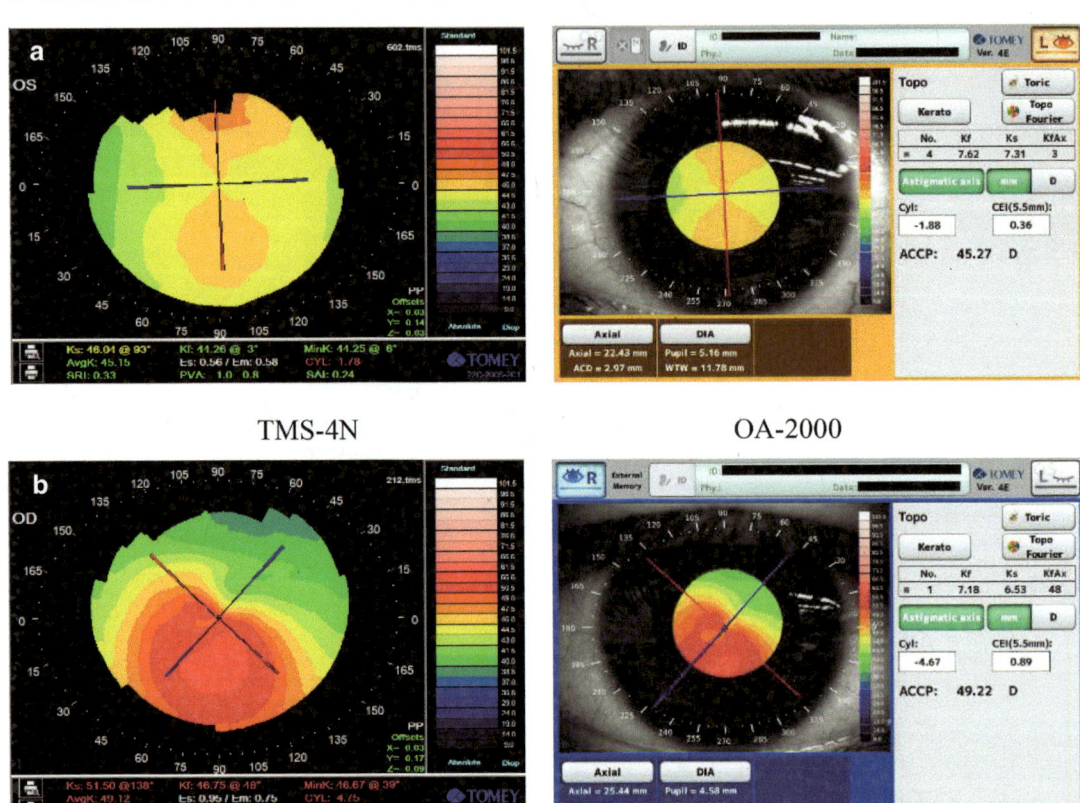

Fig. 21.10 Comparison between TMS-4N and OA-2000 on topography. (**a**) Topography of with-the-rule astigmatism eye. (**b**) Topography of keratoconus eye

Important Indices of Cornea for Cataract Surgery

OA-2000 provides not only the corneal radius of curvature results but also important indices of KAI (Kerato-Asymmetry Index) and KRI (Kerato-Regularity Index) (Fig. 21.11). These indices are ranked with A (Low)/B (Slightly high)/C (High) which show possibility to be irregular corneal astigmatism. When KAI shows high value in B or C, the eye is suspected to be a deformed cornea such as in keratoconus. When KRI shows high value, the eye is suspected to be a corneal transplant or with CL-induced problems, etc. It can call to attention checking the topographic maps so that doctors can prevent postoperative troubles. In the case that these values are high, there is higher risk of insufficient visual recovery and it should be carefully considered to choose multifocal IOLs.

CEI (Corneal Eccentricity Index) is shown in the topographic screen (Fig. 21.12). When CEI indicates positive number, the corneal shape is prolate which is normal eye. On the other hand, when CEI indicates negative number, the corneal shape is oblate which can be observed in typical post-LASIK eyes. By checking this value, even in the case that the surgical history is unknown, doctors can realize the possibility being post-LASIK eye and adopt post-LASIK IOL formula so that they can avoid refractive surprise after surgery.

Important indices of cornea for cataract surgery

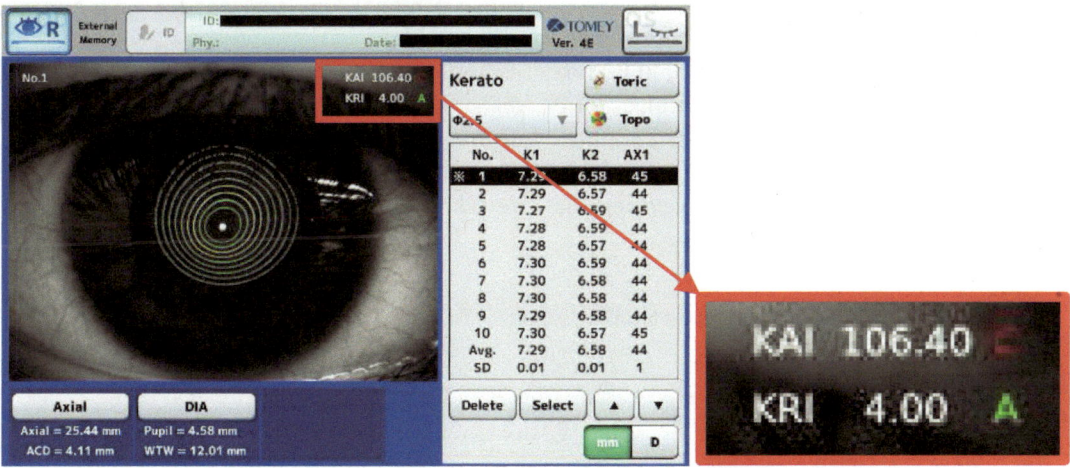

Fig. 21.11 Kerato-Asymmetry Index (KAI) and Kerato-Regularity Index (KRI)

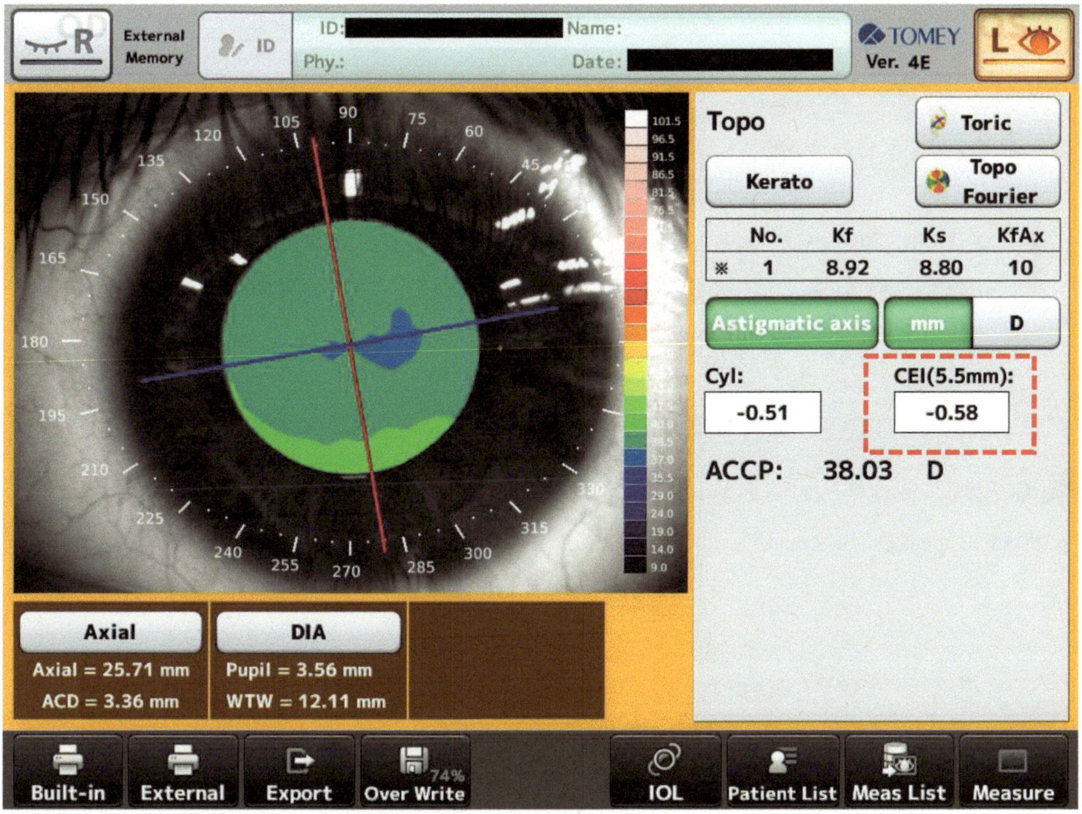

Fig. 21.12 Corneal Eccentricity Index (CEI) on post-LASIK eye

IOL Calculation and Toric Calculation

OA-2000 includes different kinds of IOL formulae, which are standard IOL formulae, toric IOL formulae, and post-Lasik IOL formulae (Table 21.1 and Fig. 21.13). In addition, function for optimization of IOL constants is included in OA-2000 and it can support to calculate personal lens constant for each surgeon (Fig. 21.14).

Toric planning function to support with axis registration is available (Fig. 21.15). It allows doctors to mark the target axis based on the reference axis of iris pattern or conjunctival blood vessels.

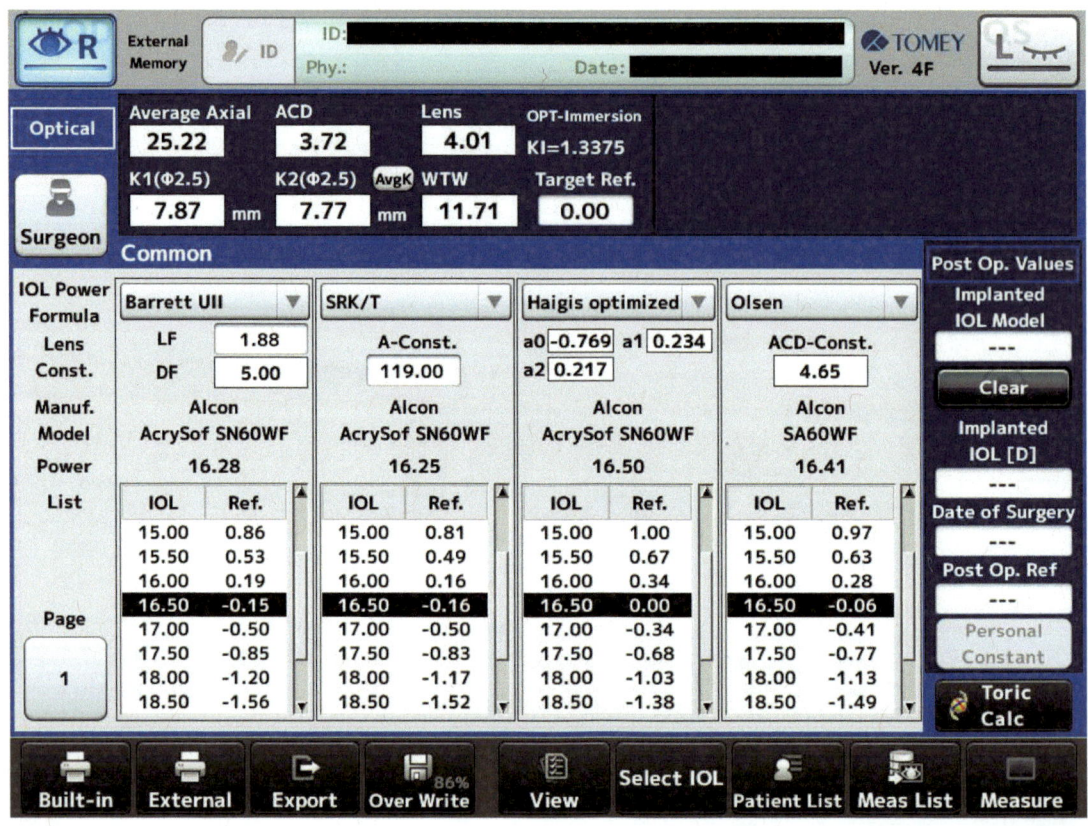

Fig. 21.13 IOL calculation screen

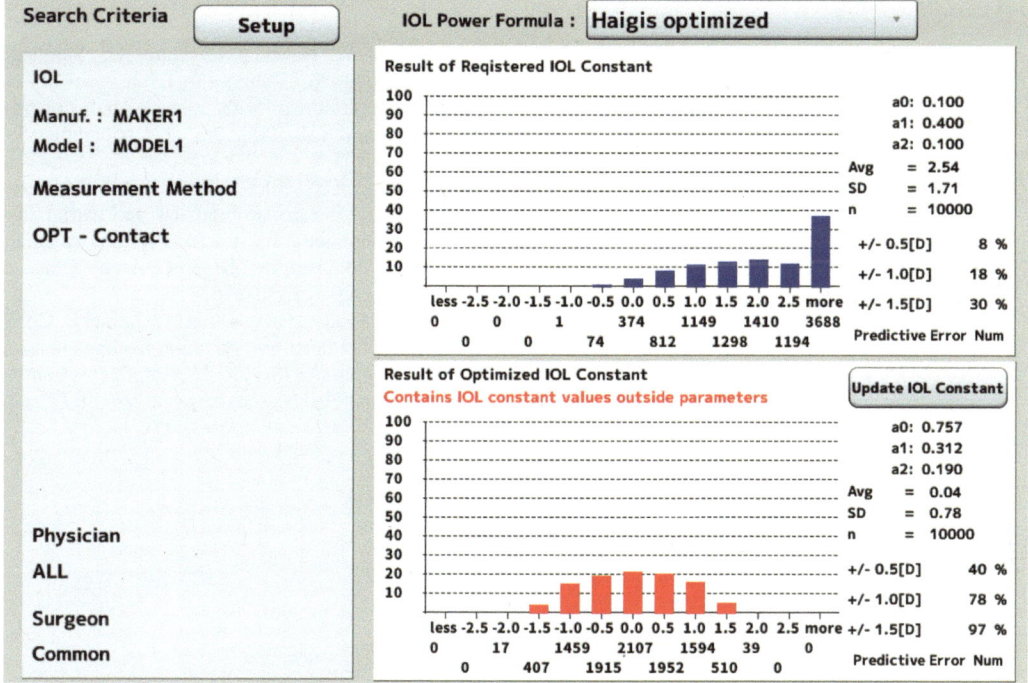

Fig. 21.14 Optimization of IOL constants

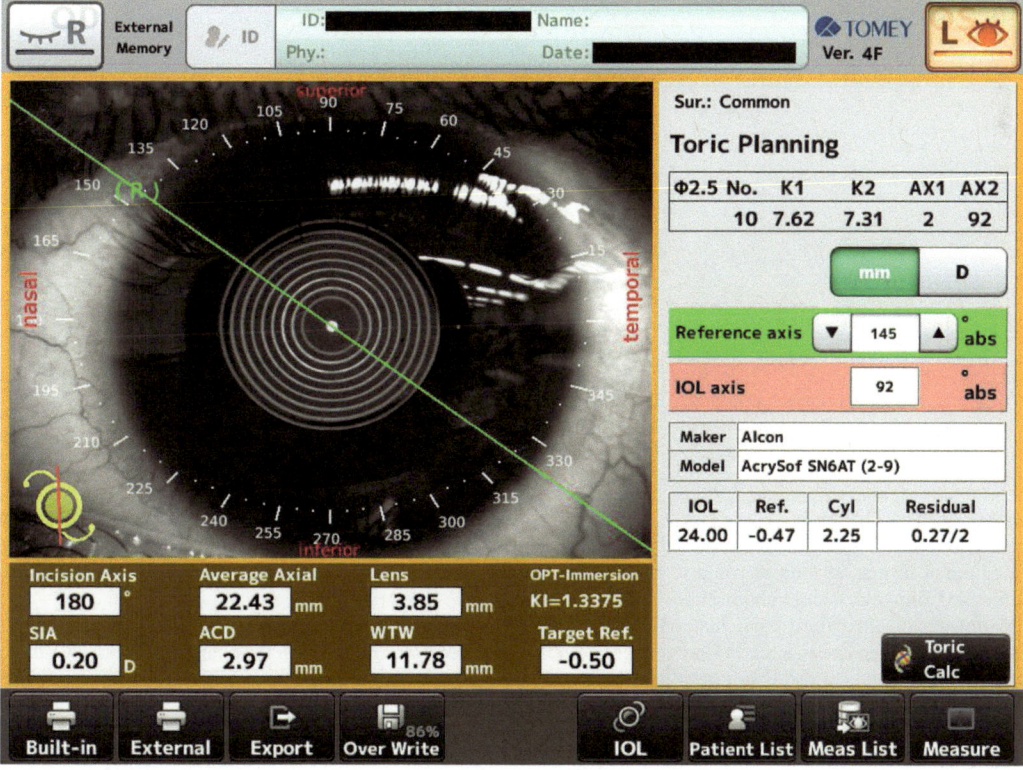

Fig. 21.15 Toric Planning screen

References

1. Savini G, Hoffer KJ, Shammas HJ, Aramberri J, Huang J, Barboni P. Accuracy of a new swept-source optical coherence tomography biometer for IOL power calculation and comparison to IOLMaster. J Refract Surg. 2017;33(10):690–5.
2. Wang W, Miao Y, Savini G, McAlinden C, Chen H, Hu Q, Wang Q, Huang J. Precision of a new ocular biometer in eyes with cataract using swept source optical coherence tomography combined with Placido-disk corneal topography. Sci Rep. 2017;7(1):13736.
3. McAlinden C, Wang Q, Gao R, Zhao W, Yu A, Li Y, Guo Y, Huang J. Axial length measurement failure rates with biometers using swept-source optical coherence tomography compared to partial-coherence inter-ferometry and optical low-coherence interferometry. Am J Ophthalmol. 2017;173:64–9.
4. Mizushima Y, Kawana K, Suto C, Shimamura E, Fukuyama M, Oshika T. Evaluation of axial length measurement with new partial coherence interferometry OA-1000. Jpn J Ophthalmic Surg. 2010;23(3):453–7.
5. Haigis W, Lege B, Miller N, Schneider B. Comparison of immersion ultrasound biometry and partial coher-ence interferometry for intraocular lens calculation according to Haigis. Graefes Arch Clin Exp Ophthalmol. 2000;238(9):765–73.
6. Guilbert E, Saad A, Grise-Dulac A, Gatinel D. Corneal thickness, curvature, and elevation readings in normal corneas: combined Placido-Scheimpflug system ver-sus combined Placido-scanning-slit system. J Cataract Refract Surg. 2012;38(7):1198–206.

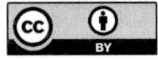

ANTERION Swept-Source OCT Biometer

Jana Schröpfer, Richard Cornwell, Sandro Gunkel, Melanie Polzer, and Steven Thomson

Background: Swept-Source OCT Imaging for the Anterior Segment of the Eye

Optical coherence tomography (OCT) has become a standard for diagnostic imaging and management of various ocular conditions. Since its introduction, OCT has gained prominence in imaging the posterior segment of the eye and developed into a relevant tool in the clinical evaluation of the cornea and anterior segment. As advances to the technology have improved the acquisition speed and enhanced the resolution of images, the impact of anterior segment OCT imaging on clinical practice has increased [1]. Anterior segment OCT imaging allows for the visualization and assessment of the cornea, conjunctiva, sclera, rectus muscles, iridocorneal angle, lens, and other ocular features [2].

With the commercial introduction of spectral-domain OCT (SD-OCT) technology, imaging of the anterior segment at high speeds with good axial resolution became feasible [1]. However, most commercial SD-OCT devices use relatively short-wavelength light sources (820–880 nm), resulting in limited image depth range and a low penetration of deeper anterior ocular structures [3]. More recently, swept-source OCT (SS-OCT) was introduced with refinements made to the illumination source and detection system. Combining SS-OCT technology with a longer wavelength light source results in an optimized approach for anterior segment image acquisition and analysis. The longer wavelength permits increased penetration depth while the SS-OCT technology ensures minimal sensitivity roll-off at this depth. This combination and the short acquisition time help reduce motion artifacts to generate high-definition images of the entire anterior chamber [1, 2].

The ability to image anterior ocular structures with high clarity and contrast provides the basis for generating clinically relevant data, such as corneal topography, corneal tomography, anterior segment analysis, and biometry. SS-OCT with a long-wavelength light source can further serve as a vital tool to measure the axial length of the human eye and has been shown to have better tissue penetration compared to partial coherence interferometry (PCI) technology [4–7]. The inherent characteristics of long-wavelength SS-OCT thus provide clinicians with the biometric data considered essential to conduct intraocular lens (IOL) power calculations that can result in accurate refractive prediction [8, 9].

J. Schröpfer · R. Cornwell · S. Gunkel · M. Polzer · S. Thomson (✉)
Heidelberg Engineering GmbH,
Heidelberg, Germany
e-mail: Jana.Schroepfer@HeidelbergEngineering.com;
Richard.Cornwell@HeidelbergEngineering.com;
Sandro.Gunkel@HeidelbergEngineering.com;
Steven.Thomson@HeidelbergEngineering.com

J. Aramberri et al. (eds.), *Intraocular Lens Calculations*, Essentials in Ophthalmology,
https://doi.org/10.1007/978-3-031-50666-6_22

Clinical Applications of Anterior Segment OCT as Implemented on ANTERION

The ANTERION® from Heidelberg Engineering is a multimodal platform optimized for the anterior segment. It makes use of the technological advantages of long-wavelength SS-OCT and combines it with proprietary features that increase image clarity, thereby enabling the generation of precise measurements needed in cataract and anterior segment surgery. Acquiring high-resolution OCT scans at a relatively long wavelength of 1300 nm, ANTERION is well suited for imaging structural details in the anterior segment as well as performing corneal topography, tomography, anterior segment biometry, axial length measurements, and IOL calculations. By combining these measurements and examinations in one upgradable device, ANTERION caters to multiple clinical applications. The platform is designed to increase patient care by streamlining clinical workflows, saving on space in the examination room and minimizing patient chair time. ANTERION's most common application areas to date include cataract surgery with IOL power calculations, refractive surgery, cornea diagnostics, structural imaging for anterior chamber angle evaluation, and anterior segment imaging for various ocular conditions. To adapt to the workflow needs of each clinical discipline, ANTERION can be configured with different "Apps": Imaging App, Cornea App, Cataract App, and Metrics App.

The **imaging application (Imaging App)** is included in every configuration of the device. It acquires OCT scans with an axial resolution of less than 10 μm, a lateral scan length of up to 16.5 mm, and a scan depth range of 14 ± 0.5 mm. ANTERION's eye tracking technology on the corneal vertex increases the imaging capabilities as it offers geometric alignment of OCT scans along the fixation axis. This also allows for automated quality checks such as eye movement, blinking, and surface segmentation (see Table 22.1 for more technical specifications).

The resulting high-resolution images allow for the evaluation of the anterior segment, with the ability to visualize all structures of interest in

Table 22.1 Technical specifications for ANTERION

Technical specifications	
Technology	Swept-source OCT with eye tracking
Wavelength	1300 nm
A-scan rate	50,000 Hz
OCT image size (width/depth)	16.5/14 ± 0.5 mm
Axial resolution (in tissue)	<10 μm
Lateral resolution	≥30 μm
Corneal topographic measurement points	16,640 (for both anterior and posterior surface)
Corneal measurement time	<1 s
Corneal diameter	8 mm (for both anterior and posterior surface)
Biometry (technology)	Optical (swept-source OCT; 1300 nm)
Data format	DICOM

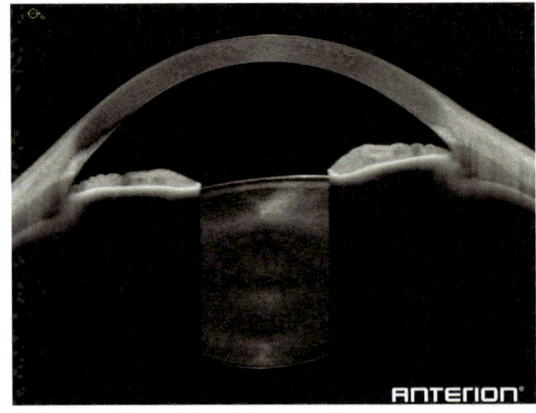

Fig. 22.1 ANTERION image of a healthy eye

one image (see Fig. 22.1). The Imaging App includes customizable scan patterns and can also be used for corneal, scleral, iridocorneal angle, and peripheral imaging, supporting the diagnosis of diseases in these locations.

The imaging capabilities assist clinicians in the diagnosis of anterior segment anomalies and provide visual confirmation of any measured parameters. ANTERION thus provides precise eye measurements as well as additional information for surgical planning and follow-up, such as the visualization of phakic lenses, IOLs, ICLs, or corneal rings.

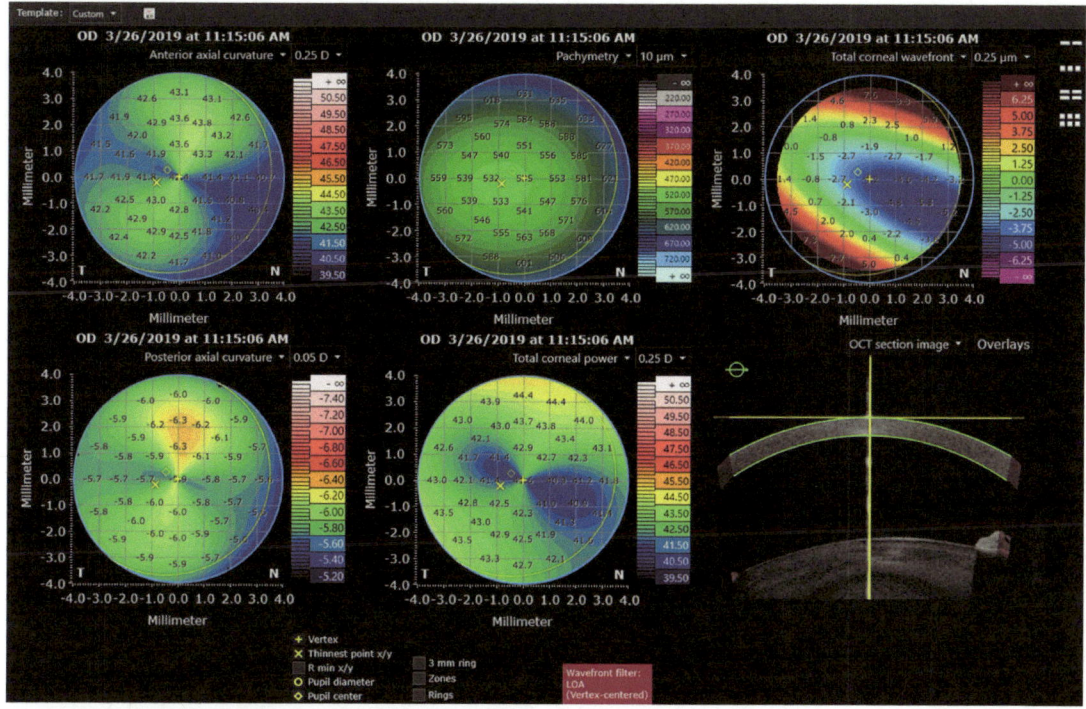

Fig. 22.2 ANTERION Cornea App: Corneal topography and tomography maps as well as corneal imaging for an eye with astigmatism and cataract. **Image Courtesy:** Damien Gatinel, MD, PhD, Paris, France

ANTERION's **cornea application (Cornea App)** scans the cornea in detail, providing a comprehensive analysis that is required in cornea diagnostics, anterior segment surgery, and IOL power calculations. The cornea data is acquired using 65 radial OCT scans (256 A-scans per B-scan), with an acquisition time of <1 s. This provides a total of 16,640 data points that contribute to the calculation of corneal maps and reports within an 8-mm zone. ANTERION's optimized SS-OCT technology considers both the anterior and the posterior corneal surface, providing important corneal topography and tomography data. The maps in the Cornea App include anterior and posterior axial curvature, tangential curvature, elevation, pachymetry, posterior/anterior corneal curvature radii ratio, total corneal power, as well as anterior and total corneal wavefront. Parameters such as pupil diameter, angle kappa, corneal vertex, thinnest point, or minimum radius can be overlaid onto the corneal maps. Due to the high-resolution imaging of the cornea, ANTERION also offers the possibility to

verify the segmentation of the corneal surfaces in the accompanying OCT images. The Cornea App templates can be customized to display all clinical information: operators can select their preferred maps and data in a multi-view template, conduct a comparison of both eyes with differential maps, and use a layout for follow-up examinations that automatically calculates progression analysis for selective measurements (see Fig. 22.2 for a customized Cornea App template). This diagnostic tool will support clinicians in the investigation of various keratopathies and ectatic disease along with refractive and other corneosurgical involvement. Beyond that, ANTERION's comprehensive corneal data is used to augment refractive cataract surgery and populate IOL power calculations.

For assessing **anterior chamber biometry and angle metrics**, ANTERION offers the **Metrics App.** With one acquisition, it provides six OCT images of the anterior chamber in a radial view (each B-scan consisting of 768 A-scans). These high-resolution OCT images provide the basis for freehand measurements and for calculating relevant angle metrics. The segmentation lines for the corneal surfaces, lens surfaces, and the iris are automatically displayed but can also be adjusted by the operator. The ability to acquire high-contrast images of the anterior chamber allows for the qualitative visualization of its architecture and the quantitative assessment of all relevant parameters. Besides iridocorneal angle assessment (anterior chamber angle, angle-opening distance, trabecular-iris space area, and scleral spur angle), the Metris App also provides measurements of the anterior chamber, cornea, and lens. Among these values are anterior chamber volume, spur-to-spur and angle-to-angle distance, central corneal thickness, corneal diameter, lens thickness, and lens vault. The ability to measure these structures while visualizing the anterior chamber at various angles can serve as a complementary tool to gonioscopy considering that the OCT technique offers the additional benefit of being non-contact [10]. The ANTERION Metrics App can therefore support in the assessment and monitoring of anterior chamber and angle closure disease. Furthermore, it can generate information useful in the evaluation of cataract surgery, anterior and posterior chamber phakic lens implantation, and other surgical procedures (see Fig. 22.3).

Finally, ANTERION offers the **Cataract App** for the **streamlined planning of cataract surgery and IOL calculation**. It combines key biometric measurements with a suite of IOL power calculation methods. The optimized SS-OCT technology provides accurate axial and surface measurements and offers visual confirmation with high-resolution images. The ability to identify eyes that have unusual geometry and to integrate total corneal power into the IOL prediction further supports the selection of the most suitable IOL.

The following chapter section presents the Cataract App in detail and summarizes all functionalities that make ANTERION a valuable tool for optical biometry and complex IOL power calculations.

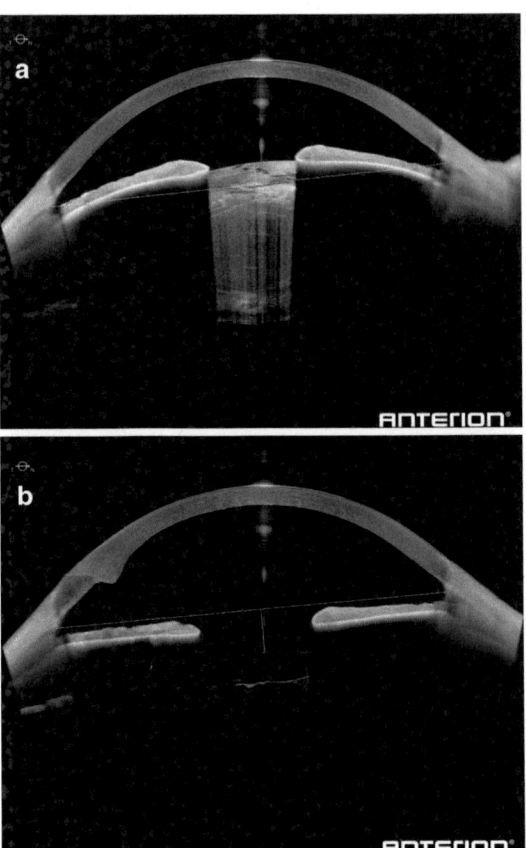

Fig. 22.3 ANTERION Metrics App: Evaluation of the same eye before (**a**) and after (**b**) cataract surgery including selected measurement overlays for anterior chamber angles, spur-to-spur distance, and lens vault. **Image Courtesy:** Damien Gatinel, MD, PhD, Paris, France

Biometry and IOL Power Calculations with ANTERION

ANTERION serves as a relevant tool for optical biometry and IOL power calculations due to its SS-OCT technology combined with high-definition topography and tomography.

Effective IOL power calculations require accurate biometry, with axial length (AL) and keratometry being two of the primary components. Improved refractive prediction accuracy can be achieved when additional variables such as anterior chamber depth (ACD), lens thickness (LT), and corneal indices are considered.

ANTERION calculates ACD from both central corneal thickness (CCT) and aqueous depth (AQD). Clear OCT images of the anterior segment significantly contribute to improved refractive accuracy by facilitating precise preoperative measurements. ANTERION generates all relevant parameters based on its precise SS-OCT imaging and sets itself apart by providing a much more comprehensive corneal analysis. Keratometry measurements, for example, are based on 16,640 data points over an 8-mm zone and detail both anterior and posterior corneal curvature (see Table 22.2 for more ANTERION parameters and features for IOL power calculation).

It is well accepted that postoperative refractive errors in IOL power calculations are typically ascribed to inaccurate preoperative AL measurements [11]. Rozema et al. [12] presented that the threshold of the AL and ACD to change the IOL power by 0.250 D for cataract surgery is 0.074 and 0.6 mm, respectively, when applied to the Haigis calculation. With the Cataract App, ANTERION measures AL with a high number of scans and calculates their standard deviation to provide clinicians with an objective rationale for evaluating the patient's fixation quality and overall reliability. The AL measurement is displayed alongside high-quality OCT section images. This includes an A-scan graph that shows the OCT signal intensity of the cornea, lens, and retina. The retinal pigment epithelium peak reflection is displayed and can be manually adjusted by the user. Furthermore, the software provides a comprehensive data display for both standard and premium IOL selection with additional anterior segment values. This includes corneal diameter, lens thickness, pupil dimeter, pupil center (kappa angle), as well as spherical aberration and higher order aberration summary. Any asymmetry between the right and left eye is automatically displayed, thus can help to identify errors and irregularities (see Fig. 22.4 for data displayed in the Cataract App).

One of the major benefits of ANTERION is the ability to combine essential parameters with an integrated IOL calculator menu. The spherical and toric IOL calculators provide various calculation methods, with IOL constants populated

Table 22.2 ANTERION parameters and features for IOL power calculation

Imaging		Infrared camera and swept-source OCT
Essential parameters	Cornea	Anterior and posterior axial and tangential curvature
		Anterior and posterior elevation
		Total corneal power
		Anterior and total corneal wavefront
		Pachymetry
		Kappa angle
		Corneal vertex
		Thinnest point
		Steepest radius
		Posterior/anterior ratio
		Corneal diameter
	Anterior chamber	Anterior chamber depth and volume
		Angle-to-angle distance
		Spur-to-spur distance
		ACA, AOD, TISA, SSA
		Pupil diameter
	Lens	Lens thickness
		Lens vault
	Axial length	Axial length including A-scan profile
Additional features	Viewing	Information for 4 segments and 2 zones
		Both eyes (OU) layout with differential maps
		Follow-up layout with differential maps
		Progression analysis
		Multi-view layout
		360° anterior chamber angle diagram
	IOL calculation	Spheric and toric IOL calculator
		IOL formulas: *Barrett universal II, Barrett true K, Haigis, Hoffer® Q, Holladay 1, SRK/T*
		OKULIX raytracing interface
	IOL databases	*ULIB* and *IOL con* database support
		Personal IOL database

ACA anterior chamber angle; *AOD* angle-opening distance; *TISA* trabecular-iris space area; *SSA* scleral spur angle

from either *IOL Con* or *ULIB*. Alternatively, this information can be entered manually with the preferred constants of the surgeon. Importantly,

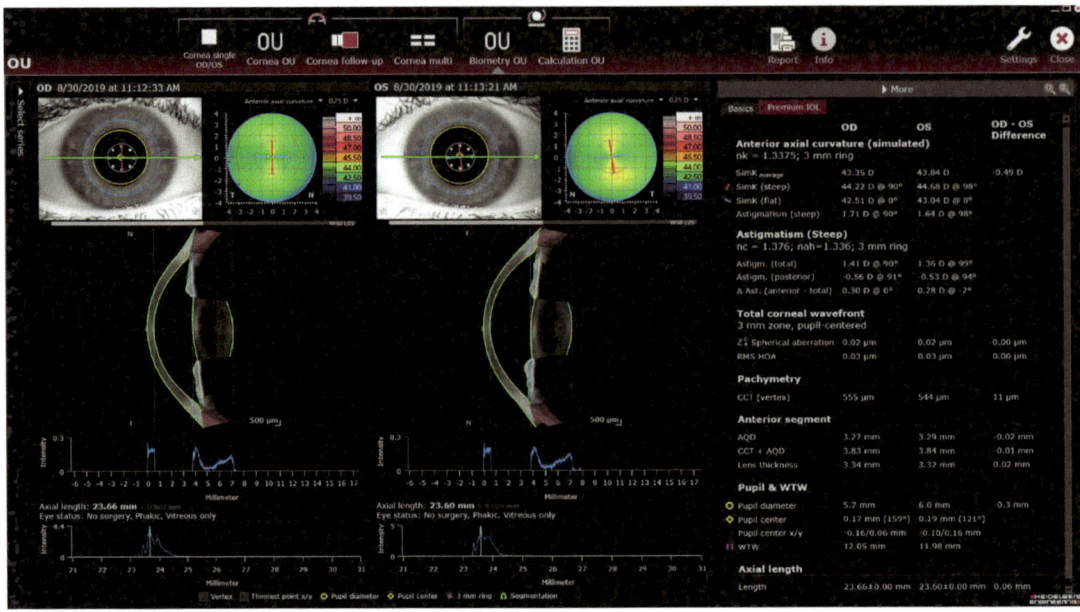

Fig. 22.4 ANTERION Cataract App: Both eyes (OU) view showing anterior axial curvature maps, OCT section images and intensity graphs, axial length diagrams, and parameters for cataract surgery planning

the patient's eye status can be edited to consider histories of refractive surgery, previous IOLs, aphakia, or vitreous surgery.

Traditionally, toric IOL calculations were based on keratometry measurements of the anterior surface of the cornea. More recently, estimation algorithms have been introduced that consider the posterior surface curvature, resulting in significant improvements in toric IOL power calculation [13–17]. ANTERION offers a toric IOL calculator, taking the incision location and surgically induced astigmatism (SIA) into account, as well as enabling the surgeon to choose either corneal astigmatism derived from anterior corneal curvature or total corneal power (see Fig. 22.5). Using preoperative crystalline lens measurements to predict potential postoperative tilt of toric IOLs may provide additional refractive improvements [18]. Ray tracing models can also be employed with these measurements to improve the postoperative refractive outcomes of toric IOLs [3]. ANTERION offers various approaches to IOL power calculation in an attempt to provide an interface that can adapt to new developments as they become available. Within its IOL power calculation section, for

example, ANTERION provides an interface to the *OKULIX* IOL ray tracing application. The *OKULIX* prediction utilizes both anterior and posterior corneal measurements and considers ACD and LT as important variables when calculating IOL power. Recent studies have suggested that *OKULIX,* populated with ANTERION data, is capable of providing surgical outcomes at a high level [19].

It should be noted that the high-resolution SS-OCT images from ANTERION provide the basis for accurate biometric measurements while aiding in the visualization of the anterior segment (including the crystalline lens). The images can be used to confirm the postoperative IOL location, including posterior chamber phakic lenses. Furthermore, visualizing and documenting cataracts with SS-OCT has been deemed a useful approach to identify those eyes symptomatic of having haze, glare, or haloes. Surgeons performing anterior cortical cataract cases may find this additional information particularly relevant [3].

The combination of ANTERION's multiple tools and apps offers clinicians and surgeons a precise evaluation of the patient's individual eye geometry and a dedicated tool for complex IOL

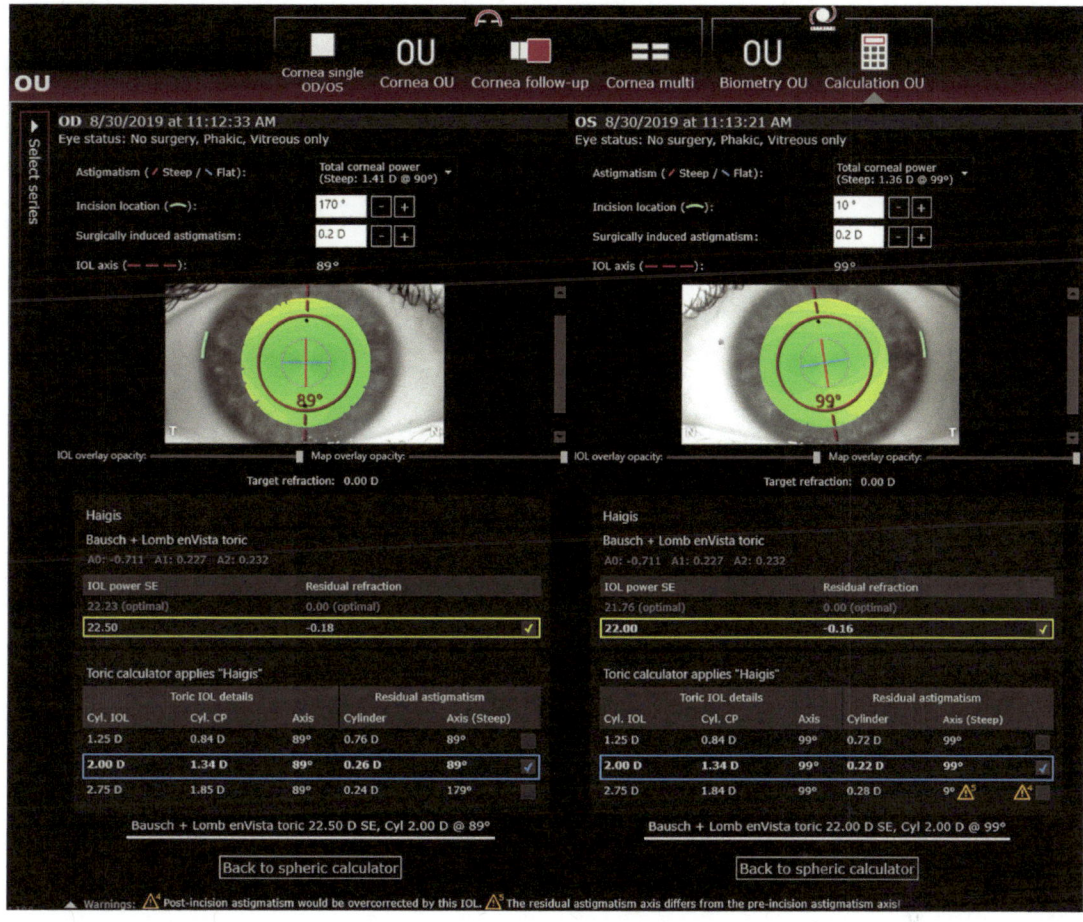

Fig. 22.5 ANTERION Cataract App: OU toric IOL calculator accounting for corneal astigmatism, incision location, and surgical-induced astigmatism

calculations. Numerous studies (detailed below) have further confirmed the precision of ANTERION and its agreement to established devices.

Study Results

Various studies have reported on the repeatability of ANTERION in both healthy eyes and in eyes undergoing cataract surgery (see Table 22.3). The repeatability of a device to provide precise measurements cannot be overlooked.

Several authors have evaluated the ANTERION in healthy eyes. Montés-Micó et al. [22] measured 69 Caucasian eyes for corneal diameter (CD), angle-to-angle (ATA), spur-to-

spur (STS), and lens vault distances. Eyes were measured five times with both horizontal and vertical meridians. Repeatability was good for the variables evaluated. Within-subject standard deviation (Sw) values were low and ranged from 0.01 to 0.07. Coefficient of repeatability (CoR) values showed a similar pattern being larger for those metrics measuring angles. Coefficient of variation (CoV) values were reported as very small for CD, ATA, and STS distances (0.16–0.57%). Intraclass correlation coefficient (ICC) values for all parameters analyzed were >0.97. An ICC < 0.75 indicates a poor correlation, whereas an ICC > 0.90 indicates a high correlation between the measurements obtained [25]. The study found no statistically significant difference in any of the repeated measurements. While

Table 22.3 Repeatability of ANTERION measurements across selected studies

ANTERION measurements		Shetty et al. [20]			Schiano-Lomoriello et al. [21]			Montés-Micó et al. [22] Tañá-Rivero et al. [23] Ruiz-Mesa et al. [24]		
		Sw	CoV %	ICC	Sw	CoV %	ICC	Sw	CoV %	ICC
Keratometry	SimK (D)	0.104 ± 0.094	0.252	0.9967	0.11	0.26	0.998	0.071	0.16	0.999 [23]
	Kmin (D)	0.134 ± 0.157	0.307	0.9947	–	–	–	–	–	–
	Kmax (D)	0.114 ± 0.093	0.258	0.9976	–	–	–	–	–	–
	TCP (D)	–	–	–	0.16	0.36	0.996	0.081	0.19	0.999 [24]
Biometry	AL (mm)	0.015 ± 0.059	0.058	0.9984	0.01	0.04	1.000	0.004	0.02	1.000 [24]
	AQD (mm)	0.004 ± 0.004	0.135	0.9999	0.10	3.48	0.987	0.051	1.78	0.999 [24]
	CD (mm)	0.051 ± 0.092	0.386	0.9839	–	–	–	0.01	0.16	1.000 [22]
	LT (mm)	0.007 ± 0.012	0.156	0.9995	0.01	0.33	0.977	0.049	1.21	0.999 [24]
	CCT (μm)	1.418 ± 1.647	0.311	0.9952	3.89	0.72	0.996	0.688	0.13	1.000 [24]

Sw within-subject standard deviation; *CoR* coefficient of repeatability; **CoV** coefficient of variation; *ICC* intraclass correlation coefficient; *SimK* simulated keratometry; *Kmin* flat axis keratometry; *Kmax* steep axis keratometry; *TCP* total corneal power; *AL* axial length; *AQD* aqueous depth; *CD* corneal diameter; *LT* lens thickness; *CCT* central corneal thickness (in μm)

the authors did find lens vault distance about 10% compared to CD, ATA, or STS distances about 0.5% (CoV), indicating these measurements were more variable, the values were clinically negligible.

Tañá-Rivero et al. [23] prospectively evaluated 74 phakic eyes (74 patients) and considered average, steep and flat keratometry (K), astigmatism for anterior, posterior, and total at 3 mm, average K and astigmatism at 6 mm, anterior and posterior eccentricity, higher order and spherical aberration, and anterior and posterior best fit sphere (BFS) at 8 mm. All eyes had five consecutive measurements taken over the course of the same session. Subjects in this study had a baseline mean spherical equivalent of −0.43 ± 1.43 D (range, 1.50 to −4.50 D). Sw values were <0.09, varying from 0.035 (posterior average K at 6 mm) to 0.0878 (anterior flat K at 3 mm). CoV values were also low and were similar among most parameters (from 0.08% to 0.21%), except for anterior, posterior, and total astigmatism (from 2.25% to 8.46%). The study concluded that cor-

neal measurements with ANTERION are highly repeatable and, in some cases, superior to other devices.

Ruiz-Mesa et al. [24] prospectively evaluated 74 healthy eyes, analyzing corneal thickness (central and at 2, 4, and 6 mm diameters), AQD, LT, anterior chamber volume (ACV), AL, and pupil (diameter and position) in five consecutive measurements taken during one visit. In this evaluation, there were no statistically significant differences between repeated measurements ($P > 0.05$). The mean difference for corneal thickness was between −0.08 and 0.28 μm. For AQD and LT, the difference was 0.004 and −0.004 mm, respectively. The mean ACV difference was −0.03 mm^3, and the mean AL difference was 0.001 mm. Pupil diameter and position mean differences ranged between −0.008 and 0.009 mm. Overall, most measurements had a Sw < 1 and a CoR < 2 in their respective units, and an ICC > 0.92, again indicating good repeatability for different ocular biometric measurements.

Table 22.4 Comparison between ANTERION and other optical biometers

		Schiano-Lomoriello et al. [21]		Fişuş et al. [26]		Shetty et al. [20]
		ANTERION IOLMaster 500		ANTERION IOLMaster 700		ANTERION Lenstar LS 900 IOLMaster 700
		95% LoA	ICC	95% LoA	MAD	ICC
Keratometry	SimK	−0.68 to +0.70 D	0.987	–	–	0.994
	Kmin	–	–	−0.12 to +0.07 mm	0.04 mm	0.993
	Kmax	–	–	−0.14 to +0.10 mm	0.04 mm	0.993
Biometry	AL (mm)	−0.06 to +0.05	1.000	−0.04 to +0.06	0.02	0.997
	ACD (mm)	−0.50 to +0.57	0.888	−0.16 to +0.01	0.07	0.996
	LT (mm)	–	–	−0.17 to +0.05	0.07	0.992
	CD (mm)	–	–	–	–	0.889
	CCT (μm)	–	–	−6.10 to +17.42	6.47	0.995

LoA limits of agreement; *ICC* intraclass correlation coefficient; *MAD* mean absolute difference; *SimK* simulated keratometry; *Kmin* flat axis keratometry; *Kmax* steep axis keratometry; *AL* axial length; *ACD* anterior chamber depth; *LT* lens thickness; *CD* corneal diameter; *CCT* central corneal thickness (in μm)

There are several studies to date that compared ANTERION to other biometers (see Table 22.4).

Schiano-Lomoriello et al. [21] assessed the repeatability of the ANTERION Cataract App to a Placido-disk corneal topography device (MS-39), using the IOLMaster 500 as the control in 96 healthy eyes (96 patients). Parameters analyzed included SimK average, keratometric astigmatism, posterior keratometry average, total corneal power (TCP), TCP astigmatism, central corneal thickness (CCT), corneal diameter, AQD, LT, and AL. Images were acquired three times for both the ANTERION and MS-39, and once for the IOLMaster 500 (or until a good quality measurement could be acquired). In this analysis, ICC was >0.98 for all variables except astigmatism (0.963) and all measurements (excluding astigmatism) showed a CoV < 1%. Repeatability improved significantly when only eyes with astigmatism >1.0 D were considered. This is a key point as keratometric astigmatism measurements are used to calculate toric IOLs that are usually not implanted in patients with low astigmatism. Importantly, it is noted that the only significant difference between measurements with the ANTERION and the IOLMaster 500 was in corneal diameter. These results add to findings that the ANTERION has high repeatability and are among the first to suggest the device also has interchangeability.

Shetty et al. [20] compared the repeatability of the ANTERION to the Lenstar LS 900 and the IOLMaster 700 to determine impact on predicted IOL power calculations. This study evaluated 127 eyes (76 patients) with established cataract. Repeatability of all measurements for a given device were excellent (ICC > 0.9, low CoV and Sw). The agreement of parameters between the biometers was very good (ranging from 0.93 to 0.99). The predicted IOL power differed statistically between the devices ($P < 0.05$), but the difference was clinically insignificant between the three biometers (ICC > 0.99 for repeat calculation of IOL power). The best agreement between the biometers was obtained for AL and least for CD. Shetty et al. further found all scans had good penetration through the lens – even in cases of mature cataracts. The authors concluded that cataract surgery outcomes using ANTERION would be comparable to other commonly used biometers, even though other devices use different wavelengths for AL, different designs for keratometry measurements, and have different axial resolutions.

Fişuş et al. [26] evaluated 389 cataractous eyes (209 subjects) that underwent measurements (keratometry, CCT, ACD, LT, and AL) on the same day with both the ANTERION and the IOLMaster 700. Overall, the study found good agreement, with a minor offset for ACD and LT measurements. However, this group recommended that these two devices could not be used interchangeably, even although these key parameter differences were small. The mean absolute difference between the keratometry data of the two devices was 0.04 ± 0.05 mm (7.80 ± 0.26 mm for the IOLMaster 700 and 7.82 ± 0.26 mm for the ANTERION; $P < 0.0001$) for the steep meridian keratometry readings and 0.04 ± 0.04 mm (7.63 ± 0.26 mm and 7.65 ± 0.25 mm; $P < 0.0001$) for the flat meridian keratometry readings. For ACD and LT, the mean absolute difference was 0.07 ± 0.04 mm and 0.07 ± 0.04 mm. The mean absolute difference for AL was 0.02 ± 0.03 mm (23.55 ± 1.18 mm for the IOLMaster 700 and 23.54 ± 1.18 mm for the ANTERION; $P < 0.0001$). The mean difference in AL found in the Fisus study (0.01 mm) correlates to about 0.03 D refraction error, which is not considered clinically relevant.

Table 22.4 summarizes the findings of Schiano-Lomoriello et al. [21], Shetty et al. [20], and Fişuş et al. [26], who compared ANTERION to other optical biometers. It indicates the agreement between the respective devices for biometric measurements and keratometry data.

Collectively, these studies confirm that ANTERION measurements show a high repeatability and a good agreement with those acquired by established devices. Future studies and publications that incorporate the ANTERION will allow for direct comparison of outcomes.

Summary

SS-OCT technology combined with a longer wavelength light source provides a strong basis for high-resolution anterior segment imaging, optical biometry, and other anterior segment measurements. It is possible that this combination will replace previous technologies and, in the future, further improvements to IOL power prediction and new application areas that enhance diagnostics and support clinical decision-making will emerge and evolve. The SS-OCT device ANTERION will help streamline cataract and refractive surgery and can also assist in the management of corneal diseases and glaucoma. This latest technology provides high-resolution images, precise biometric measurements, and comprehensive corneal data that can be used to augment refractive cataract surgery and populate IOL power calculations. Furthermore, it may prove particularly helpful in the selection of toric and multifocal IOLs and in assessing eyes with previous laser vision correction treatments. ANTERION presents an all-in-one solution which can substantially improve the workflows in busy practices and clinics by reducing the need for multiple devices. The examinations and calculations are performed at high speed and with a small footprint, thus facilitating improvements to efficiency and logistics.

References

1. Ang M, Baskaran M, Wekmeister RM, Chua J, Schmidl D, Aranha Dos Santos V, Garhöfer G, Mehta JS, Schmetterer L. Anterior segment optical coherence tomography. Prog Retin Eye Res. 2018;66:132–56.
2. Venkateswaran N, Galor A, Wang J, Karp CL. Optical coherence tomography for ocular surface and corneal diseases: a review. Eye Vis (Lond). 2018;12(5):13.
3. Sousa Asam J, Polzer M, Tafreshi A, Hirnschall N, Findl O. Anterior segment OCT. In: Bille JF, editor. High resolution imaging in microscopy and ophthalmology: new frontiers in biomedical optics. Springer; 2019. p. 285–99.
4. Hirnschall N, Varsits R, Doeller B, Findl O. Enhanced penetration for axial length measurement of eyes with dense cataracts using swept source optical coherence tomography: a consecutive observational study. Ophthalmol Ther. 2018 Jun;7(1):119–24.
5. Srivannaboon S, Chirapapaisan C, Chonpimai P, Loket S. Clinical comparison of a new swept-source optical coherence tomography-based optical biometer and a time-domain optical coherence tomography-based optical biometer. J Cataract Refract Surg. 2015;41(10):2224–32.
6. Shammas HJ, Ortiz S, Shammas MC, Kim SH, Chong C. Biometry measurements using a new large-coherence-length swept-source optical coherence tomographer. J Cataract Refract Surg. 2016;42(1):50–61.

7. Chirapapaisan C, Srivannaboon S, Chompimai P. Efficacy of swept-source optical coherence tomography in axial length measurement for advanced cataracts. Optom Vis Sci. 2020;97(3):186–91.

8. Whang WJ, Jung BJ, Oh TH, Byun YS, Joo CK. Comparison of postoperative refractive outcomes: IOLMaster versus immersion ultrasound. Ophthalmic Surg Lasers Imaging. 2012;43:496–9.

9. Yeu E. Agreement of ocular biometry measurements between 2 biometers. J Cataract Refract Surg. 2019;45:1130–4.

10. Rigi M, Bell NP, Lee DA, Baker LA, Chuang AZ, Nguyen D, Minnal VR, Feldman RM, Blieden LS. Agreement between gonioscopic examination and swept source fourier domain anterior segment optical coherence tomography imaging. J Ophthalmol. 2016;2016:1727039.

11. Olsen T. Calculation of intraocular lens power: a review. Acta Ophthalmol Scand. 2007 Aug;85(5): 472–85.

12. Rozema JJ, Wouters K, Mathysen DG, Tassignon MJ. Overview of the repeatability, reproducibility, and agreement of the biometry values provided by various ophthalmic devices. Am J Ophthalmol. 2014 Dec;158(6):1111–20.

13. Koch DD, Jenkins RB, Weikert MP, Yeu E, Wang L. Correcting astigmatism with toric intraocular lenses: effect of posterior corneal astigmatism. J Cataract Refract Surg. 2013;39(12):1803–9.

14. Koch DD, Ali SF, Weikert MP, Shirayama M, Jenkins R, Wang L. Contribution of posterior corneal astigmatism to total corneal astigmatism. J Cataract Refract Surg. 2012;38(12):2080–7.

15. Abulafia A, Hill WE, Franchina M, Barrett GD. Comparison of methods to predict residual astigmatism after intraocular lens implantation. J Refract Surg. 2015;31(10):699–707.

16. Abulafia A, Koch DD, Wang L, Hill WE, Assia EI, Franchina M, Barrett GD. New regression formula for toric intraocular lens calculations. J Cataract Refract Surg. 2016;42(5):663–71.

17. Hoffmann PC, Abraham M, Hirnschall N, Findl O. Prediction of residual astigmatism after cataract surgery using swept source Fourier domain optical coherence tomography. Curr Eye Res. 2014;39(12):1178–86.

18. Hirnschall N, Buehren T, Bajramovic F, Trost M, Teuber T, Findl O. Prediction of postoperative intraocular lens tilt using swept-source optical coherence tomography. J Cataract Refract Surg. 2017;43(6):732–6.

19. Gjerdrum B, Gundersen KG, Lundmark PO, Aakre BM. Refractive precision of ray tracing IOL calculations based on OCT data versus traditional IOL calculation formulas based on reflectometry in patients with a history of laser vision correction for myopia. Clin Ophthalmol. 2021;15:845–57.

20. Shetty N, Kaweri L, Koshy A, Shetty R, Nuijts R, Roy AS. Repeatability of biometry measured by IOLMaster 700, Lenstar LS 900 and Anterion, and its impact on predicted intraocular lens power. J Cataract Refract Surg. 2020 Nov 23.

21. Schiano-Lomoriello D, Hoffer KJ, Abicca I, Savini G. Repeatability of automated measurements by a new anterior segment optical coherence tomographer and biometer and agreement with standard devices. Sci Rep. 2021 Jan 13;11(1):983.

22. Montés-Micó R, Tañá-Rivero P, Aguilar-Córcoles S, Ruiz-Mesa R. Assessment of anterior segment measurements using a high-resolution imaging device. Expert Rev Med Devices. 2020 Sep;17(9):969–79.

23. Tañá-Rivero P, Aguilar-Córcoles S, Ruiz-Mesa R, Montés-Micó R. Repeatability of whole-cornea measurements using a new swept-source optical coherence tomographer. Eur J Ophthalmol. 2020 Jul 18;31(4):1120672120944022.

24. Ruiz-Mesa R, Aguilar-Córcoles S, Montés-Micó R, Tañá-Rivero P. Ocular biometric repeatability using a new high-resolution swept-source optical coherence tomographer. Expert Rev Med Devices. Jun 2020;17(6):591–7.

25. Muller R, Buttner P. A critical discussion of intraclass correlation coefficients. Stat Med. 1994 Dec 15–30;13(23–24):2465–76.

26. Fişuş AD, Hirnschall ND, Findl O. Comparison of two swept-source optical coherence tomography-based biometry devices. J Cataract Refract Surg 2020 Aug 5.

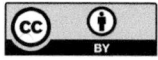

The NIDEK Cataract Suite: The OPD-Scan III Multifunction Diagnostic Device and the AL-Scan Optical Biometer

23

Farrell C. Tyson, Stefan Pieger, and Harkaran S. Bains

The NIDEK Cataract Suite includes the OPD-Scan III multifunction diagnostic device and the AL-Scan optical biometer. In this chapter, we present the use of each of these devices for diagnostics, cataract surgery, premium intraocular lens (IOL) selection, IOL calculations, and postoperative assessment.

OPD-Scan III

The OPD-Scan III is a fundamental device for cataract diagnostics (Fig. 23.1). This device measures corneal topography, wavefront aberrations, autorefraction, keratometry, pupillometry, and pupillography on the same axis. This unique combination of measurements allows comprehensive preoperative and postoperative assessment of cataract surgery patients. The measurement of topography and whole eye wavefront allows separation of corneal and internal aberrations for rapid assessment of the refractive and optical effects of the cornea, physiologic lens, or an intraocular lens (IOL) (Fig. 23.2) [1].

The OPD-Scan III measures aberrations using a unique method called dynamic spatial skiascopy [1]. This method utilizes optically conjugate projecting and receiving systems to measure aberration data in refractive diopters. A slit of infrared light is projected into the eye and rotated at 1° increments over 360°. Simultaneously, photodetectors rotate at the same rate and meridian as the projecting system and the time difference to stimulate individual photodetectors is converted into refractive power data (OPD maps).

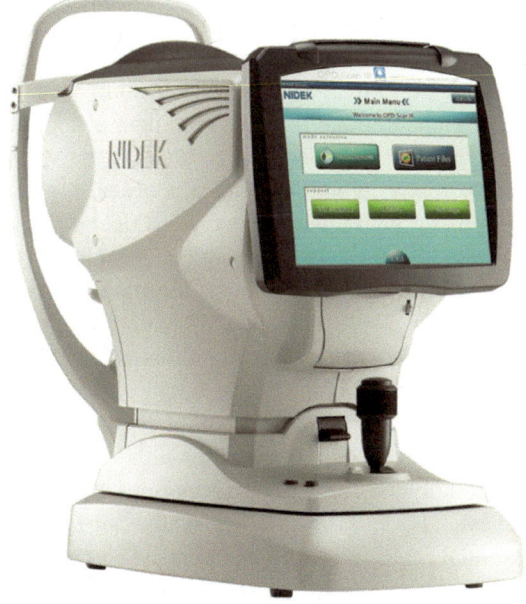

Fig. 23.1 OPD-Scan III

F. C. Tyson (✉)
Tyson Eye, Cape Coral, FL, USA

S. Pieger
Ingenieurbüro Pieger GmbH, Wendelstein, Germany
e-mail: stefan@pieger.net

H. S. Bains
Sight By Design, Edmonton, AB, Canada

© The Author(s) 2024
J. Aramberri et al. (eds.), *Intraocular Lens Calculations*, Essentials in Ophthalmology,
https://doi.org/10.1007/978-3-031-50666-6_23

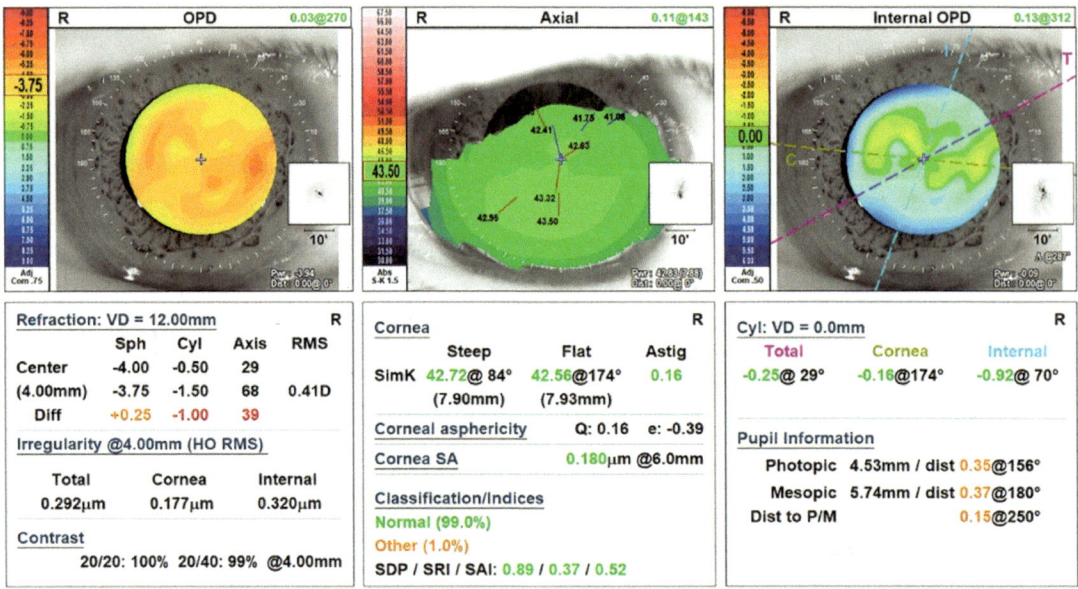

Fig. 23.2 Overview summary for preoperative evaluation of a patient with cataract. The top row presents the OPD map (top row left), axial corneal topography (top row, middle), and the Internal OPD map (top row, right).

On the OPD and Internal OPD maps, cooler colors indicate hyperopia power, warmer colors indicate myopia, and green indicates emmetropia

The refractive power is then converted to traditional wavefront data (wavefront maps). The advantage of this method is a high range of measurement (−20 D to +22 D) and the ability to measure highly aberrated eyes. The OPD-Scan III measures 2520 data points and plots aberrations for pupil diameters up to 9.50 mm, out to the eighth Zernike order. The diameter and Zernike order are selectable to address the variability in physiologic pupil size. Corneal topography is measured with Placido disk technology that uses 33 rings to cover the corneal surface utilizing 11,880 data points. Multiple studies have verified the accuracy, repeatability, and reproducibly of the various functions of the OPD-Scan III [2–5].

Preoperatively, evaluation of the Placido mires during corneal topography allows the detection of subtle ocular surface abnormalities that may indicate dry eye. A pristine ocular surface is essential for accurate preoperative measurements to generate excellent postoperative outcomes. Distortions in the Placido mires can alert the surgeon to investigate for dry eye or other corneal pathology. A recent study from the US indicates that 80% of patients presenting for a cataract evaluation had objective signs of dry eye, yet only a small proportion had been previously diagnosed [6]. The OPD-Scan III includes a neural network module that screens the cornea for pathology such as keratoconus, keratoconus suspects, and pellucid marginal degeneration and classifies eyes that have undergone refractive surgery.

Corneal pathology such as anterior membrane dystrophy and Salzmann's nodules can cause irregular astigmatism that often warrants regularization of the cornea prior to IOL surgery. The combination of corneal, internal, and whole eye maps more readily facilitates patient discussion by showing the optical effects of corneal versus internal aberrations using the point spread function and Internal OPD maps. In patients with irregular corneal astigmatism undergoing IOL implantation, the PSF can be used to educate patients that there is preexisting pathology that is distorting vision and will not be corrected by cataract surgery and will prevent them from achieving optimal vision postoperatively (Fig. 23.3).

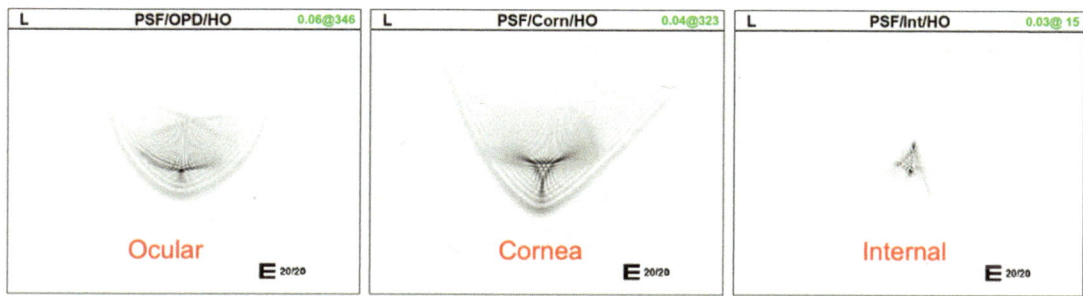

Fig. 23.3 Point spread function (PSF) from the higher-order aberrations of the entire eye (right, PSF/OPD/HO), cornea (middle, PSF/Corn/HO), and internal aberrations (left, PSF/OPD/HO) of a patient with pellucid marginal degeneration and cataract. The ocular and corneal PSF patterns are very similar and can used for patient education to explain the source of visual phenomena

The extensive data and multiple maps facilitate preoperative evaluation, surgical planning, and postoperative assessment from normal eyes to complex cases. The Overview summary presents information on refraction, corneal topography, the OPD (the whole eye), Internal OPD (everything behind the front corneal surface), pupil size, corneal astigmatism, and image quality (Fig. 23.1). This summary can be used as a screening tool for most patients. The Overview layout allows evaluation of whether corneal or internal pathology (cataract) is present and the effect on the whole eye. For example, in Fig. 23.1, the axial topography map indicates less than 0.25 D of corneal astigmatism and the Classification/Indices indicates a normal cornea. However, the OPD map and the Internal OPD maps are irregular with patterns that are similar to each other (Fig. 23.2). Additionally, the Internal OPD has −0.92 D of cylinder whereas the total and corneal astigmatism is relatively small (Fig. 23.2). Taken together, these observations indicate the source of irregularity and higher order aberrations are from the internal aspects of the eye, most likely a cataract. Clinical examination verified a visually significant cataract. The changes in the Internal OPD can be used to follow the development of the cataract and used for patient education. The Internal OPD is an excellent way to evaluate the position or possible rotation of a toric IOL.

In addition to qualitative assessment, the OPD-Scan III generates multiple values that are required for IOL calculations, surgical planning, and astigmatism management. These values include refraction, simulated keratometry (simKs), corneal spherical aberration, and Corneal Diameter (Table 23.1). The flat and steep meridians of the cornea are marked for surgical planning, including toric IOL alignment, placement of the incisions, and placement of limbal relaxing incisions. To address the accuracy of keratometry in cases with irregular corneal astigmatism, the average pupillary power (APP) is a potential alternative to simK values. The APP is the average of all the keratometry values within the photopic or mesopic pupil or at a selectable diameter, whereas the simK value is an average of 2 orthogonal keratometry values. In post-refractive surgery cases, the effective central corneal power (ECCP), developed by Jack Holladay MD, corrects traditional keratometry values by using the central mean 4.5 mm corneal refractive power and data from the unchanged corneal periphery to estimate the amount of refractive correction. The ECCP avoids the keratometric refractive index error in cases of post-myopic refractive surgery cases. In post-myopic ablation cases, the average simK values are too high leading to selection of an IOL power that results in a hyperopic outcome. In post-hyperopic ablation cases, the simK values are too low resulting in a myopic outcome after IOL implantation. Hence if conventional IOL calculation formulas are used, the ECCP can be a more appropriate keratometry value for IOL selection in post-refractive surgery cases. ECCP should not be used in post-refractive surgery formulas such as

Table 23.1 OPD-Scan III metrics used for intraocular lens selection and centration

Metric	Use in intraocular lens calculations
Simulated keratometry	Normal, virgin eye
Average pupillary power (APP)	Keratometry for irregular corneal astigmatism
Effective central corneal power (ECCP)	Keratometry for post-refractive surgery eyes
Corneal spherical aberration	Aspheric lens selection
Horizontal corneal diameter	Used in some fifth generation formulas and for phakic intraocular lens selection
Refraction	Selection of lens power
Axis of astigmatism	Toric IOL implantation, incision placement
Intraocular lens centration landmarks	Photopic angle kappa (Chord μ) Mesopic angle kappa Angle alpha (LDist on the OPD-Scan III) Photopic line of sight (pupil center) Mesopic line of sight
Photopic and mesopic pupil diameters	Multifocal lens selection
Corneal higher order aberrations	Multifocal lens selection

Haigis L, Shammas PL, or Barrett True K as the keratometric index error is internally compensated for in these formulas and using ECCP would result in double compensation.

The advent of premium IOLs has resulted in stringent tolerances for centration and alignment. To address these criteria, the OPD-Scan III includes multiple IOL centration landmarks (shown on multiples map and images) including the photopic and mesopic angle kappa (Chord μ), angle alpha, and the photopic and mesopic line of sight (pupil center) (Table 23.1). Centration landmarks can assist with IOL selection. For example, patients with photopic angle kappa (Chord μ) values greater than 0.5 mm may be poor candidates for some multifocal IOL implants. Some have advocated angle alpha (LDist value on the OPD-Scan III, Table 23.1) as a better predictor of postoperative IOL centration.

Other indices and displays for IOL selection criteria include corneal spherical aberration, Corneal Diameter, pupillometry, and pupillography. For example, patients with small physiologic pupils or misshaped pupils may not be candidates for premium presbyopic IOLs. Corneal spherical aberration is routinely used to select the appropriate aspheric IOLs for implantation. In post-hyperopic ablation cases, the increased negative spherical aberration generally indicates a spherical monofocal is more appropriate as implantation of an IOL with negative spherical aberration increases the overall magnitude of spherical aberration resulting in visual degradation akin to keratoconic corneas.

The most common summary map sets for assessing candidates for cataract surgery include the Daya Cataract Summary (developed by Sheraz Daya MD) and the Cataract Summary. Both of these predefined map sets allow quick evaluation of a candidate for cataract surgery addressing, whether the cornea is normal, the relevant corneal power values, optical quality of the cornea, corneal spherical aberration, corneal higher order aberrations, corneal cylinder, and landmarks for IOL centration. Hence, these summaries allow quick assessment of many of the relevant screening parameters for cataract surgery. Figure 23.3 presents the use of the Cataract Summary in a patient referred for cataract assessment. In this case, the corneal astigmatism was oblique, the corneal power was on the high end of normal yet within normal limits. However, the corneal screening software classified this patient as a keratoconus suspect, alerting the surgeon to delay surgery and observe the patient for signs of progression. The Cataract Summary also includes the predicted visual acuity (PVA) of the cornea for uneventful surgery with a well-centered monofocal IOL (Fig. 23.4). As this case was a keratoconus suspect, the corneal changes were too subtle to effect optical quality at presentation as indicated by the PVA (20/20) and corneal higher order visual acuity simulation chart (Fig. 23.4).

Postoperative assessment of an excellent outcome after multifocal IOL implantation is presented in Fig. 23.5. In this case of a well-centered

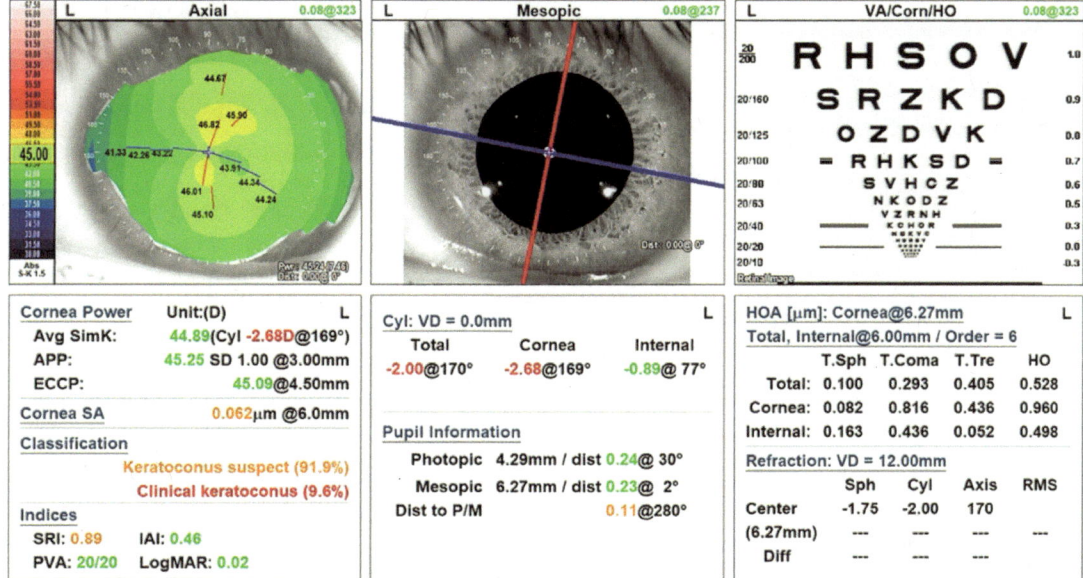

Fig. 23.4 Cataract summary of a keratoconus suspect, showing the axial topography map (top row, left) the pupil image (top row, middle) marked with the flat (blue) and steep (red) meridians on corneal topography and the simulation of corneal visual quality (top row, right). The corneal screening neural network (bottom row, left) classified this patient as a keratoconus suspect

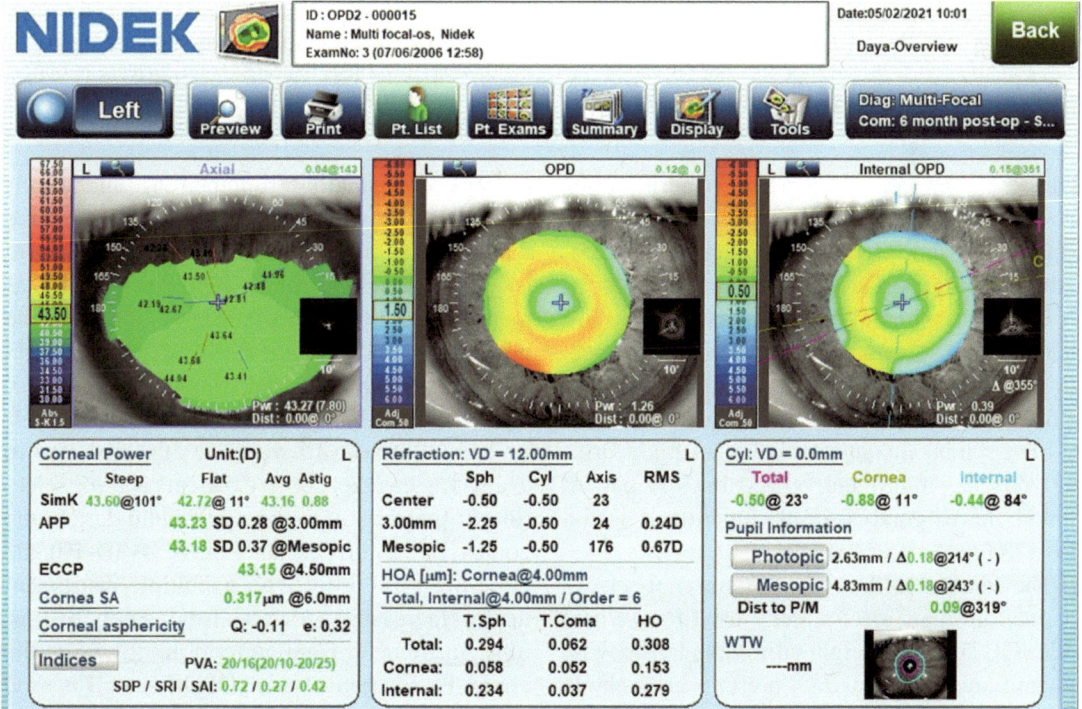

Fig. 23.5 Example of OPD-Scan III measurement of a multifocal intraocular lens implant. Showing axial corneal topography (top row, left), OPD map (top row, middle), and Internal OPD map (top row, right). On both OPD maps, the cooler colors indicate hyperopic powers, the warmer colors indicate myopic powers, and green indicates emmetropia. The central refraction in this case (bottom row, center box) was −0.50-.05X23° indicating an excellent outcome

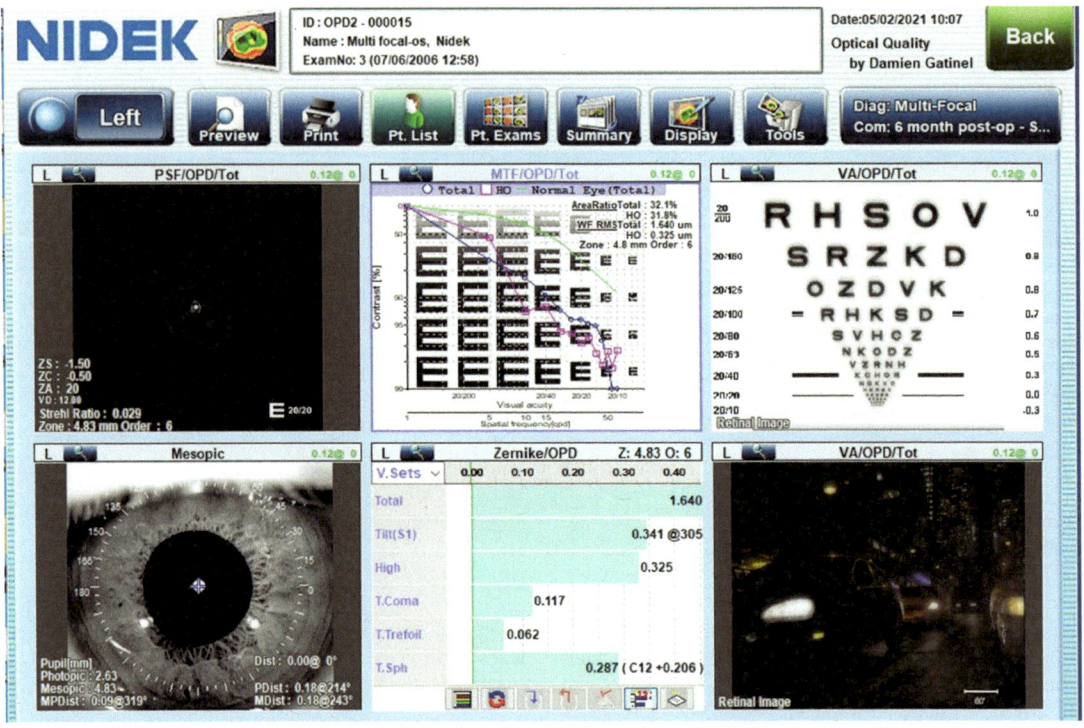

Fig. 23.6 Optical Quality summary of an eye with a multifocal intraocular lens implant with a residual refraction of −0.50-.05X23°. The modulation transfer function indicates a mild decrease in visual performance of the uncorrected (dark blue curve) and corrected eye (pink curve) compared to a that of an average curve of emmetropic patients with excellent visual quality (green curve). The point spread function (top row, left), visual acuity chart simulation (top row, right), and retinal image of night driving (bottom row, right) indicate a mild decrease in optical quality. Overall, this patient is expected to have good functional vision for the range of daily living activities

IOL, the alternating, ring-like pattern corresponds to the effect of the multifocal IOL power on the OPD and Internal OPD maps (Fig. 23.5). Using the Optical Quality summary (developed by Damien Gatinel MD PhD) to assess this case indicates an expected diminution in visual performance (modulation transfer function) and optical quality (visual acuity simulation chart and the retinal image simulation of night driving) due the multifocal optics, but the patient should have good overall functional vision (Fig. 23.6).

The Internal OPD, toric summary, or retroillumination maps are routinely used to evaluate toric IOL alignment, light adjustable lens power, tilt, and torque. Figure 23.4 presents an example of a retroillumination image for a misaligned IOL. The total refractive cylinder was 1 D after toric IOL implantation, and the internal cylinder was 1.95 D indicating that most of the cylinder power was originating from the IOL. The retroillumination image allowed assessment of the magnitude of misalignment (Fig. 23.7). Prior to surgery, toric IOL placement can be digital marked with the Toric summary by aligning the green line with a prominent iris crypt or scleral vessel and saving a digital copy of the image (or a printout) for the operating room.

The OPD-Scan III represents the first step in evaluating cataract surgery patients and for selection of premium IOL surgery candidates. In the context of the current pandemic (COVID-19), the OPD-Scan III is effectively a multiple-instrument device, increasing patient and staff safety by limiting movement from unit to unit within the clinic. Postoperatively, the OPD-Scan III is used to assess visual performance, toric IOL alignment, and IOL centration. This device can also be used to determine the source of visual phenomena if is refractive or optical.

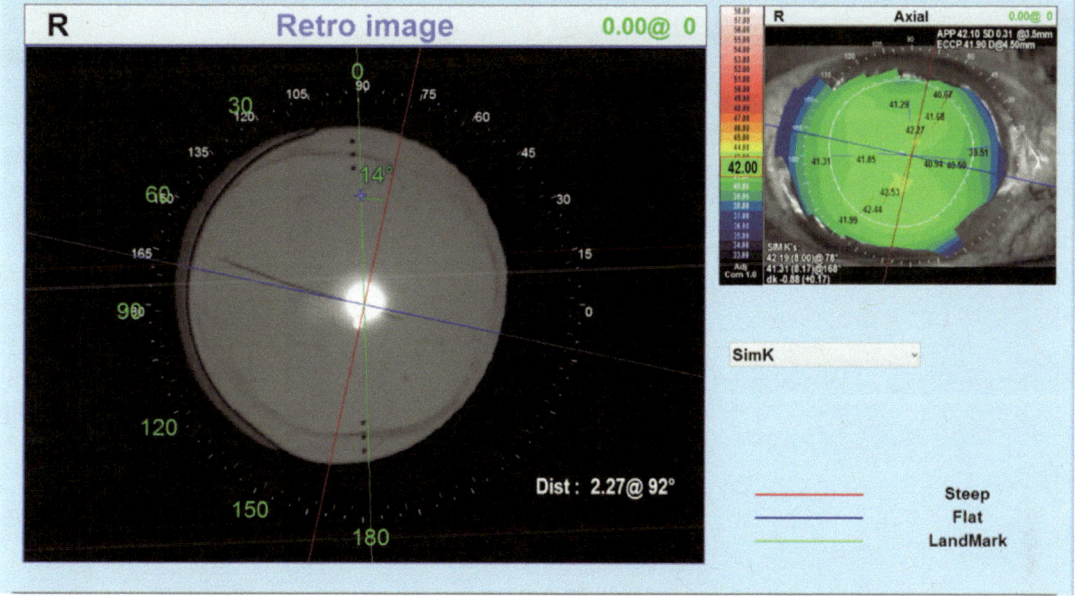

Fig. 23.7 Retroillumination image from the OPD-Scan III showing a misaligned toric intraocular lens. The red line denotes the steep corneal meridian, where the IOL should have been alignment and the blue line denotes the flat meridian. The green line can be rotated to display the difference from the steep axis (14° in this case). The inset to the top right displays the axial corneal topography

AL-Scan Optical Biometer

The AL-Scan is an optical biometer with Scheimflug imaging. Optical biometry is performed using partial coherence interferometry with an 830-nm super-luminescent diode. Scheimflug imaging is performed centrally to measure corneal thickness and anterior chamber depth. The combined functions present data on axial length, keratometry, anterior chamber depth, central corneal thickness, Corneal Diameter, pupillometry, and pupillography. The device includes a three-dimensional eye tracker and autoshot function (that can be turned on/off) to perform all the measurements within 10 s per eye, increasing office efficiency and patient flow (Fig. 23.8). The accuracy, repeatability, and reproducibility of the AL-Scan have been previously documented [7–9]. Two recent comparisons of the AL-Scan to swept source optical coherence tomography have reported clinically insignificant differences between devices [10, 11].

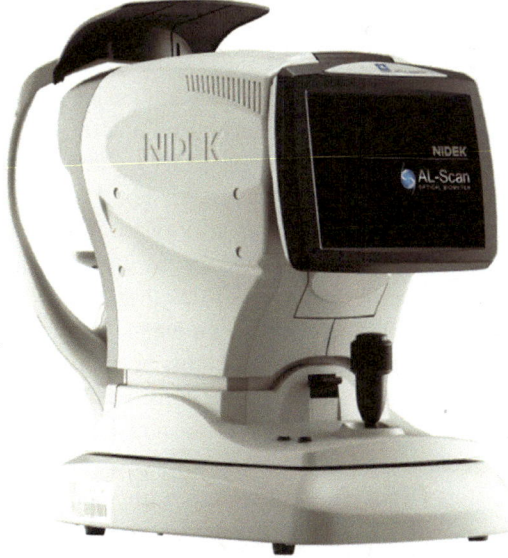

Fig. 23.8 AL-Scan

Axial length values are generated using multiple readings and selecting the one with the highest signal-to-noise ratio. Generally, the higher the signal-to-noise ratio, the more reliable the measure-

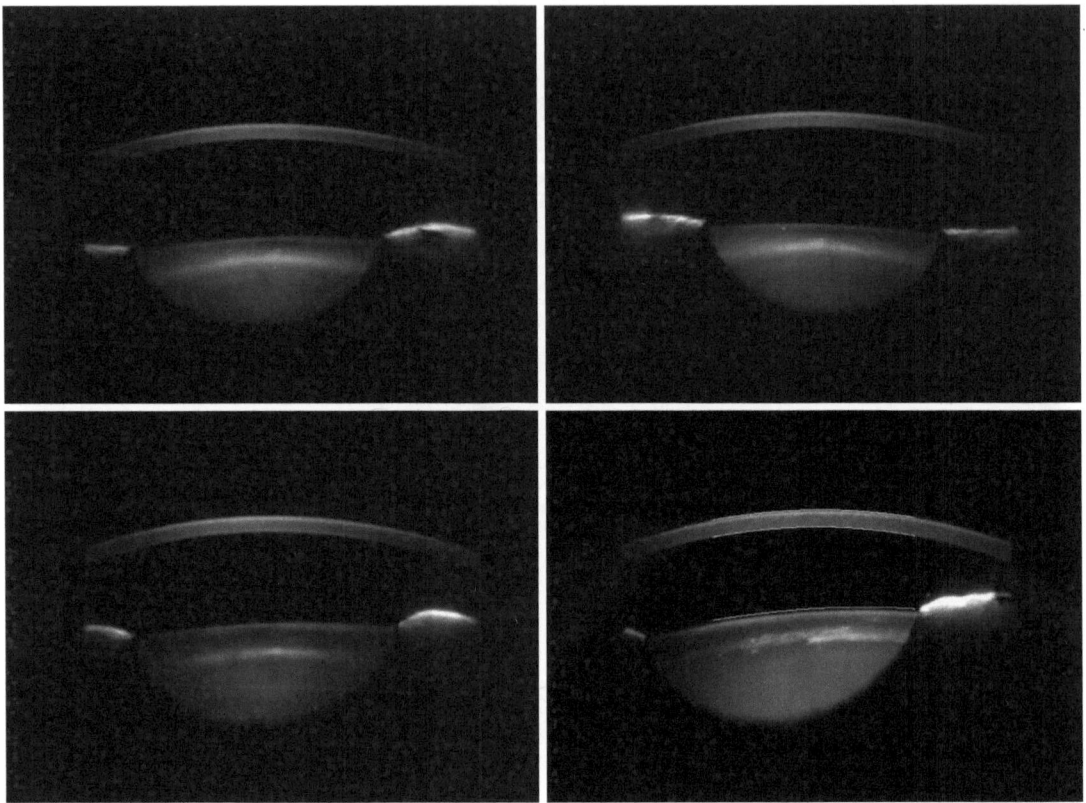

Fig. 23.9 Sample Scheimpflug images of the anterior chamber using the AL-Scan optical biometer

ment. In cases with dense cataracts, axial length can be measured by acquiring multiple readings and averaging the readings using algorithms to enhance the signal-to-noise ratio. For extremely dense cataracts, a built-in ultrasound A-scan is available with the device and can be used without having to transfer the patient to another device.

The keratometry measurements are performed with over 300 data points at each of two diameters at 2.4 mm and 3.3 mm. Historically, keratometers and optical biometers have measured corneal power at 2.4 mm diameter and IOL constants have been optimized for this diameter; hence, NIDEK elected to measure values at this diameter. Autorefractors/keratometers generally measure corneal power at 3.3 mm and IOL constants for contact ultrasound biometry are based on 3.3 mm diameter; hence, this diameter was selected for consistency to historic norms. In our experience, ptosis may yield differing delta K

values between the two diameters. In cases with poor eye exposure due to lid laxity, we generally use the 2.4 mm values. For toric IOL implantation, only the 2.4 mm values are strongly recommended. The IOL calculation in the device allows selection of optical and immersion ultrasound IOL constants.

Pupil size and Corneal Diameter are automatically measured using the captured image. Manual measurement can be performed in cases with iris or conjunctival pathology. Anterior Scheimpflug imaging captures an image of the anterior chamber to automatically measure central corneal thickness and anterior chamber depth (ACD) (Fig. 23.9). Along with visual inspection of the image, ACD imaging quality checks are included to allow the user to ensure a good image was acquired.

A Toric Assist Function is available in the device to plan toric IOL alignment and for the

Table 23.2 Intraocular lens calculation formulas in the AL-Scan and Viewer software for normal and post-refractive surgery

IOL calculation formula	Comment/remarks	Post-refractive surgery
Barrett suite	Barrett universal II	
	Barrett Toric formula	
	Barrett true-K formula Post-myopic and post-hyperopic LASIK History and no history method Can be used for post-RK cases	✓
Holladay I		
Haigis	Full benefit only through triple optimization	
	With ECCP from OPD-scan III	✓
SRK	SRK/T	
	SRK II (not recommended for use, replaced by SRK/T)	
	SRK (not recommended for use, replaced by SRK/T)	
Binkhorst	Binkhorst (not recommended for use)	
Hoffer Q		
Camellin-Calossi	History and no history method Can be used for post-RK cases	✓
Shammas PL	Only for post-myopic LASIK	✓

LASIK laser in situ keratomileusis, *ECCP* effective central corneal power, *RK* radial keratotomy

Barrett Toric formula, an image is presented of the ideal rotational lens position incorporating surgically induced astigmatism due to the incision axis. As with all biometers, the device will automatically calculate the ideal IOL power without requiring additional data.

Table 23.2 presents the IOL calculation formulas available for normal unoperated corneas and post-refractive surgery eyes on the AL-Scan and the Viewer add-on software.

In our experience, a major advantage of the AL-Scan is the ease of use and the rapid acquisition of data. Using the assumption of 100 patients exams a day and that most of the other biometry devices take at least 30 s (or longer) per eye to acquire data, the AL-Scan frees up 1 h 40 min during the day. In summary, the AL-Scan increases patient flow and includes a comprehensive complement of IOL calculations for addressing normal, unoperated eyes and eyes that have undergone excimer laser surgery or radial keratotomy.

Putting It All Together

Using the OPD-Scan III, AL-Scan and related software packages provide a number of advantages. Clinically, the devices can serve as a double check on each other for measurements such as keratometry, pupil size, pupil shape, and IOL alignment. In the era of premium lens surgery, this is especially important as patients demand excellent postoperative outcomes. For premium IOL selection, preoperative patient education is fundamental and the OPD-Scan III is ideal with the various visual acuity performance simulations of the cornea and internal aspects of the eye (Fig. 23.10). The use of corneal power values such as the APP and ECCP allow treatment of complex cases such as irregular corneal astigmatism and post-LASIK eyes, respectively. Additionally, the multifunction utility of both devices, ease of use, and quick data acquisition make them ideal for in-office efficiency and patient safety. The combination of both devices is ideal for the entire patient (and surgeon) journey from preoperatively, surgical planning to postoperatively.

IOL Selection & Simulation

Simulation Optics by <u>Cyl. Axis</u>, <u>Lens Position</u> and <u>Pupil size</u>

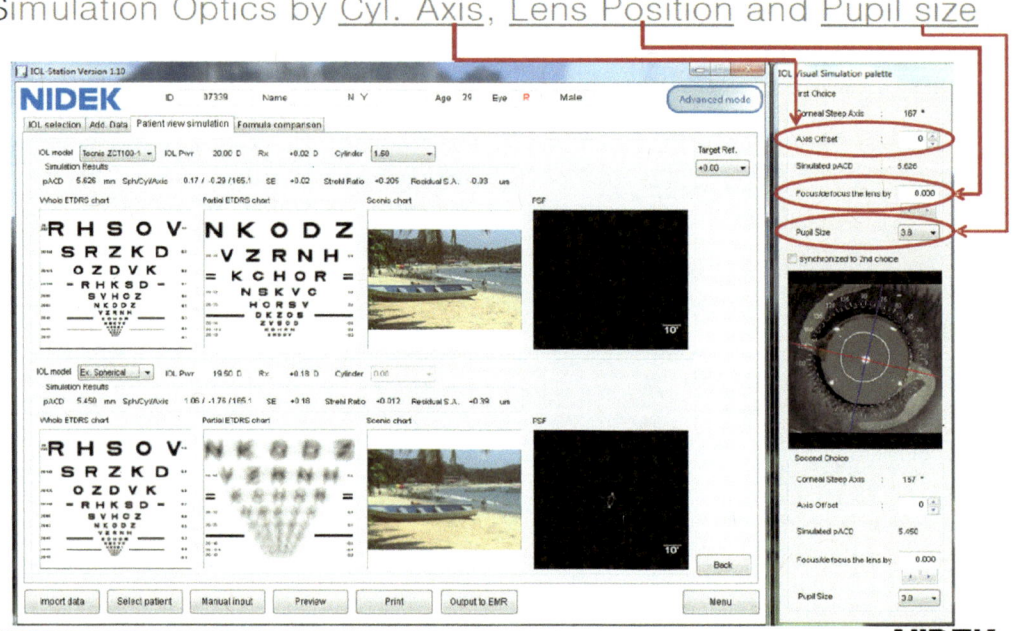

Fig. 23.10 IOL Station software that selects the ideal lens based on cornea spherical aberration and corneal cylinder and simulates the visual performance based on the lens selection (the selections can be modified). The visual acuity simulations, scenery, and point spread function can be used for patient education

References

1. MacRae S, Fujieda M. Slit skiascopic-guided ablation using the Nidek laser. J Refract Surg. 2000;16(5):S576–80.

2. Asgari S, Hashemi H, Jafarzadehpur E, Mohamadi A, Rezvan F, Fotouhi A. OPD-Scan III: a repeatability and inter-device agreement study of a multifunctional device in emmetropia, ametropia, and keratoconus. Int Ophthalmol. 2016;36(5):697–705.

3. McGinnigle S, Naroo SA, Eperjesi F. Evaluation of the auto-refraction function of the Nidek OPD-Scan III. Clin Exp Optom. 2014;97(2):160–3.

4. Guilbert E, Saad A, Gatinel D. AcuTarget measurements: repeatability and comparison to OPD-Scan III. J Refract Surg. 2014;30(3):180–5.

5. Schultz M, Oberheide U, Kermani O. Comparability of an image-guided system with other instruments in measuring corneal keratometry and astigmatism. J Cataract Refract Surg. 2016;42(6):904–12.

6. Gupta PK, Drinkwater OJ, VanDusen KW, Brissette AR, Starr CE. Prevalence of ocular surface dysfunction in patients presenting for cataract surgery evaluation. J Cataract Refract Surg. 2018;44(9):1090–6.

7. Kaswin G, Rousseau A, Mgarrech M, Barreau E, Labetoulle M. Biometry and intraocular lens power calculation results with a new optical biometry device: comparison with the gold standard. J Cataract Refract Surg. 2014;40(4):593–600.

8. Srivannaboon S, Chirapapaisan C, Chonpimai P, Koodkaew S. Comparison of ocular biometry and intraocular lens power using a new biometer and a standard biometer. J Cataract Refract Surg. 2014;40(5):709–15.

9. Suto C, Shimamura E, Watanabe I. Comparison of 2 optical biometers and evaluation of the Camellin-Calossi intraocular lens formula for normal cataractous eyes. J Cataract Refract Surg. 2015;41(11):2366–72.

10. Gebhart F. Swept source biometry results similar to partial coherent interferometry; 2019. Ophthalmology Times. https://usa.nidek.com/wp-content/uploads/2020/02/swept_source_biometry.pdf

11. Chan TCY, Wan KH, Tang FY, Wang YM, Yu M, Cheung C. Repeatability and agreement of a swept-source optical coherence tomography-based biometer IOLMaster 700 versus a Scheimpflug imaging-based biometer AL-scan in cataract patients. Eye Contact Lens. 2020;46(1):35–45.

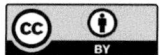

Aladdin Optical Biometer

Alessandro Foggi

Introduction

The Aladdin is an optical biometer, developed and manufactured by Visia Imaging S.r.l. and distributed by Topcon (Fig. 24.1).

The Aladdin biometer consists of the following:

- A time-domain low-coherence interferometer for measuring the main biometric parameters of the eye: axial length, anterior chamber depth, crystalline lens thickness, and central corneal thickness. These parameters need to be measured in order to calculate the power of the IOL.
- A high-precision keratometer that employs interferometry to detect the position of the corneal vertex and uses the reflection of four rings of a Placido disk to accurately measure corneal curvature at 1024 points and then combine these data to perform keratometry calculations.
- A corneal topographer that uses the reflection of a 24-ring Placido disk with a working distance of 80 mm to measure corneal curvature

at 6144 points and generate a corneal map to evaluate the regularity of the corneal surface, with a contour of approximately 10 mm in diameter.

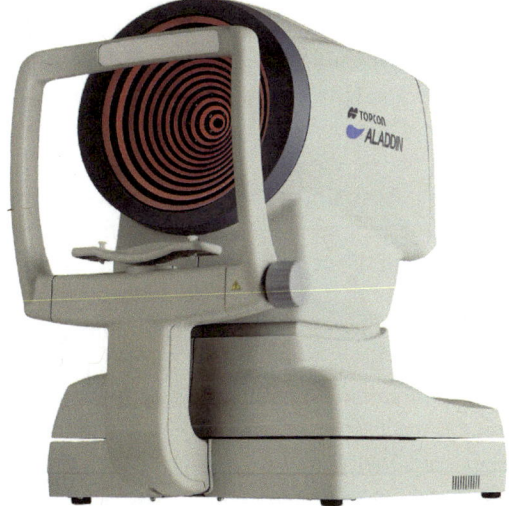

Fig. 24.1 Aladdin optical biometer

A. Foggi (✉)
Visia Imaging, San Giovanni Valdarno AR, Italy
e-mail: afoggi@topcon.com

J. Aramberri et al. (eds.), *Intraocular Lens Calculations*, Essentials in Ophthalmology,
https://doi.org/10.1007/978-3-031-50666-6_24

- A pupillometer featuring NIR LEDs, as well as two white LEDs for inducing photopic contraction in the pupil. The pupillometer is equipped with a high frame rate camera, which can dynamically measure pupil diameter and pupil decentering under both mesopic and photopic light conditions.

A good optical biometer should perform two main tasks: guiding the surgeon in the choice of the best type of intraocular lens (IOL) to implant and calculating the power of the IOL correctly by accurately measuring eye parameters and applying a wide range of calculation formulas to those measurements.

Over time, technological evolution has led to the appearance of new kinds of IOLs, generally referred to as premium IOLs, on the market. These lenses have been created for the purpose of correcting complex visual defects that cannot be corrected with conventional spherical IOLs. The most common types of premium lenses are toric lenses for correcting astigmatism. However, the use of premium lenses requires first checking the regularity of the corneal surface so that all the consequences of the use of the lenses may be accurately assessed. And it is important to note that in the case of premium IOLs, just measuring keratometry in the central zone is not enough.

The purpose of the Aladdin biometer is to provide the surgeon with the best possible support in choosing the best suitable lens for the patient, paying particular attention to two fundamental elements that are responsible for the quality of the patient's vision: the regularity of the corneal surface and the size of the pupil in different light conditions. In order to calculate the power of the IOL, in addition to the axial length and the anterior chamber depth (for some of the formulas), the corneal keratometry needs to be measured. But to be able to decide what type of IOL to implant (i.e., spherical, aspherical, or toric), it is also necessary to know the curvature of the cornea at every point that contributes to quality of vision in different lighting conditions. That is why it is very important to have access to a cor-

neal topographer. It allows to measure corneal curvature over a large area of the cornea, so as to obtain information that will be useful for appropriately assessing the regularity of the corneal surface. The impact of the corneal surface on vision quality depends on the diameter of the pupil, which varies with the ambient light conditions. For this reason, the corneal topographer must be combined with a pupillometer that measures variations in pupil diameter both statically and dynamically, correlates these variations with the curvature of the cornea, and provides a reliable assessment of vision quality. All of this relates to assessing the corneal wavefront as the pupil diameter changes, decomposing the wavefront into all of its aberration components.

In the next few pages, we will describe how the Aladdin biometer measures the patient's eye, assesses corneal regularity, carries out a screening assessment for keratoconus, performs a pupillometric analysis and evaluates its impact on quality of vision, chooses the type of IOL to implant, and calculates what the power of the IOL should be.

Measuring of Eye Parameters

The main criterion for judging the quality of a biometer is how well it measures eye parameters. In other words, a good biometer should provide highly precise and repeatable measurements, should measure a large number of parameters, should be able to penetrate the densest cataracts well, and should be easy and quick to use. In general, an interferometer should be used to ensure that the measurements of the biometric parameters—especially the axial length—are precise. But, a good interferometer should also be equipped with software featuring complex algorithms capable of always correctly identifying the retinal peak on which the measurements should be carried out. It is well known that an interferometer's axial trace may show more than one peak in retinal response. Usually the most pronounced peak is associated with the reflection

Fig. 24.2 Keratometry
area diameters

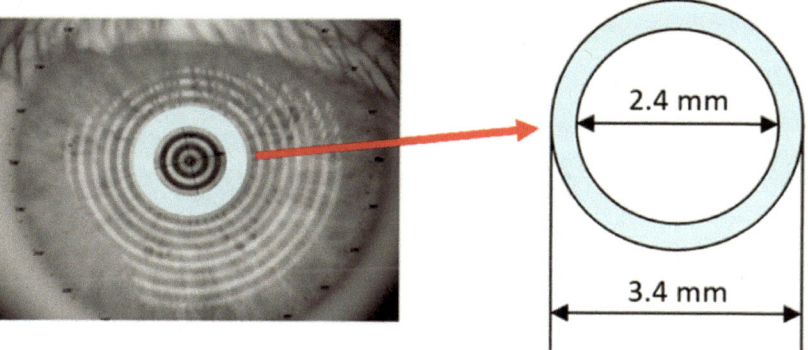

of the retinal pigment epithelium (RPE) which is the peak addressed for the calculation of axial length in optical biometry. In some cases, an interferometer trace may indicate that the highest retinal peak is found at the reflection associated with the inner limiting membrane (ILM), and this will cause the axial length to erroneously be understated by 150–350 microns. However, for the Aladdin biometer this kind of errors are intercepted and corrected by the biometer's advanced algorithms. All the formulas for the IOL power calculation are based on the value of axial length measured by an ultrasound biometer as the distance between corneal epithelium and ILM. If the axial length is measured using an optical biometer, then it is required a conversion factor. The first correlation was introduced by Professor Wolfgang Haigis in 2000 with the transformation of optical path lengths into geometrical distances. The Aladdin biometer uses a regression formula inspired to the work of Prof. Haigis to express the axial length value to be used for IOL calculation.

Keratometry must be measured very precisely, since any measurement error can lead to a miscalculation of the power of the IOL. The Aladdin biometer's keratometry measurements are based on a very precise assessment of the position of the corneal vertex, which is carried out by means of interferometric measurement. Combining the position of the corneal vertex with an image generated by the corneal reflection of a 24-ring Placido cone (i.e., a Purkinje image) yields a very accurate, point-by-point measurement of corneal curvature. Keratometry is measured on the reflection of four rings of the cone, and this permits

Table 24.1 Parameters measured by Aladdin

Item	Measurement
1	Keratometry (K1, K2, axis)
2	Axial length (AL)
3	Anterior chamber depth (ACD)
4	Lens thickness (LT)
5	Central corneal thickness (CCT)
6	Corneal topography (anterior corneal map)
7	Photopic pupil
8	Mesopic pupil
9	Corneal diameter

corneal curvature to be measured at 1024 different points distributed on a central corneal ring having an average diameter of roughly 3 mm (Fig. 24.2).

The Aladdin biometer measures nine eye parameters that are relevant for IOL power calculations (Table 24.1):

With the Aladdin biometer, acquisition takes place semi-automatically. First, a camera captures the image of the Placido cone reflected by the cornea, and special software analyzes the individual photo frames and indicates in real time the correct position for acquisition. The manual part of the acquisition process consists of using a joystick to center the live image displayed on the screen. When the conditions for acquisition are acceptable, the software displays four green arrows on the screen (Fig. 24.3).

The user then pushes a button on the joystick to start the acquisition and measurement process. When the acquisition process—which altogether takes about 20 s for a single eye—is complete, the software interface visually displays a summary of the measured parameters. If

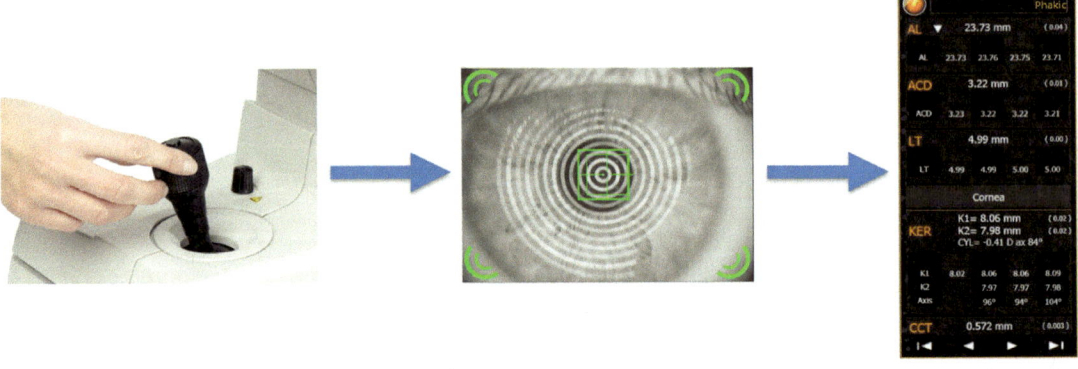

Fig. 24.3 Aladdin measurement process

Table 24.2 Number of measurements per parameter for each acquisition

Parameter	Sequence for a single acquisition
Keratometry (K1, K2, axis)	4 successive measurements
Axial length (AL)	6 successive measurements
Anterior chamber depth (ACD)	10 successive measurements
Lens thickness (LT)	10 successive measurements
Central corneal thickness (CCT)	10 successive measurements
Corneal topography (anterior corneal map)	4 successive measurements
Photopic pupil	1 measurement
Mesopic pupil	1 measurement
Corneal diameter	1 measurement

a parameter is measured multiple times, the standard deviation for the parameter in question will be displayed. A single acquisition consists of one or more measurements, as indicated in Table 24.2.

In short, the Aladdin biometer makes it possible to measure each eye parameter a large number of times in just a few seconds, and the acquisitions that consist of multiple measurements are highly precise and repeatable.

Repeatability and Reproducibility

For the Aladdin biometer, a prospective multi-operator/multi-device precision study was con-ducted by involving 66 subjects (1 eye for each subject, including 12 eyes with cataract). This study was performed to evaluate the precision in the measurement of the following ocular parameters:

- Axial length (AL).
- Anterior chamber depth (ACD).
- Keratometry at the flattest meridian (Kf).
- Keratometry at the steepest meridian (Ks).
- Lens thickness (LT).
- Central corneal thickness (CCT).
- Corneal diameter (CD).

The results for the precision analysis are reported in Table 24.3.

- Repeatability SD: Repeatability Standard Deviation, includes variation due to measurement error.
- Repeatability limit: 2.8 × Repeatability SD.
- Repeatability % COV = (Repeatability SD/abs(overall mean)) × 100.
- Reproducibility SD: Reproducibility Standard Deviation, includes variations due to the device, the operator, the interaction between device and subject, the interaction between operator and subject, the interaction between device and operator, the interaction between device, operator and subject, and measurement error.
- Reproducibility limit: 2.8 × Reproducibly SD.
- Reproducibility % COV = (Reproducibility SD/abs(overall mean)) × 100.

Table 24.3 Repeatability and reproducibility of different parameters in a prospective study ($n = 66$ eyes)

Parameter	Overall mean	Repeatability			Reproducibility		
		SD	Limit	% COV	SD	Limit	% COV
AL [mm]	24.04	0.020	0.056	0.084	0.024	0.068	0.100
Kf [D]	43.16	0.077	0.217	0.179	0.082	0.230	0.191
Ks [D]	44.26	0.121	0.339	0.274	0.127	0.355	0.286
ACD [mm]	3.67	0.026	0.073	0.708	0.026	0.074	0.721
LT [mm]	3.67	0.031	0.086	0.833	0.032	0.090	0.878
CCT [mm]	0.555	0.005	0.013	0.837	0.005	0.013	0.858
CD [mm]	12.27	0.066	0.184	0.536	0.066	0.186	0.541

Assessing of Corneal Surface Regularity

Once the acquisition process is complete, it is always good practice to assess the surface regularity of the patient's cornea in order to be able to choose the right type of IOL to implant. Most ocular biometers measure no more than central keratometry, because this measurement, along with axial length and anterior chamber depth (for some of the formulas), is necessary in order to calculate the power of the IOL. However, keratometry by itself cannot provide information on the geometry or regularity of the patient's cornea and in particular cannot provide information that would be useful for answering two questions that are critical when choosing what type of IOL to implant:

- If the cornea suffers from astigmatism, is the astigmatism regular or irregular? It is best practice to implant a toric IOL only if the astigmatism is regular.
- If the patient previously underwent refractive surgery, how is the patient's mesopic pupil positioned with respect to the optic zone that underwent surgery? The choice of what type of lens to implant, and of what kind of formula to use to calculate the lens power, is highly dependent on the geometry of the cornea.

The Aladdin biometer comes with a number of tools and evaluation indices, which are based on the analysis of the topography of the patient's cornea.

On the first screen of the measurement viewing environment, general information on corneal topography is shown, such as a map of corneal curvature—either axial or tangential and on either an absolute or normalized scale—that shows keratometry data for the three principal zones: 3 mm, 5 mm, and 7 mm. This first view provides qualitative information on the regularity of the corneal surface. For instance, in the case of a normal cornea, the axial map on an absolute scale will exhibit few of the colors from the color scale (the step sizes on the absolute color scale being 1.5 diopters). If more colors are used, the axial map may assume the classic butterfly shape of regular corneal astigmatism or it may be irregular, in which case viewing the map tangentially will permit the results to be directly associated with the real shape of the cornea (Fig. 24.4).

When a case of keratoconus is analyzed using a traditional biometer, with only keratometry being considered, generally there will be very high astigmatism at 3 mm, which might suggest to use a toric IOL. However, this type of cornea also requires topographic analysis, which will absolutely prevent such an error.

In addition to topographic analysis, the Aladdin biometer also offers a number of indices for expressing corneal surface regularity and measuring its progression over time. In detail, they are as follows.

- *Astigmatism at 3 mm and 5 mm*: This expresses the astigmatism value and the astigmatism axis in the 3 mm corneal zone and the 5 mm corneal zone, which correspond to the photopic pupil and the mesopic pupil, respectively.

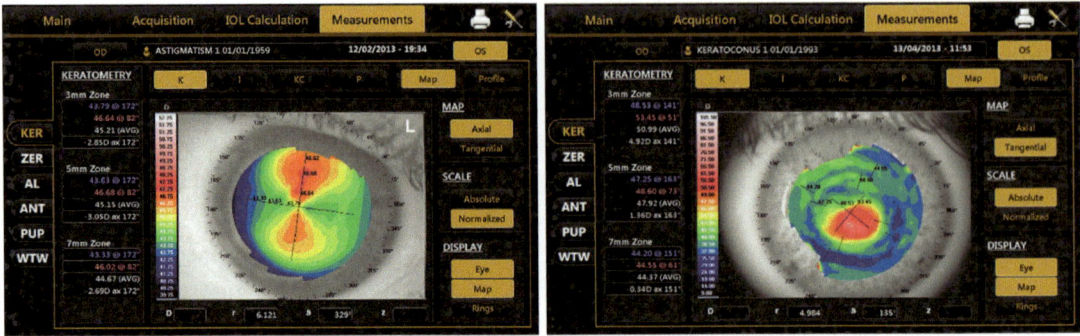

Fig. 24.4 Topographic maps: regular astigmatism and keratoconic pattern

Fig. 24.5 Topographic indices

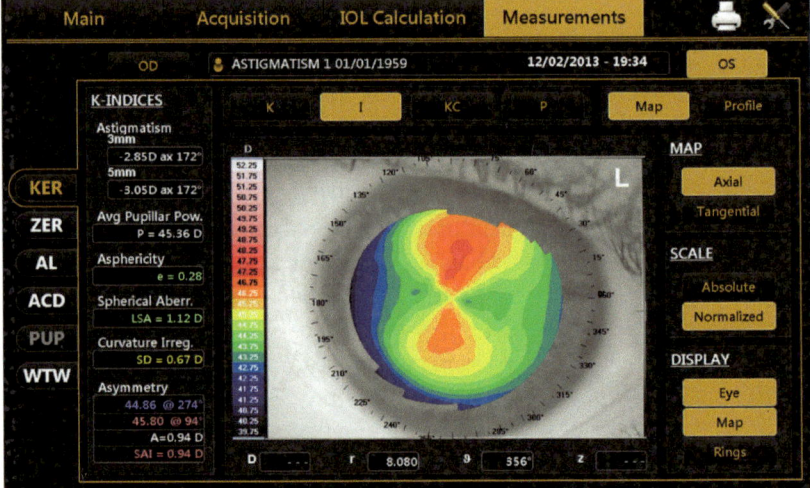

In the case of high astigmatism, it is important to consider the values and axes of the astigmatism in both these zones in order to decide whether the lens to be implanted should be toric or spherical (in the event that there are significant differences between the two zones).

- *Average pupil power*: This represents the power of the cornea as measured on an entrance pupil diameter fixed at 4.5 mm.
- *Asphericity*: This expresses how much the profile of the cornea differs from a spherical profile, and it can be set in any one of the following parameters: e, p, Q, and SF. The asphericity value is related to the amount of spherical aberration, and the value inverts in a cornea that has undergone myopic refractive surgery that has given it an oblate shape.

- *Longitudinal spherical aberration*: This represents the spherical aberration as measured along the optical axis that corresponds to a pupil with an entrance of 4.5 mm.
- *Irregularity of curvature*: This is linked to point-to-point variation in corneal curvature, and it is defined as the standard deviation of the axial curvature inside a circular pupil area with a diameter of 4.5 mm.
- *Symmetry index*: This index is represented by the dioptric power difference between the two corneal hemispheres that are most different in power.

These indices can be viewed by accessing Section I of the corneal topography software (Fig. 24.5).

Keratoconus Screening

In addition to indices of corneal surface regularity, the Aladdin biometer also offers a section dedicated to keratoconus screening. This section shows three indices (Calossi–Foggi indices) calculated using point-to-point tangential curvature in the keratoconus area, and it also shows an index of probability, obtained from the above indices, which indicates whether or not the topography is compatible with keratoconus (Fig. 24.6). If the topography is compatible with keratoconus, the software displays the geometric parameters of the keratoconus as obtained from the topographic map in order to assess the progression of the keratoconus over time.

Let us consider in detail how these calculations are carried out. First, the software searches for any keratoconus area on the map of the cornea. Algorithms are applied to the map of tangential curvature, which is the best indicator of the shape of the corneal surface. If an area is identified as being potentially keratoconus, a set of geometric and refractive parameters are calculated for that area. An index is obtained from this set of parameters, which indicates the probability that the topography is compatible with the topography of keratoconus. The software visually presents a diagnostic summary of the keratoconus screening, which displays three specific indices (Calossi–Foggi indices) whose values can be associated with the degree of severity of the keratoconus. Let us look at them in detail.

Fig. 24.6 Keratoconus analysis software

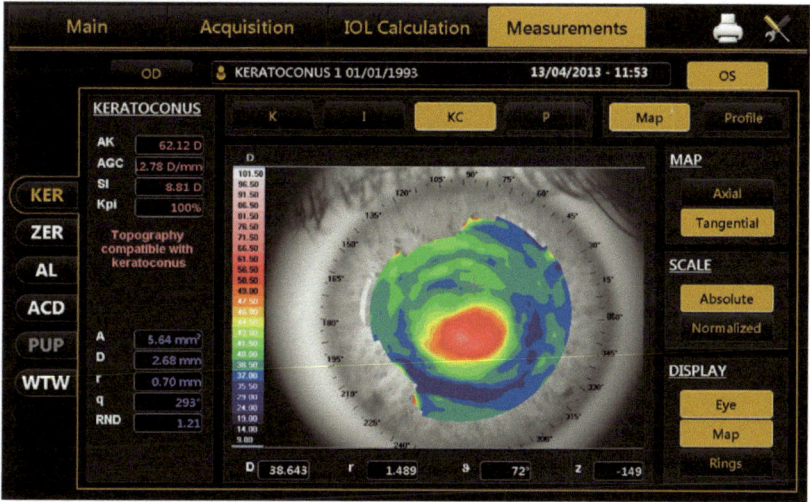

AK—Apex curvature: This represents the tangential curvature at the apex of the keratoconus, the apex being identified as the point of maximum curvature of the keratoconus.

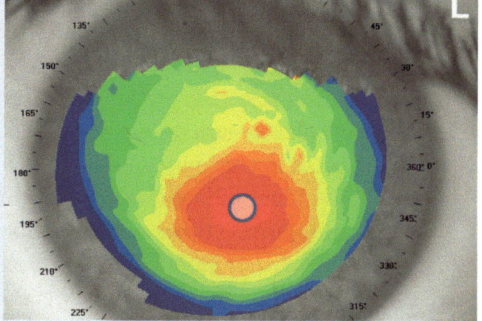

AGC—Apex gradient of curvature: This index quantifies the average difference per length unit of the corneal power in relation to the apical power.

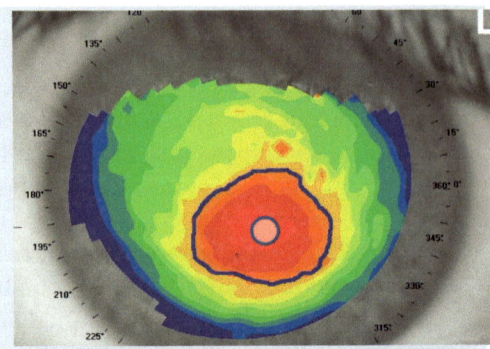

SI—Symmetry index: This represents the difference between the average tangential curvature of two symmetrical circular areas of 3 mm diameter situated on the lower hemisphere and the upper hemisphere, respectively.

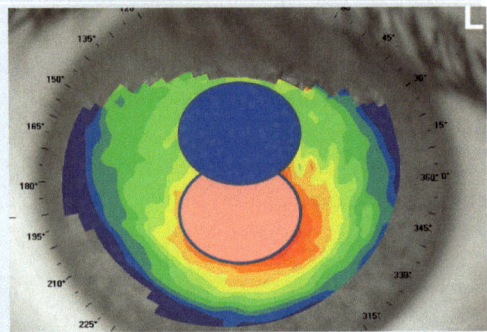

In the event that keratoconus is detected, the software provides geometric information on the keratoconus, such as its area, diameter, center of gravity, and roundness.

The keratoconus screening and indices serve as an additional source of information on the regularity of the corneal surface.

Pupillometric Analysis

The Aladdin biometer includes an advanced pupillometer which is used for static and dynamic analysis of pupil diameter and decentering, and plots the changes of the pupil's response to light stimuli over time. The Aladdin biometer has four infrared LEDs to generate the ambient lighting necessary for the camera to take photographs when the pupil is not being stimulated, plus two white LEDs to induce photopic contraction in the pupil at appropriate times. Acquisition of dynamic and static pupillometric information is carried out manually. First, the joystick is used to center the cornea's reflections of the four infrared LEDs on a grid superimposed on the live image displayed. Then the button on the joystick is used to start and stop the recording of video and storage of the individual frames, on which the pupillometric analysis is carried out. When the analysis process is complete, the following pupil parameters are displayed (Fig. 24.7):

- *Dynamic pupillometry.*
  - Minimum pupil diameter and the pupil decentering at that diameter.
  - Maximum pupil diameter and the pupil decentering at that diameter.
  - A graph of pupil decentering vs. diameter.
  - A graph, over time, of the change in pupil diameter and of the corresponding response time to light stimuli.
- *Static pupillometry.*
  - Average pupil diameter in photopic light conditions, and average pupil decentering at that diameter.
  - Average pupil diameter in mesopic light conditions, and average pupil decentering at that diameter.

Fig. 24.7 Pupillometry analysis

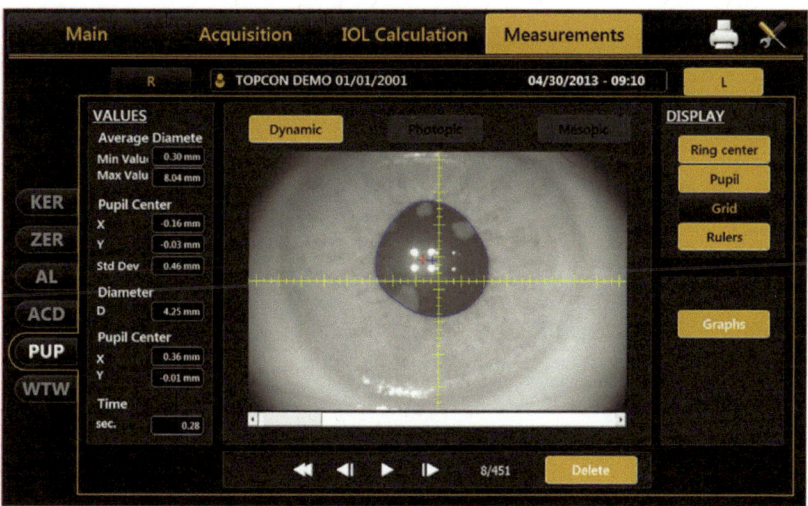

Analysis of Corneal Quality of Vision

Combining corneal topography with the diameter of the pupil in photopic and mesopic conditions makes it possible to analyze the cornea's quality of vision in the different ambient light conditions. This analysis starts with an examination of the corneal wavefront and how it is decomposed into the main aberration components introduced by the cornea. In particular, Zernike polynomial decomposition is used to obtain detailed information on astigmatism, spherical aberration, coma, and high-order aberrations as the pupil diameter changes. Additional information is provided by the software with regard to the point spread function (PSF), the spot diagram, the pyramid of Zernike coefficients, and the simulation of the corrected visus.

All this information helps provide a more comprehensive picture of the cornea's refractive characteristics, since the analysis is not limited to the keratometric value, which is basically the only need in order to calculate the power of the IOL. Instead, the analysis also includes an assessment of corneal surface regularity and of the associated impact on quality of vision in different ambient light conditions. Such information is necessary for determining the type of lens to be implanted and selecting the calculation formula for the power that will have the best vision performance for the patient in question. Figure 24.8 shows how aberrations are displayed on the Aladdin biometer in the case of a cornea with keratoconus (left) and in the case of a cornea that has undergone myopic refractive surgery (right) which has a small, decentered optic zone. Both are calculated with the entrance of the pupil being 5 mm (i.e., mesopic pupil).

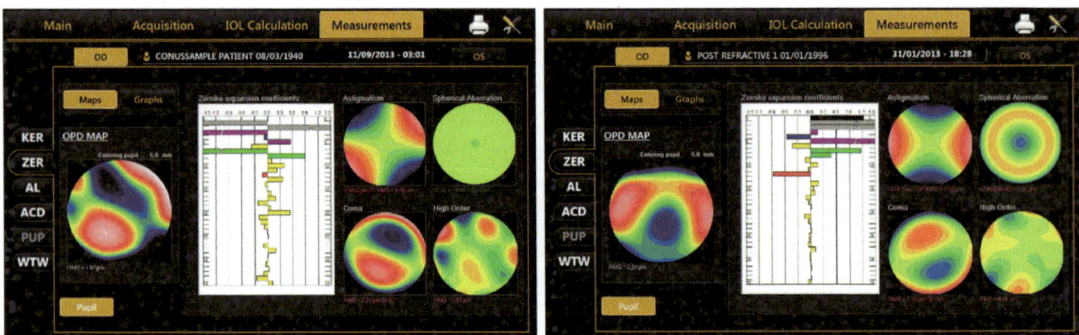

Fig. 24.8 Corneal aberrometry analysis

Fig. 24.9 IOL power
calculations table

Formulas for Calculating the Power of the IOL

The Aladdin biometer comes with a complete set of formulas for calculating the power of any type of IOL. These formulas can be accessed in a special work area that is divided into sections according to the requirements involved (Fig. 24.9). We will now describe each of the sections.

Conventional Formulas for Calculating the Power of Spherical Lenses

In this section, up to five different calculation panels can be displayed at once, each of them being associated with a particular lens and a specific calculation formula. The following calculation formulas are available:

- SRK/T.
- Haigis.
- Hoffer® Q.
- Holladay.
- Barrett Universal II.
- Olsen.

Each of the formulas uses one or more specific constants, which are optimized for each IOL model on a statistical basis. The Aladdin biometer has a complete database of the main IOLs on the market, including the optimized constants for each calculation formula as indicated in the ULIB/IOLcon database. The surgeon can modify the values for the constants for each IOL so as to customize his/her set of lenses and even create new lens models. The biometer can be used by more than one surgeon, and each surgeon can maintain his/her own separate, customized database of IOLs.

Toric Lens Calculator

The Aladdin biometer has a generic calculator for toric lenses (Fig. 24.10). This calculator first calculates the spherical equivalent power based on one of the main calculation formulas and then performs advanced calculations of the toricity of the lens, its positioning axis, and the expected refraction and residual astigmatism. To calculate the toric lens more precisely, Abulafia-Koch correction can be applied in order to take the posterior corneal surface into account on a statistical basis. In addition, the calculation can include the potential astigmatism that the surgery may cause depending on where the surgical incision is made. The biometer also offers a simulation tool for estimating the refractive error and the residual astigmatism in the event of an error in the positioning of the toric lens.

Fig. 24.10 Toric IOL calculations

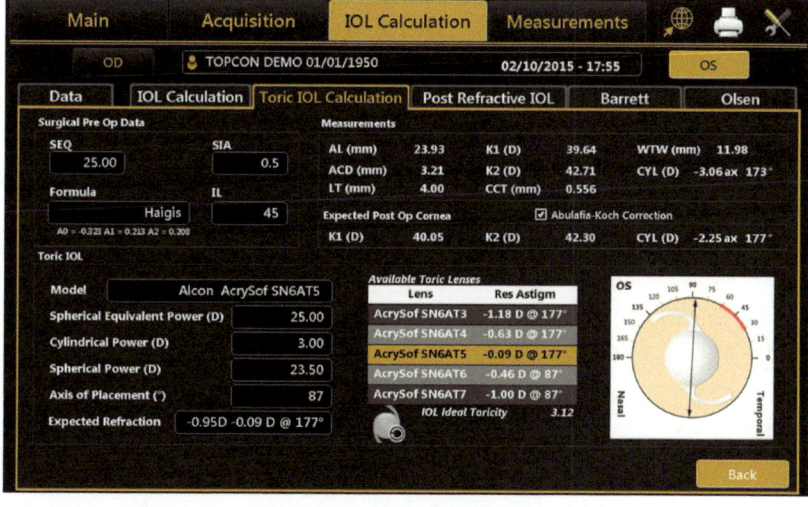

Special Formulas for Calculating Lens Power in the Case of Patients Who Have Undergone Refractive Surgery

In the case of patients who have gone through refractive surgery, the use of conventional formulas to calculate the power of the IOL is not recommended. That is because variation in the anterior surface of the cornea induced by the refractive surgery will cause conventional formulas to incorrectly estimate the effective lens position (ELP), which will reduce the accuracy of the power calculation for the IOL. For such patients, the Aladdin biometer offers the Camellin-Calossi formula and the Shammas-PL formula. In the Camellin-Calossi formula, the SIRC (or else the central and peripheral pachymetry values) must be input, but if information on previous refractive surgery is not available, then the Shammas-PL (or "No History") formula should be used.

Barrett Calculator

This is an advanced, structured calculator that can calculate the power of an IOL regardless of the type of lens or the situation of the eye. This calculator has five different types of formulas (Fig. 24.11):

- Barrett Universal II, for virgin eyes.
- True-K, for post-myopic, hyperopic, or RK (used for cases in which the SIRC is known and for no-history cases).
- Toric, for toric IOLs.
- True-K Toric, for post-myopic, hyperopic, or RK.
- RX Formula, when the use of a repositioning (rotating) toric IOL is recommended, when a change of lenses is involved, or when a piggyback (add-on) IOL is to be added.

Olsen Calculator

This is an advanced calculator based on the paraxial ray tracing method. It includes a sophisticated algorithm for estimating the ELP, and it uses a proprietary method to take into account the effect of the posterior surface of the cornea. To perform a calculation using ray tracing, one needs not only the keratometry measurements, the axial length, and the anterior chamber depth but also an accurate measurement of the thickness of the crystalline lens. Accurate execution of this calculation requires detailed knowledge of a number of design parameters for IOLs, and these parameters are included in the lens database that comes with the Aladdin biometer (Fig. 24.12).

Fig. 24.11 Barrett IOL calculations suite

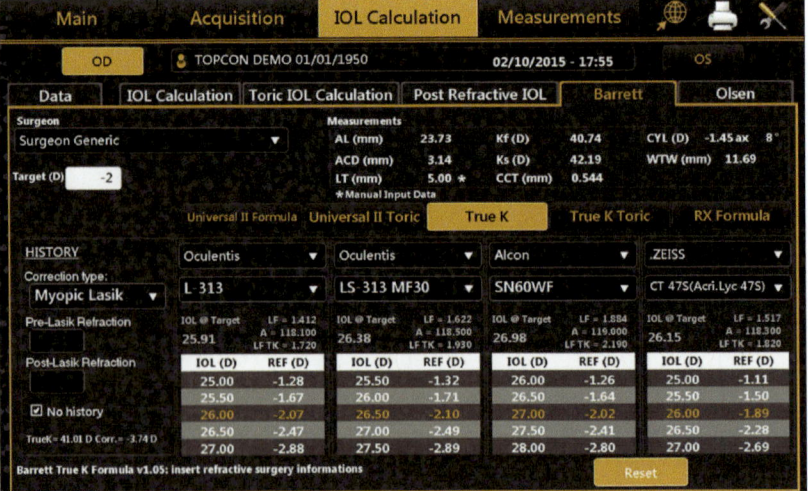

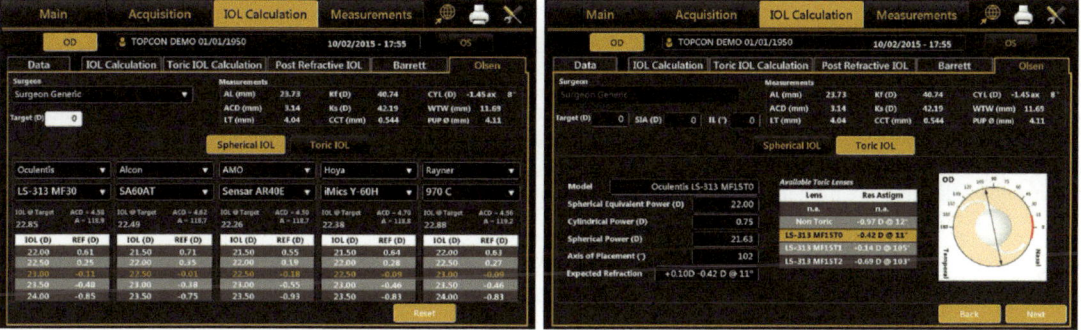

Fig. 24.12 Olsen formula

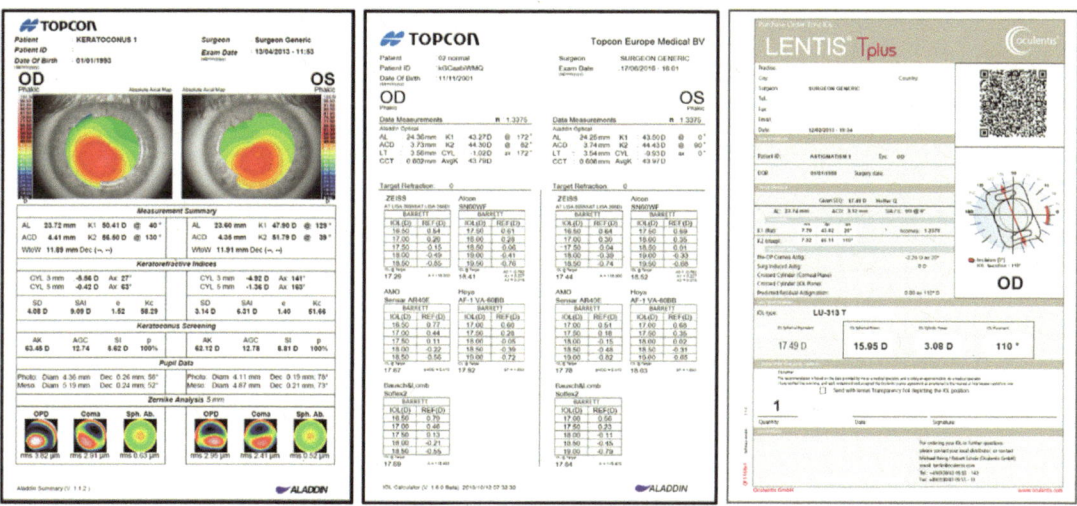

Fig. 24.13 Aladdin printouts

The Olsen calculator can be used to calculate the power of spherical or toric IOLs for any type of patient.

Printed Reports

The Aladdin biometer offers an extensive set of printed reports, with a report for each of the main work areas (Fig. 24.13):

- A summary report of all measurements made.
- A diagnostic report regarding corneal surface regularity.
- A report on the power of IOLs.
- A summary report regarding toric lenses.

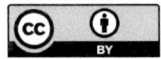

Haag-Streit Biometers: Eyestar 900 and Lenstar 900

25

Thomas Bütler

Introduction

With the Eyestar 900, as the introduction of a complete swept-source OCT-based eye analyzer, Haag-Streit is opening a new chapter in measuring, imaging, and diagnosing the human eye. The Eyestar 900 features swept-source OCT technology, enabling precise measurement, as well as topographic assessment, of the front and back corneal surface and the anterior chamber, including the lens, as well as imaging of all these structures. It also includes cornea-to-retina biometry of the entire eye (Fig. 25.1).

The swept-source OCT-based technology provides topography of the front and back corneal surface, pachymetry maps, biometry, and both A- and B-scan imaging, in a single measuring procedure, on a single device. All data is based on swept-source OCT, enabling precise measurements, stunning imaging, and excellent cataract penetration in a single, fully automated, and rapid data acquisition process. The device also features well-established dual-zone reflective keratometry, specifically for cataract applications, providing precise and IOL-constant compatible keratometry and astigmatism measurements. The pooled information enables the eyecare specialist to improve outcomes of surgical interventions (e.g., cataract surgery), diagnose diseases (e.g., keratoconus) quickly and reliably, and document eye status and surgical outcomes (Fig. 25.2).

The Eyestar 900 is powered by EyeSuite, the intuitive software tool that enables seamless integration of the device into any practice environment. It also includes the often-copied, never-equalled EyeSuite IOL cataract planning software, for excellent planning of cataract interventions based on latest-generation IOL calculation methods, such as Hill-RBF, Barrett, and Olsen.

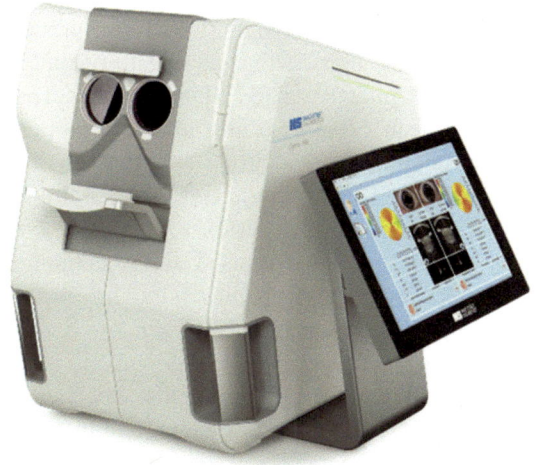

Fig. 25.1 Eyestar, the fully automated swept-source OCT-based eye analyzer by Haag-Streit

T. Bütler (✉)
Haag-Streit AG, Koeniz, Switzerland
e-mail: thomas.beutler@haag-streit.com

© The Author(s) 2024
J. Aramberri et al. (eds.), *Intraocular Lens Calculations*, Essentials in Ophthalmology,
https://doi.org/10.1007/978-3-031-50666-6_25

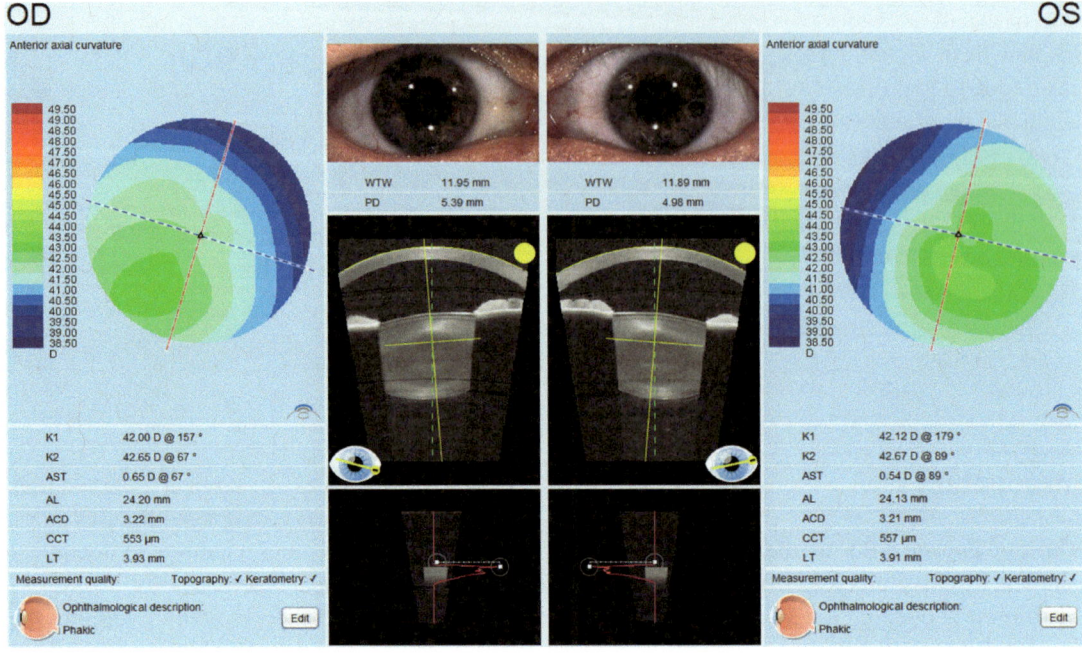

Fig. 25.2 Comprehensive overview screen of a measurement result in the Eyestar Cataract Suite, featuring all information necessary for successful cataract planning, from standard mono-focal- to premium multifocal- and/or toric IOL

Swept-Source OCT-Based Biometry and Tomography with Mandala Scan Technology

One of the challenges of OCT-based tomography, and even more for topography, is the compensation of artifacts due to eye motion. With Eyestar, Haag-Streit is introducing new and patented scanning technology, called Mandala Scan. The Mandala-Scan system features all OCT motion compensation, independent of any video-based eye-tracking. Classical systems use multiple radial scans across the vertex to scan the eye (Fig. 25.3). The vertex is used as the common scan location. This enables straightforward motion compensation based on standard video eye-tracking technology. The downside is a potential latency time between the video eye-tracking and the OCT scan system, and that the line-scan may be regarded as motion-free. In contrast, the Mandala Scan technology uses a series of circular scans of the eye. The optimized distribution of intersections in the Mandala Scan allows for mathematical identification and com-

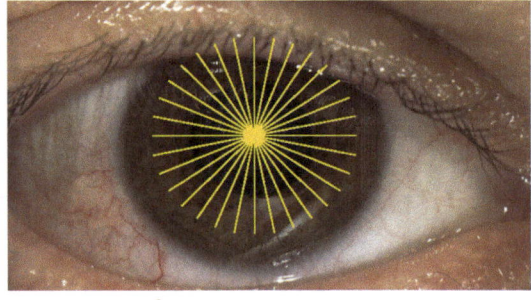

Fig. 25.3 Classical radial scan pattern, with vertex as the common point and decreasing scan densitiy to the perifery

pensation of motion with high spatial and temporal resolution, and zero latency (Fig. 25.4). This furthermore leads to very dense surface scanning, incorporating 64,000 A-scans.

The advantage of the high-density scans is improved quality of the topography, as well as the derived measurement parameters e.g. SimK, enabling the creation of virtual cross sections (B scans) of any direction and pattern in the scan volume, as well as high-resolution latency-free motion correction (Fig. 25.5). A positive side effect of the all OCT motion compensation of the Mandala Scan technology is an improved scan density due to micromotion of the eye during the high-speed scanning of the eye.

The result is an evenly distributed, high density of A-scans in the entire scan volume, thereby enabling the creation of virtual B-scans at any location and of any trajectory in the scan volume acquired.

Using swept-source OCT for the Eyestar enables the creation of robust A-scans of the entire eye, without the need for stitching of scan sections, which is inherent with, for example, standard Fourier-domain OCT systems. These full-eye A-scans allow high-precision biometry of the entire eye, from the cornea to the retina. Swept-source OCT also already demonstrates improved cataract penetration capabilities, when compared to standard time domain systems, which are still in widespread use for cataract planning. This improved cataract penetration rate leads to more comfort for the patient, with a reduced need for ultrasound examinations, which are uncomfortable for the patient and demanding on the examiner's skills.

Swept-Source OCT Biometry of the Entire Eye

With the Lenstar optical biometer, Haag-Streit has pioneered biometry of the entire eye, introducing measurement of the central corneal thickness, as well as the lens thickness with laser interferometric measurement precision. The Eyestar follows this paradigm but provides valuable additional information such as swept-source OCT B-scans and topography (Fig. 25.6).

In the Cataract Suite, Eyestar services 16 radial virtual B-scans from the cornea to the retina. This information is combined with the A-scan image and allows for intuitive verification of the automated measurement process, as well as identification of unusual or pathological eye configurations.

In addition to these 16 B-scans, Eyestar provides an additional virtual B-scan in the plane of maximum lens tilt (Fig. 25.7). This scan is available for the natural crystalline lens of a patient or an implanted IOL after cataract removal. The scans include the angle of maximum lens tilt to the optical axis. This information may be used to identify unusual extensive lens tilt that might limit the efficacy of a premium IOL when implanted or might help to explain a non-optimum refractive result after the operation.

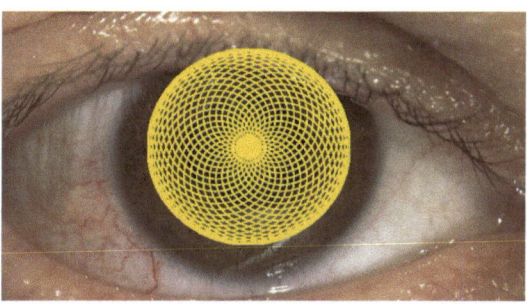

Fig. 25.4 Mandalay Scan pattern providing high scan density and a high number of intersections

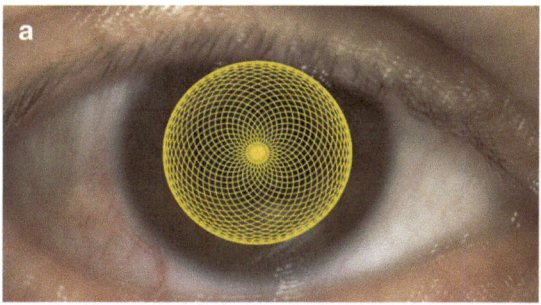
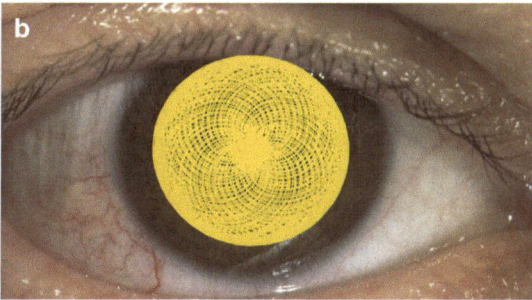

Fig. 25.5 Image (**a**) shows the scan pattern and density without the motion correction, depicted by the displaced images of the eye and image blur. Image (**b**) shows the scan pattern and density of the motion-corrected scan. The micromotion of the eye throughout the scan duration leads to an improved density of A-scans in the scan volume

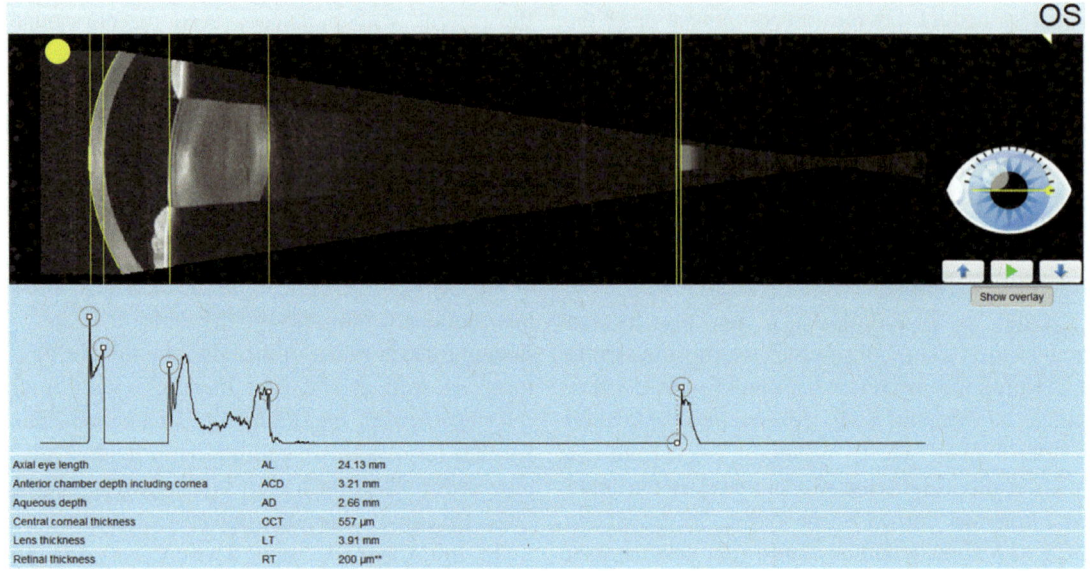

Fig. 25.6 Combined A- and B-scan display for greater confidence in the biometry measurements. In the B-scan section, the user may toggle through 16 predefined radial B-scans or play them as a video

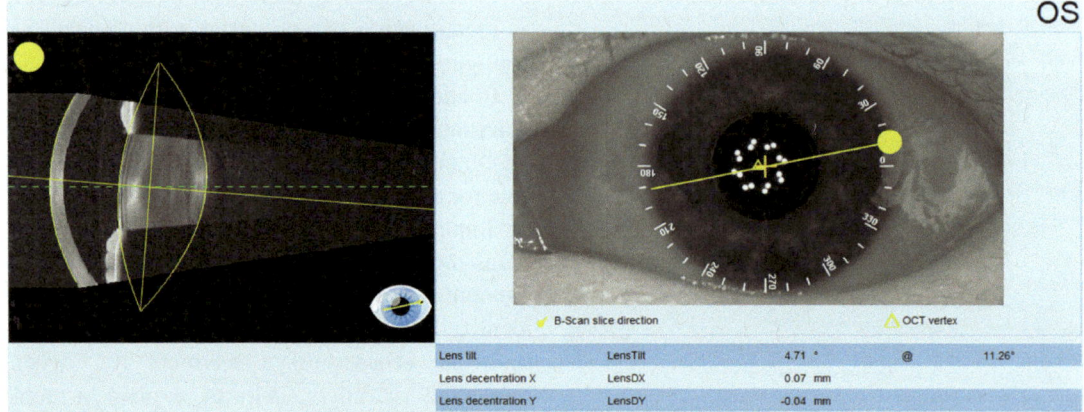

Fig. 25.7 Lens tilt display with the orientation of the maximum lens tilt, the extent, and the decentration of the lens, with respect for the corneal vertex

Swept-Source OCT Topography

Biometry based on swept-source OCT provides the user with far more than just axial length measurements and keratometry. Detailed information on the cornea front and back surfaces gives the potential to significantly improve cataract planning for astigmatic and post-refractive patients. The topography maps allow the surgeon to screen for signs of corneal pathologies that may limit the patient's post-cataract surgery visual potential. In toric candidates, the symmetry and regularity of the astigmatism on the cornea front and back are readily available, allowing for a thorough assessment of the patient's eligibility for a premium IOL.

Eyestar's cataract suite serves a wide range of topography maps, with a diameter of 7.5 mm, as well as a pachymetry covering the same area. Furthermore, the anterior topography complies with the normative requirements of a Class A topographer, ensuring excellent visualization, as

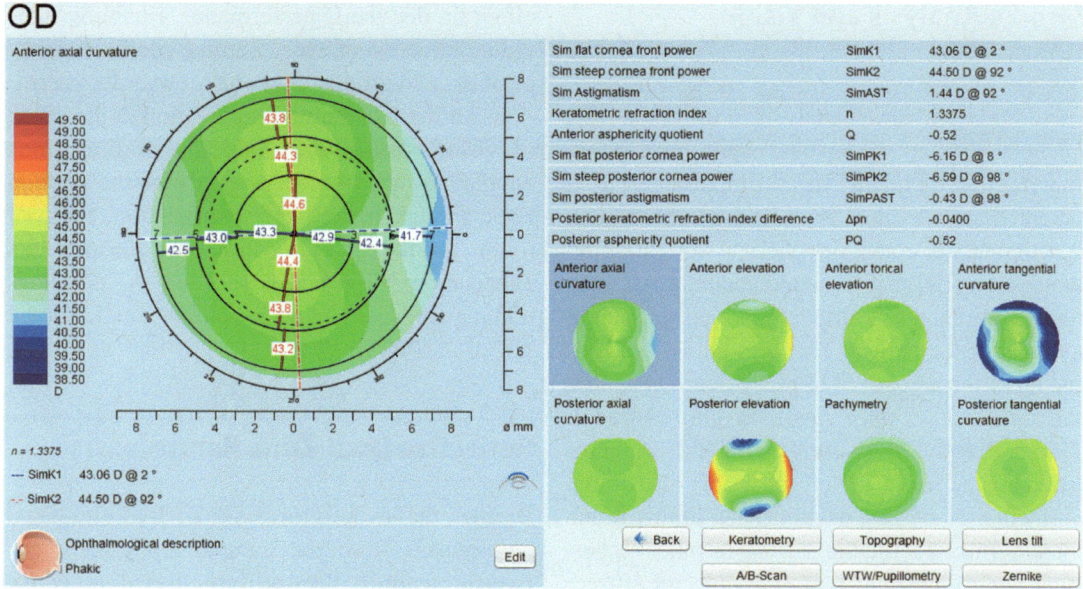

Fig. 25.8 Topography display of the Eyestar's Cataract Suite, providing thumbnail previews for all maps provided, as well as details of the selected map enriched with selected measurements tailored to the needs of the cataract surgeon. In this image, the zone-based keratometry was enabled for the axial curvature display

well as measurements of the cornea. The back corneal topography, like the front, is based on swept-source OCT, which is one of the leading technologies in providing precise measurements and high-quality imaging.

EyeSuite IOL, as part of the Cataract Suite software package on the Eyestar, takes advantage of the combined information from the cornea front and back and provides these measurements for the latest generation of IOL calculation formulae. Besides standard IOL calculation formulae like Haigis, Hoffer Q, Holladay, and SRK/T, it also features the latest developments such as the Olsen Formula, the Barrett Suite with calculation methods for every different kind of eyes, and IOL designs and Hill RBF as the first artificial intelligence-based IOL calculation method, featuring not only IOL power information for the user but also a quality index for the reliability of the predicted IOL power (Fig. 25.8).

The information from the individual topographic maps is enriched with simulated keratometry measurement information of the front and back cornea, as well as information on the sphericity of the cornea. The curvature maps for the front and back cornea also feature zone-based keratometry. This feature provides information on keratometry in the central 3-mm, the intermediate 3 to 5-mm and the more peripheral 5 to 7-mm optical zones of the cornea front and back. The zone-based keratometry does not follow the standard keratometry's paradigm of solely providing information on a steep and a flat meridian, perpendicular to each other, but on up to four (two steep and two flat meridians), with independent orientation for each zone. In a perfect astigmatic eye, the zone-based and the standard simulated keratometry will match perfectly, but the more an eye differs from being a perfect astigmatic eye, the more the information on the individual zones will differ from the simulated keratometry. Simulated keratometry is a valuable tool for assessing the symmetry of the astigmatism in different areas of the eye and may support the eyecare specialist in the decision-making process for a toric IOL.

Zernike Analysis and Vision Simulation

The Zernike wavefront analysis of the cornea is a valuable tool to understand and, even more important, to explain visual impairment to a patient. The individual Zernike parameters such as astigmatism, coma, or spherical aberration, to name just a few, enable an understanding of what visual limitation is caused by which geometric anomaly of the cornea. This also allows for estimation of the amount of improvement a potential corrective action may entail, as glasses and/or IOLs currently only correct for the defocus, astigmatism, and some spherical aberration. Correction of corneal asymmetries shown in the coma Zernike coefficient, as well as other higher-order aberrations, are not accessible for correction by these standard means. The information from the Zernike wavefront analysis is combined with a simulated display of how the letter E or Landolt ring on a vision Chart may be seen by the patient. On-the-fly adjustment of the covered area of the analysis enables simulation of different lighting conditions and how the diameter of the patent's pupil may have a positive or negative effect on the visual performance. Enabling individual selection of every Zernike coefficient and/or of the two groups' high- and low-order aberrations allows for intuitive explanation of the effect of vision-corrective actions and of limitations entailed by the corneal anatomy of the patient. Even though it is solely a simulation, the tool might be of high value in setting the patient's expectations right and supporting the decision-making process for the optimal implant-type selection (Fig. 25.9).

Reflective Dual-Zone Keratometry

Besides the swept-source OCT-based simulated keratometry from the corneal topography, the Eyestar features the well-established reflective dual-zone keratometry, specifically for cataract applications, providing precise and IOL-constant compatible keratometry and stigmatism measurements.

Why does a high-precision OCT device like the Eyestar need reflective keratometry in addition to the simulated keratometry form the corneal topography? The answer is simpler than

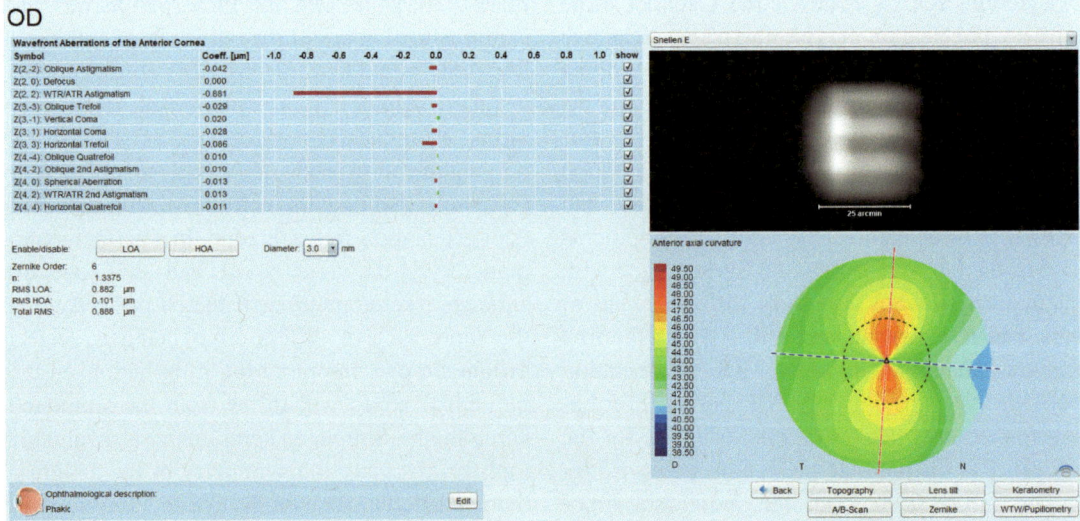

Fig. 25.9 Zernike analysis and vision simulation, with the display featuring all individual Zernike coefficients to the fourth order, as well as root mean square for the low-order aberrations (RMS LOA), and one for the high-order aberrations (RMS HOA), as well as the overall aberrations (total RMS). The vision simulation may be altered between the letter E and Landolt ring display

expected. The two modalities feature completely different baseline information. While reflective keratometry is based on video imaging of the corneal reflection of 32 infrared LED markers, located in two concentric rings covering 1.65 and 2.3 mm on an average cornea, showing the geometric deviation of the cornea from a sphere by a distorted reflection pattern of the projected LED points, the simulated keratometry of the OCT topography is based on elevation/height information for the corneal surface covered by the scan. This height information is then mathematically converted to SimK values. Even though the two modalities may provide the same information on average, there might be significant differences between the modalities for the individual patient due to the different baseline information on which they rely when providing keratometry readings.

Specifically, for the cataract application, it is key for the surgeon to have excellent keratometry information, since any error in this measurement parameter 1:1 promotes the visual performance of the patient postoperatively. This is the reason why Haag-Streit chooses to complement the Eyestar's swept-source OCT measurement technology with the well-established and over the years clinically proven dual-zone keratometry also used by its predecessor, Lenstar. Compared to the Lenstar, the Eyestar's dual-zone reflective keratometry was improved with a slightly adapted LED pattern and new analysis algorithms showing an overall improvement in measurement performance, as compared to the already excellent information provided by the Lenstar.

Other Standard Parameters and Displays

Like most other devices, the Eyestar Cataract Suite also provides information on the Corneal Diameter, as well as the pupil diameter. This measurement information is complemented with the eccentricity values of the respective diameter centers to the apex. In some literature, these eccentricity values are also referred to as angle Alpha and Kappa, even though the values displayed with

the Eyestar are in mm and refer to the offset of the circular fit of the pupil and Corneal Diameter to the apex. The measurements are displayed in high-resolution images of the patient's eye under whitelight illumination, as well as infrared illumination, depicting eye structures such as iris details or conjunctival vessels in detail.

Usability and Patient Comfort

Apart from the comprehensive measurement palette with excellent performance, the Eyestar was also developed to provide a new and improved measurement experience for the user, as well as for the patient. The all-in-one design of the Eyestar is fully self-contained and, apart from the height adjustment of the chin rest, does not feature any parts that move outside the housing. The measurement process is rapid and fully automated. In typically less than 40 s all data is acquired on both eyes, including OCT tomography, topography, keratometry, biometry, and imaging. The rapid acquisition reduces patient fatigue, leading to improved patient cooperation and making the measurement more convenient for the technician running the device.

AC Suite and More

The Cataract Suite presented here is just the first in a range of application suites for use with the Eyestar 900 that will soon be available.

The first extensions focuses on topography and anterior chamber analysis in more detail. The topography maps are extended to 12 mm diameter, and analysis tools such as higher order Zernike wavefront and vision simulation, keratoconus screening and progression views are included.

The extension of imaging enables the user to create custom B-scan images of the anterior chamber, including the lens in the 18-mm anterior corneal scan volume. This tool may serve as a diagnostic aide and for documentation purposes.

Other extensions in the pipeline will focus on the chamber angle for glaucoma diagnosis and further improvements to the Cataract Suite, for example, an analysis tool for refractive surprises or outcome documentation for phakic IOL.

Summary

The Eyestar Precision OCT/Cataract Suite provides ambitious cataract surgeons with all the information they need, enabling excellent results and optimum patient satisfaction (Table 25.1).

Table 25.1 Technical specifications

Technology	Swept-source OCT
Wavelength	1060 nm
Scan speed	30,000 Hz
OCT imaging range (cataract/AC suite/ imaging)	Ø 7.5 mm/12 mm/up to 18 mm on the anterior cornea covering the entire AL scan range
Central corneal thickness (CCT)	300–800 µm (±1.5 µm)
Anterior chamber depth (ACD)	1.8–6.3 mm (±0.014 mm)
Lens thickness (LT)	0.5–6-5 mm (±0.015 mm)
Axial length (AL)	14–38 mm (±0.005 mm)
Keratometry anterior cornea (K)	32.1–67.5 dpt (±0.067 dpt)
Keratometry posterior cornea (SimPK)	3.9–9.5 dpt (±0.025 dpt)
Topography	EN ISO 19980:2012 for corneal topography systems, type A compliant
Corneal topography measurement points:	64,000 A-scans (anterior and posterior cornea)
Corneal topography diameter Cataract suite/AC suite	Ø 7.5 mm/12 mm
Corneal Diameter (CD)	7–16 mm (±0.079 mm)
Supported EMR interfaces	DICOM, GDT, EyeSuite script language, EyeSuite command line Interface

Lenstar, the All-in-One Cataract Planning Platform

Introduction

Back in 2008, Haag-Streit redefined and broadened optical biometry with the introduction of the Lenstar optical biometer, featuring laser interferometry biometry of the entire eye from the cornea to the retina with measurements of all the segments (CCT, ACD, LT, and AL) of the

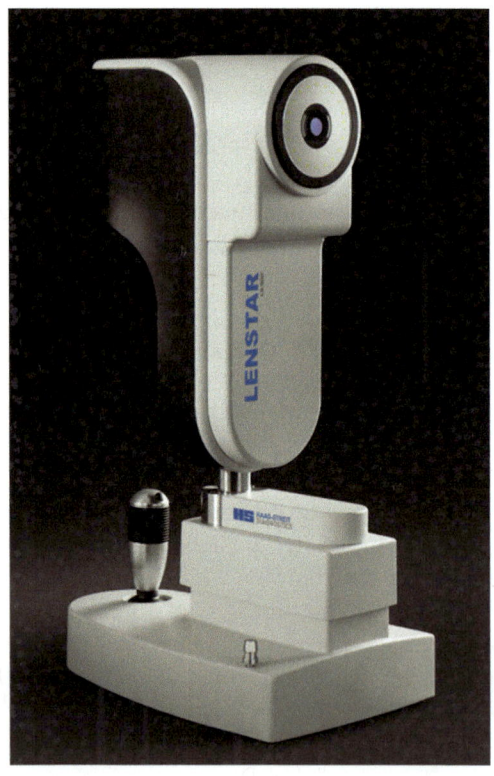

Fig. 25.10 Lenstar provides highly accurate laser optic measurements for every section of the eye—from the cornea to the retina—and was the first commercially available optical biometer on the market that could measure the thickness of the crystalline lens

human eye (Fig. 25.10). Due to the long period this device has served the cataract market with its excellent measurements and design features, many book chapters have been written about its clinical benefits, so that this section will solely summarize some of the key features of this workhorse biometer.

Even though the Lenstarhas been around for more than a decade, with no change in its exterior appearance or naming, this does not mean that this is an outdated device. On the contrary, Haag-Streit has continuously improved the device and kept it at the forefront of optical biometry for cataract application. The automated positioning system, APS, available as an option, significantly improves the usability of the device by automatization of the fine alignment and eye-tracking during the measurement process. The cataract penetration was improved with the introduction of DCM (Dense Cataract Measurement Mode), and studies published at the ESCRS by Hirnshall et al. have demonstrated that the Lenstar can play in the group of newly introduced swept-source devices. Finally, the Lenstar can be complemented with real-type B-Placido-based corneal topography, if the optional T-Cone is used. The additional topography information may serve as a valuable tool in the selection of optimal implant design.

For IOL planning, the user can rely on the latest-generation IOL calculation methods such as Olsen, the Barrett Suite, and Hill RBF. All of them consider the posterior cornea for the calculation of toric implants. Another useful addition is the option to create a planning sketch of a toric implantation on high-resolution whitelight images of the patient's eye, nicely showing the iris and conjunctival details.

Summary

Despite its age, the Lenstar still provides excellent measurement information for everyday cataract planning in a busy practice (Table 25.2).

Table 25.2 Technical specifications

Technology	OLCR Optical low coherence interferometry
Wavelength	1060 nm
Central corneal thickness (CCT)	300–800 µm (±2.3 µm)
Anterior chamber depth (ACD)	1.5–6.5 mm (±0.04 mm)
Lens thickness (LT)	0.5–6-5 mm (±0.08 mm)
Axial length (AL)	14–32 mm (±0.035 mm)
Keratometry anterior cornea (R)	5–10.5 mm (±0.03 mm)
Topography with the T-cone (option)	EN ISO 19980:2012 for corneal topography systems, type B compliant
Corneal topography diameter	Ø 6.0 mm
Corneal Diameter (CD)	7–16 mm (±0.04 mm)
Supported EMR interfaces	DICOM, GDT, EyeSuite script language, EyeSuite command line Interface

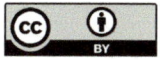

The Pentacam Family

26

Jörg Iwanczuk

Introduction

Cataract surgery is the most frequently performed eye surgery today—and IOL power calculation is a fascinating discipline in Ophthalmology!

May we introduce, your partners:

The use of the Pentacam family (Fig. 26.1) in modern cataract surgery can be described like a continues process (Fig. 26.2):

A few topics as listed below should be touched in this chapter:

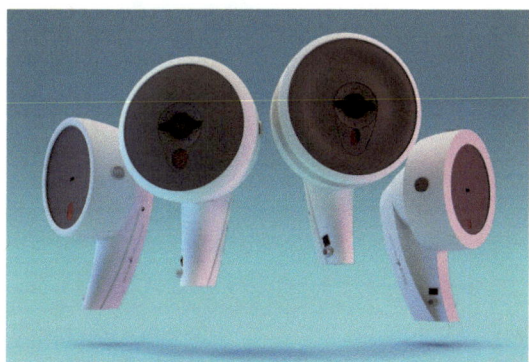

Fig. 26.1 Pentacam Family

- Pentacam history and basic principle.
- Some basic questions.
- Every patient is an individuum = customization.
- IOL power calculation formulas in the Pentacam.
- Post-op visual assessment.

History and Basic Principle

The Pentacam family was born in 2002 and further expanded by the Pentacam HR in 2006. Both devices are based on a rotating Scheimpflug camera (Fig. 26.3), capturing high-resolution pictures of the anterior eye segment, from the cornea, down to the crystalline lens. The benefits of this technology are the snapshot-capturing of the single images, highest density in the corneal center, full cornea and scleral coverage, and a minimum of nose shadow.

The Pentacam contains since day one, a second camera, the iris camera, detecting eye motions during the scan process. The captured Scheimpflug images, up to 100, are composed to

J. Iwanczuk (✉)
OCULUS Optikgeräte, Wetzlar, Germany
e-mail: j.iwanczuk@oculus.de

© The Author(s) 2024
J. Aramberri et al. (eds.), *Intraocular Lens Calculations*, Essentials in Ophthalmology,
https://doi.org/10.1007/978-3-031-50666-6_26

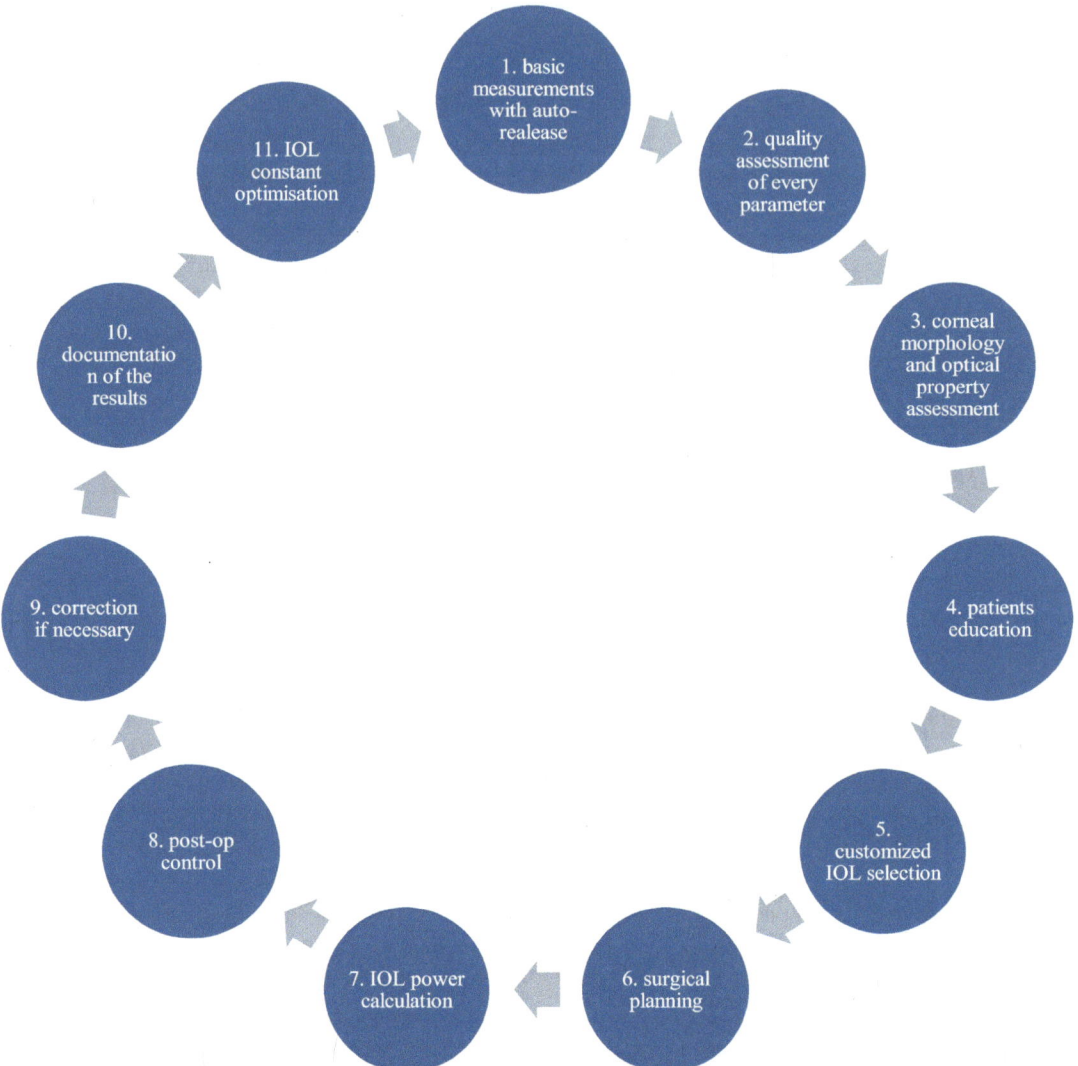

Fig. 26.2 Modern cataract surgery process

a three-dimensional model of the anterior eye segment in which the eye motions are corrected. A quality specification informs the user regarding the quality of the exam (Table 26.1).

This proven concept is reflected by its highest repeatability of keratometry [1–4], the most influential component in IOL power calculation. This might be due its tear film independency since Scheimpflug tomography does not require an intact tear film to reflect Placido rings or keratometry LEDs. No artificial tears should be applied before the measurements since this might change the normal conditions of the cornea. Moreover, objective crystalline lens density analysis [5] and grading of the nucleus [6] are possible.

In 2015, the Pentacam AXL was launched, combining the proven Scheimpflug tomography with optical biometry based on PCI technology and its comparability to the gold standard was proven [7]. This model includes the IOL calculator, containing IOL power calculation formulas for almost every cornea status, including IOL constant optimization. The IOL database is included, so no time-wasting collection of whatever IOLs are necessary. It contains up to 500 different IOL models from up to 35 manufactures who provided all details. Moreover, the IOL geometries are included for many IOLs, allowing total ray-traced-based IOL power calculation using the Olsen [8] formula.

The Pentacam AXL Wave launched in 2019 contains, besides the Scheimpflug tomography and optical biometry, a Hartmann–Shack wavefront sensor and retroillumination. These two features allow an assessment of the total eye visual performance, including objective refraction and high-order aberration analysis, and a post-op assessment of the IOL position in the human eye. The true separation of the internal wavefront from the total corneal wavefront (not possible with Placido technology) is the basis for a better understanding of individual visual quality and possible reasons for visual disturbance.

Some Basic Questions

Is Pure Keratometry and Axial Length Enough for IOL Power Calculation Today?

The most often used IOL power formulas like SRK/T [9], Haigis [10], Hoffer Q [8], and Holladay 1 [10] use axial length and keratometry for the calculation of the IOL power and for the prediction of the position of the IOL in the pseudophakic eye—whereby the Haigis formula uses the anterior chamber depth, measured from the epithelium as well. Every IOL formula has at least two components, the calculation of the power and the prediction of its position in the pseudophakic eye, and the second component is of highest interest and the biggest source of errors today. To improve this, many more factors are taken into account like HCD (corneal diameter), thickness of the human lens, and others are necessary. To achieve low prediction errors and less post-op surprises, more parameters have to be considered like the Barrett Universal 2 [11].

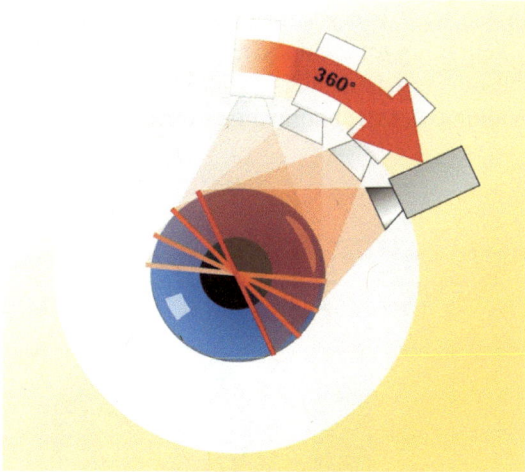

Fig. 26.3 Pentacam rotating Scheimpflug Scan

Table 26.1 Pentacam model specifications

Model Specs	Pentacam®	Pentacam® HR	Pentacam® AXL	Pentacam® AXL wave
Camera	Digital CCD camera			
Light source	Blue LED (475 nm UV-free)			
Speed	50 images in 2 s	100 images in 2 s [a]		
Axial length	–	–	14–40 mm	
Curvature	3–38 mm/9–99 D			
Precision	±0.2 D	±0.1 D		
Reproducibility	±0.2 D	±0.1 D		
Operating distance	80 mm/3.1 inch			

[a] Cornea fine scan

Does One Formula for Every Purpose Exist?

One formula for every purpose which should achieve best results no matter what the cornea look like may still not exist today. Many formulas exist for corneas after laser refractive interventions [11–15], for keratoconus [8], for the correction of astigmatism [16, 17] and ray tracing formulas for every corneal shape, including corneal transplants and all the odd corneal shapes like corneal transplants and others.

Every IOL for Every Patient?

The development of different IOL designs to improve our patients' visual performance is a blessing but requires careful patients selection. Our patients are entitled to understand about the possibilities and limitations to adjust expectations and avoid disappointments after surgery.

Every Patient Is an Individuum = Customization

Considering the fact that just keratometry and axial length is not enough to achieve top- outcome, that individual formulas might be necessary and patients selection is key to success [18], more than just a pure standard optical biometer is necessary.

The OCULUS Pentacam addresses this in particular (Fig. 26.4):

Corneal Morphology Assessment

Corneal Tomography = total cornea assessment has its benefit over pure corneal topography [19]. The total cornea is analyzed and described like a thick lens: anterior and posterior surface and its thickness at every single position are known. Scheimpflug tomography analyzes the cornea in almost every detail and provides important information to detect abnormalities and diseases:

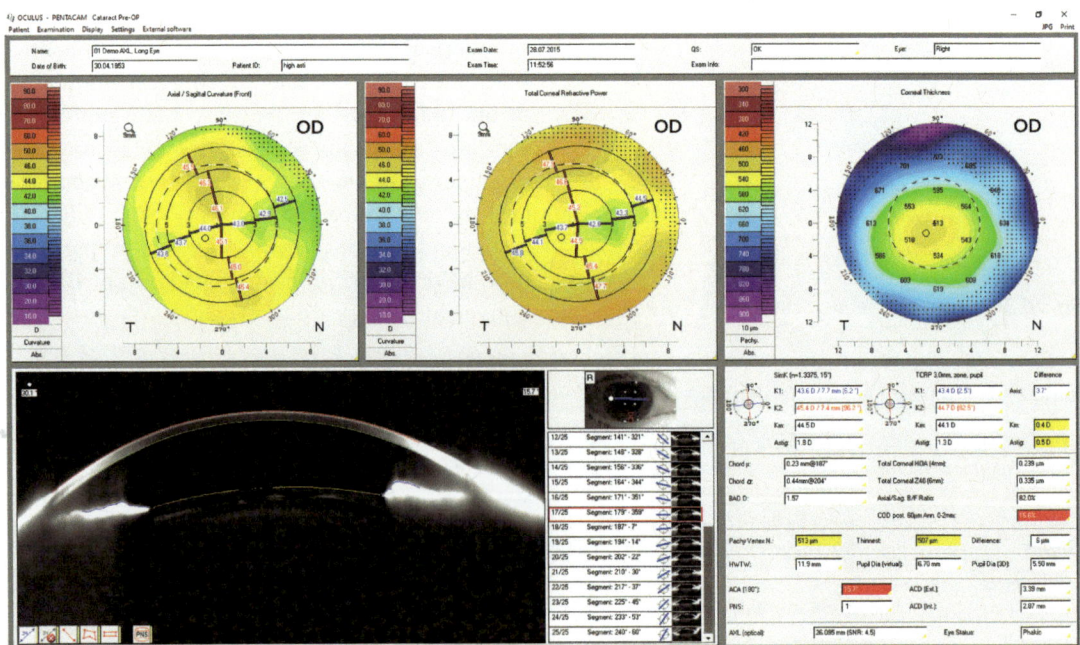

Fig. 26.4 Cataract pre-op display

- The keratometry and the assessment of the corneal astigmatism is basic knowledge. Moreover, the low astigmatism and the consideration of the posterior surface providing Total Corneal Refractive Astigmatism without any assumptions is a step forward [15, 16].
- The topography maps of the anterior and posterior surface highlights irregular corneal shape [20].
- The analysis regarding possible laser refractive or other surgical interventions using tomography, the B/F-ratio (back to front ratio) of the cornea, which is for normal eyes around 82% [21], plays an important role too. This factor is lower for post-myopic and higher for post-hyperopic laser surgery and for post-RK (radial keratotomy).
- The Belin/Ambrosio Enhanced Ectasia separates normal from abnormal patients and supports in the detection of corneal ectasia while having a final color-coded parameter, the "D"-value [20].

- The early detection of Endothelium Fuchs Dystrophy became more important. It is a progressive disease which requires sooner or later a posterior cornea transplant (DMEK or DSEK). The Pentacam supports in the early detection [22]. This often results in a post-op hyperopic shift. Arising questions are first, the best surgical planning, combined or in two steps and second the formula which should be used after the corneal transplant. A good option could be the Olsen ray tracing formula.

The More Complex Corneas: How to Deal with It?

These corneas, often after refractive surgery or other surgical interventions, are always a challenge in IOL power calculation. The corneal power distribution display is a powerful assessment tool for these cases. But not only these challenging cases might be of interest, it just starts with the assessment of the astigmatisms (Fig. 26.5):

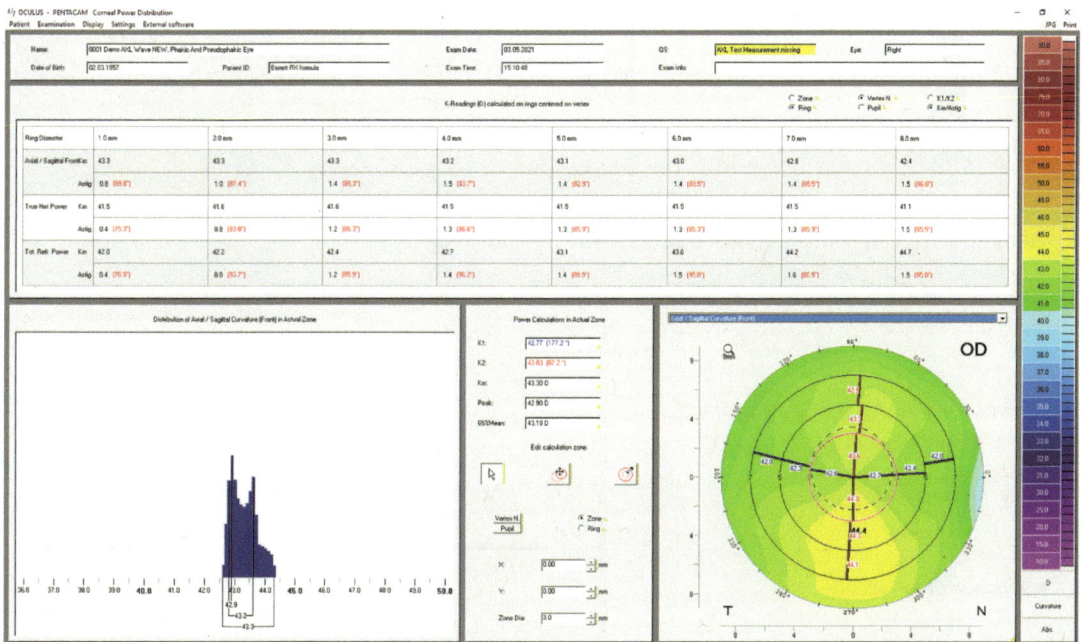

Fig. 26.5 Corneal power distribution of a regular astigmatism

– Is the magnitude and the axis in the central zone same or different compared to the periphery?
– Does it change and if yes how much?
– How is this related to the pupil diameter, does it matter?
– What about the orientation of the axis of the astigmatism, for a WTR (with the rule), ATR (against the rule), or oblique astigmatism?

– What about the influence of the posterior corneal surface in terms of possible axis shifts? Does it matter and if yes, which IOL formula approach should be used?

The example below shows a patient after LASIK with a homogenous ablation zone and a small corneal power distribution (Fig. 26.6).

On the other hand, an example of a post-LASIK patients with a decentered ablation and flap problems (Fig. 26.7).

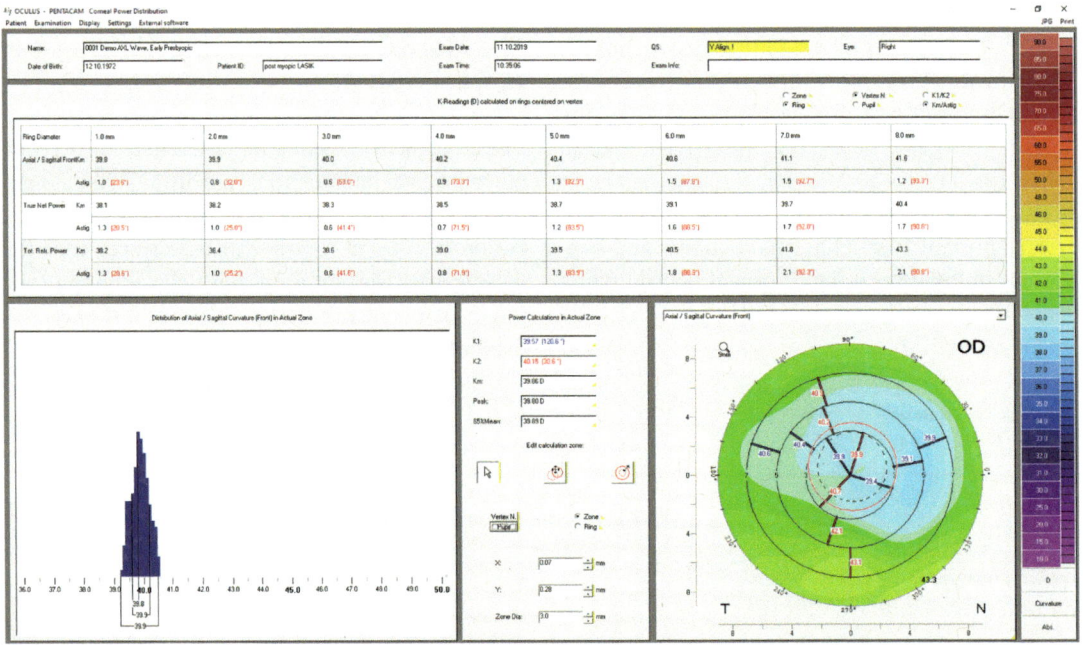

Fig. 26.6 Small corneal power distribution after LASIK

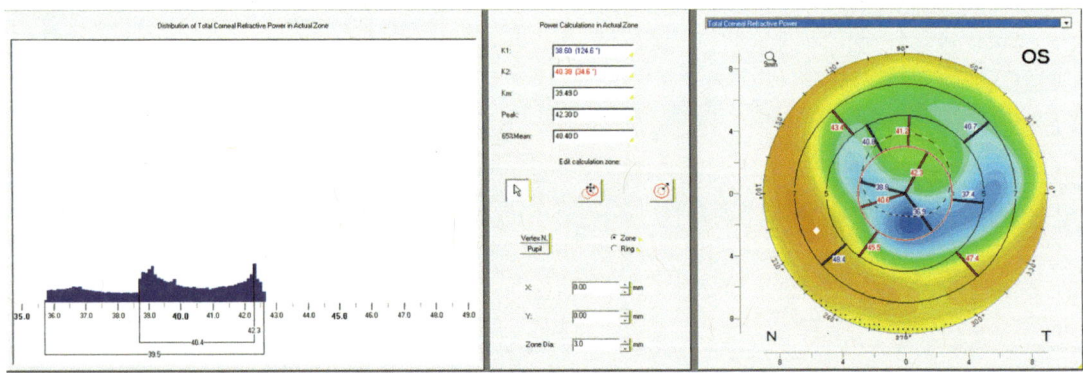

Fig. 26.7 Huge corneal power distribution after LASIK

Corneal Optical and Anterior Chamber Properties Assessment

The human eye is not an optical bench. Hence, it requires individual assessment of corneal optical and anterior chamber properties which are "solid-factors" for IOL selection.

The Pentacam tomography calculates the total corneal wavefront, considering the posterior surface.

- The total spherical aberrations, which are often associated with halos, starburst, ghost images, and loss of contrast sensitivity, are important to measure. This supports the selection of an aspherical or an aberration-neutral IOL design. Normative values are provided [23].
- Increased coma, which causes an optical effect like a comet tail and may result in double-vision, might be contraindication for multifocal IOLs.
- Increased trefoil, which spreads the light in three directions, is important to quantify as well.

They do not occur individually, and they are limiting factors for the visual performance per se. The Pentacam provides all these values, including cut-off suggestions, supporting in the selection of multifocal IOLs.

The Pentacam provides the anterior chamber depth, measured form the epithelium as well as the anterior chamber depth measured from the endothelium. angle is calculated in every Scheimpflug image and is used for the selection if a patient might be suitable for a pIOL implantation. Please note that for pseudophakic eyes the anterior chamber depth should be double-checked.

Centration of Optical Elements and Pupil Diameter

Pentacam tomography provides parameters associated with the optical path of the individual eye.

The vectorial distance between the vertex normal—the reference for all Pentacam measurements—and the pupil center, called chord μ and chord α which is the distance between vertex normal and the corneal geometric center. If they are high, there might be a risk for reduced visual performance.

The Pentacam AXL Wave provides the pupil diameter under day and night conditions. In combination with the corresponding refraction, additional support for cataract refractive surgery is provided.

Total Eye Visual Performance

The Pentacam AXL Wave with its built-in Hartmann–Shack sensor for total eye wavefront has the ability to display the source, or the reasons for visual impairments. The example below (Fig. 26.8) shows an early presbyopia case of a female aged 47 with a previous myopic LASIK. The reason for her typical problems, like driving at night or when it is rainy and foggy, is the crystal lens. This picture helps her understand immediately the reason.

The example below shows a patient with previous RK (Fig. 26.9) having high expectations in the cataract surgery. No matter which lens you are going to implant, the visual quality will never be as good as expected. The patient understood—the image told more than 1000 words.

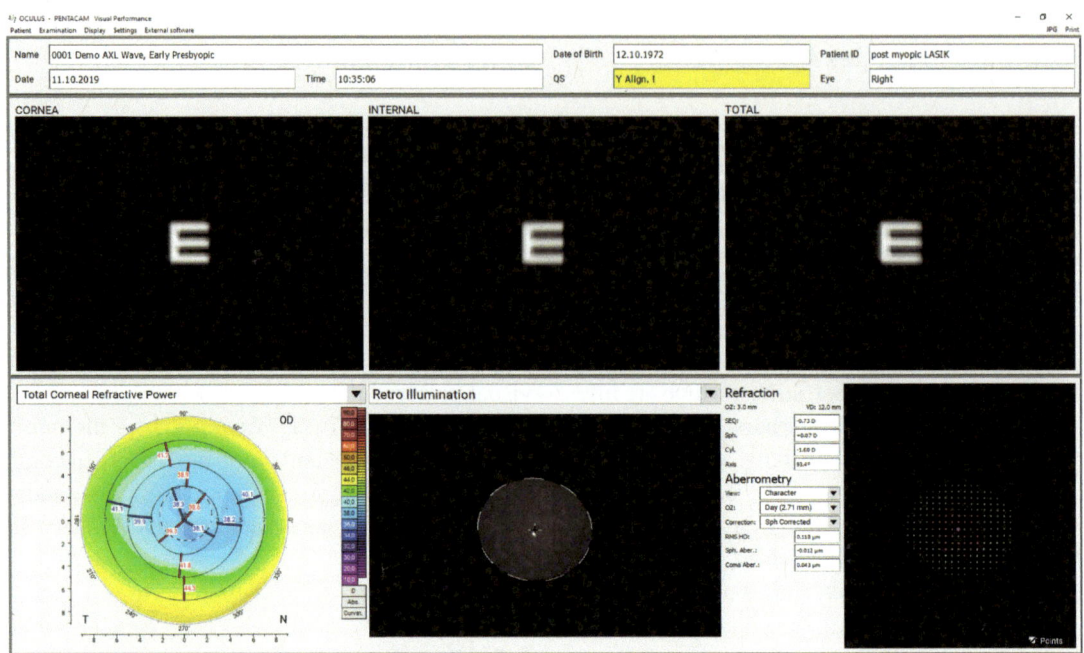

Fig. 26.8 Myopic LASIK patient, early presbyopia

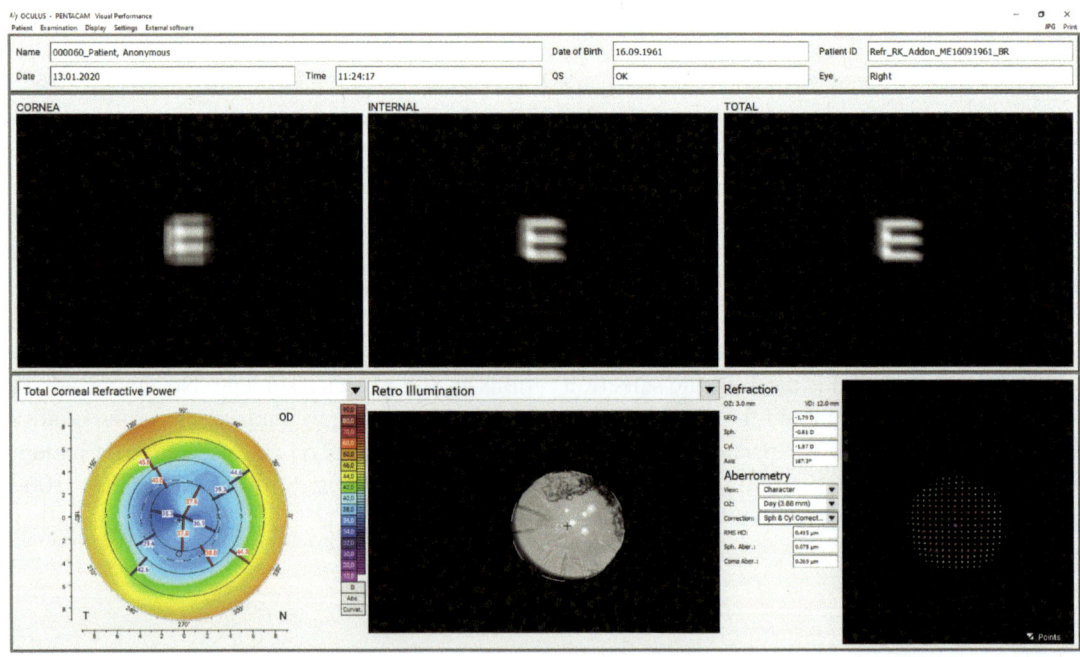

Fig. 26.9 Patient after RK (radial keratotomy)

IOL Power Calculation Formulas in the Pentacam

The improvement of IOL power calculation formulas is a process. The IOL calculator built into the Pentacam AXL and Pentacam AXL Wave includes IOL power calculation formulas for almost every purpose and the IOL database—ready to use. No online calculators have to be assessed.

The Pentacam keratometry was proven to be most accurate, for normal and abnormal corneas [2, 4, 12]. Combined with precise axial length and other required parameter, the basis is made to achieve very good refractive outcomes [21].

Every single surgeon in a bigger clinic can have his/her own profile with individual combinations of IOLs with IOL power calculation formulas. For the calculation of toric IOLs, the SIA (surgical-induced astigmatism) has to be entered and is considered in the respective formulas. The IOL calculator displays the standard parameters as well as total corneal spherical and high-order aberrations. Abnormal values are highlighted to inform the user (Fig. 26.10).

Monofocal IOL Formulas for Virgin Corneas

The IOL formulas for monofocal IOLs are intuitively organized and contain the most common standard and modern IOL formulas (Figs. 26.11 and 26.12).

Toric IOL Formulas for Virgin Corneas

The IOL power calculation for toric IOLs offers formulas (Fig. 26.13) with measured and with estimated posterior surface. The estimated post-op refraction as well as the orientation of the toric implant are shown (Fig. 26.14).

IOL Formulas for Patients After Corneal Laser Refractive Surgery and RK (Radial Keratotomy)

This is still a challenge today. The IOL calculator offer customized formulas [13, 14] for the Pentacam (Fig. 26.15) as well as the Barrett

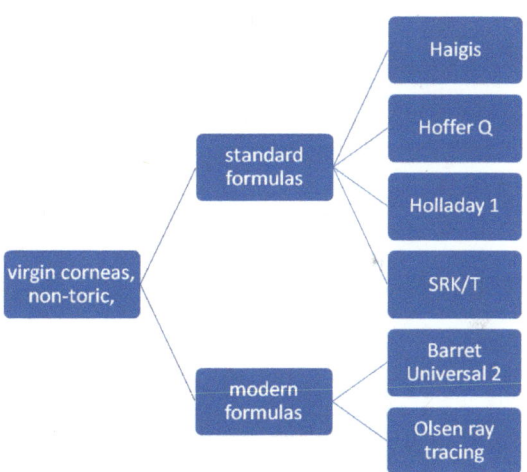

Fig. 26.11   Standard and modern IOL formulas

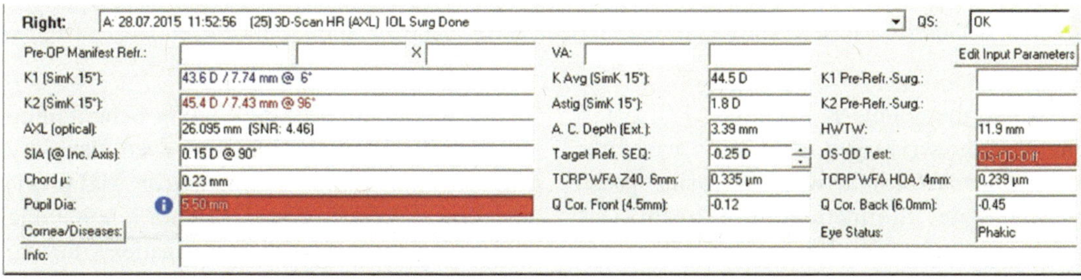

Fig. 26.10   Parameters in the IOL Calculator

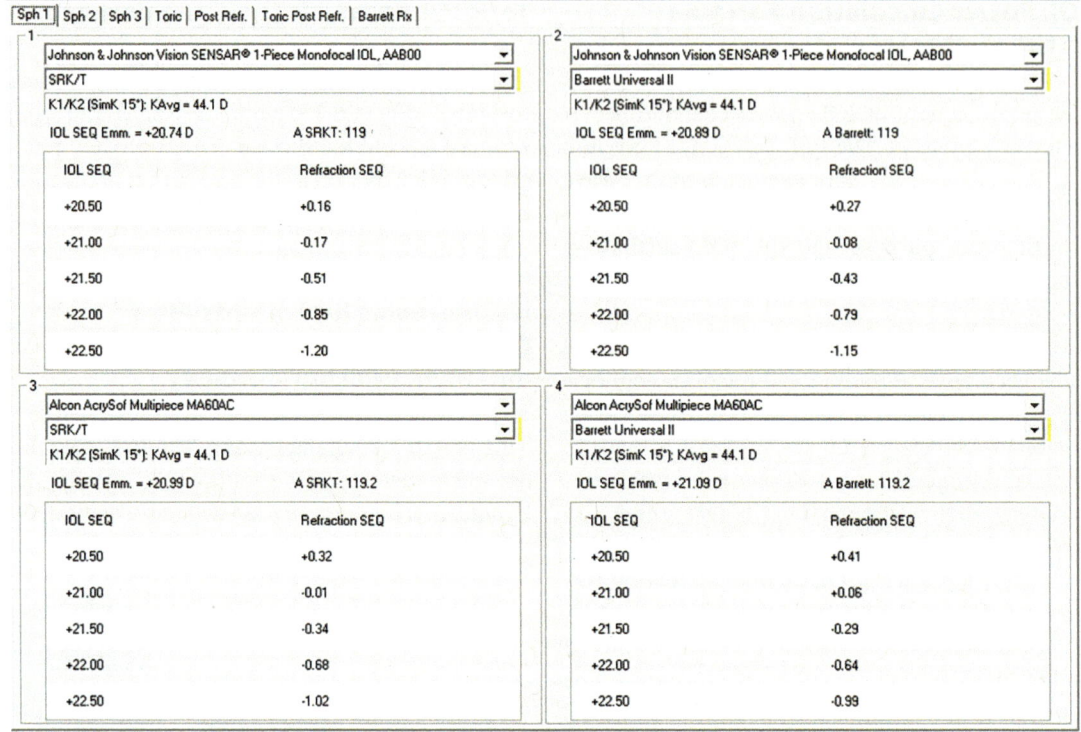

Fig. 26.12 IOL formulas for monofocal IOLs in the IOL Calculator

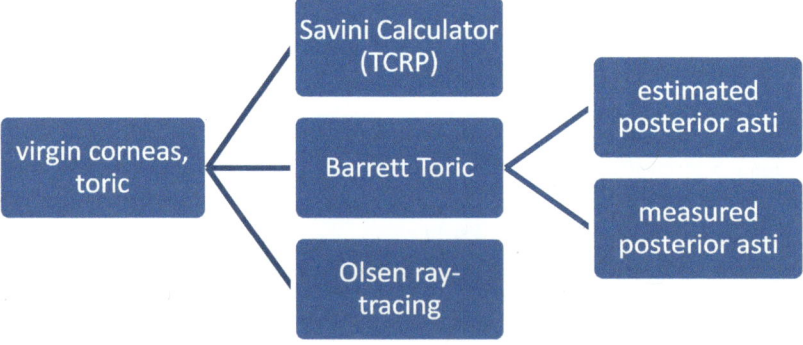

Fig. 26.13 IOL formulas for toric IOLs

True K and the double-K formulas [17]. Latest study has shown very good results using the Barrett True K formula with increasing precision the more information prior history are available [24]. On the other hand, the Olsen ray tracing formula is fully independent of any information prior refractive surgery [25] (Fig. 26.16).

The Pentacam with its rotating Scheimpflug tomography allow to measure even the very irregular corneas. For patients having had previous corneal refractive surgery with a remaining high astigmatism as well as for patients having had PKP (penetrating keratoplasty), the Olsen formula can be used (Fig. 26.17).

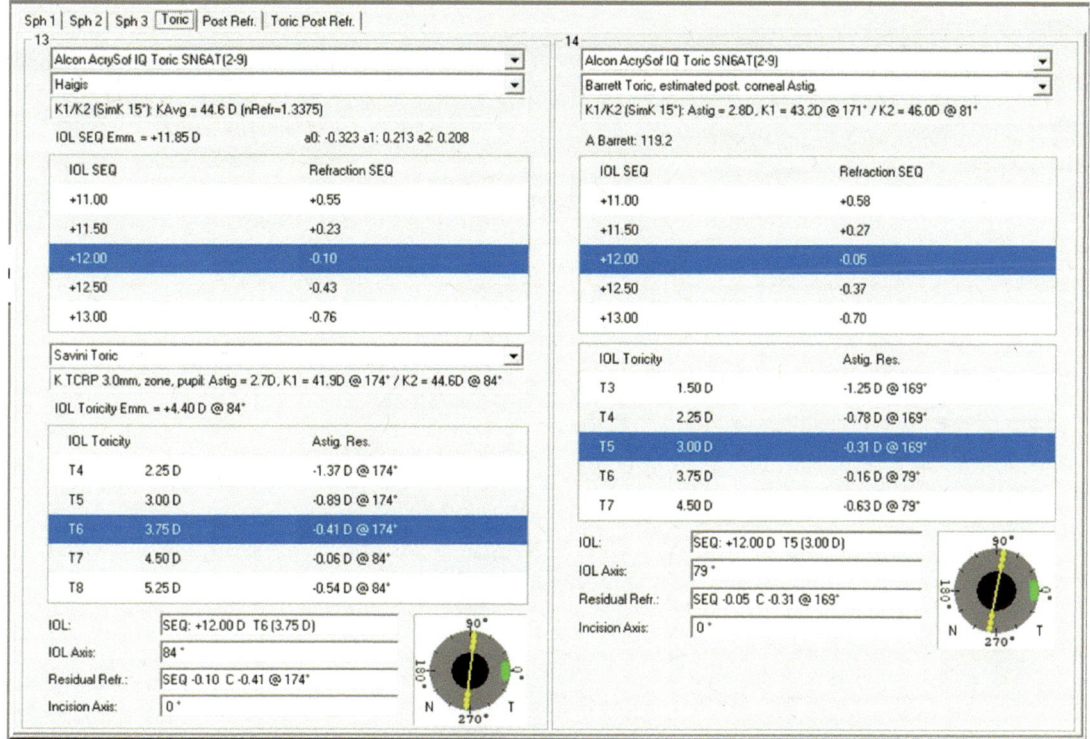

Fig. 26.14 Toric IOL formulas for virgin eyes in the IOL calculator

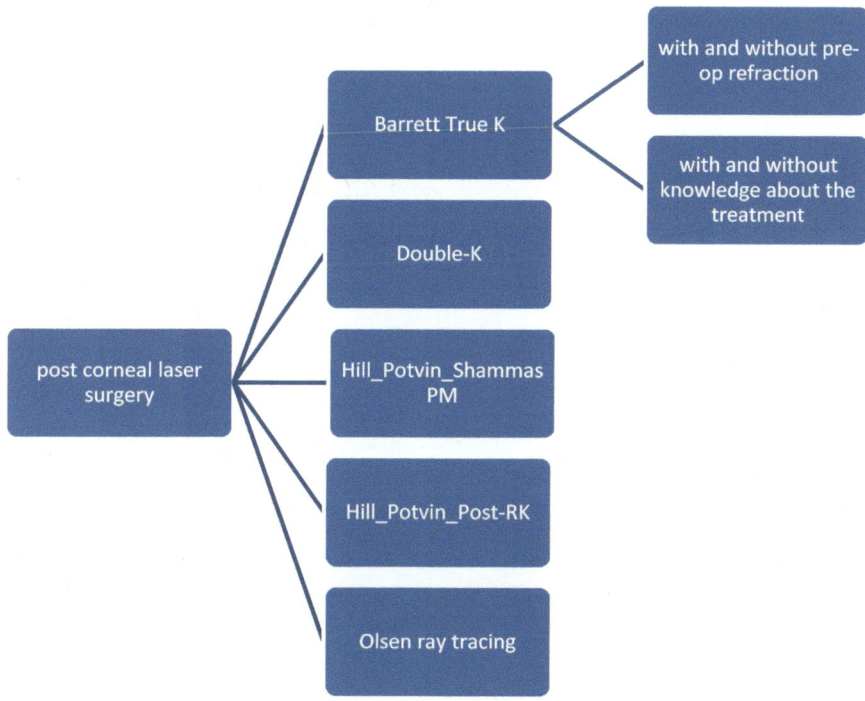

Fig. 26.15 IOL formulas for patients after refractive surgery and RK

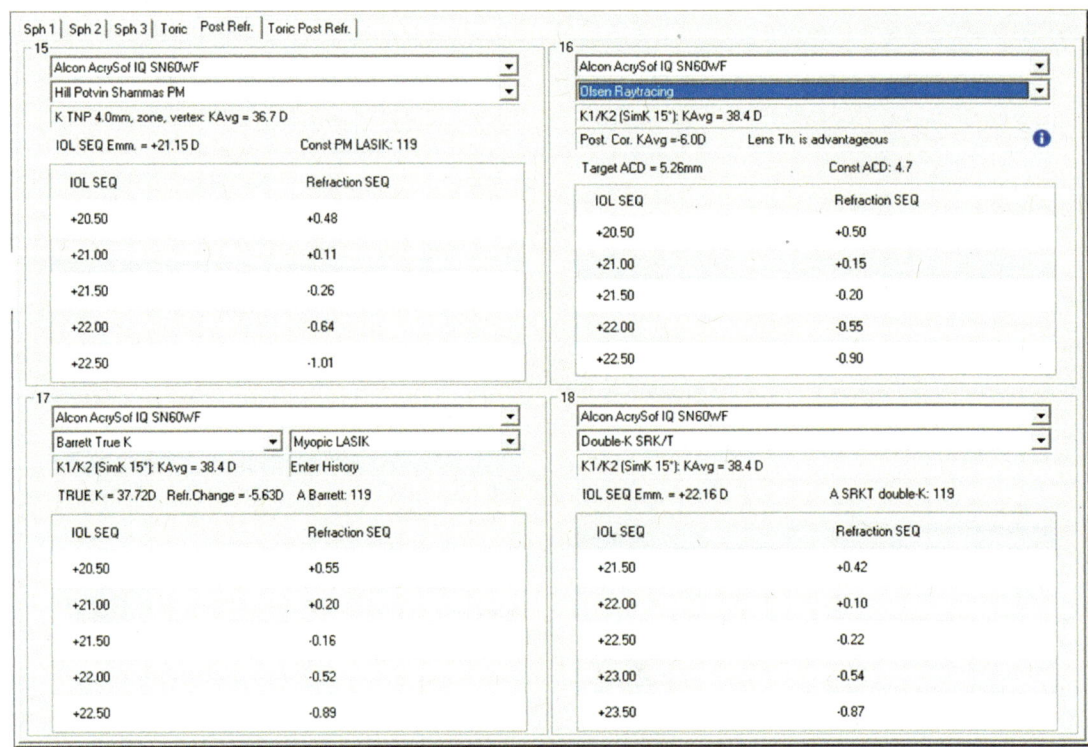

Fig. 26.16 IOL formulas for patients after refractive surgery in the IOL calculator

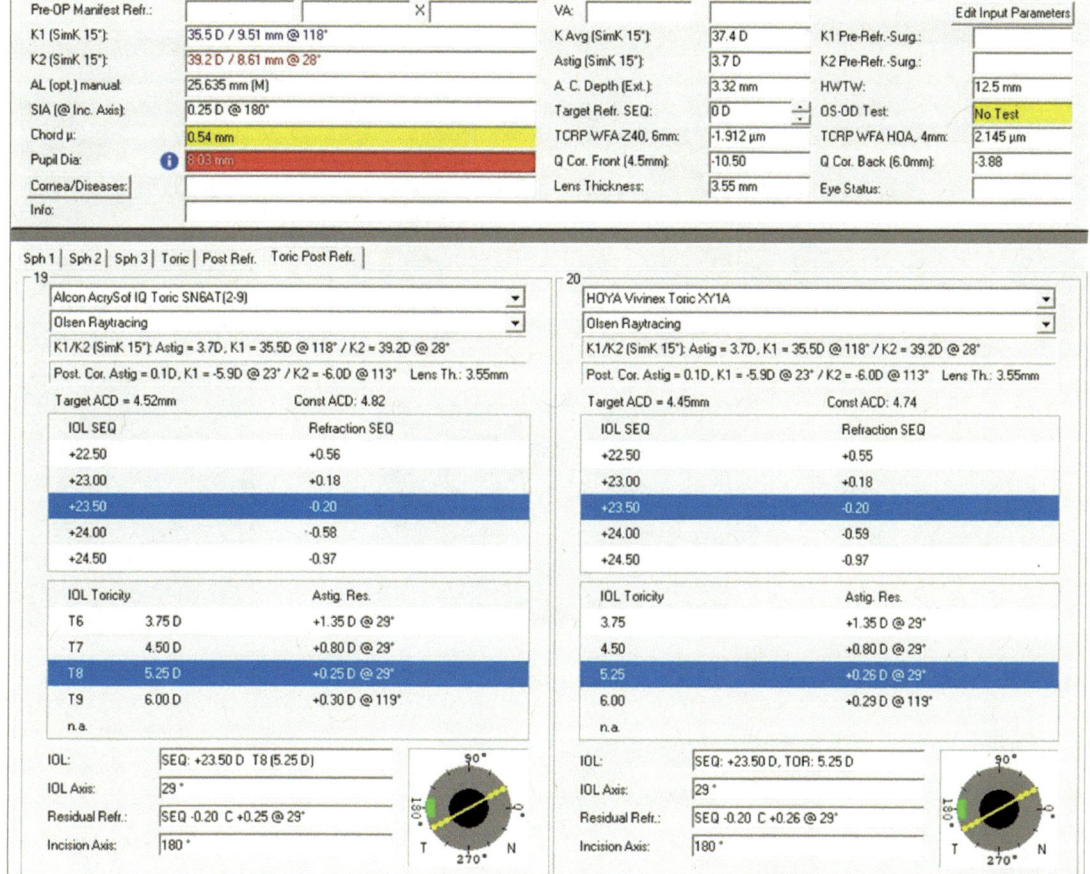

Fig. 26.17 Olsen ray tracing formula in the IOL Calculator

The Post-op Visual Assessment

The post-op visual assessment for documentation, quality assessment, and continuous improvement is a must today in modern cataract surgery.

The subjective refraction is one parameter combined with the slit-lamp exam, and a final short talk to the patients is routine anyway. But, what to do and how to handle unhappy patients? We all heard about the "20/20 unhappy patients." Here, the Pentacam can be of help again.

The Pentacam AXL Wave performs total eye wavefront, objective refraction, biometry, and tomography, providing a solid basis for further diagnosis—before the physicians starts the conversation with the patient.

The first example shows a happy patient after multifocal-toric implantation (Fig. 26.18). The refraction is almost plano, the Total Visual Performance is very good, and the IOL is on axis.

The example below is an example of an unhappy patient with bad visual quality after cataract surgery (Fig. 26.19). The Pentacam AXL Wave shows the Total Visual Performance and the refraction at a glance.

The retroillumination image below gives the answer, and it is a decentered IOL (Fig. 26.20).

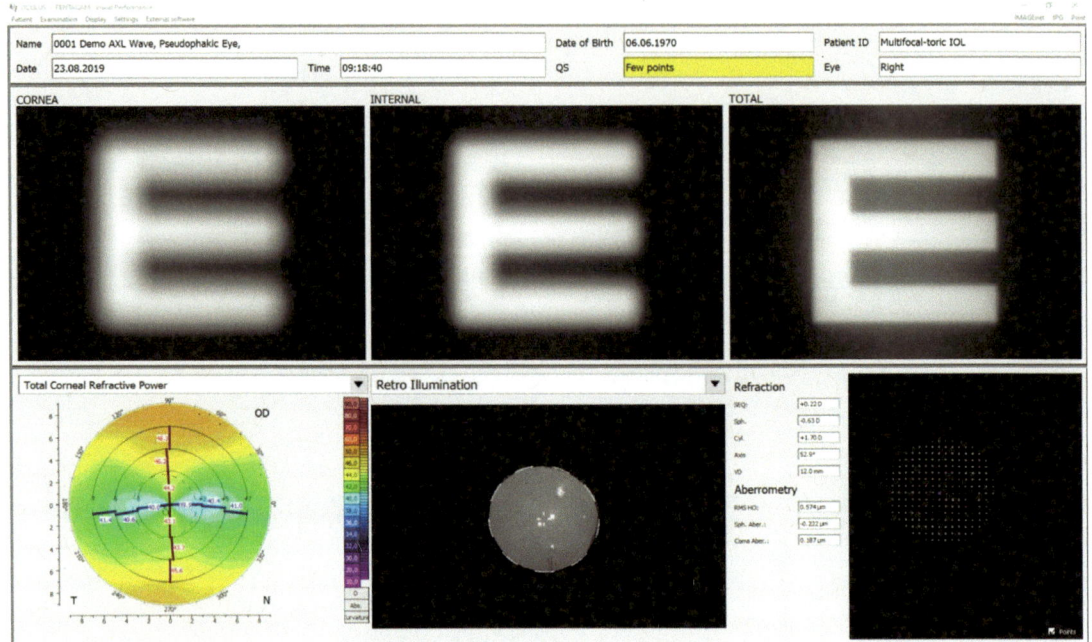

Fig. 26.18 Visual performance after multifocal toric implantation

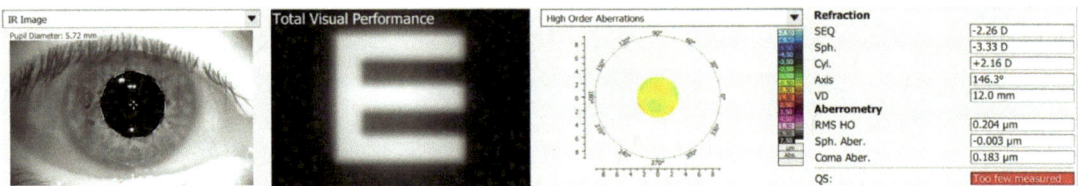

Fig. 26.19 Refraction and visual performance, decentered IOL

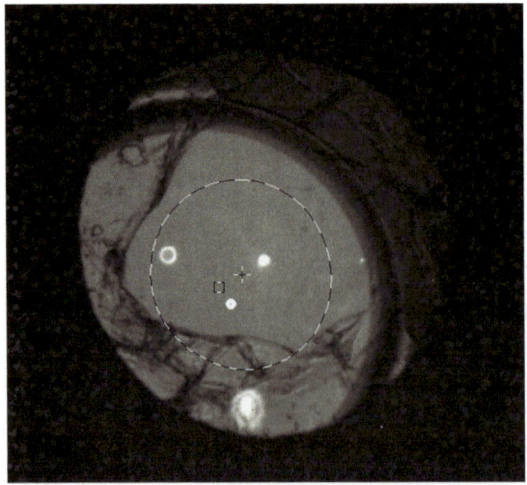

Fig. 26.20 Decentered IOL in the retroillumination image

Summary and Take-Home Message

The Pentacam AXL as well as the Pentacam AXL Wave offer the full-capacity performing IOL power calculation on the highest level. Besides this, it offers so many other clinical applications, making it the "swiss-army-knife" for every eye clinic.

References

1. Rozema JJ, Wouters K, Mathysen DGP, Tassignon M-J. Overview of the repeatability, reproducibility, and agreement of the biometry values provided by various ophthalmic devices. Am J Ophthalmol. 2014;158(6):1111–1120.e1. http://www.ncbi.nlm.nih.gov/pubmed/25128596

2. Shetty R, Arora V, Jayadev C, Nuijts RMMA, Kumar M, Puttaiah NK, Kummelil MK. Repeatability and agreement of three Scheimpflug-based imaging systems for measuring anterior segment parameters in keratoconus. Invest Ophthalmol Vis Sci. 2014;55(8):5263–8. http://www.ncbi.nlm.nih.gov/pubmed/25074774

3. Visser N, Berendschot TTJM, Verbakel F, de Brabander J, Nuijts RMMA. Comparability and repeatability of corneal astigmatism measurements using different measurement technologies. J Cataract Refract Surg. 2012;38(10):1764–70. http://www.ncbi.nlm.nih.gov/pubmed/22999600

4. Fityo S, Bühren J, Shajari M, Kohnen T. Keratometry versus total corneal refractive power: analysis of measurement repeatability with 5 different devices in normal eyes with low astigmatism. J Cataract Refract Surg. 2016;42(4):569–76. http://www.ncbi.nlm.nih.gov/pubmed/27113880

5. Weiner X, Baumeister M, Kohnen T, Bühren J. Repeatability of lens densitometry using Scheimpflug imaging. J Cataract Refract Surg. 2014;40(5):756–63. http://www.ncbi.nlm.nih.gov/pubmed/24767909

6. Nixon DR. Preoperative cataract grading by Scheimpflug imaging and effect on operative fluidics and phacoemulsification energy. J Cataract Refract Surg. 2010;36(2):242–6. http://www.ncbi.nlm.nih.gov/pubmed/20152604

7. Shajari M, Cremonese C, Petermann K, Singh P, Müller M, Kohnen T. Comparison of axial length, corneal curvature, and anterior chamber depth measurements of 2 recently introduced devices to a known biometer. Am J Ophthalmol. 2017;178:58–64. http://www.ncbi.nlm.nih.gov/pubmed/28263734

8. Olsen T, Jeppesen P. Ray-tracing analysis of the corneal power from Scheimpflug data. J Refract Surg. 2018;34(1):45–50. http://www.ncbi.nlm.nih.gov/pubmed/29315441

9. Haigis W, Lege B, Miller N, Schneider B. Comparison of immersion ultrasound biometry and partial coherence interferometry for intraocular lens calculation according to Haigis. Graefes Arch Clin Exp Ophthalmol. 2000;238:765–73.

10. Hoffer KJ. The Hoffer Q formula: a comparison of theoretic and regression formulas. J Cataract Refract Surg. 1993;19(11):700–12. Errata: 1994;20(6):677 and 2007;33(1):2–3.

11. Aramberri J. Intraocular lens power calculation after corneal refractive surgery: Double-K method. J Cataract Refract Surg. 2003;29(11):2063–8. http://www.sciencedirect.com/science/article/pii/S088633500300957X

12. Camellin M, Savini G, Hoffer KJ, Carbonelli M, Barboni P. Scheimpflug camera measurement of anterior and posterior corneal curvature in eyes with previous radial keratotomy. J Refract Surg. 2012;28(4):275–9. http://www.ncbi.nlm.nih.gov/pubmed/22386371

13. Savini G, Hoffer KJ, Barrett GD. Results of the Barrett True-K formula for IOL power calculation based on Scheimpflug camera measurements in eyes with previous myopic excimer laser surgery. J Cataract Refract Surg. 2020;46(7):1016–9. https://pubmed.ncbi.nlm.nih.gov/32271267/

14. Potvin R, Hill W. New algorithm for post-radial keratotomy intraocular lens power calculations based on rotating Scheimpflug camera data. J Cataract Refract Surg. 2013;39(3):358–65. http://www.ncbi.nlm.nih.gov/pubmed/23337527

15. Potvin R, Hill W. New algorithm for intraocular lens power calculations after myopic laser in situ keratomileusis based on rotating Scheimpflug camera data. J Cataract Refract Surg. 2015;41(2):339–47. http://www.ncbi.nlm.nih.gov/pubmed/25661127

16. Savini G, Næser K. An analysis of the factors influencing the residual refractive astigmatism after cataract surgery with toric intraocular lenses. Invest Ophthalmol Vis Sci. 2015;56(2):827–35. https://doi.org/10.1167/iovs.14-15903.

17. Savini G, Næser K, Schiano-Lomoriello D, Ducoli P. Optimized keratometry and total corneal astigmatism for toric intraocular lens calculation. J Cataract Refract Surg. 2017;43(9):1140–8. http://www.ncbi.nlm.nih.gov/pubmed/28991609

18. Donaldson K, Fernández-Vega-Cueto L, Davidson R, Dhaliwal D, Hamilton R, Jackson M, et al. Perioperative assessment for refractive cataract surgery. J Cataract Refract Surg. 2018;44(5):642–53. http://www.ncbi.nlm.nih.gov/pubmed/29891157

19. Tonn B, Klaproth OK, Kohnen T. Anterior surface–based keratometry compared with Scheimpflug tomography–based total corneal astigmatism. 2015. http://iovs.arvojournals.org/article.aspx?articleid=2212759

20. Villavicencio OF, Gilani F, Henriquez MA, Izquierdo L, Ambrósio RR. Independent population validation of the Belin/Ambrósio enhanced ectasia display: implications for keratoconus studies and screening. Int J Keratoconus Ectatic Corneal Dis. 2014;3(1):1–8. https://doi.org/10.5005/jp-journals-10025-1069.

21. Ho J-D, Tsai C-Y, Tsai RJ-F, Kuo L-L, Tsai I-L, Liou S-W. Validity of the keratometric index: evaluation by the Pentacam rotating Scheimpflug camera. J Cataract Refract Surg. 2008;34(1):137–45. https://pubmed.ncbi.nlm.nih.gov/18165094/

22. Ní Dhubhghaill S, Rozema JJ, Jongenelen S, Ruiz Hidalgo I, Zakaria N, Tassignon MJ. Normative values for corneal densitometry analysis by Scheimpflug Optical Assessment. Invest Ophthalmol Vis Sci. 2014;55:162–8. http://iovs.arvojournals.org/article.aspx?articleid=2128026

23. Klaproth OK, Buehren J, Otto K, Kohnen T. Repeatability of the corneal wavefront measure-

ments with Pentacam HR. 2011. https://iovs.arvojournals.org/article.aspx?articleid=2356309

24. Taroni L, Hoffer KJ, Barboni P, Schiano-Lomoriello D, Savini G. Outcomes of IOL power calculation using measurements by a rotating Scheimpflug camera combined with partial coherence interferometry.

J Cataract Refract Surg. 2020;46(12):1618–23. https://pubmed.ncbi.nlm.nih.gov/32818357/

25. Barrett GD. An improved universal theoretical formula for intraocular lens power prediction. J Cataract Refract Surg. 1993;19(6):713–20. https://doi.org/10.1016/S0886-3350(13)80339-2.

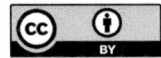

GALILEI G6 Lens Professional

27

Gregor Schmid

Overview

The GALILEI G6 is a noninvasive, noncontact optical diagnostic system designed for the assessment of the anterior segment of the eye by means of processed images taken with an integrated rotating Dual-Scheimpflug tomography and Placido topography system. The Dual-Scheimpflug system (two opposite cameras instead of one) allows significant reduction in measurement time without losing data coverage and automatic compensation of measurement decentration. Optical A-scans based on time-domain partial-coherence interferometry enables the precise measurement of axial, intraocular distances, thereby adding the information needed to perform IOL power calculation. The precise acquisition of posterior corneal surface data reduces the risk of postoperative surprises. Together with the complete set of biometry data, including lens thickness measurement, the full dataset for making the optimal decision for surgeons and their patients is available.

G. Schmid (✉)
Ziemer Ziemer Ophthalmic Systems AG,
Port, Switzerland
e-mail: Gregor.schmid@ziemergroup.com

Hardware

The GALILEI G6 is composed of a measurement head containing Placido disk and Dual-Scheimpflug optics/mechanics/electronics, a main monitor, a PC, an elevation table, and an optical A-scan accessory (Fig. 27.1).

The measurement head includes an optical front end for coupling the light beam from the optical A-scan accessory into the eye, optics for Placido and Dual-Scheimpflug imaging, mechanics to rotate the cameras, as well as electronics for controlling measurement head rotation, light sources, and image acquisition. For data collection, the measurement head is rotated about the central instrument axis by 180°. During the rotation, a series of Scheimpflug, Placido, and Topview images are taken of the cornea, iris, pupil, limbus, anterior chamber, and crystalline lens and transferred to the PC for processing and display. Topography and anterior segment tomography are then calculated from those images. Figures 27.2 and 27.3 show examples of a Dual-Scheimpflug image pair and a Topview/Placido image, respectively.

The scanning process acquires an adjustable number (between 7 and 30, default: 17) of Scheimpflug and Topview images, including two Placido Topview images at 54° apart. On the Scheimpflug images, edges are detected (anterior cornea, posterior cornea, anterior lens, and iris). On the Placido images, the ring edges are

J. Aramberri et al. (eds.), *Intraocular Lens Calculations*, Essentials in Ophthalmology,
https://doi.org/10.1007/978-3-031-50666-6_27

Fig. 27.1 GALILEI G6
Lens Professional

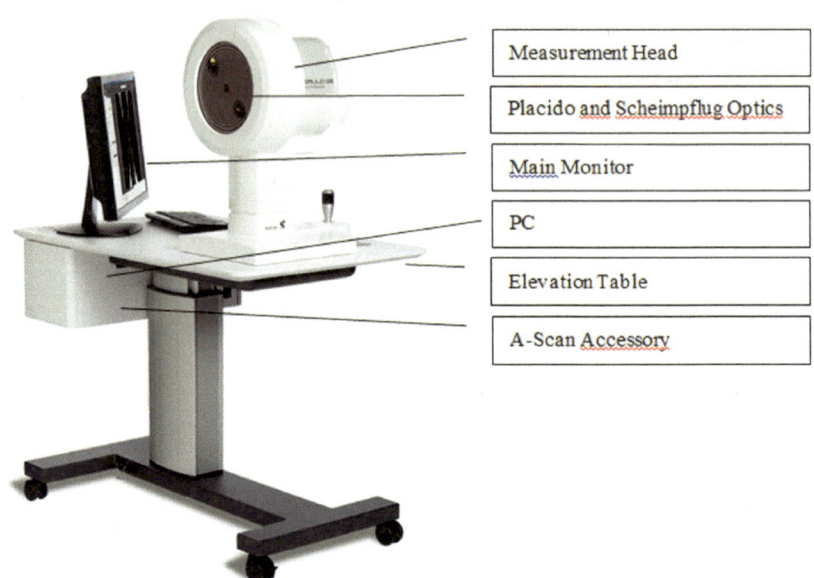

Measurement Head

Placido and Scheimpflug Optics

Main Monitor

PC

Elevation Table

A-Scan Accessory

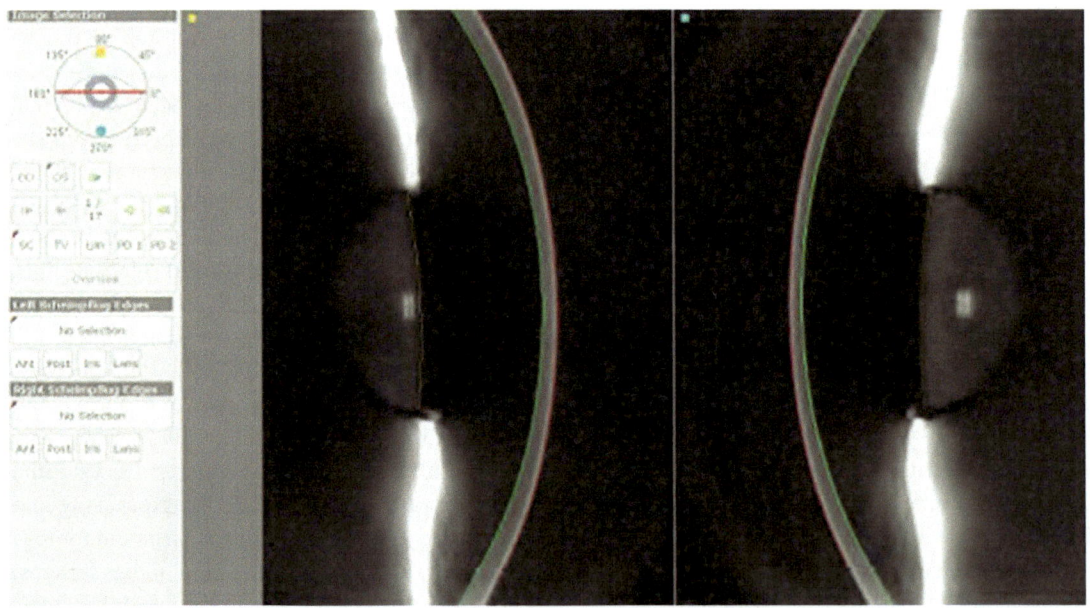

Fig. 27.2 Pair of Dual-Scheimpflug images

detected. In a separate process, the limbus and pupil are detected from a Topview image. The limbus and pupil do not influence any other calculations performed by the system. From the Scheimpflug edges, height data is determined. The slope data from the Placido images are transformed into conforming height data. Scheimpflug and Placido data are thereafter merged based on respective quality using a proprietary merging algorithm. The merged data are then used to create surface fits from where indices are calculated and maps are generated. In addition, a color Topview camera permits taking color images of the front view of the eye (Fig. 27.4).

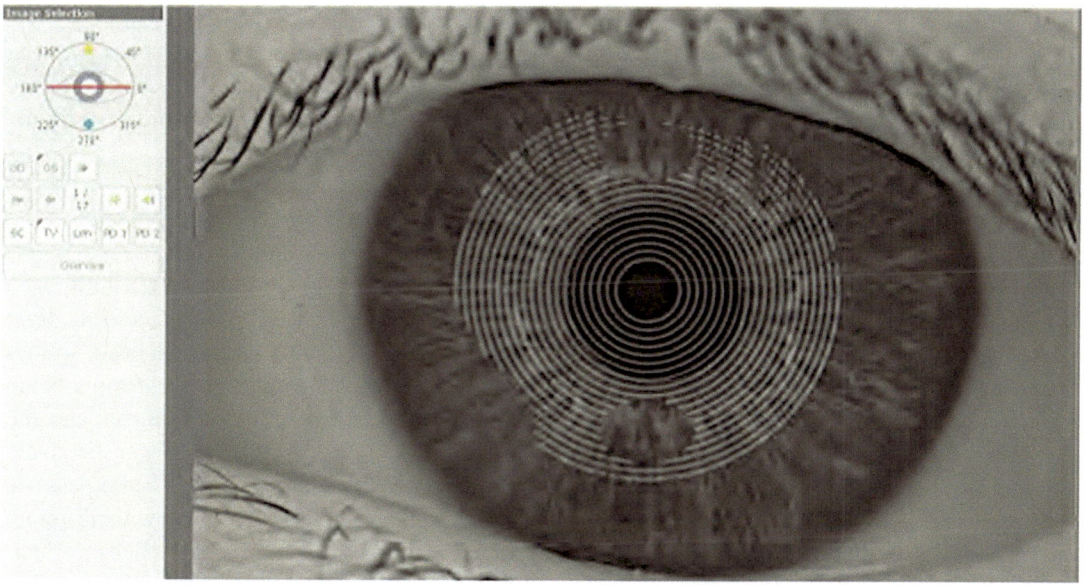

Fig. 27.3 Topview image of Placido ring reflection

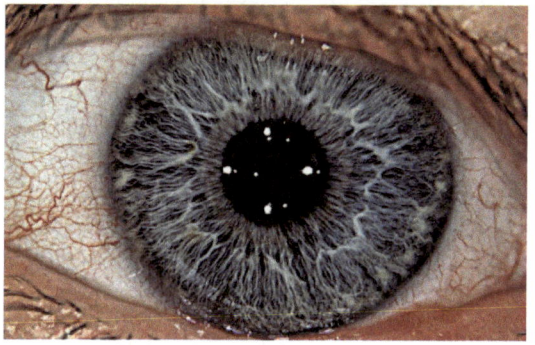

Fig. 27.4 Color Topview image

Dual-Scheimpflug Concept

Figure 27.5 illustrates how decentration and eye motion during a measurement can affect height data of the posterior surface, which directly affects pachymetry, as pachymetry is determined from anterior and posterior height data. When the slit light is well centered on the cornea, the left and right Scheimpflug cameras view the same corneal thickness as outlined by the blue and green lines. In the case of decentration to either side, the two Scheimpflug cameras view different

Fig. 27.5 Decentration affecting the images as viewed by the two Scheimpflug cameras

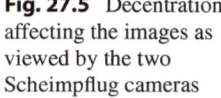
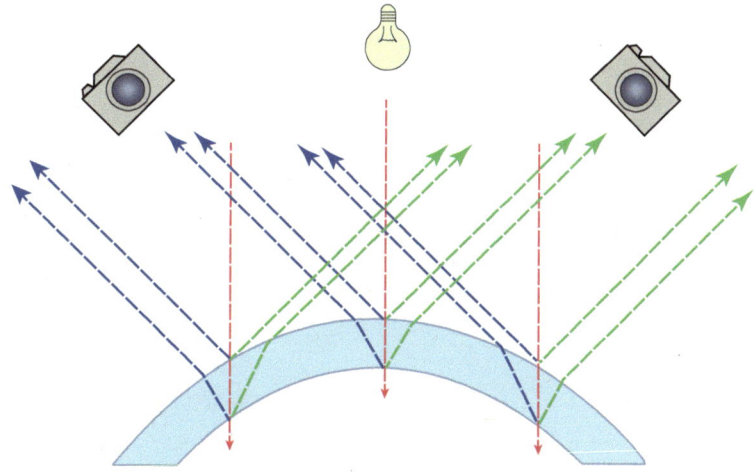

corneal thicknesses. Note: the difference in separation of the blue and green line pairs depends on the camera angle and the direction of displacement from the center of the cornea.

Combining the two camera views using ZIEMER's patented Dual-Scheimpflug solution, the systematic error in the original captured image is automatically corrected by averaging the two opposed camera images. Averaging the two images corrects the decentration error caused by eye motion or misalignment, making the measurement of the posterior edge independent of eye motion, allowing for accurate pachymetry and elevation data.

Accurate anterior surface calculations technically require only one of the two Scheimpflug images, along with the Placido image. However, for posterior surfaces, both Scheimpflug images are needed to compensate for decentration due to eye motion. Therefore, accurate determination of corneal pachymetry, anterior chamber depth, and posterior corneal surface requires complete Dual-Scheimpflug images. Loss of one of the two means that the corresponding image will be discarded and the Scheimpflug quality percentage will drop accordingly.

Comparing the GALILEI to a single Scheimpflug device, Aramberri et al. [1] reported that, while repeatability and reproducibility were good with both devices for all parameters and agreement was good with some relevant exceptions, the single-camera device was more precise for curvature, astigmatism, and corneal wavefront error measurements, and the dual-camera device was more precise for pachymetry measurements.

Axial Biometry by Optical A-Scan

Within the optical A-scan accessory, a collimated beam of an infrared, super-luminescent light emitting diode (SLED) is split by a beam splitter (BS) into a reference beam and a sample beam that are directed to a reference mirror and the patient's eye along its visual axis, respectively (Fig. 27.2). Whenever the sample beam passes a transition between ocular layers with different refractive indices (e.g., corneal surfaces, crystalline lens surfaces, and retinal surfaces), a portion of the light is reflected back toward the beam splitter. The optical path length of the light reflected from ocular surfaces is compared to the optical path length of light that is reflected from the reference mirror which is adjusted by moving the reference mirror at a constant velocity (V). When these optical lengths match to within the coherence length (CL) of the SLED, an interference signal is generated whose intensity is recorded with a detector and plotted as a function of the mirror position. The sample position is then deduced from the location on the plot's x-axis of the interference peak (Fig. 27.6).

Fig. 27.6 Time-domain, partial coherence interferometry for precisely measuring axial, intraocular distances

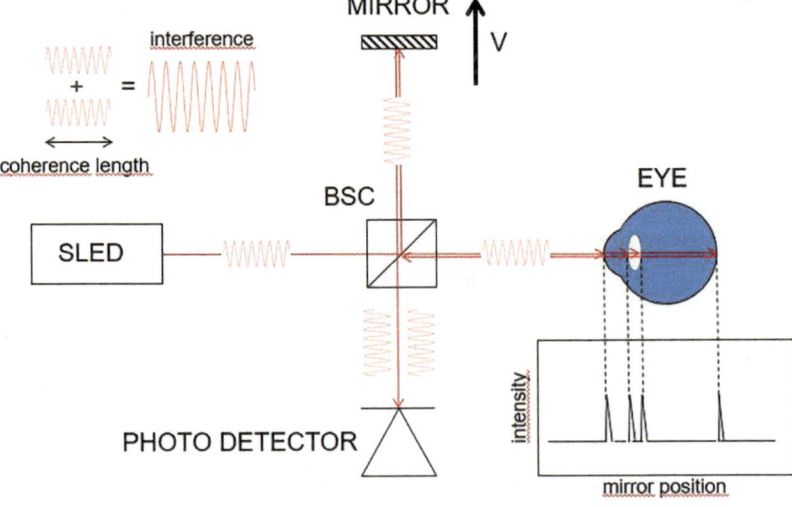

Conversion of Optical Distances to Geometrical Distances

Optical biometers, including the GALILEI G6, measure optical distances that represent geometrical (actual) distances multiplied with the measured material's refractive index. Thus, optical distances are converted to geometrical distances through division by the material's refractive index. When converting optical axial length (AL) to geometrical AL, one faces the challenge that the components along the measurement axis (cornea, anterior chamber, crystalline lens, vitreous chamber) have different refractive indices, and that refractive indices are dependent on the wavelength of the measuring light. With some optical biometers, the surfaces of the crystalline lens cannot be determined, such that an average refractive index must be employed for the conversion of optical AL to geometrical AL. This works reasonably well if the measured AL is within a certain range of normal AL. For very long or very short ALs, however, significant measurement errors may result because of altered refractive index contributions of the various axial components to the average refractive index. Such errors can be prevented by dividing the components' optical distances separately by their respective refractive indices and then adding the resulting, separate geometrical distances to obtain geometric AL. The Galilei G6 is capable of determining the surfaces of the crystalline lens, thereby measuring lens thickness, and therefore capable of converting optical distances segment-wise to geometrical distances. Two different AL are calculated and displayed by the GALILEI G6:

1. Total AL (tAL) that is converted segment-wise using component-specific, wavelength-adjusted, group refractive indices. It is defined as the distance from the anterior cornea to the posterior retina and designed for specific IOL equations that employ optical approaches such as ray tracing.

2. AL that is converted using an average refractive, wavelength-adjusted, group refractive index. It is defined as the distance from the anterior cornea to the anterior retina as is the case with ultrasound AL and matched to AL as measured with the IOLMaster. It is used with standard, empirical IOL equations.

Total Corneal Power (TCP)

Three types of TCP are computed with the GALILEI: TCP1, TCP2, TCP_IOL. They differ from each other in terms of what reference surface (anterior or posterior cornea) is used to determine the total focal length (f') of the cornea, and what refractive index (n; either that of the cornea or that of the aqueous) is used to convert the total focal length of the cornea to the total power of the cornea ($D = n/f'$).

- TCP1 is calculated using the corneal index of refraction ($n_{cornea} = 1.376$), and f' is referenced to the anterior corneal surface.
- TCP2 is calculated using the aqueous index of refraction ($n_{aqueous} = 1.336$), and f' is referenced to the anterior corneal surface, as is the case with TCP1.
- TCP_IOL is calculated using the aqueous index of refraction ($n_{aqueous} = 1.336$), and f' is referenced to posterior corneal surface.

TCP1 was the original value incorporated in the GALILEI G1 and carried forward in subsequent device iterations. TCP2 was introduced to try to better estimate true corneal power, and finally this too was replaced by TCP_IOL, though all options remain on current devices to allow users to customize individual preferences.

Technical Specifications (Table 27.1)

Table 27.1 Technical specifications of the GALILEI G6 Lens Professional

Measurement principle tomography/topography	Rotational Dual-Scheimpflug tomography/topography merged with Placido disk topography
Measurement principle biometry	Partial coherence interferometry (optical A-scan)
Measurement time tomography/topography	<1 s
Measurement time biometry	≈ 30–40 s per eye (3 consecutive scans in anterior segment and retina)
Placido disk geometry	20 rings, ranging in diameter from 20 mm to 200 mm
Number of cameras	3 (2 Scheimpflug, 1 Topview)
Number of measurement points	Up to 100,000 (Scheimpflug and Placido)
Displayed map coverage	10 mm maximum
Measurement ranges	Keratometry: 25–75 D (4.5–13.5 mm) Central corneal thickness: 250–800 μm Pupillometry: 0.5–10 mm Corneal Diameter: 6–14 mm Anterior chamber depth: 1.5–6.5 mm Lens thickness: 0.5–6.5 mm Axial length: 14–40 mm (default: 18–35 mm)
Measurement precision (standard deviation of repeated measurements). In brackets: Typical precision in normal eyes	SimK: ≤0.25 D (0.05 D) Angle of flattest meridian: ≤10° for astigmatism >0.5 D (2.9°) CCT: ≤3.00 μm; (1.2 μm) Pupillometry: ≤50 μm (6 μm) CD: ≤50 μm (16 μm) ACD: ≤50 μm (15 μm) LT: ≤100 μm (29 μm) AL: ≤50 μm (17 μm)
Illumination wavelengths	Scheimpflug: 470 nm (UV-free LED) Topview: 810 nm (IR LED) Placido: 810 nm (IR LED) Fixation target: 617 nm (LED) Biometry: 880 nm (SLED)

Study Results

A clinical study in adult subjects was performed to assess repeatability and reproducibility in the parameters indicated in Table 27.2 as measured by the GALILEI G6 Lens Professional (G6) in 20 normal, adult eyes. Measurements were repeated on the same eye and on the same device under the same conditions. To obtain reproducibility values, measurements were taken and compared for different operators using the same device. All parameters showed repeatability with coefficients of variation comparable to those reported with a predicate device, the Pentacam® AXL (PAXL; OCULUS Optikgeraete GmbH, Muenchholzhaeuser Str. 29, 35,582 Wetzlar, Germany), where only normal eyes were assessed.

In the same clinical study, parameters indicated in Table 27.3 measured by the G6 to those obtained by the PAXL. A total of 105 eyes were measured, 49 being right eyes and 56 being left eyes. Only one eye of each subject was measured, and 20 eyes were measured to represent each of the following five eye populations: (1) normal eyes (phakic eyes without cataracts or corneal disease), (2) eyes with varying degrees of cataract, (3) eyes with high myopia, (4) eyes with high hyperopia, and (5) eyes with postkeratorefractive surgery). The additional five eyes analyzed were two eyes with severe keratoconus and three eyes with prior cross-linking treatment. The G6 demonstrated agreement with the PAXL for the assessment of AL, CCT, R flat, R steep, Rm, CC, A flat, and ACD in eyes with normal eyes, eyes with cataracts, eyes with high myopia

Table 27.2 Repeatability and reproducibility with the GALILEI G6 in 20 normal eyes

Parameter	Nr of eyes	Mean	Repeatability		Reproducibility	
			SD	CV [%]	SD	CV [%]
AL (mm)	20	23.82	0.02	0.08	0.02	0.08
CCT (um)	20	543	1.49	0.27	1.49	0.27
R flat (mm)	20	7.76	0.01	0.18	0.01	0.18
R steep (mm)	20	7.63	0.02	0.22	0.02	0.22
R mean (mm)	20	7.69	0.01	0.16	0.01	0.16
CC (D)	20	0.75	0.12	16.07	0.12	16.07
A flat (deg)	20	163	4.52	2.78	4.52	2.78
ACD (mm)	20	3.63	0.01	0.35	0.01	0.35
CD (mm)	20	12.19	0.02	0.20	0.02	0.20

Table 27.3 Differences between GALILEI G6 and Pentacam AXL (PAXL) in 105 eyes, including eyes with severe keratoconus or prior cross-linking treatment

Parameter	G6 mean (SD)	PAXL mean (SD)	Mean diff (SD)	95% CI for mean diff	Paired t-test p-value
AL (mm)	23.96 (1.74)	23.95 (1.78)	0.05 (0.04)	0.05, 0.06	<0.001
CCT (um)	532.73 (43.82)	536.50 (41.91)	−3.77 (7.71)	−5.26, −2.28	<0.001
R flat (mm)	7.88 (0.44)	7.89 (0.46)	−0.01 (0.07)	−0.03, 0.00	0.07
R steep (mm)	7.66 (0.47)	7.66 (0.50)	−0.00 (0.10)	−0.02, 0.02	0.65
R mean (mm)	7.77 (0.45)	7.78 (0.47)	−0.01 (0.08)	−0.03, 0.01	0.18
CC (D)	1.28 (1.10)	1.36 (1.47)	−0.09 (0.65)	−0.21, 0.04	0.18
A flat (deg)	140.56 (63.26)	142.27 (62.24)	−1.71 (12.43)	−4.12, 0.70	0.16
ACD (mm)	3.54 (0.37)	3.50 (0.38)	0.04 (0.07)	0.03, 0.06	<0.001
CD (mm)	12.16 (0.40)	11.81 (0.39)	0.33 (0.07)	0.32, 0.34	<0.001

or hyperopia, eyes with postkeratorefractive surgery, and eyes with prior cross-linking treatment. Demonstration of agreement in eyes with severe keratoconus was limited by inherent difficulties in assessing the above parameters both by the G6 and the PAXL. The difference in CD between G6 and PAXL is due to differences between the devices—as well as between other devices for CD measurement on the market—in the definition of the transition zone between sclera and cornea, the modality used for the measurement, the measurement geometry, the wavelength of the measuring light source, and assumptions in ocular refractive indices.

Comparing the GALILEI G6 to the IOLMaster 700 swept-source optical biometer, Soyeon et al. [2] reported that the two biometers showed high repeatability and relatively good agreement. Supiyaphun et al. [3] compared anterior segment parameters and axial length using the G6 and the Pentacam AXL and found good repeatability of corneal curvature, ACD, and AL in both devices. Most parameters obtained from the Pentacam AXL were statistically significantly different from those obtained from GALILEI G6, except for steep meridians and ACD. Savini et al. [4] assessed the refractive outcomes of intraocular lens power calculation using different corneal power measurements with the GALILEI G6. They demonstrated that biometric measurements provided by the GALILEI G6 can be used to accurately calculate IOL power. Simulated K and TCP led to similar outcomes after constant optimization. Jung et al. [5] compared biometry and postoperative refraction in cataract patients between GALILEI G6 and IOL Master 500. The study revealed that ocular biometric measurements and prediction of postoperative refraction using GALILEI G6 were as accurate as with IOL Master 500. Jae et al. [6] reported that the GALILEI G6 provided precise ocular biometrics that were well correlated with results from standard biometers, and in particular, obtained accurate ACD measurements compared to AS-OCT. Furthermore, prediction of postoperative refraction using GALILEI G6 was comparable to the IOL-Master 500. Wang et al. [7] demonstrated that GALILEI G6 Dual-Scheimpflug measurements of corneal power, pachymetry, ACD, and corneal aberrations for Zernike terms in the middle of the Zernike tree showed excellent repeatability.

Software

Axial, intraocular distances, including axial length and lens thickness, are precisely measured with a series of optical A-scans (Fig. 27.7). Peak locations within the interference curve, and hence intraocular distances, are determined with customized peak detection algorithms. Automatically detected lens surfaces positions may be manually adjusted to allow for specific individual assessment (red arrows). Optical distances are converted to geometrical distances segment-wise: axial length is determined by dividing optical distances of each segment along the measurement axis by its respective refractive index and then adding the resulting geometrical distances.

For accurate biometry in an eye filled with silicon oil, the option "Silicon" may be selected prior to data collection to account for the difference in refractive indices.

Several IOL power calculation formulas are readily available on the GALILEI G6 to determine the adequate power of a given IOL in a given patient during cataract surgery. These formulas include Haigis, Holladay 1, HofferQ, SRK/T, SRK II, Shammas post-LASIK,

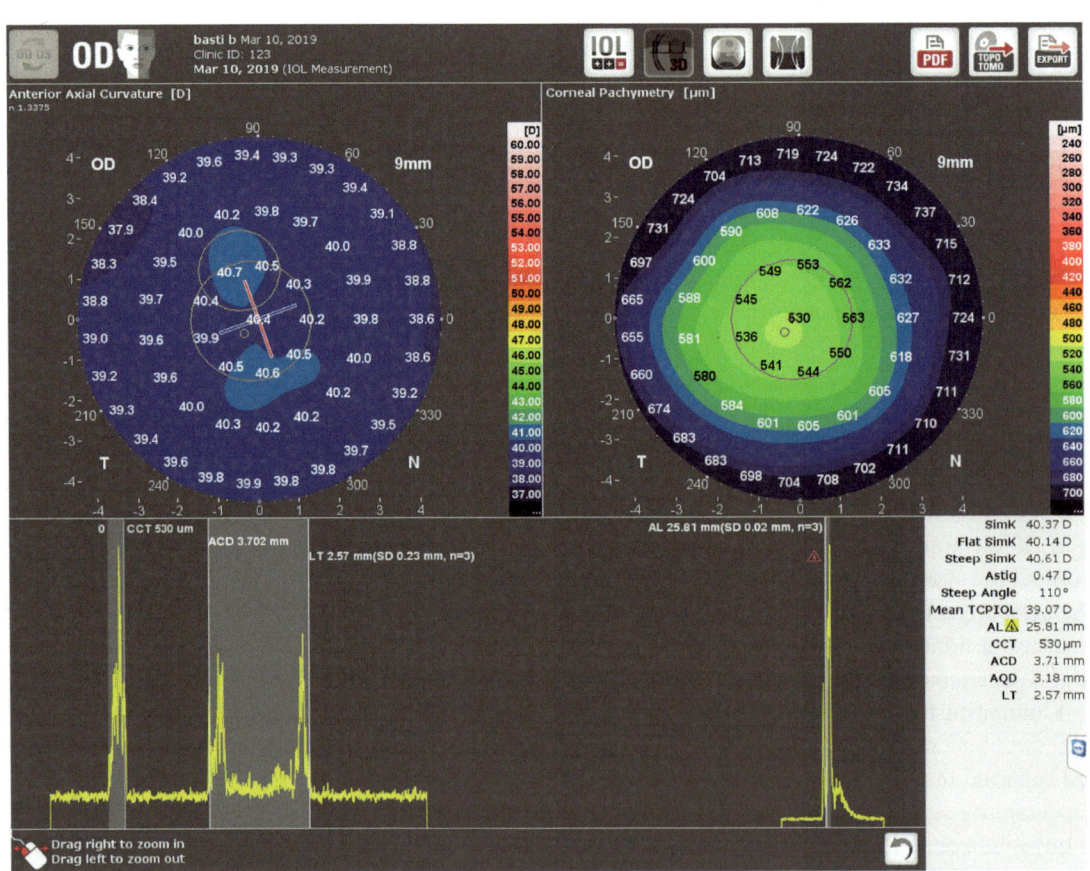

Fig. 27.7 Biometry display with interference curve, detected peak locations, indices, and selectable maps

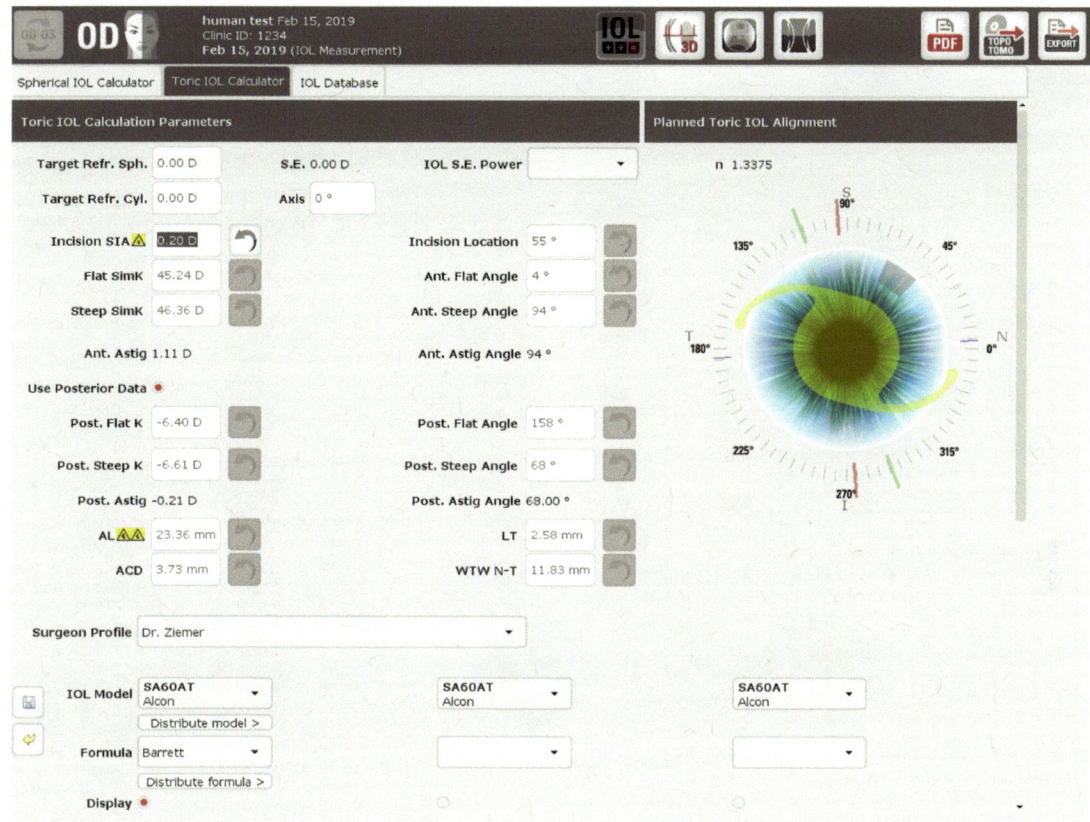

Fig. 27.8 Barrett Toric Calculator (top of display)

Barrett Universal II, and Barrett Toric (Figs. 27.8 and 27.9). A data export to the Holladay IOL Consultant Software and Panacea IOL & Toric Calculator Application will soon be released.

Through direct export and computation on the GALILEI G6, the ray-tracing IOL calculator OKULIX is optionally available. The ray-tracing IOL calculator PhacoOptics is being fine-tuned for the GALILEI G6 and will be released shortly.

An essential display for decision-making in cataract surgery planning is the Advanced IOL Display (Fig. 27.10). The anterior and posterior curvature data minimize the risk of postoperative surprises. The coma map allows a quick assessment of aberrations due to coma, which is an indicator whether premium IOLs are suitable in a given eye.

Other displays containing specific maps and indices may be used for cataract and refractive surgery planning and the detection of ocular diseases that have the potential to negatively affect the outcome of such surgeries. Various displays are available with the GALILEI G6 for that purpose by switching to the Topo/Tomo software (link via logo at top right):

- The expanded Cone Location and Magnitude Index (CLMI.X) Display searches for asymmetries that are typically related to keratoconus and computes an overall index that represents a clinically established keratoconus detection probability in a given eye (Fig. 27.11).
- The Comparison Display allows point-by-point subtraction of two maps and the creation of the resulting difference map for the assessment of changes over time or differences between fellow eyes (Fig. 27.12).

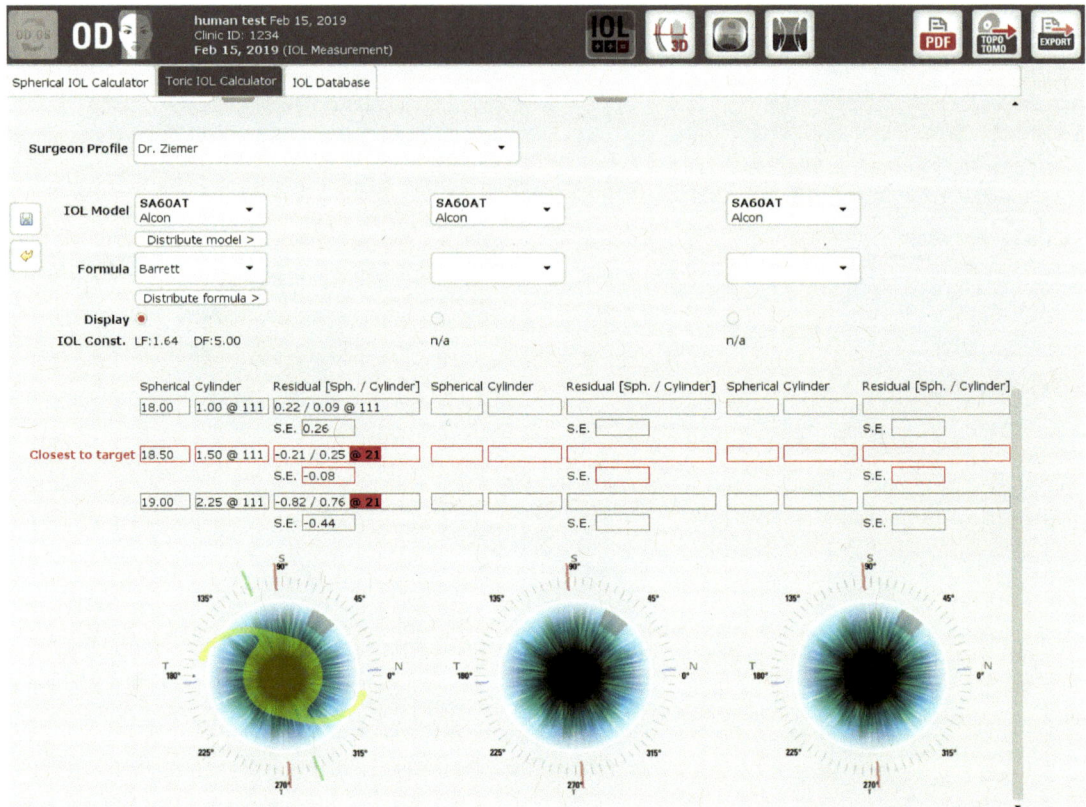

Fig. 27.9 Barrett Toric Calculator (bottom of display)

- The Wavefront Display (Fig. 27.13) illustrates corneal aberration of lower and higher orders, up to the eighth order, in terms of Zernike coefficients, equivalent diopters, and total RMS. Centration is selectable between Purkinje I, pupil center, limbus center or custom (entry of x and y in mm), and assessment zone diameter is selectable between 3 mm and 10 mm. The dominating type of aberration can easily be identified with the help of a pie chart and is another source of information for preoperative planning. The computation and display of anterior asphericity Q as assessed over a corneal area of 8 mm in diameter allow improving cataract planning involving premium IOLs as well as refractive surgery planning.

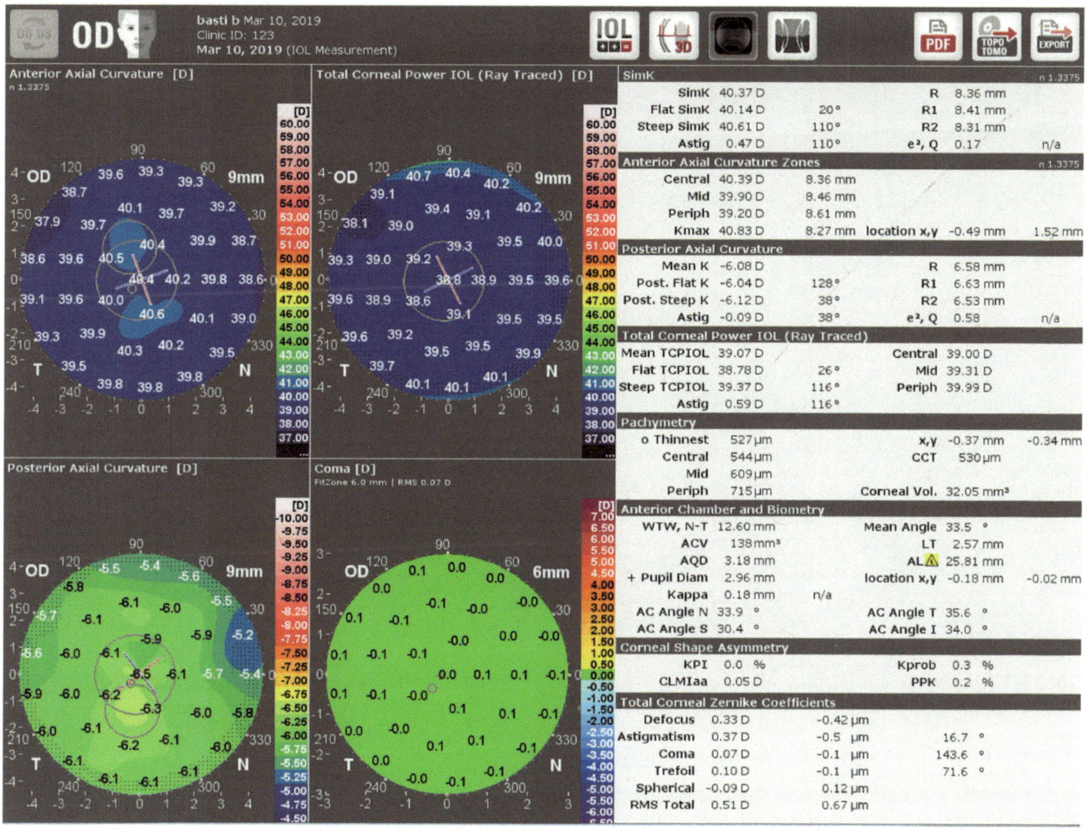

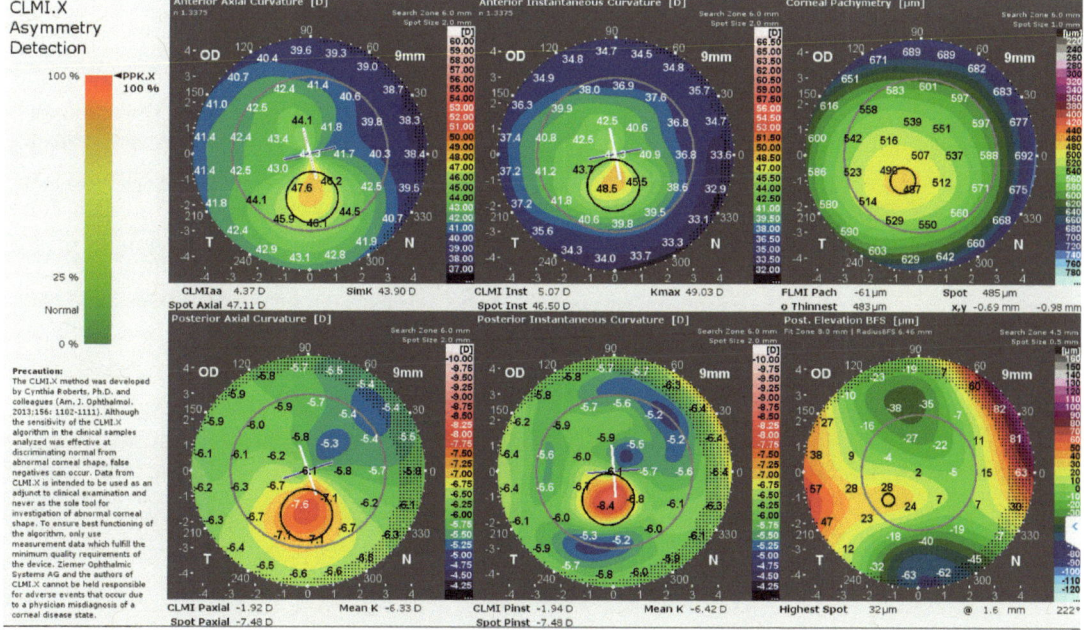

Fig. 27.10 Advanced IOL Display with selectable maps and indices

Fig. 27.11 Expanded Cone Location and Magnitude Index (CLMI.X) Display indicating keratoconus detection probability

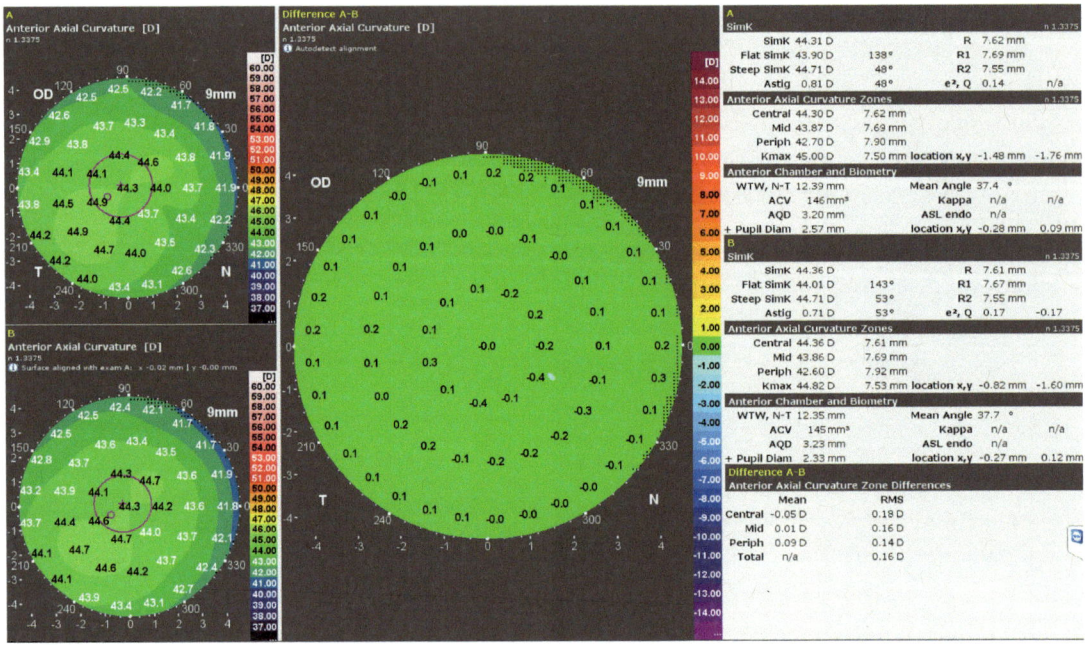

Fig. 27.12 Comparison Display allowing the assessment of differences or changes between two maps by means of point-by-point subtraction

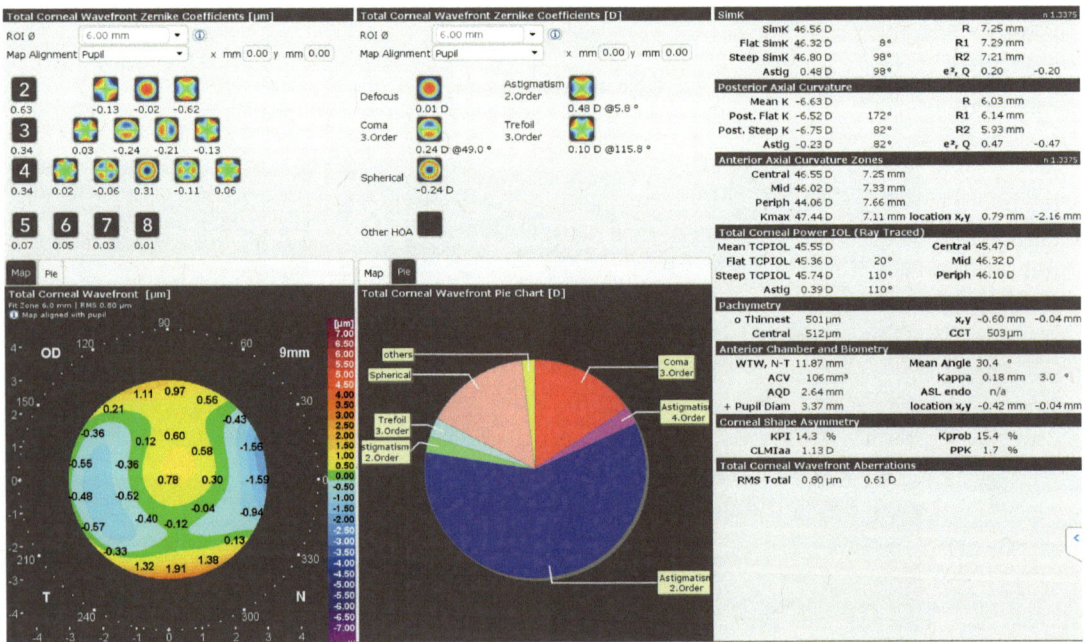

Fig. 27.13 Wavefront Display illustrating corneal aberrations of lower and higher orders

Summary

The combination of Dual-Scheimpflug tomography with high-resolution Placido topography and precise, optical A-scan biometry enables the following features of the GALILEI G6 Lens Professional:

- Short topography/tomography measurement time of less than 1 s, as with the Dual-Scheimpflug system only a half-full-circle measurement head rotation is needed to cover all meridians without losing data coverage.
- Insensitivity to measurement head decentration and eye motion because data of two opposite Scheimpflug cameras is averaged, thereby elimination decentration and eye motion errors.
- High precision and high resolution in keratometry at both central and peripheral areas due to Placido–Scheimpflug combination.
- Accurate and precise axial length and lens thickness measurement by optical A-scan regardless of eye size due to segment-wise conversion from optical to geometrical distances.
- Improved IOL power calculation and reduction in refractive error due to the availability of posterior cornea data and its inclusion in the IOL power calculation.
- Direct printing capability of every display and IOL calculation report directly from the GALILEI G6 device.
- Availability of additional information and explanation from the E-Learning Center.

References

1. Aramberri J, Araiz L, Garcia A, et al. Dual versus single Scheimpflug camera for anterior segment analysis: precision and agreement. J Cataract Refract Surg. 2012;38(11):1934–49.
2. Soyeon J, Hee SC, Na RK, Kang WL, Ji WJ. Comparison of repeatability and agreement between swept-source optical biometry and dual-Scheimpflug topography. J Ophthalmol. 2017;2017:1516395.
3. Supiyaphun C, Rattanasiri S, Jongkhajornpong P. Comparison of anterior segment parameters and axial length using two Scheimpflug devices with integrated optical biometers. Clin Ophthalmol. 2020;14:3487–94.
4. Savini G, Negishi K, Hoffer KJ, Lomoriello DS. Refractive outcomes of intraocular lens power calculation using different corneal power measurements with a new optical biometer. J Cataract Refract Surg. 2018;44(6):701–8.
5. Jung WL, Seung HP, Min CS, Min HK. Comparison of ocular biometry and postoperative refraction in cataract patients between GALILEI-G6® and IOL master. J Korean Ophthalmol Soc. 2015;56(4):515–20.
6. Jae YH, Hyun GK, Hyung KL. Comparison of the ocular biometry and intraocular lens power measured by a new optical biometry device and standard biometers. Invest Ophthalmol Vis Sci. 2018;59:2202.
7. Li Wang L, Shirayama M, Koch DD. Repeatability of corneal power and wavefront aberration measurements with a dual-Scheimpflug Placido corneal topographer. J Cataract Refract Surg. 2010;36(3):425–43.

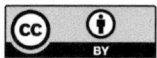

CASIA2: Anterior Segment 3D Swept-Source OCT

Naoko Hara, Kathrin Benedikt,
and Hirofumi Owaki

Introduction

CASIA2 (Fig. 28.1) was launched in 2015 from Tomey Corporation (Nagoya, Japan) as the successor to SS-1000 which was the world's first commercialized swept-source 3D optical coherence tomography in 2008. CASIA2 achieves deeper penetration and wider image by adopting the higher scanning speed light source with 1310 nm wavelength (Table 28.1), and it can acquire high-quality 3D images from the anterior surface of cornea to the back surface of the crystalline lens in short time in noncontact and noninvasive at one measurement (Fig. 28.2). CASIA2 can also provide the reliable quantitative evaluation by the stable scanning system.

The touch alignment system same as OA-2000 is employed. It can provide a stable measurement and a high reproducibility between operators because CASIA2 align itself automatically to patient eye once an operator only touches the center of the pupil on the screen. Operators can capture optical coherence tomography (OCT) image easily without any special skills.

The latest model of CASIA2 employs the color observation camera. Additionally, it makes possible observing the toric axis marking dots directly on the front camera images by optimization of the optical performance. CASIA2 is continually advancing.

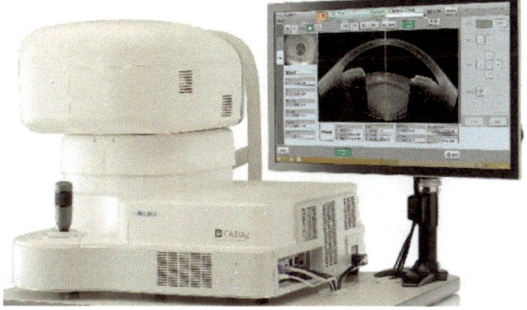

Fig. 28.1 Anterior segment swept-source 3D OCT CASIA2

Table 28.1 Specifications of CASIA2

	Type	Swept-source laser
Light source	wavelength principal	1310 nm Fourier domain
Resolution	Axial (depth) Transverse	10 μm or less (in tissue) 30 μm or less (in tissue)
Scan speed	50,000 A-scans/s	
Scan range	16 × 16 × 13 mm	

N. Hara · K. Benedikt · H. Owaki (✉)
Tomey Corporation, Nagoya, Japan
e-mail: kathrin@tomey.de; matsu@tomey.co.jp

© The Author(s) 2024
J. Aramberri et al. (eds.), *Intraocular Lens Calculations*, Essentials in Ophthalmology,
https://doi.org/10.1007/978-3-031-50666-6_28

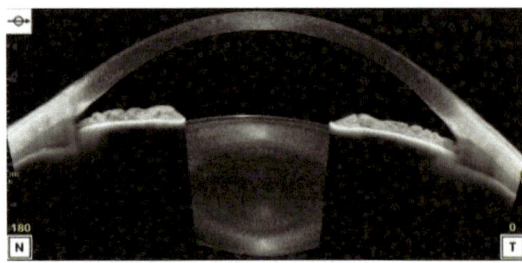

Fig. 28.2 OCT image of normal eye by CASIA2

Various Functions for Cataract Surgery

The deep and wide 3D images (Fig. 28.3) from the anterior surface of cornea to the back surface of the crystalline lens provides various functions, especially for pre- and post-operative cataract surgery.

CASIA2 has an application suite named CICS (CASIA IOL Cataract Surgery) which can sup-

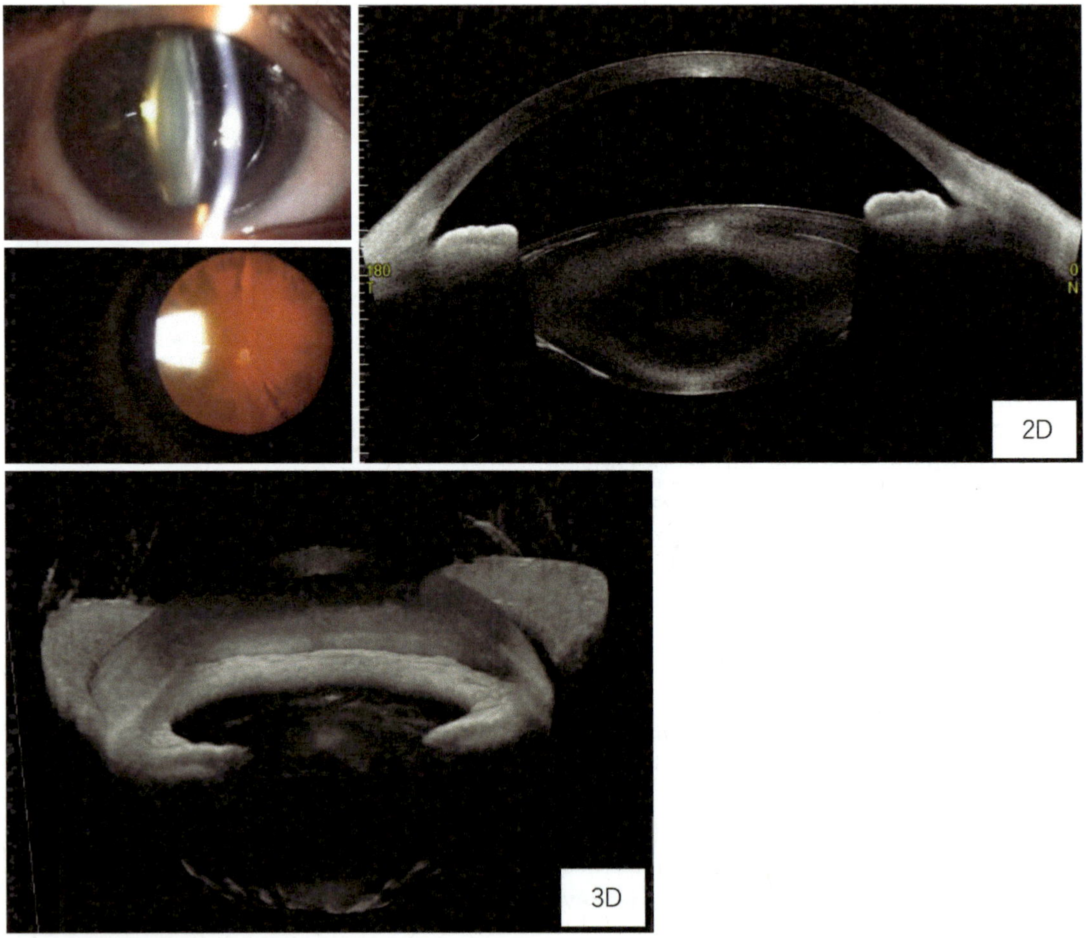

2D

3D

Fig. 28.3 Observation of a cortical cataract eye by 3D view function of CASIA2. Cortex opacity condition can be observed in 3D. Data are provided by Dr. Yuta Ueno, Department of Ophthalmology, Institute of Clinical Medicine, University of Tsukuba

port users on cataract surgery. CICS includes pre-op cataract and post-op cataract applications so that doctors can perform a perfect cataract surgery from planning to post-operative evaluation.

IOL Screening on Pre-op Cataract

Intraocular lens (IOL) screening display (Fig. 28.4) provides various analysis results on the anterior segment of the eye including useful information to select premium IOLs. Topography maps and basic indices of corneal shape (Fig. 28.4a), indices to select IOLs including corneal regular astigmatism and irregular astigmatism (high-order aberrations [HOAs], spherical aberration [SA]) (Fig. 28.4b), OCT image (Fig. 28.4c), indices-related anterior chamber (Fig. 28.4d), and the simulated retinal image of Landolt ring based on corneal HOAs (Fig. 28.4e)

are displayed on one report. The indices are indicated in yellow or red when they are outside of normal range.

To ensure efficient screening of corneal topography in candidates of cataract surgery, Goto and Maeda propose four steps for the interpretation of the results [1] (Table 28.2).

First, check for corneal irregular astigmatism. When HOAs are high as indicated in yellow or red on Fig. 28.4f, there is higher risk of insufficient visual recovery. Multifocal IOLs should be avoided.

Second, check the abnormal topographic pattern caused by refractive surgery. Figure 28.5 shows IOL screening report of a post-Lasik eye. Axial power map shows the central flattening pattern (Fig. 28.5a) and pachymetric map shows thinner pattern (Fig. 28.5b). Average K (AvgK) and central corneal thickness (CCT) are also indicated in red (Fig. 28.5c, d). In the case of

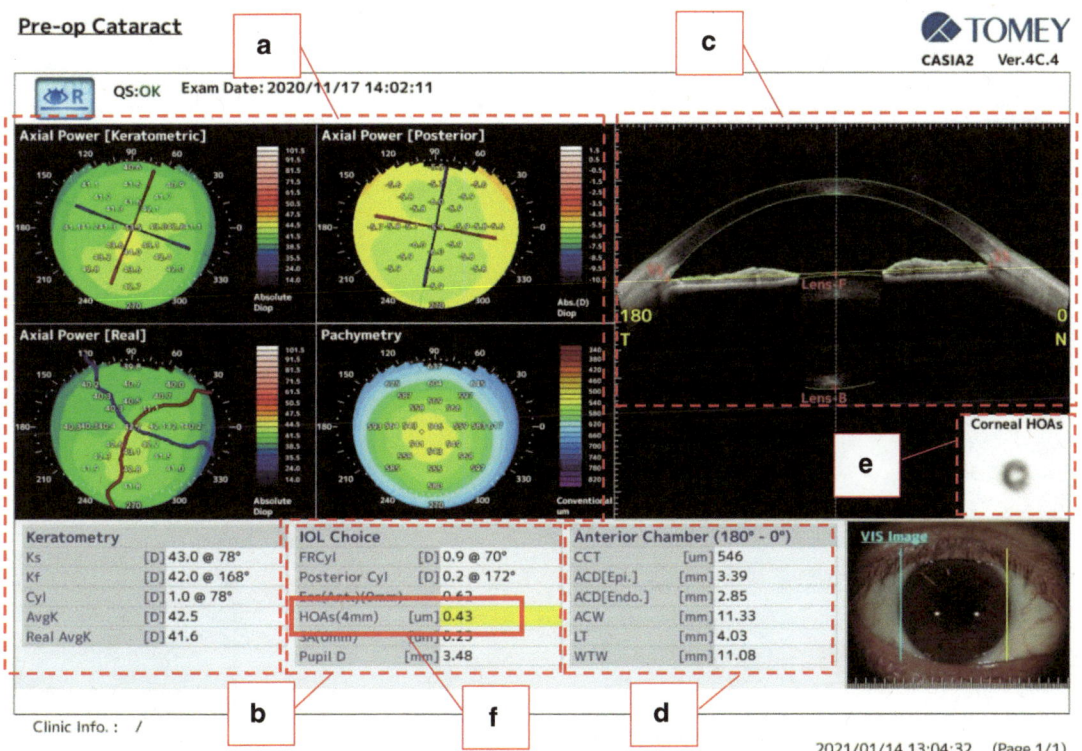

Fig. 28.4 IOL screening report, which is developed under supervision of prof. Naoyuki Maeda, Department of Ophthalmology, Osaka University Graduate School of Medicine and Associate Prof. Kazuhiko Onuma, Center for Frontier Medical Engineering, Chiba University

such a typical post-Lasik eye, IOL formula for post-Lasik should be used instead of standard formulae to prevent post-operative hyperopia surprise.

Table 28.2 Four steps in corneal topography for screening before cataract surgery [1]

Step 1: Corneal higher-order aberration (HOAs)
If corneal HOA is abnormal, multifocal or toric intraocular lens (IOLs) should be avoided and informed consent should be conducted for irregular astigmatism.
Step 2: Topographic pattern
If topographic pattern indicates post-refractive surgery, special IOL formula should be used in place of routinely used formula.
Step 3: Corneal astigmatism
If topographic pattern indicates regular astigmatism without asymmetry for both surfaces, toric IOL can be considered.
Step 4: Corneal spherical aberration
If corneal spherical aberration shows negative values, spherical IOLs should be considered.

Third, check regular astigmatism. Figure 28.6 is an example of IOL screening report for with-the-rule astigmatism. The anterior and posterior topography maps show the bowtie pattern without asymmetry (Fig. 28.6a). The indices in red are only for the anterior cylinder (Fig. 28.6b, Cyl) and the total cylinder (Fig. 28.6b, FRCyl), and other indices are in the normal range. In such case, toric IOL would be a good choice, and also multifocal and aspherical IOL can be considered.

Fourth, check for corneal spherical aberration. Figure 28.7 is an example of IOL screening report for a typical keratoconus eye. Spherical aberration (Fig. 28.7a, SA) is indicated in red with negative number. Implanting an aspherical IOL into such eye may increase irregular astigmatism, so the use of a spherical IOL should be considered.

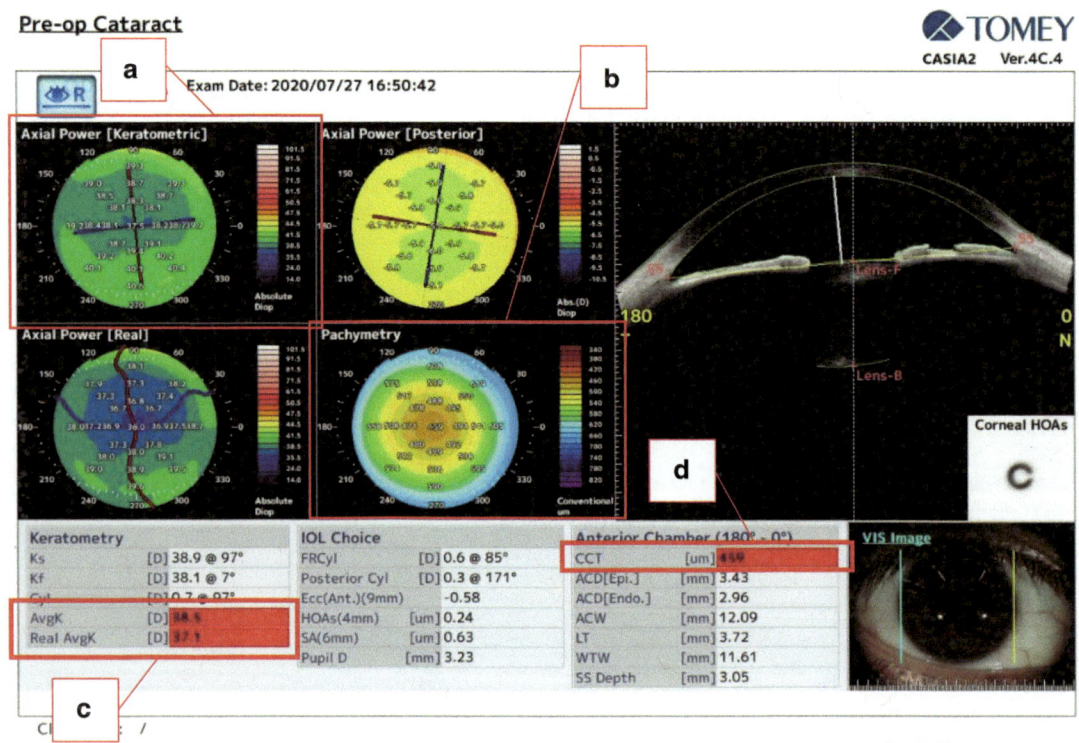

Fig. 28.5 IOL screening report of post-Lasik eye

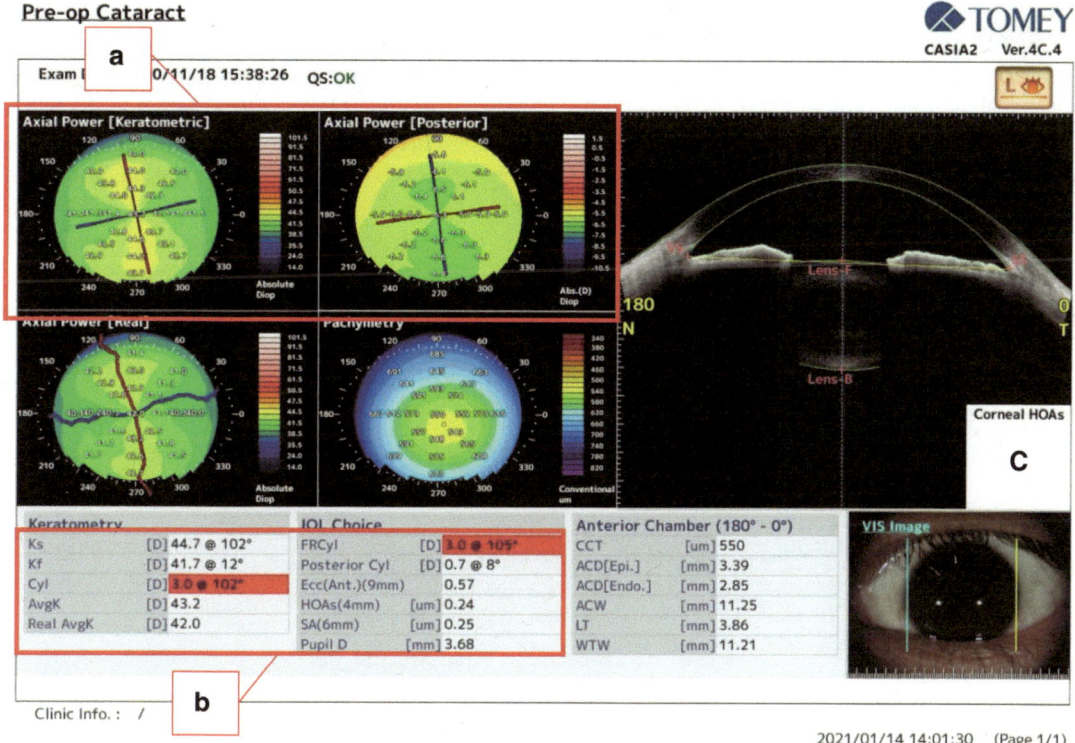

Fig. 28.6 IOL screening report of regular astigmatism eye

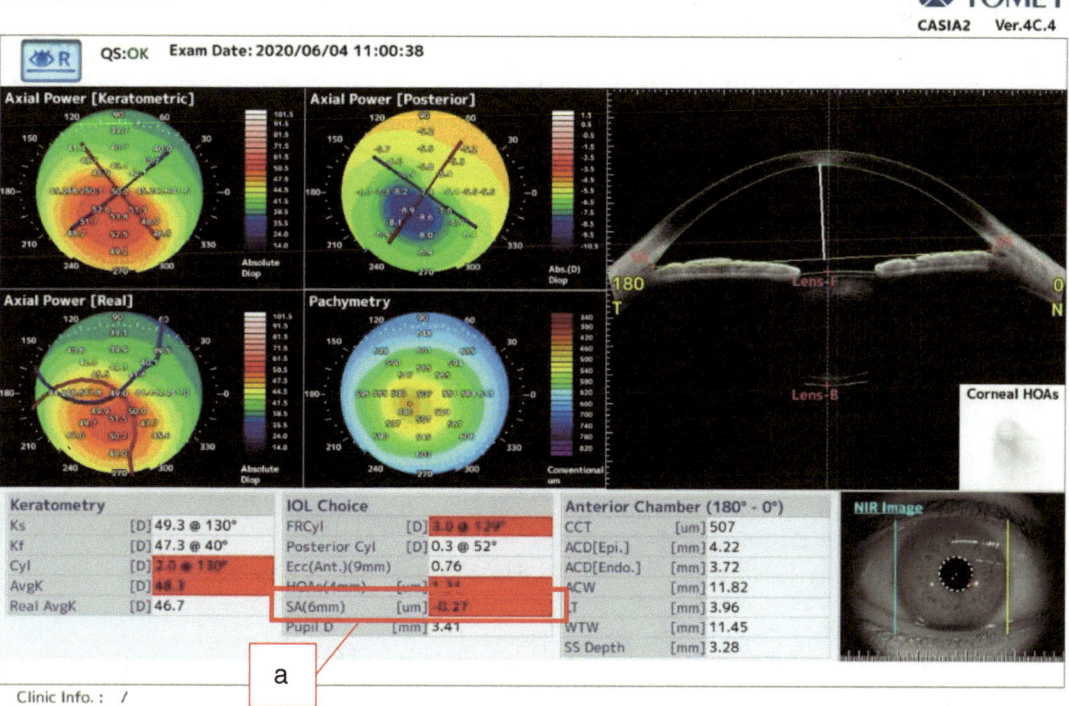

Fig. 28.7 IOL screening report of keratoconus

IOL Power Calculation on Pre-op Cataract

Pre-op cataract app includes IOL power calculation function (Fig. 28.8). Different kinds of IOL formulae, which are standard IOL formulae, toric IOL formulae and post-Lasik IOL formulae, are available on CASIA2 (Table 28.3). Other various new IOL formulae using parameters (posterior cornea, ACD, Lens thickness, ATA, etc.) obtained by anterior segment OCT are proposed [2–4]. It is expected that new concept IOL formulae will be put into practical use near future. Function for optimization of IOL constants is included in CASIA2, and it can support users to calculate personal lens constant for each surgeon. CASIA2 can connect with OA-2000 (Fig. 28.9), measurement results of axial length and corneal power by OA-2000 are automatically transferred to CASIA2 based on patient ID, and IOL calculation results can be obtained with these values.

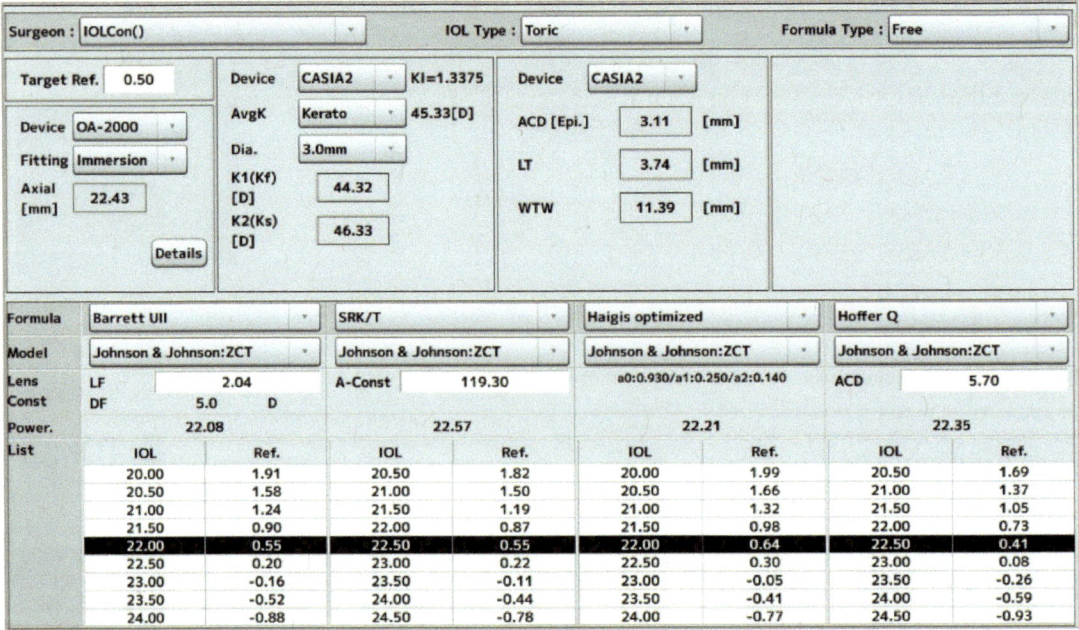

Fig. 28.8 IOL power calculation screen

Table 28.3 Available IOL formulae on CASIA2

Standard IOL formulae
Barrett Universal II, Haigis standard, Haigis optimized, Hoffer® Q, Holladay 1, SRK/T, OKULIX[a]
Toric IOL formulae
CASIA Toric (simple vector calculation), Barrett Toric Calculator, Barrett True K Toric Calculator, OKULIX[a]
IOL formulae for post-Lasik
Barrett True K, Shammas-PL, A-P method, OKULIX[a]

[a]Optional, depending on sales area

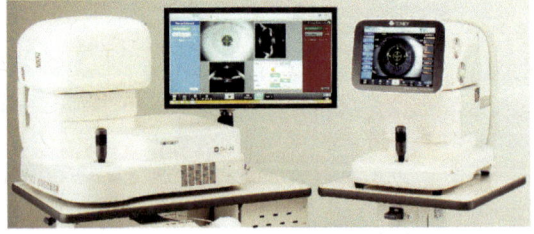

Fig. 28.9 Data linkage with OA-2000

Toric IOL Calculation and Axis Registration Support on Pre-op Cataract

Pre-op Cataract app includes toric planning function with toric calculator and axis registration function. It can support surgeons to mark the target axis based on the reference axis of iris pattern or conjunctival blood vessels. The color front image is available on the latest CASIA2, and blood vessel as reference points can be observed clearly (Fig. 28.10, The color front image is available on the newest hardware.).

Lens Analysis Function

Crystalline lenses are analyzed in 3D, its curvature of radius for front and back surfaces, tilt, and decentration are calculated automatically by lens analysis function (Fig. 28.11).

Kimura reports that a strong correlation was found between the average tilt and decentration values of the crystalline lens and the IOL. These results suggest that an aspherical lens should not be chosen for the IOL if there is a significant tilt or decentration of the crystalline lens before surgery [5].

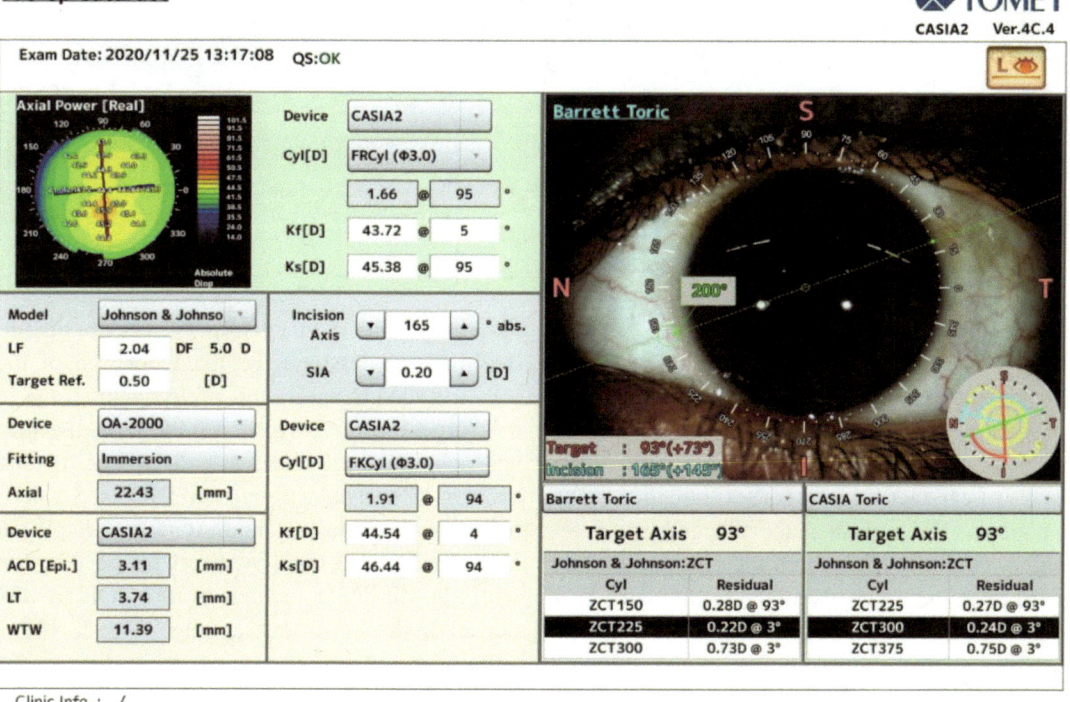

Fig. 28.10 Toric calculation and planning report

Lens Analysis

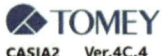

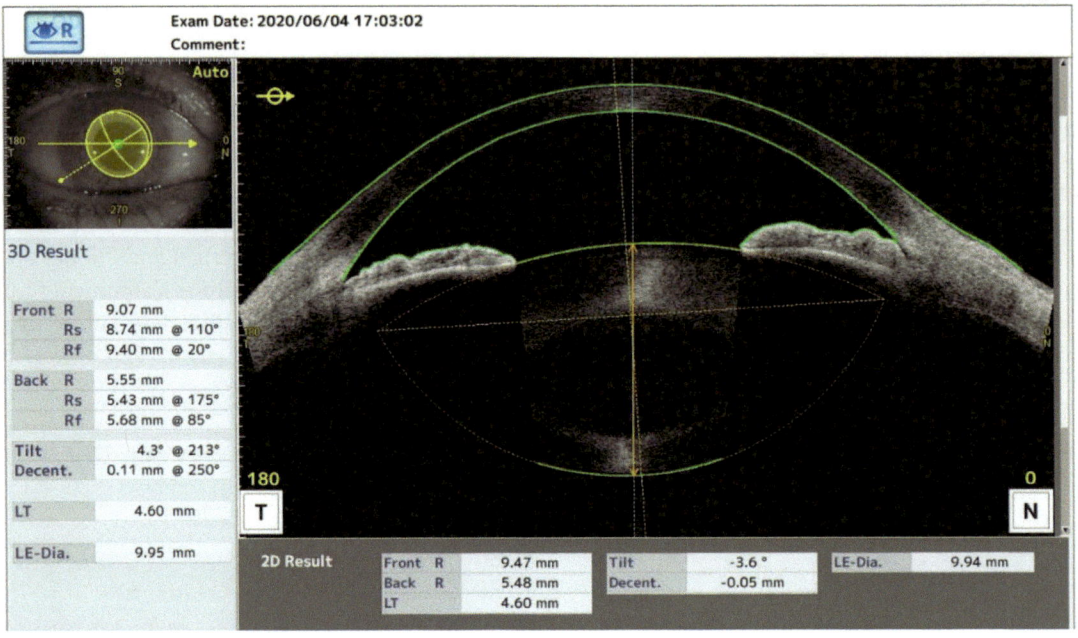

Fig. 28.11 Lens analysis report

Post-op Cataract

Post-op cataract (Fig. 28.12) is an application to compare data between pre- and post-operative. It can support doctors to evaluate, analyze the results of cataract surgery, and explain the results to patients. The corneal shape change by cataract surgery can be confirmed on the differential map of the total corneal map and the pachymetry map (Fig. 28.12a). By superimposing OCT image before and after cataract surgery, it is possible to intuitively understand the fixed position of the IOL and the change in the angle opening due to the surgery (Fig. 28.12b). In addition, the pre- and post-operative and that's difference of total average K, corneal astigmatism, HOAs, SA, lens tilt, lens decentration, and ACD are displayed numerically, and the IOL-fixed image diagram with IOL tilt in 3D and axis of toric IOL are displayed on the front camera image (Fig. 28.12c).

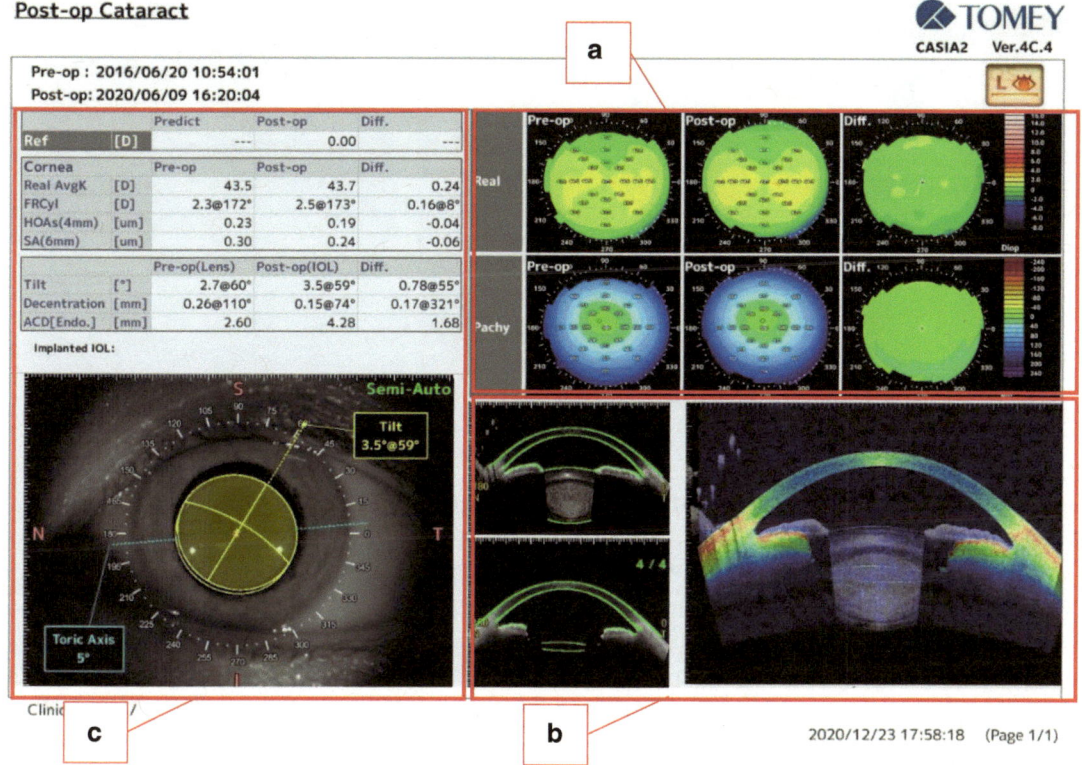

Fig. 28.12 Post-op cataract report

Direct Observation of Toric Axis Marking Dots

Toric axis marking dots of implanted IOL can be observed directly on the latest CASIA2 by optimization of optical performance (Fig. 28.13, red arrows. It is available on the newest hardware). Doctors can measure toric axis directly, and it is useful for identifying the cause when astigmatism correction is unsatisfied.

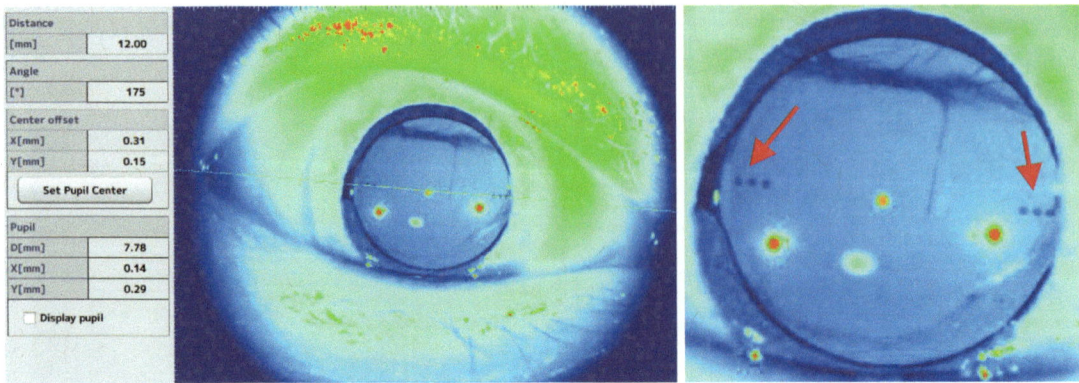

Fig. 28.13 Observation of toric axis marking dots by latest CASIA2

Various Functions for Other Clinical Fields

In addition to pre- and post-cataract examinations, CASIA2 is equipped with applications to support daily practice in various clinical fields such as corneal diseases, refractive correction, and glaucoma.

Functions for ICL®

CASIA2 includes two ICL® size determination formulae which calculate predicted vaults after surgery and optimal ICL® size using the distance between scleral spurs (NK formula [6]) or angle-to-angle (KS formula [7]) obtained from AS-OCT image (Fig. 28.14a). In addition, function to measure vaults of ICL-implanted eyes is included,

and it supports doctors for post-operative management (Fig. 28.14b). In the recent study, Gonzalez-Lopez reports importance of vaulting under light-induced maximum miosis and proposes a new method of vault dynamic assessment using CASIA2 [8].

Trend Analysis

The change over time in corneal shape is displayed using a topography map and a graph of indices so that it can be grasped intuitively on the trend analysis function (Fig. 28.15). By using the corneal thickness, the best fit sphere on the posterior surface of the cornea, Kmax (Keraometric), etc., it supports analysis of keratoconus progression and judgment of performing cross-linking treatment.

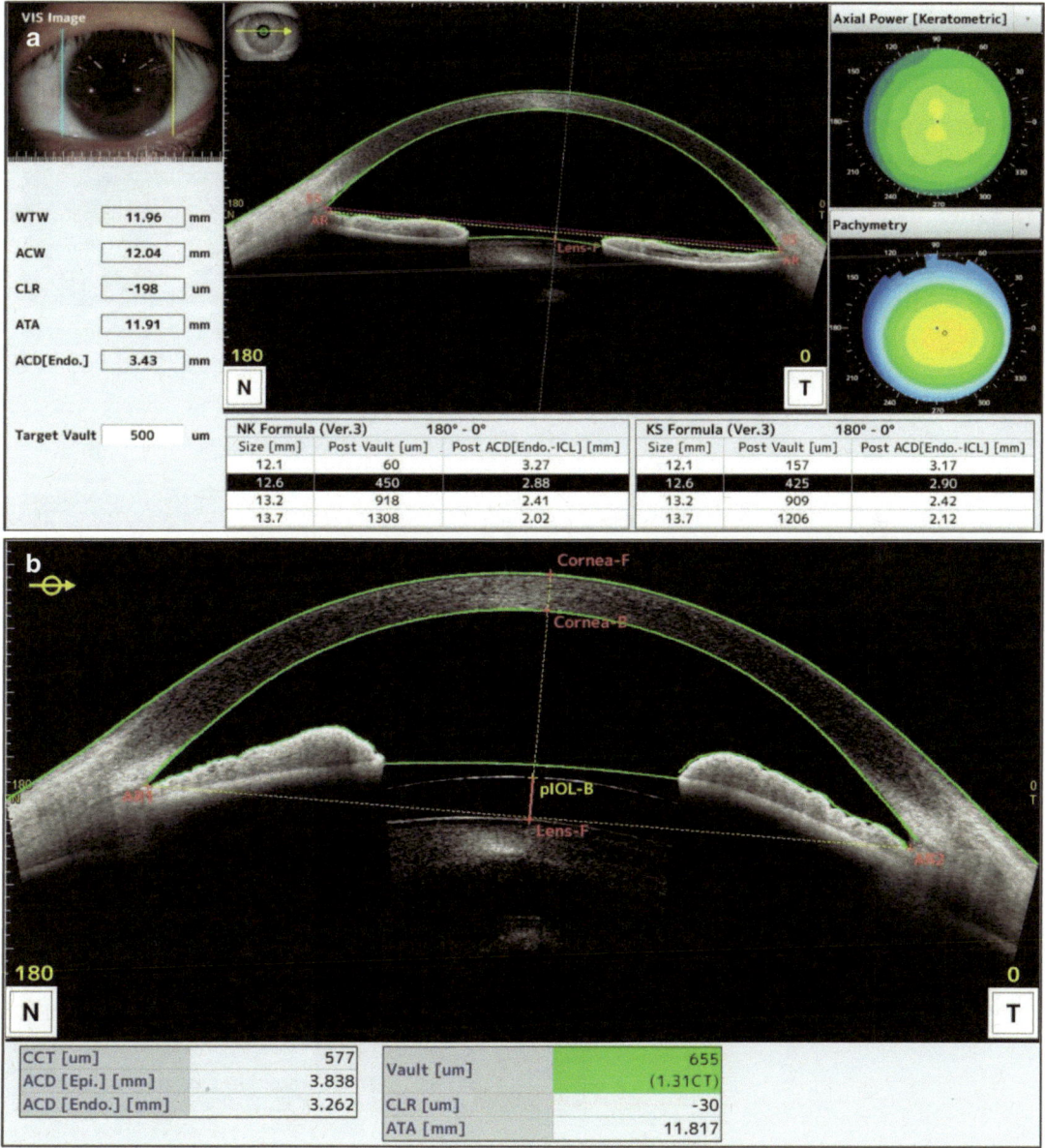

Fig. 28.14 Application for ICL®. (**a**) ICL® sizing app, (**b**) Measurement of vaulting

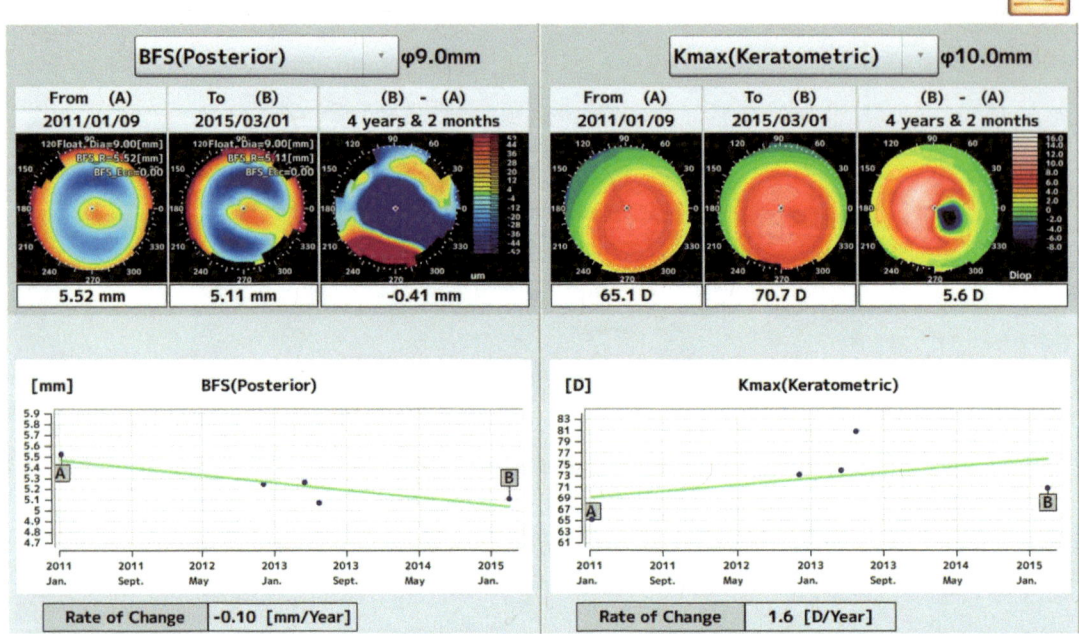

Fig. 28.15 Trend analysis on progressive keratoconus eye

Fig. 28.16 Observation of implanted tube shunt by wide averaging image of CASIA2. Provided by Dr. Hideo Nakanishi, Department of Ophthalmology, Eye Center, Hidaka Medical Center, Toyooka Hospital

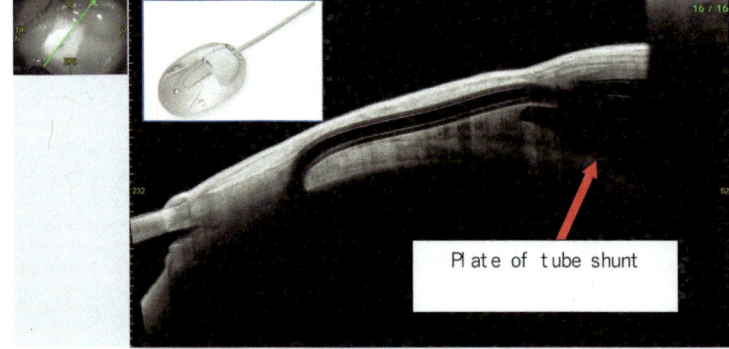

Wider and Deeper Image with Averaging

CASIA2 provide wider and deeper image with averaging technique due to the higher scan speed, which can reduce noise and enhanced signal. Figure 28.16 is an example of a wide range image of CASIA2. It can be observed clearly from angle to plate of implanted tube shunt and tissue structure.

STAR360°

STAR360° (Scleral spur Tracking for Angle analysis and Registration 360°) analyzes the whole 360° of anterior camber angle (ACA), describes various ACA parameters such as *iridotrabecular contact* (ITC) and angle opening distance (AOD) with visual chart, and calculates 360° quantitative indices (Fig. 28.17).

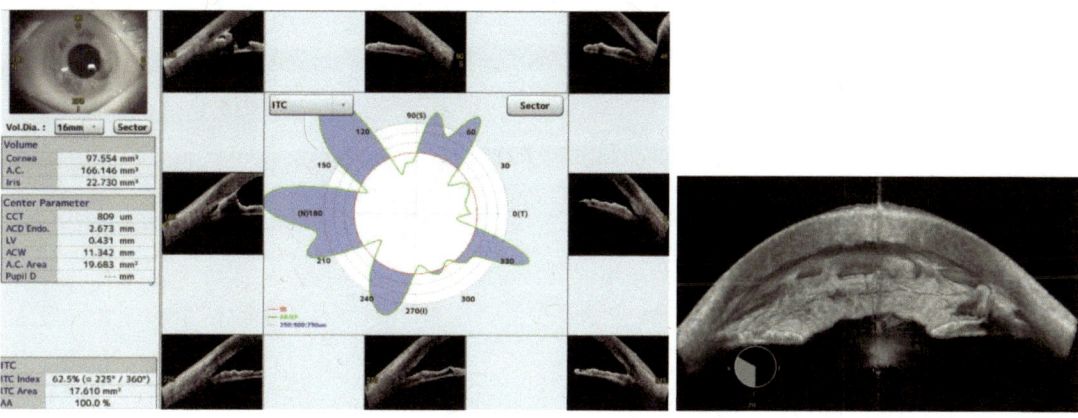

Fig. 28.17 ITC chart on STAR360°. Data provided by Dr. Hideki Mori, Department of Ophthalmology, Tokyo medical university

This application is developed under supervision of Prof. Christopher Leung MD, MB ChB, Department of Ophthalmology, The University of Hong Kong [9].

References

1. Goto S, Maeda N. Corneal topography for intraocular lens selection in refractive cataract surgery. Ophthalmology. 2021;128(11):e142–52.
2. Olsen T. Prediction of the effective postoperative (intraocular lens) anterior chamber depth. J Cataract Refract Surg. 2006;32(3):419–24.
3. Goto S, Maeda N, Koh S, Ohnuma K, Hayashi K, Iehisa I, Noda T, Nishida K. Prediction of postoperative intraocular lens position with angle-to-angle depth using anterior segment optical coherence tomography. Ophthalmology. 2016;123(12):2474–80.
4. Satou T, Shimizu K, Tsunehiro S, Igarashi A, Kato S, Koshimizu M, Niida T. Development of a new intraocular lens power calculation method based on lens position estimated with optical coherence tomography. Sci Rep. 2020;10(1):6501.
5. Kimura S, Morizane Y, Shiode Y, Hirano M, Doi S, Toshima S, Fujiwara A, Shiraga F. Assessment of tilt and decentration of crystalline lens and intraocular lens relative to the corneal topographic axis using anterior segment optical coherence tomography. PLoS One. 2017;12(9):e0184066.
6. Nakamura T, Isogai N, Kojima T, Yoshida Y, Sugiyama Y. Implantable collamer lens sizing method based on swept-source anterior segment optical coherence tomography. Am J Ophthalmol. 2018;187:99–107.
7. Igarashi A, Shimizu K, Kato S, Kamiya K. Predictability of the vault after posterior chamber phakic intraocular lens implantation using anterior segment optical coherence tomography. J Cataract Refract Surg. 2019;45(8):1099–104.
8. Gonzalez-Lopez F, Bouza-Miguens C, Tejerina V, Mompean B, Ortega-Usobiaga J, Bilbao-Calabuig R. Long-term assessment of crystalline lens transparency in eyes implanted with a central-hole phakic collamer lens developing low postoperative vault. J Cataract Refract Surg 2020.
9. Leung CK. Optical coherence tomography imaging for glaucoma - today and tomorrow. Asia Pac J Ophthalmol (Phila). 2016;5(1):11–6.

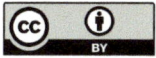

CSO MS-39: Principles and Applications

29

Gabriele Vestri, Francesco Versaci, and Giacomo Savini

Introduction

Tomographers based on Scheimpflug technology had the undoubted merit of extending the diagnostic capabilities of Placido corneal topographers, which were limited to an accurate automated measurement in one single shot of a large area of the anterior corneal surface. Indeed, they enabled the imaging of whole anterior segment sections, thus adding visual and quantitative information on the posterior corneal surface and on the anterior chamber (iris, angles, and anterior part of the crystalline lens). With these advancements, clinicians were able to get new information about their patients: elevation maps of the anterior and posterior corneal surfaces and pachymetric maps to detect keratoconus and ectasia, posterior and total corneal astigmatism to plan toric intraocular lenses (IOLs) implantation, calculation of total corneal power by ray tracing to compute IOL power after corneal refractive surgery. Nevertheless, the main limitations of Scheimpflug technology were the low resolution, the poor quality of anterior segment scans, and the presence of artefacts due to an excessive

G. Vestri (✉) · F. Versaci
CSO s.r.l., Florence, Italy
e-mail: g.vestri@csoitalia.it; f.versaci@csoitalia.it

G. Savini
IRCCS Bietti Foundation, Rome, Italy

Studio Oculistico d'Azeglio, Bologna, Italy
e-mail: giacomo.savini@startmail.com

amount of tissue scattering. MS-39 was conceived to overcome the previous limitations thus allowing for the acquisition of high-quality angle-to-angle images of the anterior segment. The superior quality of the images, in particular the improved detail of corneal layers, offers the clinician new opportunities for early keratoconus detection, preoperative and postoperative management of corneal transplantations, refractive surgery, and orthokeratology.

Technical Features of MS-39

MS-39 is a topographer-tomographer (Fig. 29.1), which puts together a Placido disc [1] and a FD-OCT (Fourier domain optical coherence tomography) system [2–4]. Placido disc is solely

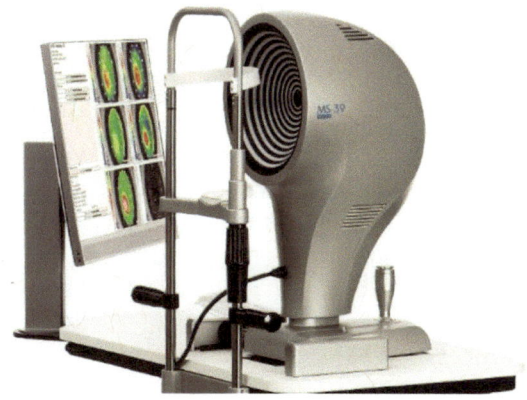

Fig. 29.1 CSO srl, MS-39

© The Author(s) 2024

J. Aramberri et al. (eds.), *Intraocular Lens Calculations*, Essentials in Ophthalmology,
https://doi.org/10.1007/978-3-031-50666-6_29

used for the topography of the anterior corneal surface, while the OCT system is used for the topography and tomography of the anterior ocular segment. The Placido technology is based on the principle of reflection of a known pattern of rings on a curved mirror, which is the anterior corneal surface. A proper processing of their reflected image on the corneal surface allows for an accurate measurement of its shape.

The OCT system is specifically a SD-OCT (spectral domain), which is based on the interference of two beams of a broadband infrared radiation coming from a reference arm and a sample arm. The basic scheme of a SD-OCT (Fig. 29.2) system is made up of a broadband radiation source, an interferometer with four arms, a spectrometer for collecting the interference signal, a processing unit that transforms the interference signal into a tomographic image. One arm of the interferometer is the entry of the broadband radiation. A second arm (reference arm) is used for creating a reference in distance and for generating one of the interfering beams. The third arm (sample arm) is for launching the radiation toward the sample and for collecting its backscattered beam. The fourth one (detection arm) is for collecting the interference of the beams coming from the reference and sample arms into a spectrometer.

In MS-39, the broadband source is an infrared superluminescent diode (SLD) emitting a radiation centered around 850 nm. This is splitted by the interferometer toward the reference and sample arms. At the end of the reference arm, a fixed mirror reflects the beam back toward the detection arm where the spectrometer collects it. Similarly, the radiation transmitted to the sample arm is pointed toward a certain direction outside the instrument by an X–Y scanning system and, then, backscattered by the ocular tissues toward the detection arm, where it interferes with the beam back-reflected by the reference arm. For each wavelength available in the source, the sensor of the spectrometer collects the intensity of a beam generated by the constructive, destructive, or partially constructive interference of the two

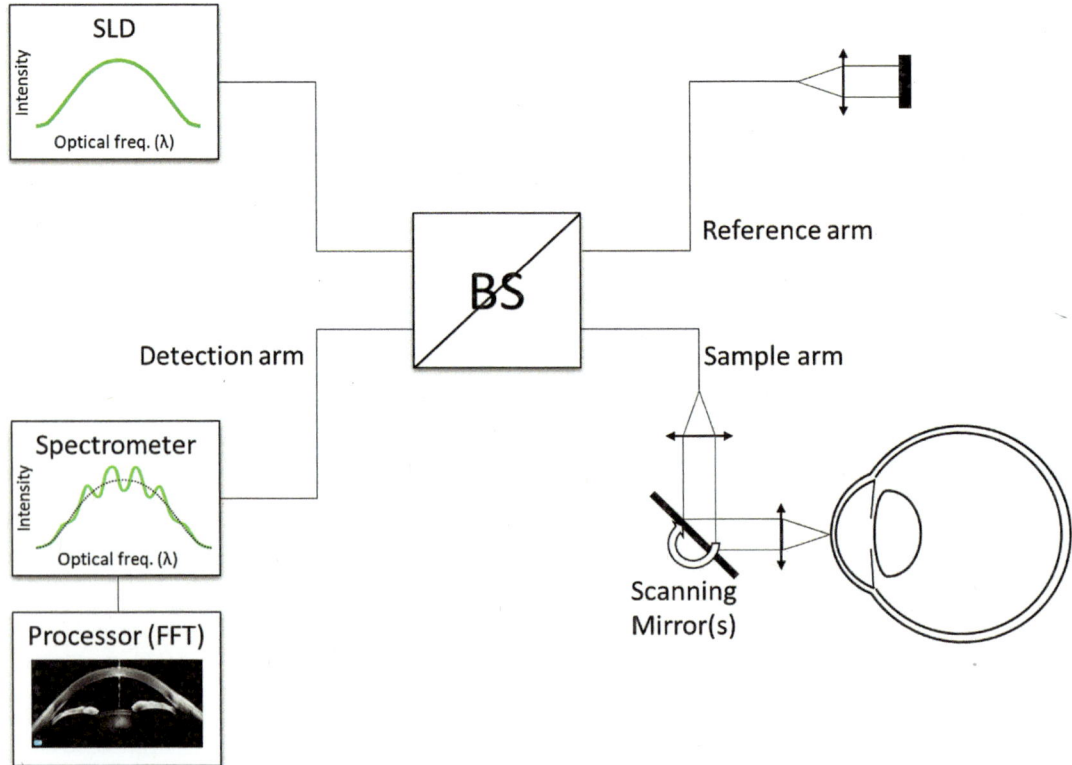

Fig. 29.2 Basic scheme of SD-OCT

beams coming from the reference and sample arms. The set of these values at various wavelengths is processed with a proprietary algorithm, basically containing a Fourier transformation, to obtain the reflectivity profile of the sample along the axis of the scanning beam. Therefore, in a single shot, the sensor of the spectrometer collects the spectrum necessary to determine the profile of reflectivity along one axis of the sample. The spectrometer inside the instrument collects an interval of wavelengths of about 80 nm thus ensuring an axial pixel size of 4.8 μm in air (about 3.5 μm in tissue) and an imaging depth of about 10 mm in air. The scanning system is based on two galvanometric mirrors, which deviate the beam according to the numerous preset trajectories, and allows a maximum transversal field of 16 mm and a transversal resolution of 35 μm.

SD-OCT technology was chosen for the MS-39 instead of the SS-OCT (Swept Source), even though the latter has already shown some undeniable advantages like a higher scan rate and a greater imaging depth because it allows for an axial resolution that is less than half that of the best SS-OCT systems (5 μm instead of 13 μm,

respectively). High-resolution Scheimpflug cameras can hardly provide an axial resolution at least double than the one of SS-OCT instruments. To the best of our knowledge, the axial pixel size of the MS-39 is currently the highest of all the OCT instruments available on the market, be they designed for the anterior segment or retina. It has to be emphasized that this feature is extremely important to resolve details in corneal layers, in particular for the epithelium. The imaging depth of the MS-39 is also the highest of all the ophthalmic SD-OCT instruments on the market.

Even though the axial resolution of the OCT system is high, it was necessary to integrate it with a Placido disc to get a reliable measurement of the height and curvature of the anterior corneal surface. To explain better this choice, let us consider the height profile of two spheres with curvatures of 42.50 D and 42.75 D (7.94 and 7.89 mm), i.e., differing by 0.25 D in curvature. The height difference between two meridional sections of the two spheres is about 0.06 μm at 0.4 mm from the center, 0.6 μm at 1 mm, 1.6 μm at 2 mm (Fig. 29.3). If these values are compared with the axial pixel size of the OCT system in air and if

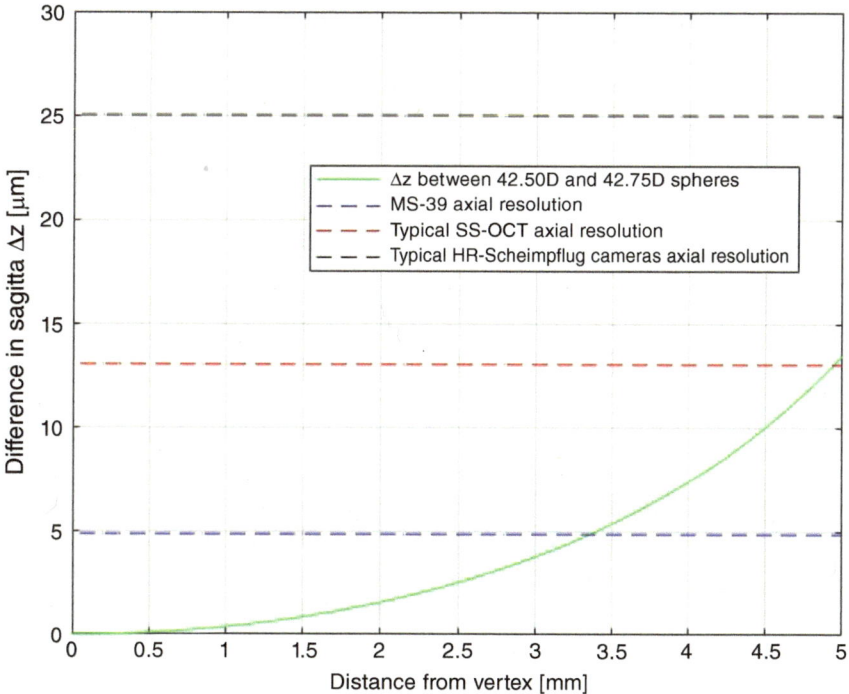

Fig. 29.3 Difference in the height profile of two spheres with curvatures of 42.50 D and 42.75 D (7.94 μm and 7.89 μm)

we consider that one of the primary purposes of the instrument is the accurate measurement of corneal surfaces, the need to add a Placido disc immediately becomes clear. In MS-39 software, for all cases where the keratoscopy is available and reliable (i.e., the anterior corneal surface is not very irregular or damaged), the measurement of the anterior surface obtained with Placido disc is preferred to the measurement done with the OCT system.

As regards the wavelength choice, MS-39 adopts a radiation source centered around 850 nm instead of the longer wavelength 1310 nm used in anterior segment OCT devices of other competitors. It was preferred to improve the image detail in corneal layers rather than the penetration into tissues, which would have had the advantage of imaging deeper structures such as the scleral spur or the posterior surface of the iris. At 850 nm the corneal epithelial layer is perfectly delineated, as it is the case for the transition from cornea to conjunctiva in the limbal region. Details of the normal structure of the stroma, including minimal changes of transparency approaching the limbal area, can be fully appreciated thanks to the 850 nm wavelength of the instrument, close to that of visible light. The iridocorneal angle and the iris stroma down to the posterior pigmented epithelium, as well as the crystalline lens within the pupillary aperture, can be visualized in fine detail. Unfortunately, no OCT can penetrate the eye beyond the iris pigmented epithelium, even those utilizing longer wavelengths, leaving the investigation of other ocular structure (e.g., ciliary body tumors) to other more invasive means, including ultrasounds, CT, and MRI.

Acquisition

MS-39 offers a wide range of different acquisition modalities, which allow the clinician to fully exploit the diagnostic potential of the instrument.

Section

This important modality recalls the use of the slit lamp, but with the fundamental difference that the captured images, based on OCT scanning technology, can be suitable for accurate measurements.

Two options are available for choosing the image quality:

- High definition: several images of the same section are captured in order to calculate an average image where the presence of the speckle is drastically reduced.
- Raw image: this option is faster than the previous one as there is no averaging of multiple pictures; it is useful when the patient is not very cooperative in order to reduce the acquisition time.

The sectional images can be acquired at various orientations (Fig. 29.4a) by selecting the angle through a rotating wheel on the top of the joystick or by clicking the desired direction on the enface corneal image shown on the screen.

The width of the transversal field of view can be chosen by the user between two options 10 and 16 mm, respectively, dedicated to the analysis of details in the layers of a limited corneal portion and to the overall view of the anterior segment.

In order to influence the pupil dilation, three illuminating conditions of the eye are available during the acquisition: scotopic, mesopic, and photopic.

In order to speed up the daily workflow of a clinical practice, some preset scanning patterns are made available:

- 2×: two sections at 90° degrees are acquired, one in the horizontal and one in the vertical direction (Fig. 29.4b).
- 4×: four sections are acquired at equispaced angular orientations, one at 0°, one at 45°, one at 90°, and one at 135°(Fig. 29.4c).

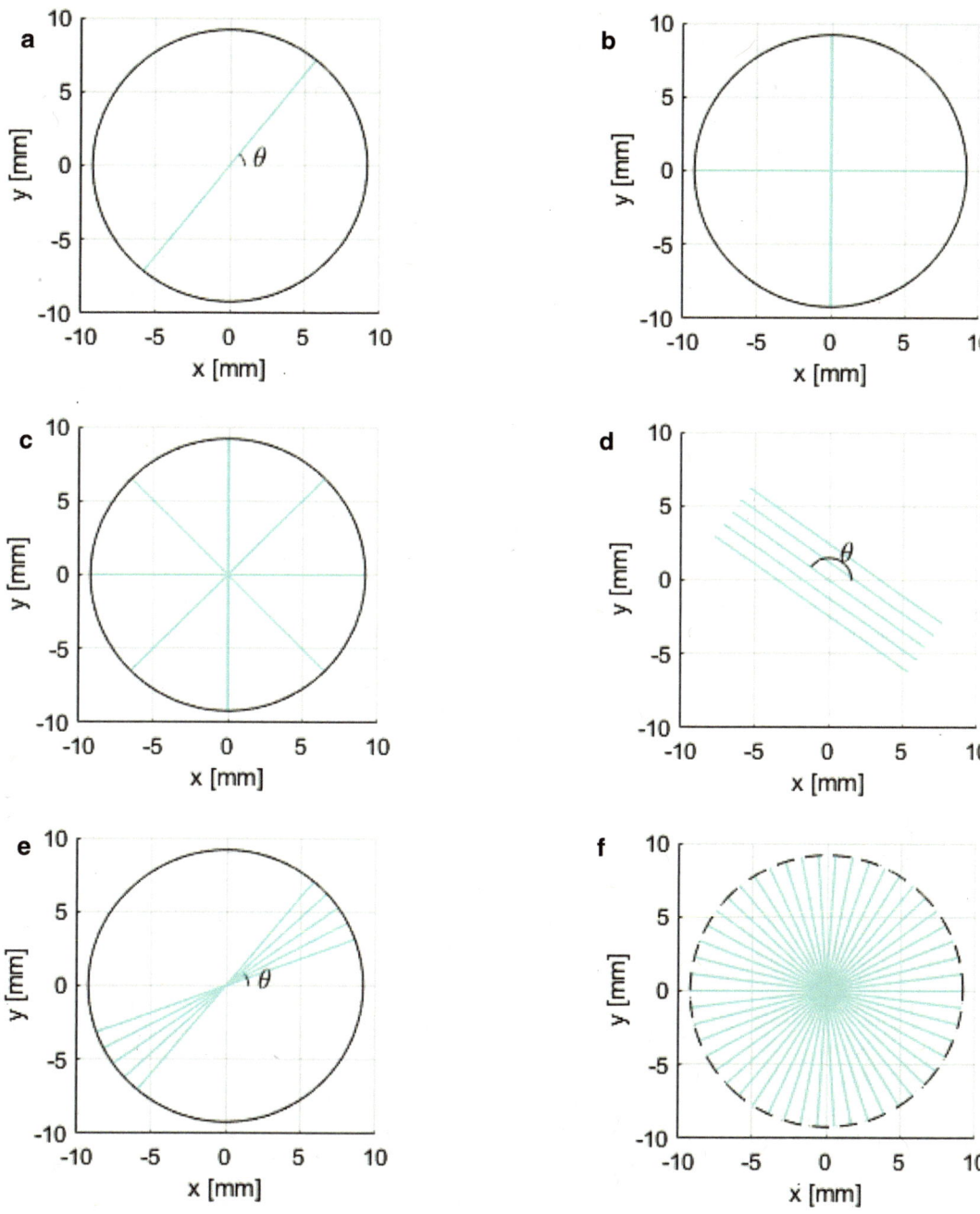

Fig. 29.4 *Scanning patterns*: (**a**) Line scanning, (**b**) horizontal and vertical lines (2×), (**c**) four meridians (4×), (**d**) raster scanning with 5 lines and interdistance equal to 1 mm, (**e**) sector scanning with 5 lines, (**f**) star scanning for topography (25 sections)

- Raster: an odd number of sections (from 3 to 7) are captured at an orientation and interline distance chosen by the user. The interline distance can be adjusted from 0.3 to 1 mm (Fig. 29.4d).
- Sector: an odd number of images (from 3 to 7) can be captured at equispaced angles within a sector, whose orientation and angular amplitude can be chosen by the user (Fig. 29.4e).

In cataract surgery, this exam may be important for detecting possible conditions which would be not clearly visible with other instruments like slit lamps or Scheimpflug tomographers, e.g., endothelial detachments, secondary cataracts, corneal oedemas, and capsular bag distension syndromes. Some interesting examples are reported in Figs. 29.5, 29.6 and 29.7.

Last but not least, a section video modality is made available for capturing nonstationary phenomena. It can be helpful, for instance, in analyzing the iris motion and the possible closure of the irido-corneal angle (dynamic gonioscopy), the ICL vaulting changes at standardized luminous

conditions or to document the presence of floating elements in the aqueous (e.g., fibrins after cataract surgery), as shown in Fig. 29.8.

Lens Biometry

This acquisition mode is for the analysis of the crystalline lens. In this case, two sections, one horizontal and the other vertical, are acquired over a width of 16 mm. This exam is used to check the lens transparency, detect possible cataracts, and for measuring the lens thickness and estimating the position of its equatorial plane. These measurements can be useful as input data for those IOL calculation formulas, which require the knowledge of the crystalline lens for the prediction of the IOL position.

Pupillography

MS-39 offers a specific examination for the measurement of pupil position and diameter in several light conditions: scotopic, mesopic, photopic, and dynamic (i.e., during the transition from a high-photopic to a scotopic condition). This exam, often underestimated or completely neglected in the clinical practice, is very important for the assessment of the optical quality of the anterior ocular segment particularly in com-

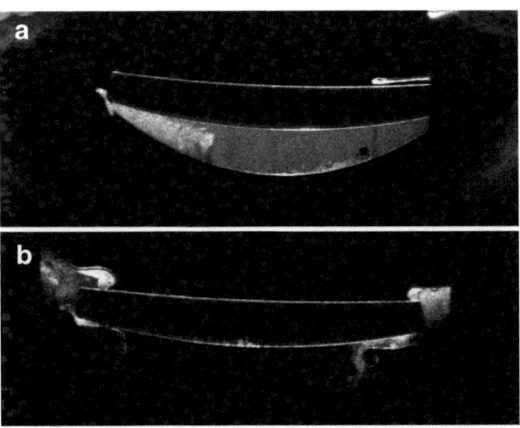

Fig. 29.5 (**a**) the AS-OCT shows the hyperscattering material between the IOL and the posterior capsule, which is distended towards the vitreous. This image helps the clinician to differentiate the capsular bag distension syndrome from a more common posterior capsule opacification. (**b**) After Nd:Yag laser capsulotomy, the milky liquid immediately disappeared. The patient's refraction changed from −0.75 D to plano and uncorrected visual acuity changed from 20/50 to 20/20

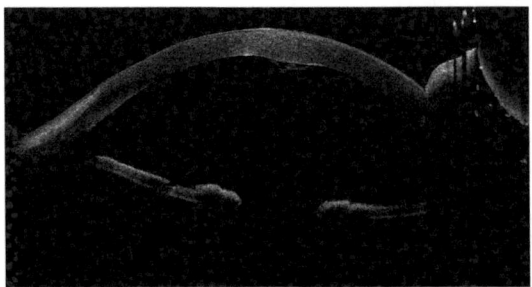

Fig. 29.6 A post-traumatic flap of the corneal endothelium is clearly imaged by the AS-OCT scan. Serial follow-up enabled the clinician to see the progressive recovery of the endothelium, which was fully adherent to the stroma after air injection into the anterior chamber

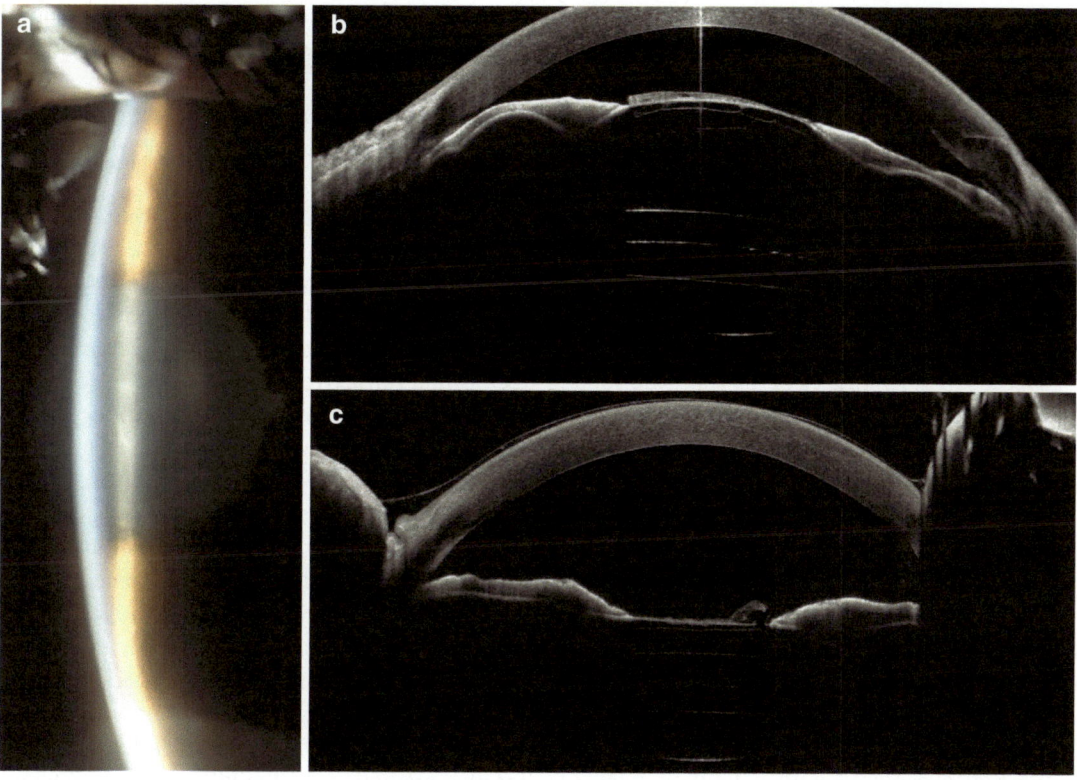

Fig. 29.7 (**a**, **b**) Pupillary block due to fibrin subsequent to TASS in a patient that received an add-on IOL in the sulcus. (**c**): Immediately after YAG laser application on the fibrin membrane, the block resolved and the anterior chamber depth returned physiological. The hole caused by the laser can be observed on the right of the scan

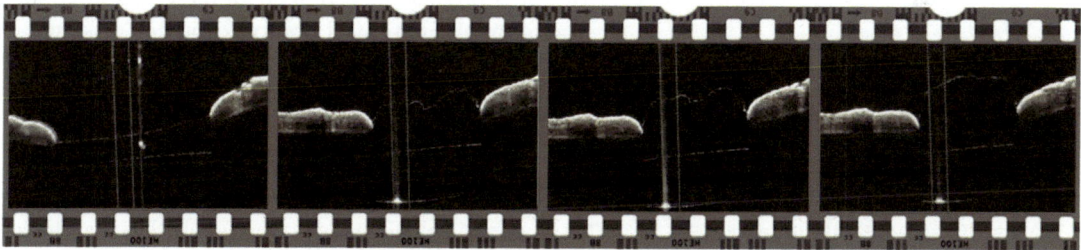

Fig. 29.8 A thin fibrin membrane occluding the whole pupillary area the first day following cataract surgery can be visualized, and its movements observed while protruding in the anterior chamber when pupillary constriction is elicited by light

bination with a corneal topography. Specific applications can be the pre-operative evaluation of a candidate for refractive surgery or the decision on whether to implant a multifocal or an aspheric IOL or the postoperative evaluation of the optical zone after refractive surgery.

Topography

The topography acquisition modality is for collecting the images necessary for the measurement of the anterior ocular segment, i.e., for the calculation of the classical curvature, power, and height maps of the corneal surfaces and of the anterior chamber depth.

Three options are available for the OCT star scanning pattern of meridional sections at equally spaced angular positions:

1. 25 B-scans, each made up of 1024 A-scans, of 16 mm sections captured in a time lapse of about 1 s (Fig. 29.4f).
2. 12 B-scans over a width of 16 mm, each made up of 1024 A-scans and resulting from the average of the 2 images of the same meridian, captured in a time lapse of about 1 s.
3. 12 B-scans over a width of 10 mm, each made up of 600 A-scans and resulting from the average of 5 images of the same meridian, captured in a time lapse of about 1.5 s.

The second and third options can be used to produce higher-quality images over the full transverse field or a reduced central portion of it.

During the OCT scan, two frontal images of the eye, one for keratoscopy and the other of the iris, are also captured with a field of view of about 14.1 × 10.6 mm.

As an evolution of the CSO Sirius topographer-tomographer, the MS-39 is able to measure all the classical maps of the anterior ocular segment (Fig. 29.6):

- Axial and tangential curvature maps of both anterior and posterior corneal surfaces
- Altimetric difference maps of both anterior and posterior corneal surfaces respect to a reference spherical, conicoidal, or toric surface
- Refractive power maps for both corneal surfaces alone and for the whole cornea
- Corneal thickness
- Anterior chamber depth
- Gaussian curvature maps for the anterior and posterior corneal surfaces
- Wave front error maps for the whole cornea and its components due to the anterior and posterior corneal surfaces

Accurate topographic maps may be useful in cataract surgery planning in order to discriminate between a normal case, where third- and fourth-generation IOL formulas are sufficiently reliable, and a complex case, where it is necessary to adopt an eye model more refined than simple keratometries and a ray tracing calculation for the choice of the best IOL. Topographic maps are also necessary for planning a refractive retreatment, when the optical quality of cornea should be improved before cataract surgery in order to have a satisfactory visual quality after the IOL implant. This is, for example, the case of eyes with a decentered optical zone due to an imperfect former refractive surgery or in some cases of corneal irregularity due, for instance, to corneal grafts.

In MS-39 software topographic maps are accompanied by a great number of synthetic indices. Some of them refer to corneal morphology (keratometries and shape indices), some other to corneal optical quality (refractive indices), and some other to generic features of the anterior segment. Among them, the software offers the measurement of the horizontal tilt component of the iris plane. This can be useful in cataract surgery for the prediction of the tilt of the implanted IOL. Tilt of intraocular lenses has a negative effect on optical performance, especially for aspheric, toric, and multifocal IOLs and lead to less predictable astigmatism outcomes after surgery. An improved ability to predict postoperative tilt would help determine the best IOL for a patient and potentially improve long-term outcomes.

By exploiting its superior imaging capability in resolving corneal layers, the MS-39 is also able to calculate the epithelial and stromal thickness maps over a diameter of 8 mm (Fig. 29.9). It is by now widely acknowledged that epithelial thickness maps can be used as an adjunctive tool to improve the sensitivity and specificity of keratoconus screening [5–10].

During preoperative assessment for refractive surgery, epithelial thickness mapping can be very valuable at least in two situations. First, it can correctly detect or confirm a keratoconus diagnosis for those patients where their anterior surface topography may be clinically judged within normal limits and their posterior surface topography is outside normal limits. Epithelial information

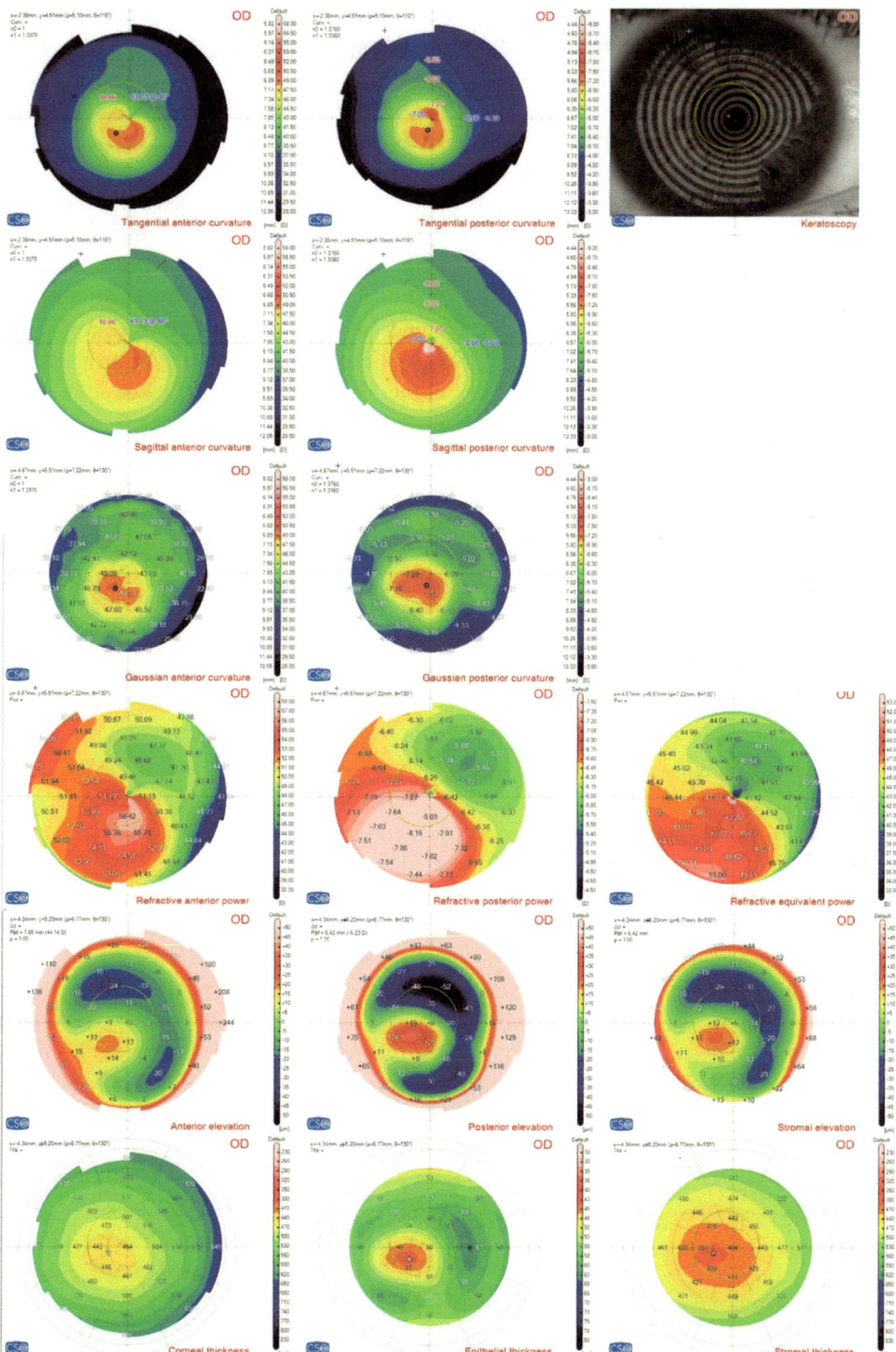

Fig. 29.9 Maps of a keratoconic eye. From top left corner: tangential anterior curvature, tangential posterior curvature, keratoscopy, sagittal anterior curvature, sagittal posterior curvature, Gaussian anterior curvature, Gaussian posterior curvature, refractive anterior power, refractive posterior power, refractive equivalent power, anterior elevation, posterior elevation, stromal elevation, corneal thickness, epithelial thickness, and stromal thickness

allows a more solid earlier diagnosis of keratoconus, as epithelial changes precede changes on the anterior corneal surface. An epithelial doughnut pattern, characterized by epithelial thinning surrounded by an annulus of thicker epithelium [7, 8], coincident with the bulging zone of the posterior elevation and the steepening of the posterior corneal surface, is consistent with keratoconus and it reinforces its diagnosis. Second, epithelial thickness profiles may be helpful in excluding a misdiagnosis of keratoconus when the topography of anterior corneal surface is suspect. An epithelial thickening over an area of topographic steepening implies that the steepening is due to the epithelium and not to an underlying ectatic surface. Asymmetrical topographic patterns and focal anterior steepening can sometimes be secondary to corneal warpage: analysis of the epithelial layer with high-resolution AS-OCT allows for direct detection of the abnormality rather than just supposing it.

In addition to keratoconus screening, corneal epithelial mapping provides a practical tool in a variety of other clinical applications. It allows for the measurement of corneal epithelial thickness changes following laser ablative myopic surgeries, such as LASIK [11–17], PRK [18–21], and small incision lenticule extraction (SMILE) [22]. Studies have suggested that epithelial thickening is associated with myopic regression after LASIK as well as PRK, although the wound healing process would be quite different in the two procedures [12, 18, 20]. It also allows for the quantitative analysis of the effects of an orthokeratology treatment [23–27] or the anatomical evaluation of corneal changes induced by intracorneal ring segments implantation [28].

IOL Module

CSO's method for IOL calculation is an attempt to apply the most advanced engineering method used for optical system design and analysis to IOL calculation. The method is intended to keep a good accuracy not only with normal eyes but also with eyes, which underwent refractive surgery or with a heavy amount of astigmatism or

with even more irregular corneas (keratoconic eyes or post-graft eyes after DMEK or DSAEK). The measured data of the anterior segment, i.e., the altimetric data of the anterior and posterior corneal surfaces and of the iris are used in combination with the altimetric data of the intraocular lens to build a three-dimensional model of the eye. In this way, the corneal surfaces are considered with their possible asymmetry, inclination, mutual decentration, and irregularities. The intraocular lens is modeled using the nominal parameters provided by its manufacturer. Possible aspherical profiles can be taken into account as well as possible torical shapes.

Ray tracing is used in order to simulate the path of light inside the eye. The calculation is done by the software for each available power of the selected IOL model. For the lens, which best satisfy the requirement of target equivalent sphere chosen by the surgeon, the following results are shown:

- refraction (sphere, cylinder, axis, and spherical equivalent)
- wave front aberrations
- refractive map
- point spread function (PSF)
- defocus chart

These results can also be consulted by the user for those lenses whose powers are included in an interval centred around the power of the best lens. If the IOL model is toric, the software makes the results available for each of the available IOL cylinders. Further details about CSO's method for IOL calculation will be given in a dedicated chapter of this book.

Toric IOL Marker

CSO's software also offers the clinician a useful tool (Camellin's marker) for marking the axis of a toric IOL and some reference points on a frontal image of the eye, which can be printed and used as a reference for the IOL alignment during surgery (Fig. 29.10). The basic idea is to use a frontal colour image of the eye captured by the

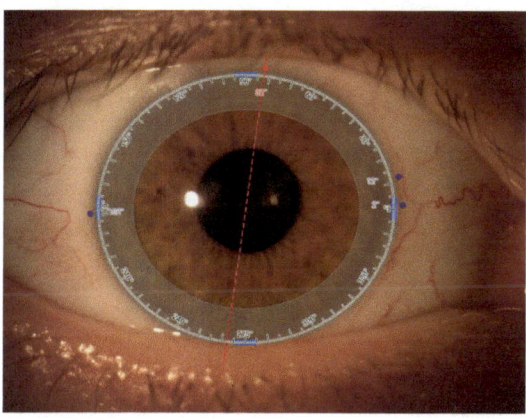

Fig. 29.10 Toric marker: the axis of the IOL is represented by the dotted red line; the violet circles are the reference points

slit lamp. For a correct use of the toric marker, it is necessary to use the 10x magnification lens in CSO slit lamp microscope. This is the only magnification, which allows the user to see the entire eye. The user has to translate and deform a goniometer so that it matches the limbus of the eye (Fig. 29.7). The goniometer will be used as a reference for the angular position of the IOL axis.

After that, the user has to place 3 small violet discs near some reference vessels on the sclera and rotate the axis of the IOL at the desired angle. Of course, it is also necessary to choose an image of the eye where the vessels are well visible on the sclera.

The toric marker is accessible from both the slit lamp environment and the IOL module. In the IOL module, the user can also associate an axial map to the picture of the toric marker.

References

1. Mejía-Barbosa Y, Malacara-Hernández D. A review of methods for measuring corneal topography. Optom Vis Sci. 2001;78(4):240–53.
2. Huang D, et al. Optical coherence tomography. Science. 1991;254(5035):1178–81.
3. Wojtkowski M, Leitgeb R, Kowalczyk A, Bajraszewski T, Fercher AF. In vivo human retinal imaging by Fourier domain optical coherence tomography. J Biomed Opt. 2002;7:457–63.
4. Vakhtin AB, Kane DJ, Wood WR, Peterson KA. Common-path interferometer for frequency-domain optical coherence tomography. Appl Opt. 2003;42:6953–8.
5. Scroggs MW, Proia AD. Histopathological variation in keratoconus. Cornea. 1992;11:553–9.
6. Aktekin M, Sargon MF, Cakar P, Celik HH, Firat E. Ultrastructure of the cornea epithelium in keratoconus. Okajimas Folia Anat Jpn. 1998;75:45–53.
7. Reinstein DZ, Archer TJ, Gobbe M. Corneal epithelial thickness profile in the diagnosis of keratoconus. J Refract Surg. 2009;25:604–10.
8. Reinstein DZ, Gobbe M, Archer TJ, Silverman RH, Coleman DJ. Epithelial, stromal, and total corneal thickness in keratoconus: three-dimensional display with Artemis very high-frequency digital ultrasound. J Refract Surg. 2010;26:259–71.
9. Temstet C, Sandali O, Bouheraoua N, Hamiche T, Galan A, El Sanharawi M, Basli E, Laroche L, Borderie V. Corneal epithelial thickness mapping using Fourier-domain optical coherence tomography for detection of form fruste keratoconus. J Cataract Refract Surg. 2015;41(4):812–20.
10. Li Y, et al. Corneal epithelial thickness mapping by Fourier-domain optical coherence tomography in normal and Keratoconic eyes. Ophthalmology. 2012;119(12):2425–33.
11. Kanellopoulos AJ, Asimellis G. Longitudinal postoperative Lasik epithelial thickness profile changes in correlation with degree of myopia correction. JRefract Surg. 2014;30:166–71.
12. Lohmann CP, Güell JL. Regression after LASIK for the treatment of myopia: the role of the corneal epithelium. Semin Ophthalmol. 1998;13:79–82.
13. Reinstein DZ, Silverman RH, Sutton HF, Coleman DJ. Very high-frequency ultrasound corneal analysis identifies anatomic correlates of optical complications of lamellar refractive surgery: anatomic diagnosis in lamellar surgery. Ophthalmology. 1999;106:474–82.
14. Spadea L, Fasciani R, Necozione S, Balestrazzi E. Role of the corneal epithelium in refractive changes following laser in situ keratomileusis for high myopia. J Refract Surg. 2000;16:133–9.
15. Erie JC, Patel SV, McLaren JW, Ramirez M, Hodge DO, Maguire LJ, Bourne WM. Effect of myopic laser in situ keratomileusis on epithelial and stromal thickness: a confocal microscopy study. Ophthalmology. 2002;109:1447–52.
16. Patel SV, Erie JC, McLaren JW, Bourne WM. Confocal microscopy changes in epithelial and stromal thickness up to 7 years after LASIK and photorefractive keratectomy for myopia. J Refract Surg. 2007;23:385–92.
17. Reinstein DZ, Srivannaboon S, Gobbe M, Archer TJ, Silverman RH, Sutton H, Coleman DJ. Epithelial thickness profile changes induced by myopic LASIK as measured by Artemis very high-frequency digital ultrasound. J Refract Surg. 2009;25:444–50.
18. Lohmann CP, Patmore A, Reischl U, Marshall J. The importance of the corneal epithelium in excimer-laser photorefractive keratectomy. Ger J Ophthalmol. 1996;5:368–72.

19. Gauthier CA, Holden BA, Epstein D, Tengroth B, Fagerholm P, Hamberg-Nyström H. Role of epithelial hyperplasia in regression following photorefractive keratectomy. Br J Ophthalmol. 1996;80:545–8.

20. Lohmann CP, Reischl U, Marshall J. Regression and epithelial hyperplasia after myopic photorefractive keratectomy in a human cornea. J Cataract Refract Surg. 1999;25:712–5.

21. Chen X, Stojanovic A, Liu Y, Chen Y, Zhou Y, Utheim TP. Postoperative changes in corneal epithelial and stromal thickness profiles after photorefractive keratectomy in treatment of myopia. J Refract Surg. 2015;31:446–53.

22. Luft N, Ring MH, Dirisamer M, Mursch-Edlmayr AS, Kreutzer TC, Pretzl J, et al. Corneal epithelial remodeling induced by small incision Lenticule extraction (SMILE). Invest Ophthalmol Vis Sci. 2016;57:176–83.

23. Reinstein DZ, Gobbe M, Archer TJ, Couch D, Bloom B. Epithelial, stromal and corneal pachymetry changes during orthokeratology. Optom Vis Sci. 2009;86:E1006–14.

24. Swarbrick HA, Wong G, O'Leary DJ. Corneal response to orthokeratology. Optom Vis Sci. 1998;75:791–9.

25. Lu F, Simpson T, Sorbara L, Fonn D. Malleability of the ocular surface in response to mechanical stress induced by orthokeratology contact lenses. Cornea. 2008;27:133–41.

26. Sridharan R, Swarbrick H. Corneal response to short-term orthokeratology lens wear. Optom Vis Sci. 2003;80:200–6.

27. Haque S, Fonn D, Simpson T, Jones L. Epithelial thickness changes from the induction of myopia with CRTH RGP contact lenses. Invest Ophthalmol Vis Sci. 2008;49:3345–50.

28. Reinstein DZ, Srivannaboon S, Holland SP. Epithelial and stromal changes induced by intacs examined by three-dimensional very high-frequency digital ultrasound. J Refract Surg. 2001;17:310–8.

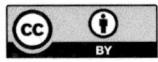

IOL Power Calculations with ORA Intraoperative Aberrometer

Tom Padrick

Intraoperative aberrometry allows measurements of an eye's refractive power when the eye is "aphakic". The results of these measurements are used to assess total corneal astigmatism (with contributions from both the anterior and posterior corneal surfaces) and the aphakic spherical equivalent which is used for calculation of the IOL power. The ORA system consists of an optical head that contains the aberrometer (discussed below). The optical head is mounted to the surgical microscope and is designed to be used during cataract surgery. Wavefront data is obtained, analyzed, and presented to the user via a cart mounted LCD touch screen (see Fig. 30.1) and in the surgeon's ocular of the microscope within a period of time that does not impede the surgical procedures.

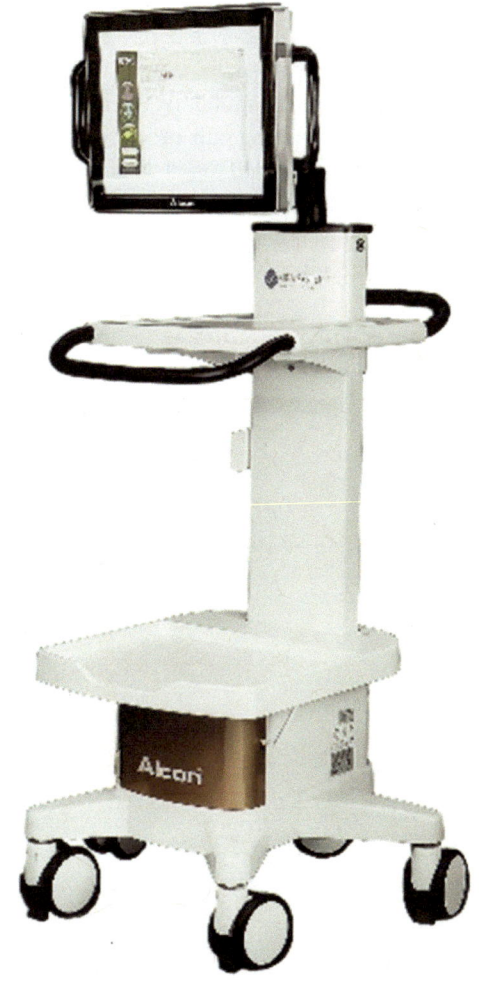

Fig. 30.1 ORA operating room cart

T. Padrick (✉)
Alcon Vision, LLC, Fort Worth, TX, USA

© The Author(s) 2024

J. Aramberri et al. (eds.), *Intraocular Lens Calculations*, Essentials in Ophthalmology,
https://doi.org/10.1007/978-3-031-50666-6_30

Talbot-Moiré Aberrometer

The development of the ORA intraoperative aberrometer began in 2005 at WaveTec Vision. The first commercial system was installed in the summer of 2008. Many hardware and software iterations have occurred over the years to improve performance, but the basic principal of the Talbot-Moiré aberrometer has remained the same. The schematic diagram shows the layout of the Talbot-Moiré aberrometer used in the ORA system (Fig. 30.2). A thin laser beam or superluminescent light emitting diode (SLED) beam is directed into the eye and reflects off the back of the eye. The light reflected from the back of the eye fills the pupil diameter and passes through the cornea. The pupil image is relayed onto a pair of Ronchi gratings separated by 1 Talbot distance. The Ronchi grating pair produces a fringe pattern which is recorded on a CCD array. A Fourier transform [1] of the fringe pattern is preformed and then translated using proprietary software into the refractive state of the eye being measured.

A more detailed description of the Ronchi gratings is shown in Fig. 30.3. The crossed Ronchi gratings are as shown, i.e., a crossed pattern of lines which create a pattern of openings. Light passing through the openings is diffracted. The refracted light emerging from each opening in the grating interferes with the light from neighboring openings causing further diffraction. For large grating periods (space between lines), the image reproduced at the Talbot distance can be captured by a CCD camera and easily analyzed. To increase the resolution, finer grating periods can be used, and a second grating is placed at a Talbot distance. At a Talbot distance, a high contrast pattern of the image produced at the exit of the first grating is imaged onto the front surface of the second grating. As light passes through the second grating, additional diffraction occurs. Rotating the second grating with respect to the first grating creates a Moiré effect which further increase resolution. Thus, the name of the aberrometer is Talbot-Moiré.

Once the fringe pattern is captured, it is converted from spatial domain to frequency domain using a fast Fourier transform function [1]. Because the fringe patterns have similar frequencies, peaks are generated in the Fourier transform of the image. Two of the primary peaks are used in the "Peaks Method" of analysis. The relative position of two peaks versus the position for a

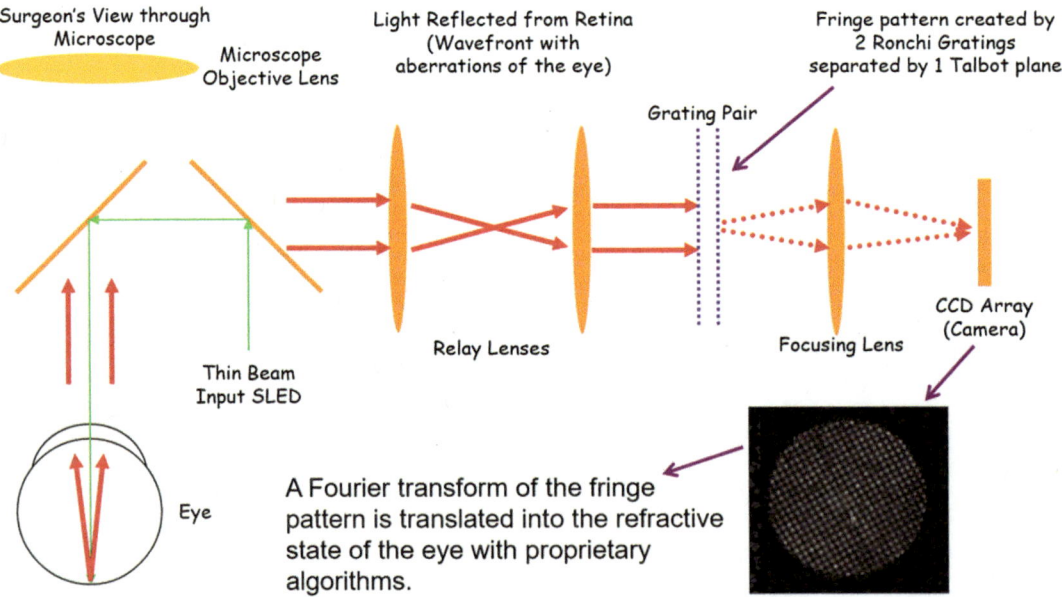

Fig. 30.2 Schematic diagram of ORA intraoperative aberrometer

Fig. 30.3 Ronchi gratings and the Talbot distance

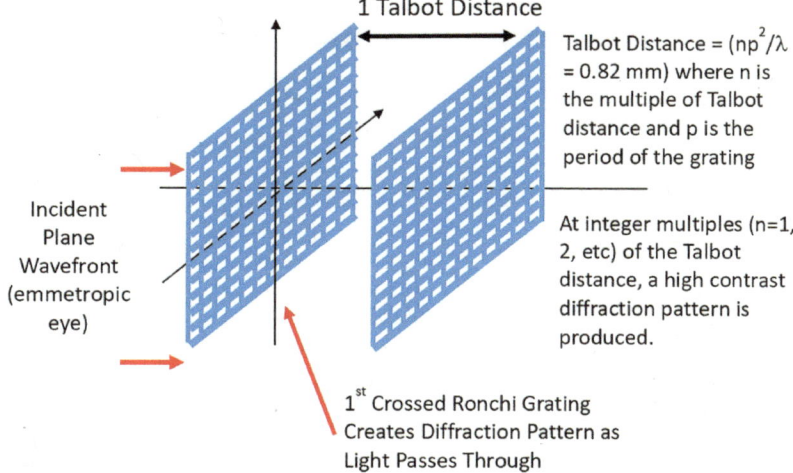

1 Talbot Distance

Talbot Distance = $(np^2/\lambda$ = 0.82 mm) where n is the multiple of Talbot distance and p is the period of the grating

At integer multiples (n=1, 2, etc) of the Talbot distance, a high contrast diffraction pattern is produced.

Incident Plane Wavefront (emmetropic eye)

1st Crossed Ronchi Grating Creates Diffraction Pattern as Light Passes Through

Fig. 30.4 Fast Fourier transform and the peaks method to determine sphere, cylinder, and axis

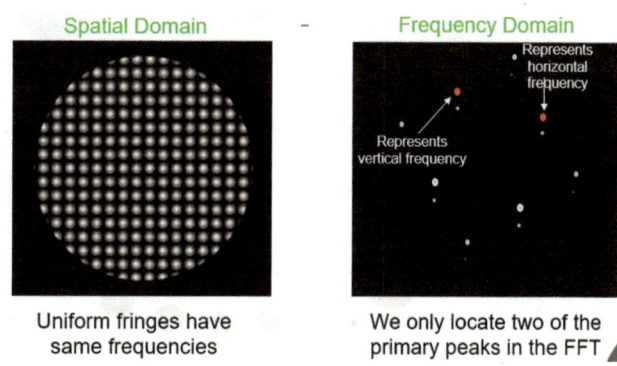

Spatial Domain   –   Frequency Domain

Represents horizontal frequency

Represents vertical frequency

Uniform fringes have same frequencies

We only locate two of the primary peaks in the FFT

known power yields the sphere, cylinder, and axis for the measurement. Subpixel image analysis locates small movements in the peaks. This method is shown in Fig. 30.4.

Increasing myopia rotates the peaks counter clockwise, and increasing hyperopia rotates the peaks clockwise. Difference in the amount of rotation of the two primary peaks determines the cylinder of the measurement.

All ORA carts in the field are connected to a secure server maintained by Alcon. After each surgery, the preoperative and surgical data (aphakic SE, IOL model, and power implanted, predicted postop SE, etc.) are uploaded to the server. The data is saved in the AnalyzOR database, which is used by R&D for optimization of lens constants (described below) and for development of improved IOL power calculations and optimization methods. The AnalyzOR database can also

be used by surgeons to look at their specific outcomes, generate reports, and compare their results to those of the larger database.

IOL Power Calculation

After the sphere, cylinder and axis of the aphakic measurement have been calculated, and the system can use that information to calculate the IOL power. Many of the current IOL power formulas calculate IOL power using the vergence formula. This is a simple optics formula that can determine the power of a lens to achieve the desired post op refractive outcome if one knows the curvature of the cornea, the length of the eye and relative position of the IOL with respect to the corneal surface and back of the eye. This position is referred to as the effective lens position or ELP.

Fig. 30.5 Refractive
vergence formula

Refractive Vergence Formula

$$\text{IOL Power} = \cfrac{1336}{\cfrac{1336}{\cfrac{1336}{1000}} - \text{ELP}} - \cfrac{1336}{\cfrac{1336}{\cfrac{1336}{1000}} - \text{ELP}}$$

ORA Aphakic SE   DPostOp Rx

The primary difference in IOL power formulas is how the ELP is estimated [exceptions are the Olsen C and the Hill RBF which do not have an ELP term (other formulas may also fall in this category)].

The ORA approach is to use the refractive vergence formula (Fig. 30.5) introduced by Jack Holladay, MD for calculation of the power in a piggyback lens implanted to address unplanned ametropia after cataract surgery [2]. This formula does not use axial length but a refraction value. Rather than the patient's pre piggyback surgery manifest refraction the ORA formula uses the aphakic SE as shown below.

The ORA formula still requires an average corneal curvature K and the ELP. For the "average" eye, the ELP is equal to the lens constant. As an eye deviates from the "average," the various IOL power formulas calculate a term which adds or subtracts from the lens constant to determine the ELP for the patient.

$$\text{ELP} = \text{Lens Constant} + \text{Patient} - \text{Specific Factor}$$

For many of the formulas that depend on ELP, the patient-specific factor is estimated from their formula specific combination of the axial length and the corneal K value. Since the ORA measured aphakic SE is only a function of average K and axial length (a theoretical aphakic SE is 1336/axial length—average K), the ORA formula obtains its estimate of ELP from the measured aphakic SE. ORA uses a quadratic equation derived from plotting the theoretical aphakic SE versus calculated ELPs from various IOL power formulas. (ORA uses a different formula for post myopic LASIK >26 mm axial length). This equation has subsequently been updated using actual ORA aphakic SE measurements and back calcu-

lated ELP for the outcome achieved. Using the ORA equation for ELP, it has been determined that an aphakic SE = 12.5D would yield a zero patient specific factor. Whereas an aphakic SE of 5D (long eye) would yield a patient specific factor of +0.99. Likewise for a short eye an aphakic SE of 18D would yield a patient specific factor of −0.62. The basic refractive vergence formula with the measured aphakic SE, the derived ELP and average K value yields respectable results, but these results can be improved by regression analysis. When we have a sufficient number of cases with preoperative, intraoperative and post op data have been entered into AnalyzOR for a particular IOL lens model, and the lens constant is iterated to yield a zero mean prediction error (prediction error = measured post-operative SE—formula predicted post-operative SE for IOL power implanted). For an IOL model with sufficient number of cases, we know the prediction error after the lens constant has been optimized. This prediction error is regressed against the axial length, average K, White to White (WTW), and a term we refer to as Delta SE (theoretical aphakic SE minus measured aphakic SE). This regression analysis produces a set of coefficients for each of the four terms. For a new patient, their respective preoperative terms and measured aphakic SE (provides ELP and Delta SE term) are multiplied by these coefficients to produce a "correction factor," which is added to the predicted post op SE from the basic refractive vergence formula for a given IOL power.

Prior to lens models having sufficient data for optimization (>100 cases), these nonoptimized models are grouped together. The lens constants for each IOL are still the manufacturer's suggested value, but this group is regressed as above

Fig. 30.6 Changes in outcomes as regression steps are added to the process

Alcon SN60WF		
808 Eyes - 36 Surgeons		**72 Eyes**
Basic Refractive Vergence Formula w/Optimized Lens Constant	**With Regression Coefficents Applied**	**Single Surgeon With Surgeon Optimized Lens Constant**
MAE = 0.469 D	0.360 D	0.259 D
Std Dev = 0.378 D	0.300 D	0.188 D
%<0.5 D = 66.63%	79.03%	91.67%
%<1.0 D = 91.81%	96.28%	100.00%
Median = 0.377 D	0.290 D	0.237 D

Axial Length Range = 21.01mm to 28.72mm
K Range = 38.16 D to 49.16 D
IOL Power Range = 10.0 D to 29.5 D

generating regression coefficients for this group of lens models, this improves outcomes until sufficient number of cases are available to generate the ORA optimized lens constants and regression coefficients for an individual IOL model.

The optimization process was started with basic linear regression, but a different approach is now being used. RANdom SAmple Consensus (RANSAC) [3] is a computational algorithm that estimates one or more parameters of a mathematical model from a set of observed data. This program randomly selects a set of data (predetermined number of cases) from the database, performs a linear regression on that set, and then applies the generated regression coefficients to the entire dataset. It does this (up to a total of 60,000 times) until the preset variable is maximized or minimized. For ORA, the target variable is % ≤0.50D, so a maximum for this parameter is being sought. The coefficients that yield this maximum are then used for future patients with this IOL model.

It was observed early on that our results for long eyes and short eyes were not optimal compared to results for average eyes. Therefore, it was decided to employ a cluster approach for the regression analysis. The dataset is divided into axial length clusters, a minimum of 2 clusters with 50 cases each and a maximum of 20 clusters (cluster size can vary form 50 cases to several thousand cases). A RANSAC regression is performed on each cluster. When a new patient is

entered, their axial length determines that regression coefficients are applied. If a new axial length is near a boundary between clusters, we utilize a blend function to determine the appropriate regression coefficients. This combination of RANSAC regressing axial length clusters of data has greatly improved ORA outcomes for long and short eyes.

Once a particular lens model has been optimized (both lens constant and regression coefficients), results can be further improved for a single surgeon by optimizing the lens constant to minimize the mean prediction error for the surgeon's data. The surgeon's data is isolated (>30 cases with a particular lens model), and then the lens constant is personaslized to reduce the mean prediction error to zero. This surgeon specific lens constant is then applied with the global regression coefficients only to that surgeon's new cases using that lens model. Below is an example of the effect of each of these steps (Fig. 30.6).

Using ORA

To use ORA, a patient file is created by securely (proper password) logging into the practice on AnalyzOR from any computer. After the patient's personal information is entered, the surgery information is entered. This includes the surgery date, the surgeon, the facility, whether they have had refractive surgery, keratometry measurements, axial length, white to white, and target refraction. On the day of surgery, all cases scheduled that day at a particular surgery facility (a practice can have multiple surgery locations) are downloaded from AnalyzOR to the cart in the operating room (Fig. 30.7).

Clicking on the patient's name from the list of patients opens the patient's data file as shown in the screen shot above right. After clicking "Begin Surgery" the screen below is shown (Fig. 30.8).

Most frequently the "Power Calculation" button under Aphakic is clicked to begin data acquisition. Looking at the monitor on the cart (Fig. 30.9), the surgeon sees the patient's eye which allows the surgeon to verify that the lid speculum is not near the cornea causing pressure that would impact the cylinder measurement. The fringe pattern generated by the aberrometer is to the right of the screen, and the alignment box is on the lower right. Viewing the fringe pattern

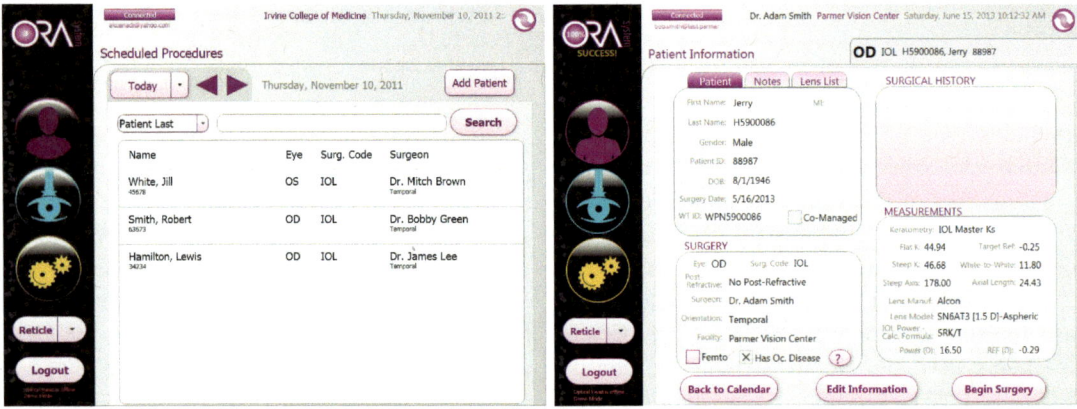

Fig. 30.7 List of patients scheduled for surgery on a given day and a selected patient's data

Fig. 30.8 Measurement type selection screen

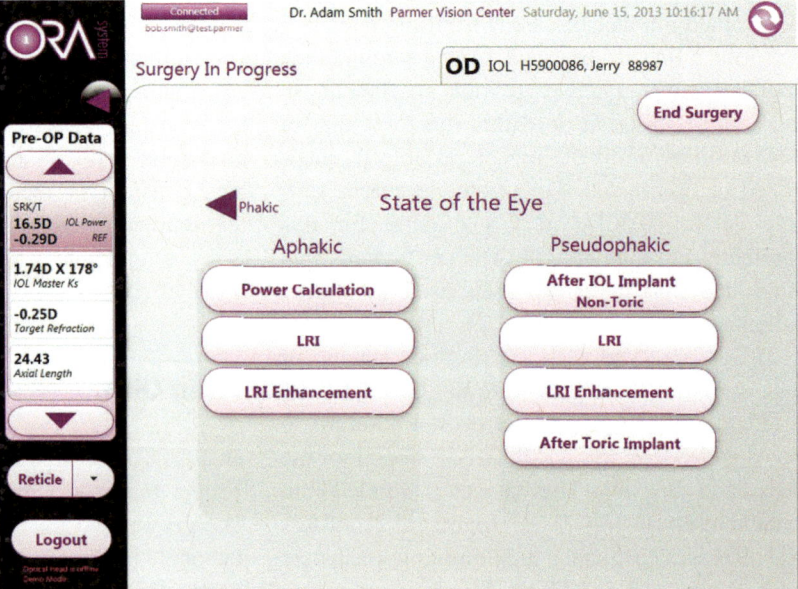

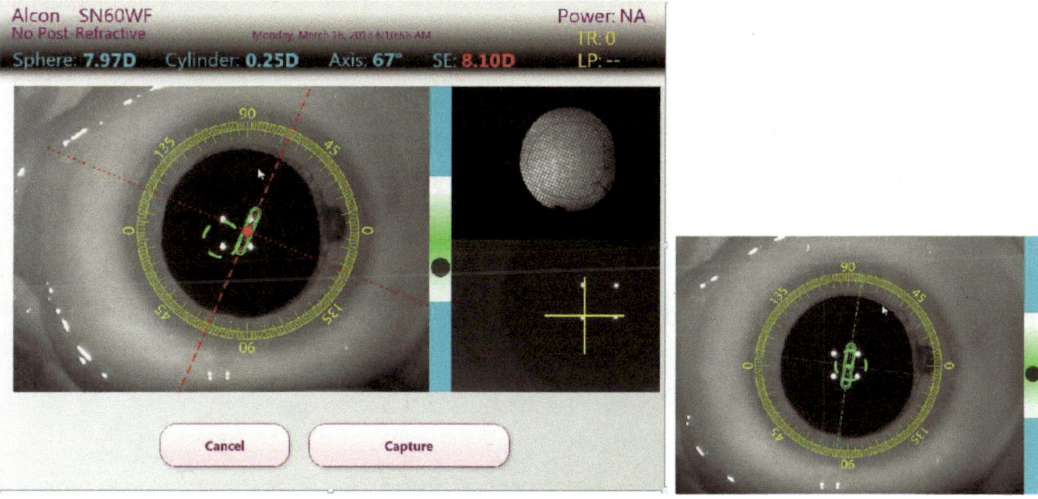

Fig. 30.9 The screen seen by the surgeon for alignment and capture of the aphakic refraction

allows the surgeon to know if there are air bubbles or crystalline lens residue (dark areas in fringe pattern) or if excessive incision hydration (dark shadow in fringe pattern) are causing an error in the measurement. Across the top of the screen is the real time refraction. In the screen on the left, we see a red dot in the center indicating that the system is not aligned. While the patient fixates, the surgeon moves the patient's head either laterally or by tilting to achieve the proper alignment as shown in the right image with a green dot inside the green circle. Focus is indicated by the vertical bar with the black dot. When the eye is in correct focus, the black dot will be within the green range shown. The image on the right is properly aligned and focused. When this occurs the system automatically captures 40 frames in a few seconds.

After capturing the 40 frames of the fringe pattern and analyzing, the screen in Fig. 30.10 appears. On the right hand side of the screen, the aphakic sphere, cylinder, and axis (+SE) are shown. In the center of the screen are selected lens models and predicted post op SE for a given IOL power. Clicking on the second lens choice

would result in new predicted post op SE for various IOL powers. The IOL power in bold font shows is the power with the predicted post op SE closest to the target refraction entered when the patient file was created. Using the scroll function to the right of the IOL power column changes, the IOL power choices for the full range of IOL powers associated with that particular lens model.

If a toric IOL is used, once the IOL power is selected (desired post op SE), and the screen in Fig. 30.11 is displayed. This screen shows the predicted residual cylinder for various cylinder power IOLs. The amount of cylinder correction at the corneal plane is dependent upon the spherical power of the IOL and the ELP (a toric IOL closer to the cornea will correct more than the manufacturers specified amount and likewise an IOL further from the cornea will correct less cylinder). The ORA system takes these factors into account. When you select the spherical power, we have calculated our expected ELP for the patient. The anticipated cylinder for the toric IOL models is calculated for the specific patient undergoing surgery based on their measured

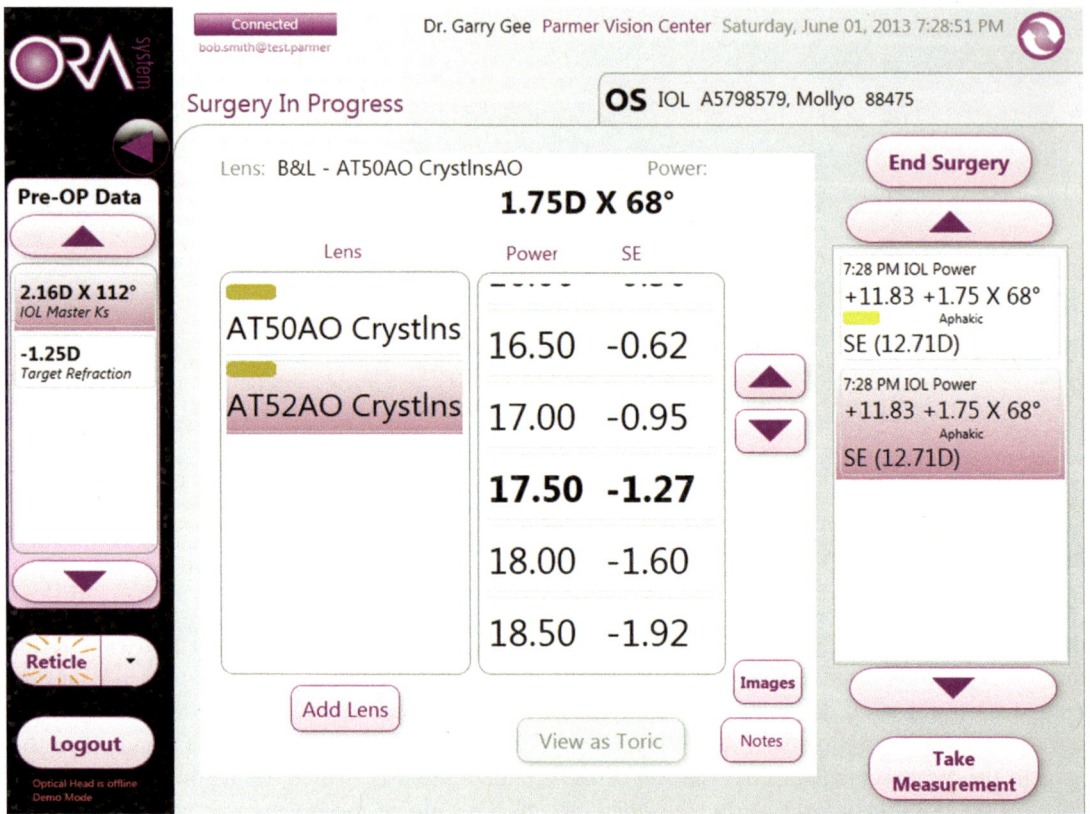

Fig. 30.10 Display of aphakic refraction and predicted post op SE for various IOL powers

aphakic cylinder, the spherical power of the IOL chosen by the surgeon, and the ORA calculated ELP for that patient.

Once the toric IOL is implanted, it must be aligned to the measured cylinder axis in order to achieve the minimum residual cylinder. Following a pseudophakic measurement, if the measured cylinder is not less than 0.5D, ORA directs the surgeon to rotate the IOL clockwise or counterclockwise in small increments until the measured cylinder is less than 0.50D. The recommendation

for rotation is based on the axis of the residual cylinder. Because of the effect of crossed cylinders, the direction of rotation is opposite of what is expected. For example, if the true axis of astigmatism is at 85 degrees and the measured pseudophakic cylinder axis is at 90, the correct recommended direction of rotation is clockwise. When the measured pseudophakic cylinder is <0.5D, the screen shows NRR (no rotation recommended).

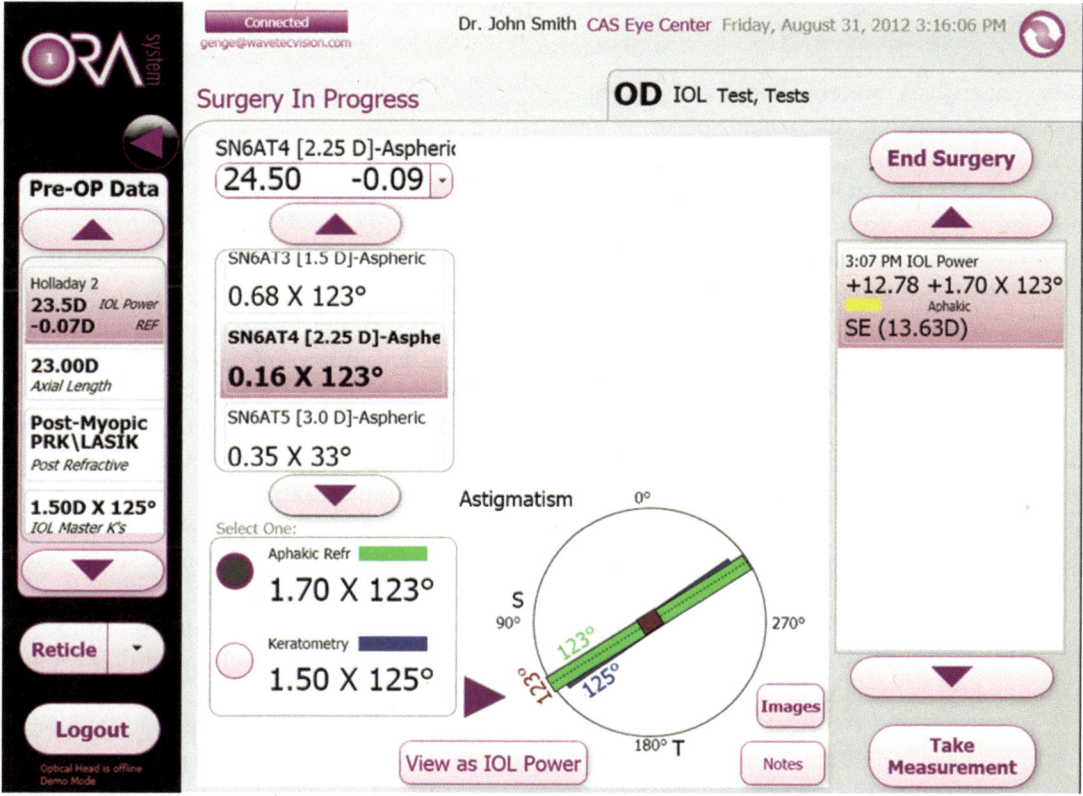

Fig. 30.11 Selecting toric cylinder power to achieve minimum residual astigmatism

Results

Many papers have been published and presentations made detailing the results of using the ORA intraoperative wavefront aberrometry (IWA) to calculate IOL power. ORA IWA is used most frequently for standard cataract surgery involving the implantation of advanced technology IOLs, but has also been proven to be highly effective in calculating IOL power for patients who previously had refractive surgery. Beyond the scope of this paper is the use of ORA to determine total corneal astigmatism and alignment of the toric IOL on the axis of that astigmatism. I will summarize some of the results using the ORA system for IOL power for standard cataract patients and for post refractive surgery patients.

A retrospective study of 32,189 eyes was published by Cionni et al. [4] in 2018. This study looked only at outcomes of patients implant with Alcon IOL models. The basic characteristics of cohort is shown in Table 30.1:

The outcomes data were analyzed by comparing the mean absolute prediction error (MAPE) and the %MAPE ≤ 0.5D for the ORA data and the results based on the preoperative formula planning. The prediction error is defined as the difference between the actual manifest postop

Table 30.1 Baseline characteristics of patients in the aberrometer database

Characteristic	$n(\%)$, N
Sex	
Female	14,235 (58.4), 24,375
Male	10,140 (41.6), 24,375
IOL Type	
Non-toric	21,429 (66.6), 32,189
Toric	10,760 (33.4), 32,189

refraction SE and the formula predicted post op SE for the IOL power implanted. The results of this analysis are shown in Fig. 30.12.

The difference between the ORA PE and the preoperative planning PE was even greater when the IOL power implanted was different from the preoperative planned IOL power (the surgeon chose a IOL power different than their preoperative plan based on the ORA measurement). These results are shown in Fig. 30.13.

It was stated in the Cionni et al. article [3] that "One limitation of the current study is that the preoperative formulas used were not standardized (surgeons used whichever preoperative formula they preferred). However, this study's database provides a very large source of real world data from a wide variety of surgical centers and surgeons, which allows in-depth comparison between preoperative and ORA IWA calculations in a real-world setting."

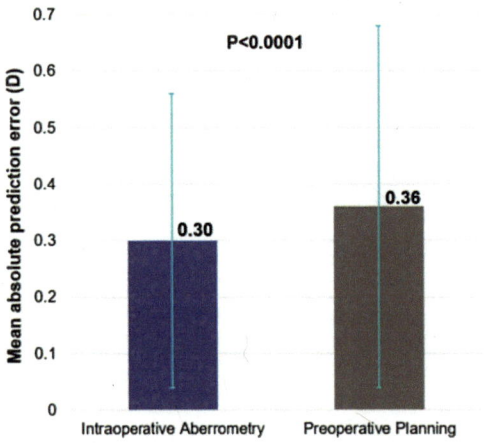
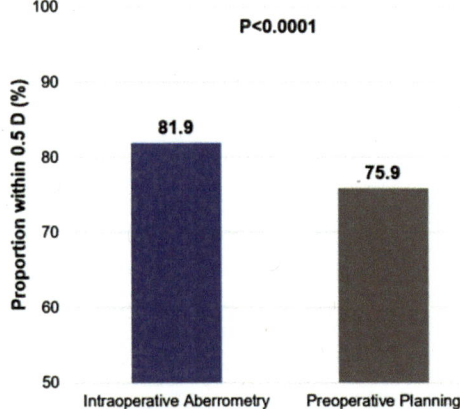

Fig. 30.12 Comparison of ORA outcomes versus preop planning for 32,189 eyes

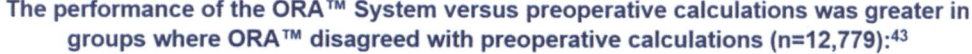

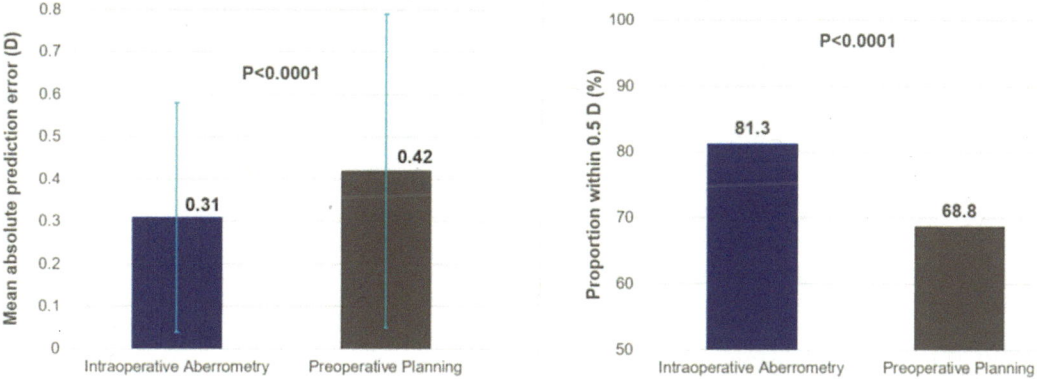

Fig. 30.13 Comparison of ORA outcomes versus preop planning in subgroup of patients where the implanted IOL power was different than the preoperative planned IOL power

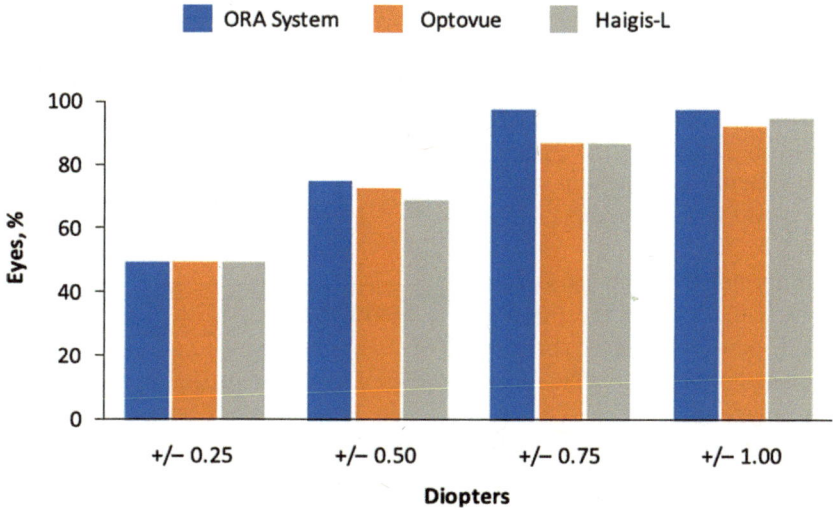

Fig. 30.14 Percentage of eyes within certain refractive IOL power prediction errors (eye without historical data ($n = 39$))

The ORA system has also proven to be an effective approach to IOL power calculations in post refractive cases, especially cases without historical data. The ORA system divides post refractive cases into several subgroups, and each subgroup is optimized separately producing regression coefficients for that subgroup. ORA does separate regressions for post myopic LASIK greater than 26 mm axial length, post myopic LASIK less than or equal to 26 mm axial length,

post hyperopic LASIK, post RK 4 cuts, and post RK 8 cuts. Fram et al. [5] compared the outcomes of the ORA system to those using a traditional post LASIK formula, the Haigis-L and a new formula based on Fourier-domain OCT measurements. The results are shown in Fig. 30.14.

Another paper by Ianchuliev et al. [6] describes outcomes of a retrospective study of 246 eyes of 215 patients and found a similar benefit using ORA versus conventional methods of

Table 30.2 Refractive outcomes in all eyes ($N = 246$)

Refractive outcomes	IA (ORA™ System)	Conventional preoperative methodology (Surgeon best choice)	Haigis L method	Shammas method
MedAE, D (95% CI)	0.35[a] (0.35 – 0.43)	0.60 (0.58 – 0.73)	0.53 (0.52 – 0.65)	0.51 (0.50 – 0.60)
MAE ± SD (D)	0.42 ± 0.39[b]	0.71 ± 0.56	0.65 ± 0.58	0.59 ± 0.52
% within ± 0.50 D	67[b]	46	48	50
% within ± 0.75 D	85[b]	63	66	72
% within ± 1.00 D	94[b]	76	80	87

CI confidence interval, *D* diopters, *MAE* mean absolute error, *MedAE* median absolute error, *SD* standard deviation

[a]$P < 0.0001$ for IA versus Surgeon Best Choice, IA versus Haigis L, and IA versus Shammas (2-sided binomial proportion test)

[b]$P < 0.0001$ for IA versus Surgeon Best Choice, IA versus Haigis L, and IA versus Shammas (repeated measures analysis of variance)

performing IOL power calculations in post myopic LASIK patients. The results are shown in Table 30.2.

Surgeon Benefits

While the ORA system can be and is used as a standalone IOL power calculator, most surgeons use the ORA in conjunction with their preoperative IOL formula or formulas. ORA provides the surgeon with an added level of confirmation of the IOL power to achieve the desired refractive outcome. In the AnalyzOR database when outcomes reports are generated, there is a column which list one of three possible scenarios. These are ORA Confirms Surgeon Choice, ORA Influenced Surgeon Choice, or Surgeon Pre-Op Calc Chosen. ORA Confirms means that the ORA suggested IOL Power was equal to the preoperative formula recommended IOL power. ORA Influenced means that the IOL power implanted was different from the Surgeon preop power. It could be the actual ORA recommended power or a value different from either the ORA suggested of the Surgeon Pre-OP power. The ORA measurement and suggested power caused the surgeon to deviate from their preoperative plan, ORA Influence the choice of the implanted

power. The Surgeon Pre-Op Calc Chosen is self-explanatory.

In Fig. 30.13, the results from a dataset in which 40% of the cases were ORA Influenced Surgeon Choice. As was pointed out above, the impact of ORA on outcomes is greater in these situations where the implanted IOL power was different from the preoperative formula planned IOL power.

Summary

The ORA system (hardware and software) has now been used in over two million cataract surgeries worldwide. ORA has proven to be invaluable to surgeons as a means of providing confidence at the time of surgery that the correct IOL power is being implanted. Because of axial length clustering of the data prior to generation of the regression coefficients, ORA can provide nearly uniform outcomes across the axial length range. ORA has also proven to be invaluable for post refractive cases—myopic, hyperopic, and RK. Because the aphakic SE which is used in the power calculation is done through the entire cornea (front and back surfaces), the changes in the corneal shape do not have to be calculated from the amount of refractive correction by the LASIK or RK procedure performed; no pre refractive surgery information is needed. As mentioned earlier, it is beyond the scope of this chapter, but ORA has proven to be a valuable way to measure total astigmatism and to properly align the implanted toric IOL to minimize the residual cylinder.

The ORA hardware and software has continued to evolve from 2005 to the present. In addition to quarterly optimizations of lens constants and regression coefficients, new approaches to improving outcomes are under development. The ORA system and IOL power calculations are not static but dynamic.

References

1. Cooley JW, Turkey JW. Math Comput. 1955;19:297–301.
2. Holladay JT. Am J Ophthalmol. 1993;116:63–6.
3. Fischler M, Bolles R. Commun ACM. 1981;24:381–95.
4. Cionni RJ, Dimalanta R, Breen M, Hamilton C. J Cataract Refract Surg. 2018;44:1230–5.
5. Fram NR, Masket S, Wang L. Ophthalmology. 2015;122:1096–101.
6. Ianchulev T, Hoffer KJ, Yoo SH, Chang DF, Breen M, Padrick T, Tran DB. Ophthalmology. 2014;121:56–60.

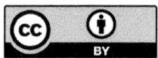

Cassini Corneal Topographer

31

Joris Snellenburg, Maarten Huijbregtse,
Benhur Ortiz-Jaramillo, Masmei Ginting,
and Ernst Serfontein

Introduction

Cassini provides cataract surgeons with an accurate and detailed description of the cornea, helping them to improve their surgical outcomes, reducing the number of postoperative surprises, and cutting the number of patients requiring follow-up corrective laser treatments. Cassini addresses the most important sources of corneal errors in cataract surgery, using a unique reflection-based technology, with color and infrared LED illumination (Fig. 31.1).

Over the past two decades, surgeons have been able to improve the outcomes of cataract procedures considerably due to more sophisticated IOL power formulas, as well as more advanced optical biometers. Despite these advancements, even today, the accuracy of the refractive predictions is still far from perfect even for virgin corneas [1]. In an endeavor to further reduce postoperative errors, reliable preoperative corneal measurements are essential, particularly of the first refractive layer: the tear film. As the cornea accounts for about two-thirds of the total

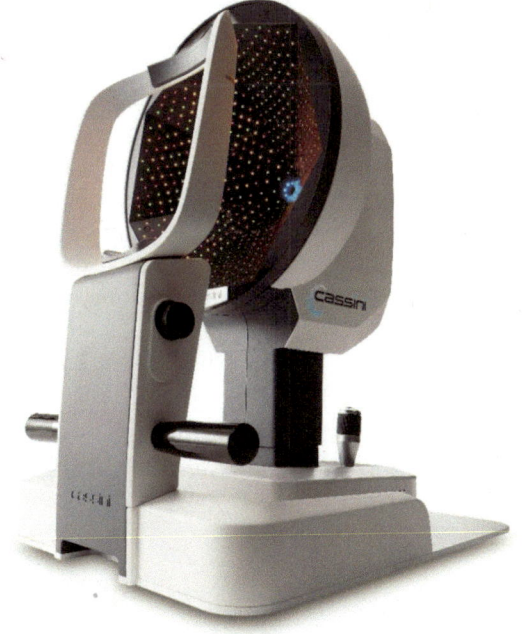

Fig. 31.1 The Cassini Device

dioptric power of the eye, small variations in the measured corneal shape can have a large effect on the recommended power of an IOL [2].

Cassini uses reflection-based technology to measure the shape and state of the tear film. The quality of the tear film layer can be assessed by analyzing the appearance of the reflected LEDs: sharp reflections indicate a smooth tear film layer, while distorted reflections indicate a disrupted tear film layer.

J. Snellenburg (✉) · M. Huijbregtse ·
B. Ortiz-Jaramillo · M. Ginting · E. Serfontein
Cassini Technologies B.V.,
The Hague, The Netherlands
e-mail: j.snellenburg@cassini-technologies.com;
m.huijbregtse@cassini-technologies.com;
b.ortiz-jaramillo@cassini-technologies.com;
n.ginting@cassini-technologies.com;
e.serfontein@cassini-technologies.com

© The Author(s) 2024

J. Aramberri et al. (eds.), *Intraocular Lens Calculations*, Essentials in Ophthalmology,
https://doi.org/10.1007/978-3-031-50666-6_31

In addition to assessing the quality of the tear film, it is important to consider the *entire* shape of the surface to judge the accuracy of the displayed K-readings. Unlike the K-readings may suggest, the shape of the cornea is far more intricate than the toric model described by these two radii of curvatures. Irregular features and the aspheric shape of the cornea can have a large impact on the K-readings and limit their validity as an approximation of the entire corneal shape. Cassini measures the entire shape of the anterior surface of the cornea, including the peripheral zone, using hundreds of LEDs. A quick assessment of the topographic maps will highlight irregular features such as cones and irregular astigmatism. If present, surgeons should carefully assess the reliability of the displayed K-readings before using them to calculate the power of an IOL.

Cassini is a pioneer in measuring the shape of the posterior corneal surface using LED technology. The anterior and posterior corneal data can be used together to determine the corneal ratio, helping surgeons by indicating the risk of a myopic or hyperopic shift. Also, planning for toric IOLs can be improved using total corneal astigmatism.

Altogether, the Cassini corneal shape analyzer helps surgeons to make the right decisions for their patients. Cassini connects to the latest surgical devices, exporting reliable preoperative data into surgery and allowing surgeons to maintain high accuracy while speeding up their procedures.

Cassini's mission is to offer highly accurate, personalized data for each patient undergoing cataract surgery to enable the best possible outcomes, even for those patients with challenging corneas.

Cassini Basic Principle

Cassini employs a dual modality system for imaging of the human eye in both the visible and infrared spectrum. A multitude of colored and infrared LEDs serve as illumination sources, as well as data points for its topography modules that measure the anterior and posterior surfaces of the cornea.

The anterior surface is measured by projecting the signature pattern of color LEDs onto the eye. The emitted light reflects off the convex mirror constituted by the tear film of the anterior corneal surface, toward the RGB camera inside the Cassini device (Fig. 31.2). The shape of the cornea is modeled as a linear combination of Zernike

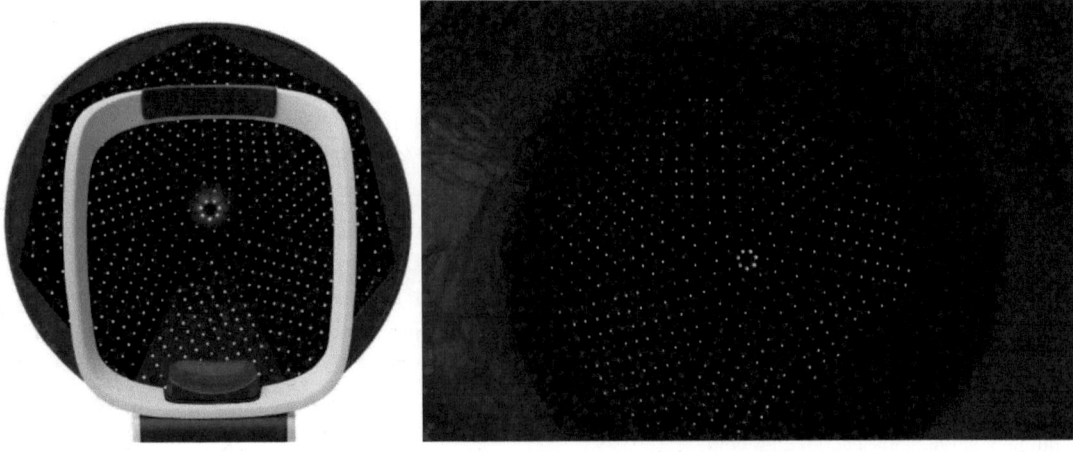

Fig. 31.2 Cassini's signature, color-coded LED pattern (left) and its reflection off an eye as imaged by the RGB camera (right)

polynomials, where the polynomial coefficients are iteratively updated using ray tracing until the differences between the angles of incidence and the angles of reflection are minimized in a least squares sense [3]. Color coding of the LED pattern ensures a direct relationship between each image point and a corresponding source point. Skew ray errors are thus avoided and, in combination with the sampling density, this allows for highly detailed and accurate surface measurements—especially considering the axis of astigmatism and higher-order aberrations [4].

A small fraction of the source light will not directly reflect off the anterior surface, but traverse through the cornea and reflect off the posterior surface instead—an effect that is enhanced in the infrared spectrum and utilized by Cassini to determine the global posterior surface shape with its infrared imaging system. Source light emitted from multiple infrared LEDs is captured by an infrared camera after reflecting off the corneal surfaces (Fig. 31.3). Ray tracing and an extended corneal model—including the anterior and posterior surface separated by a corneal thickness—are combined to determine the posterior toric shape that best fits the image data in a least squares sense. The posterior measurement captures the relevant information to investigate the effects of the posterior surface on the total corneal power and astigmatism.

In addition to the topographic capabilities, Cassini's imaging system can be used to derive other ocular metrics like tear film dynamics, horizontal visible iris diameter, and pupil sizes under various lighting conditions.

Acquired data is presented in a concise, yet complete overview in the Cassini software GUI (Fig. 31.4). Customizable settings for, e.g., color keys, units, and overlays allow for data interpretation in a personalized manner. Cassini's printing suite transfers the data in a similarly concise format to a variety of reports tailored to the surgical plan under consideration—whether pertaining to astigmatism correction, multifocal IOL, FLACS, or any combination thereof.

Fig. 31.3 Infrared image of an eye, showing the infrared LED reflections from the anterior surface (1) and posterior surface (2)

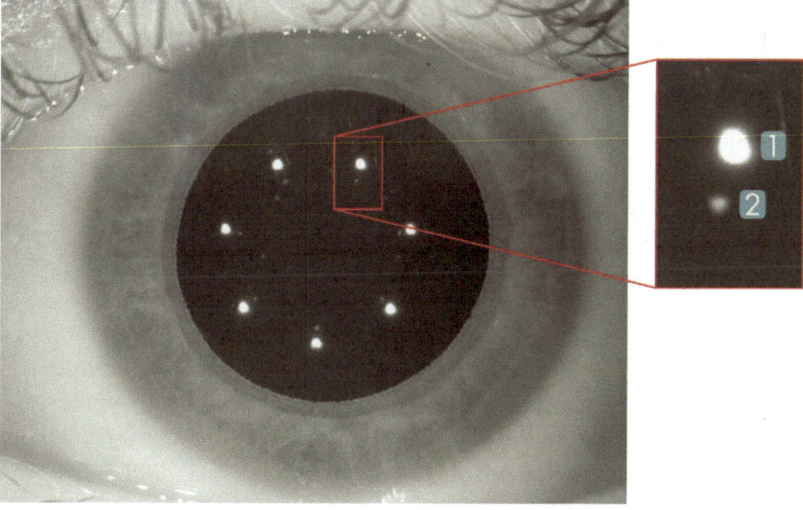

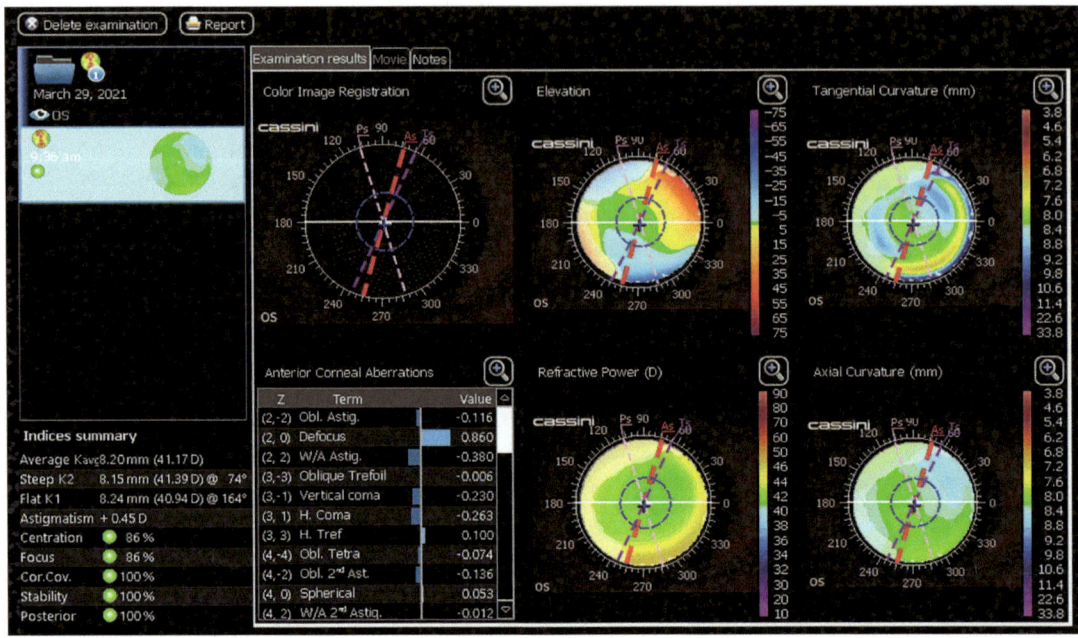

Fig. 31.4 Cassini's highly customizable layout featuring, e.g., color scales, custom ordering in the 6-up view, opening in a detailed 1-up view, printing reports, or writing notes

Surgical Planning with Cassini

Monofocal IOLs

All IOL power formulas, even the latest and most sophisticated models, strongly rely on the flat and steep K-readings [5]. These two K-readings summarize the power distribution of the entire anterior corneal surface into a simplistic toric representation. It is therefore important that the K-readings plugged into the IOL power calculators are a reliable representation of the true anterior surface of the cornea, which is typically far more complex. Care must be taken especially for post-refractive corneas and poor tear film layers. To avoid postoperative surprises, Cassini users are advised to review the preoperative data thoroughly. Deleting and repeating a bad measurement before surgery is always preferable to avoid postoperative surprises, conducting refractive touch-ups and disappointed patients [6].

The key aspect to evaluate whether the displayed K-readings are a correct representation of the true shape of the cornea is to look at the overall shape of the cornea. Cassini measures the entire corneal surface and displays its true shape in a series of topographic maps. Astigmatism (bow tie), irregular features (cones) and post-refractive eyes (flattened) have characteristic forms that are easy to identify. Also, in each untreated cornea, the central region is steeper and therefore more powerful than the outer regions of the cornea. Altogether, the magnitude of the K-readings is strongly influenced by the selected corneal region. Care must be taken if devices base their K-readings on just a few measuring points as they might miss relevant information from other regions. Cassini measures the entire corneal surface, revealing important irregularities and helping surgeons to interpret the reliability of the K-readings. Even a quick assessment of these maps will inform the surgeon if the shape is normal or irregular and consequently, if the two K-readings are representative for the entire cornea and can therefore be trusted.

Recent findings by Wang et al. [7] emphasize the significant role of the posterior corneal surface in total corneal refraction, challenging the longstanding assumption that the anterior surface solely dictates corneal power. Traditionally, cataract surgeons relied on a simulated K-reading derived from the anterior surface, based on the presumed constancy of the posterior-to-anterior corneal ratio. However, Wang et al. discovered varying ratios: 0.81 and 0.82 for normal corneas, 0.76 for eyes post-myopic LASIK/PRK, and 0.86 for post-hyperopic LASIK/PRK. These findings highlight the necessity of considering both corneal surfaces in refraction calculations, particularly in eyes that have undergone refractive surgeries, which significantly alter the corneal shape and, consequently, the corneal ratio. Next to modified eyes, studies show the spread in corneal ratio among normal corneas is also significant; to conclude that surgeons cannot use the anterior surface of the eye only to predict the total power of the cornea [8]. Cassini measures both the anterior and posterior surface of the cornea and determines the corneal ratio to indicate whether the simulated corneal readings fit the IOL-power calculations model or not (Fig. 31.5).

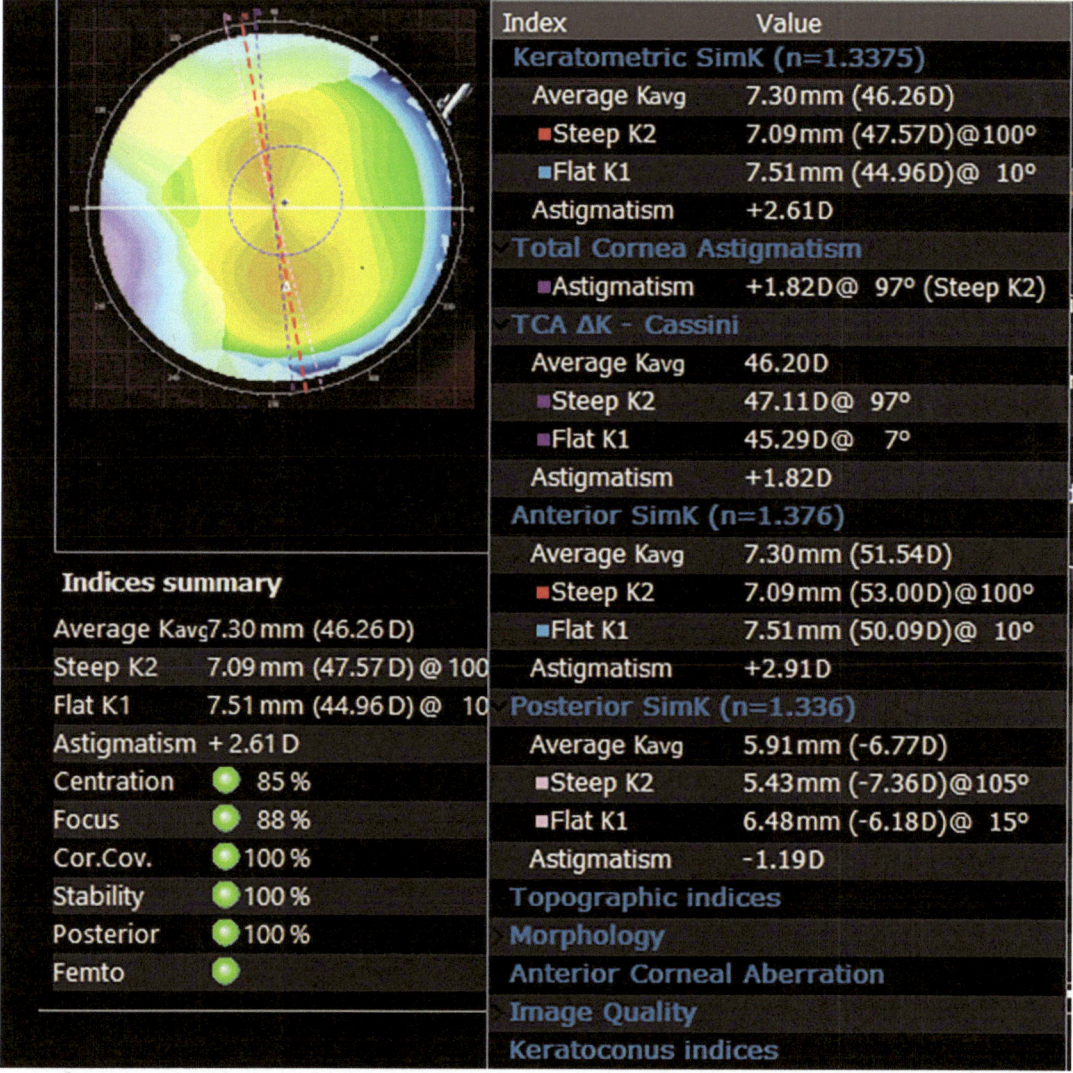

Fig. 31.5 Indices summary with traditional K-readings, examination quality factors and when expanded a host of other properties, including information on the posterior surface and eye morphology

Toric IOLs

Astigmatism is even more sensitive to corneal irregularities. Even nonastigmatic features such as a conic surface will lead to a difference in steep and flat K-readings (astigmatism magnitude), and therefore a false assumption of astigmatism.

The astigmatism-per-zone overlay on Cassini's topographic maps provides insight into the regularity of astigmatism (Fig. 31.6). Regular

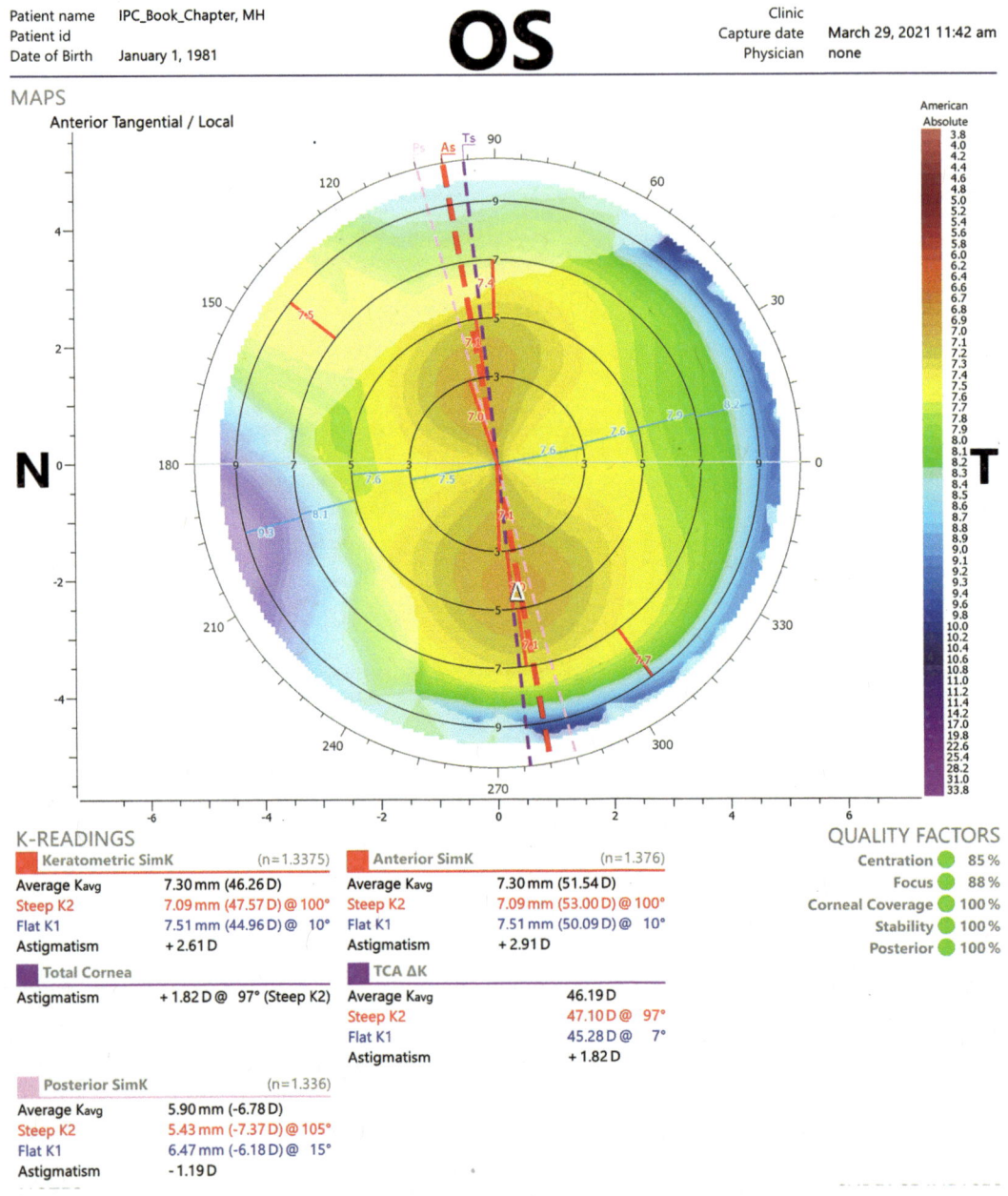

Fig. 31.6 Astigmatism per zone overall featuring a nice symmetric bow tie. Note a significant amount of posterior astigmatism, significantly reducing the total cornea astig-matism resulting in spectacle-free day vision for this healthy volunteer's eye

astigmatism is characterized by a highly symmetric bow tie, whereas irregular astigmatism is characterized by skewed radial axes or an asymmetric bow tie, or both.

In 2012, D. Koch et al. published a study on the contribution of the posterior corneal astigmatism to the total corneal astigmatism [9]. The study played an important role in the awareness of the posterior corneal astigmatism and its prominent effect on corneal astigmatism management. Ignoring the contribution of the posterior corneal astigmatism may lead to an overcorrec-

tion in eyes that have with-the-rule astigmatism and undercorrection in eyes that have against-the-rule astigmatism. A few examples are shown in Fig. 31.7. This new insight led to the Baylor Nomogram, which helps surgeons to adjust the power of astigmatism by incorporating population-based averages for the posterior surface [10].

This led to better results on average; however, results are not optimal for all patients due to the weak correlation between the anterior and posterior corneal astigmatism. Cassini directly measures the posterior corneal astigmatism and combines this

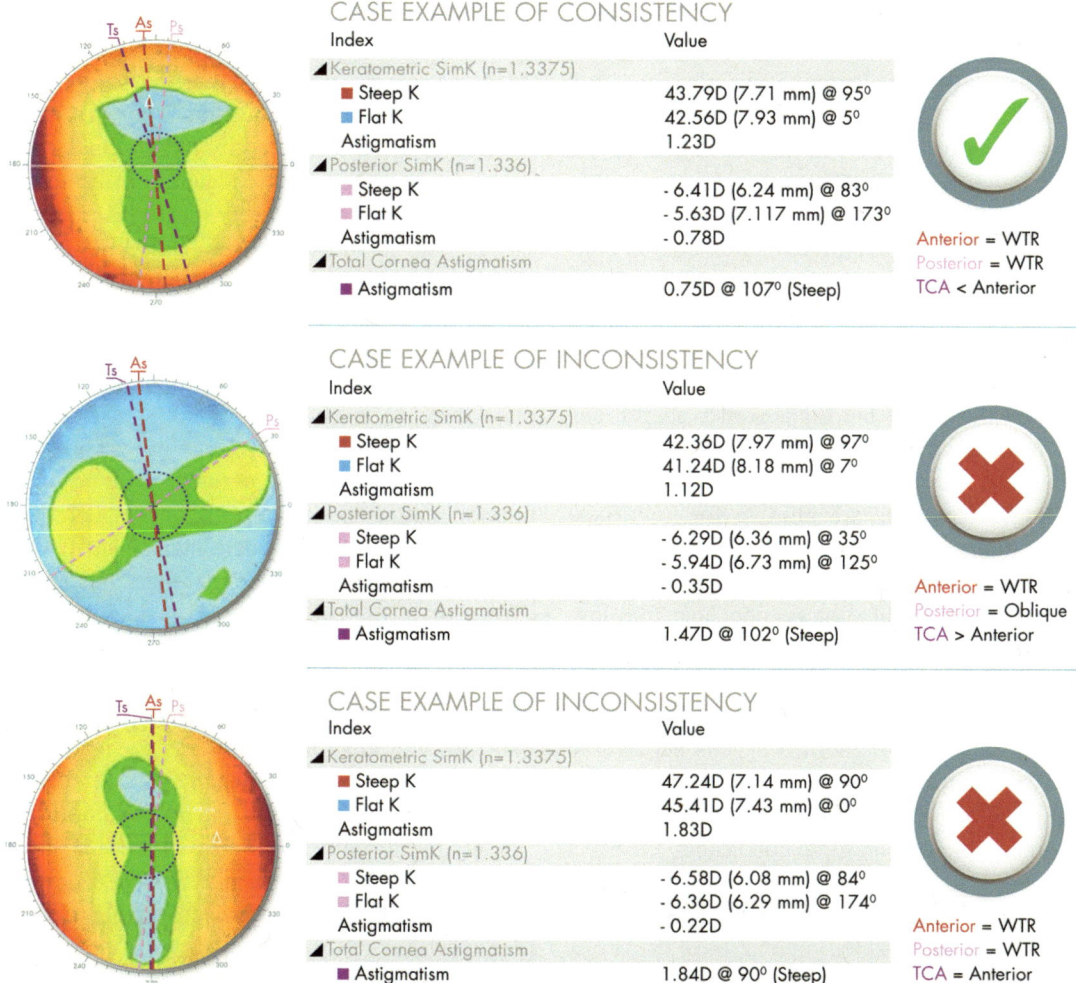

CASE EXAMPLE OF CONSISTENCY

Index	Value
▲ Keratometric SimK (n=1.3375)	
■ Steep K	43.79D (7.71 mm) @ 95°
■ Flat K	42.56D (7.93 mm) @ 5°
Astigmatism	1.23D
▲ Posterior SimK (n=1.336)	
■ Steep K	- 6.41D (6.24 mm) @ 83°
■ Flat K	- 5.63D (7.117 mm) @ 173°
Astigmatism	- 0.78D
▲ Total Cornea Astigmatism	
■ Astigmatism	0.75D @ 107° (Steep)

Anterior = WTR
Posterior = WTR
TCA < Anterior

CASE EXAMPLE OF INCONSISTENCY

Index	Value
▲ Keratometric SimK (n=1.3375)	
■ Steep K	42.36D (7.97 mm) @ 97°
■ Flat K	41.24D (8.18 mm) @ 7°
Astigmatism	1.12D
▲ Posterior SimK (n=1.336)	
■ Steep K	- 6.29D (6.36 mm) @ 35°
■ Flat K	- 5.94D (6.73 mm) @ 125°
Astigmatism	- 0.35D
▲ Total Cornea Astigmatism	
■ Astigmatism	1.47D @ 102° (Steep)

Anterior = WTR
Posterior = Oblique
TCA > Anterior

CASE EXAMPLE OF INCONSISTENCY

Index	Value
▲ Keratometric SimK (n=1.3375)	
■ Steep K	47.24D (7.14 mm) @ 90°
■ Flat K	45.41D (7.43 mm) @ 0°
Astigmatism	1.83D
▲ Posterior SimK (n=1.336)	
■ Steep K	- 6.58D (6.08 mm) @ 84°
■ Flat K	- 6.36D (6.29 mm) @ 174°
Astigmatism	- 0.22D
▲ Total Cornea Astigmatism	
■ Astigmatism	1.84D @ 90° (Steep)

Anterior = WTR
Posterior = WTR
TCA = Anterior

Fig. 31.7 Three example cases where ignoring the posterior contribution may lead to unexpected surprises, specifically when anterior astigmatism is with-the-rule, but posterior is not

with the anterior corneal astigmatism to calculate the total corneal astigmatism (TCA). This does not only lead to the correct power of astigmatism but also to the correct angle of astigmatism. Modern IOL calculators could increase their accuracy by allowing the inclusion of such a parameter within their calculations. Meanwhile, a corneal astigmatism planning report allows surgeons to make use of the information provided by TCA, to be used in conjunction with standard online toric calculators.

Multifocal IOLs

Multifocal intraocular lenses can offer patients spectacle-free vision. Planning multifocal IOLs require detailed preoperative examinations that go beyond the power and astigmatism considerations described above. Irregular features of the cornea such as coma and higher-order aberrations as well as the quality of the tear film become even more important for multifocal IOLs. Loss of contrast and sensitivity associated with multifocal IOLs will become more apparent if the ocular surface is not smooth and the generic shape of the cornea is far from uniform. Cassini calculates the contribution of the higher-order aberrations (HOA) and displays each Zernike component separately. Surgeons can use this information to judge if patients are eligible for multifocal IOLs. Increased higher-order aberrations are common to corneas that have undergone refractive surgery, corneal surgery, poor tear film layers, and conic corneas [11]. Also, the pupil size, shape, and centration significantly influence the quality of vision. Light distribution through the various zones of the multifocal lens depends to a large extent on the size and centration of the pupil. Cassini displays these pupil features under both photopic and mesopic conditions. Incorrect assessment of these parameters may lead to photophobia phenomena like glare and halo. Centration of the multifocal lens in relation to the vertex

position of the cornea may also play an important role in the occurrence of unwanted visual effects. The distance between the corneal vertex—or more correctly: "the subject-fixated coaxially sighted corneal light reflex" and pupil center is described by chord mu [12], and historically labeled as Angle KAPPA. The distance between the corneal vertex and the center of the limbus is labeled as Angle Alpha. Cassini reports Angle KAPPA and Angle Alpha for both the photopic and mesopic pupil conditions (Fig. 31.8).

FLACS

Femtosecond laser-assisted cataract surgery (FLACS) can be used to assist the surgeon in managing patient astigmatism. The structural features of the iris, defined by its muscular configuration, can be used to determine the exact location of the preoperatively measured angle of astigmatism in surgery. The so-called iris registration algorithm uses these fingerprint-like features of the iris to compensate for well-known errors such as cyclotorsion, which can be more than 10 degrees [13]. Manual marking, which often leads to the blurring of ink spots, can be eliminated as well, thereby removing yet another source of error. For the correction of minimal to moderate amounts of astigmatism, FLACS can be used to create arcuate incisions. FLACS can also be used to create radial markings in the cornea or in the capsulorrhexis to identify axis alignment of toric IOLs. Cassini preoperative iris imaging and astigmatism diagnostics allows for increased accuracy in the placement of arcuate incisions and identification marks for toric IOL alignment. Automatic connectivity will reduce manual transcription errors and procedure time.

Cassini currently interfaces with Johnson & Johnson Vision's CATALYS Precision Laser System and the LENSAR Laser System by LENSAR (Fig. 31.9).

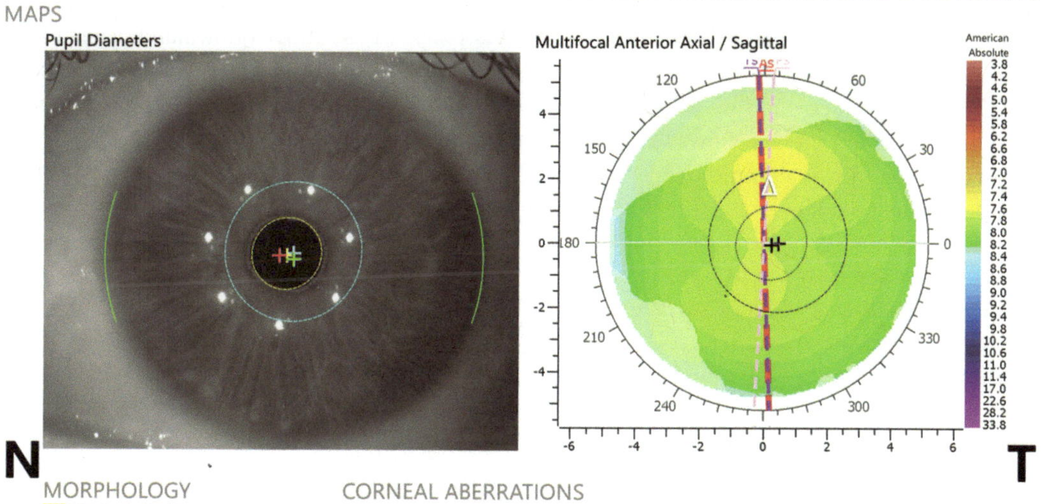

MAPS
Pupil Diameters
Multifocal Anterior Axial / Sagittal
American
Absolute
3.8
4.2
4.6
5.0
5.4
5.8
6.2
6.6
6.8
7.0
7.2
7.4
7.6
7.8
8.0
8.2
8.4
8.6
8.8
9.0
9.2
9.4
9.8
10.2
10.6
11.0
11.4
17.0
22.6
28.2
33.8
N
T

MORPHOLOGY

Photopic Pupil

Diameter	2.24 mm
Angle KAPPA	0.24 mm @ 360°

Mesopic Pupil

Diameter	4.37 mm
Angle KAPPA	0.45 mm @ 7°

Limbus Morphology

W2W	12.0 mm
Angle Alpha	0.48 mm @ 345°

Visual Axis

CORNEAL ABERRATIONS

#Z	Term	Photopic zone (2.24mm)	Mesopic zone (4.37mm)	Surgeon zone (6.00mm)
3(2,-2)	Oblique Astigmatism	-0.012	-0.015	0.058
4(2, 0)	Defocus	0.015	0.295	1.109
5(2, 2)	With/Against Astigmatism	-0.144	-0.602	-1.190
6(3,-3)	Oblique Trefoil	-0.004	-0.044	-0.127
7(3,-1)	Vertical coma	0.010	0.082	0.220
8(3, 1)	Horizontal coma	0.004	0.020	0.050
9(3, 3)	Horizontal Trefoil	0.006	0.035	0.068
10(4,-4)	Oblique Tetrafoil	-0.002	-0.023	-0.056
11(4,-2)	Oblique 2nd astigmatism	0.001	0.012	0.048
12(4, 0)	Spherical Aberration	0.005	0.085	0.301
13(4, 2)	With/Against 2nd Astigmatism	-0.002	-0.016	-0.024
14(4, 4)	Horizontal Tetrafoil	0.001	0.008	-0.005
	HOA	0.014	0.136	0.412

Fig. 31.8 Multifocal IOL Planning Report; showcasing a case with a relatively large-angle KAPPA and a less likely candidate for a multifocal IOL

Cassini Corneal Analyzer™
Preoperative Undilated Eye
LENSAR Laser Iris Registration
Docked Dilated Eye

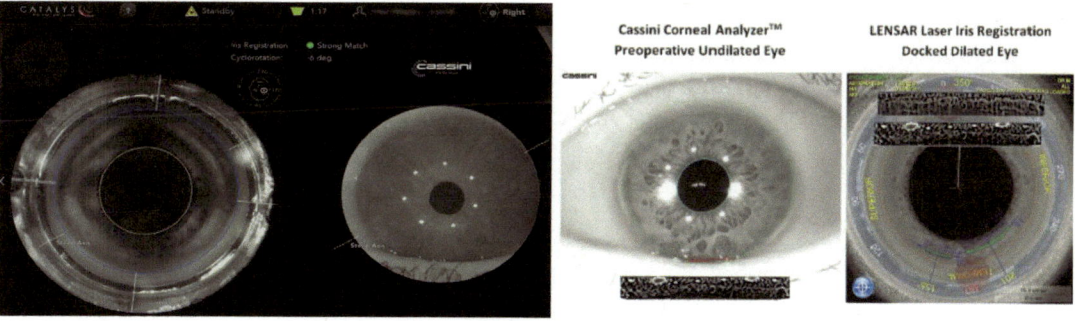

Fig. 31.9 Cassini Connects CATALYS [14] and Cassini Streamlines LENSAR [15]

Ocular Surface Diagnostics (Tear Film)

The ocular surface is covered by a few microns thin liquid film called the tear film. The composition of the tear film is complex and plays an essential role in nourishing and protecting the cornea. The tear film has three distinct layers: (1) the hydrophobic top layer (lipid layer) made of a thin sheet of lipids that reduces surface tension and helps to spread the tears after each blink; (2) the aqueous layer, which is the thickest layer of the tear film and plays, among others, an important role in the oxygenation of the cornea; and (3) the mucous layer, which compensates for corneal unevenness and reduces friction during blinking [16]. Optically, the role of the tear film layer is to form a smooth refractive surface over the uneven corneal surface. At each blink, the tear film layer is being refreshed and goes through a dynamic tear buildup phase to form a tear film layer. The lipid top layer protects the underlying aqueous layer from evaporation. Local rupture in the lipid top layer exposes the aqueous layer directly to air leading to high evaporation rates that potentially produces rupture of the tear film [17]. The time between the formation of the tear film (buildup) and breakup of the tear film depends strongly on the quality of the tear film (mix of lipids and water), the environmental conditions and the pathology of the cornea. The period immediately after the tear buildup phase and before the tear breakup can vary from just a few to more than 20 seconds [18]. Measuring the shape of

the first reflective ocular layer should occur in this phase of the inner blink period. Reflection-based technologies, such as Cassini, can use the smoothness of the reflective surface to extract the quality of the tear film layer. Dysfunctional tear glands, wearing of contact lenses and environmental conditions may affect the quality of the tear film. Healthy tear film layers are very even and reflect light like a convex mirror. Tear film layers which tend to breakup, or evaporate quickly, become very uneven, leading to a distortion of the reflective points. From a vision point of view, light crossing these uneven surfaces gets refracted in a similarly uneven way, leading to higher-order aberrations which diminish the image quality at the retina. From a K-reading point of view, instable tear films affect the measured radius of curvature significantly [19]. In this context, Cassini can be used to assess the dynamics (stability) of the tear film by recording the corneal reflection of its projected LED pattern over time. When the surface of the cornea is smooth, each projected color LED appears regular in the image forming a circle-like shape. However, during the inner blink period the tear film changes dynamically: producing localized "dry" regions that leads to distorted shapes of the projected color LEDs in the image (see Fig. 31.10 for comparison). To capture the transition from a circle-like shape to distorted reflection, Cassini processes every frame and monitors the uniformity of every reflected color LED. The distorted LED reflections are marked to indicate potential dry regions.

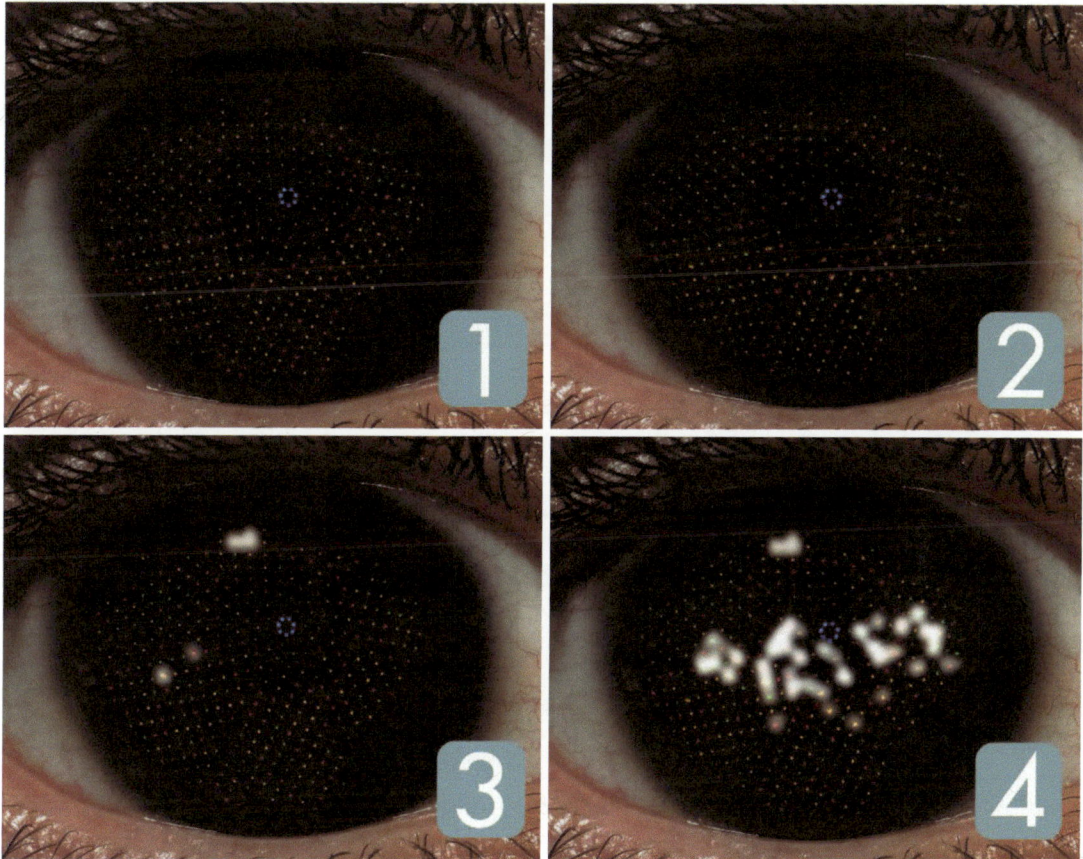

Fig. 31.10 Projected corneal reflection into the colour camera captured with a Cassini device: (1) no degradation of the first Purkinje image and (2) first Purkinje image degraded. (3, 4) Lower 2 images are processed images where the degradation is highlighted in white

Conclusion

Reflection-based corneal topography is not something new, but Cassini's distinct and unique measuring principle sets it apart from other technologies. With close to 700 multicolor LEDs, as well as the ability to measure the posterior surface of the cornea by means of second Purkinje reflections, Cassini has taken the "proven" point-measurement system to a new level (Fig. 31.11). It is therefore a clearly differentiating platform with its primary application in the field of cataract surgery.

CASSINI
SPECIFICATIONS

Submicron accuracy with up to 700 ambient multicolor LEDs combined with 2nd Purkinje raytracing technology

Anterior axis repeatability within 3 degrees [8]

Keratometric data display of Steep, Flat and Average in Diopters and millimeters for anterior, posterior and Total Corneal Astigmatism (TCA)

Topographic indices: Shape factor (E), eccentricity (e), Asphericity (Q) and form factor (p)

Topography mapping: Axial, Refractive, Tangential and Elevation

Multiple color keys for topography map customization

Keratoconus screening indices: Surface Asymmetry Index (SAI) and Surface Regularity Index (SRI)

Corneal aberrations with individual Zernike terms and total HOA parameter display

Multifocal IOL suitability module with White-to-White, Pupillometry, Angle Alpha and Angle KAPPA

External Ocular Photography

Seamless ocular surface screening and visualization module

Automated and manual capturing with joystick positioning on visual axis

Accuracy verification with Quality Factors

Incorporated Iris Registration for Femtosecond Laser Assisted Cataract Surgery (FLACS)

Encrypted patient management with various clinical report export options: DICOM, USB, Wi-Fi, PDF, JPG and PNG

Fig. 31.11 Cassini specifications

References

1. Koch DD, Hill W, Abulafia A, Wang L. Pursuing perfection in intraocular lens calculations: I. Logical approach for classifying IOL calculation formulas. J Cataract Refract Surg. 2017;43(6):717–8.
2. Larkin H. Bright path ahead: Examining six requirements for reducing errors and eliminating 'refractive surprise'. Eurotimes Stories; 2017. https://www.eurotimes.org/refractions/
3. Snellenburg JJ, Braaf B, Hermans EA, van der Heijde RGL, Sicam VADP. Forward ray tracing for image projection prediction and surface reconstruction in the evaluation of corneal topography systems. Opt Express. 2010;18(18):19324–38.
4. Klein SA. Corneal topography reconstruction algorithm that avoids the skew ray ambiguity and the skew ray error. Optom Vis Sci. 1997;74(11):945–62.
5. Savini G, Taroni L, Hoffer KJ. Recent developments in intraocular lens power calculation methods - update 2020. Ann Transl Med. 2020 Jul;8(22):1–9.
6. Hill WE, Abulafia A, Wang L, Koch DD. Pursuing perfection in intraocular lens calculations. II. Measuring foibles: Measurement errors, validation criteria, IOL constants, and lane length. J Cataract Refract Surg. 2017;43(7):869–70.
7. Li Wang, Ashraf M. Mahmoud, Betty Lise Anderson, Douglas D. Koch, Cynthia J. Roberts; Total Corneal Power Estimation: Ray Tracing Method versus Gaussian Optics Formula. Invest. Ophthalmol. Vis. Sci. 2011;52(3):1716–22.
8. Haigis W, Hoffer KJ, Holladay JT, Olsen T. The Creator's Forum: IOL power calculations for postrefractive surgery eyes. CRSTEurope 2012 MayE.
9. Koch DD, Ali SF, Weikert MP, Shirayama M, Jenkins R, Wang L. Contribution of posterior corneal astigmatism to total corneal astigmatism. J Cataract Refract Surg. 2012;38(12):2080–7.
10. Koch DD, Jenkins RB, Weikert MP, Yeu E, Wang L. Correcting astigmatism with toric intraocular lenses: effect of posterior corneal astigmatism. J Cataract Refract Surg. 2013;39(12):1803–9.
11. Taskov G, Taskov T. Higher order aberrations (HOA) changes after Femto-LASIK in topography and wavefrontguided treatments. Folia Med. 2020;62:331.
12. Chang DH, Waring GO. The subject-fixated coaxially sighted corneal light reflex: a clinical marker for centration of refractive treatments and devices. Am J Ophthalmol. 2014 Nov;158(5):863–74.
13. Febbraro JL, Koch DD, Khan HN, Saad A, Gatinel D. Detection of static cyclotorsion and compensation for dynamic cyclotorsion in laser in situ keratomileusis. J Cataract Refract Surg. 2010;36(10):1718–23.
14. Internal Image Collection. 2021. Collected by Trey Bishop, MD. Bishop Eye Center, Hilton Head, South Carolina.
15. Cataract & Refractive Surgery Today: Intelligent Integration for Optimal Outcomes, Cataract Surgery Feature Stories. July 2015. Mark Packer, MD, CPI.
16. Anga M, Baskaran M, Werkmeister RM, Chua J, Schmidl D, dos Santos VA, Garhöfer G, Mehta JS, Schmetterer L. Anterior segment optical coherence tomography. Prog Retin Eye Res. 2018;66:132–56.
17. King-Smith PE, Fink BA, Nichols JJ, Nichols KK, Hill RM. Interferometric imaging of the full thickness of the precorneal tear film. J Opt Soc Am A Opt Image Sci Vis. 2006;23(9):2097–104.
18. Willcox M, Argüeso P, Georgiev HJ, Laurie G, Millar T, Papas E, Rolland J, Schmidt T, Stahl U, Suarez T, Subbaraman L, Uçakhan O, Jones L. TFOS DEWS II tear film report. Ocul Surf. 2017;15:369–406.
19. Doğan A, Gürdal C, Köylü M. Does dry eye affect repeatability of corneal topography measurements? Turk J Ophthalmol. 2017;48:57–60.

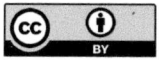

Part IV

Calculation Methods

An Overview of Intraocular Lens Power Calculation Methods

32

Han Bor Fam

Cataract surgery is refractive surgery. Besides removing the dysfunctional cataract, cataract surgery restores and corrects the refractive status of the eye. The success of modern-day cataract surgery is dependent on the refractive outcome. Postoperative refractive surprise is unnecessarily disappointing and frustrating to everyone.

In prescribing the correct glasses, accurate refraction is key to that outcome. In laser cornea refractive surgery, again good preoperative refraction, whether objectively, subjectively, or wavefront-driven, is imperative to a happy result. In cataract surgery, good biometry coupled with good intraocular lens power calculation is crucial to ensure good eventuality. It is akin to accurate refraction in cornea refractive surgery.

In 1949, Harold Ridley implanted a plastic lens in a patient. Despite the less than favorable initial results, he had ushered in a new era of intraocular lenses and indirectly lead to the subsequent development of the science of intraocular lens power calculation.

In the past, IOL power calculation formulas are categorized by generation. However, this can be confusing as formulas evolved and newer methods are being developed. As aptly described by Koch et al., it is opportune to adopt a newer classification based on methodology [1, 2]. However,

this has recently been more thoroughly updated by Savini, Hoffer and Kohnen in a recent JCRS Editorial [2].

Historical Methods

Standard Lens Method

Learning from the poor outcomes of the pioneering implantations, the dioptric power of the early lens implants was adjusted to an improved single-lens power for all patients, depending on what type IOL was used (Prepupillary, Iris Plane or Anterior Chamber). The initial gross refractive errors were reduced. This lasted for almost two decades. This overly simplistic method is obsolete due to the inherently poor outcomes.

The Refraction Method

Among the first attempts at calculating IOL power was a simple refraction-based method. The power of the IOL was adjusted by a factor of the preoperative refraction.

$$\text{IOL Power} = 18.00 + 1.25^* \text{ preoperative refraction.}$$

The refraction method has poor outcomes as preoperative refraction with a cataract present is an imprecise method of determining the power

H. B. Fam (✉)
National Healthcare Group Eye Institute, Tan Tock Seng Hospital, Singapore, Singapore

of the lens. The cataract itself may induce index refractive error that confounds the preoperative refraction.

Theoretical Formulas

In 1967, Fyodorov and Kolonko [3] presented their theoretical formula based on geometric optics. The formula utilizesd keratometry and axial length which was measured with A-scan ultrasonography. That marked the nascency of today's geometrical optics or theoretical formulas.

The eye is essentially a 2-lens system. It consists of the cornea as the first lens that contributes about two-third of the refractive power of the eye; and the crystalline lens that accounts for the remaining one-third of the refracting power of the eye (Fig. 32.1). Theoretical formulas using vergence formulas are based on Gaussian optics.

The geometric formulas of Fyodorov and Kolonko [3] and the other early workers, notably Colenbrander [4], Thijssen [5], Van der Heijde [6], Hoffer [7] and R Binkhorst (Binkhorst, The optical design of intraocular lens calculation [8]) are all applied to schematic eyes using theoretical constants. Basically, these formulas use different correction factors but utilize identical vergence concept of:

$$P = \frac{n}{AL - ACD} - \frac{n}{\dfrac{n}{K} - ACD}$$

Where P is the IOL power; n is aqueous and vitreous refractive index; and ACD the estimated anterior chamber depth that is adjusted by the individual formulaic correction factors.

The early formulas were good with normal axial lengths of around 23.5 mm (22–24.5 mm) but were less precise with short (<22 mm) or long (>2.5 mm) axial length eyes. Further development on regression and theoretical formulas involved improvement in outcomes in eyes with an expanded range of axial lengths.

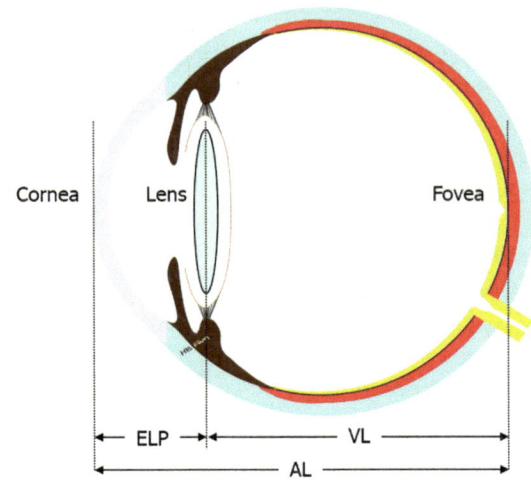

Fig. 32.1 A schematic optical diagram of the eye depicting the 2-lens system of the eye. *ELP* effective lens position (commonly known as the predicted postoperative anterior chamber depth), vl vitreous length (optical vitreous length), *AL* axial length (optical axial length)

The early generation of theoretical formulas assumed fixed postoperative anterior chamber depths. A second generations of theoretical formulas was introduced by Hoffer in 1982, which includes a sub-equation for ELP that mathematically predicts the postoperative effective lens position (ELP) as a function of axial length. The sub-equation (ELP=2.92*AL-2.93) was based on one IOL model and would be best for that model. R. Binkhorst followed with another iteration. (Binkhorst, Intraocular lens power calculation manual: A guide to the Author's TICC-40 Programs, Edition 3 [9], [10] (Hoffer, The effect of axial length on posterior chamber lenses and posterior capsule position [11, 12]). The main difference between these second-generation formulas lies in its prediction of the postoperative effective lens position.

The third generation of theoretical formulas utilizes both AL and keratometry as predictors of preoperative anterior chamber depth (Olsen, Prediction of intraocular lens position after cataract extraction [13]), hence the ELP [14, 15]. All these formulas are based on the Gullstrand eye model.

2-Variables Thin-Lens Vergence Formula: Third Generation Theoretical Formulas

For the last 3 decades, modern theoretical formulas were the commonly used formulas. These were Hoffer Q, the Holladay, and the SRK/T formulas. These 3 formulas make use of the radius of curvature of the anterior cornea and axial length to predict the ELP. Olsen first introduced the use of more variable such as the ACD and LT. Later, Holladay introduced his Holladay 2 (Holladay, Holladay IOL Consultant User's Guide and Reference Manual [16]) which uses up to 7 variables to predict the ELP. Besides corneal radius and axial length, these include preoperative ACD, phakic lens thickness, the corneal diameter (CD), and the patient's age. Hoffer and Savini later introduced gender and race in their Hoffer H-5 formula.

Hoffer Q and Hoffer QST

This formula was published by Kenneth J Hoffer in 1993 (Hoffer KJ, The Hoffer Q formula: a comparison of theoretic and regression formulas [17]). The core vergence formula is the basic Hoffer formula (a major modification of Colenbrander's formula) but with a new ELP prediction equation he called the Q formula which predicted the ELP based on the AL and the Tangent of the K.

Thanks to the studies by Melles [18, 19], Hoffer, Savini, and Taroni have further developed a new formula, the Hoffer QST. This is an evolution of the 1993 Hoffer Q formula with the use of AI to enhance the prediction of ELP and algorithms to improve accuracy in the long eyes. There are several studies now showing the Hoffer QST to be as good or better than all the modern formulas depending on the criteria chosen (MAE, MedAE, SD, %+/-0.50 D, etc) [20]. It is freely available on its website www.HofferQST.com with a Research page allowing lens constant (pACD) optimization and IOL power studies on your data.

Holladay 1 and Holladay 2 Formulas

Holladay's first formula (Holladay 1) is a 3-part formulation [14]. The first part is a set of screening criteria for data. The purpose is to identify the improbable axial length and keratometry measurements and to alert the users to validate the measurements and the possibility of untoward outcomes. He used the Hoffer AJO 1980 study of 7,500 eyes for normal differences in bilateral eyes [21]. This set of useful checklists has persisted and is now part of most biometry systems but with some modifications with the changing times. The second part is the formula proper; this is a further modification of the second-generation theoretical formula to improve on the prediction of the ELP using Fyodorov's Corneal Height equation (using AL and K). Finally, a personalized "surgeon factor" (SF) (his lens constant) compensates for any systematic bias in the individual surgeon's postoperative outcome.

Holladay's Data Screening Criteria [14] to identify unusual measurement and require further validation. Repeat measurement if:

1. Axial length < 22.0 mm or > 25.0 mm
2. Average corneal power < 40.0 Diopters or > 47.0 Diopters
3. Calculated emmetropic IOL power > 3.0 Diopters of average power* for the specific lens type
4. Between eyes, the difference in.
   (a) Average corneal power > 1.0 Diopter
   (b) Axial length > 0.3 mm
   (c) Emmetropic IOL power > 1.0 Diopter

The Holladay 2 formula is unpublished but is available for purchase as part of the Holladay IOL Consultant program (Fig. 32.2). It requires inputs of, besides AL and K, phakic preop ACD, LT, CD and patient's age. Having more parameters enabled the Holladay 2 to appreciate the nuances of disproportionate eyes and render the calculation appropriately.

	Short	Normal	Long
Small	Nanophthalmia(1.8%)	Microcornea(1.5%)	Microcornea + Axial Myopia (0%)
Normal	Axial Hyperopia(6.9%)	Normal(73.4%)	Axial Myopia(13.5%)
Large	Megalocornea + Axial Hyperopia (0%)	Megalocornea(1.5%)	Buphthalmia(1.5%)

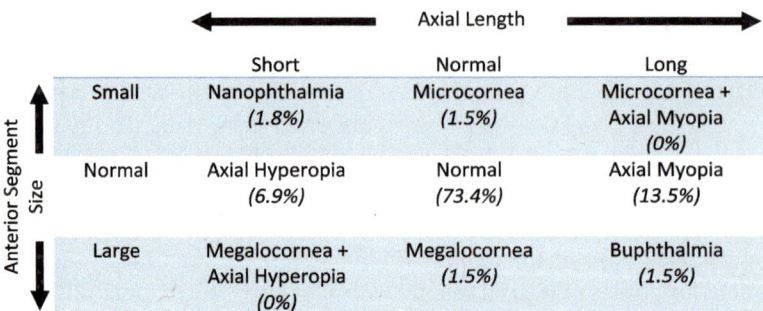

Fig. 32.2 Holladay JT MD. has categorized human eyes into nine categories (Fig. 32.2). This illustrates that the human is not necessarily proportional. This disparity poses a challenge to IOL power calculation, particularly in unusual eyes. Fortunately, most of the eyes are normal. Modern IOL power calculation formulas factored in the above into their algorithms

SRK/T

Using the Holladay 1 formula as a base but modifying so it will use the A constant of the SRK formula, Retzlaff published the SRK/T formula [15] in 1990. The SRK/T is a theoretical formula based on Fyodorov's Corneal Height formula [1] for the postoperative ELP prediction. The retinal thickness correction factor and the corneal refractive index are likewise optimized.

Relationship Between the Third-Generation Formulas and Axial Length

While most third-generation formulas perform well in normal eyes with axial lengths between 22.0 mm to 25.0 mm, these formulas perform less favorably beyond these confines. These formulas tend to have a higher percentage of hyperopic prediction errors in longer axial lengths and conversely, myopic outcomes in shorter axial lengths (Fig. 32.3).

Fam Adjusted

In 2009, Fam et al. [22] published a paper to optimize the relationship between the predicted refractive outcomes and axial lengths as measured by PCI biometry. The concept was based on 2 readjustments. The first readjustment, OAL1, was to reverse the initial calibration by Haigis [23] of the PCI against ultrasound biometry and thereby using the 'actual' optical axial length as measured by the PCI biometer. The second adjustment, OAL2, was converting 'actual optical axial length' to 'true optical path length' using the mean refractive index proposed by Olsen [24]. The smaller annulus keratometry measurement with the PCI biometer was also calibrated to the slightly larger mire of auto-keratometry. With these adjustments, the performance of the third-generation formulas on longer eyes improved (Fig. 32.4).

Wang-Koch Adjustment

Wang et al., in 2011 [25], proposed a set of adjustment equations to optimize the outcomes in eyes longer than 25 mm. The adjustments were shown to reduce the risk of hyperopic outcomes in patients with long eyes. It has been modified since then.

The T2 Formula

The T2 formula was described by Sheard, in 2010 [26]. Using a larger and more up-to-date database, Sheard was able to correct the non-physiological behavior of the quadratic function of the corneal height prediction of SRK/T first pointed out by Hoffer and then Haigis [27].

Haigis Formula

Haigis realized the importance of lens geometry on the ELP [28]. Thin lens formulas, by having just a single constant, neglect the effect of changing lens geometry with different IOL power, curvatures, thickness, and styles. In unusual eyes where the almost linear relationship between the ELP and axial length starts to deviate, the perfor-

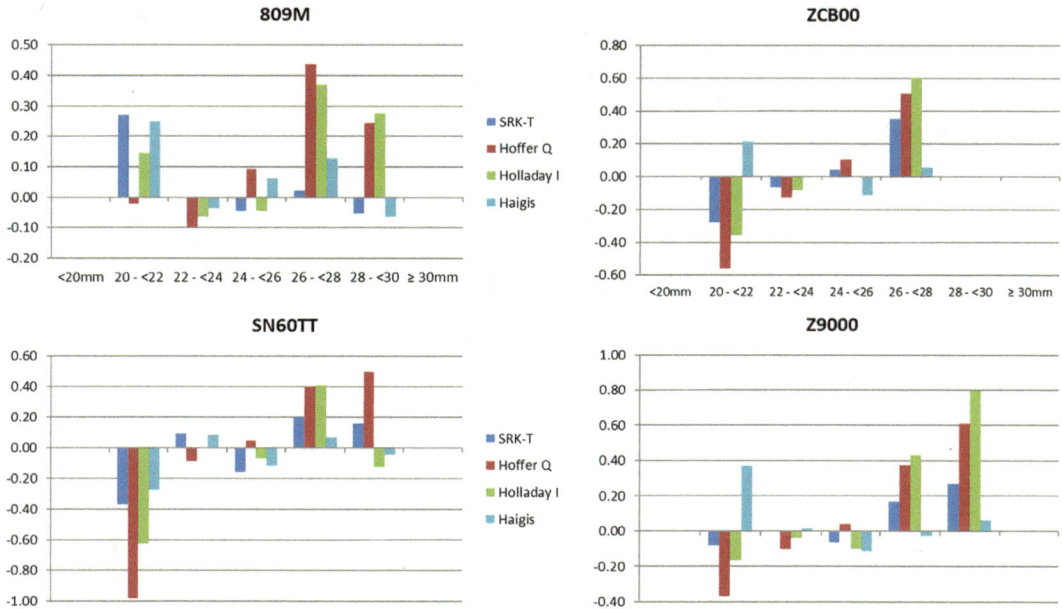

Fig. 32.3 The effect of axial lengths on the prediction errors of 4 theoretical formulas on 4 different IOLs. 3 of the 4 formulas showed hyperopic prediction errors with long axial lengths. Conversely, the same 3 formulas showed myopic tendency with shorter axial lengths with 3 IOLs

mances of these formulas start to falter. The Haigis formula, without resorting to the complexity of thick lens formulas, uses 3 lens constants (a_0, a_1 a_2) instead of one; and using the preoperative measured ACD instead of K as a variable which overcomes some of the problems of thin lens vergence formulas with short and long eyes.

In the Haigis formula, there are 2 types of constant optimization:

1. Classical optimization where one constant a_0 is optimized but not the other two. In this case, the formula performs as good, if not better than the other popular thin lens vergence formulas.
2. Full optimization where all three constants are optimized. This is when the full potential of the formula for wider ALs and lens types is achieved.

Regression Versus Theoretical Models

Regression formulas are entirely based on regression with a large database of postoperative outcomes. The larger the database, the better their predictability. More importantly, are the quality and integrity of the database. In theoretical formulas, regression with real-world postoperative results is utilized to refine its predictability. This is notably so in predicting the effective lens position and is embedded in the constants and correction factors of the formulas. Pure regression formulas (SRK and SRK II) are no longer recommended or used today.

Thin Lens Formula

The popular 3rd generation formulas for IOL power calculation like the Hoffer Q, Holladay 1, and the SRK/T are based on thin lens optics. A normal lens has a thickness and two refracting surfaces. In thin lens optics, the thickness of the lens is ignored, and its two refracting surfaces are reduced to a single plane thin lens. It is assumed that all refractions of light occur in that single plane. The advantage of the thin lens formula is that it simplifies the calculation and circumvents the difficulty of measuring certain parameters often not obtainable.

The popular formulas of Hoffer Q [17], Holladay 1 [14], and SRK/T [15] are based on thin

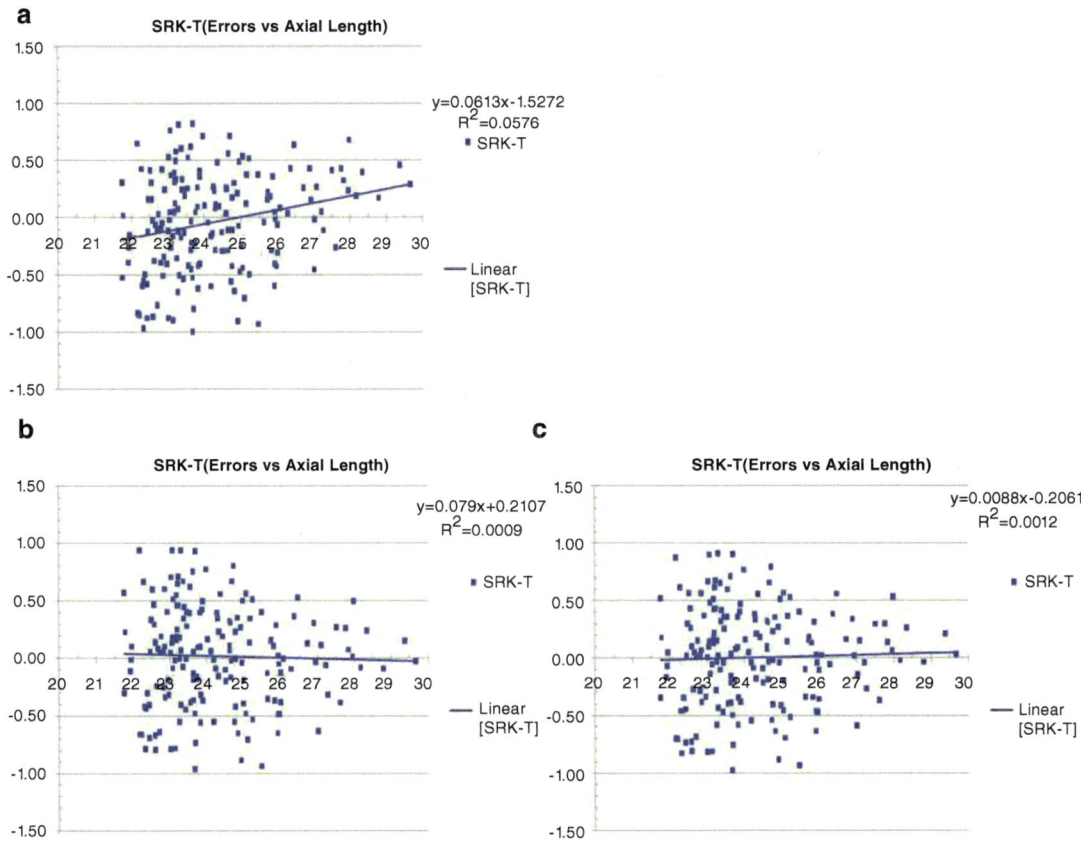

Fig. 32.4 (**a**) SRK/T outcomes with inputs from PCI. (**b**) SRK/T outcomes with OAL1-K readjustment and (**c**) SRK/T outcomes with OAL2-K readjustment. The abscissas are axial length in mm and the ordinates the prediction error

lens optics. Haigis [28] subsequently developed an improved thin lens formula by using a thick lens algorithm and regressing the ELP with pre-operative data. Unlike the other 3 formulas, Haigis' ELP is derived ELP from the measured axial length and the preoperative anterior chamber depth.

The Impact of Optical Biometry

In ultrasound biometry, axial length measurement error alone accounted for 54% to 68% of the total prediction error according to Olsen [29]. With the availability of optical biometry, the source of error from axial length measurement decreased substantially from 0.65 D to 0.43 D or 30 to 40% of the total prediction error according to Olsen [30]. The repeatability of optical biometry was

reduced from an SD of ±0.11 mm to ±0.03 mm [31]. Despite the improvement in AL measurement, this precision is not reflected in reducing prediction error according to Olsen [30]. This less than encouraging improvement was probably overshadowed and supplanted by the ACD prediction error, a function of IOL power calculation formulas [31].

Newer formulas can leverage the ever improving accuracy of biometric measurement and the quantum leap improvement in computational power to improve the precision and sophistication toward better outcomes and predictability.

In the last decade, many new and better formulas have emerged, making use of the heightened accuracy of the newer biometers and increasing computational power. It is not feasible to go through all the formulas and this article does not claim to be exhaustive.

Ladas Super Formula (LSF) 1.0

The Hoffer Q, Holladay 1, and SRK/T formulas have different optimal ranges for better outcomes, first proven and published by Hoffer in 1993. The Ladas Super Formula blends the proven popular formulas of Hoffer Q, Holladay 1 (with and without Wang-Koch adjustment [25], Haigis and SRK/T using a 3-dimensional model to determine the best power for each eye [32] based on its 2 to 3 variables inputs. This formula was originally developed by Ladas and subsequently included Siddiqui, Devgan, and Jun. The method has now been enhanced with artificial intelligence. www.iolcalc.com.

Kane Formula

Developed by Jack X Kane, [33–35] the Kane formula is an unpublished formula based on theoretical optics with refinements through both regression and artificial intelligence. It was developed using approximately 30,000 eyes from various cataract practices. The required parameters are AL, K, ACD, and gender with LT and CCT being optional. Various studies have reported excellent outcomes with this formula. The formula is available on www.iolformula.com.

Panacea

This is a thin lens vergence formula developed by David Flikier. It is a 5-variable calculator using AL, K, ACD, LT; and to date the only formula that can utilize the asphericity Q value of the anterior corneal curvature and the anterior-to-posterior corneal curvature ratio [36]. It uses a demographic to statistically data screen the quality of the various inputs. This formula is available only for downloading at www.panaceaiolandtoriccalculator.com.

VRF-G

The VRF is a published vergence-based thin lens formula by Voytsekivskyy [37]. The VRF-G is a newer improved unpublished formula [38, 39]. The latter formula is based on theoretical optics with ray-tracing components; further refined through regression. This is an 8-variables formula.

Castrop

Castrop is a hybrid thin and thick lens formula [40]. It considers the cornea as a thick lens. It uses a constant like the Olsen C constant and readjusts the axial length based on Cooke's sum-of-segments approach. Finally, besides the IOL constant that is integral to the equation, it uses a second constant, offset R to the final dioptric power. The formula requires mandatory AL, ACD, and K inputs, with CCT and Post K being optional.

Thick Lens Formula

The third-generation formulas are simple thin lens formulas that do not require complex calculations. A simple calculator would be sufficient for the formula to be executed. Thin lens formulas are based on the Gullstrand eye model that assumed a fixed ratio of anterior to posterior corneal curvature and a keratometric index of refraction of 1.3375. The systematic deviations of these thin lens assumptions are compensated by the IOL constants. A thin lens formula assumed all the IOL powers of the same IOL model to have the same lens constant. This works reasonably well for the average eye requiring the average IOL power. Despite being the same IOL model, as the IOL power changes: its two curvatures, the ratio of its curvatures, and the lens thickness change. These changes will shift the ELP of the IOL.

Similarly, as the measuring devices become more accurate and comprehensive, more parameters can be measured accurately and be included in the computation of IOL power, without the risk of increasing the errors of propagation.

Barrett Universal II and EVO are thick lens formulas. In simpler terms, these formulas, like the third-generation formulas, predict the ACD of the IOL in the eye. After determining the initial ACD for the eye, the formulas iterate to determine the final ELP and thence the final IOL power for the eye. These iterative calculations are far more complex and require the power of modern-day computers.

Barrett Universal II (BUII) Formula

The concept behind the Barrett Universal formula was first described by Barrett himself in 1987 [41] and further elucidated in 1993 [42]. The Barrett Universal II (BUII) is a further refinement of the Barrett Universal formula and includes the use of more variables such as ACD, LT, and radius of curvature of the posterior cornea. These latter additional parameters have reached a high level of precision (with today's optical biometers) to be used confidently.

The BUII heralded in a new era of IOL power calculation formulas, with improved and consistent performances [43]. AL and K inputs are mandatory with ACD, LT, and CD being optional. With the accessibility to corneal thickness (CCT) and posterior corneal curvature (PK) in newer biometers, these variables are now additional optional variables for the formula.

Næser Formula

Conceptualized by Kristian Næser, this is a paraxial, step-along formula that considers the IOL a thick lens. The difference between Næser 1 [44] and Næser 2 [45] are on the source of the IOL architecture. Næser 1 uses the available information on the IOL architecture from the manufacturers (Cutting Card), whereas Næser 2 derived this information from open, commercial but nonproprietary sources. Also, the measured AL is optimized for different axial lengths.

EVO

Emmetropia Verifying Optical (EVO) formula is a thick lens formula developed by TK Yeo. The formula is based on the emmetropization concept of a normal eye and is constantly updated and improved. Presently, it requires mandatory AL and K inputs, with ACD, LT and CCT being optional, has recently been updated to include posterior cornea curvature.

PEARL-DGS

This is a thick lens IOL formula that relies on artificial intelligence of machine learning and modeling to predict ELP and fine-tuning of outputs for extreme biometric values. This formula

was developed by G. Debellemanière, D. Gatinel and A. Saad. The formula is accessible at iol-solver.com.

Ray Tracing

Ray tracing is a method for calculating the path of individual rays through the various elements in an optical system. These various elements, with their surfaces and refractive indices, bend and change the passing light path. These individual rays are traced and calculated as they are refracted at each of these surfaces according to Snell's law [46]. Ray tracing may be limited to just the paraxial rays or cover any area on the pupil. The former neglects higher-order aberration, while the latter takes account of them and allows predicting the IOL power that provides the best visual quality.

Olsen Formula

First published by Olsen in 1987 [47], this formula has undergone many upgrades and refinement over the years [48, 49]. The latest is based on thick-lens ray-tracing optics. The uniqueness of this formula is the C constant concept [50] that generates the ELP based on the preoperative measurements of ACD and LT but can be additionally tweaked by AL and K, if desirable. The Olsen formula is available as an option in the LenStar biometer or as a standalone PhacoOptics program for purchase (www.phacooptics.net). The Olsen formula (Olsen2P = Olsen 2 parameters) that is preinstalled in biometers uses 2 parameters: ACD and LT to predict the C constant. The Olsen formula (Olsen4P) in the standalone PhacoOptics program uses 4 parameters, besides ACD and LT, AL, and K as well.

Okulix

Okulix is a standalone computer program that calculates IOL power based on ray-tracing the optical path of single rays that pass through the ocular structure. It uses measured parameters that are fed directly via computer interfacing from the biometers and corneal tomographers. Parameters can also be entered manually, where interfacing is not available. The program includes a compilation of IOL geometry of commonly used IOLs.

CSO Method

Two corneal tomographers (developed by the Italian company CSO) include a software module that performs IOL power calculations based on exact ray tracing: Sirius is a Scheimpflug-Placido device, and MS 39 is an OCT-Placido instrument. Corneal surfaces as well as actual IOL data are raytraced to calculate the optical performance of the eye and select the IOL power that will produce the targeted refraction or the best visual quality.

Regression Methods

To improve the accuracy of the early 2nd generation (R Binkhorst, regression formulas were born). The regression formulas are derived empirically from analyzing the relationship between the preoperative biometric measurements and the postoperative refractive outcomes. Using a large outcomes database, the relationship below was established.

$$P \propto A + bK + c\text{AL}$$

Where P is the IOL power, A is the A constant; b and c are constants; K is the keratometry power and AL is the axial length.

It was first introduced by Thomas Lloyd (a technician with James Gills) [51] and followed first by John Retzlaff [52, 53] and then by Donald Sanders [54] & Manus Kraff. After the latter 3 combined forces, the SRK formula by Sanders, Retzlaff, and Kraff became the most established regression formula. It underwent subsequent revision (SRK II by Sanders) to compensate for the non-linear relationship between the intraocular lens power and the axial length. The SRK II was popular during the 1980s. It was superseded by the later more accurate 3rd generation theoretical formulas.

Artificial Intelligence (AI)

AI examines huge data efficiently and differently from how we humans do; it identifies relationships, patterns, and trends that escape us. AI has been used in medicine, but these are mainly for image classification and object recognition. IOL power calculation is now benefiting from AI as well.

Critical to the success of AI is a large and sound "training" dataset. AI learns from its dataset through interpreting and unraveling, to achieve the desired goal. An accurate and consistent dataset is indispensable to good machine learning. With a large and accurate dataset, AI can figure out the complex relationships between the many biometric parameters that may not fit traditional eye models or Gaussian optics.

Datasets from different devices may have to be interpreted differently, or at the very least adjusted and optimized to the device. Newer IOLs with novel optical structures that have yet to attain a sufficient sizable dataset may pose a challenge for AI. As AI learning capabilities improve, it may be able to adapt to parameters from different devices and bridge newer IOLs.

Despite these challenges, the future of AI is bright. It has already markedly improved outcomes as shown by some formulas such as RBF 3.0, Hoffer QST and PEARL-DGS. As the datasets get larger, these formulas improve further as typified by the version numbers. More and more parameters are being utilized as the neuronal circuits are refined and expanded.

Radial Basis Function (RBF)

Developed by Hill and his team, this formula is based on radial basis function (RBF), a machine-learning form of artificial intelligence. RBF with its multidimensions pattern recognition and adaptive neural learning process is appropriate to these real-world challenges of IOL power calculation. The formula is constantly being updated as more and more data is available to refine the process. At last look, the formula has been updated to version 3.0 with an expanded domain.

RBF is available as an option on some devices as well as online at www.rbfcalculator.com. The required variables are AL, K, and ACD with LT, CCT, and CD as options.

BART

This update on the development of Bayesian Additive Regression Trees (BART) [55] was described by Clarke et al. in 2020. This is an AI method using a machine-learned algorithm that sums decision trees. It gauges its accuracy using Monte Carlo simulations and generates intervals of possible lens powers with a probability density. Over a fivefold cross-validation process, the result of BART was an SD of 0.242 D compared to 0.416 (Holladay 1), 0.569 D (RBF 1.0), 0.575 D (SRK/T), 0.936 D (Hoffer Q), and 1.48 D (Haigis). The results were without optimizing the constants (which might be unfair to some of the formulas). MedAE was 0.204 D (BART), 0.416 D (Holladay 1), 0.676 D (RBF 1.0), 0.714 D (SRK/T), 0.936 D for Hoffer Q, and 1.204 D for Haigis. BART prediction achieved 89.5% within +/-0.50 D of prediction error, RBF 1.0 was 61.4%, and SRK/T with 52.0%.

Ladas Super Formula (LSF) 2.0

This formula uses machine learning algorithms to refine the prediction of the original LSF 1.0. using AL, K, and ACD as inputs. In a sample of 101 eyes implanted with the same IOL Taroni found in 2020, that this formula was one of the best performers among several modern formulas with a median absolute error of 0.22 D [56].

Intraoperative Aberrometry

ORA

Optiwave Refractive Analysis (ORA) is a methodology first proposed by Ianchulev in 2005 [57, 58]. This intraoperative Talbot-Moiré interferom-etry measures the ocular wavefront aberrations after removal of the crystalline lens in surgery. The captured real-time wavefront information is used to determine the aphakic spherical equivalent of the eye and thence calculate the proper desired IOL power. The system is independent of AL and K.

Conclusion

Today, there is an explosion of new IOL power calculation formulas and methods. This is a welcome development, as today patients are expecting better refractive outcomes. The newer formulas have shown to be more accurate than the once eminently popular third-generation formulas. As the hardware and computational power improve, we can expect even better formulas [1].

References

1. Koch D, Hill W, Abulafia A, Wang L. Pursuing perfection in intraocular lens calculations: 1. Logical approach for classifying IOL calculation formulas. J Cataract Refract Surg. 2017;43:717–8.
2. Savini G, Hoffer KJ, Kohnen T. IOL power formula classifications (Guest Editorial). J Cataract Refract Surg. 2024;50(2):105. https://doi.org/10.1097/j.jcrs.0000000000001378.
3. Fyodorov S, Kolonko A. Estimation of optical power of the intraocular lens. Vestnik Oftalmologic (Moscow). 1967;4:27.
4. Colenbrander M. Calculations of the power of an iris clip lens for distance vision. Br J Ophthalmol. 1973;57:735–40.
5. Thijssen J. The emmetropic and iseikonic implant lens: Computer calculation of the refractive power and its accuracy. Ophthlmologica. 1976;171:467–86.
6. van der Heijde G. The optical correction of unilateral aphakia. Trans Am Academy Ophthalmol Otolaryngol. 1976;81:80–8.
7. Hoffer KJ. Intraocular lens calculation: the problem of the short eye {Hoffer Formula}. Ophthalmic Surg. 1981;12(4):269–72.
8. Binkhorst R. The optical design of intraocular lens calculation. Arch Ophthalmol. 1981;99:1819–23.
9. Binkhorst, R. (1984). Intraocular lens power calculation manual: A guide to the Author's TICC-40 Programs, Edition 3. New York.
10. Shammas H. The fudged formula for intraocular lens power calculations. J Cataract Refract Surg. 1982;8:350–2.

11. Hoffer K. The effect of axial length on posterior chamber lenses and posterior capsule position. Curr Concept Ophthalmol Surg. 1984a;1:20–2.

12. Hoffer K. The effect of axial length on posterior chamber lenses and posterior capsule position. Curr Concept in Ophthal Surg. 1984b;1:20–2.

13. Olsen T. Prediction of intraocular lens position after cataract extraction. J Cataract Refract Surg. 1986;12(7):376–9.

14. Holladay J, Prager T, Chandler T, Musgrove K. A three-part system for refining intraocular lens power calculations. J Cataract Refract Surg. 1988;14:17–24.

15. Retzlaff JA, Sanders DR, Kraff MC. Development of the SRK/T intraocular lens power calculation formula. J Cataract Refract Surg. 1990;16:333–40. Errata: 1990;16:528 and 1993;19(5):444–446

16. Holladay J. Holladay IOL consultant user's guide and reference manual. Houston: Holladay LASIK Institute; 1999.

17. Hoffer KJ. The Hoffer Q formula: A comparison of theoretic and regression formulas. J Cataract Refract Surg. 1993;19(11):700–12. Errata: 1994;20(6):677 and 2007;33(1):2–3

18. Melles R, Holladay J, Chang W. Accuracy of intraocular lens calculation. Ophthalmol. 2018;125:169–78.

19. Melles R, Kane J, Olsen T, Chang W. Update on intraocular lens calculation formulas. Ophthalmol. 2019;1226:1334–5.

20. Savini G, Di Maita M, Hoffer K, Næser K, Schiano-Lomoriello D, Vagge A, et al. Comparison of 13 formulas for IOL power calculation with measurments from partial coherence interferometry. Br J Ophthalmol. 2021;105(4):484–9. https://doi.org/10.1136/bjophthalmol-2021-316193.

21. Hoffer KJ. Biometry of 7,500 cataractous eyes. Am J Ophthalmol. 1980;90(3):360–8., Erratum: 1980;90(6):890. https://doi.org/10.1016/S0002-9394(14)74917-7.

22. FAM H, Lim K. Improving refractive outcomes at extreme axial lengths with the IOLMaster: the optical axial length and keratometric transformation. Br J Ophthalmol. 2009;93:678–83.

23. Haigis W, Lege B, Miller N. Comparison of immersion ultrasound biometry and partial coherence interferometry for intraocular lens calculation according to Haigis. Graefes Arch Clin Exp Ophthalmol. 2000;238:765–73.

24. Olsen T, Thorwest M. Calibration of axial length measurements with Zeiss IOLMaster. J Cataract Refract Surg. 2005;31:1345–50.

25. Wang L, Shirayama M, Ma X. Optimizing intraocular lens power calculations in eyes with axial lengths above 25mm. J Cataract Refract Surg. 2011;37:2018–27.

26. Sheard R, Smith G, Cooke D. Improving the prediction accuracy of the SRK/T formula: the T2 formula. J Cataract Refract Surg. 2010;36:1829–34.

27. Haigis W. Occurrence of erroneous anterior chamber depth in the SRK/T formula. J Cataract Refract Surg. 1993;19:442–6.

28. Haigis W, Waller W, Duzanec Z, Voeske W. Postoperative biometry and keratometry after posterior chamber lens implantation. Eur J Implant Ref Surg. 1990;2:191–202.

29. Olsen T. Sources of error in intraocular lens power calculations. J Cataract Refract Surg. 1992;18:125–9.

30. Olsen T. Improved accuracy of intraocular lens power calculation with the Zeiss IOLMaster. Acta Ophthalmol Scand. 2007;85:84–7.

31. Norrby S. Sources of error in intraocular lens power calculation. J Cataract Refract Surg. 2008;34:368–76.

32. Ladas J, Siddiqui A, Devgan U. A 3-D "Super Surface" combining modern intraocular lens formulas to generate a "Super Formula" and maximize accuracy. JAMA Ophthalmol. 2015;133:1431–6.

33. Kane J, van Heerden A, Atik A, Petsoglou C. Intraocular lens power formula accuracy: comparison of 7 formulas. J Cataract Refract Surg. 2016;42:1490–500.

34. Kane J, van Heerden A, Atik A, Petsoglou C. Accuracy of 3 new methods for intraocular lens power selection. J Cataract Refract Surg. 2017;43:333–9.

35. Reitblat O, Gali H, Chou L, Bahar I, Weinreb R, Afshari N, Sella R. Intraocular lens power calculation in the elderly population using the Kane formula in comparison with existing methods. J Cataract Refract Surg. 2020;46:1501–7.

36. Savini G, Taroni L, Hoffer K. Recent developments in intraocular lens power calculation methods - update 2020. Ann Transl Med. 2020c;8(22):1553.

37. Voytsekhivskyy O. Development and clinical accuracy of a new intraocular lens power formula (VRF) compared to other formulas. Am J Ophthalmol. 2018;185:56–67.

38. Hipólito-Fernandes D, Luis M, Gil P, Maduro V, Fejiao J, Yeo T, et al. VRF-G, a new intraocular lens power calculation formula: a 13 formulas comparison study. Clin Ophthalmol. 2020a;14:4395–402.

39. Hipólito-Fernandes D, Luis M, Serras-Pereira R, Gil P, Maduro V, Feijóão J, Alves N. Anterior chamber depth, lens thickness and intraocular lens calculation formula accuracy: nine formulas comparison. Br J Ophthalmol. 2020b;0:1–7.

40. Wendelstein J, Hoffmann P, Hirnschall N, Fischinger I, Mariacher S, Wingert T, et al. Project hyperopic power prediction: accuracy of 13 different concepts for intraocular lens calculation in short eyes. Br J Ophthalmol. 2021;0:1–7.

41. Barrett G. Intraocular lens calculation formulas for new intraocular lens implants. J Cataract Refract Surg. 1987;13:389–96.

42. Barrett G. An improved universal theoretical formula for intraocular lens power prediction. J Cataract Refract Surg. 1993;19:713–20.

43. Turnbull A, Hill W, Barrett G. Accuracy of intraocular lens power calculation methods when targeting low myopia in monovision. J Cataract Refract Surg. 2020;46:862–6.

44. Naeser K. Intraocular lens power formula based on vergence calculation and lens design. J Cataract Refract Surg. 1997;23:1200–7.

45. Naeser K, Savini G. Accuracy of thick-lens intraocular lens power calculation based on cutting-card or calculated data for lens architecture. J Cataract Refract Surg. 2019;45:1422–9.

46. Preussner P, Wahl J, Lahdo H, Burkhard D, Findl O. Ray tracing for intraocular lens calculation. J Cataract Refract Surg. 2002;28:1412–9.

47. Olsen T. Theoretical approach to intraocular lens calculation using Gaussian optics. J Cataract Refract Surg. 1987;13:141–5.

48. Olsen T, Corydon L, Gimbel H. Intraocular lens power calculation with an improved anterior chamber depth prediction algorithm. J Cataract Refract Surg. 1995;21:313–9.

49. Olsen T. Prediction of effective postoperative (intraocular lens) anterior chamber depth. J Cataract Refract Surg. 2006;32:419–24.

50. Olsen T. C Constant: new concept for ray tracing-assisted intraocular lens power calculation. J Cataract Refract Surg. 2014;40:764–73.

51. Gills J. Minimizing postoperative refractive error. Cont Intraocular Lens Med J. 1980;6:56–9.

52. Retzlaff J. A new intraocular lens calculation formula. J Cataract Refract Surg. 1980a;6:148–52.

53. Retzlaff J. Posterior chamber implant power calculation: regression formulas. J Cataract Refract Surg. 1980b;6:268–70.

54. Sanders D. Improvement of intraocular lens power calculation using empirical data. J Cataract Refract Surg. 1980;6:263–7.

55. Clarke G, Kapelner A. The Bayesian Additive Regression Trees formula for safe machine learning-based intraocular lens predictions. Front Big Data. 2020;3:572134.

56. Taroni LHK-L. Outcomes of IOL power calculation using measurements by a rotating Scheimpflug camera combined with partial coherence interferometry. J Cataract Refract Sur. 2020;46(12):1618–23.

57. Ianchulev T, Salz J, Hoffer K. Intraoperative optical refractive biometry for intraocular lens power estimation without axial length and keratometry measurements. J Cataract Refract Surg. 2005;31:1530–6.

58. Raufi N, James C, Kua A, Vann R. Intraoperative aberrometry vs preoperative formulas in predicting intraocular lens power. J Cataract Refract Surg. 2020;46:857–61.

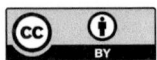

Outcomes Review of Intraocular Lens Power Calculation Formulas

33

Han Bor Fam

Acronyms

AE	Absolute error
ME	Mean (numerical) prediction error
MAE	Mean absolute error
MedAE	Median absolute error
OLCR	Optical low-coherence reflectometry (Lenstar LS900, Haag-Streit AG, Kõniz, Switzerland)
Olsen2P	Device preinstalled Olsen (utilizing 2 parameters, ACD and LT to determine ELP
Olsen4P	Standalone Olsen from PhacoOptics (4 determinants, ACD, LT, AL, and K, of ELP)
P_{emme}	Emmetropic IOL power for the specific eye
PCI	Partial coherence interferometry
PI	Performance Index
PE	Prediction error (numerical)
SS-OCT	Swept-source optical coherence tomography
WK	Formula specific Wang-Koch adjustment for axial length for long eye

H. B. Fam (✉)
National Healthcare Group Eye Institute, Tan Tock Seng Hospital, Singapore, Singapore

In Memory of Wolfgang Haigis

The late Wolfgang Haigis proposed a concept of quality metrics of measuring the performance IOL power calculation formulas. The final index is known as the IOL formula performance index, **PI**. This is a quantitative analysis. For a good and fair comparison, the constants should be optimized before analyzing their performances. This eliminates the bias of the lens constant that was chosen for the analysis. After optimizing the constants, the formulas are compared on their standard deviation, SD_{ME}, of prediction (numerical) error; the median absolute error, **MedAE**; the dependency of prediction error on axial length, **m**, and; finally, the reciprocal of the percentage of predicted refraction within ±1.00 D, **n10**.

A good formula comparison is when, ME = 0:

1. $SD_{ME} \rightarrow 0$
2. $MedAE \rightarrow 0$

3. $|m| = \dfrac{\Delta PE}{\Delta AL} \rightarrow 0$

4. $\dfrac{1}{n_{10}} \rightarrow 0$

*where **ME** is the Mean (numerical) prediction error of the formula and should be zero when the constant is optimized. PE is the prediction error. **SD**_{ME} is the standard deviation of prediction (numerical) error; **MedAE** is the median absolute*

© The Author(s) 2024
J. Aramberri et al. (eds.), *Intraocular Lens Calculations*, Essentials in Ophthalmology, https://doi.org/10.1007/978-3-031-50666-6_33

*error; |m| is the absolute gradient of the relationship of prediction error with axial length; and finally, **n**10 is the percentage of eyes within ±1.00 D of predicted spherical equivalent refraction target.*

Thereafter, $f = \text{SD}_{ME} + \text{MedAE} + 10 * |m| + 10 * (n_{10})^{-1}$

Finally, the IOL formula performance index, PI

$$PI = \frac{1}{f} = \frac{1}{\text{SD}_{ME} + \text{MedAE} + 10 * |m| + 10 * (n_{10})^{-1}}$$

The metrics $|m|$ and **n10**−1 were amplified by a factor of 10 because of their small values. Absolute values are used to prevent false reduction of outcomes. In any case, a good formula should be independent of axial length. Whether positive or negative gradient would denote dependency of formula on axial length.

Modification

Wolfgang Haigis first presented the above metric in an ESCRS Meeting and it is available to view on the ESCRS website. It was updated and published in JCRS in 20 [1] which is the only publication of it to date. Today [1], the newer formulas have become more accurate and therefore some updates to his original concept are due to allow for better resolution. There is an increasing emphasis on the importance of MAE, and rightly so, since this should be included as a metric. Besides n_{10}, n_5 is added also is. n_5 which is defined as the reciprocal of the percentage of correctly predicted refractions within ±0.50 D. This should provide a better resolution. n_{10} is kept as a safety metric. n_5 and n_{10} are normalized by multiply by 20.

Besides having a dependency on AL, some formulas also exhibit bias against K. For more detailed analysis, the relationship between prediction outcomes and K is also included as a metric in the modified Haigis index.

With the additional metrics to the equation, the PI becomes:

$$f = \text{SD}_{ME} + \text{MAE} + \text{MedAE} + 10 * |m| + 3 * |k| + 20 * (n_5)^{-1} + 20 * (n_{10})^{-1}$$

$$PI = \frac{1}{f} = \frac{1}{\text{SD}_{ME} + \text{MAE} + \text{MedAE} + 10 * |m| + 3 * |k| + 20 * (n_5)^{-1} + 20 * (n_{10})^{-1}}$$

where $|k|$ is the gradient, $\left(\dfrac{\Delta PE}{\Delta k}\right)$ of prediction *error against keratometry. **MAE** is the mean absolute error.*

Application

It must be noted at the outset of evaluating these formulas, that the author of the Hoffer Q formula [2, 3] recommended it primarily for short eyes (<22.0 mm) and never for eyes with an AL greater than 24.5 mm and definitely not for very long eyes (>26.0 mm), yet most of these studies evaluated the Hoffer Q over the full range of ALs, thus insuring it's rating would be rather low.

In 2017, Fam presented a paper at the annual conference of the Asia-Pacific Association of Cataract and Refractive Surgeons (APACRS) [4]. The paper detailed the outcomes of a single IOL, ZCB00. A total of 291 eyes from 291 patients with preoperative biometry measured with partial coherent interferometry (PCI) (IOLMaster 500) and postoperative refractions carried out between 4 and 6 weeks. All the third-generation formulas are calculated using constants from a previous pool of patients. Barrett Universal II (BUII) [5, 6], EVO, and RBF are based on using an optimized A constant from the same pool of patients. BUII, EVO 1.0, and RBF 1.0 were more accurate than the third-generation theoretical formulas. The Haigis formula, both with personalized triple optimization and ULIB constants, did also very well (see Fig. 33.1, Table 33.1).

Using the modified Haigis' quality metrics on IOL power calculation formula, as described in Table 33.1, the following f values and performance indices are generated for the above data. These values are tabulated in Table 33.2 and featured in Fig. 33.2.

Unfortunately, the bias of the prediction errors against K and AL were not available in most studies in this review and therefore have to be omitted as metrics. Ideally, only optimized constants should be used when comparing formulas. In this review, not all studies were based on optimized constants, especially in subgroup analyses. In this review, ME would be omitted in the ranking of formulas in general studies across ALs. This is to avoid a systematic error. For subgroup analyses, PE would be included as a metric to capture bias against the subgroup.

For analysis of the general group, the following metrics would be included:

1. Standard deviation of prediction error SD_{ME} 0
2. Mean absolute error MAE 0
   Mean Absolute Error MedAE 0
3. Percentage of error within ±0.5D $n_5^{-1} = \dfrac{1}{n_5}0$
4. Percentage of error within ±1.0D $n_{10}^{-1} = \dfrac{n_5^{-1}}{n_{10}}0$

f is the sum of all the above metrics:

$$f = SD_{ME} + MAE + MedAE + 20*(n_5)^{-1} + 20*n_{10}^{-1}$$

and finally **PI**, the **performance index:**

$$PI = \frac{1}{f} = \frac{1}{SD_{ME} + MAE + MedAE + 20*(n_5)^{-1} + 20*(n_{10})^{-1}}$$

The following metrics will be used for analyzing subgroup studies:

1. Absolute mean numerical prediction error [ME] 0
2. Standard deviation of prediction error SD_{ME} 0
3. Mean absolute error MAE 0
4. Median absolute error MedAE 0
5. Percentage of error within ±0.50 D $n_5^{-1} = \dfrac{1}{n_5}0$
6. Percentage of error within ±1.00 D $n_{10}^{-1} = \dfrac{n_5^{-1}}{n_{10}}0$

f is the sum of all the above metrics:

$$f = |ME| + SD_{ME} + MAE + MedAE + 20*(n_5)^{-1} + 20*n_{10}^{-1}$$

and finally **PI$_{sub}$**, the **performance index (subgroup):**

$$PI_{sub} = \frac{1}{f} = \frac{1}{|ME| + SD_{ME} + MAE + MedAE + 20*(n_5)^{-1} + 20*(n_{10})^{-1}}$$

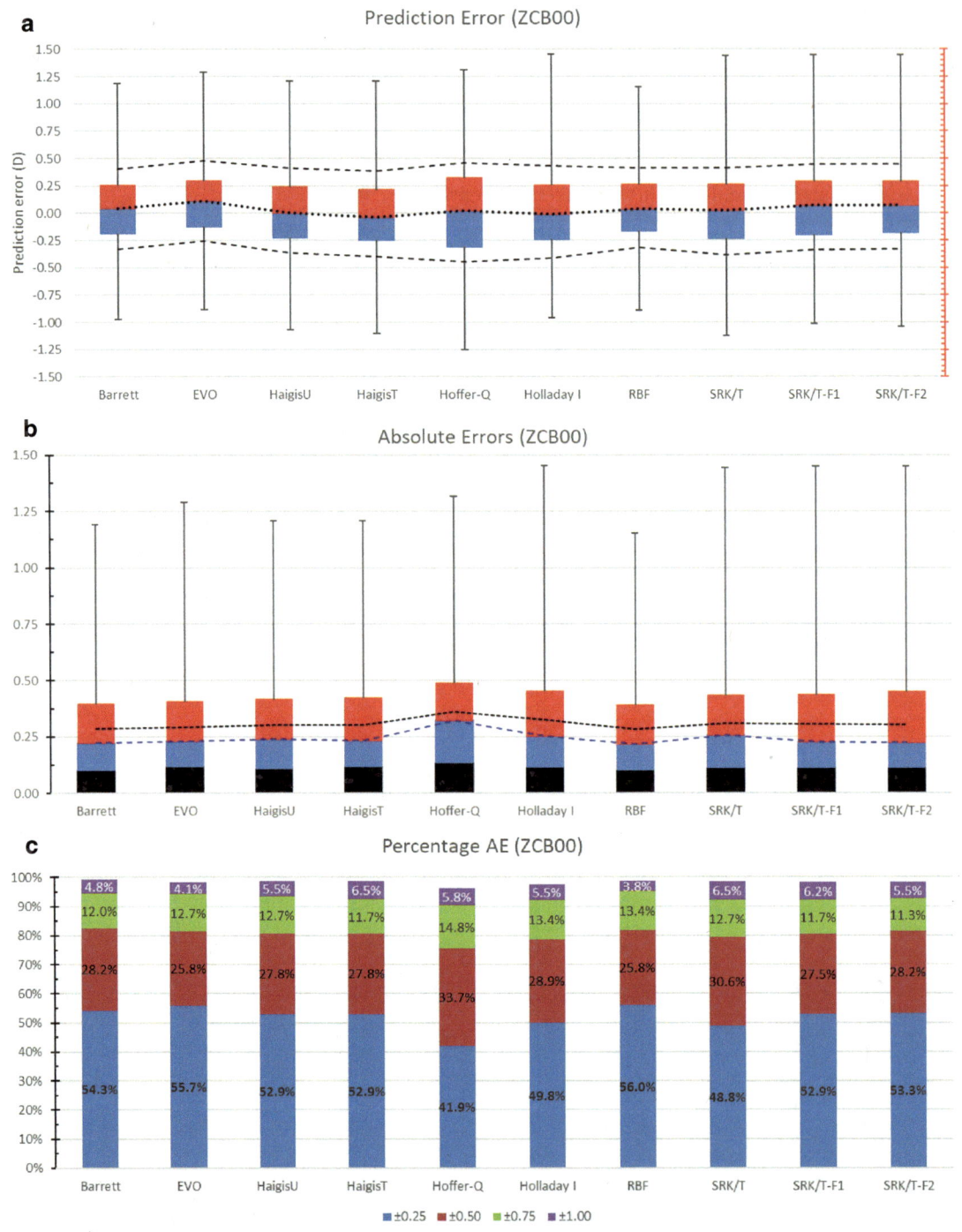

Fig. 33.1 This Figure and Table 33.1 depict the outcomes of the various formulas. (**a**) The spread of the prediction errors of the eyes of the different formulas. The bottom and top error plots represent the lower and upper quartiles while the blue and red boxes, the second and third quartiles. The dotted line is the mean prediction errors and the dashed lines, the lower and upper SDs. (**b**) is a graph showing the absolute errors of the formulas. The MAE and MedAE are represented by the dotted line and blue dashed lines, respectively. Chart (**c**) is a stacked histogram showing the percentage of eyes within a predicted spherical equivalent (SE) (EVO is EVO 1.0; HaigisT is Haigis with personalized triple optimization; HaigisU is Haigis with ULIB constants; RBF is RBF 1.0. SRK/T-F1 [10–12] and SRK/T-F2 are the Fam-adjusted SRK/T formulas [13] (Fam, The Formula1 of IOL Power Calculation [7])

Table 33.1 This table shows the results of the various formulas (EVO is EVO 1.0; HaigisT is Haigis with personalized triple optimization; HaigisU is Haigis with ULIB constants; RBF is RBF 1.0) [7]. The ±0.50 D is in bold and important clinically, as are ±1.00 D

Formula	n	MeanPE	SD E	MAE	MedAE	±0.25 D	±0.50 D	±0.75 D	±1.00 D
Barrett	291	0.04	0.37	*0.28*	*0.22*	54.3%	**82.5%**	94.5%	**99.3%**
EVO	291	0.11	0.37	*0.29*	*0.23*	55.7%	**81.4%**	94.2%	**98.3%**
HaigisT	291	−0.01	0.39	*0.30*	*0.23*	52.9%	**80.8%**	92.4%	**99.0%**
HaigisU	291	0.02	0.39	*0.30*	*0.24*	52.9%	**80.8%**	93.5%	**99.0%**
Hoffer Q	291	0.01	0.46	*0.36*	*0.32*	41.9%	**75.6%**	90.4%	**96.2%**
Holladay I [8, 9]	291	0.01	0.42	*0.32*	*0.25*	49.8%	**78.7%**	92.1%	**97.6%**
RBF	291	0.05	0.36	*0.28*	*0.22*	56.0%	**81.8%**	95.2%	**99.0%**
SRK/T	291	0.02	0.40	*0.31*	*0.26*	48.8%	**79.4%**	92.1%	**98.6%**
SRK/T-F1	291	0.05	0.39	*0.31*	*0.23*	52.9%	**80.4%**	92.1%	**98.3%**
SRK/T-F2	291	0.06	0.39	*0.30*	*0.22*	53.3%	**81.4%**	92.8%	**98.3%**

Table 33.2 This table shows the values of the Haigis quality metrics based on the data from the previous table

Formula	±0.50	±1.00	mAL	mK	f	PI
Barrett	0.012	0.010	0.046	−0.027	**1.757**	**0.569**
EVO	0.012	0.010	−0.004	−0.019	**1.334**	**0.750**
HaigisT	0.012	0.010	−0.011	0.093	**1.663**	**0.601**
HaigisU	0.012	0.010	0.007	0.082	**1.590**	**0.629**
Hoffer-Q	0.013	0.010	0.162	0.002	**3.134**	**0.319**
Holladay I	0.013	0.010	0.142	−0.045	**2.907**	**0.344**
Hill-RBF	0.012	0.010	0.042	−0.009	**1.654**	**0.604**
SRK/T	0.013	0.010	0.089	−0.105	**2.521**	**0.397**
SRK/T-F1	0.012	0.010	0.079	−0.091	**2.336**	**0.428**
SRK/T-F2	0.012	0.010	0.065	−0.088	**2.172**	**0.460**

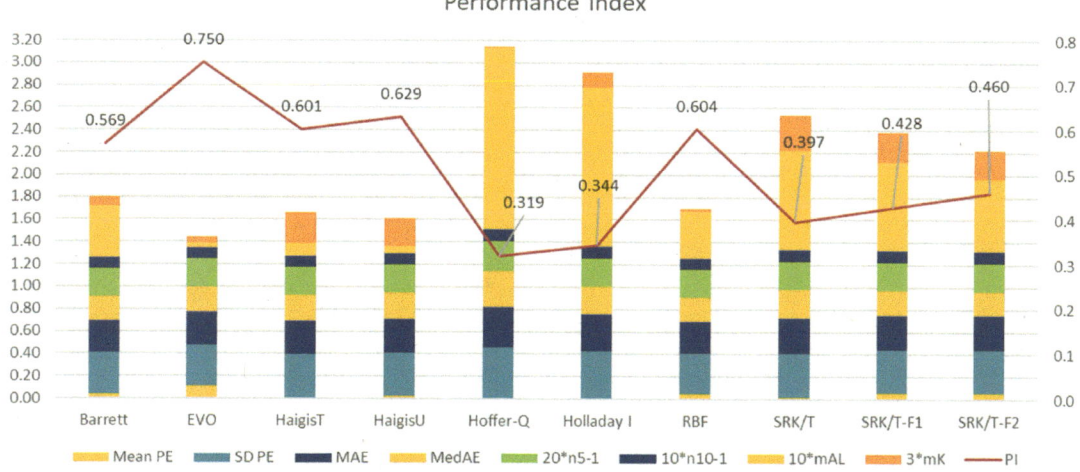

Fig. 33.2 The stacked histogram depicts the values of individual metrics, based on the previous table. The lower the individual component and overall height f of the stacked histogram the better. The scale for the stacked histogram f is on the left. The red line graph depicts the performance indices of the formulas. The performance index is the reciprocal of the total value of the stacked column. The higher, the better is the performance. The scale for the performance index is on the right. As illustrated, the best performing formula is EVO followed by the 2 Haigis, RBF 1.0, and BUII. These 4 formulas performed much better than the other formulas

Not all studies detailed all of the above metrics. For this review, we will only rank formulas in studies, in both general and subgroups, that have more than 3 of the above 6 metrics.

Further Review

There have been numerous studies published comparing the outcomes of the newer formulas, as well as against the established 3rd generation theoretical formulas. We will review some of these published articles and papers presented during recent conferences. A summary of the review is tabulated in Table 33.3.

Table 33.3 is a summary of outcomes in the literature as well as papers presented at conferences. The orders of the formula for each source are sorted in an order based on a modification of the Haigis performance index (PI) for comparing IOL power calculation formulas as explained above. The parameters used in this modified quality metrics are the SD, MAE, and MedAE, percentage of absolute error within ±0.50 D and ±1.00 D. The inverse of the percentage of absolute error are used and these are normalized by

amplifying by 20 for ±0.50 D and ±1.00 D, respectively. All the parameters are added up quantitatively. All the 4 to 6 parameters are summed up. The lower the sum the better. The reciprocal of that sum is the PI. The order above was sorted in decreasing performance index. The outcome is quite similar to that employed by Cooke et al. The formulas are ranked within the same study and not between studies, as the available parameters and clinical situations may be different.

The stacked histogram (Fig. 33.3) shows how the formulas fare in 17 articles, of which sixteen are ranked. Each box indicates the frequency the formula is ranked first, second, third, and fourth based on their PI. These are denoted by blue for 1st; magenta for 2nd; turquoise for 3rd and yellow for 4th. The line graph represents the number of ranked studies the formula was being compared. BUII was the most quoted and had performed well with most studies ranking it as first. EVO and Kane had also done well, with Kane having a relatively high proportion as best performing formula while EVO 2.0 had the highest proportion of being featured as one of the top 4 ranked formulas.

Table 33.3 ME, SD, MAE, and MedAE refer to mean numerical prediction error, the standard deviation of prediction error, mean absolute error, and median absolute error, respectively. BUII-noACD and EVO 2.0-no ACD signify ACD values were omitted in the related formulas. Holladay 2 PreSurgRef and Holladay 2 NoRef refer to Holladay 2 formula with and without preoperative refractions, respectively. Holladay 2018 and Holladay 2019 pertains to the versions of the Holladay 2 formula. Holladay 2-ALadj is a non-linear AL adjustment available as an option in the Holladay 2 program for eyes that are longer than 24.0 mm. LSF stands for Ladas Super Formula. Olsen2P and Olsen4P are Olsen formula using 2 parameters and 4 parameters to determine ELPs, respectively. Olsen2P is preinstalled in biometers while Olsen4P is also known as Olsen standalone and is available in the program, PhacoOptics. SRK/T-F1 and SRK/T-F2 are SRK/T with Fam-adjustment to the ALs and Ks. When specified, ULIB implies using the constants from the ULIB website. _WK indicates Wang-Koch adjustment

Article	Formula	ME	SD	MAE	MedAE	± 0.50	± 1.00	PI	Rank
Cooke and Cooke [14]	Olsen4P	0.000	0.361	0.284	0.225	83.7	99.1	*0.763*	1
1079 eyes/1079	BUII	0.000	0.365	0.285	0.230	82.9	99.2	*0.756*	2
LS-900	Olsen2P	0.000	0.378	0.296	0.245	82.0	98.6	*0.732*	3
SN60WF	T2	0.000	0.397	0.313	0.262	79.6	98.8	*0.701*	4
	Haigis	0.000	0.393	0.314	0.268	80.4	98.7	*0.701*	5
	Holladay 2 NoRef	0.000	0.404	0.318	0.261	79.0	98.1	*0.694*	6
	LSF	0.000	0.403	0.321	0.269	79.1	98.4	*0.690*	7
	Holladay 1	0.000	0.408	0.320	0.268	79.1	98.6	*0.689*	8
	Holladay 2 PreSurgRef	0.000	0.423	0.336	0.288	76.6	98.4	*0.662*	9
	Hoffer Q	0.000	0.428	0.340	0.285	77.8	97.4	*0.660*	10
	SRK/T	0.000	0.433	0.342	0.289	75.7	98.1	*0.653*	11

Article	Formula	ME	SD	MAE	MedAE	± 0.50	± 1.00	PI	Rank
Cooke and Cooke [14]	BUII	0.000	0.387	0.306	0.255	80.6	99.3	*0.716*	1
1079 eyes/1079	T2	0.000	0.404	0.319	0.265	79.0	98.7	*0.693*	2
IOLMaster3.02	Haigis	0.000	0.401	0.319	0.271	79.8	98.7	*0.692*	3
SN60WF	LSF	−0.060	0.410	0.326	0.275	79.9	98.3	*0.683*	4
	Holladay 1	0.000	0.414	0.326	0.270	79.5	98.4	*0.683*	5
	Holladay 2 NoRef	0.000	0.417	0.331	0.287	79.3	97.7	*0.670*	6
	Hoffer Q	0.000	0.432	0.341	0.281	77.0	97.4	*0.658*	7
	Holladay 2 PreSurgRef	0.000	0.432	0.346	0.297	75.2	98.1	*0.647*	8
	SRK/T	0.000	0.440	0.346	0.290	75.1	98.1	*0.647*	9
	Olsen4P	0.010	0.446	0.348	0.285	75.1	97.1	*0.645*	10
Kane et al., Intraocular	Barrett	−0.190		0.385	0.305	72.3	99.9	*0.857*	1
lens power formula	Holladay 1	0.000		0.408	0.326	69.4	99.6	*0.818*	2
accuracy: Comparison of	T2	−0.030		0.407	0.330	70.0	99.7	*0.817*	3
7 formulas [15]	SRK/T	−0.010		0.413	0.335	69.6	99.7	*0.809*	4
3241 eyes/3241	Haigis	0.010		0.420	0.337	68.3	99.6	*0.800*	5
IOLMaster 5.4	Holladay 2	0.000		0.420	0.341	67.4	99.7	*0.795*	6
SN60WF	Hoffer Q	−0.010		0.427	0.347	67.2	99.6	*0.786*	7
Kane et al., Accuracy of	BUII	−0.020		0.381	0.300	72.8	94.8	*0.857*	1
3 new methods for	Holladay 1	−0.010		0.398	0.321	70.1	94.3	*0.822*	2
intraocular lens power	T2	−0.030		0.398	0.330	70.8	94.4	*0.818*	3
selection [16]	LSF	−0.040		0.402	0.325	69.8	94.3	*0.816*	4
3122 eyes/3122	SRK/T	−0.010		0.402	0.330	70.4	94.4	*0.814*	5
IOLMaster 5.4	RBF 1.0	−0.130		0.407	0.330	69.6	94.3	*0.809*	6
SN60WF	Haigis	0.000		0.409	0.334	69.2	93.6	*0.803*	7
	Holladay 2	−0.010		0.410	0.337	68.2	94.4	*0.799*	8
	Hoffer Q	−0.020		0.417	0.344	67.9	93.5	*0.788*	9
	FullMonte IOL	−0.110		0.428	0.351	66.6	93.0	*0.773*	10
Fam, 7 good habits of	RBF 1.0	0.047	0.365	0.283	0.220	81.8	99.0	*0.760*	1
IOL power calculations	BUII	0.040	0.368	0.284	0.220	82.5	99.3	*0.760*	2
[17]	EVO	0.113	0.366	0.294	0.230	81.4	98.3	*0.747*	3
291 eyes/291	SRK/T-F2	0.057	0.387	0.303	0.220	81.4	98.3	*0.736*	4
IOLMaster 5.4	Haigis	−0.008	0.392	0.303	0.230	80.8	99.0	*0.728*	5
ZCB00	SRK/T-F1	0.053	0.391	0.306	0.230	80.4	98.3	*0.725*	6
	Haigis (ULIB)	0.022	0.388	0.301	0.240	80.8	99.0	*0.725*	7
	SRK/T	0.015	0.400	0.309	0.260	79.4	98.6	*0.702*	8
	Holladay 1	0.010	0.421	0.324	0.250	78.7	97.6	*0.688*	9
	Hoffer Q	0.008	0.455	0.360	0.320	75.6	96.2	*0.622*	10
Naeser [18] & Savini,	BUII	0.020	0.310	0.240	0.180	89.0	100.0	*0.866*	1
Accuracy of thick-lens	Næser 1	0.010	0.320	0.240	0.180	89.0	99.0	*0.857*	2
intraocular lens power	Næser 2	0.000	0.320	0.240	0.180	89.0	99.0	*0.857*	2
calculation based on	Haigis	0.000	0.340	0.240	0.190	87.0	99.0	*0.832*	4
cutting-card or calculated	SRK/T	−0.020	0.340	0.270	0.230	86.0	99.0	*0.785*	5
data for lens architecture	Hoffer Q	−0.060	0.360	0.280	0.230	85.0	99.0	*0.765*	6
[19]									
151 eyes/151									
Aladdin optical biometer									
SN60WF									

(continued)

Table 33.3 (continued)

Article	Formula	ME	SD	MAE	MedAE	± 0.50	± 1.00	PI	Rank
	Holladay 1	−0.060	0.360	0.290	0.250	85.0	100.0	*0.749*	7
Melles (Melles Ophth 2019) Melles et al. [20, 21] 18,501 eyes/18,501 LS900 SA60AT, SN60WF	Kane	0.000	0.384	0.295	0.236	83.0	98.3	*0.736*	1
	Olsen4P	0.000	0.394	0.302	0.244	81.7	98.0	*0.720*	2
	BUII	0.000	0.404	0.311	0.252	80.9	97.8	*0.705*	3
	EVO	0.000	0.409	0.315	0.255	80.2	97.9	*0.698*	4
	Olsen2P	0.000	0.424	0.325	0.258	78.7	97.4	*0.682*	5
	RBF 2.0	0.000	0.421	0.325	0.266	78.9	97.6	*0.680*	6
	Holladay 22019	0.000	0.429	0.332	0.269	78.0	97.4	*0.670*	7
	Haigis	0.000	0.437	0.338	0.275	77.0	97.3	*0.660*	8
	Holladay 1_WK	0.000	0.439	0.340	0.275	76.6	97.2	*0.658*	9
	Holladay 2018	0.000	0.450	0.350	0.285	75.4	97.0	*0.642*	10
	Holladay 1	0.000	0.453	0.351	0.287	75.0	96.8	*0.639*	11
	SRK/T	0.000	0.463	0.360	0.292	74.1	96.6	*0.628*	12
	Hoffer Q -WK	0.000	0.461	0.360	0.295	74.0	96.5	*0.628*	13
	SRK/T-WK	0.000	0.467	0.363	0.295	73.6	96.5	*0.623*	14
	Hoffer Q	0.000	0.473	0.369	0.303	73.0	96.2	*0.615*	15
	Haigis-WK	0.000	0.490	0.383	0.318	71.0	95.6	*0.595*	16
Darcy et al. [22] 10,930 eyes/10,930 SA60AT, 920H, 970C, AO	Kane	0.000		0.377	0.302	72.0	95.2	*0.857*	1
	RBF 1.0	0.000		0.387	0.310	71.2	94.9	*0.841*	2
	Olsen	0.000		0.388	0.309	70.6	94.9	*0.840*	3
	Holladay 2	0.000		0.390	0.312	71.0	94.9	*0.837*	4
	BUII	0.000		0.390	0.314	70.7	94.7	*0.835*	5
	Holladay 1	0.000		0.397	0.321	69.6	94.4	*0.822*	6
	SRK/T	0.000		0.403	0.323	69.1	93.9	*0.814*	7
	Haigis	0.000		0.405	0.327	69.0	94.3	*0.810*	8
	Hoffer Q	0.000		0.410	0.332	68.1	94.0	*0.801*	9
Savini et al. [23] 155 eyes/155 OA-2000 SN60WF	EVO	0.000	0.306	0.205	0.240	90.7	100.0	*0.854*	1
	BUII	0.005	0.323	0.202	0.253	88.0	100.0	*0.830*	2
	T2	0.001	0.328	0.200	0.257	88.7	100.0	*0.826*	3
	RBF 1.0	0.037	0.335	0.205	0.252	90.7	99.3	*0.824*	4
	Olsen4P	−0.010	0.326	0.209	0.256	89.3	100.0	*0.823*	5
	Kane	0.000	0.342	0.200	0.257	90.0	100.0	*0.819*	6
	Holladay 2-ALadj	−0.076	0.325	0.225	0.266	89.3	99.3	*0.806*	7
	VRF	0.000	0.340	0.210	0.262	86.0	99.3	*0.803*	8
	SRK/T	0.001	0.344	0.221	0.262	84.7	100.0	*0.792*	9
	Olsen2P	0.013	0.378	0.240	0.294	84.0	98.7	*0.739*	10
	Holladay 2	−0.020	0.417	0.228	0.279	86.7	98.0	*0.736*	11
	Hoffer Q	0.000	0.395	0.248	0.307	85.3	97.3	*0.719*	12
	Haigis	0.002	0.400	0.254	0.307	84.7	98.0	*0.714*	13
	Holladay 1	0.000	0.407	0.249	0.306	85.3	96.7	*0.713*	14
	Panacea	−0.006	0.413	0.248	0.314	80.0	96.7	*0.698*	15

Table 33.3 (continued)

Article	Formula	ME	SD	MAE	MedAE	± 0.50	± 1.00	PI	Rank
Cheng et al. [24] 410 eyes/410 IOLMaster700 MX60	Kane	0.000	0.451	0.348	0.286	77.1	100.0	*0.647*	1
	Olsen	0.000	0.456	0.349	0.283	75.9	100.0	*0.645*	2
	EVO 2.0	0.000	0.460	0.354	0.293	74.6	100.0	*0.635*	3
	BUII	0.000	0.470	0.362	0.283	75.2	100.0	*0.633*	4
	Holladay 2	0.000	0.482	0.378	0.325	72.6	100.0	*0.602*	5
	RBF 2.0	0.000	0.492	0.385	0.314	73.4	100.0	*0.601*	6
	T2	0.000	0.500	0.391	0.317	72.0	100.0	*0.593*	7
	PEARL-DGS	0.000	0.515	0.388	0.305	71.0	100.0	*0.592*	8
	Haigis	0.000	0.521	0.404	0.322	68.8	100.0	*0.575*	9
	SRK/T	0.000	0.548	0.426	0.371	66.4	100.0	*0.542*	10
	Hoffer Q	0.000	0.612	0.465	0.379	63.0	100.0	*0.507*	11
	Holladay 1	0.000	0.611	0.478	0.376	60.5	100.0	*0.501*	12
Fernandez et al. [25] 3519 eyes/3519 IOLMaster700 POD-F, POD-FGF	Hoffer Q					84.3	97.1		
	Haigis					82.9	95.7		
	Pearl-DGS					81.4	95.7		
	BUII					77.1	97.1		
	EVO					78.6	95.7		
	Kane					84.3	92.9		
	SRK/T					77.1	95.7		
	Holladay 2					81.4	94.3		
	RBF 1.0					74.3	95.7		
Turnbull et al. [26] 176 eyes/88 SN6ATT	BUII	0.000	0.235	0.268	0.200	86.9	98.9	*0.881*	1
	RBF 2.0	−0.080	0.232	0.286	0.228	84.1	98.9	*0.843*	2
	Haigis	0.000	0.263	0.308	0.240	77.3	97.7	*0.785*	3
	SRK/T	0.000	0.255	0.327	0.268	76.7	98.9	*0.762*	4
	Holladay 1	0.000	0.302	0.355	0.282	75.0	97.2	*0.709*	5
	Hoffer Q	0.000	0.303	0.368	0.297	69.9	96.0	*0.684*	6
Zhao et al. [27] 53 eyes/41 IOLMaster SBL-3	EVO	0.000	0.600	0.430	0.300	69.8	88.7	*0.543*	1
	BUII	0.000	0.610	0.440	0.310	67.9	88.7	*0.532*	2
	Kane	0.000	0.610	0.450	0.310	67.9	88.7	*0.529*	3
	Haigis	0.000	0.600	0.450	0.330	66.0	90.6	*0.525*	4
	RBF 2.0	0.000	0.610	0.460	0.360	62.3	90.6	*0.507*	5
	Holladay 1	0.000	0.620	0.460	0.380	67.9	90.6	*0.506*	6
	Hoffer Q	0.000	0.610	0.470	0.360	60.4	86.8	*0.500*	7
	SRK/T	0.000	0.620	0.460	0.400	64.2	90.6	*0.497*	8

(continued)

Table 33.3 (continued)

Article	Formula	ME	SD	MAE	MedAE	± 0.50	± 1.00	PI	Rank
Savini et al. [28]	BUII-noACD	−0.058	0.343	0.262	0.218	88.0	99.0	*0.799*	1
205 eyes/205	Kane	−0.001	0.348	0.265	0.214	86.5	99.0	*0.794*	2
AL-Scan	T2	0.000	0.347	0.269	0.228	88.5	99.0	*0.786*	3
SI255	EVO 2.0-(noACD	0.000	0.348	0.267	0.225	87.0	98.5	*0.786*	4
	BUII	−0.045	0.353	0.268	0.218	85.5	99.0	*0.784*	5
	RBF 2.0	−0.003	0.356	0.272	0.215	85.0	99.5	*0.782*	6
	Holladay 1	0.000	0.355	0.275	0.232	88.5	99.0	*0.775*	7
	EVO 2.0	0.000	0.357	0.276	0.233	83.5	99.0	*0.765*	8
	SRK/T	0.000	0.365	0.287	0.223	86.0	98.0	*0.762*	9
	VRF	0.000	0.372	0.280	0.235	84.5	99.5	*0.755*	10
	Pearl-DGS	0.000	0.366	0.286	0.238	84.5	98.5	*0.752*	11
	Hoffer Q	0.000	0.388	0.295	0.229	84.0	99.5	*0.740*	12
	Holladay 2-Aladj	0.000	0.387	0.297	0.228	83.0	98.5	*0.737*	13
	Haigis	−0.012	0.402	0.306	0.240	82.0	98.5	*0.717*	14
	Næser 2	0.027	0.409	0.313	0.256	80.0	99.0	*0.699*	15
Szalai et al. [29]	Haigis	−0.013		0.273	0.200	78.0	98.0	*1.071*	1
95 eyes/95	LSF	0.011		0.387	0.330	62.0	89.0	*0.791*	2
Anterion	Hoffer Q	0.175		0.424	0.290	63.0	84.0	*0.788*	3
690AB, AO, SA60AT,	Holladay 1	0.125		0.424	0.310	59.0	88.0	*0.769*	4
SN60WF, Clareon	Kane	−0.070		0.346	0.500	79.0	86.0	*0.751*	5
	RBF 2.0	−0.065		0.400	0.410	61.0	89.0	*0.734*	6
	BUII	−0.037		0.449	0.370	60.0	88.0	*0.725*	7
	SRK/T	0.161		0.449	0.370	55.0	88.0	*0.709*	8
Reitblat et al. [30]	BUII	0.030	0.590	0.440	0.330	72.2	92.2	*0.54*	1
90 eyes/90	Kane	0.020	0.610	0.460	0.350	72.2	90.0	*0.52*	2
IOLMaster 5.21	SRK/T	−0.020	0.630	0.480	0.380	61.1	98.9	*0.50*	3
SN60WF	Haigis	−0.010	0.630	0.490	0.370	65.6	86.7	*0.49*	4
	Holladay 1	−0.080	0.610	0.470	0.390	58.9	90.0	*0.49*	5
	Hoffer Q	−0.050	0.650	0.490	0.370	61.1	90.0	*0.49*	6
Hipolito-Fernandes et al. [31]	Kane	0.000	0.418	0.324	0.274	79.3	97.7	*0.679*	1
828 eyes/828	VRF-G	0.000	0.423	0.332	0.273	79.5	97.1	*0.673*	2
LS-900	EVO 2.0	0.000	0.419	0.329	0.282	78.5	97.6	*0.671*	3
SN60WF	BUII	0.000	0.429	0.339	0.291	77.8	97.2	*0.657*	4
	RBF 2.0	0.000	0.433	0.342	0.291	76.7	97.6	*0.653*	5
	PEARL-DGS	0.000	0.436	0.344	0.290	76.9	97.2	*0.651*	6
	VRF	0.000	0.440	0.347	0.293	76.7	97.0	*0.646*	7
	T2	0.000	0.441	0.346	0.291	75.5	97.1	*0.646*	8
	SRK/T	0.000	0.454	0.356	0.303	75.1	97.2	*0.631*	9
	Næser 2	0.000	0.455	0.357	0.309	74.9	96.3	*0.627*	10
	Holladay 1	0.000	0.461	0.361	0.299	74.3	96.1	*0.626*	11
	Haigis	0.000	0.459	0.359	0.309	74.5	95.4	*0.623*	12
	Hoffer Q	0.000	0.489	0.383	0.317	69.9	95.7	*0.594*	13

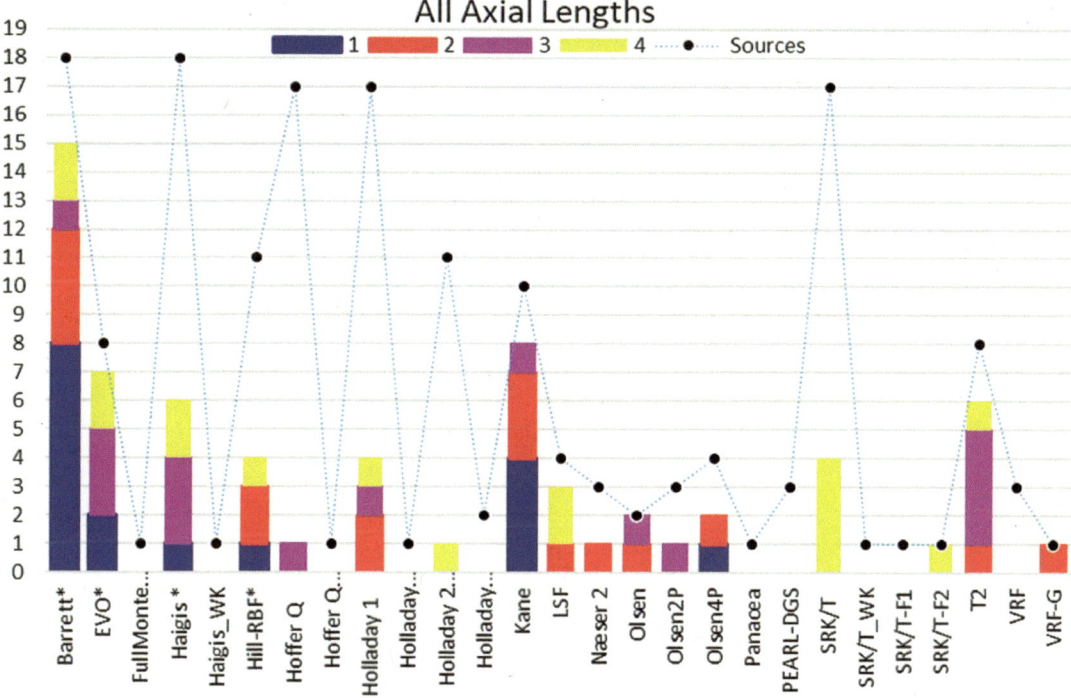

Fig. 33.3 Stacked histogram showing the performance indices of the various formulas in the literature

Subgroup Analyses

The third-generation theoretical formulas are good but are noted to have a bias against AL and K. In the past, different formulas were recommended for different ALs and Ks as first recommended and published by Hoffer in 1993. For normal, these older formulas function well. Against this backdrop, newer formulas must show improvement in longer and shorter axial lengths and extreme corneal curvatures.

The Long and Short of It

Short Eyes

A short eye is generally defined as an eye that is 22.0 mm in AL or shorter. IOL power calculation in short eyes is always a challenge. The biometric measurements have to be more precise. The IOL powers are of higher iopter and are consequently more sensitive to even small variations in

ELP. Hence, the prediction errors are generally higher than in normal eyes.

The charts (Fig. 33.4) and Table 33.4 showed the accuracy of the different formulas in short eyes (≤22.0 mm). IOL constants for the third-generation formulas were from the greater pool of patients and IOLs. ULIB constants were used for Haigis as some IOLs did not have sufficient numbers for triple optimization. 8 different IOLs are used in this study. BUII, EVO, and RBF were calculated with the optimized A-constant. Fig. 33.4a shows the prediction errors of the formulas, while Fig. 33.4b, c show the absolute errors and percentage of absolute errors.

From Fig. 33.4 and Table 33.4, BUII, Haigis (ULIB), RBF 1.0 and EVO had better outcome metrics than the other formulas. BUII, Haigis, RBF 1.0, and EVO 1.0 had lower than 0.40 D and 0.30 D of MAE and MedAE, respectively, and more than 70% within ±0.5 D of expected refraction. All four formulas scored better than 0.60 on the performance index.

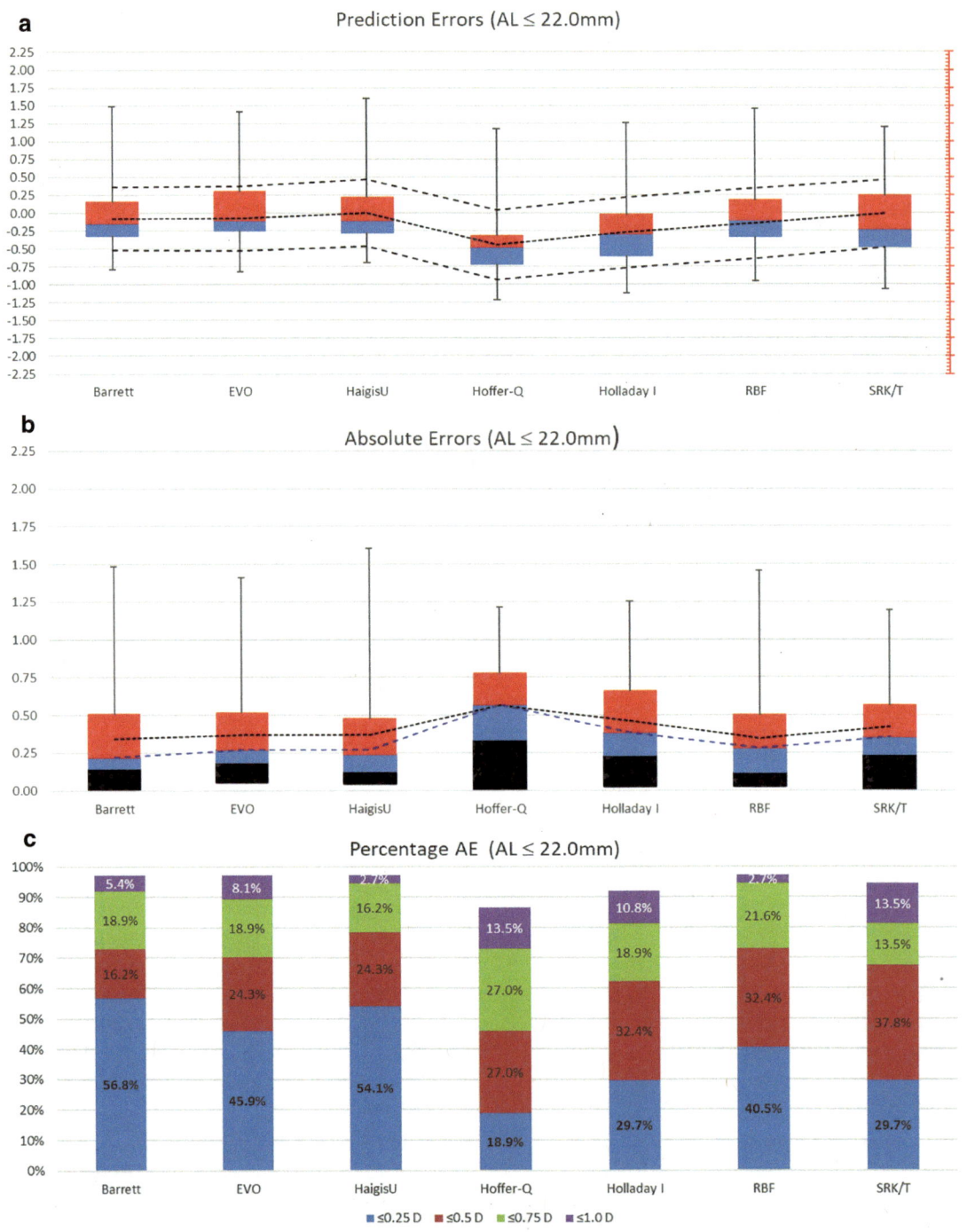

Fig. 33.4 Chart (**a**) displays the prediction error of the formulas. The dual colored boxes in chart (**a**) represent the 2nd and 3rd quartiles of the spread of prediction errors. The error plots are the 1st and 4th quartiles. The line graphs are the upper and lower SDs. Chart (**b**) shows the absolute error of the formulas. The tri-colored boxes are the 1st, 2nd, and 3rd quartiles while the error plot is the last quartile. The blue and black dashed lines are the MedAEs and MAEs. Chart (**c**) is a stacked histogram showing the percentage of eyes within ±0.25, ±0.50, ±0.75, and ±1.00 D of the refraction target

Table 33.4 This table shows the modified Haigis performance indices of the various formulas (EVO is EVO 1.0; RBF is RBF 1.0) [32]

Formula	n	ME	SD	MAE	MedAE	±0.50 D	±1.00 D	PI	Rank
BUII	37	−0.077	0.452	0.344	0.220	73.0	97.3	*0.668*	1
Haigis	37	0.002	0.466	0.342	0.240	78.4	97.3	*0.663*	2
RBF 1.0	37	−0.079	0.445	0.342	0.280	73.0	97.3	*0.646*	3
EVO	37	−0.015	0.471	0.369	0.270	70.3	97.3	*0.625*	4
SRK/T	37	−0.149	0.496	0.424	0.350	67.6	94.6	*0.563*	5
Holladay 1	37	−0.274	0.490	0.459	0.380	62.2	91.9	*0.535*	6
Hoffer Q	37	−0.444	0.490	0.565	0.570	45.9	86.5	*0.436*	7

Review (Short Axial Lengths)

Table 33.5 is a summary of outcomes in the literature as well as papers presented at conferences on short eyes. As with the above table, the order of the formulas for each source are sorted in order based on a modification of Haigis "Quality metrics for comparing IOL calculation formulas."

The stacked histogram (Fig. 33.5) shows how the formulas fare in 8 ranked datasets of 11 articles. Each box indicates the number of times the formula is being ranked based on its PI. Blue is for 1st ranking; magenta for 2nd; turquoise for 3rd and yellow for 4th. The line graph represents the frequency of ranked studies the formula was being compared. Most of the new formulas performed reasonably well. PEARL-DGS was ranked 1st in both studies quoted. Holladay 1 and Barrett were the two most featured formulas. Both had performed reasonably well with most studies ranking it as among the top 4. Among the older theoretical formulas, Haigis and Holladay 1 stand out.

Wendelstein et al. did a study to look at the accuracy of 13 different concepts in extreme short eyes [4]. 150 eyes of 150 patients were recruited for this study and 2 IOL models (SA60AT and ZCB00) were used. The constants were optimized from a separate patient cohort. Biometry was measured with either LenStar LS 900 or IOLMaster 700 (Carl Zeiss Meditec AG, Jena, Germany). Postoperative refraction was done at 4 weeks. They concluded that PEARL-DGS, Okulix [43], Kane, and Castrop showed the lowest MAE.

From the graph (Fig. 33.6), Castrop had good accuracy for both groups. PEARL-DGS was the most accurate for the >28.5 D group and was also good for the ≤28.5D group. Okulix had also performed well with the subgroup performance index of above 0.60.

Medium Axial Length

Medium AL is the range of a AL where most eyes are found. It is generally taken to be between 22.0 mm to 24.5 mm, with minor variations. Most formulas perform well in these eyes.

Review (Medium Axial Lengths)

Table 33.6 is a summary of outcomes in the literature as well as papers presented at conferences on medium AL eyes. As with the earlier tables, the orders of the formula for each source are sorted in order based on a modification of Haigis "Quality metrics for comparing IOL calculation formulas."

The stacked histogram (Fig. 33.7) shows how the formulas fare in 6 ranked datasets in 9 papers. Each box indicates the frequency the formula is being ranked based on PI. Blue for 1st; magenta for 2nd; turquoise for 3rd; and yellow for 4th. The dotted line joins the number of ranked studies the formula was being compared to. There were far fewer studies specifically focused on this range. This chart mirrored that of all ALs, as most of the eyes fall into this group. The performances in this range of ALs were quite spread out. This is not surprising as most formulas perform well in this "normal" range. BUIIt and Holladay 1 were the most quoted and had the highest number of top 4 rankings. RBF 2.0, Kane, and Olsen were next.

Table 33.5 ME, SD, MAE, and MedAE refer to mean numerical prediction error, the standard deviation of prediction error, mean absolute error, and median absolute error, respectively. Holladay 2 PreSurgRef and Holladay 2 NoRef refer to Holladay 2 formula with and without preoperative refractions, respectively. LSF stands for Ladas Super Formula [33]. Olsen2P and Olsen4P are Olsen [34–41] using 2 parameters and 4 parameters to determine ELPs, respectively. Olsen2P is preinstalled in biometers while Olsen4P is also known as Olsen standalone and is available in the program, PhacoOptics. When specified, ULIB implies using the constants from the ULIB website

Article	Formula	ME	SD	MAE	MedAE	±0.50	±1.00	PI	Rank
Cooke et al. [14]	Olsen4P	−0.070	0.402	0.322	0.225	75.6	100.0	*0.674*	1
LS 900	BUII	−0.150	0.417	0.338	0.260	78.0	95.1	*0.613*	2
SN60WF	Haigis	0.000	0.460	0.390	0.308	65.9	100.0	*0.602*	3
≤22.0	Olsen2P	0.080	0.453	0.380	0.325	70.7	97.6	*0.579*	4
	SRK/T	−0.150	0.494	0.407	0.327	68.3	95.1	*0.532*	5
	Holladay 1	−0.250	0.457	0.397	0.302	75.6	92.7	*0.530*	6
	T2	−0.230	0.474	0.407	0.341	70.7	95.1	*0.514*	7
	LSF	−0.290	0.472	0.426	0.320	75.6	92.7	*0.503*	8
	Holladay 2 PreSurgRef	−0.270	0.445	0.426	0.397	70.7	92.7	*0.491*	9
	Holladay 2 NoRef	−0.350	0.430	0.437	0.345	58.5	90.2	*0.470*	10
	Hoffer Q	−0.440	0.455	0.500	0.493	53.7	90.2	*0.403*	11
Cooke et al. [14]	Haigis	−0.020	0.509	0.407	0.311	68.3	95.1	*0.571*	1
IOLMaster3.02	BUII	−0.150	0.483	0.392	0.295	78.0	92.7	*0.558*	2
SN60WF	Holladay 1	−0.210	0.486	0.389	0.269	80.5	92.7	*0.550*	3
≤ 22.0	SRK/T	−0.110	0.508	0.402	0.301	68.3	95.1	*0.548*	4
	T2	−0.190	0.493	0.394	0.296	73.2	95.1	*0.539*	5
	LSF	−0.230	0.479	0.401	0.283	80.5	92.7	*0.538*	6
	Olsen4P	−0.020	0.565	0.458	0.370	61.0	95.1	*0.513*	7
	Holladay 2 PreSurgRef	−0.240	0.472	0.427	0.395	65.9	92.7	*0.487*	8
	Holladay 2 NoRef	−0.330	0.467	0.443	0.402	73.2	87.8	*0.467*	9
	Hoffer Q	−0.410	0.493	0.483	0.383	63.4	87.8	*0.432*	10
Fam (Fam, Approaching	Haigis-ULIB	0.002	0.466	0.342	0.240	78.4	97.3	*0.662*	1
atypical eyes with	BUII	−0.077	0.452	0.344	0.220	73.0	97.3	*0.636*	2
confidence [32])	EVO	−0.015	0.471	0.369	0.270	70.3	97.3	*0.619*	3
59 eyes	RBF	−0.079	0.445	0.342	0.280	73.0	97.3	*0.615*	4
IOLMaster3.02 eyes/	SRK/T	−0.149	0.496	0.424	0.350	67.6	94.6	*0.519*	5
IOLMaster5.4	Holladay 1	−0.274	0.490	0.459	0.380	62.2	91.9	*0.467*	6
8 IOLs	Hoffer Q	−0.444	0.490	0.565	0.570	45.9	86.5	*0.366*	7
≤ 22.0									
Kane et al., Intraocular lens	Haigis	−0.090		0.473	0.334	62.8	100.0	*0.706*	1
power formula accuracy:	Holladay 1	−0.070		0.453	0.377	63.5	99.4	*0.706*	2
Comparison of 7 formulas	SRK/T	−0.040		0.458	0.397	59.6	99.4	*0.698*	3
[15]	Holladay 2	−0.070		0.466	0.383	61.5	100.0	*0.692*	4
IOLMaster 5.4	T2	−0.100		0.459	0.415	60.3	99.4	*0.664*	5
SN60WF	BUII	−0.260		0.469	0.395	62.2	100.0	*0.608*	6
≤ 22.0	Hoffer Q	−0.220		0.499	0.441	55.8	100.0	*0.582*	7
Accuracy of 3 new methods for IPC	Holladay 1	−0.090		0.417	0.360	66.4	95.6	*0.726*	1
Kane, JCRS 2017; 43:333–339	RBF	−0.150		0.423	0.360	66.4	95.6	*0.693*	2
	LSF	−0.140		0.433	0.370	63.5	94.9	*0.681*	3
IOLMaster 5.4	BUII	−0.280		0.451	0.400	63.5	94.2	*0.603*	4

Table 33.5 (continued)

Article	Formula	ME	SD	MAE	MedAE	±0.50	±1.00	PI	Rank
SN60WF	FullMonte IOL	−0.250		0.513	0.462	55.5	89.1	*0.553*	5
IPC in short eyes	RBF	0.050	0.470	0.360	0.310	70.9	96.5	*0.595*	1
Gökce, [42]	BUII	−0.040	0.490	0.390	0.320	68.6	95.3	*0.574*	2
86 eyes eyes/67	Holladay 1	−0.040	0.500	0.390	0.340	70.9	97.7	*0.569*	3
LS900	Holladay 2	−0.250	0.460	0.400	0.330	69.8	91.9	*0.514*	4
SN60WF, SN6AT, SA60AT, ZCB00, ZCT	Haigis	−0.090	0.540	0.420	0.390	68.6	90.7	*0.512*	5
	Hoffer Q	−0.220	0.490	0.440	0.390	64.0	94.2	*0.484*	6
	Olsen	0.270	0.510	0.460	0.410	59.3	91.9	*0.454*	7
Melles et al. [20, 21]	Kane			0.345					
LS900	Olsen4P			0.360					
SA60AT, SN60WF	BUII			0.377					
< 22.5 mm	RBF			0.382					
	EVO			0.384					
	Holladay 1			0.400					
	Haigis			0.402					
	Holladay 2			0.416					
	SRK/T			0.417					
	Hoffer Q			0.448					
Darcy et al. [22]	Kane				0.441				
IOLMaster	Holladay 2				0.458				
SA60AT, 920H, 970C, AO	Olsen				0.459				
≤ 22.5 mm	Hill-RBF 2.0				0.470				
	Holladay 1				0.493				
	BUII				0.461				
	Hoffer Q				0.478				
	Haigis				0.486				
	SRK/T				0.492				
Cheng et al. [24]	PEARL-DGS			0.378	0.278	70.8	95.8	*0.872*	1
IOLMaster700	Hoffer Q			0.409	0.273	70.8	91.7	*0.846*	2
MX60	Holladay 1			0.420	0.352	70.8	91.7	*0.786*	3
	Kane			0.472	0.417	62.5	87.5	*0.696*	4
	RBF 2.0			0.608	0.579	41.7	83.3	*0.524*	5
Hipolito-Fernandes et al. [31]	VRF-G			0.345					
LS-900	EVO 2.0			0.347					
SN60WF	Kane			0.348					
	VRF			0.365					
	BUII			0.367					
	RBF 2.0			0.368					
	PEARL-DGS			0.368					
	Næser 2			0.380					
	SRK/T			0.384					
	Haigis			0.397					
	T2			0.400					
	Holladay 1			0.409					
	Hoffer Q			0.478					

(continued)

Table 33.5 (continued)

Article	Formula	ME	SD	MAE	MedAE	±0.50	±1.00	PI	Rank
Wendelstein et al. [4]	Pearl-DGS	0.030	0.420	0.330	0.260	80.0	96.7	*0.668*	1
150 eyes/150	Castrop	−0.040	0.420	0.330	0.270	74.7	99.3	*0.654*	2
LS-900, IOLMaster700	Okulix	−0.040	0.420	0.340	0.300	79.3	98.7	*0.643*	3
SA60AT, ZCB00	Kane	−0.010	0.450	0.350	0.300	78.7	96.0	*0.636*	4
< 21.5 mm; Pemme>28.5D	Olsen2P	0.030	0.500	0.400	0.330	70.0	96.7	*0.571*	5
	Haigis	−0.060	0.490	0.390	0.320	68.0	95.3	*0.567*	6
	RBF 2.0	−0.100	0.490	0.380	0.320	73.3	95.3	*0.564*	7
	Holladay 1	0.030	0.530	0.410	0.340	66.7	94.0	*0.549*	8
	EVO 2.0	0.220	0.440	0.390	0.300	70.0	96.7	*0.543*	9
	Holladay 2	−0.260	0.490	0.430	0.380	66.0	92.0	*0.481*	10
	BUII	−0.200	0.640	0.490	0.330	62.7	84.7	*0.451*	11
	SRK/T	0.250	0.600	0.500	0.420	76.9	94.9	*0.446*	12

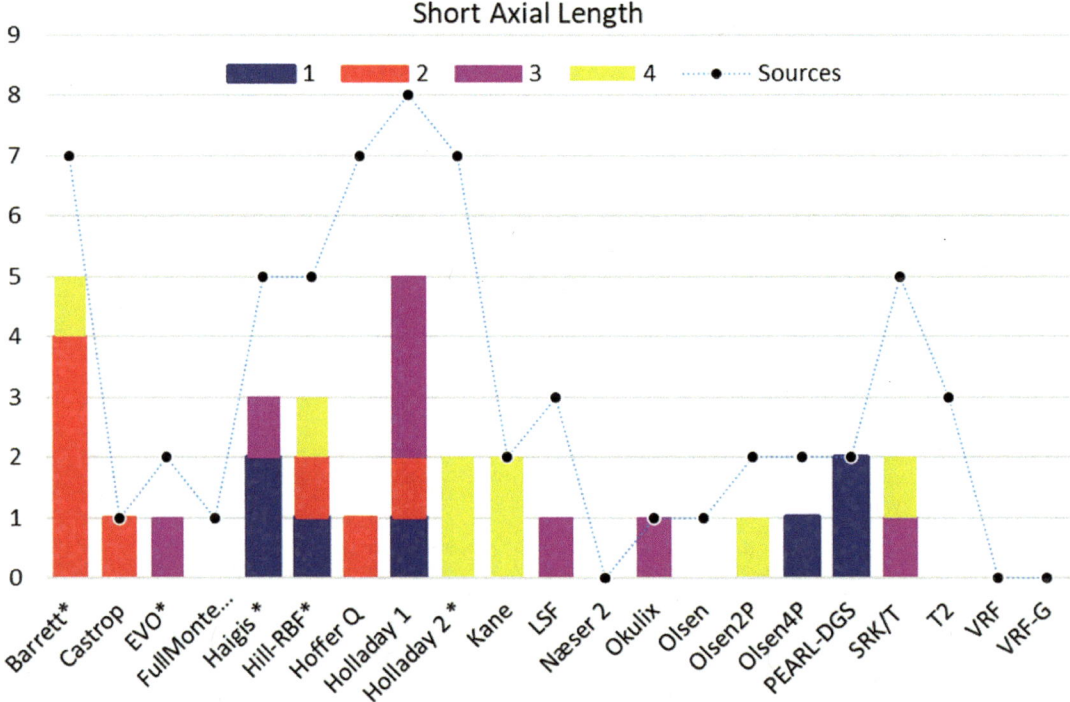

Fig. 33.5 Stacked histogram showing the performance indices of the various formulas for short axial length

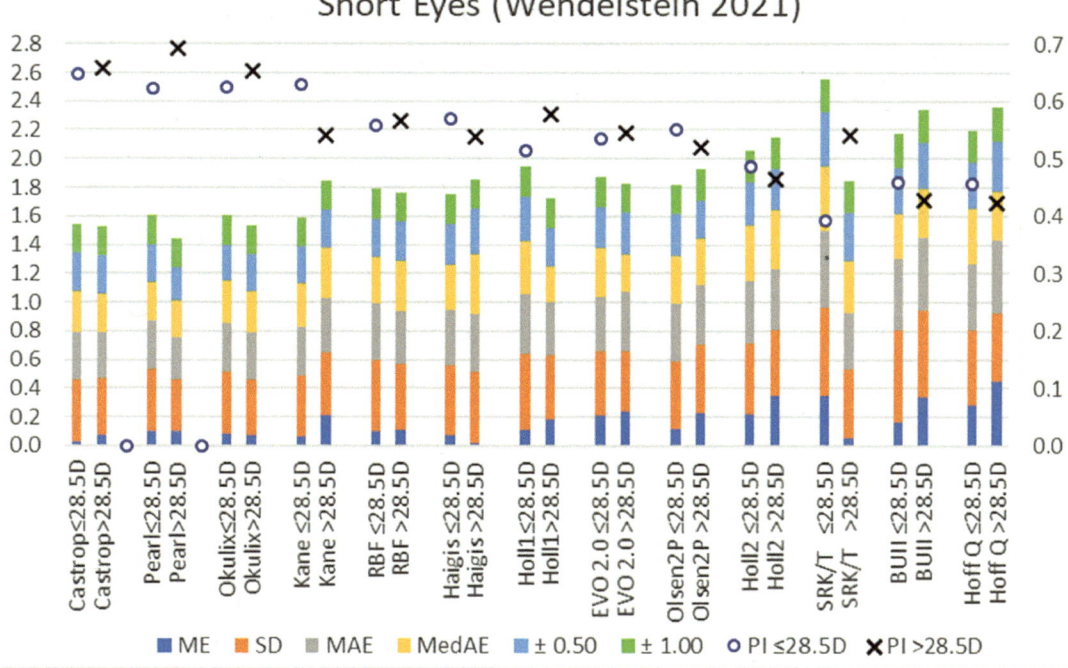

Fig. 33.6 The stacked histograms show the quality metrics f of the formulas in extremely short eyes [4]. Each formula is divided into 2 groups (1. Emmetropic IOL power ≤ 28.5D and 2. Emmetropic IOL power >28.5D). The scale for the stacked histogram f is on the left. The lower the stacked histogram, the better is the formula performance. The circles and triangles represent the PI. The scale for PI is on the right. The higher the PI score, the better. *BUII* = Barrett, *Hai* = Haigis, *HoffQ* = Hoffer Q, *Holl1* = Holladay 1, Holl2 = Holladay 2, *PEARL* = PEARL-DGS, *RBF* = RBF 2.0.

Very Long Axial Length (>26.0 mm)

The threshold for medium long AL is from 24.5 mm to 26.0 mm. Very long ALs are defined as >26.0 mm.

At the 2016 APACRS annual conference in Bali, Fam presented his findings on the performances of the various formulas for eyes with very long ALs [32]) (Fig. 33.8, Table 33.7).

In long eyes, the third-generation formulas underestimated the dioptric powers and the resultant refractions were hyperopic. The newer formulas such as BUII, EVO, and RBF 2.0 were more accurate in their calculations. EVO was the most accurate in both datasets. The Fam and Wang-Koch adjustment compensated well for the

otherwise hyperopic outcomes of Holladay 1. The hyperopic errors and inconsistencies were more apparent and exacerbated in the low dioptric lens powers.

Review (Long Axial Lengths)

Table 33.8 is a summary of outcomes in the literature as well as papers presented at conferences on long eyes. As with the earlier tables, the orders of the formula for each source are sorted in order based on a modification of Haigis "Quality metrics for comparing IOL calculation formulas."

The stacked histogram (Fig. 33.9) shows how the formulas fare in 16 articles, of which sixteen are ranked. Each box indicates the number of

Table 33.6 ME, SD, MAE, and MedAE refer to mean numerical prediction error, the standard deviation of prediction error, mean absolute error, and median absolute error, respectively. LSF stands for Ladas Super Formula. Olsen2P and Olsen4P are Olsen using 2 parameters and 4 parameters to determine ELPs, respectively. Olsen2P is preinstalled in biometers, while Olsen4P is also known as Olsen standalone and is available in the program, PhacoOptics. SRK/T-F1 and SRK/T-F2 are SRK/T with Fam-adjustment to the ALs and Ks. When specified, ULIB implies using the constants from the ULIB website

Article	Formula	ME	SD	MAE	MedAE	± 0.50	± 1.00	PI	Rank
Kane et al., Intraocular lens power formula accuracy: Comparison of 7 formulas [15] IOLMaster 5.4 SN60WF 22.0 < AL < 24.5 mm	Holladay 1	−0.010		0.404	0.323	69.8	99.7	*0.817*	1
	SRK/T	−0.020		0.408	0.329	70.8	99.8	*0.807*	2
	Haigis	−0.010		0.415	0.335	69.0	99.6	*0.800*	3
	T2	−0.030		0.405	0.330	69.5	99.7	*0.798*	4
	Holladay 2	−0.020		0.416	0.337	68.1	99.7	*0.789*	5
	Hoffer Q	−0.020		0.420	0.339	68.1	99.6	*0.785*	6
	BUII	−0.200		0.386	0.300	71.3	99.9	*0.732*	7
Kane et al., Intraocular lens power formula accuracy: Comparison of 7 formulas [15] IOLMaster 5.4 24.5 £ AL < 26.0 mm	BUII	−0.130		0.338	0.270	76.6	100.0	*0.834*	1
	T2	0.030		0.385	0.305	71.2	99.7	*0.832*	2
	Holladay 1	0.050		0.385	0.316	71.2	99.7	*0.811*	3
	Holladay 2	0.120		0.405	0.334	67.2	99.7	*0.737*	4
	SRK/T	0.120		0.414	0.341	66.7	99.7	*0.727*	5
	Haigis	0.130		0.409	0.347	68.5	99.5	*0.725*	6
	Hoffer Q	0.140		0.415	0.357	68.8	99.5	*0.712*	7
Kane et al., Accuracy of 3 new methods for intraocular lens power selection [16] IOLMaster 5.4 SN60WF 22.0 < AL < 24.5 mm	LSF	−0.010		0.400	0.320	70.5	94.2	*0.816*	1
	Holladay 1	−0.010		0.400	0.321	70.1	94.0	*0.814*	2
	BUII	−0.200		0.383	0.300	72.5	94.4	*0.730*	3
	RBF 2.0	−0.140		0.412	0.330	69.1	93.8	*0.722*	4
	FullMonte IOL	−0.120		0.426	0.347	67.2	92.8	*0.711*	5
Kane et al., Accuracy of 3 new methods for intraocular lens power selection [16] IOLMaster 5.4 SN60WF 24.5 ≤ AL < 26.0 mm	RBF 2.0	−0.010		0.370	0.305	75.0	96.8	*0.863*	1
	Holladay 1	0.030		0.374	0.313	72.4	95.6	*0.832*	2
	BUII	−0.140		0.333	0.270	77.9	97.9	*0.831*	3
	FullMonte IOL	−0.090		0.385	0.306	69.7	96.8	*0.785*	4
	LSF	−0.110		0.398	0.328	68.5	95.3	*0.747*	5
Melles et al. [20, 21] LS900 SA60AT, SN60WF 22.5 £ AL £ 25.5 mm	Kane			0.291					
	Olsen4P			0.297					
	BUII			0.304					
	EVO			0.305					
	RBF 22.0			0.319					
	Holladay 2			0.325					
	Haigis			0.332					
	Holladay 1			0.328					
	SRK/T			0.351					
	Hoffer Q			0.348					
Darcy et al. [22] IOLMaster SA60AT, 920H, 970C, AO 22.0 < AL < 26.0 mm	Kane				0.375				
	Holladay 2				0.387				
	Olsen				0.384				
	RBF 2.0				0.382				
	Holladay 1				0.385				
	BUII				0.387				
	Hoffer Q				0.401				
	Haigis				0.402				
	SRK/T				0.399				

Table 33.6 (continued)

Article	Formula	ME	SD	MAE	MedAE	± 0.50	± 1.00	PI	Rank
Cheng et al. [24] IOLMaster700 MX60 22.0 < AL < 24.5 mm	Olsen			0.347	0.255	76.5	95.7	*0.932*	**1**
	Kane			0.351	0.271	76.9	95.7	*0.917*	**2**
	EVO 2.0			0.353	0.280	75.2	95.3	*0.902*	**3**
	BUII			0.361	0.281	75.6	96.2	*0.897*	**4**
	PEARL-DGS			0.356	0.292	74.4	95.7	*0.888*	**5**
Cheng et al. [24] IOLMaster700 MX60 24.5 ≥ AL < 26.0 mm	Kane			0.350	0.338	78.5	98.5	*0.873*	**1**
	BUII			0.357	0.308	72.3	96.9	*0.871*	**2**
	Olsen			0.353	0.337	75.4	96.9	*0.861*	**3**
	RBF 2.0			0.368	0.334	76.9	96.9	*0.856*	**4**
	EVO 2.0			0.358	0.355	72.3	96.9	*0.836*	**5**
Hipolito-Fernandes et al. [31] LS-900 SN60WF 22.0 < AL <26.0 mm	Kane			0.323					
	EVO 2.0			0.329					
	VRF-G			0.333					
	BUII			0.338					
	RBF 2.0			0.339					
	PEARL-DGS			0.339					
	VRF			0.346					
	Næser 2			0.357					
	Haigis			0.357					
	Holladay 1			0.339					
	Hoffer Q			0.357					

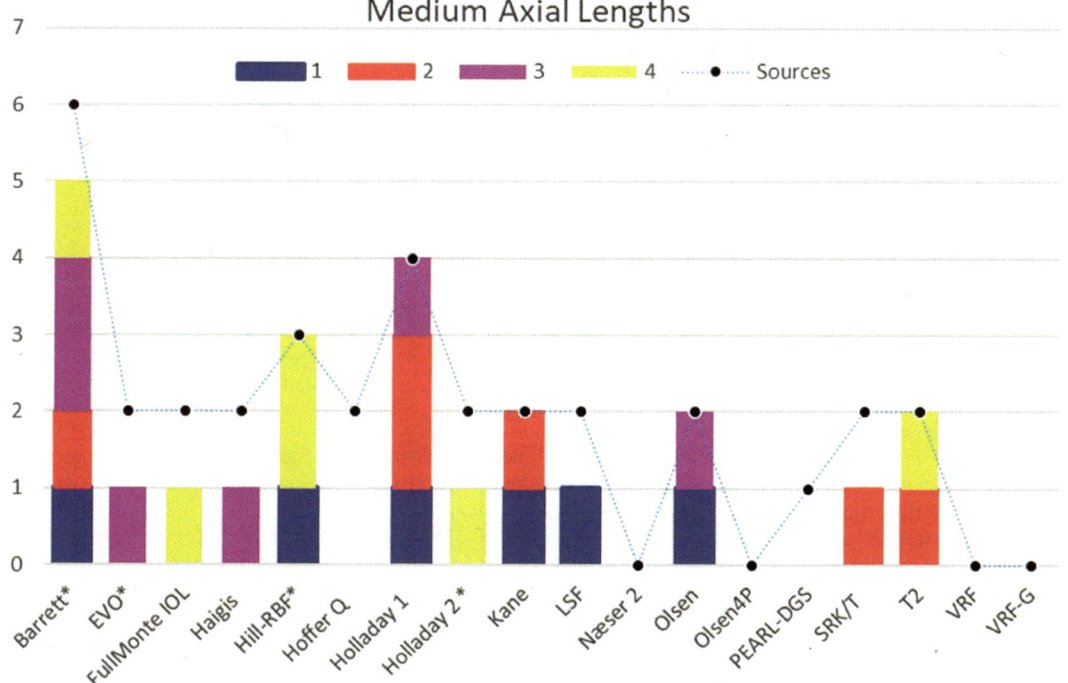

Fig. 33.7 Stacked histogram comparing the performance indices of the various formulas for medium ALs

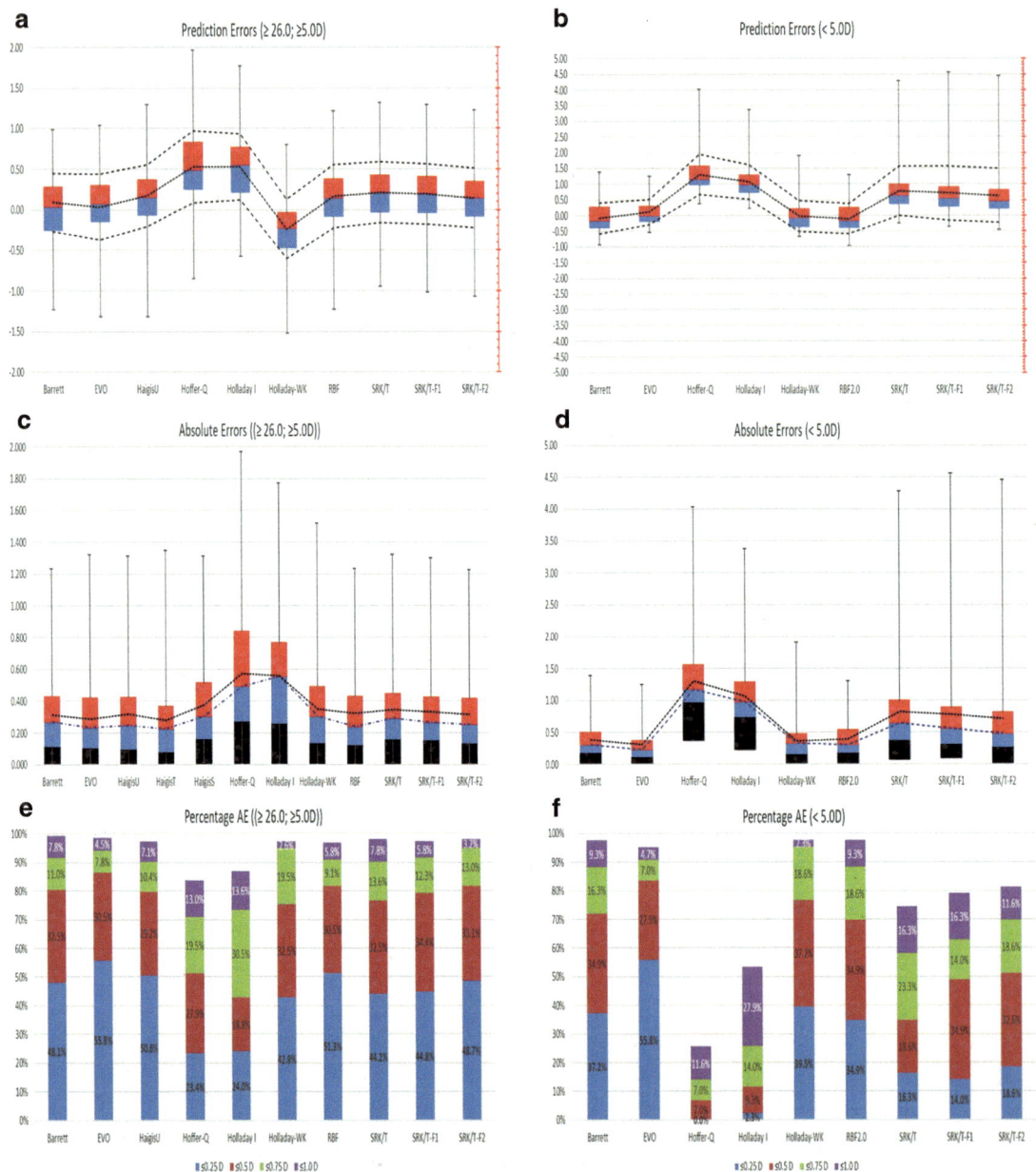

Fig. 33.8 The charts and Table 33.7 depict the outcomes for very long eyes (≥26.0 mm). Charts on the left column were for eyes 26.0 mm and longer and implanted with IOL ≥ 5.0D. 11 different IOLs were used in this study. IOL constants for the third-generation formulas were from the greater pool of patients and IOLs. ULIB constants were used for Haigis as some IOLs did not have sufficient numbers for triple optimization. BUII, EVO, and RBF 2.0 were calculated with the optimized A-constant of SRK/T. The charts on the right column show outcomes for eyes 26.0 mm and longer, and implanted with IOL <5.0D. 7 different IOLs were included in the study; most of these were special very low or negative-diopter IOLs. Figure (**a**, **b**) display the numerical prediction errors of the formulas, while Figs. (**c**, **d**) depict the absolute errors; and (**e**, **f**) the percentage of absolute errors. Most of these eyes were out of the domain for RBF 1.0. RBF in the original presentation was updated to RBF 2.0 in these charts. The formulas in Table 33.7 are arranged in order of their subgroup PI ranking. *n* is for the number of eyes. ME and SD are the means and standard deviations of numerical prediction errors, respectively. MAE and MedAE are the mean and median absolute errors. ±0.50 D and ±1.00 D are the percentage of eyes within those ranges of target refractions, respectively

Table 33.7 This table shows the modified Haigis performance indices of the various formulas (EVO is EVO 1.0; RBF is updated to RBF 2.0) [32]

>26.0 mm	n	ME	SD E	MAE	MedAE	±0.50	±1.00	PI	Rank
EVO	154	0.092	0.361	0.288	0.230	86.4	98.7	*0.761*	1
SRK/T-F2	154	0.144	0.369	0.313	0.250	81.8	98.1	*0.724*	2
RBF 2.0	154	0.168	0.388	0.324	0.240	81.8	96.8	*0.713*	3
Haigis	154	0.174	0.381	0.317	0.250	79.9	97.4	*0.712*	4
SRK/T-F1	154	0.193	0.371	0.333	0.260	79.2	97.4	*0.703*	5
BUII	154	0.030	0.406	0.316	0.270	80.5	99.4	*0.694*	6
SRK/T	154	0.212	0.376	0.346	0.290	76.6	98.1	*0.677*	7
Holladay1WK	154	−0.237	0.365	0.348	0.310	75.3	97.4	*0.670*	8
Hoffer Q	154	0.530	0.440	0.571	0.500	51.3	83.8	*0.467*	9
Holladay 1	154	0.526	0.404	0.560	0.560	42.9	87.0	*0.450*	10
>26.0 mm;<5.0D	**n**	**ME**	**SD E**	**MAE**	**MedAE**	**± 0.50**	**± 1.00**	**PI**	**Rank**
EVO	43	0.110	0.402	0.303	0.230	83.7	95.4	*0.723*	1
Holladay1WK	43	−0.025	0.490	0.365	0.330	76.7	97.7	*0.606*	2
BUII	43	−0.088	0.484	0.388	0.310	72.1	97.7	*0.601*	3
RBF 2.0	43	−0.107	0.482	0.396	0.310	69.8	97.7	*0.596*	4
Haigis	43	0.575	0.509	0.596	0.510	48.8	83.7	*0.442*	5
SRK/T-F2	43	0.636	0.852	0.716	0.480	51.2	81.4	*0.372*	6
SRK/T-F1	43	0.714	0.859	0.778	0.560	48.8	79.1	*0.350*	7
SRK/T	43	0.788	0.780	0.821	0.650	34.9	74.4	*0.323*	8
Holladay 1	43	1.068	0.553	1.068	0.980	11.6	53.5	*0.213*	9
Hoffer Q	43	1.308	0.634	1.308	1.170	7.0	25.6	*0.148*	10

times the formula is being ranked according to the color: blue for 1st; magenta for the 2nd; turquoise for 3rd and yellow for 4th. The dotted line joins the number of ranked studies the formula was being compared to. BUII was the most quoted and had performed well. EVO 2,0 was quoted in 6 articles but had a proportionately higher number of first ranking. RBF 2.0 and Haigis had also done well.

We will look deeper into the accuracy of the formulas in long axial length but between low-diopter and even lower-diopter eyes.

The 2 charts (Fig. 33.10) illustrate the difference in formula precision as the ALs approach low diopter or negative diopter territory. Chart A is by Abulafia [44] and Chart B by Fam [32]. Abulafia used 6 D while Fam used 5 D as thresholds. The newer formulas such as EVO 2.0, BUII, and RBF 2.0 showed good precisions throughout both groups, as demonstrated by the high subgroup PIs. Wang-Koch adjustments also showed good results, especially with the Holladay 1.

Table 33.8 ME, SD, MAE, and MedAE refer to mean numerical prediction error, the standard deviation of prediction error, mean absolute error, and median absolute error, respectively. Barrett-noACD and EVO 2.0-no ACD signify ACD values were omitted in the related formulas. Holladay 2 PreSurgRef and Holladay 2 NoRef refer to Holladay 2 formula with and without preoperative refractions, respectively. Holladay 2018 and Holladay 2019 pertain to the versions of the Holladay 2 formula. Holladay 2-ALadj is a nonlinear AL adjustment available as an option in Holladay 2 program for eyes that are longer than 24.0 mm. LSF stands for Ladas Super Formula. Olsen2P and Olsen4P are Olsen using 2 parameters and 4 parameters to determine ELPs, respectively. Olsen2P is preinstalled in biometers, while Olsen4P is also known as Olsen standalone and is available in the program, PhacoOptics. SRK/T-F1 and SRK/T-F2 are SRK/T with Fam-adjustment to the axial lengths and corneal powers. -AL1, AL2, and nonlinear AL indicate the first and second linear versions and the non-linear version of Wang-Koch axial length adjustments, respectively. CMAL pertains to the Cook-modified AL. When specified, ULIB implies the constants from the ULIB website are being used in the calculations. _WK indicates ALs with Wang–Koch adjustments

Article	Formula	ME	SD	MAE	MedAE	± 0.50	± 1.00	PI	Rank
Abulafia et al. [44]	Haigis (ULIB)	−0.030	0.320	0.270		89.5	100.0	*0.958*	1
106 eyes/68	Olsen	0.060	0.320	0.260		88.6	100.0	*0.938*	2
IOLMaster5.4	SRK/T (ULIB)	−0.040	0.350	0.280		86.8	100.0	*0.909*	3
MA60MA, SA60AT,	SRK/T	−0.050	0.350	0.280		86.8	100.0	*0.901*	4
SN60TT, SN60WF,	BUII	−0.100	0.320	0.280		89.5	100.0	*0.890*	5
SN6AD1, SN6ATT	Haigis	−0.170	0.350	0.310		78.9	100.0	*0.779*	6
>26.0 mm; ≥6.0D	Holladay 2	0.220	0.380	0.340		83.0	95.7	*0.719*	7
	Holladay 1_WK	−0.270	0.320	0.360		69.7	100.0	*0.696*	8
	Hoffer Q (ULIB)	0.270	0.370	0.360		71.1	98.7	*0.674*	9
	Hoffer Q	0.290	0.370	0.370		71.1	97.4	*0.659*	10
	SRK/T-WK	−0.310	0.360	0.410		65.8	100.0	*0.631*	11
	Holladay 1 (ULIB)	0.330	0.360	0.380		64.5	97.4	*0.631*	12
	Hoffer Q-WK	−0.350	0.350	0.420		67.1	98.7	*0.617*	13
	Holladay 1	0.350	0.360	0.400		63.2	97.4	*0.613*	14
	Haigis-WK	−0.720	0.330	0.730		23.7	77.6	*0.347*	15
Abulafia et al. [44]	Haigis-WK	−0.030	0.400	0.320		86.7	96.7	*0.842*	1
106 eyes/68	BUII	0.100	0.390	0.300		83.3	96.7	*0.808*	2
IOLMaster5.4	Holladay 1-WK	0.070	0.420	0.320		80.0	96.7	*0.789*	3
MA60MA, SA60AT,	SRK/T-WK	0.020	0.490	0.390		66.7	96.7	*0.711*	4
SN60TT, SN60WF,	Hoffer Q-WK	0.170	0.480	0.390		63.3	96.7	*0.640*	5
SN6AD1, SN6ATT	Haigis (ULIB)	0.120	0.580	0.480		60.0	86.7	*0.573*	6
>26.0 mm; <6.0D	Olsen	0.460	0.400	0.490		57.1	90.5	*0.520*	7
	SRK/T (ULIB)	0.140	0.670	0.550		53.3	86.7	*0.509*	8
	Holladay 1 (ULIB)	0.180	0.840	0.720		40.0	76.7	*0.400*	9
	Haigis	0.670	0.410	0.690		40.0	76.7	*0.395*	10
	SRK/T	0.820	0.530	0.840		30.0	70.0	*0.318*	11
	Hoffer Q (ULIB)	0.230	1.000	0.880		26.7	53.3	*0.309*	12
	Holladay 2	1.130	0.470	1.130		3.3	50.0	*0.109*	13
	Holladay 1	1.210	0.410	1.210		3.3	33.3	*0.105*	14
	Hoffer Q	1.420	0.490	0.370		3.3	16.7	*0.105*	15

Table 33.8 (continued)

Article	Formula	ME	SD	MAE	MedAE	± 0.50	± 1.00	PI	Rank
Cooke et al. [14] LS 900 SN60WF ≥26.0	Olsen4P	−0.020	0.325	0.250	0.190	85.2	100.0	*0.820*	1
	Olsen2P	−0.050	0.312	0.249	0.183	85.2	100.0	*0.814*	2
	Haigis	0.000	0.351	0.259	0.208	83.3	98.1	*0.792*	3
	BUII	0.050	0.355	0.274	0.218	83.3	100.0	*0.748*	4
	T2	0.030	0.388	0.293	0.251	83.3	96.3	*0.709*	5
	LSF	−0.220	0.388	0.335	0.278	72.2	96.3	*0.586*	6
	Holladay 1-WK	−0.220	0.388	0.335	0.278	72.2	96.3	*0.586*	6
	Holladay 2 NoRef	0.270	0.382	0.382	0.325	74.1	98.1	*0.546*	8
	SRK/T	0.200	0.444	0.392	0.344	77.8	94.4	*0.541*	9
	Holladay 2 PreSurgRef	0.260	0.400	0.394	0.352	72.2	98.1	*0.530*	10
	Hoffer Q	0.320	0.436	0.435	0.405	61.1	96.3	*0.469*	11
	Holladay 1	0.430	0.431	0.505	0.479	53.7	94.4	*0.412*	12
Cooke et al. [14] IOLMaster3.02 SN60WF ≥26.0	Haigis	−0.010	0.366	0.280	0.168	81.5	98.1	*0.785*	1
	Olsen4P	−0.140	0.352	0.290	0.198	83.3	98.1	*0.702*	2
	BUII	0.030	0.379	0.303	0.255	75.9	98.1	*0.697*	3
	T2	0.000	0.401	0.319	0.269	81.5	98.1	*0.695*	4
	LSF	−0.250	0.404	0.348	0.291	75.9	96.3	*0.567*	5
	Holladay 1-WK	−0.250	0.404	0.348	0.291	75.9	96.3	*0.567*	5
	SRK/T	0.170	0.454	0.399	0.368	75.9	98.1	*0.538*	7
	Holladay 2 NoRef	0.230	0.407	0.390	0.353	68.5	98.1	*0.533*	8
	Holladay 2 PreSurgRef	0.220	0.426	0.407	0.377	68.5	98.1	*0.519*	9
	Hoffer Q	0.300	0.445	0.430	0.388	63.0	96.3	*0.479*	10
	Holladay 1	0.400	0.446	0.495	0.473	55.6	92.6	*0.418*	11
Fam (Fam, Approaching atypical eyes with confidence [32]) 154 eyes eyes/146 IOLMaster3.02 eyes/ IOLMaster5.4 11 IOLs ≥26.0 mm; ≥ 5.0D	EVO	0.092	0.361	0.288	0.230	86.4	98.7	*0.712*	1
	BUII	0.030	0.406	0.316	0.270	80.5	99.4	*0.679*	2
	SRK/T-F2	0.144	0.369	0.313	0.250	81.8	98.1	*0.656*	3
	RBF	0.168	0.388	0.324	0.240	81.8	96.8	*0.637*	4
	Haigis (ULIB)	0.174	0.381	0.317	0.250	79.9	97.4	*0.634*	5
	SRK/T-F1	0.193	0.371	0.333	0.260	79.2	97.4	*0.619*	6
	SRK/T	0.212	0.376	0.346	0.290	76.6	98.1	*0.592*	7
	Holladay 1-WK	−0.237	0.365	0.348	0.310	75.3	97.4	*0.578*	8
	Hoffer Q	0.530	0.440	0.571	0.500	51.3	83.8	*0.375*	9
	Holladay 1	0.526	0.404	0.560	0.560	42.9	87.0	*0.364*	10

(continued)

Table 33.8 (continued)

Article	Formula	ME	SD	MAE	MedAE	± 0.50	± 1.00	PI	Rank
Fam (Fam, Approaching atypical eyes with confidence [32]) 43 eyes/40 7 type of IOLs ≥26.0 mm; < 5.0D	EVO	0.110	0.402	0.303	0.230	83.7	95.4	*0.669*	1
	Holladay-WK	−0.025	0.490	0.365	0.330	76.7	97.7	*0.597*	2
	Barrett	−0.088	0.484	0.388	0.310	72.1	97.7	*0.571*	3
	RBF 2.0	−0.107	0.482	0.396	0.310	69.8	97.7	*0.560*	4
	Haigis	0.575	0.509	0.596	0.510	48.8	83.7	*0.352*	5
	SRK/T-F2	0.636	0.852	0.716	0.480	51.2	81.4	*0.301*	6
	SRK/T-F1	0.714	0.859	0.778	0.560	48.8	79.1	*0.280*	7
	SRK/T	0.788	0.780	0.821	0.650	34.9	74.4	*0.258*	8
	Holladay 1	1.068	0.553	1.068	0.980	11.6	53.5	*0.174*	9
	Hoffer Q	1.308	0.634	1.308	1.170	7.0	25.6	*0.124*	10
Kane et al., Intraocular lens power formula accuracy: Comparison of 7 formulas [15] SN60WF IOLMaster 5.4 ≥26.0	SRK/T	0.060		0.484	0.419	62.7	97.3	*0.672*	1
	T2	−0.050		0.498	0.440	64.0	100.0	*0.666*	2
	BUII	−0.200		0.435	0.370	62.7	100.0	*0.656*	3
	Haigis	0.210		0.526	0.392	57.3	98.7	*0.595*	4
	Holladay 2	0.220		0.544	0.404	57.3	97.3	*0.581*	5
	Holladay 1	0.380		0.586	0.441	57.3	97.3	*0.510*	6
	Hoffer Q	0.340		0.589	0.467	53.3	98.7	*0.507*	7
Accuracy of 3 new methods for IPC Kane, JCRS 2017; 43:333–339 SN60WF IOLMaster 5.4 ≥26.0	RBF	−0.070		0.373	0.310	68.1	95.7	*0.796*	1
	SRK/T	−0.080		0.365	0.358	66.0	97.9	*0.763*	2
	BUII	−0.290		0.375	0.325	76.6	95.7	*0.685*	3
	LSF	−0.410		0.503	0.435	55.3	93.6	*0.520*	4
	FullMonte IOL	0.470		0.576	0.511	46.8	87.2	*0.452*	5
Melles et al. [20, 21] SA60AT, SN60WF LS900 25.5 > AL ≥ 28.5 mm	Kane			0.283					
	Olsen			0.289					
	BUII			0.298					
	Holladay 2			0.307					
	RBF			0.314					
	EVO			0.319					
	Haigis			0.320					
	SRK/T			0.365					
	Hoffer Q			0.428					
Melles et al. [20, 21] SA60AT, SN60WF LS900 >28.5 mm	Holladay 1			0.438					
	Kane			0.284					
	Olsen4P			0.288					
	Holladay 2			0.317					
	BUII			0.340					
	RBF			0.340					
	EVO			0.380					
	Haigis			0.420					
	SRK/T			0.502					
	Hoffer Q			0.828					

Table 33.8 (continued)

Article	Formula	ME	SD	MAE	MedAE	± 0.50	± 1.00	PI	Rank
Accuracy and precision of IOL Calculation	Holladay 1			0.978					
Wan, Am J Ophthalmol 2019; 205:66–73									
127 eyes/127	BUII		0.390		0.210	86.6	98.4	*0.967*	1
ZCB00, AR40E, SN60WF, SA60WF, SA60AT, MA60MA, MX60	RBF 2		0.400		0.200	86.6	96.9	*0.964*	2
IOLMaster500	Haigis		0.440		0.280	83.5	97.6	*0.859*	3
≥26.0 mm	Holladay 1-WK		0.410		0.310	71.7	96.1	*0.828*	4
	SRK/T		0.490		0.270	82.7	95.3	*0.825*	5
	Holladay 1		0.500		0.300	70.9	94.5	*0.773*	6
	SRK/T-WK		0.450		0.370	70.1	95.3	*0.760*	7
	Hoffer Q		0.540		0.330	73.2	94.5	*0.738*	8
	Hoffer Q-WK		0.440		0.490	51.2	92.9	*0.651*	9
	Haigis-WK		0.440		0.770	22.8	70.1	*0.422*	10
Darcy et al. [22]	Kane				0.329				
SA60AT, 920H, 970C, AO	Holladay 1				0.338				
	Holladay 2				0.352				
IOLMaster	Olsen				0.352				
≥26.0 mm	RBF 2.0				0.352				
	Haigis				0.359				
	SRK/T				0.363				
	Hoffer Q				0.454				
Savini et al. [45]	BUII				0.475				
SN60WF	EVO 2.0	0.042	0.306	0.168	0.211	89.5	100.0	*0.869*	1
OA-2000	Kane	−0.075	0.310	0.200	0.220	94.7	100.0	*0.822*	2
> 26.0 mm	BBUII	−0.011	0.323	0.202	0.253	84.2	94.7	*0.808*	3
	RBF 2.0	0.068	0.301	0.230	0.244	94.7	100.0	*0.797*	4
	Olsen4P	−0.076	0.308	0.209	0.256	89.5	100.0	*0.786*	5
	Haigis	−0.017	0.382	0.253	0.298	84.2	100.0	*0.721*	6
	T2	−0.049	0.378	0.270	0.311	89.5	100.0	*0.699*	7
	Holladay 2-ALadj	−0.142	0.345	0.265	0.296	84.2	100.0	*0.673*	8
	SRK/T	0.173	0.371	0.313	0.312	84.2	100.0	*0.622*	9
	VRF	−0.240	0.387	0.196	0.344	68.4	94.7	*0.599*	10
	Olsen2P	0.194	0.509	0.205	0.338	84.2	94.7	*0.590*	11
	Hoffer Q	0.346	0.439	0.248	0.397	73.7	89.5	*0.519*	12
	Panacea	−0.331	LT ≤ 4.19 mm	0.345	0.415	63.2	94.7	*0.499*	13

(continued)

Table 33.8 (continued)

Article	Formula	ME	SD	MAE	MedAE	± 0.50	± 1.00	PI	Rank
Cheng et al. [24]	Holladay 2	0.428	0.672	0.260	0.483	73.7	79.0	*0.422*	14
87 eyes/87	Holladay 1	0.567	0.454	0.436	0.582	57.9	79.0	*0.379*	15
IOLMaster700	Kane			0.306	0.248	80.5	98.9	*0.995*	1
MX60	EVO 2.0			0.315	0.250	78.2	97.7	*0.975*	2
≥26.0 mm	BUII			0.341	0.247	77.0	96.6	*0.948*	3
Zhang et al. [46]	RBF 2.0			0.345	0.251	74.7	97.7	*0.936*	4
164 eyes/164	PEARL-DGS			0.475	0.325	60.9	86.2	*0.735*	5
IOLMaster700	EVO 2.0	0.000	0.460	0.350	0.270	79.3	96.3	*0.649*	1
MX60	Holladay 1-AL1	0.000	0.480	0.350	0.270	74.4	95.7	*0.634*	2
≥26.0 mm	EVO-CMAL	0.000	0.470	0.360	0.280	76.2	95.7	*0.632*	3
	Holladay 1-nonlinear AL	0.000	0.470	0.360	0.280	75.0	95.7	*0.631*	4
	BUII	0.000	0.490	0.380	0.280	73.2	93.9	*0.611*	5
	SRK/T-AL1	0.000	0.500	0.380	0.290	76.2	94.5	*0.608*	6
	BUII-CMAL	0.000	0.500	0.380	0.300	70.1	93.9	*0.596*	7
	LSF-CMAL	0.000	0.540	0.400	0.290	72.0	93.3	*0.581*	8
	Holladay 1-AL2	0.000	0.510	0.400	0.330	68.9	95.1	*0.575*	9
	SRK/T-CMAL	0.000	0.540	0.400	0.310	72.6	92.7	*0.574*	10
	SRK/T-AL2	0.000	0.530	0.420	0.360	69.5	93.9	*0.552*	11
	Holladay 1-CMAL	0.000	0.550	0.420	0.350	68.9	94.5	*0.549*	12
Hipolito-Fernandes et al. [31]	LSF	0.000	0.570	0.430	0.320	68.3	91.5	*0.546*	13
828/828	SRK/T	0.000	0.580	0.430	0.350	66.5	93.3	*0.533*	14
LS-900	Holladay 1	0.000	0.620	0.480	0.400	63.4	92.1	*0.492*	15
SN60WF	Kane			0.301					
4 weeks	EVO 2.0			0.308					
Optimized	VRF-G			0.309					
≥26.0 mm	BBUII			0.319					
	Næser 2			0.319					
	RBF 2.0			0.325					
	VRF			0.329					
	T2			0.339					
	Haigis			0.352					
	SRK/T			0.364					

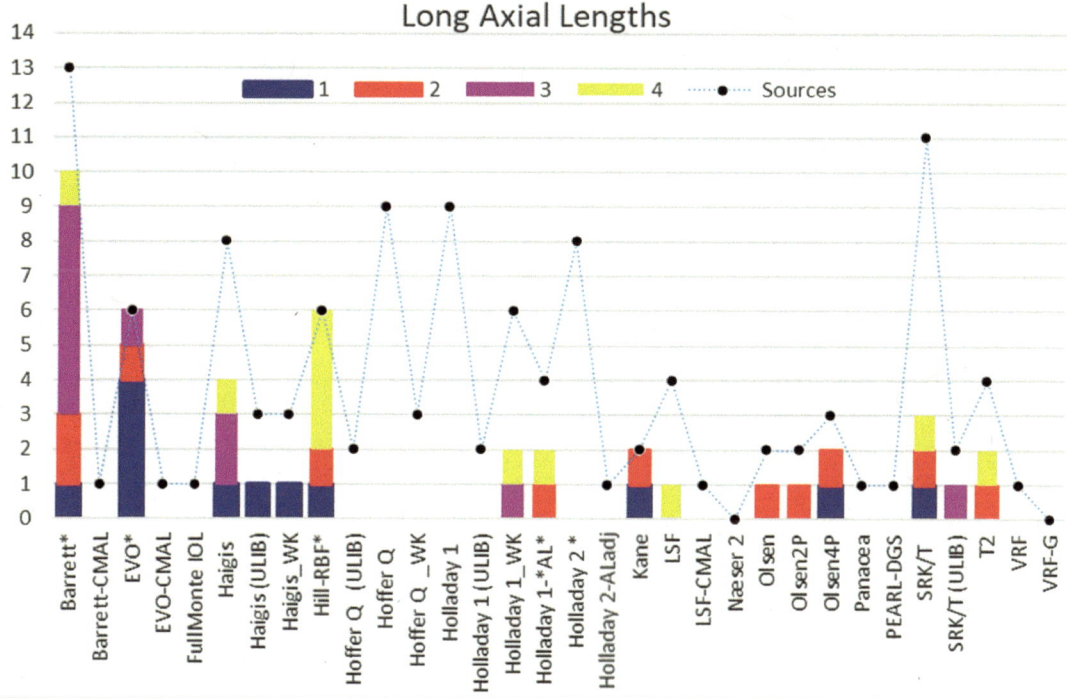

Fig. 33.9 Stacked histogram comparing the performance indices of the various formulas for long axial lengths (≥26 mm)

Other Parameters

Flat Cornea (<42.0D) & Steep Cornea (>48.0D)

The charts (Figs. 33.11 and 33.12) and Table 33.9 depict the extremes of cornea curvatures. These were virgin eyes without any history of corneal refractive surgery. Charts on the left column were for a flat cornea (<42.0D) and on the right column for a steep cornea (>48.0D). 7 different IOLs were used for flat eyes and 8 different IOLs for steep eyes. IOL constants for the third-generation formulas were from the larger pool of patients. ULIB constants were used for Haigis as some IOLs did not have enough numbers for triple optimization. BUII, EVO 2.0, and RBF 2.0 were calculated with the optimized A-constant. Fig. 33.11a, b shows the prediction errors of the formulas while Fig. 33.11

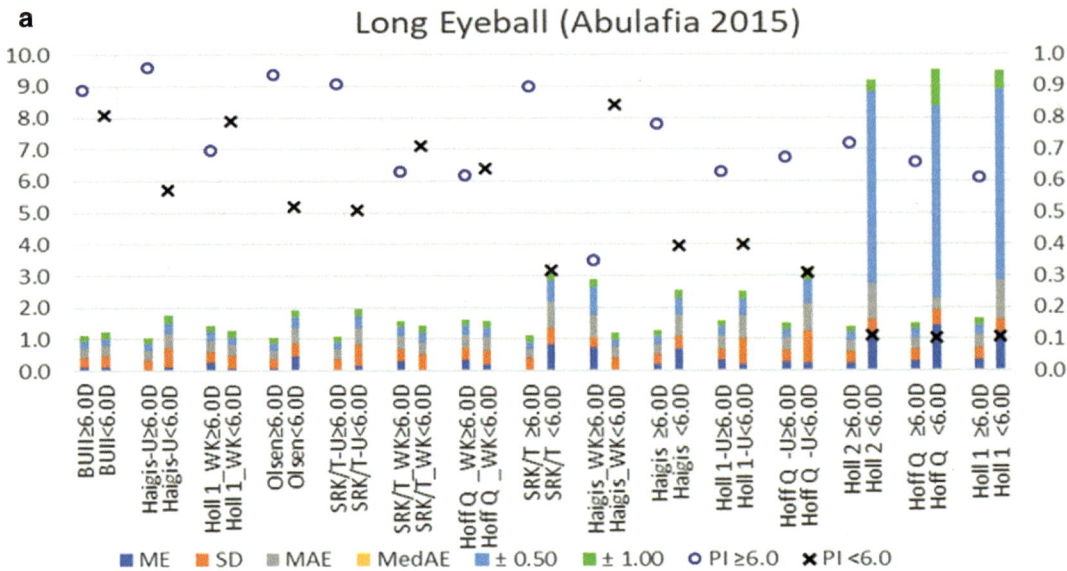

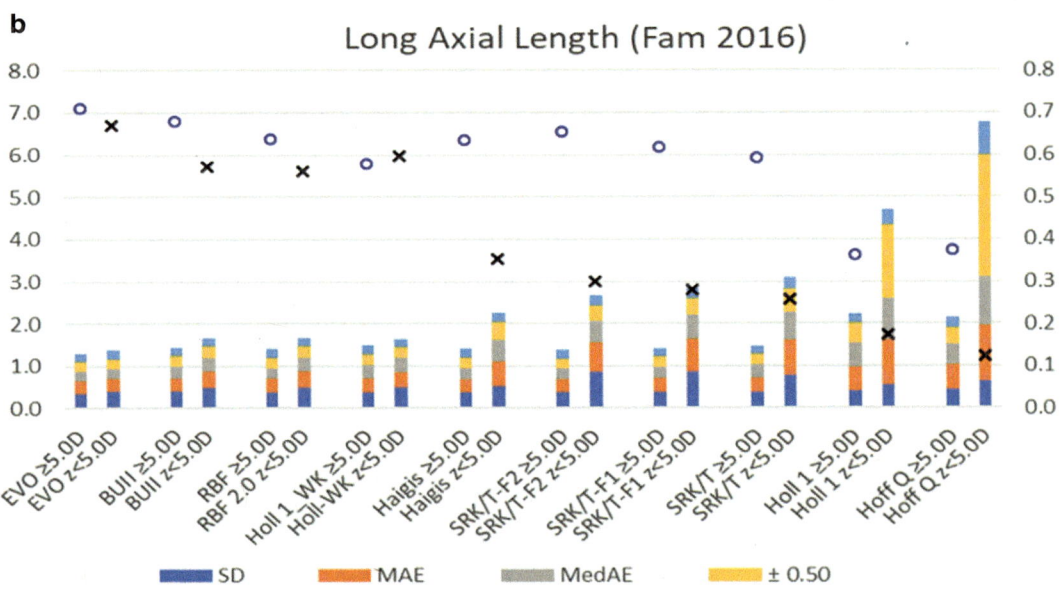

Fig. 33.10 Stacked histograms depicting the components of quality metrics and the line charts showing the subgroup Performance Indices, PI of the formulas for very long axial lengths. (**a**) is from the study by Abulafia [44] (**b**) is from Fam [32]. The circles are for higher diopter PIs, while the crosses are for lower diopter PIs. The scales for the stacked histograms *f* are on the left while the scales for PIs are on the right. BUII is Barrett. Holl and Hoff are short for Holladay and Hoffer Q respectively. SRK/T-F1 and SRK/T-F2 are Fam adjusted ALs [13]. -WK is with the Wang-Koch adjustments to the AL

Flat Cornea (< 42.0D) & Steep Cornea (> 48.0D)

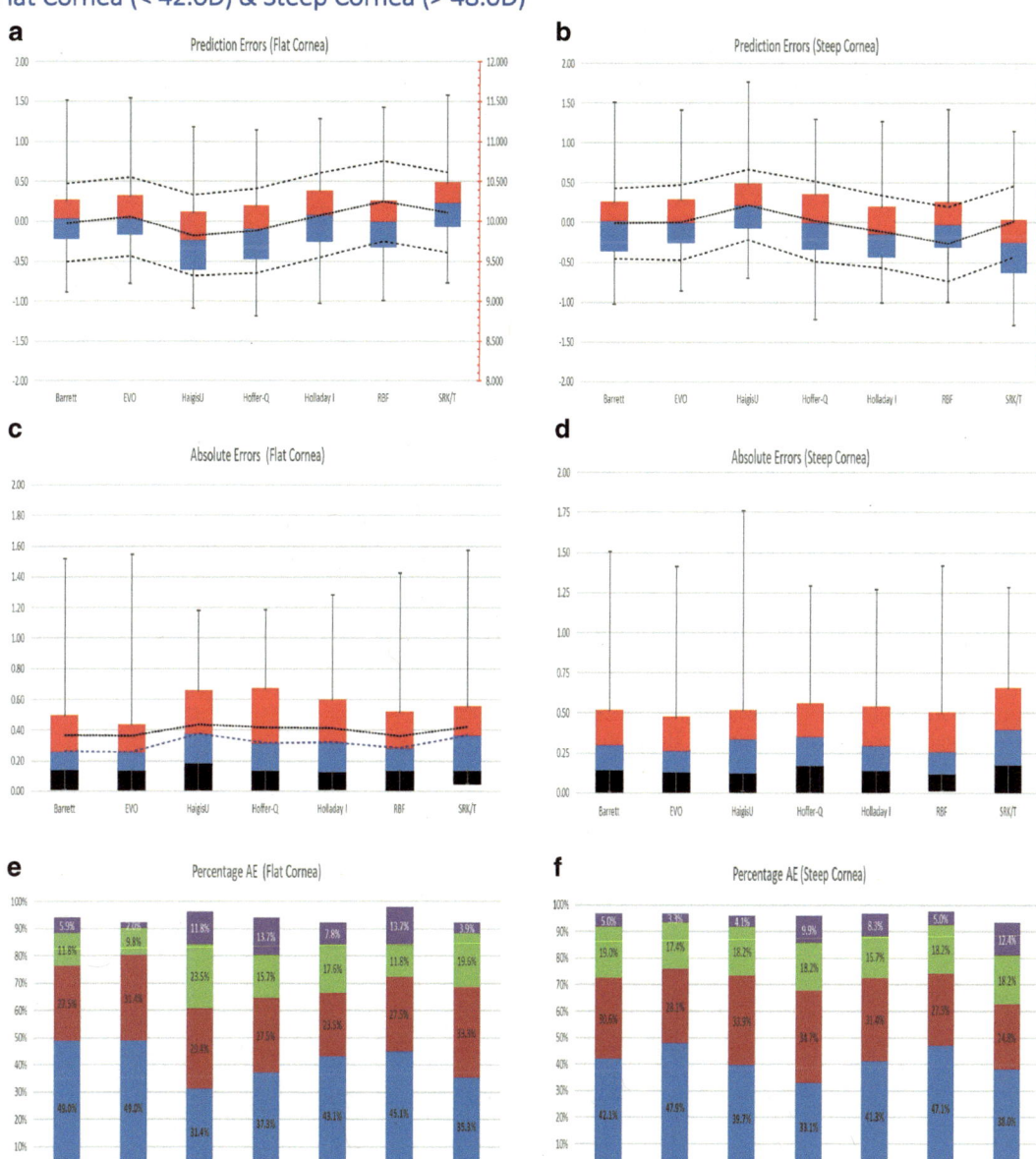

Fig. 33.11 The charts and Table 33.7 depict the outcomes for flat (<42.0D) and steep corneas (>48.0D). Charts on the left column were for flatter corneas and the right for steeper corneas. (**a, b**) Display the numerical prediction errors of the formulas. The colored boxes are for the 2nd and 3rd quartiles, while the error plots are for the 1st and 4th quartiles. The 2 dashed lines are the upper and lower SD. (**c, d**) depict the absolute errors. The tri-colored boxes are the 1st, 2nd, and 3rd quartiles, and the black and blue dashed lines are the MAEs and MedAEs. (**e, f**) The percentage of absolute errors

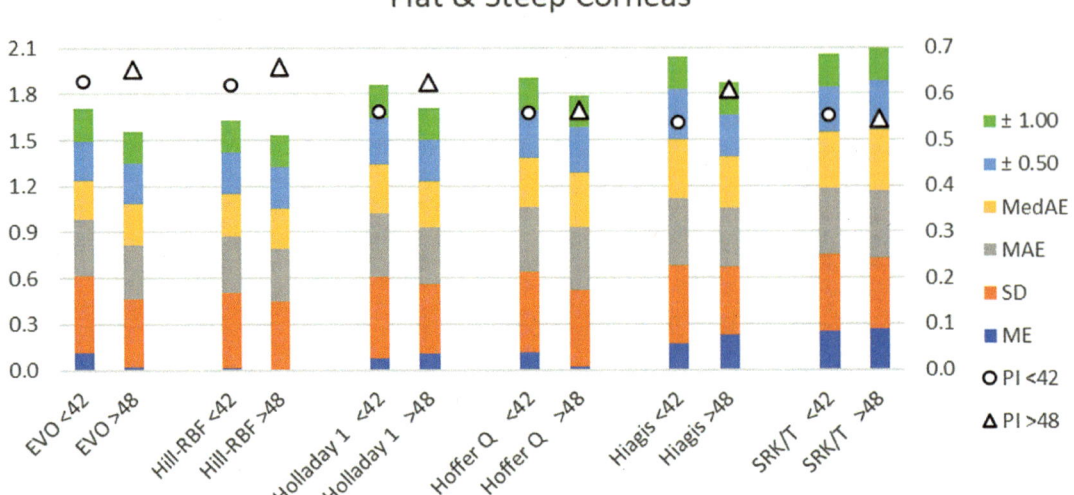

Flat & Steep Corneas

Fig. 33.12 The stacked histogram shows the quality metrics of the formulas with different corneal powers. <42 is for a corneal power of less than 42 D and >48 is for a corneal power of greater than 48 D. The scale for the stacked histogram is on the left. The lower the stacked histogram, the better is the formula. The circles and triangles are for the performance indices (PI). The scale for PI is on the right. The higher the PI score, the better. The formulas in Table 33.9 are arranged in order of their subgroup PI ranking. n is for the number of eyes. ME and SD are the means and standard deviations of numerical prediction errors, respectively. MAE and MedAE are the mean and median absolute errors. ±0.50 and ±1.00 are the percentage of eyes within ±0.50 D and ±1.00 D target refractions, respectively

Table 33.9 This table shows the modified Haigis performance indices of the various formulas (EVO is EVO 1.0; RBF is RBF 1.0) [32]

<42.0D	n	ME	SDE	MAE	MedAE	±0.50	±1.00	PI	Rank
RBF	51	−0.015	0.487	0.366	0.280	72.5	98.0	*0.615*	1
BUII	51	0.057	0.495	0.368	0.270	76.5	94.1	*0.601*	2
EVO	51	0.114	0.502	0.364	0.260	80.4	92.2	*0.586*	3
Holladay 1	51	0.078	0.530	0.413	0.320	66.7	92.2	*0.538*	4
Hoffer Q	51	−0.115	0.527	0.419	0.320	64.7	94.1	*0.526*	5
Haigis	51	−0.174	0.509	0.436	0.380	60.8	96.1	*0.491*	6
SRK/T	51	0.252	0.502	0.425	0.370	68.6	92.2	*0.486*	7
>48.0D	n	ME	SD E	MAE	MedAE	±0.50	±1.00	PI	Rank
RBF	121	−0.008	0.443	0.343	0.260	74.4	97.5	*0.654*	1
EVO	121	0.023	0.446	0.343	0.270	76.0	96.7	*0.644*	2
BUII	121	0.002	0.472	0.367	0.300	72.7	96.7	*0.616*	3
Holladay 1	121	−0.106	0.455	0.366	0.300	72.7	96.7	*0.585*	4
Hoffer Q	121	0.018	0.503	0.405	0.360	67.8	95.9	*0.559*	5
Haigis	121	0.225	0.443	0.382	0.340	73.6	95.9	*0.534*	6
SRK/T	121	−0.263	0.468	0.433	0.400	62.8	93.4	*0.477*	7

c, d show the absolute errors. Figure 33.11e, f are the percentage of absolute errors. Furthers details on the outcomes are in the following tables. Formulas had different accuracy in flat (<42.0D) and steep (>48.0D) eyes. Using the Haigis Quality Metrics, EVO 2.0 and BUII performed the best for flat corneas while RBF 2.0 and EVO 2.0 for steep corneas. In these extremes of curvatures, Haigis and SRK/T were biased and were oppositely affected. Haigis overestimated while SRK/T underestimated for the flat cornea. The converse was true for the steep cornea. From graph G, most formulas were slightly better with a steep cornea than with a flat, except for SRK/T. However, this may not be conclusive, as the comparison was not with the same number of eyes. The above paper was presented in APACRS 2016 in Bali [32].

The bias or neutrality of formulas with AL and K was reflected with the many charts above and below. This trend was also noted by Melles et al. [20, 21].

Ametropia

At the APACRS annual conference in Hangzhou, Fam presented his finding on ametropia outcomes [7]. The study included 111 eyes with 3 different IOLs. The IOL constants were opti-

mized for the third-generation formulas from a larger pool. The BUIIt was calculated using the optimized A-constant. The targeted refraction ranged from −1.00 D to −5.00 D with the average at −2.00 D.

The charts (Fig. 33.13) and Table 33.10 detailed the outcomes for the ametropia study. IOL constants for the third-generation formulas were optimized from the larger pool of patients. HaigisT was Haigis with triple optimization. BUII and EVO were calculated with the optimized A-constant. Figure 33.13a, b show the prediction (numerical) errors and the absolute errors of the formulas, respectively, while Fig. 33.13c is a stacked histogram depicting the percentage of

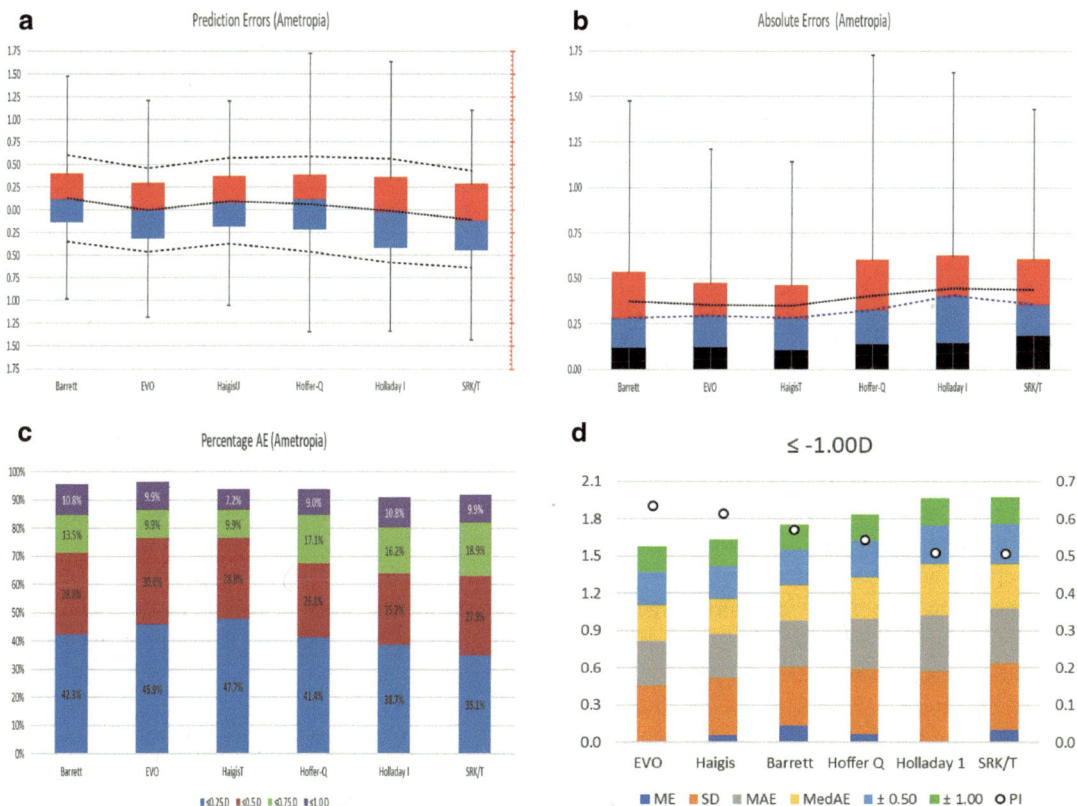

Fig. 33.13 The charts present the numerical prediction error (**a**), absolute error (**b**), the percentage of eyes within the specified prediction errors (**c**), and the quality metrics (**d**). The colored boxes in (**a**) are for the second and third quartiles while the error plot are for the first and fourth quartiles. The 2 dashed lines are the upper and lower standard deviations. The 3 colored boxes in (**b**) are the first, second, and third quartiles and the black and blue dashed lines are the mean and median absolute errors. The stacked histograms in (**d**) are the components of quality metrics.

The lower the total column the better. The circles represent the subgroup PI. The higher the better. The details of the charts are tabulated in Table 33.10. The formulas in Table 33.10 are arranged in order of their subgroup PI ranking. *n* is for the number of eyes. ME and SD E are the means and standard deviations of numerical prediction errors, respectively. MAE and MedAE are the mean and median absolute errors. ± 0.50 and ± 1.00 are the percentage of eyes within 0.5 and 1.0D target refractions, respectively

Table 33.10 This table shows the modified Haigis performance indices of the various formulas [7]

≤-1.00D	n	ME	SD E	MAE	MedAE	±0.50	±1.00	PI	Rank
EVO	111	0.000	0.460	0.355	0.290	76.6	96.4	*0.635*	1
Haigis	111	0.061	0.459	0.353	0.280	76.6	93.7	*0.615*	2
BUII	111	0.131	0.477	0.376	0.280	71.2	95.5	*0.570*	3
Hoffer Q	111	0.067	0.524	0.408	0.330	67.6	93.7	*0.544*	4
Holladay 1	111	−0.008	0.570	0.446	0.410	64.0	91.0	*0.508*	5
SRK/T	111	−0.102	0.536	0.440	0.360	63.1	91.9	*0.507*	6

Table 33.11 ME, SD, MAE, and MedAE refer to mean numerical prediction error, the standard deviation of prediction error, mean absolute error, and median absolute error, respectively

Article	Formula	ME	SD	MAE	MedAE	±0.50	±1.00	PI	Rank
Turnbull et al. [26]	*BUII*	−0.02	0.195	0.241	0.197	87.5	100	*0.925*	1
176/88	*Haigis*	−0.03	0.211	0.284	0.218	85.2	100	*0.849*	2
SN6ATT	*RBF 2.0*	−0.1	0.202	0.271	0.225	86.4	100	*0.813*	3
Distance	*SRK/T*	0.01	0.221	0.307	0.277	83	100	*0.796*	4
	Holladay 1	0.01	0.267	0.334	0.268	78.4	98.9	*0.748*	5
	Hoffer Q	0.01	0.265	0.344	0.289	75	98.9	*0.726*	6
Near (−1.00D)	*BUII*	0.01	0.26	0.298	0.235	86.4	97.3	*0.806*	1
	RBF 2.0	−0.06	0.258	0.3	0.233	81.8	97.7	*0.769*	2
	SRK/T	−0.02	0.294	0.356	0.261	70.5	97.7	*0.705*	3
	Haigis	0	0.311	0.351	0.26	69.3	95.5	*0.704*	4
	Holladay 1	−0.01	0.329	0.392	0.32	71.6	95.5	*0.649*	5
	Hoffer Q	−0.03	0.341	0.415	0.319	64.8	93.2	*0.614*	6

eyes within a specified Diopter range of predicted spherical equivalent. Figure 33.13d is the stacked histogram of the quality metrics for each of the formulas. The circle represents the subgroup performance index, PI. The table shows the details of Haigis' Quality Metrics. EVO was the highest-ranking followed by Haigis and Barrett. All three formulas have performance indices that were better than 0.6.

Monovision is a fairly common practice to reduce spectacles dependency. Turnbull et al. looked at the accuracy of various formulas when targeting ametropia [26]. They used a single IOL (SN6ATx) with the constants optimized for the entire dataset. 88 patients planning for monovision were recruited for the study with one eye targeting distance and the other for −1.25 D for near (Table 33.11, Fig. 33.14). Postoperative refractions were done 4 weeks postoperatively.

The formulas perform better when targeting emmetropia than they do for ametropia. BUII and RBF 2.0 were similar in their accuracy and had the least difference between targeting emmetropia and targeting for near. BUII had 87.5% and 86.4%, while RBF had 86.4% and 81.8% within ±0.50 D for distance and near respectively. While Haigis and SRK/T had more than 80% (Haigis, 85.2% and SRK/T, 83.0%) within ±0.50 D for distance, that figure dropped down to 69.3% and 70.5% for near respectively. The differences were statistically significant. Holladay 1 and Hoffer Q had less than 70% for both distance and near eyes. The paper highlighted the decrease in accuracy when targeting ametropia as opposed to emmetropia in IOL power calculation. BUII and RBF were the least affected by this phenomenon.

In the year following his earlier study on short eyes, Gökce et al. published another paper looking into the accuracy of 8 different formulas with different ACDs in patients with normal ALs [47]. Gökce et al. stratified the ACD into 3 groups: ≤3.0 mm, >3.0 to <3.5 mm, and finally ≥3.5 mm.

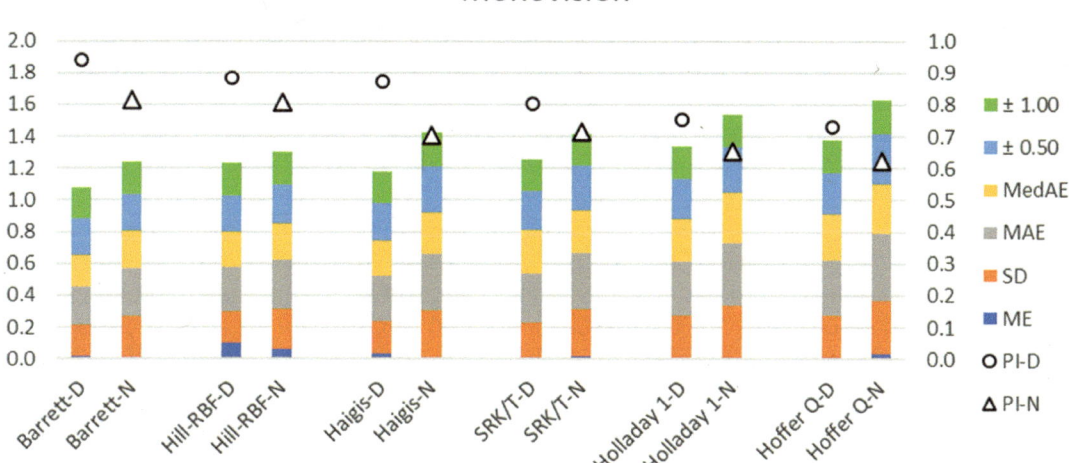

Fig. 33.14 The stacked histogram shows the quality metrics of the formulas with a different refractive target. -D is for distance target and -N for near (−1.00D). The scale for the stacked histogram is on the left. The lower the stacked histogram, the better is the formula. The circles and triangles are for the performance index (PI). The scale for PI is on the right. The higher the PI score, the better

Only patients with AL between 22.0 and 25.0 mm were recruited in this study. For the medium ACD group, all formulas had mean prediction error values that were close to zero. In the shallow ACD and deep ACD groups, BUII, Holladay 2, Haigis, and Olsen$_{4P}$ had mean prediction errors that were not significantly deviated from zero. BUII had the lowest MAE in all 3 ACD groups. It had the lowest MedAE (0.18 D) in the shallow ACD group and next to the lowest (0.21 D) in the deep ACD group. BUII, Haigis, and Holladay 2 (with and without refraction) were noted to have no bias against ACD. RBF 2.0 was good for medium and large ACD groups. Olsen$_{4P}$ was good for shallow and deep ACD groups. The study noted that when the mean numerical PE for each formula for the dataset was optimized to zero, the MedAE for BUII, Haigis, Holladay 1 and 2, Olsen, and RBF 2.0 were found to have no differences. The paper inferred that ACD was an important variable in the accuracy of IOL power calculation and that multiple-variable formulas were more accurate than 2-variable formulas (3rd generation).

Hipólito-Fernandez also looked at the impact of ACD and LT on the accuracy of the formulas [48]. Like Gökce, they divide the ACD into 3 similar groups. They included ALs between 22.0 and 26.0 mm. This is a single IOL (SN60WF) with LenStar LS900 (Haag-Streit AG, Köniz, Switzerland) as the preoperative biometer. 695 eyes of 695 patients were recruited. Postoperative refraction was done at 4 weeks. Their conclusion was the new generation formulas, particularly Kane, PEARL-DGS and EVO 2.0 were more reliable and robust across the various ACD and LT combinations.

From the 2 stacked histograms, the newer formulas such BUII, Kane, PEARL-DGS, and EVO 2.0 were more precise and robust than the third-generation theoretical formulas (Table 33.12, Fig. 33.15). For normal ACD (3.0 to 3.5 mm) most formulas perform well. It was in the shallow and deeper ACDs that we see the new formulas perform more consistently better. Without requiring ACD as a parameter, most of the third-generation formulas were unable to take ACD variation into account.

Table 33.12 ME, SD, MAE, and MedAE refer to mean numerical prediction error, the standard deviation of prediction error, mean absolute error, and median absolute error respectively. Holladay 2 PreSurgRef and Holladay 2 NoRef refer to Holladay 2 formula with and without preoperative refractions, respectively. Olsen2P and Olsen4P are Olsen using 2 parameters and 4 parameters to determine ELPs, respectively. Olsen2P is preinstalled in biometers, while Olsen4P is also known as Olsen standalone and is available in the program, PhacoOptics

Article	Formula	ME	SD E	MAE	MedAE	± 0.50	± 1.00	PI	Rank
Gokce et al. [47] LS-900 ZCB00, ZCT 270eyes/270 ACD ≤ 3.0 mm	BUII	0.000	0.320	0.240	0.180	90.2	99.0	*0.859*	1
	Holladay 2 NoRef	0.010	0.360	0.290	0.250	86.3	100.0	*0.745*	2
	Olsen4P	0.060	0.350	0.280	0.240	87.3	100.0	*0.736*	3
	Holladay 2 PreSurgRef	−0.010	0.370	0.300	0.280	83.3	100.0	*0.714*	4
	RBF	−0.100	0.380	0.300	0.220	83.3	99.0	*0.693*	5
	Haigis	0.000	0.390	0.320	0.300	81.4	99.0	*0.686*	6
	Holladay 1	−0.140	0.360	0.300	0.230	80.4	99.0	*0.675*	7
	Olsen2P	0.100	0.380	0.320	0.280	79.4	100.0	*0.653*	8
	Hoffer Q	−0.200	0.410	0.360	0.300	74.5	98.0	*0.574*	9
	RBF	0.030	0.330	0.280	0.270	87.1	100.0	*0.746*	1
	BUII	−0.010	0.360	0.290	0.250	85.9	98.8	*0.743*	2
ACD > 3.0 mm ACD < 3.5 mm	Holladay 2 NoRef	−0.010	0.370	0.300	0.280	88.2	98.8	*0.720*	3
	Holladay 1	0.020	0.360	0.290	0.280	83.5	98.8	*0.718*	4
	Haigis	0.020	0.380	0.300	0.250	83.5	97.7	*0.717*	5
	Olsen4P	0.000	0.390	0.310	0.260	80.0	97.7	*0.707*	6
	Hoffer Q	0.020	0.370	0.320	0.290	85.9	97.7	*0.696*	7
	Holladay 2 PreSurgRef	−0.030	0.390	0.310	0.280	84.7	97.7	*0.689*	8
	Olsen2P	0.000	0.410	0.330	0.280	80.0	97.7	*0.678*	9
	BUII	0.010	0.300	0.240	0.210	88.0	100.0	*0.842*	1
	Olsen4P	−0.070	0.320	0.250	0.200	83.1	100.0	*0.781*	2
	Holladay 2 NoRef	0.020	0.320	0.270	0.270	88.0	100.0	*0.765*	3
ACD ≥ 3.5 mm	RBF	0.100	0.300	0.260	0.220	86.8	100.0	*0.763*	4
	Holladay 2 PreSurgRef	0.030	0.330	0.280	0.260	88.0	100.0	*0.753*	5
	Haigis	−0.020	0.350	0.280	0.260	86.8	100.0	*0.746*	6
	Holladay 1	0.150	0.300	0.270	0.260	89.2	100.0	*0.712*	7
	Olsen2P	−0.140	0.350	0.290	0.230	78.3	100.0	*0.682*	8
	Hoffer Q	0.210	0.330	0.320	0.320	81.9	98.8	*0.615*	9
Hipolito-Fernandes et al. [48] 695eyes/695 LS900 SN60WF	Kane	0.010	0.400	0.316	0.277	80.2	98.7	*0.687*	1
	PEARL-DGS	−0.020	0.400	0.322	0.270	81.1	99.1	*0.685*	2
	BUII	0.020	0.410	0.331	0.290	78.0	98.7	*0.662*	3
	EVO 2.0	0.030	0.410	0.327	0.297	78.0	97.8	*0.656*	4
	RBF 2.0	−0.010	0.430	0.337	0.280	74.9	98.7	*0.655*	5
	SRK/T	−0.090	0.440	0.348	0.292	76.7	97.4	*0.611*	6
	Haigis	−0.040	0.450	0.361	0.313	72.7	97.4	*0.608*	7
ACD ≤ 3.00 mm	Holladay 1	−0.150	0.420	0.344	0.289	74.4	97.4	*0.596*	8
	Hoffer Q	−0.200	0.420	0.365	0.295	71.8	96.5	*0.566*	9
	Kane	0.000	0.400	0.315	0.276	81.6	97.3	*0.694*	1
	PEARL-DGS	−0.020	0.420	0.321	0.270	79.9	97.3	*0.673*	2
	Holladay 1	0.000	0.410	0.343	0.288	79.3	97.0	*0.667*	3
ACD > 3.00 ACD < 3.50	RBF 2.0	0.000	0.420	0.337	0.280	77.9	97.0	*0.667*	4
	EVO 2.0	−0.020	0.410	0.327	0.297	80.6	97.3	*0.663*	5
	BUII	−0.010	0.420	0.331	0.290	79.6	97.0	*0.663*	6
	SRK/T	0.000	0.430	0.348	0.292	77.9	97.3	*0.653*	7
	Hoffer Q	0.020	0.430	0.365	0.295	78.6	97.0	*0.637*	8
	Haigis	−0.010	0.450	0.360	0.313	76.6	94.6	*0.623*	9
	EVO 2.0	−0.050	0.440	0.345	0.285	75.7	97.9	*0.630*	1

(continued)

Table 33.12 (continued)

Article	Formula	ME	SD E	MAE	MedAE	± 0.50	± 1.00	PI	Rank
ACD ≥ 3.50	RBF 2.0	0.010	0.450	0.363	0.320	77.5	98.2	*0.623*	**2**
	Kane	−0.050	0.460	0.351	0.286	76.3	97.6	*0.620*	**3**
	BUII	−0.020	0.460	0.363	0.310	76.9	96.4	*0.617*	**4**
	PEARL-DGS	−0.040	0.460	0.359	0.310	74.0	95.3	*0.606*	**5**
	Haigis	−0.010	0.480	0.378	0.319	75.7	95.3	*0.602*	**6**
	Holladay 1	0.100	0.440	0.367	0.326	75.7	98.2	*0.588*	**7**
	SRK/T	0.080	0.470	0.386	0.370	71.6	97.6	*0.559*	**8**
	Hoffer Q	0.190	0.460	0.399	0.347	67.5	95.9	*0.526*	**9**

From Fig. 33.16, the newer formulas such as Kane, EVO 2.0, PEARL-DGS, and BUII show remarkable robustness between the 3 subgroups of LT (≤4.19 mm; 4.20–4.76 mm; ≥4.77 mm) and show good precision overall. The third-generation formulas were sensitive to thin and thick lens thickness.

Ray Tracing and Intraoperative Aberrometry

Hoffmann et al. looked at the benefits of raytracing IOL power calculation for 3 aspheric-correcting IOLs in 2013 [49]. The study compared the outcomes of 308 eyes of 185 patients using Okulix ray-tracing software (version 8.79) with Hoffer Q, Holladay 1, and SRK/T. All preoperative measurements were done with LenStar and the one-month postoperative refractions were used. The constants of the third-generation formulas were optimized. The ray-tracing calculation with offset correction (mean error adjust to zero) had the lowest SD/MAE/MedAE of 0.37D/0.30D/0.24D compared to the third-generation formulas. Raytracing with offset correction had the highest percentage (81.1%) of eyes within ±0.50 D of prediction error. The paper commented that raytracing reduced the number of outliers in calculating IOL powers.

Raufi et al. published a paper looking into the outcomes of intraoperative aberrometry and comparing it with BUII and RBF [50]. 949 virgin eyes of 949 patients with 4 different IOLs were included in this study. Preoperatively, all eyes were measured with Lenstar LS 900, and postoperatively, all eyes were refracted no earlier than one month. Overall, BUII had the lowest MAE/MedAE with 0.29 D and 0.23 D, respectively. BUII had the highest percentage of eyes within ±0.50 D, 84.0%. They concluded that there was no significant difference between ORA [51] and the 2 preoperative IOL formulas.

The accuracy of intraoperative aberrometry in short eyes was studied by Sudhakar et al. [52]. Using ULIB constants, the subjects in the retrospective study were implanted with 6 different IOLs. Preoperatively, measurements were done with IOLMaster 500 PCI, and refractions were done between 20 and 60 days postoperatively. Except for Haigis (+0.26 D), most of the formulas had mean prediction errors that were insignificantly different from zero. RBF and ORA had the lowest MAE with 0.49 D and 0.48 D and the highest percentage of eyes within ±0.50 D, 60.8%, and 58.8%, respectively. The conclusion was that ORA was equivalent to the best preoperative IOL formulas.

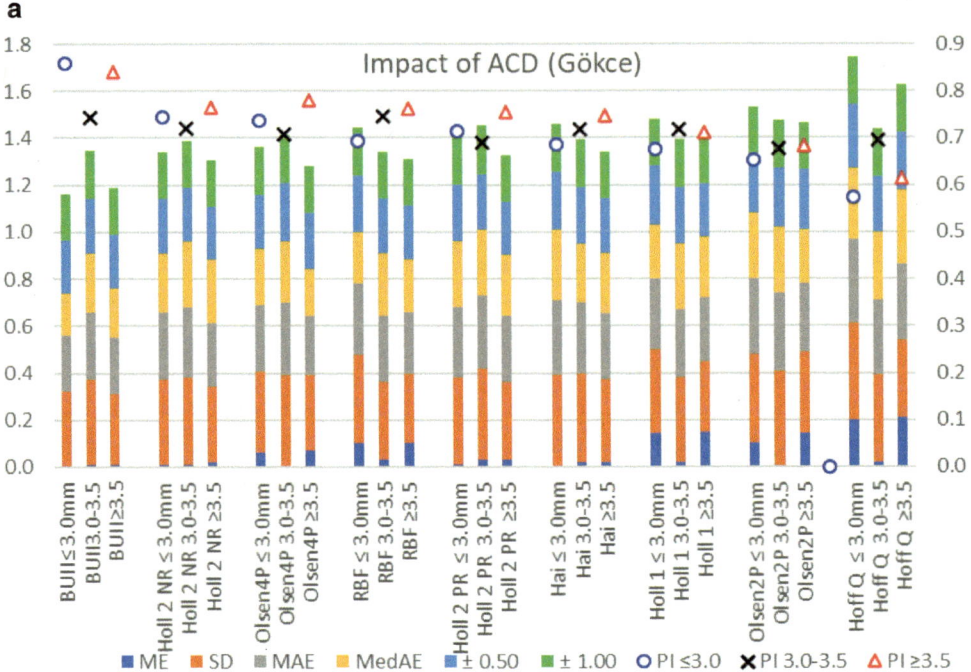

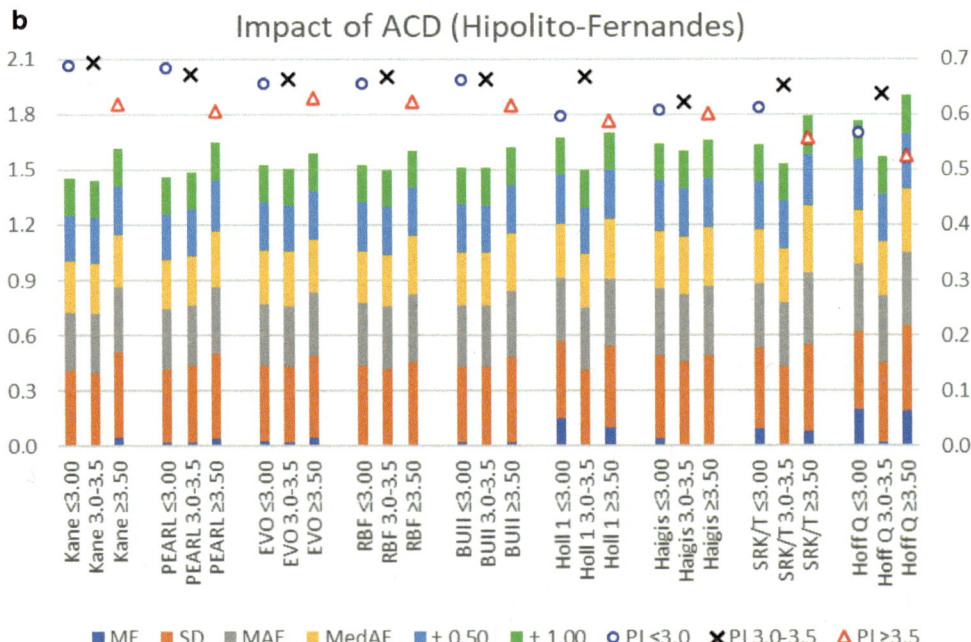

Fig. 33.15 The stacked histograms show the quality metrics of the formulas with different ACDs. Chart (**a**) and (**b**) are based on Gökce et al. [47] and Hipólito-Fernandez et al. [48] respectively. Each formula is divided into 3 ACD groups (≤3.00 mm; 3.00 to 3.50 mm; ≥3.50 mm). The scale for the stacked histogram is on the left. The lower the stacked histogram, the better is the formula performance. The circles and triangles represent the performance index (PI). The scale for PI is on the right. The higher the PI score, the better. BUII = Barrett Universal II, Hai = Haigis, Hoff = Hoffer Q, Holl = Holladay 1, PEARL = PEARL-DGS, RBF = RBF 2.0

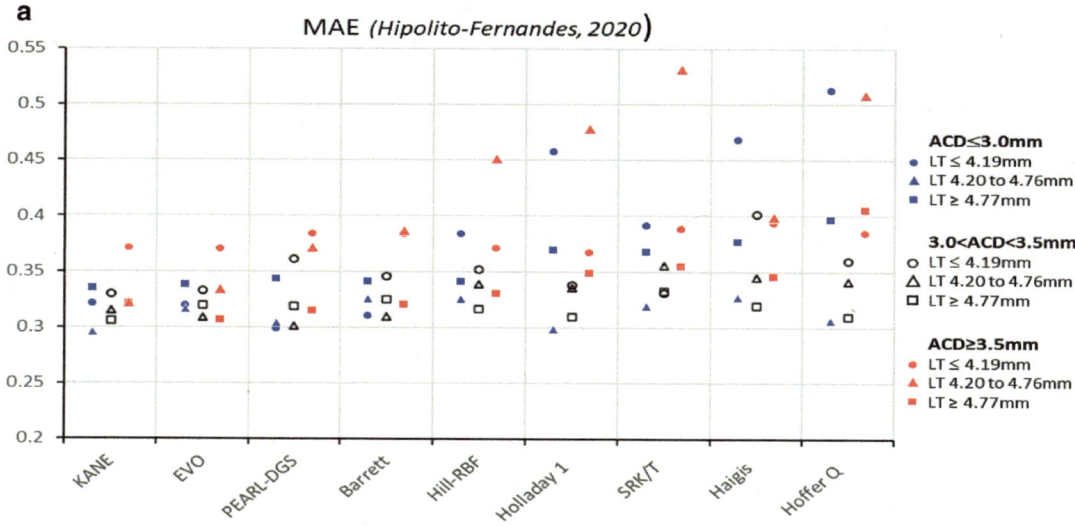

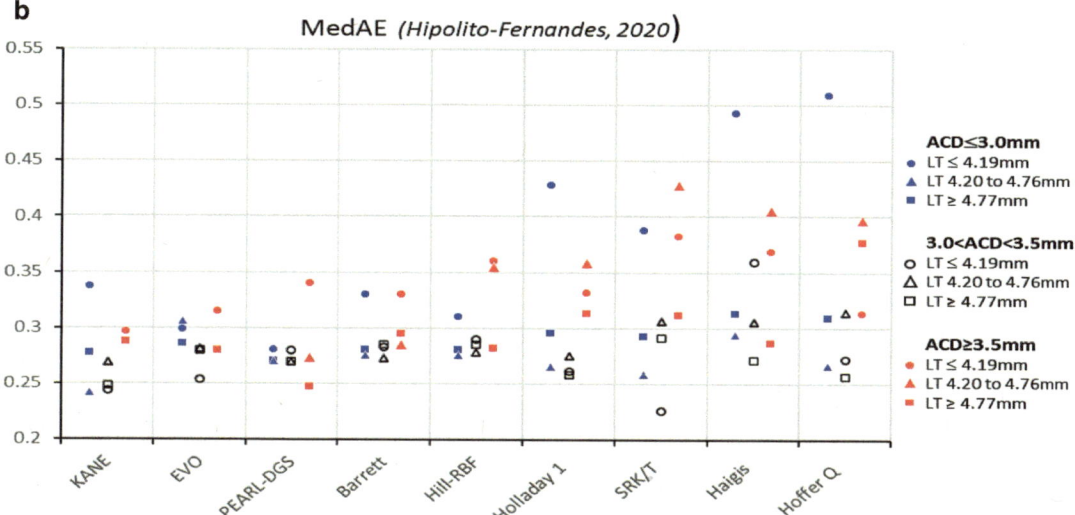

Fig. 33.16 The line graphs show the relationship of the mean (**a**) and median (**b**) absolute errors with varying ACDs and LTs. *BUII* = Barrett, *Hai* = Haigis, *Hoff* = Hoffer Q, *Holl* = Holladay 1, *PEARL* = PEARL-DGS, *RBF* = RBF 2.0

Even More Parameters

Table 33.13 is a summary of outcomes in the literature as well as papers presented at conferences on other parameters affecting IOL power calculation. As with the earlier table, the orders of the formula for each source are sorted in order based on a modification of Haigis "Quality metrics for comparing IOL calculation formulas."

The stacked histogram (Fig. 33.17) shows how the formulas fare in 4 articles, all of which are ranked. Each box indicates the number of times the formula is being ranked. Blue is for 1st; magenta for 2nd ranking; turquoise for 3rd, and yellow for 4th. The dotted line joins the number of ranked studies the formula was being compared tp. BUII was the most quoted and had dem-

Table 33.13 ME, SD, MAE, and MedAE refer to mean numerical prediction error, the standard deviation of prediction error, mean absolute error, and median absolute error respectively

Article	Formula	ME	SD E	MAE	MedAE	± 0.50	± 1.00	PI	Rank
Hoffmann & Lindemann, Intraocular lens calculation for aspheric intraocular lenses [49] 308eyes/185 iMics1, SN60WF, Tecnis	Okulix 8.79 (corrected)	0.000	0.370	0.300	0.240	81.1	99.7	*0.737*	1
	AL selected	0.000	0.410	0.310	0.260	79.8	97.7	*0.697*	2
	Holladay	0.000	0.410	0.310	0.260	79.2	97.4	*0.695*	3
	Hoffer Q	0.000	0.410	0.320	0.280	76.6	98.4	*0.678*	4
	SRK/T	0.000	0.430	0.340	0.280	78.8	98.1	*0.663*	5
	Okulix 8.79	0.040	0.410	0.340	0.300	76.2	99.4	*0.644*	6
Hirnschall et al. [53] 40Eyes/40 409 M/MP IOLMaster 700	Ray		0.320	0.320	0.270	80	95	*0.730*	1
	BUII		0.290	0.370	0.330	75	98	*0.685*	2
	RBF 2.0		0.310	0.390	0.300	73	93	*0.672*	3
	Haigis		0.360	0.420	0.330	55	93	*0.592*	4
	SRK/T		0.390	0.520	0.450	70	93	*0.537*	5
Raufi et al. [50] 949eyes/603 LS-900	BUII	−0.018		0.290	0.230	84	97	*1.018*	1
	RBF 2.0	0.047		0.310	0.240	83	97	*0.958*	2
	ORA	−0.041		0.310	0.250	82	97	*0.951*	3
Sudhakar [52] 51eyes/38 IOLMaster AO60, AF-1 FY60AD, SA60AT, ZCT, ZKB00, ZLB00	IA	0.000		0.480		58.8	88.2	*0.955*	1
	RBF 2.0	0.070		0.490		60.8	90.2	*0.900*	2
	BUII	0.110		0.510		52.9	86.3	*0.813*	3
	Hoffer Q	−0.080		0.540		49	86.3	*0.794*	4
	Holladay 2	−0.140		0.530		43.1	88.2	*0.735*	5
	Haigis	0.260		0.600		52.9	80.4	*0.673*	6

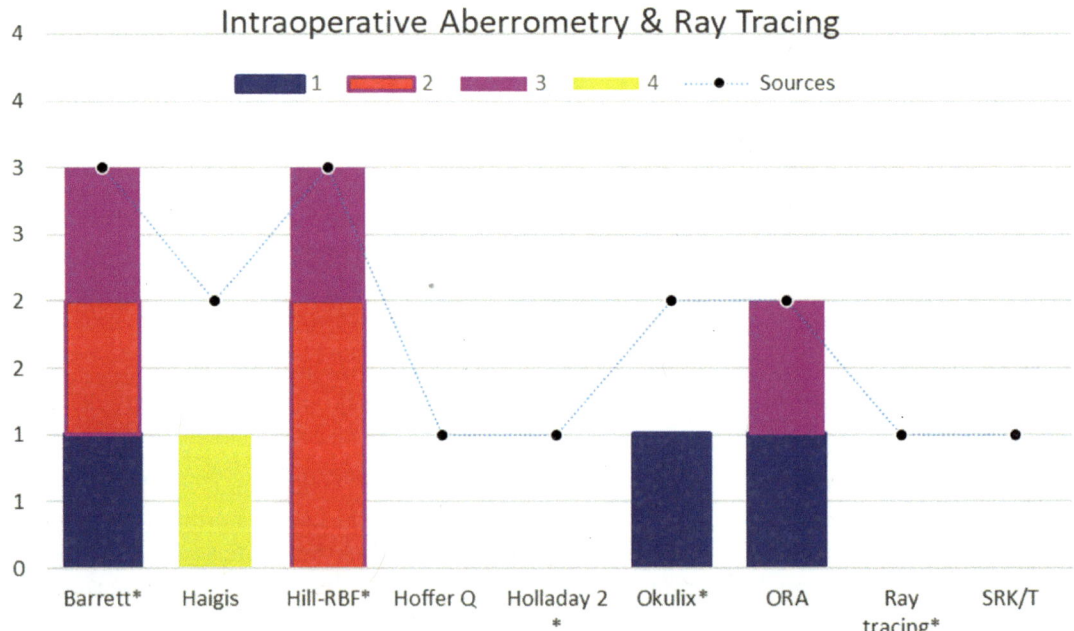

Fig. 33.17 Stacked histogram comparing the performance indices intraoperative aberrometry, ray tracing methods with the more more popular formulas of determining IOL power

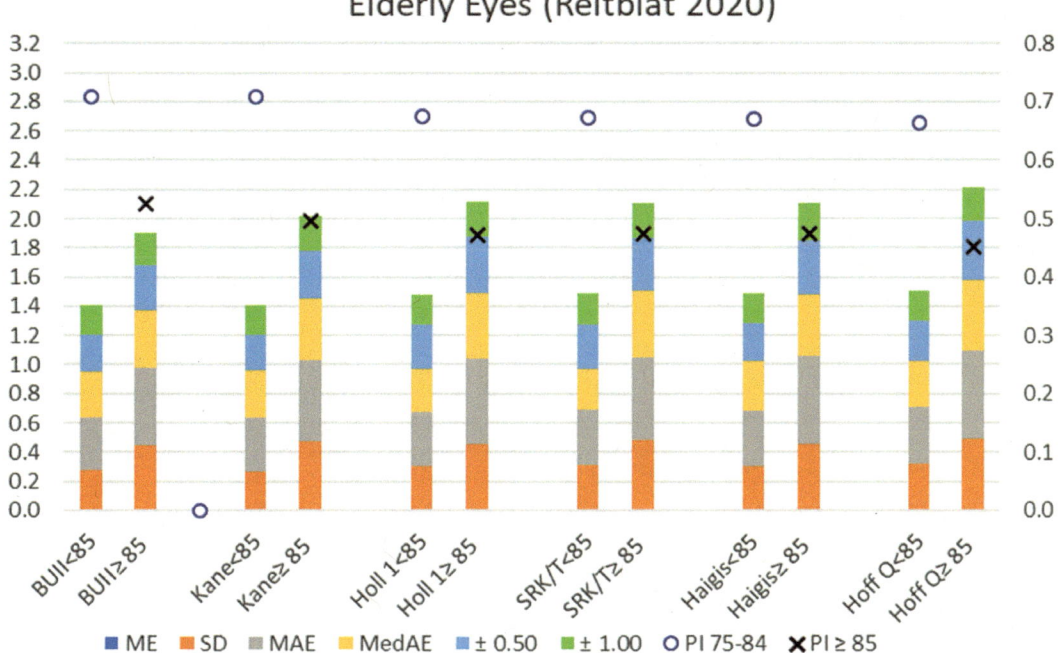

Fig. 33.18 The stacked histograms show the quality metrics of the formulas on different age groups (75–84 and ≥ 85) [30]. The scale for the stacked histogram is on the left. The lower the stacked histogram, the better is the formula. The circles and triangles represent the performance index (PI). The scale for PI is on the right. The higher the PI score, the better. BUII = Barrett Universal II, Hoff = Hoffer Q, Holl = Holladay 1, PEARL = PEARL-DGS, RBF=RBF 2.0.

onstrated good precision. Ray tracing (including Okulix) and intraoperative aberrometry (ORA) had shown results as good but not better than the newer formulas.

Elderly

The impact of the formulas on elderly patients was investigated by Reitblat et al. [30]. Her cohort of 90 eyes from 90 patients was measured with IOLMaster PCI. All patients were implanted with SN60WF and postoperative refractions were carried out at 1 to 3 months postoperatively. There were 2 arms to the study; one for the age group of 75–84 years old and the other was 85 years old or older. For both age groups, BUII, with MAE/MedAE of 0.36D/0.31D and 0.53D/0.39D and Kane, 0.37D/0.32D and 0.56D/0.42D, respectively, were found to be the most accurate. The percentage errors within ±0.5 D for Kane were 78.26% and 65.91%; and for BUII, 82.61% and 61.36% for the younger and older age group, respectively. The rest of the formulas were Haigis, Hoffer Q, Holladay 1 and SRK/T. All formulas showed lower accuracy in the more elderly group.

The graph (Fig. 33.18) and Table 33.14) shows quite clearly that all formulas performed worse in the more elderly age group. The drops in PIs were consistent throughout the formulas. BUII and Kane were the more accurate formulas in this study.

Table 33.14 ME, SD, MAE, and MedAE refer to mean numerical prediction error, the standard deviation of prediction error, mean absolute error, and median absolute error, respectively. This table is a summary of outcomes from Reitblat et paper [30]. As with the earlier tables, the orders of the formula for each source are sorted in order based on a modification of the Haigis "Quality metrics for comparing IOL calculation formulas"

Article	Formula	ME	SD E	MAE	MedAE	±0.50	±1.00	PI	Rank
Reitblat et al. [30]	BUII		0.280	0.360	0.310	78.3	97.8	*0.709*	1
90/90	Kane		0.270	0.370	0.320	82.6	95.7	*0.709*	2
IM 5.21	Holladay 1		0.300	0.370	0.300	65.2	97.8	*0.675*	3
SN60WF	SRK/T		0.310	0.380	0.280	65.2	95.7	*0.673*	4
75–84	Haigis		0.300	0.380	0.340	76.1	95.7	*0.670*	5
	Hoffer Q		0.320	0.390	0.310	71.7	95.7	*0.663*	6
	BUII		0.450	0.530	0.390	65.9	86.4	*0.525*	1
	Kane		0.470	0.560	0.420	61.4	84.1	*0.497*	2
≥85	Haigis		0.460	0.600	0.420	54.6	77.3	*0.475*	3
	SRK/T		0.480	0.570	0.460	56.8	81.8	*0.475*	4
	Holladay 1		0.460	0.580	0.450	52.3	81.8	*0.472*	5
	Hoffer Q		0.490	0.600	0.490	50.0	84.1	*0.451*	6

Conclusion

The third-generation theoretical formulas were popular in the past. Hoffer Q, Holladay 1 and 2, Haigis, and SRK/T were commonly used. These were good formulas. In the last decade, newer formulas began emerging. Barrett Universal II, Hoffer QST, Kane and then RBF 2.0 are the more prominent among these newer formulas. Subsequently, more and more formulas emerged and are still emerging. These formulas, unlike the third generation, are constantly being upgraded and enhanced. These are reflected by the changing version numbers.

Generally, the newer formulas are more accurate than the third-generation formulas. BUII, EVO, RBF 3.0, Hoffer QST and Kane are more frequently being quoted and have been shown to perform better, almost across all ALs, Ks, and ACDs. The other newer formulas also show promise. With these more accurate formulas, cataract surgery is becoming truly a refractive surgery. These will also allow for newer concepts of optical design to be developed.

The above reviews are by no means, exhaustive. The rankings method used here is a modification of the Haigis quality metrics. There are other ways of ranking but this, in my opinion, is an objective and quantitative way of ranking the formulas. The parameters used are limited to the data that were made available in the papers and presentations. Finally, these reviews were on virgin eyes. Post-corneal refractive surgery, keratoconus, etc. are beyond the scope of this chapter.

References

1. Hoffer KJ, Savini G. Update on intraocular lens power calculation study protocols: the better way to design and report clinical trials. Ophthalmol. 2021;128(11):e115–20. https://doi.org/10.1016/j.ophtha.2020.07.005.
2. Hoffer K. The effect of axial length on posterior chamber lenses and posterior capsule position. Curr Concept Ophthal Surg. 1984;1:20–2.
3. Hoffer KJ. The Hoffer Q formula: A comparison of theoretic and regression formulas. J Cataract Refract Surg. 1993;19(11):700–12. Errata: 1994;20(6):677 and 2007;33(1):2–3
4. Wendelstein J, Hoffmann P, Hirnschall N, Fischinger I, Mariacher S, Wingert T, et al. Project hyperopic power prediction: accuracy of 13 different concepts for intraocular lens calculation in short eyes. Br J Ophthalmol. 2021;0:1–7.
5. Barrett G. Intraocular lens calculation formulas for new intraocular lens implants. J Cataract Refract Surg. 1987;13:389–96.
6. Barrett G. An improved universal theoretical formula for intraocular lens power prediction. J Cataract Refract Surg. 1993;19:713–20.
7. Fam H. The formula1 of IOL power calculation. Hangzhou: Asia-Pacific Association of Cataract and Refractive Surgeons; 2017b.
8. Holladay J. Holladay IOL consultant user's guide and reference manual. Houston: Holladay LASIK Institute; 1999.

9. Holladay J, Prager T, Chandler T, Musgrove K. A three-part system for refining intraocular lens power calculations. J Cataract Refract Surg. 1988;14:17–24.

10. Retzlaff J. A new intraocular lens calculation formula. AIOIS J. 1980a;6:148–52.

11. Retzlaff J. Posterior chamber implant power calculation: regression formulas. AIOIS J. 1980b;6:268–70.

12. Retzlaff JA, Sanders DR, Kraff MC. Development of the SRK/T intraocular lens power calculation formula. J Cataract Refract Surg. 1990;16:333–40. Errata: 1990;16:528 and 1993;19(5):444–446

13. FAM H, Lim K. Improving refractive outcomes at extreme axial lengths with the IOLMaster: the optical axial length and keratometric transformation. Br J Ophthalmol. 2009;93:678–83.

14. Cooke D, Cooke T. Comparison of 9 intraocular lens power calculation formulas. J Cataract Refract Surg. 2016;42:1157–64.

15. Kane J, van Heerden A, Atik A, Petsoglou C. Intraocular lens power formula accuracy: comparison of 7 formulas. J Cataract Refract Surg. 2016;42:1490–500.

16. Kane J, van Heerden A, Atik A, Petsoglou C. Accuracy of 3 new methods for intraocular lens power selection. J Cataract Refract Surg. 2017;43:333–9.

17. Fam H (2017a) 7 good habits of IOL power calculations. Hangzhou.

18. Næser K. Intraocular lens power formula based on vergence calculation and lens design. J Cataract Refract Surg. 1997;23:1200–7.

19. Næser K, Savini G. Accuracy of thick-lens intraocular lens power calculation based on cutting-card or calculated data for lens architecture. J Cataract Refract Surg. 2019;45:1422–9.

20. Melles R, Holladay J, Chang W. Accuracy of intraocular lens calculation. Ophthalmology. 2018;125:169–78.

21. Melles R, Kane J, Olsen T, Chang W. Update on intraocular lens calculation formulas. Ophthalmology. 2019;1226:1334–5.

22. Darcy K, Gunn D, Tavassoli S, Sparrow J, Kane J. Assessment of the accuracy of new and updated intraocular lens power calculation formulas in the 10 930 eyes from the UK National Health Service. J Cataract Refract Surg. 2020;46:2–7.

23. Savini G, Di Maita M, Hoffer K, Næser K, Schiano-Lomoriello D, Vagge A, et al. Comparison of 13 formulas for IOL power calculation with measurments from partial coherence interferometry. Br J Ophthalmol. 2020a;0:1–6.

24. Cheng H, Kane J, Liu L, Li J, Cheng B, W, M. Refractive predictability using the IOLMaster 700 and artificial intelligence-based IOL power formulas compared to standard formulas. J Refract Surg. 2020;36(7):466–72.

25. Fernandez J, Rodriguez-Vallejo M, Poyales F, Burguera N, Garzòn N. New method to assess the accuracy of intraocular lens power calculation formulas according to ocular biometric parameters. J Cataract Refract Surg. 2020;46:849–56.

26. Turnbull A, Hill W, Barrett G. Accuracy of intraocular lens power calculation methods when targeting low myopia in monovision. J Cataract Refract Surg. 2020;46:862–6.

27. Zhao J, Liu L, Cheng H, Li J, Han X, Liu Y, Wu M. Accuracy of eight intraocular lens power calculation formulas for segmented multifocal intraocular lens. Int J Ophthalmol. 2020;13(9):1378–84.

28. Savini G, Hoffer K, Balducci N, Barboni P, Schiano-Lomoriello D. Comparison of formula accuracy for intraocular lens power calculation based on measurements by a swept-source opticl coherence tomography optical biometer. J Cataract Refract Surg. 2020b;46:27–33.

29. Szalai E, Toth N, Kolkedi Z, Varga C, Csutak A. Comparison of various intraocular lens formulas using a new high-resolution swept-source optical coherence tomographer. J Cataract Refract Surg. 2020;46:1136–41.

30. Reitblat O, Gali H, Chou L, Bahar I, Weinreb R, Afshari N, Sella R. Intraocular lens power calculation in the elderly population using the Kane formula in comparison with existing methods. J Cataract Refract Surg. 2020;46:1501–7.

31. Hipolito-Fernandes D, Luis M, Gil P, Maduro V, Fejiao J, Yeo T, et al. VRF-G, a new intraocular lens power calculation formula: a 13 formulas comparison study. Clin Ophthalmol. 2020;14:4395–402.

32. Fam H. Approaching atypical eyes with confidence. Bali: Asia-Pacific Association of Cataract and Refractive Surgeons; 2016.

33. Ladas J, Siddiqui A, Devgan U. A 3-D "Super Surface" combining modern intraocular lens formulas to generate a "Super Formula" and maximize accuracty. JAMA Ophthalmol. 2015;133:1431–6.

34. Olsen T. Prediction of intraocular lens position after cataract extraction. J Cataract Refract Surg. 1986;12(7):376–9.

35. Olsen T. Theoretical approach to intraocular lens calculation using Gaussian optics. J Cataract Refract Surg. 1987;13:141–5.

36. Olsen T. Sources of error in intraocular lens power calculations. J Cataract Refract Surg. 1992;18:125–9.

37. Olsen T. Prediction of effective postoperative (intraocular lens) anterior chamber depth. J Cataract Refract Surg. 2006;32:419–24.

38. Olsen T. Improved accuracy of intraocular lens power calculation with the Zeiss IOLMaster. Acta Ophthalmol Scand. 2007;85:84–7.

39. Olsen T. C Constant: new concept for ray tracing-assisted intraocular lens power calculation. J Cataract Refract Surg. 2014;40:764–73.

40. Olsen T, Thorwest M. Calibration of axial length measurements with Zeiss IOLMaster. J Cataract Refract Surg. 2005;31:1345–50.

41. Olsen T, Corydon L, Gimbel H. Intraocular lens power calculation with an improved anterior chamber

depth prediction algorithm. J Cataract Refract Surg. 1995;21:313–9.

42. Gõkce S, Zeiter J, Weikert M, Koch D, Hill W, Wang L. Intraocular lens power calculations in short eyes using 7 formulas. J Cataract Refract Surg. 2017;43:892–7.

43. Preussner P, Wahl J, Lahdo H, Burkhard D, Findl O. Ray tracing for intraocular lens calculation. J Cataract Refract Surg. 2002;28:1412–9.

44. Abulafia A, Barrett G, Rotenberg M, Kleinmann G, Levy A, Reitblat O, et al. Intraocular lens power calculation for eyes with axial length greater than 26.0mm: Comparison of formulas and methods. J Cataract Refract Surg. 2015;41:548–56.

45. Savini G, Taroni L, Hoffer K. Recent developments in intraocular lens power calculation methods - update 2020. Ann Transl Med. 2020c;8(22):1553.

46. Zhang J, Tan X, Wang W, Yang G, Xu J, Ruan X, et al. Effect of axial length adjustment methods on intraocular lens power calculation in highly myopic eyes. Am J Ophthalmol. 2020;214:110–8.

47. Gokce S, De Oca I, Cooke D, Wang L, Koch D, Al-Mohtaseb Z. Accuracy of 8 intraocular lens calculation formulas in relation to anterior chamber depth in patients with normal axial lengths. J Cataract Refract Surg. 2018;44:362–8.

48. Hipólito-Fernandes D, Luis M, Serras-Pereira R, Gil P, Maduro V, Feijóão J, Alves N. Anterior chamber depth, lens thickness and intraocular lens calculation formula accuracy: nine formulas comparison. Br J Ophthalmol. 2020;0:1–7.

49. Hoffmann P, Lindemann C. Intraocular lens calculation for aspheric intraocular lenses. J Cataract Refract Surg. 2013;39:867–72.

50. Raufi N, James C, Kua A, Vann R. Intraoperative aberrometry vs preoperative formulas in predicting intraocular lens power. J Cataract Refract Surg. 2020;46:857–61.

51. Ianchulev T, Salz J, Hoffer K. Intraoperative optical refractive biometry for intraocular lens power estimation without axial length and keratometry measurements. J Cataract Refract Surg. 2005;31:1530–6.

52. Sudhakar S, Hill D, King T, Scott I, Mishra G, Ernst B, Pantanelli S. Intraoperative aberrometry versus preoperative biometry for intraocular lens power selection in short eyes. J Cataract Refract Surg. 2019;45:719–24.

53. Hirnschall N, Buehren T, Trost M, Findl O. Pilot evaluation of refractive prediction errors associated with a new method for ray-tracing-based intraocular lens power calculation. J Cataract Refract Surg. 2019;45:738–44.

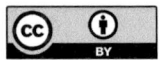

ELP Estimation

Lens Power Calculation Formulas

Thomas Olsen

ELP Estimation

The first-generation IOL power formulas were the so-called thin-lens formulas where the cornea and the IOL are regarded as single refracting planes. Examples of the thin-lens approach include the Fyorodov [1], Colenbrander [2], Binkhorst [3], Hoffer [4], Holladay [5], SRK/T [6], Haigis [7], and others. The basic formula is

$$P = \frac{n}{Ax - ELP} - \frac{1}{1/K - ELP/n} \quad (34.1)$$

where P = IOL power of emmetropia, n = refractive index of aqueous/vitreous, Ax = axial length, K = corneal power, and ELP = estimated lens plane of the IOL. The logic of the formula is to subtract the vergence in front of the IOL (second term) from the vergence behind the IOL (first term) to give the IOL power needed for emmetropia.

Some caution should be taken about the term "ELP." The estimated lens plane (ELP) is often used to denote the value for the IOL plane to be used with the old thin-lens formulas. It is important to know that this need not be the physical position of the IOL but rather the value that predicts the observed refraction with that formula. Because the ELP in this way is a back-calculated value it becomes a virtual distance that may work

to absorb any other off-set errors in the system, much like the A-constant works for the SRK formulas. To distinguish between the ELP as a virtual distance and the actual, physical position, it has been suggested to use alternate terms like the physical lens position (PLP) or the actual lens position (ALP).

Apart from questions about the K-reading and the axial length, the obvious unknown in Eq. (34.1) is of course the final location of the IOL in the eye after surgery. All right, we know the placement of the IOL is often in-the-bag (Fig. 34.1), but the exact location cannot be predicted on theoretical grounds. Factors like optic and haptic design [8], surgical technique, size of the capsular opening, capsular bag shrinkage, and possible change over time add uncertainty to the prediction. Remember that ±0.7 mm axial displacement of the IOL is the equivalent to a ±1 D shift in IOL power in a normal sized eye. The effect is, however, very dependent on the axial length of the eye as shown in Fig. 34.2, where the Rx error per mm change in ELP (IOL position) has been calculated in a real-world simulation dataset of 2870 eyes and plotted against the axial length. As can be seen the error amounts to about 1.4 D/mm for a 24 mm eye but doubles for an eye shorter than 20 mm and approaches zero for a long eye. The minus value in some of the very long eyes is due to the minus powered IOL. Note, however, that the accuracy of the IOL position does not matter much for a long eye because the IOL power is low.

T. Olsen (✉)
Aros Private Hospital, Aarhus N, Denmark

© The Author(s) 2024
J. Aramberri et al. (eds.), *Intraocular Lens Calculations*, Essentials in Ophthalmology,
https://doi.org/10.1007/978-3-031-50666-6_34

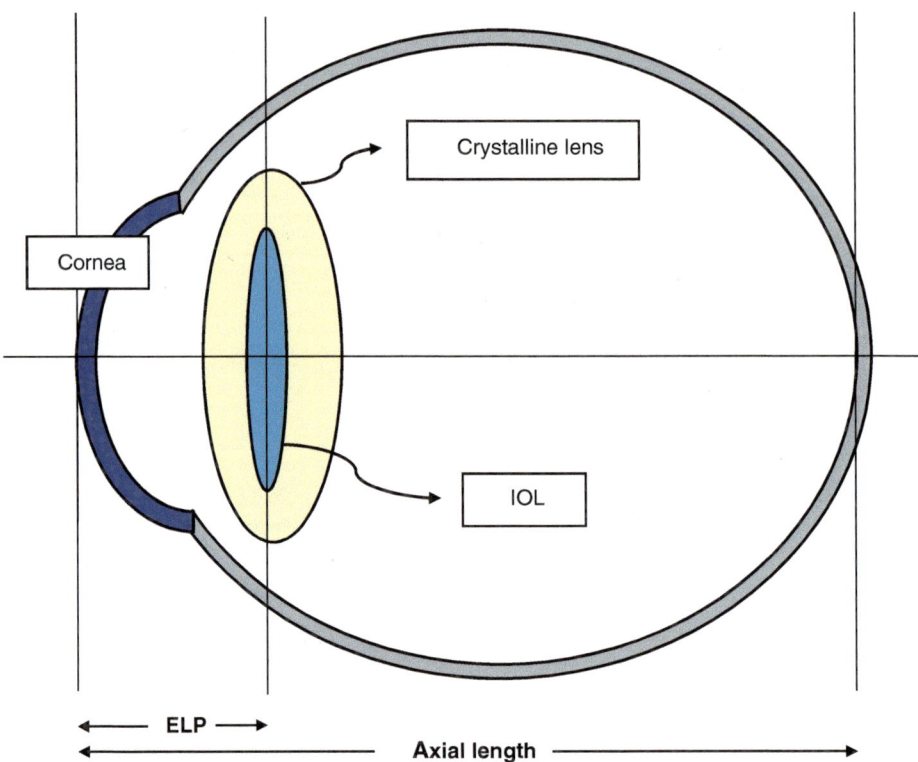

Fig. 34.1 The estimated lens plane (ELP) refers to the plane of the IOL after surgery

Fig. 34.2 The Rx error per mm change in ELP (IOL position) calculated in a clinical dataset of 2870 eyes

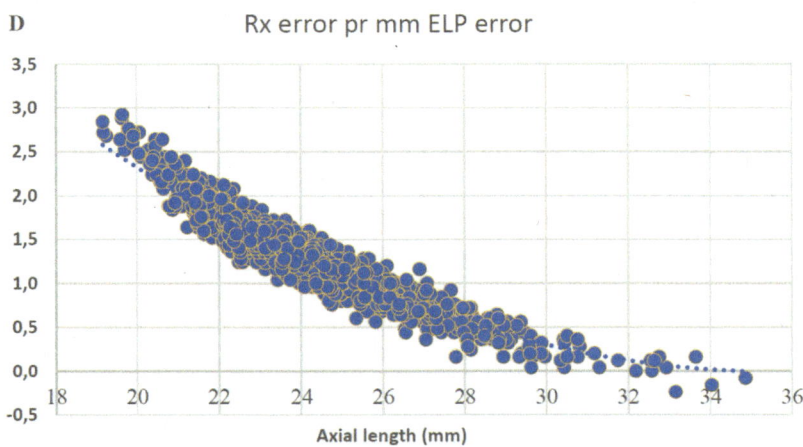

Methods to Estimate the ELP

The first IOL power formula in the world was described by S Fyodorov in 1967 [8] in a Russian paper and 1975 republished in Invest Ophthalmol [9]. To estimate the ELP, he used the height of the corneal dome from the iris plane based on Pythagoras theorem:

$$ELP = r - \sqrt{r^2 - d^2/4} \qquad (34.2)$$

where r = corneal radius, d = corneal diameter (taken as the corneal diameter plus 10%). This method was developed for iris-clip lenses after intracapsular extraction which was popular at that time. The idea of using the K-reading and corneal diameter has later been taken up by several authors as one of the predictors for the ELP for modern posterior chamber IOLs. Now, more than 50 years since the paper by Fyodorov, you can still find this ELP concept inside the SRK/T and the Holladay formulas.

A common procedure of many formulas has been to back-calculate for the ELP based on the actual outcome: In each case, the ELP is solved that gives the actual outcome, and statistical analysis is applied to find the covariation with possible predictors in a representative sample. The statistical ELP dependence—typically a regression equation—is then incorporated into the formula. In this way, the formula can be made to work even if the optical model of the formula may not be correct! For example, what happens if the corneal power is input as the K-reading (and we know this may be a falsely high value)? The formula would need to move the ELP a little further back to work. This underlines the fact that the ELP calculated in this way is not a physical distance but rather a virtual distance which cannot be verified by direct measurement of the IOL position.

It has been common practice for IOL manufacturers to state the ELP on the IOL label along with the A-constant. As far as the author knows, this ELP refers to the old Binkhorst formula. The reader may have noticed that the labeled "ELP" value typically reads more than 5 mm, which is higher than the real position found after surgery from actual measurements. The explanation is the K-reading issue as mentioned above (Binkhorst uses keratometer index 1.3333 rather than 1.3375 originally advocated to account for some flattening of the cornea after surgery). Some of this confusion may be avoided if the formula does not take the K-value directly from standard keratometry but takes the corneal radius as a parameter. Still, the radius needs to be converted to a corneal power inside the formula.

Many methods have been suggested to model the ELP prediction and each formula has its own. In the early days of IOL power formulas, the ELP was expressed as a function of the K-reading (Fyodorov) and the axial length (Binkhorst) with various mathematical representation. As more clinical data became available in larger series, other parameters like corneal diameter, anterior chamber depth, lens thickness, and other factors like age, sex, and refraction have been tried. Table 34.1 is a summary of some of the suggested predictors of the ELP in the various formulas.

Table 34.1 ELP predictors used by different authors of some optical formulas

Formula	Axial length	K-reading	ACD	Lens thickness	Other
Fyodorov	–	X	–	–	–
Binkhorst	X	–	–	–	–
SRK/T	X	X	–	–	–
Hoffer Q	X	X	–	–	–
Holladay I	X	X	–	–	
Holladay II	X	X	X	X	CD [a], Rx [a], age [a]
Haigis	X	–	X	–	–
Olsen	(x)	(x)	X	X	–
Preussner	X	X	X	X	
Barrett II	X	X	X	X [a]	CD [a], Rx
Kane	X	X	X	X [a]	Gender, CCT [a]

ACD preoperative anterior chamber depth, *CD* corneal diameter, *Rx* preoperative refraction, *CCT* central corneal thickness
[a] Optional

Beware the Unusual Eyes!

As mentioned, for optimization purposes, the ELP is often back-calculated as the value that will "predict" the outcome with a given formula. When this virtual distance is correlated with all available parameters like axial length, K-reading, ACD, lens thickness, corneal diameter distance, corneal thickness, refraction, gender, age, shoe size (sorry, not published), and subjected to a data cruncher, it often happens that small correlations are found that will tend to improve the refractive predictions with a small statistical significance. However, as is the case with statistical analysis, the correlations are strictly speaking only valid for the dataset on which the analysis was performed, and care has to be taken when we move outside the normality.

A classic example is the post-LASIK cases where the anatomy of the cornea has changed so that the K-reading is not representative of the true corneal power in the first place but also cannot be used as a predictor for the ELP in the second place as the Fyodorov "height" formula (used by the SRK/T and the Holladay formulas) is based on a normal anterior segment. For such cases, it has been suggested to use the so-called double K method principle [10] where the ELP dependence is replaced by the pre-LASIK value or a standard value. These considerations also apply to keratoconus, megalocornea, keratoplasties, and other abnormal cornea with a disrupted anterior segment.

Another example is the use of the preoperative refraction for the prediction of the ELP. This variable may be shown to have a small influence in a large sample. However, what happens in case of lenticular myopia? This is outside the normal covariation between the refractive components of the eye and can lead to a gross error if included as a predictor.

So, each formula has its limitations, often to be found in the "engine room" of the formula, i.e., the ELP method. Especially methods that use multiple predictors have a risk of being misguided if one of the predictors is out-of-range. Eventually, it is up to the user to identify those outliers and maybe switch to another formula if an error is anticipated. Therefore, careful screening of patients scheduled for lens surgery is highly recommended.

The C-Constant

Optical biometry (Zeiss IOLMaster 500) was originally introduced for the measurement of axial length by partial coherence interferometry (PCI). However, the measurement of the ACD with the IOLMaster was still based on a slit-lamp technique. A decade later, Haag-Streit introduced another optical biometer called the Lenstar LS 900. The working principle of the Lenstar was optical low coherence reflectometry (OLCR) which has some advantages over PCI in the extended range of measurement, covering all the intraocular distances including the corneal thickness, the ACD, and the lens thickness.

For the prediction of the ELP, many previous studies (see section above) had shown a significant role of both the preoperative ACD and lens thickness, but those studies were mainly based on ultrasound biometry. The question that may be asked is this: given the new accuracy of the laser biometer for all intraocular distances, do we have better options for the prediction of the IOL position?

Studies were undertaken by the author to measure the actual IOL position routinely after surgery in a series of cataract cases and to establish the possible predictive value of all available predictors: K-reading, axial length, anterior chamber depth, lens thickness, Corneal Diameter distances all of which were measured by the Lenstar biometer (Fig. 34.3). For the present chapter, a reanalysis was made on the database collected over the years while working at the University department. It included the original dataset from 2014 [11] and additional 200 cases, making a total 1622 cases.

In Fig. 34.4, the position of the IOL (measured by OLCR optical biometry) has been plotted against the axial length as well as the preoperative position of the anterior and posterior capsule of

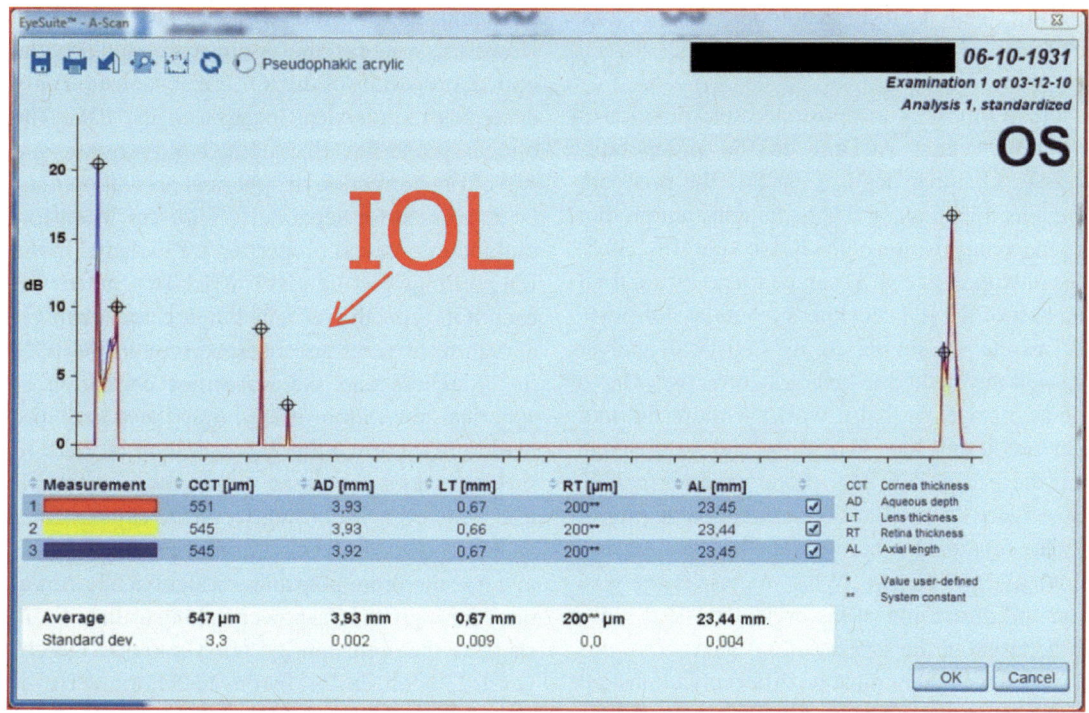

Fig. 34.3 IOL position measured by laser biometry

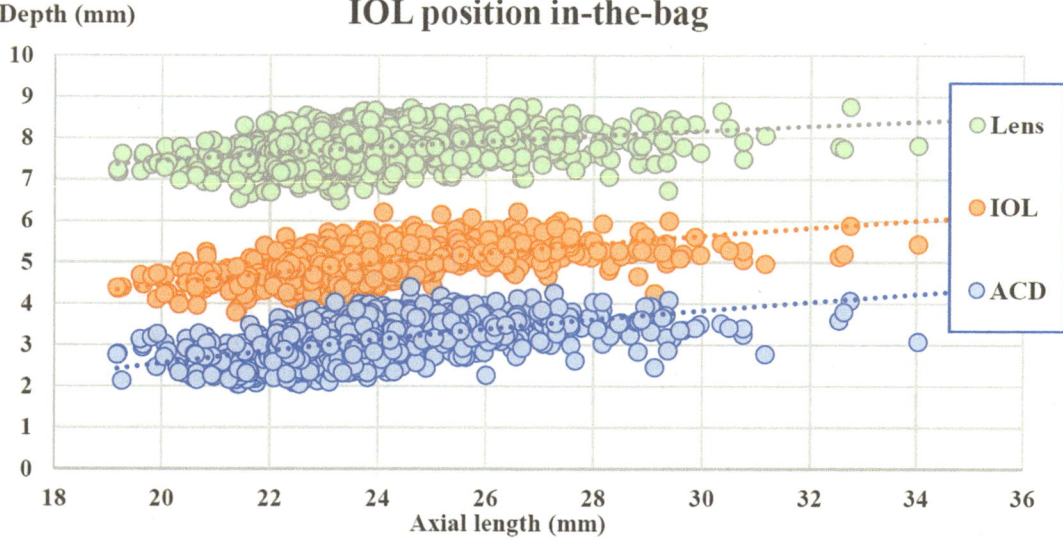

Fig. 34.4 IOL position vs axial length and located of anterior and posterior capsule of the lens

the crystalline lens. As can be seen, the postoperative IOL position was tightly connected to both the preoperative ACD and the lens thickness in a way that clearly depicted the in-the-bag placement of the IOL. The IOL appeared to locate itself at a constant fraction (around 40%) of the space between the anterior and the posterior capsule (= lens thickness), irrespective of the axial length.

Thus, the IOL position could be described as

$$IOLpost = ACDpre + C \times LensT \quad (34.3)$$

where IOLpost is the postoperative position of the IOL center, ACDpre is the preoperative anterior chamber depth, LensT is the preoperative lens thickness, and C is the constant predicting the axial position of the IOL center (Fig. 34.5). The postoperative ACD can be found by subtracting half of the IOL thickness from the IOLpost.

Despite its simple form, statistical analysis showed the method to be highly effective. One of the advantages is that it works without the indirect predictors like K-reading and axial length and the principle is less prone to abnormal K's (post-LASIK) or conditions causing a disproportionate relationship between the anterior segment and length of the eye. What matters is the position and dimension of the crystalline lens which is the target of the surgery.

Of course, there must be different C-constants for different lens types, depending on the haptics, the shape of the optic, and the behavior of the IOL inside the bag after surgery as a result of capsular contraction. Much like the A-constant summarizes the refractive effect of a given lens type, the C-constant describes the IOL-specific

anatomic relationship with the capsular bag. However, whereas the A-constant includes the optical properties of the IOL, the C-constant only describes the physical location of the IOL. The optical properties like optic configuration and wavefront correction of spherical aberration must be accounted for separately. With the Olsen formula, these optical properties are included in the IOL settings for the given IOL. This means for each IOL type, the refractive index, the (average) curvature of front and back surface of the IOL, the thickness and the wavefront correction of spherical aberration, if any, must be stated. The reader might argue that the curvature of the IOL surfaces varies according to the power and this is true. However, according to the ANSI standard, an IOL power is labeled as the paraxial power, and it is therefore possible to calculate the curvatures for a given IOL power as long as the overall shape of the optic configuration is known (biconvex 1:2, biconvex 1:1, biconvex 2:1, etc.). This is done internally by the Olsen formula from the average IOL definition. As a result, it is possible to model the exact physical properties of the IOL eye, which can be used for ray tracing and further optical analysis.

Error Propagation Model

No matter how good the biometry or the formula is, a statistical error will always be associated with the refractive predictions. You may divide this residual error into measurement errors and formula errors.

One important source of error to be considered is the measurement error of the axial length. In the old days of ultrasound biometry, this was a major source of error. What is measured is the transit time of ultrasound traveling from the corneal surface to the vitreoretinal interface. The time is translated into distance assuming a certain velocity of sound through the ocular media. Many uncertainties exist by this technique: possible indentation of the cornea, alignment issues, velocity settings, impact of the cataractous lens, retinal thickness, and the fact that there is a limit to the resolution given by wavelength of ultra-

Lens capsule pre- and postop

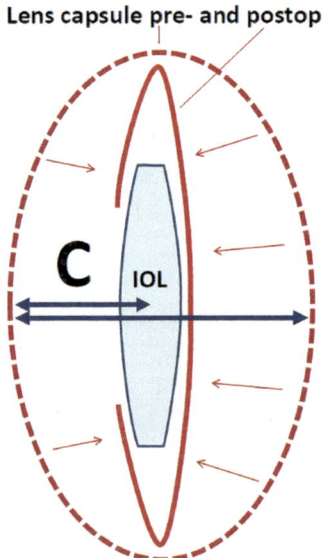

Fig. 34.5 The C-constant predicts the location of the IOL as a fraction of crystalline lens thickness

sound. According to the author's experience, the reproducibility of good ultrasound readings is typically within ±0.2 mm. Recalling that 1 mm of error in axial length amounts to 2.5 D error in the spectacle plane, the ultrasound reproducibility of 0.2 mm is the equivalent of 0.5 D error in the spectacle plane.

The introduction of optical biometry more than 20 years ago [12] was a quantum leap in the era of IOL power calculation. First, the wavelength of light is so much shorter than that of ultrasound giving an ultrahigh tissue resolution. (A laser wavelength of 1060 nm corresponds to about 800 nm in ocular tissue and 10 MHz ultrasound with velocity of 1550 m/s in the eye has a wavelength of about 0.16 mm.) Second, the measurements are performed contact free in the line of sight and the end point is the pigment epithelium. So, the measurements are less prone to alignment issues, and the off-set issues of ultrasound like deformation and the question of retinal thickness do not exist. It should be remembered, however, that the laser does not measure the geometrical distance directly. What is measured is the time—or optical path—for light to travel from the corneal to the retinal reflection. Akin to the velocity issue of ultrasound we need to assume a refractive index of the ocular media in order to translate the optical path into geometrical distance. The group refractive index used by the IOLMaster was calculated by Haigis [13] who calibrated the laser readings against the results of immersion ultrasound, assuming this was the true distance measurement. By doing this, the output reading of the IOLMaster was in reality similar to that measured by ultrasound. The advantage of this calibration was no need to change existing IOL constants based on numerous ultrasound measurements.

It has been questioned by the author whether the Haigis group refractive index of the phakic eye was indeed the most accurate. The question arose from the observation that there is a systematic difference between pre- and postoperative readings with the IOLMaster. The difference amounted to 0.08 mm shorter readings of the IOL eye as compared to the preoperative phakic eye.

There is no reason to believe that the eye shortens by the surgery so the explanation must be found in the assumed refractive indices of the ocular components, in particular the crystalline lens which is hard to examine. The author has shown that if the index of the crystalline lens is changed from the Haigis assumed value of 1.407 to 1.429, there will be consistency between the preoperative and the postoperative measurements [14]. With the Olsen calibration, the overall group refractive index of the phakic eye changes from 1.3574 to 1.3616. The difference is slight in the normal range but becomes larger in the longer eyes.

Whatever calibration of the optical biometer, the reproducibility of measurements with optical biometry is impressive and readings often fall within 0.02 mm. So, if optical biometry was the only source of error in the system, the refractive predictions would be within 0.05 D error only (!). However, as everyone knows this accuracy is not achieved in clinical work and therefore other errors must be at work.

Keratometry must also be considered as a significant source of error. Generally, autokeratometry tends to give good readings if one pays attention to the quality of the tear film, focus, alignment issues, lid pressure, contact lens wear, and other confounders. Beware the post-LASIK cases, keratoconus, high astigmatism and other odd cases. However, even "perfect" readings do have a variation and it may sometimes be wise to repeat the measurement with days apart to have consistent readings. It is not just about the spherical equivalent but also about the astigmatism that need to be assessed accurately. It is the experience of the author that the error of good, consistent K-readings should be well below 0.1 D (spherical equivalent) or better.

The most critical formula error is, however, the error associated with the prediction of the IOL position (ELP). If we were able to predict the ELP with 100% accuracy, the only source of error would be the measurement error associated with the K-reading and the axial length. It may be difficult to assess the error of ELP prediction. First of all the ELP in many formulas is not a physical distance but rather a virtual distance calculated in retrospect and therefore not directly measurable. One exception to this is the Olsen formula which was designed to use the physical dimensions all through the calculations. This includes the shape of the IOL as well as the real pseudophakic ACD.

An error propagation model of the total error associated with IOL power calculation was first published by Olsen in 1992 [15] and by Norrby in 2008 [16]. The assumption is that the total error is the sum of individual and independent components. The individual sources of error mainly consist of measurement errors from keratometry and axial length measurements. For completeness we also need to consider the process of taking the refraction itself as recommended by Norrby and probably other factors like pupil size, variations in Gullstrand ratio of the cornea, IOL tilt and IOL power tolerance. However, the most important source of error—and we shall see how important—is the error associated with the prediction of the ELP.

According to the error propagation model, if we know the error of each component, we can calculate the total error by adding the variances of each component and take the square root of the sum. In our case, we have

$$\delta\left(\text{Total}\right)=\sqrt{\delta^{2}\left(\text{Ax}\right)+\delta^{2}\left(K\right)+\delta^{2}\left(\text{ELP}\right)+\delta^{2}\left(\text{Rx}+\right)} \tag{34.4}$$

where δ(Total) = total error of the IOL power prediction as standard deviation, δ(Ax) = error of axial length, $\delta(K)$ = error of keratometry, δ(ELP) = error of ELP prediction, and δ(Rx+) = error of taking the refraction and other errors.

How do we assess the error of each component? One method would be simply to take a number of measurements and calculate the error between repeated measurements. In this way, we get the intra-session error, but this need not be the real variability because of day-to-day variation in tear film, intraocular pressure, pupil size, observer dependent bias, etc. In the attempt to estimate the total error, Olsen in his 1992 publication estimated the variation between pre- and postoperative measurements, thereby including the surgical influence. However, at that time ultrasound was used for biometry and other instrumentation like keratometry may not be representative of modern technique with optical biometry, accurate keratometry with confirmation from several devices, standardized small-incision surgery with capsulorrhexis, and in-the-bag placement of the IOL and improved ELP prediction.

As mentioned above, the difference between repeated optical biometry readings is often within 0.02 mm. So, a conservative estimate of the standard deviation might be in the region of 0.03 mm. This is the equivalent of 0.075 D in the spectacle plane. For keratometry there is one study comparing the inter-session variability of different keratometry devices [17] showing standard deviations from 0.12 D (Nidek TonoRef II) to 0.17 D (IOLMaster 500). The author has a preference of using autokeratometry and therefore a reasonable estimate might be 0.15 D for the standard deviation of keratometry.

The error predicting the IOL position can be assessed by measuring the postoperative anterior chamber depth and comparing with the predicted value. As mentioned above, this is not possible with the standard thin-lens formulas because the ELP is a virtual distance. However, with the Olsen formula, this is possible because the formula was developed to accept the physical (measurable) dimensions all through the calculations. In the paper describing the C-constant for prediction of the IOL position [18], the mean difference between the expected and the observed IOL position as measured by laser biometry (Lenstar) was 0.0 ± 0.17 mm (SD). This corresponds to 85.9% of the cases within ±0.25 mm difference. The observed error may of course include some measurement error but for now a reasonable estimate might be to use the value 0.17 mm, which corresponds to 0.28 D error in the spectacle plane.

Finally, some error will arise from taking the refraction itself and other sources. Norrby [16] cites a study on 80 patients aged 11–60 years by Bullimore [18] who found the 95% limits of agreement between automated and manual refraction ranged from −0.90 to +0.65 D with an SD of 0.39 D. To the author this seems to be a huge variability and difficult to extrapolate to a clinical setting with premium implants where patients may be intolerant to variations in the refraction of a quarter of a diopter.

The reproducibility of manifest refraction was recently reported by Taneri et al. [19], who studied the latest 2 manifest refractions of 1000 eyes obtained at 2 separate visits. The study population was mostly myopic with a median age of 35 years. They found a standard deviation of the pairwise difference of 0.19 D. One might argue that accurate refractions are more difficult in young, phakic patients as compared to pseudophakic patients. For the present study and considering the difference between phakic and pseudophakia patients, the author believes a reasonable estimate for the error to be 0.20 D (standard deviation).

Having defined the error of these four individual components, the calculation of the total error is straightforward as shown in Table 34.2. The variances in D units are calculated for each component and summed to give the total variance of the model. The total standard deviation is then found as the square root of the total variance. In the numerical example, an SD of 0.385 D was found. This corresponds to a mean absolute error (MAE) of 0.308 D with 81% of the cases within 0.5 D prediction error. This is not far from reality in the author's own clinical experience.

The relative contribution of the different components of error is shown in Fig. 34.6. Note the small contribution of the axial length and the dominant contribution of the ELP prediction accounting for more than 50% of the total error. To improve the accuracy further, we need to improve the prediction of the ELP.

The reader is asked to copy the scheme of Table 34.2 into a spreadsheet and see what impact a change in error of each of the four components will have on the total error. In this way, we can predict the limits of accuracy based on the error of each component. There is no magic.

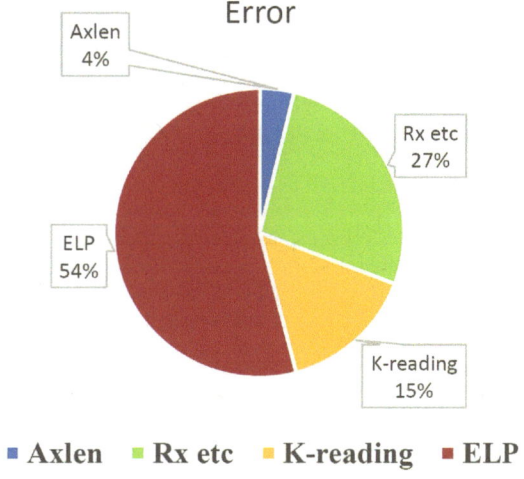

Fig. 34.6 The components of error in IOL power calculation

Table 34.2 Error propagation model of total IOL prediction error

Source of error	Error (SD)	Rx (SD)	Variance (SD^2)	Per cent
ELP, mm	0.17	0.28	0.0803	54.1
Rx, other, D	0.20	0.20	0.0225	15.2
Keratometry, D	0.15	0.15	0.0144	13.1
Axial length, mm	0.03	0.075	0,0056	3.8
Total, D	0.38	<<<	0.1484	100

References

1. Fedorov SN, Kolinko AI, Kolinko AI. Estimation of optical power of the intraocular lens [Russian]. Vestn oftalmol. 1967;80(4):27–31.
2. Colenbrander MC. Calculation of the power of an iris clip lens for distant vision. Br J Ophthalmol. 1973;57:735–40.
3. Binkhorst CD. Dioptrienzahl Künstlicher Augenlinsen. Klin Monatsbl Augenheilkd. 1973;162:354–61.
4. Hoffer KJ, Allen DR. A simple lens power calculation program for the HP-67 and HP-97 calculators. J Cataract Refract Surg. 1978;4:197–9.
5. Holladay JT, et al. A three-part system for refining intraocular lens power calculations. J Cataract Refract Surg. 1988;14:17–24.
6. Retzlaff JA, Sanders DR, Kraff MC. Development of the SRK/T intraocular lens implant power calculation formula. J Cataract Refract Surg. 1990;16:333–40. Errata: 1990;16:528 and 1993;19(5):444–446.
7. Haigis W, et al. Comparison of immersion ultrasound biometry and partial coherence interferometry for intraocular lens calculation according to Haigis. Graefes Arch Clin Exp Ophthalmol. 2000;238:765–73.
8. Norrby S. Using the lens haptic plane concept and thick-lens ray tracing to calculate intraocular lens power. J Cataract Refract Surg. 2004;30(5):1000–5.
9. Fyodorov SN, Galin MA, Linksz A. Calculation of the optical power of intraocular lenses. Investig Ophthalmol. 1975;14:625–8.
10. Aramberri J. Intraocular lens power calculation after corneal refractive surgery: Double-K method. J Cataract Refract Surg. 2003;29:2063–8.
11. Olsen T, Hoffmann P. C constant: new concept for ray tracing–assisted. Intraocular lens power calculation. J Cataract Refract Surg. 2014;40:764–73.
12. Drexler W, Findl O, Menapace R, et al. Partial coherence interferometry: a novel approach to biometry in cataract surgery. Am J Ophthalmol. 1998;126:524–34.
13. Haigis W. Pseudophakic correction factors for optical biometry. Graefes Arch Clin Exp Ophthalmol. 2005;239:589–98.
14. Olsen T, Thorwest M. Calibration of axial length measurements with the Zeiss IOLMaster. J Cataract Refract Surg. 2005;31:1345–50.
15. Olsen T. Sources of error in intraocular lens power calculation. J Cataract Refract Surg. 1992;16:125–9.
16. Norrby S. Sources of error in intraocular lens power calculation. J Cataract Refract Surg. 2008;34:368–76.
17. Laursen JVN, Jeppesen P, Olsen T. Precision of 5 different keratometry devices. Int Ophthalmol. 2016;36:17–20.
18. Bullimore MA, Fusaro RE, Adams CW. The repeatability of automated and clinician refraction. Optom Vis Sci. 1998;75:617–22.
19. Taneri S, Arba-Mosquera S, Rost A, Kießler S, Dick HB. Repeatability and reproducibility of manifest refraction. J Cataract Refract Surg. 2020;46:1659–66.

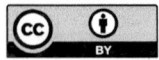

Anterior Chamber Depth and IOL Calculations

35

Oliver Findl, Nino Hirnschall, and Martin Kronschläger

In biometry, the anterior chamber depth (ACD) is defined as the distance between the central anterior corneal epithelium and the anterior lens capsule of the crystalline lens [1]) or the anterior surface of the intraocular lens (IOL) or the anterior surface of the remaining anterior capsule or anterior iris surface in aphakic eyes. The thickness of the central cornea is included. This is important since ACD is often confused with aqueous depth (AQD), which is measured as the distance between the corneal endothelium and the anterior lens capsule of the crystalline lens [1].

Many different devices are available to measure the ACD, such as optical coherence tomography (OCT), partial coherence interferometry (PCI), Scheimpflug imaging, and ultrasound and ultrasound biomicroscopy (UBM). However, Nakakura et al. showed that ACD measurements of those devices were significantly different except for OCT and PCI measurements which

were interchangeable [2]. Although good agreement was found for those devices, recent findings suggest that even in two different swept source OCT based biometry devices (Zeiss IOL Master 700 vs Heidelberg Engineering ANTERION) devices should not be used interchangeably [3]. Further, good agreement between OCT and PCI was not confirmed [4] and interchangeability might differ between phakic and pseudophakic eyes [5].

A cross-sectional study (The Singapore Chinese Eye Study) found that the determinants of ACD are mainly the lens vault (LV) and the posterior corneal arc length (PCAL) [6]. LV was defined as the perpendicular distance from the horizontal line between the 2 scleral spurs to the anterior pole of the crystalline lens, and the PCAL was defined as the arc distance of the posterior corneal border between scleral spurs.

In clinical practice, the dynamics of ACD change after cataract surgery is an essential factor for refractive outcome since 1 mm in ACD change results in a 1.44 diopter spherical equivalent change in a normal eye [7].

O. Findl (✉) · M. Kronschläger
Vienna Institute for Research in Ocular Surgery (VIROS), A Karl Landsteiner Institute, Hanusch Hospital, Vienna, Austria
e-mail: oliver@findl.at;
martin.kronschlaeger@oegk.at

N. Hirnschall
Department for Ophthalmology and Optometry, Kepler University Hospital GmbH and Medical Department Johannes Kepler University Linz, Linz, Austria
e-mail: nino@hirnschall.at

Impact of Postoperative ACD

In cataract surgery, the natural crystalline lens is replaced by an IOL. Nowadays, patients' expectations are high and cataract surgery is not only restoring vision it is also optimizing refraction.

© The Author(s) 2024
J. Aramberri et al. (eds.), *Intraocular Lens Calculations*, Essentials in Ophthalmology,
https://doi.org/10.1007/978-3-031-50666-6_35

However, between 10 and 20% [8–10] and with up-to-date formulae between 2% and 5% [11] of the patients post-operatively need a refractive correction of more than ±1 diopter (spherical equivalent). In these patients, unaided visual acuity is low, and consequently, satisfaction is reduced. Moreover, these refractive surprises are a common cause for IOL explantation [12].

Uncertainty about the refractive outcome is triggering the research field of biometry and power calculation. Investigating the error distribution of different factors on the postoperative manifest refraction, many factors were shown to have a significant impact [7] such as axial eye length [13–15], corneal anterior apical radius (mm), corneal posterior/anterior radius ratio [14, 16, 17], corneal anterior and posterior asphericity [14, 16, 17], corneal thickness [14, 16, 17] and the refractive indices of aqueous and vitreous, as well as pupil size (mm)[18], the error of the postoperative manifest subjective refraction itself [19], and most importantly the prediction of the postoperative ACD [20]. Taking into account the three variables axial eye length, corneal power, and prediction of the postoperative ACD, an impact of 36%, 22%, and 42% was found, respectively [21]. The principles of basic optics tell us that the impact of postoperative change of ACD increases with IOL power. This effect is multiplied by the fact that the relative change in ACD after cataract surgery is larger in short eyes than in long eyes [22, 23].

Postoperative ACD Prediction

Consequently, the main source of error for the refractive outcome is the prediction of the postoperative IOL position, or postoperative ACD. Today, most conventional IOL power calculation formulae are including a factor correcting for the postoperative IOL position. To estimate the postoperative IOL position/ postoperative ACD, the concept of the effective lens position (ELP) was introduced for thin lens formulas, i.e., using simplified models for the cornea and the lens. The ELP does not correspond to the anatomical IOL position and is used as a "fudge" factor to optimize the formulae for empirical data. In thick lens formulas, the total power of the IOL is not located in the ELP but is assumed to be distributed on the anterior and posterior IOL surface, therefore using powers and positions of both anterior and posterior IOL surfaces. To date, there are several approaches to estimate the postoperative IOL position/postoperative ACD:

1. Retzlaff et al. [24], Hoffer [24, 25], and Holladay et al. [26] used axial eye length (AL) and corneal power (K).
2. Haigis [27] used AL and preoperative ACD.
3. Olsen [28] developed a thick lens formula using AL, ACD, crystalline lens thickness (LT), corneal radius (CR), and preoperative refraction. Similarly, the Okulix algorithm (not published) used AL, ACD, and LT. Later, Olsen established the C-constant method, which is not dependent on the K-reading or the axial length. The C-constant defines the physical IOL position from the preoperative ACD and lens thickness [29].
4. Barrett [30] used a theoretical model eye in which ACD is related to AL and K and is also determined by the relationship between the A-constant and a "lens factor."
5. Fourth- and fifth-generation formulae use more variables.

.Olsen [28] included the LT as a predictor for the postoperative IOL position, and this was debated controversially. Initially, Norrby also incorporated the LT as a predictor for the haptic plane [31, 32]. Finally, however, Norrby et al. showed that LT was not a relevant prediction parameter [33]. In this study, Norrby et al. aimed to develop algorithms for preoperative estimation of the true postoperative IOL position. Fifty patients were implanted randomly with a 3-piece IOL model in one eye and a single-piece model in the other eye. Preoperatively, the IOLMaster was used to determine axial length, ACD, and mean corneal radius. Lens thickness and corneal width were measured with the ACMaster. Postoperative IOL position was measured with partial coherence laserinterferometry (Zeiss ACMaster). Data for both IOL models were pooled, and partial least-square regressions in various combinations of prediction parameters were calculated. It was shown that nothing was gained when including more parameters than axial length and preoperative ACD. In fact, preoperative ACD alone was a sufficient predictor. The following relationship was found (Formula 1).

$$\text{Postoperative anterior lens position} = 4.415 + 0.3587 \times \text{Preoperative ACD}$$

Formula 1 True Postoperative ACD

Postoperative ACD prediction is a challenging field of biometry, and there is only little literature on dealing with the true IOL position like Norrby et al. described it [33]. Naeser designed a formula that used the preoperative posterior lens capsule as a predictor for the postoperative IOL position/ACD [34] (Formula 2)

$$PLC = 2.4 + 0.011 \times Age + 0.171 \times ACD + 0.051 \times ALACDpostOP = PLC - LPCD - IOLTPLC$$
$$= 2.40 + 0.011 \times Age + 0.171 \times ACD + 0.051 \times ALACDpostOP = PLC - (LPCD + IOLT)$$

Formula 2 Naeser's Prediction Algorithm for the Posterior Lens Capsule (PLC) and the Postoperative ACD

PLC = postoperative posterior lens capsule.

ACD = preOP ACD

AL = axial eye length

LPCD = lens posterior capsule distance

IOLT = thickness of the IOL

Naeser et al. intended to come up with a true way of predicting the postoperative IOL position; however, it turned out to be an empirical regression model. Three factors in their models were observed to be good predictors: age, preoperative ACD, and axial eye length. And again lens thickness was identified to have almost no influence. This is most likely due to "intercorrelation" (collinearity) of the data in their study. That applies to lens thickness and age, but also to ACD (inversely). Moreover, weaker zonules in the elderly population could cause a more posterior position of the posterior lens capsule resulting in a deeper ACD.

Norrby picked up the idea of predicting a true way of the postoperative IOL position/post-operative ACD and further developed this concept by introducing the lens haptic plane concept for normal looped lenses (LHP) [31, 32, 35]. The LHP is defined as the plane through the vertices of the loops approximating the equator of the lens. Since the measurement of this position was not possible, the LHP was estimated (Formula 3).

LHP = lens haptic plane ≈ equator of the lens capsule

ACD = preOP ACD

$PLC = 2.4 + 0.011 \times Age + 0.171 \times ACD + 0.051 \times AL$

$ACDpostOP = PLC - LPCD - IOLT$

$PLC = 2.40 + 0.011 \times Age + 0.171 \times ACD + 0.051 \times AL$

$ACDpostOP = PLC - (LPCD + IOLT)$

$LHP = ACD + Const \times LEN$

LEN = Lens thickness (preOP)

Formula 3 Lens Haptic Plane Formula

The LHP defines the haptic plane but does not predict the position of the anterior IOL surface. Therefore, the term "compressed vault height" was suggested to describe the distance between the LHP and the anterior IOL surface. Major forces that have an impact on the position of the anterior IOL surface are postoperative shrinkage of the lens capsule and the IOL haptics, which will be described later. To overcome the LHP estimation, intraoperative optical coherence tomography (OCT) scans of the anterior lens capsule of the aphakic eye enable measurements of a position close to the theoretical LHP. This new approach was introduced by us [36, 37]. Figure 35.1 shows the significant change of ACD before and after removing the crystalline lens.

The best intraoperative prediction factor for the postoperative IOL position/ postoperative ACD in this study was the anterior lens capsule after implanting a capsular tension ring (CTR_A) (Fig. 35.2), followed by the anterior lens capsule without a CTR (aphak_a). Overall, the posterior lens capsule was a poor predictor.

Moreover, we showed that the intraoperative optical coherence tomography mea-

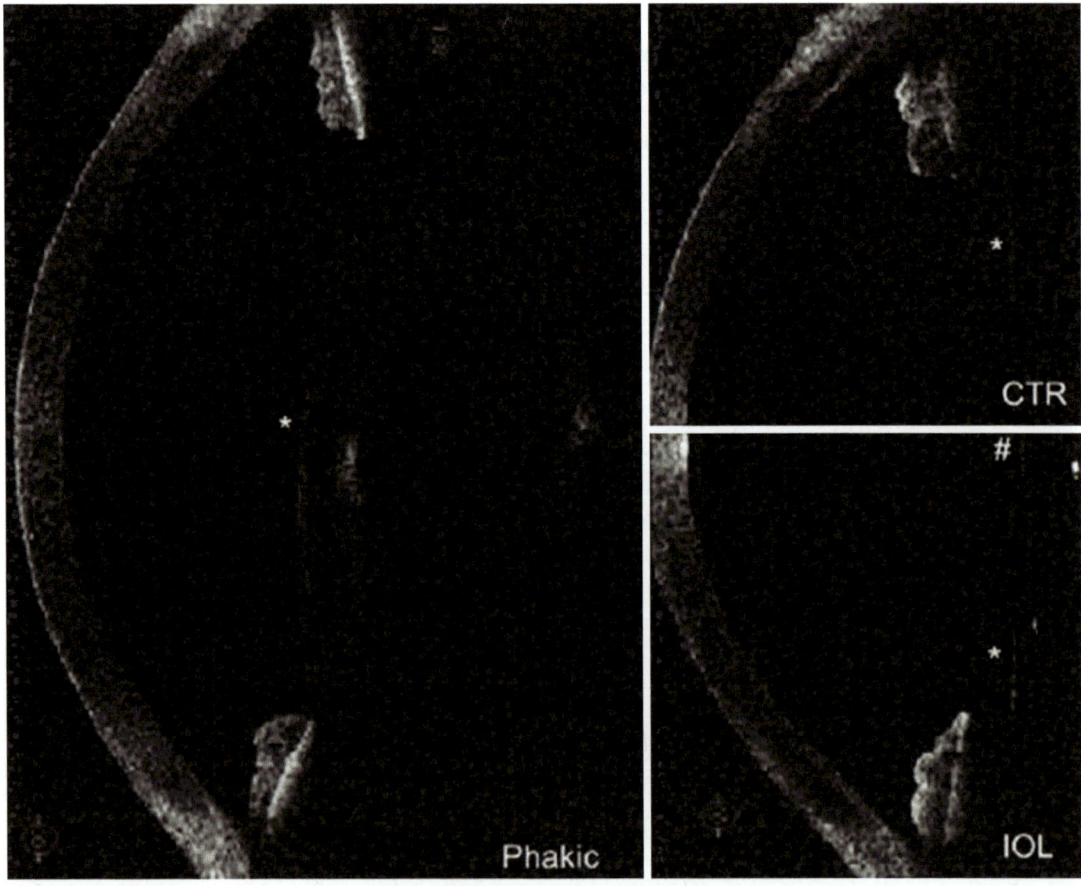

Fig. 35.1 OCT of the anterior segment before cataract surgery and intraoperative after phacoemulsification and capsular tension ring (CTR) implantation [36, 37]. * Anterior lens capsule # center of the anterior surface of the IOL

Fig. 35.2 Influence of intraoperative measurements (explanatory variables) on the postoperative ACD (dependent variable) (Hirnschall, Amir-Asgari, et al. 2013). Anterior lens capsule after implanting a capsular tension ring (CTR_A), anterior lens capsule without a CTR (aphak_a), posterior lens capsule after implanting a capsular tension ring (CTR_P), posterior lens capsule without a CTR (aphak_p)

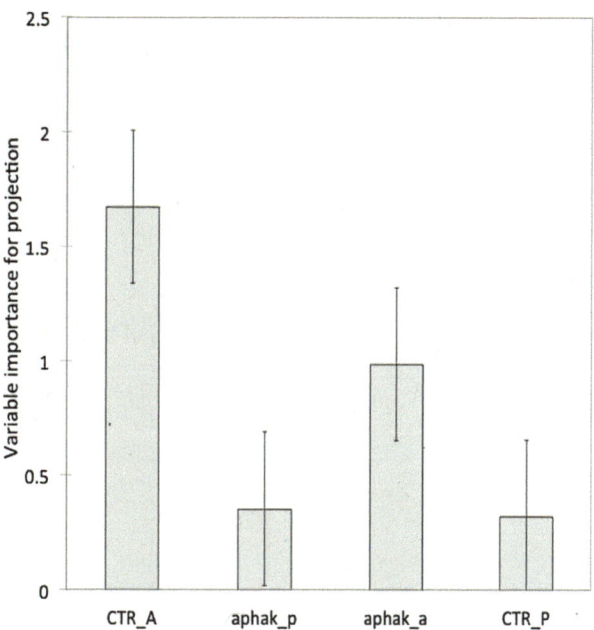

surements of the anterior capsule are a better predictor of the postoperative IOL position/ postoperative ACD compared with preoperatively measured factors (Fig. 35.3). This is especially true in the first hours after lens extraction and then becomes less obvious (but in total still significant) 3 months after cataract surgery due to a further shift of the ACD that is probably more due to lens capsule shrinkage than due to the overall anterior segment anatomical situation [36, 37].

As a consequence, using the intraoperative aphakic ACD for lens power calculation helps to better predict the refractive outcome [38]

Reflecting on our concept measuring the anterior lens capsule after CTR implantation it might be possible that CTR implantation by itself could alter ACD. However, CTR implantation had no significant influence on the postoperative axial IOL position (Fig. 35.4) [39]. Moreover, Weber et al. showed that there was no effect of a CTR on the A-constant for the SRK/T for-

mula (predicting ELP instead of the real IOL position).

Recently, we confirmed that intraoperative aphakic ACD (time-domain OCT) measurements (aphakic eye) predict the postoperative ACD better than preoperative ACD (swept source OCT) measurements [40]. This was independent of whether an open-loop IOL or plate haptic IOL was implanted. Moreover, combining intraoperative aphakic ACD measurements and preoperative ACD measurements resulted in the best postoperative ACD prediction. In detail, the combined prediction was based on partial least-square regression as follows (Formula 4 + Formula 5). Furthermore, a corrected intraoperative ACD value was obtained by adding the mean difference between the 2-month ACD and intraoperative ACD to the intraoperative ACD. The corrected intraoperative ACD value was then calculated to 0.699 ± 0.502 mm. Table 35.1 demonstrates the predictive power of each formula and the effect on the refractive outcome.

$$\text{Postop ACD} = 2.86 + 0.31 \times \text{Intraoperative ACD} + 0.2 \times \text{Preoperative ACD}$$

Fig. 35.3 Variable importance for projection on the ACD (1 h after surgery: upper graph; 3 month after surgery: lower graph) [36, 37]

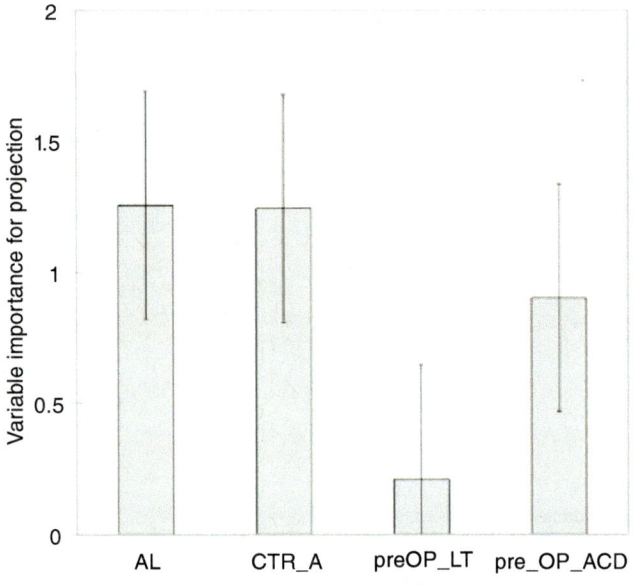

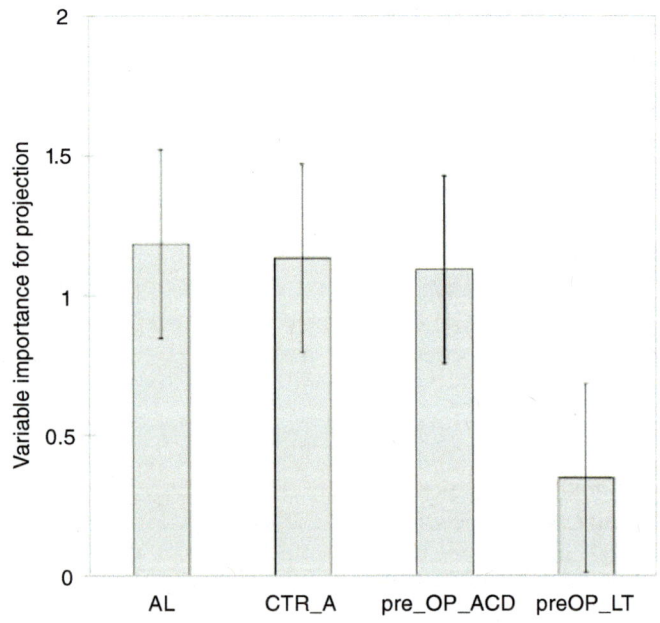

Fig. 35.4 Correlation of the postoperative ACD in eyes with and without a CTR in mm [39]

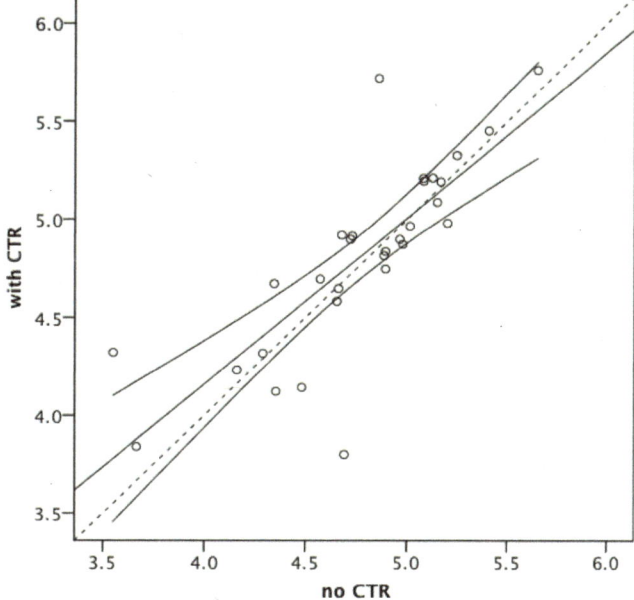

Table 35.1 Influence of the Formulas 4–6 on postACD prediction and the effect on postoperative refraction [40]

	Absolute difference to 3-month ACD (mm) mean (SD); median (max)	Influence on refraction (D) mean (SD); median (max)
PreACD	1.64 (0.56); 1.49 (3.83)	2.75 (1.23); 2.46 (9.06)
intraopACD	0.72 (0.48); 0.48 (2.19)	1.15 (0.79); 0.93 (3.79)
Formular 4 (partial least square regression)	0.35 (0.30); 0.27 (1.37)	0.56 (0.48); 0.41 (2.36)
Formular 5 (no constant)	0.37 (0.38); 0.25 (1.64)	0.59 (0.62); 0.38 (2.82)
Formular 6 (corrected intraopACD)	0.37 (0.34); 0.26 (1.49)	0.58 (0.54); 0.42 (2.58)

Formula 5 Postoperative ACD prediction Without Constant

$$\text{Postop ACD} = 0.92 \times \text{Intraoperative ACD} + 0.31 \times \text{Preoperative ACD}$$

Formula 6
Corrected Intraoperative ACD

Problems of Intraoperative ACD Measurements

Still unsolved is the problem of intraoperative hydration of the vitreous. As a consequence of vitreous hydration, the anterior chamber is artificially shallow and therefore interfering with the aphakic ACD measurements. Following a washout phase of some hours to days after surgery the hydration vanishes, though leaving a discrepancy between the intraoperatively measured ACD and the postoperatively measured ACD.

Formula 4 Postoperative ACD Prediction with Constant

$$\text{Postop ACD} = 2.86 + 0.31 \times \text{Intraoperative ACD} + 0.20 \times \text{Preoperative ACD}$$

Intraoperative accuracy could be improved by using a swept source OCT since until now it was limited to time-domain OCT.

Postoperative ACD Shift

Within the first weeks of cataract surgery, the ACD shifts. This is because of the interaction of forces between the collapsing and then shrinking lens capsule and as well as the memory of the IOL haptics. So far, lens capsule shrinking is not preventable. Therefore, the only remaining variable that is controllable is lens haptic design. Today, three main lens haptic types are on the market: plate haptics, single-piece open-loop haptics, and three-piece open-loop haptics.

ACD Shift in Plate Haptics IOL Vs Standard Three-Piece Open-Loop Haptics IOL of the Same Acrylic Material [36, 37]

We demonstrated that plate haptics IOL showed a slight backward shift in the first month after surgery that was not found to be significantly different compared to the standard three-piece open-loop haptics IOL (Fig. 35.5). At the one-year follow-up visit, the ACD was similar in both groups.

The tendency for backward shifts in plate haptics is supported by Findl et al. for another plate haptic IOL [41].

Fig. 35.5 ACD shift haptic dependance: standard three-piece open-loop haptic IOL (gray) and plate haptic IOL (black) [36, 37]

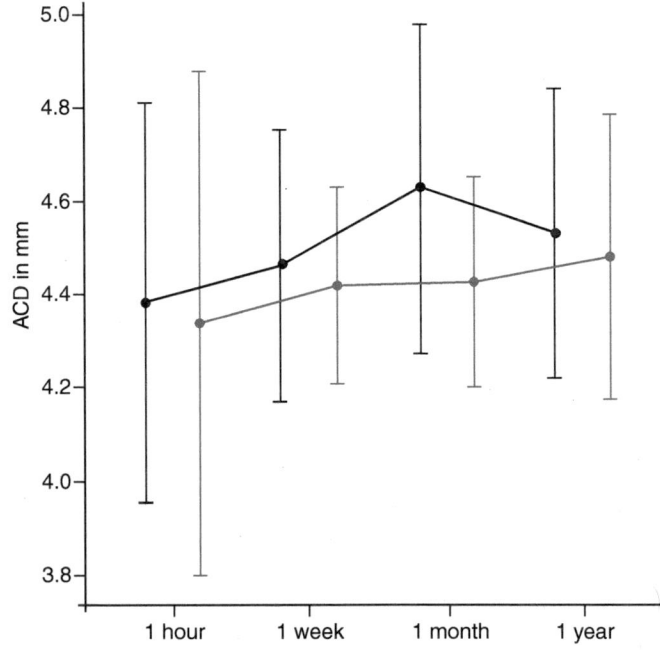

ACD Shift in Single-Piece Open-Loop haptics IOL Vs Three-Piece Open-Loop Haptics IOL of the Same Acrylic Material [42]

Findl et al. showed that angulated three-piece open-loop haptics IOL have a slightly more pronounced ACD shift compared to single-piece IOLs (Fig. 35.6).

The more pronounced ACD shift in 3 piece open loops haptics was recently confirmed by Sato et al. [43] and was also found in multipiece haptics [44]. Moreover, analyzing different open-loop haptic IOLs with a different haptic thickness, no significant difference regarding ACD was observed [45].

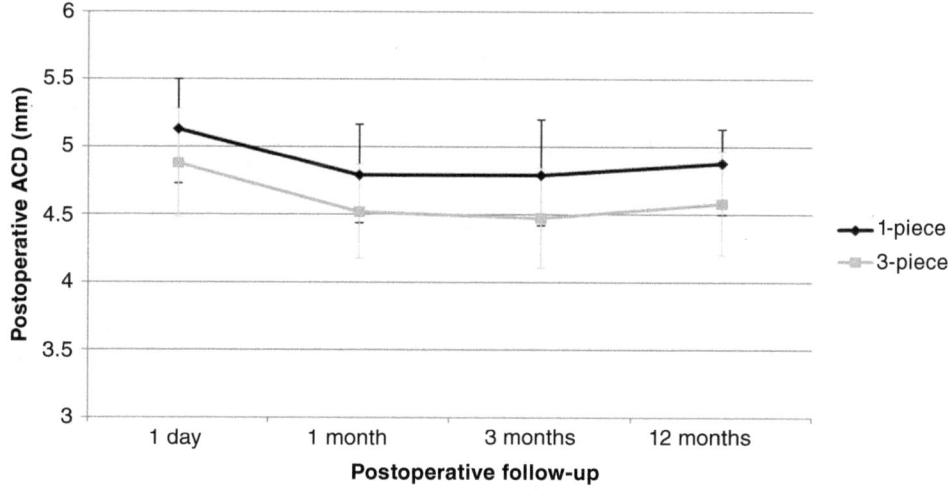

Fig. 35.6 ACD changes in mm between the first postoperative day and 1 year for a 1-piece open-loop and a 3-piece IOL [42]

Fig. 35.7 ACD changes in mm between the first postoperative week (W1), first month (M1) and 4–6 months (M4–6) for a single-piece open-loop (blue) and plate haptic IOL (orange) [46]

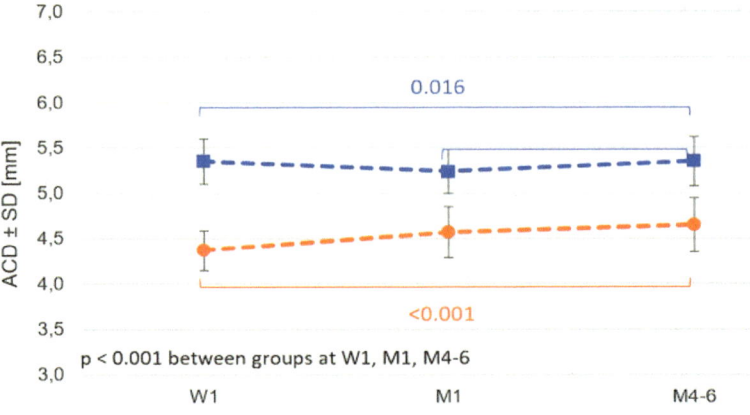

ACD Shift in Single Piece Open-Loop Haptics IOL Vs Plate Haptics IOL of the Same Acrylic Material [46]

Hienert et al. reported that single-piece open-loop haptics IOL and plate haptics IOL resulted in significantly different ACD values at all time points from the first postoperative to 4–6 months after surgery (Fig. 35.7). The overall IOL shift was 0.25 ± 0.16 mm for the plate haptics and 0.14 ± 0.09 mm for the open-loop haptics. Although ACD was shifting, there was no impact of ACD on manifest refraction at any follow-up visit.

Postoperative ACD Shift and Rhexis Shape and Size

Size and shape of the manual continuous curvilinear capsulorrhexis (CCC) could play a major role in determining the postoperative ACD shift. Findl et al. investigated manual CCC and rhexis size and shape [47]. They defined RSF as the rhexis shape factor (1.0 is a perfect circle and a lower value describes the imperfection of the roundness), A as the area in mm^2 of the rhexis and C as the circumference of the rhexis in mm (Formula 7).

$$RSF = A/((\llbracket\llbracket C \wedge 2\rrbracket \_ /4\pi\rrbracket^\wedge))$$

Formula 7 Rhexis Shape Factor (RSF) Formular

A = Area of rhexis $\left(mm^2\right)$

C = Circumference of the rhexis $\left(mm\right)$

No difference concerning postoperative ACD shift was found between those eyes with a perfect rhexis and those patients with an eccentric, or small rhexis (Figs. 35.8 and 35.9). However, patients with an incomplete rhexis-IOL overlap had a higher risk of postoperative unexpected large ACD. Cekic demonstrated in their study that the postoperative ACD shifted significantly, when comparing a 4.0 mm rhexis and a 6.0 mm rhexis [48]. Major weaknesses of that study were that it was not randomised and that an older PMMA IOL design was used. Consequently, it is not clear whether their finding holds true for more modern IOLs.

Assuring a 100% rhexis-IOL overlap like in precision pulse capsulotomy was shown to result in an overall reduction of variability in ACD shift [49], thus creating more axial stability.

Fig. 35.8 ACD in mm for eyes with normal eccentric and small rhexis (<4.5 mm) eyes [47]

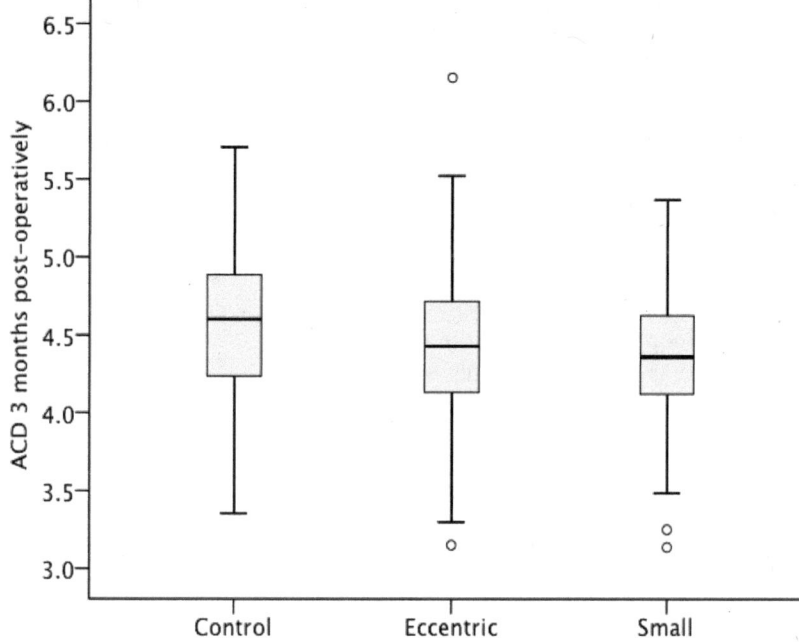

Fig. 35.9 ACD shift in mm for eyes with normal eccentric and small rhexis (<4.5 mm) eyes [47]

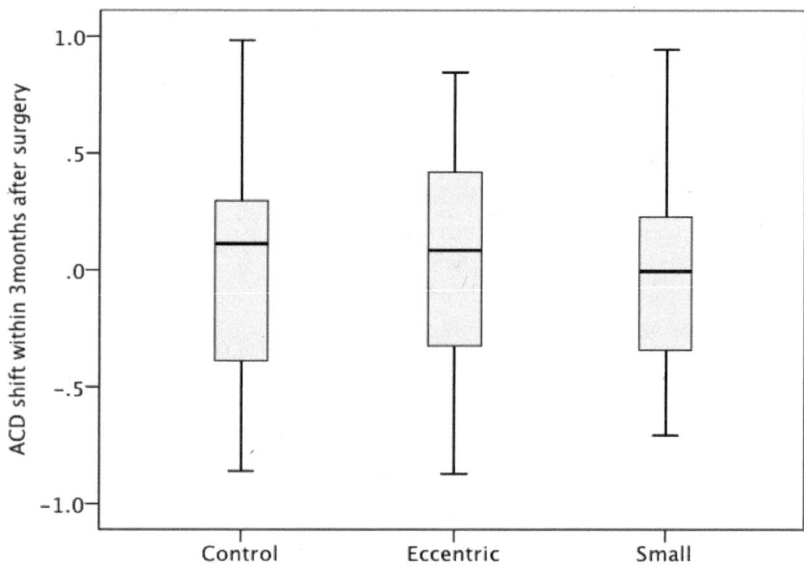

Postoperative ACD Shift and Capsular Shrinkage

Besides haptic design, a major factor responsible for postoperative axial IOL movement is capsular bag shrinkage. Strenn et al. introduced a CTR as a measuring device for quantification of capsular bag diameter (CBD) and postoperative capsular shrinkage [50]. We found that CBD within the first postoperative month after implanting a three-piece open-loop haptics IOL and a CTR shrank by 0.29 ± 0.15 mm (range 0.55 to 0.07 mm) ($P < 0.005$). This shrinkage of the capsule significantly correlated (0.67; ($P < 0.005$) with the postoperative change of ACD [51].

Summary

ACD has become a major player in the field of biometry and power calculation due to the increasing demands of good refractive outcomes. Measurements of ACD with one device should not be used interchangeably with other devices. Referring to refractive outcomes, postoperative ACD is the most influencing parameter. Intraoperative measurements of aphakic ACD have shown to significantly improve estimations of postoperative ACD especially when combined with preoperative ACD measurements. Postoperative ACD stabilizes in the first months, and postoperative ACD shift is dependent on IOL haptic design as well as the extent of capsule shrinkage. Postoperative ACD shift is most prominent in three piece IOL haptics followed by plate IOL haptics and is least pronounced in single piece open-loop IOL haptics. Finally, postoperative ACD shift seems not to be dependent of rhexis size, centering, and shape as long as there is a complete rhexis-IOL overlap. However, there remains some variability of ACD shift probably due to patient factors such as zonule insertion and integrity as well as differences in capsule shrinkage after surgery.

References

1. Hoffer KJ. Definition of ACD. Ophthalmology. 2011;118(7):1484.
2. Nakakura S, Mori E, Nagatomi N, Tabuchi H, Kiuchi Y. Comparison of anterior chamber depth measurements by 3-dimensional optical coherence tomography, partial coherence interferometry biometry, Scheimpflug rotating camera imaging, and ultrasound biomicroscopy. J Cataract Refract Surg. 2012;38(7):1207–13.
3. Fişuş AD, Hirnschall ND, Findl O. Comparison of two swept-source optical coherence tomography-based biometry devices. J Cataract Refract Surg. 2021;47(1):87–92. https://doi.org/10.1097/j.jcrs.0000000000000373.
4. Yang CM, Lim DH, Kim HJ, Chung T-Y. Comparison of two swept-source optical coherence tomography biometers and a partial coherence interferometer. PLoS One. 2019;14(10):e0223114.
5. Hamoudi H, Christensen UC, la Cour M. Agreement of Phakic and Pseudophakic anterior chamber depth measurements in IOLMaster and Pentacam. Acta Ophthalmol. 2018;96(3):e403.
6. Sng CC, Foo L-L, Cheng C-Y, Allen Jr JC, He M, Krishnaswamy G, Nongpiur ME, Friedman DS, Wong TY, Aung T. Determinants of anterior chamber depth: the Singapore Chinese eye study. Ophthalmology. 2012;119(6):1143–50.
7. Norrby S. Sources of error in intraocular lens power calculation. J Cataract Refract Surg. 2008;34(3):368–76.
8. Elder MJ. Predicting the refractive outcome after cataract surgery: the comparison of different IOLs and SRK-II v SRK-T. Br J Ophthalmol. 2002;86(6):620–2.
9. Liu B, Liang X, Wang YX, Jonas JB. Prevalence of cataract surgery and postoperative visual outcome in greater Beijing: the Beijing eye study. Ophthalmology. 2009;116(7):1322–31. https://doi.org/10.1016/j.ophtha.2009.01.030.
10. Lundström M, Barry P, Henry Y, Rosen P, Stenevi U. Evidence-based guidelines for cataract surgery: guidelines based on data in the European registry of quality outcomes for cataract and refractive surgery database. J Cataract Refract Surg. 2012;38(6):1086–93.
11. Melles RB, Holladay JT, Chang WJ. Accuracy of intraocular lens calculation formulas. Ophthalmology. 2018;125(2):169–78.
12. Fernández-Buenaga R, Alió JL. Intraocular lens Explantation after cataract surgery: indications, results, and Explantation techniques. Asia Pac J Ophthalmol (Phila). 2017;6(4):372–80.
13. Haigis W, Lege B, Miller N, Schneider B. Comparison of immersion ultrasound biometry and partial coher-

ence interferometry for intraocular lens calculation according to Haigis. Graefes Arch Clin Exp Ophthalmol. 2000;238(9):765–73.

14. Norrby S. Multicenter biometry study of 1 pair of eyes. J Cataract Refract Surg. 2001;27(10):1656–61.

15. Rainer G, Petternel V, Findl O, Schmetterer L, Skorpik C, Luksch A, Drexler W. Comparison of ultrasound Pachymetry and partial coherence interferometry in the measurement of central corneal thickness. J Cataract Refract Surg. 2002;28(12):2142–5.

16. Dubbelman M, Weeber HA, van der Heijde RGL, Völker-Dieben HJ. Radius and Asphericity of the posterior corneal surface determined by corrected Scheimpflug photography. Acta Ophthalmol Scand. 2002;80(4):379–83.

17. Dubbelman M, Sicam VADP, Van der Heijde GL. The shape of the anterior and posterior surface of the aging human cornea. Vis Res. 2006;46(6-7):993–1001.

18. Cheng ACK, Rao SK, Cheng LL, Lam DSC. Assessment of pupil size under different light intensities using the Procyon Pupillometer. J Cataract Refract Surg. 2006;32(6):1015–7.

19. Shah R, Edgar DF, Rabbetts R, Harle DE, Evans BJW. Standardized Patient Methodology to Assess Refractive Error Reproducibility. Optom Vis Sci. 2009;86(5):517–28.

20. Olsen T. Sources of error in intraocular lens power calculation. J Cataract Refract Surg. 1992;18(2):125–9.

21. Olsen T. Calculation of intraocular lens power: a review. Acta Ophthalmol Scand. 2007;85(5):472–85. https://doi.org/10.1111/j.1755-3768.2007.00879.x.

22. Muzyka-Woźniak M, Ogar A. Anterior chamber depth and iris and lens position before and after phacoemulsification in eyes with a short or long axial length. J Cataract Refract Surg. 2016;42(4):563–8. https://doi.org/10.1016/j.jcrs.2015.12.050.

23. Ning X, Yang Y, Yan H, Zhang J. Anterior chamber depth — a predictor of refractive outcomes after age-related cataract surgery. BMC Ophthalmol. 2019;19(1):134. https://doi.org/10.1186/s12886-019-1144-8.

24. Retzlaff JA, Sanders DR, Kraff MC. Development of the SRK/T intraocular lens power calculation formula. J Cataract Refract Surg. 1990;16:333–40. Errata: 1990;16:528 and 1993;19(5):444–446.

25. Hoffer KJ. The Hoffer Q formula: A comparison of theoretic and regression formulas. J Cataract Refract Surg. 1993;19(11):700–12. Errata: 1994;20(6):677 and 2007;33(1):2–3.

26. Holladay JT, Musgrove KH, Prager TC, Lewis JW, Chandler TY, Ruiz RS. A three-part system for refining intraocular lens power calculations. J Cataract Refract Surg. 1988;14(1):17–24. https://doi.org/10.1016/s0886-3350(88)80059-2.

27. Haigis W. Occurrence of erroneous anterior chamber depth in the SRK/T formula. J Cataract Refract Surg. 1993;19(3):442–6.

28. Olsen T. Prediction of the effective postoperative (intraocular lens) anterior chamber depth. J Cataract Refract Surg. 2006;32(3):419–24.

29. Olsen T, Hoffmann P. C constant: new concept for ray tracing-assisted intraocular lens power calculation. J Cataract Refract Surg. 2014;40(5):764–73.

30. Barrett GD. An improved universal theoretical formula for intraocular lens power prediction. J Cataract Refract Surg. 1993;19(6):713–20.

31. Norrby S. Using the lens haptic plane concept and thick-lens ray tracing to calculate intraocular lens power. J Cataract Refract Surg. 2004;30(5):1000–5. https://doi.org/10.1016/j.jcrs.2003.09.055.

32. Norrby S, Lydahl E, Koranyi G, Taube M. Clinical application of the lens haptic plane concept with transformed axial lengths. J Cataract Refract Surg. 2005;31(7):1338–44.

33. Norrby S, Bergman R, Hirnschall N, Nishi Y, Findl O. Prediction of the true IOL position. Br J Ophthalmol. 2017;101(10):1440–6.

34. Naeser K, Boberg-Ans J, Bargum R. Biometry of the posterior lens capsule: a new method to predict Pseudophakic anterior chamber depth. J Cataract Refract Surg. 1990;16(2):202–6. https://doi.org/10.1016/s0886-3350(13)80731-6.

35. Norrby NE, Koranyi G. Prediction of intraocular lens power using the lens haptic plane concept. J Cataract Refract Surg. 1997;23(2):254–9.

36. Hirnschall N, Amir-Asgari S, Maedel S, Findl O. Predicting the postoperative intraocular lens position using continuous intraoperative optical coherence tomography measurements. Invest Ophthalmol Vis Sci. 2013a;54(8):5196–203.

37. Hirnschall N, Nishi Y, Crnej A, Koshy J, Gangwani V, Maurino V, Findl O. Capsular bag stability and posterior capsule opacification of a plate-haptic design microincision cataract surgery intraocular lens: 3-year results of a randomised trial. Br J Ophthalmol. 2013b;97(12):1565–8.

38. Hirnschall N, Norrby S, Weber M, Maedel S, Amir-Asgari S, Findl O. Using continuous intraoperative optical coherence tomography measurements of the Aphakic eye for intraocular lens power calculation. Br J Ophthalmol. 2015;99(1):7–10.

39. Weber M, Hirnschall N, Rigal K, Findl O. Effect of a capsular tension ring on axial intraocular lens position. J Cataract Refract Surg. 2015;41(1):122–5.

40. Hirnschall N, Farrokhi S, Amir-Asgari S, Hienert J, Findl O. Intraoperative optical coherence tomography measurements of Aphakic eyes to predict postoperative position of 2 intraocular lens designs. J Cataract Refract Surg. 2018;44(11):1310–6.

41. Findl O, Drexler W, Menapace R, Bobr B, Bittermann S, Vass C, Rainer G, Hitzenberger CK, Fercher AF. Accurate determination of effective lens position and lens-capsule distance with 4 intraocular lenses. J Cataract Refract Surg. 1998;24(8):1094–8.

42. Findl O, Hirnschall N, Nishi Y, Maurino V, Crnej A. Capsular bag performance of a hydrophobic acrylic 1-piece intraocular lens. J Cataract Refract Surg. 2015;41(1):90–7.

43. Sato T, Shibata S, Yoshida M, Hayashi K. Short-term dynamics after single- and three-piece acrylic intra-

ocular lens implantation: a swept-source anterior segment optical coherence tomography study. Sci Rep. 2018;8(1):10230.

44. Wirtitsch MG, Findl O, Menapace R, Kriechbaum K, Koeppl C, Buehl W, Drexler W. Effect of haptic design on change in axial lens position after cataract surgery. J Cataract Refract Surg. 2004;30(1):45–51.

45. Gangwani V, Hirnschall N, Koshy J, Crnej A, Nishi Y, Maurino V, Findl O. Posterior capsule opacification and capsular bag performance of a micro-incision intraocular lens. J Cataract Refract Surg. 2011;37(11):1988–92.

46. Hienert J, Hirnschall N, Ruiss M, Ullrich M, Zwickl H, Findl O. Prospective study to compare axial position stability following fellow-eye implantation of two distinct intraocular lens designs. J Cataract Refract Surg. 2021;47(8):999–1005. https://doi.org/10.1097/j.jcrs.0000000000000557.

47. Findl O, Hirnschall N, Draschl P, Wiesinger J. Effect of manual Capsulorhexis size and position on intraoc-

ular lens tilt, centration, and axial position. J Cataract Refract Surg. 2017;43(7):902–8.

48. Cekiç O, Batman C. The relationship between Capsulorhexis size and anterior chamber depth relation. Ophthalmic Surg Lasers. 1999;30(3):185–90.

49. Bang SP, Jun JH. Comparison of postoperative axial stability of intraocular lens and Capsulotomy parameters between precision pulse Capsulotomy and continuous curvilinear Capsulotomy: a prospective cohort study. Medicine. 2019;98(48):e18224.

50. Strenn K, Menapace R, Vass C. Capsular bag shrinkage after implantation of an open-loop silicone lens and a poly(methyl methacrylate) capsule tension ring. J Cataract Refract Surg. 1997;23(10):1543–7. https://doi.org/10.1016/s0886-3350(97)80027-2.

51. Koeppl C, Findl O, Kriechbaum K, Sacu S, Drexler W. Change in IOL position and capsular bag size with an angulated intraocular lens early after cataract surgery. J Cataract Refract Surg. 2005;31(2):348–53.

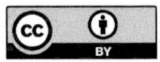

IOL Constant Optimization

36

Petros Aristodemou

Refinements in surgical technique, advances in biometry instrumentation, and the evolution of IOL power formulae have all brought about progressive improvements in predicting the refractive outcome following cataract surgery. Improving predictions depends on reducing random and systematic error, thus improving precision and accuracy, respectively.

Accuracy vs Precision

Random error refers to the degree of spread of the outcomes. The lower the random error, the tighter the spread, and the greater the precision. This is the difference of spread comparing the wide spread of hits using a regular gun (Target A) and the tight spread of hits using a sniper gun (targets B and C) (Table 36.1). Optical biometry and refinements in IOL power calculations have reduced random error and brought about improvements in the precision of refractive outcomes. Systematic error refers to results being systematically off-center on average and therefore compromising the accuracy of the outcomes. These results are amenable to correction in the same way that someone calibrates the crosshair of the sniper rifle and corrects the aim of the gun from the results of target B to the results of target C.

Optimizing the IOL constant corrects the systematic error of an IOL power formula in the same way as calibrating the crosshair of a gun. In the example above, the graph on the left side demonstrates a more diffuse spread around 0 and represents the spread of prediction error following a combination of applanation ultrasound with an appropriate IOL constant. When optical biometry is used, the spread of outcomes is tighter as the precision in axial measurement improves. Nevertheless, if the IOL constant is kept the same as for applanation ultrasound, the prediction error is systematically hyperopic (because applanation ultrasound systematically measures eyes shorter than optical biometry). The refractive outcomes in the graph with optical biometry and incorrect IOL constant are poor, worse than with applanation ultrasound (graph on left), with the average patient ending up with +0.5D hyperopia. When the appropriate IOL constant value is used, this resets the systematic error induced by the change in the biometry method, thus resetting the average prediction error to 0 [1] There is a multitude of sources of systematic error, arising from the biometry measurement to the IOL model used, so each combination of the biometry machine/IOL model yields a different IOL constant value.

P. Aristodemou (✉)
VRMCy Clinic, Limassol, Cyprus

The Cyprus Institute of Neurology and Genetics, Nicosia, Cyprus

© The Author(s) 2024

J. Aramberri et al. (eds.), *Intraocular Lens Calculations*, Essentials in Ophthalmology, https://doi.org/10.1007/978-3-031-50666-6_36

Table 36.1 Comparison of accuracy and precision in refractive outcomes

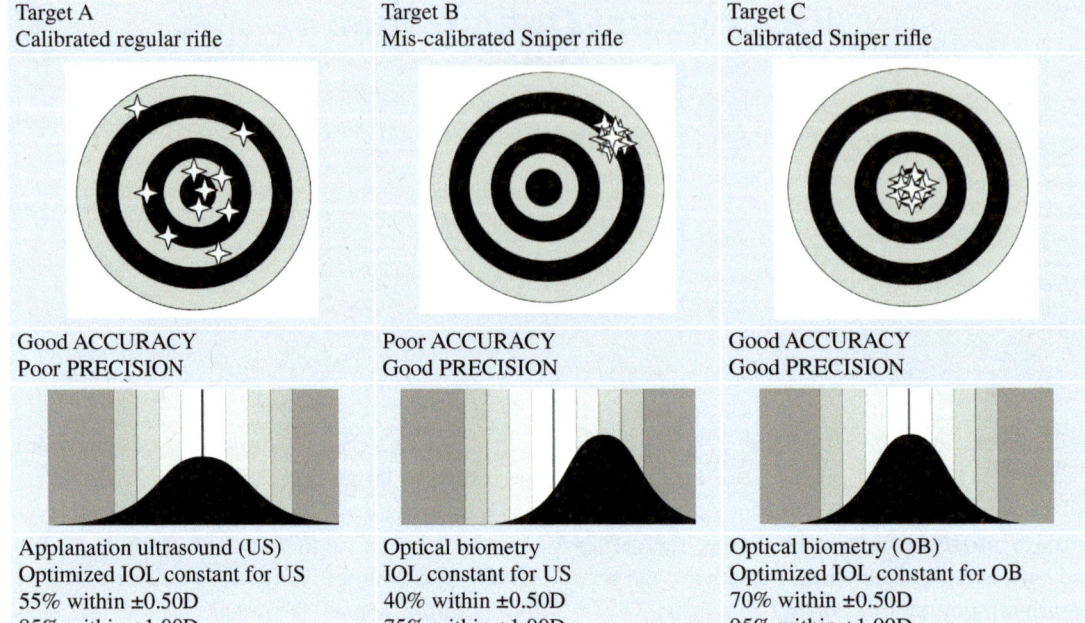

Target A Calibrated regular rifle	Target B Mis-calibrated Sniper rifle	Target C Calibrated Sniper rifle
Good ACCURACY Poor PRECISION	Poor ACCURACY Good PRECISION	Good ACCURACY Good PRECISION
Applanation ultrasound (US) Optimized IOL constant for US 55% within ±0.50D 85% within ±1.00D	Optical biometry IOL constant for US 40% within ±0.50D 75% within ±1.00D	Optical biometry (OB) Optimized IOL constant for OB 70% within ±0.50D 95% within ±1.00D

Factors That Affect the IOL Constant

Differences between IOL designs and biometry methods are all sources of systematic error and can displace the average prediction error away from 0.0D. These require an adjustment of the value (optimization) of the IOL constant in order to reset the mean prediction error to 0.0D. Therefore, each combination of the IOL model and biometry device may require a different IOL constant value.

A. The IOL Geometry

Even with in-the-bag IOL implantation, the post-operative IOL position and the location of the principal planes of the lens would depend on the geometry of the IOL. This may be related to the distribution of optical power between the anterior and the posterior IOL surfaces, the angulation of the haptics relative to the optic plane, and the shape, size, and material of the IOL(the material affects the refractive index and the softness of the material can affect the IOL thickness, eg hydrophilic acrylic is softer than hydrophobic acrylic and softer IOLs are often made thicker). Table 36.2 illustrates the location of the principal planes of a number of IOL optical designs.

The Alcon MA series (Alcon, Fort Worth, TX) is a good example of how the effective optical power varies after in-the-bag IOL implantation for the same optical power of an IOL and its impact on the IOL constant (Table 36.3).

Technical product information accessible at https://www.alcon.com/eye-care-products

B. Location of IOL implantation

Optimized constants for posterior chamber IOLs published by sites such as ULib (ocusoft. de/ulib/c1.htm) and IOL Con (iolcon.org) are specifically indicated for calculations when the IOL is implanted in the capsular bag (ULib has not been updated for some time at the time of writing this chapter). When the IOL is not implanted in the capsular bag, the optimized IOL constant may not be appropriate for that specific IOL position.

When an IOL is not implanted in the capsular bag, its anteroposterior position will affect its effective lens power. The more anterior the location of the IOL, the higher the effective power of the optic, and therefore, the nominal power of the IOL needs to be adjusted downwards in order to achieve the refractive target. This can be done in a

Table 36.2 Schematic location of principal planes with respect to the optical design of the IOL optic

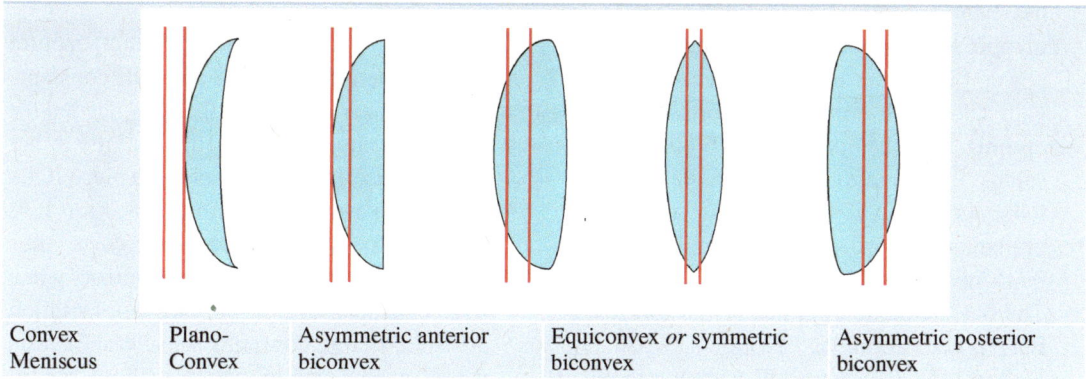

| Convex Meniscus | Plano-Convex | Asymmetric anterior biconvex | Equiconvex *or* symmetric biconvex | Asymmetric posterior biconvex |

Table 36.3 The influence of IOL design on effective lens power and IOL constant

IOL model	MA30 MA	MA60 AC	MA60 BM
Optic configuration	Asymmetric anterior biconvex	Asymmetric anterior biconvex	Asymmetric posterior biconvex
Haptic configuration	5° posterior angulation	10° posterior angulation	10° posterior angulation
Principal plane location	More anterior		More posterior
Effective lens power	Higher power		Lower power
ULIB optimized	5.46	5.67	6.08
Hoffer Q pACD, Holladay 1 sf,	1.64	1.90	2.33
SRK/T A-constant	118.7	119.2	119.8

number of ways. For anterior chamber IOLs, this is conventionally achieved by using their specific IOL constant, which is typically much lower than for posterior chamber IOLs. The same applies for iris-claw lenses, where the IOL constants for retro-pupillary fixation are higher than for fixation of the same IOL in front of the iris but lower than for other in-the-bag IOL models (iolcon.org).

When IOL constants for in-the-bag placement are used, sulcus implantation results in a myopic prediction error compared to intracapsular implantation. Various approaches have been described to address this systematic error:

(1) To reduce the IOL power by 0.5D or 1.0D for sulcus implantation in all cases: This would work in averaged-sized eyes and average powered IOLs but for high powered IOLs, the power reduction needs to be greater. The opposite applies to low-powered IOLs. By subtracting the same amount of power in all cases, this would undercorrect small eyes and overcorrect long eyes [2]. A slightly better rule of thumb is to reduce the implanted IOL power by 5% of that for in-the-bag implantation [3], but this approach is still suboptimal.

(2) To use IOL constants derived for sulcus implantation: The advantage of adjusting the IOL constant to match the new effective lens position is that the IOL power formula will predict the appropriate power adjustments with respect to the IOL power. This means that high-powered IOLs will have a greater reduction in IOL power, whereas low-powered IOLs will be affected less so. Surgeons should generate new IOL power constants for their IOL model of choice for sulcus implantation and have one calculation in their IOL calculation sheet so that the appropriate IOL power is available when sulcus implantation is indicated.

Obtaining the appropriate IOL constants for sulcus implantation can be done either by the conventional way or by collecting enough cases and performing optimization calculations [4] (see methodology), but this is often not possible as only very large centers would have the 100 or more eyes required with sulcus IOL implantation of the same IOL model. Alternatively, one can take into account the difference in average prediction error between in-the-bag implantation and sulcus implantation for the same IOL model. This has been calculated at around −0.6 D of myopic shift for the sulcus for the same IOL power [3]. In the absence of enough cases with sulcus IOL implantation for formal IOL optimization, the optimized IOL constant for sulcus implantation can be derived by reducing the IOL constant for in-the-bag implantation by 0.47 (corresponding to the 0.6D myopic shift of sulcus implantation). The 0.47 reduction applies to the following IOL power formulae: Hoffer Q (pACD), Holladay 1 (sf), Barrett UII (surgeon factor), Holladay 2 (ACD), Haigis (a0), and the Olsen (ACD). For the IOL formulae using an "A constant" (SRK-T, T2, K6, and Kane formulae), the A constant should be reduced by 0.75 to obtain an optimized A constant for sulcus implantation (see Table 36.12). For example, the Alcon MA60AC 3-piece IOL has in-the-bag IOL constants of 5.67, 1.90, and 119.2 for the Hoffer Q, Holladay 1, and SRK/T, respectively (Table 36.3). For sulcus implantation, the estimated constants for the same IOL model are 5.20, 1.43, and 118.45 for the Hoffer Q, Holladay 1, and SRK/T, respectively.

Using a specific IOL constant for sulcus implantation has two main advantages: (1) the ease of use and (2) the automatic adjustment of the IOL power with respect to its effective lens position. When one uses a triple-optimized Haigis formula with real post-op data derived from sulcus IOL implantation, further refinements in precision can be obtained as the pre-operative ACD, Ks, and AL are used to predict the sulcus diameter, which, in turn, affects the compression of the IOL haptics in the sulcus and the posterior vault distance of the IOL optic [5].

(3) Perform back calculations for sulcus placement. Please refer to the chapter on out-of-the-bag IOL implantation by Dr. Jaime Aramberri.

There are other alternative fixation techniques, including (1) sulcus IOL haptic placement with the optic captured through the anterior capsulorrhexis opening, (2) sutured scleral fixation, and (3) sutureless scleral fixation at various distances behind the limbus.

Sulcus placement with optic capture through the anterior CCC has IOL constants that are closer in value to the ones needed for in-the-bag implantation [6]. On the other hand, intrascleral fixation of three piece IOLs appears to result in a more posterior IOL location to an in-the-bag reference, thus resulting in hyperopic prediction errors when IOL constants for in-the-bag implantation are used, so IOL constants for scleral fixation would need to be higher than those for in-the-bag implantation [7, 8].

C. Biometry
a. Axial Length

Axial length (AL) measurement in the days of ultrasound biometry was considered the primary source of prediction error [9]. Applanation ultrasound had additional issues with inducing errors because of the corneal flattening during measurement as this would measure the eye shorter [10]. Manufacturer's IOL constants were typically derived using applanation ultrasound as this was the most widely used approach. Immersion ultrasound offered superior outcomes as it left the eye undistorted during measurement but this was more labor intensive, and patients did not like the immersion water bath that was required for this ultrasound technique. When Zeiss developed the IOL Master, Prof Wolfgang Haigis, who was instrumental in its development, had calibrated the axial length measurements of the IOL Master against a high-definition 40 MHz immersion ultrasound machine. These made IOL Master AL measurements on average of the same magnitude as immersion ultrasound AL measurements (albeit with a smaller standard deviation, a narrower spread, offering improved precision) [11].

When subsequent biometry machines were developed by other manufacturers, their AL measurements were calibrated against the IOLMaster in order to meet FDA and other regulatory standards, so this makes the AL measurements between different biometers have very little to no systematic difference, translating to very similar outcomes. This applies both to low coherence interferometry [12, 13] and swept-source OCT-based machines [14].

For some biometers, there are systematic differences in axial length measurement in longer eyes, and this stems from the fact that, currently, the axial length is measured as one singular measure despite it incorporates a number of media of optically different density (see Tables 36.4 and 36.5) for comparisons in axial length and ACD between biometers). When sum-of-segments axial length measurements become established in IOL power calculations, this would certainly translate to a change in IOL constant value but it may also make measurements between biometers more consistent [15] (see David Cooke's chapter on axial length measurements).

b. Keratometry

Any systematic differences in measuring corneal radii, even when they are seemingly very small, would have a disproportionate effect on shifting refractive outcomes away from an average 0.0D prediction error. This is because, in addition to measuring corneal power, keratometry measurements are used by IOL power formulae to predict the post-operative anterior chamber depth and effective lens position. Hence, systematic differences in keratometry have a double whammy effect on prediction error by both changing the corneal power and the predicted position of the IOL [44]. Therefore, any systematic difference should be factored into the IOL constant used for the specific biometry device (Table 36.6).

It must be stressed that Sim Ks from some topographers should not be used for IOL power calculations as these measurements can sometimes be very different from biometer Ks and result in a significant ametropic shift in refractive outcomes.

D. Less important factors: IOL Constant "Personalization"

Surgeons generally do not have significantly different "Personalised" IOL Constants from one another. The term "personalized IOL constant" dates back to a time when extracapsular cataract extraction (ECCE) was the standard surgical procedure [45]. For this surgical procedure, there are additional important variables and sources of error, compared to phacoemulsification with in-the-bag IOL implantation. In ECCE, surgeons typically performed a can opener capsulotomy, which was large and included radial capsular tears. Sometimes this permitted the placement of the lens in the bag and sometimes the lens was placed in the sulcus. Some surgeons were more reliable in achieving intracapsular implantation, whereas other surgeons routinely placed their IOLs in the sulcus regardless of the state of the anterior capsulotomy. The more anterior placement of the IOL causes the effective power of the IOL to increase and results in a more myopic deviation from an in-the-bag placement. This is why when using ECCE, it was important for every surgeon to determine their own "personalized" IOL constant, which would primarily depend on their routine IOL placement [46].

With phacoemulsification cataract extraction through a continuous curvilinear capsulorrhexis (CCC), IOL implantation has become more predictable, and therefore, any surgeon-derived variability has diminished [47, 48]. Provided that the CCC is smaller than the IOL optic (thus preventing any anterior optic prolapse) and that the posterior capsule remains intact at the end of the surgery, most surgeons appear to have very similar results. In a study of refractive outcomes looking at IOL constants, the IOL constants of 27 surgeons with more than 64 cases each and using the same biometer were very similar, and only one surgeon' constant deviated more than what is considered to be a clinically significant difference of IOL constant value from the average of all surgeons tested [1]. Another study used multilevel multivariate modeling to analyze 490,987 eyes of 351,864 patients, who had phacoemulsification cataract surgery by 2567 surgeons. It found that the surgeon accounted for only 4% of the variability in refractive outcomes, as opposed to 23% attributed to the patient level (patient-specific variables affecting both eyes and not attributed to the already measured biometry variables) and 73% to the eye level and other factors (e.g., biometry measurements, IOL power formula, etc) [49]. Therefore, the influence of the

Table 36.4 Comparisons in axial length measurements between different biometry machines (Refs [16–43])

Axial length	IOL Master5/500	Lenstar LS 900	AL Scan	Aladdin	Pentacam AXL	IOLMaster 700	Anterion	Argos Movu	Revo NX	Tomey OA 2000
IOL Master 5/500	X	NSDM NSDM NSDM +0.08 mm	NSDM	+0.04 mm NSDM	NSDM NSDM	NSDM NSDM Staphyloma: +0.095 mm NSDM		−0.026 mm		NSDM −0.06 −0.05
Lenstar LS 900		X	NSDM	NSDM NSDM	NSDM NSDM NSDM	Short AL: NSDM Med AL: NSDM Long AL: −0.05 mm −0.01 mm −0.01 mm	0.05 mm	−0.05 mm −0.05 mm	NSDM	0.03
AL scan			X							
Alladin				X		NSDM		−0.03		
Pentacam AXL					X	−0.07 mm		NSDM		
IOLM 700						X	NSDM −0.02 mm −0.07 mm	−0.03 mm −0.08 mm	NSDM	
HE Anterion							X			
Argos Movu								X		
Revo NX									x	
Tomey 2000										X

Numbers specify the mean difference of Top Row from Left Column, NSDM: No statistically significant difference between the means of AL

Table 36.5 Comparisons in ACD measurements between different biometry machines (Refs [16–43])

ACD	IOL Master 5/500	Lenstar LS 900	AL Scan	Aladdin	Pentacam AXL	IOLMaster 700	Anterion	Argos Movu	Revo NX	Tomey OA 2000
IOL Master 5/500	X	NSDM NSDM +0.23 mm +0.13 mm	NSDM	NSDM	+0.05	−0.065 mm NSDM		−0.061 mm +0.20 mm		+0.05 mm −0.09 mm +0.01 mm
Lenstar LS 900		X	NSDM	NSDM	NSDM	−0.03 mm −0.07 mm NSDM	+0.05 mm	−0.03 mm		+0.05 mm
AL scan			X					+0.04 mm		
Alladin				X				+0.05 mm		
Pentacam AXL					X	−0.03 mm				
IOLM 700						X	+0.08 mm	NSDM +0.1 mm		
HE Anterion							X			
Argos Movu								X		
Revo NX									x	
Tomey OA2000										X

Numbers specify the mean difference of Top Row from Left Column, NSDM: No statistically significant difference between the means of ACD

Table 36.6 Comparisons in mean keratometry measurements between different biometry machines: (Refs [16–43])

Mean keratometry	IOL Master5/500	Lenstar LS 900	AL Scan	Aladdin	Pentacam AXL	IOLMaster 700	Anterion	Argos Movu	Tomey OA 2000
IOL Master 5/500	X	−0.16D −0.12D NSDM NSDM	+0.08D NSDM	+0.16D −0.09D NSDM NSDM	−0.1 D	−0.10D −0.078D NSDM		NSDM NSDM	NSDM −0.10D −0.13D
Lenstar LS 900		X	+0.11D	−0.04D NSDM	−0.19D −0.15D	NSDM −0.02D NSDM −0.11D	−0.26D	NSDM	+0.13D
AL Scan			X			−0.2D			
Alladin				X		NSDM		0.05D	
Pentacam AXL					X	+0.04D	NSDM	+0.280D	
IOLM 700						X	−0.06D NSDM NSDM −0.14D −0.37D	+0.075D +0.17D	
HE Anterion							X		
Movu								X	
Tomey OA 2000									X

Numbers specify the mean difference of Top Row from Left Column, NSDM: No statistically significant difference between the means of mean keratometry values

individual surgeon on the IOL constant is no longer such a critical factor as long as the other important factors have been taken into consideration, namely the biometry machine used and the IOL model implanted.

E. Spurious Factors Which Can Result in Incorrect IOL Constant Values
　a. The Short Vision Lane Issue

An often overlooked source of bias is the postoperative refraction. Our IOL selection is based on a target refraction for an optical correction that achieves emmetropia, i.e., a far point at infinity. Nevertheless, our vision lanes have finite dimensions. Although the standard is set at 6 m, some vision lanes can be 4 m in length or shorter. This is another source of bias, which can affect the refractive outcomes as the refractionist tests at a far point less than 6 m. It is very important to stress that short lanes would give erroneous hyperopic outcomes, and these must NOT be used to optimize IOL constants; otherwise, these incorrect IOL constants would result in patients ending up myopic on average.

If the post-op refraction data are derived from testing at a short vision lane, the refraction can easily be adjusted to a far point at 6 m by subtracting the difference in vergence between the two far points, using the formula or Table 36.7 [50].

$$\left(\text{Spherical equivalent at 6 metres}\right) = \left(\text{Spherical equivalent at } X \text{ metres}\right) + \frac{1}{6} - \frac{1}{X}$$

b. The "Home Court Advantage" Issue

Data from subjective refraction may misleadingly show improved outcomes of the IOL formula used by the surgeon. This is because of the inherent bias of subjective refraction, as the subjectiveness of this test is also derived from the part of the refractionist. Therefore, patients with

Table 36.7 Adjustment of post-op refraction spherical equivalent derived from short lane testing

Lane length	6 m	5 m	4 m	3.5 m	3 m
Correction to 6 m	N/A	= 0.17 − 0.20 = −0.03D Subtract 0.03D	= 0.17 − 0.25 = −0.08 Subtract 0.08D	= 0.17 − 0.29 = 0.12 Subtract 0.12D	= 0.17 − 0.33 = −0.15 Subtract 0.15D

low refractive errors and small pupils who may be able to see 20/20 may be labeled as having a 0.00 D refractive error. This gives a false advantage to the IOL power formula used by the surgeon, as the surgeon often chooses the IOL power giving a target refraction closest to 0, and the refractionist may label the patient as having 0 refractions, thus erroneously matching a 0 target with a 0 refraction. Over repeated cases, the IOL formula in question would have more target refractions closer to 0 compared to other formulae that were not used thus giving the formula a "home court advantage" a term coined by Dr. David Cooke of Great Lakes Eye Care, St. Joseph, Michigan. This may explain why when comparing IOL formulae calculations, the best-performing formula is often the one actually used by the surgeon for the power calculation.

Although subjective refraction is still considered by many the gold standard, this a topic often discussed among the members of the IOL power club, and some members feel that a calibrated autorefractor may be a better approach for outcome studies as it would be less prone to the subjective sources of bias discussed above. In an ideal scenario, both subjective refraction and autorefraction would be performed with the former used for any spectacle prescriptions and the later for audit purposes and IOL constant refinement.

The Methodology for Deriving IOL Constants

Data and Sample Size Requirements

The sample of eyes used for IOL constant optimisation should have undergone uncomplicated phacoemulsification with an in-the bag IOL. The capsulorrhexis size should be smaller than the optic, with no post-operative prolapse of the IOL

optic through the bag, no corneal sutures, and a post-op visual acuity of logMAR 0.2 or better (≥7/10, ≥6/9, ≥20/30 decimal) in order to achieve accurate subjective refractions. There should be no attempt to select eyes with respect to their biometric variables (i.e., the sample should contain a non-selected and non-biased distribution of axial lengths, keratometry, ACD, etc). Care must be taken not to use cases where the IOL has been implanted back-to-front. There should be no history of refractive corneal or any other ophthalmic surgery. Significant corneal pathology, such as keratoconus, pterygium, or corneal scarring, should be excluded. All postoperative subjective refractions should ideally be refined using a red/green duochrome test. Please note the issues raised regarding the length of the vision lane, if this is shorter than 6 m, an appropriate correction should be applied for that working distance. The essential/*ideal* set of data would include (1) Axial Length, (2) K1 and K2, (3) *CCT*, (4) ACD, (5) LT, (6) *Horizontal Corneal Diameter* (HCD), (7) *Gender*, (8) IOL Model, (9) IOL Power, (10) Refraction, and (11) Vision lane distance. Some IOL power formulae require post-op biometric measurements for optimization so (12) biometrically measured post-op ACD is essential for optimizing the Olsen, Castrop, and K6. Formulae using a thick lens model can require the physical characteristics of the IOL model and for some formulae, even the variation of these across the IOL power range. It is also important to note that the same biometry machine model must be used for all cases and that the IOL derived would be specific for use with that biometry machine model.

The general consensus is that 100 eyes are enough to optimize IOL constants. It is said that 250 eyes are needed for triple optimization of the Haigis formula. Figures 36.1, 36.2, 36.3, and 36.4 show the fluctuation of IOL constants (for the Hoffer Q, Holladay 1, SRK/T, Haigis) with

Fig. 36.1 ACD (Hoffer Q) and increasing sample size

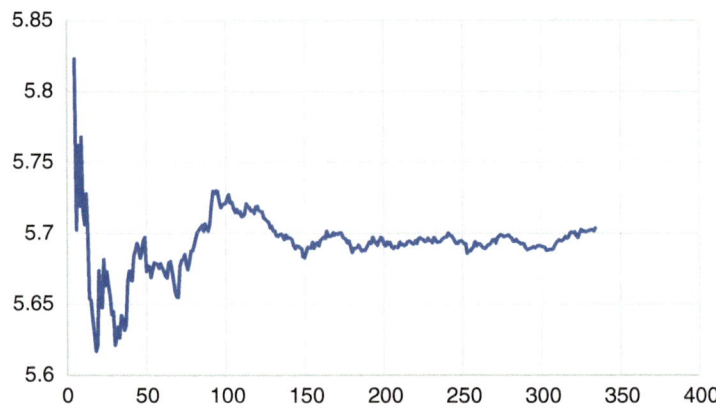

Fig. 36.2 sf (Holladay 1) and increasing sample size

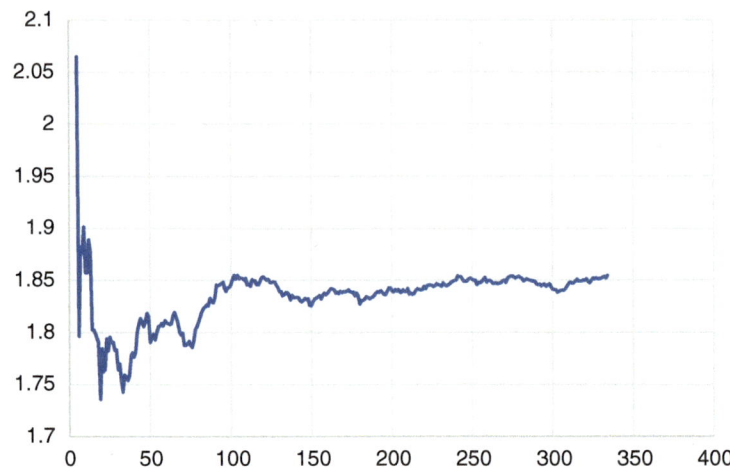

Fig. 36.3 A constant (SRK/T) and increasing sample size

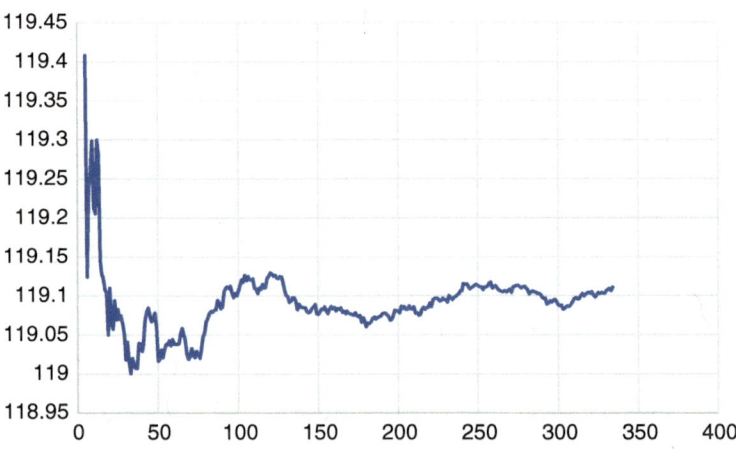

respect to an increasing sample of eyes, starting from 10 eyes up to 330 eyes. The data are from my private practice using the same IOL model, and for this process, they are analyzed in a randomized order without removing outliers from the optimization process as in reality; it is difficult to detect outliers from the outset before having a large enough sample.

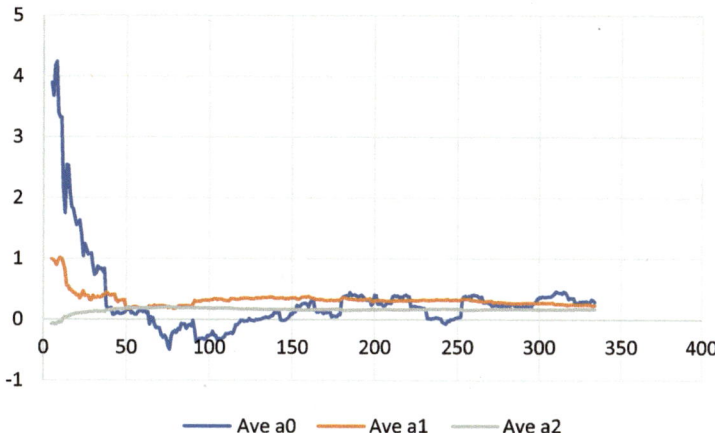

Fig. 36.4 Haigis constants (a0, a1, and a2) and increasing sample size

Previous studies on theoretical refractive outcomes suggest that for the Hoffer Q and Holladay 1, IOL constant change within ±0.05 and for the SRK/T change within ±0.10 has no significant impact on refractive outcomes [1]. Based on the above, 100 eyes should be enough to calculate IOL constants. Figure 36.4 shows the triple optimization for the Haigis may need fewer than 250 eyes. The a1 and a2 constants representing the regression coefficients (slope) for ACD and AL, respectively, are the first to stabilize, followed by the intersect (a0).

Optimization of Single-Variable IOL Power Formulae

Most IOL power formulae contain only one IOL constant. For the vast majority of single-variable formulae, the IOL constant is optimized by finding the IOL constant value for each eye in order to achieve a match between predicted refraction and post-op refraction for the IOL power used for that eye. This is repeated for all the eyes in the sample used, and the values are averaged to give the optimized IOL constant.

A. Standard Iterative Approach for Optimizing Single-Variable IOL Power Formulae

The code has been published for some IOL formulae [11, 51–53], and this can be used to perform these calculations (Please note that the orig-inal papers for the Hoffer Q, the Holladay 1, and SRK/T had typographical errors in the code, which were later corrected by published letters and errata) [54, 55]. After transcribing the code on a spreadsheet, one can use pre-op biometry measurements to calculate the IOL power for a specific refractive outcome. If surgeons choose to use this approach, they should exercise particular care to avoid any transcription errors in the formula code, which would result in incorrect calculations. Textbox 36.1 provides a calculation guide for optimizing the third generation IOL power formulae.

> **Box 36.1 Calculation Guide for Optimizing Hoffer Q, Holladay 1, SRK/T and Haigis Formulae**
> The tables below contain the code for each of the formulae Hoffer Q, Holladay 1, SRK/T and Haigis (Tables 36.8, 36.9, and 36.10). Each table represents a separate sheet in an Excel workbook (Microsoft Corporation, version 2010 or newer). Table 36.8 is to be used for third generation IOL constant optimization sheet. This sheet should be named "**Constant optimization**". Table 36.9 is for the double regression calculation for the Haigis formula optimization sheet. This sheet should be named "**Haigis optimization**". Table 36.10 is for the IOL power calculation sheet,

Table 36.8 SHEET 1: IOL Constant Optimisation Sheet [11, 44, 51–55]

Column	Row 1	Row 2
A	Case No	*Input Data (case 1,2,3,4, etc)*
B	Axial Length	*Input Data (in mm)*
C	K1	*Input Data (in D)*
D	K2	*Input Data (in D)*
E	Pre op ACD	*Input Data (in mm)*
F	Implanted IOL power	*Input Data (in D)*
G	Desired Post op SEq	*Input Data (in D)*
H	Post op Sphere	*Input Data (in D)*
I	Post Op Cylinder	*Input Data (in D)*
J	Post op Axis	*Input Data (in degrees)*
K	Post op Spherical Equivalent	=H2+(I2/2)
L	Mean K	=(C2+D2)/2
Hoffer Q Optimisation		
M	Calculated "ACD" Constant For each eye	Use the GoalSeek function in a Macro to calculate the ACD value so that the Calculated IOL power (**V**) matches the Implanted IOL power (**F**) and use the Post op RX result values (**K**) to populate the Desired Rx SE (**Q**). This will find the ACD constant for each case so that the calculated IOL power matches the IOL power used.
N	Axial length	=**B2**
O	Mean K	=**L2**
P	Vertex distance	=12 *(twelve mm is the standard vertex distance)*
Q	Post op op SE used as desired Rx	=**K2**
R	*M*	=IF(**B2**<23,1,-1)
S	*G*	=IF(**B2**<23,28,23.5)
T	Predicted ACD	=**M2**+0.3*(**N2**-23.5)+(TAN(**O2***PI()/180))^2+(0.1 ***R2***(23.5-**N2**)^2*(TAN(0.1*(**S2**-**N2**)^2*PI()/180)))-0.99166
U	Expected Rx SEq for the IOL selected	=(1.336/(1.336/(1336/(**N2**-**T2**-0.05)-**F2**)+(**T2**+0.05)/1000))-O2
V	Calculated IOL power	=(1336/(**N2**-**T2**-0.05))-(1.336/((1.336/(**O2**+**Q2**/(1-0.001***P2***Q2**)))-((**T2**+0.05)/1000)))
Holladay 1 Optimisation		
W	Calculated "SF" constant for each eye	Use the GoalSeek function in a Macro to calculate the SF value so that the Calculated IOL power (**AF2**) matches the Selected IOL power (**F2**) and use the Post op RX result values (**K2**) to populate the Desired Rx SE (**AC2**). This will find the SF constant for each case so that the calculated IOL power matches the IOL power used.
X	Axial length	=**B2**
Y	ALm	=**X2**+0.2
Z	Mean K	=**L2**
AA	R-H1	=337.5/**Z2**
AB	Vertex distance	=12 *(twelve mm is the standard vertex distance)*
AC	Post op op SE used as desired Rx	=**K2**
AD	Ag	=12.5***X2**/23.45
AE	ACD post K	=0.56+**AA2**-SQRT(**AA2**^2-**AD2**^2/4)

Table 36.8 (continued)

Column	Row 1	Row 2
AF	Calculated IOL power	=1336*(1.336***AA2**-1/3*Y2-0.001***AC2***(**AB2***(1.336***AA2**-1/3*Y2)+Y2***AA2**))/ ((Y2-**AE2**-**W2**)*(1.336***AA2**-1/3*(**AE2**+**W2**)-0.001***AC2***(**AB2***(1.336***AA2**-1/3*(**AE2**+**W2**))+(**AE2**+**W2**)***AA2**)))
AG	Expected Rx for the IOL selected	=(1336*(1.336***AA2**-(4/3-1)*Y2)-F2*(Y2-**AE2**-**W2**)*(1.336***AA2**-(4/3-1)*(**AE2**+**W2**)))/(1.336*(12*(1.336***AA2**-(4/3-1)*Y2)+Y2***AA2**)-0.001***F2***(Y2-**AE2**-**W2**)*(12*(1.336***AA2**-(4/3-1)*(**AE2**+**W2**))+(**W2**+**AE2**)***AA2**))
AH	Predicted ACD	=**W2**+**AE2**
SRK-T Optimisation		
AI	Axial Length	=**B2**
AJ	Calculated A-constant	Use the GoalSeek function in a macro to calculate the A constant value so that the calculated expected refraction (**AX2**) matches the post op refraction (**K2**). This will find the A-constant for each case so that the calculated expected refraction matches the post op refraction for the IOL power used.
AK	ACD constant	=0.62467***AJ2**-68.747
AL	Mean K	=**L2**
AM	Radius – SRK/T	=337.5/**AL2**
AN	LCOR	=IF(**AI2**>24.2,-3.446+1.716***AI2**-0.0237***AI2**^2,**AI2**)
AO	Cw	=-5.41+0.58412***AN2**+0.098***AL2**
AP	H	=**AM2**-SQRT(**AM2**^2-**AO2**^2/4)
AQ	ACD estimate	=**AP2**+**AK2**-3.336
AR	Vertex distance	=*12 (twelve mm is the standard vertex distance)*
AS	na	=1.336
AT	nc	=1.333
AU	ncm1	=0.333
AV	Retinal thickness	=0.65696-0.02029***AI2**
AW	LOPT	=**AI2**+**AV2**
AX	Expected RX for IOL selected	=(1336*(**AS2***AM2**-**AU2***AW2**)-F2*(**AW2**-**AQ2**)*(**AS2***AM2**-**AU2***AQ2**))/ (**AS2***(12*(**AS2***AM2**-**AU2***AW2**)+**AW2***AM2**)-0.001***F2***(**AW2**-**AQ2**)*(12*(**AS2***AM2**-**AU2***AQ2**)+**AQ2***AM2**))
AY	IOL for emmetropia	=(1000***AS2***(**AS2***AM2**-**AU2***AW2**))/((**AW2**-**AQ2**)*(**AS2***AM2**-**AU2***AQ2**))
Haigis Optimisation		
AZ	a0	Leave blank to populate later with the optimized a0 value – in order to ensure that the mean prediction error is 0
BA	a1	Leave blank to populate later with the optimized a1 value – In order to ensure that the mean prediction error is 0
BB	a2	Leave blank to populate later with the optimized a2 value – In order to ensure that the mean prediction error is 0
BC	Pre op ACD	=**E2**
BD	Axial length	=**B2**
BE	RC1	=((1.3375-1)/**L2**)*1000
BF	Desired Rx matched to post op Rx	=**BO2**
BG	d	Use the GoalSeek function in a macro to calculate the "d" value so that the calculated IOL power (**BM2**) matches the selected IOL power (**BP2**) *(this is the column of data used in conjunction with pre op ACD (BC) and axial length (BD) to perform double linear regression in order to calculate a0, a1 and a2)*
BH	PC	=(1331.5-1000)/**BE2**
BI	Vertex distance	=*12 (twelve mm is the standard vertex distance)*

(continued)

Table 36.8 (continued)

Column	Row 1	Row 2
BJ	Rx for VD	=BF3/(1-**BI3***0.001***BF3**)
BK	T1	=1336*(1336-**BR2***(**BD2-BG2**))
BL	T2	=1336*(**BD2-BG2**)+**BG2***(1336-**BR2***(**BD2-BG2**))
BM	Calculated IOL power	=**BK2-BL2**
BN	Z1	=1336*(1336-**BR2***(**BD2-BG2**))
BO	Z2	=1336*(**BD2-BG2**)+**BG2***(1336-**BR2***(**BD2-BG2**))
BP	Z	=**BN2/BO2**
BQ	Post op refraction	=**K2**
BR	Implanted IOL	=**F2**
DATA CHECK FOR SUCCESSFUL ITERATION AND OPTIMISED IOL CONSTANTS		
BS	PE Hoffer	=**K2-U2** **This value should be 0 in every case, if the iteration calculation was successful**
BT	PE Holladay 1	=**K2-AG2** **This value should be 0 in every case, if the iteration calculation was successful**
BU	PE SRK/T	=**K2-AX2** **This value should be 0 in every case, if the iteration calculation was successful**
BV	BLANK	
BW	Use for labels	Cell BW2: "Optimized pACD" Cell BW3: "Optimized SF" Cell BW4: "Optimized A Constant"
BX	IOL constant values	Cell BX2: =AVERAGE(**M:M**) Cell BX3: =AVERAGE(**W:W**) Cell BX4: =AVERAGE(**AJ:AJ**)

Table 36.9 SHEET 2: Double linear regression for Haigis Optimisation IOL Constant Optimisation Sheet [11, 44]

A	ACD (X_1)	copy – paste (values) column BC from sheet 1
B	Axial Length (X_2)	copy – paste (values) column BD from sheet 1
C	"d" (Y)	copy – paste (values) column BG from sheet 1
D	(X_1-avX_1) * (Y-avY)	=(A2-(AVERAGE(A:A)))*(C2-(AVERAGE(C:C))) make sure you use all the brackets as specified
F	(X_2-avX_2) * (Y-avY)	=(B2-(AVERAGE(B:B)))*(C2-(AVERAGE(C:C))) make sure you use all the brackets as specified
G	(X_1-avX_1) * (X_2-avX_2)	=(A2-(AVERAGE(A:A)))*(B2-(AVERAGE(B:B))) make sure you use all the brackets as specified
H	(X_1-avX_1)^2	=POWER((A2-(AVERAGE(A:A))),2) make sure you use all the brackets as specified
I	(X_2-avX_2)^2	=POWER((B2-(AVERAGE(B:B))),2) make sure you use all the brackets as specified
J,K	BLANK	
L	Use for labels for M values	L5: "$\sum$ (X_1-avX_1)^2 " L6: "$\sum$ (X_2-avX_2)^2" L7: etc….
M5	Cell M5 " $\sum$ (X_1-avX_1)^2 "	=sum(H:H)
M6	Cell M6 "$\sum$ (X_2-avX_2)^2 "	=sum(I:I)
M7	Cell M7 "$\sum$((X_1-avX_1) * (Y-avY))"	=sum(D:D)
M8	Cell M8 "$\sum$((X_2-avX_2) * (Y-avY))"	=sum(F:F)
M9	Cell M9 "$\sum$((X_1-avX_1) * (X_2-avX_2))"	=sum(G:G)
M10	Cell M10 "Haigis Constants"	Blank
M11	Cell M11 "a0"	=(AVERAGE(C:C))-((AVERAGE(A:A))*M12)-((Average(B:B))*M13) "the intersect on the Y axis"
M12	Cell M12 "a1"	=((M6*M7)-(M9*M8))/((M5*M6)-(M9*M9)) "the ACD coefficient"
M13	Cell M13 "a2"	=((M5*M8)-(M9*M7))/((M5*M6)-(M9*M9)) "the AL coefficient"

Table 36.10 SHEET 3: IOL Power calculations using Optimised IOL constants [11, 44, 51–55]

Column	Row 1	Row 2
Enter data		
A	Case No	*Input Data* (case 1,2,3,4, etc)
B	Axial Length	*Input Data* (in mm)
C	K1	*Input Data* (in D)
D	K2	*Input Data* (in D)
E	Pre op ACD	*Input Data* (in mm)
F	Implanted IOL power	*Input Data* (in D)
G	Desired Post op SEq	*Input Data* (in D)
H	Post op Sphere	*Input Data* (in D)
I	Post Op Cylinder	*Input Data* (in D)
J	Post op Axis	
K	Post op Spherical Equivalent	=H2+(I2/2)
L	Mean K	=(C2+D2)/2
Hoffer Q calculations with an optimised IOL constant		
M	Optimised "ACD" Constant	For every case, use the optimized ACD constant value from **Sheet 1, Cell BX2**
N	Axial Length	=**B2**
O	Mean K	=**L2**
P	Vertex Distance	=*12 (twelve mm is the standard vertex distance)*
Q	Desired Rx	=**G2**
R	*M*	=IF(**B2**<23,1,-1)
S	*G*	=IF(**B2**<23,28,23.5)
T	Predicted ACD	=**M2**+0.3*(**N2**-23.5)+(TAN(**O2***PI()/180))^2+(0.1 ***R2***(23.5-**N2**)^2*(TAN(0.1*(**S2-N2**)^2*PI()/180)))-0.99166
U	Expected Rx SEq for the IOL selected	=(1.336/(1.336/(1336/(**N2-T2**-0.05)-**F2**)+(**T2**+0.05)/1000))-O2
V	Calculated IOL Power for Desired Rx	=(1336/(**N2-T2**-0.05))-(1.336/((1.336/(**O2+Q2**/(1-0.001***P2*Q2**)))-((**T2**+0.05)/1000)))
Holladay 1 calculations with an optimised IOL constant		
W	Optimised SF constant	For every case, use the optimized SF constant value from **Sheet 1, Cell BX3**
X	Axial Length	=**B2**
Y	ALm	=**X2**+0.2
Z	Mean K	=**L2**
AA	R-H1	=337.5/**Z2**
AB	Vertex Distance	=*12 (twelve mm is the standard vertex distance)*
AC	Desired Rx	=**G2**
AD	ag	=12.5***X2**/23.45
AE	ACD post K	=0.56+**AA2**-SQRT(**AA2**^2-**AD2**^2/4)
AF	Calculated IOL Power for Desired Rx	=1336*(1.336***AA2**-1/3*Y2-0.001***AC2***(**AB2***(1.336***AA2**-1/3***Y2**)+**Y2*AA2**))/((**Y2-AE2-W2**)*(1.336***AA2**-1/3*(**AE2+W2**)-0.001***AC2***(**AB2***(1.336***AA2**-1/3*(**AE2+W2**))+(**AE2+W2**)***AA2**)))
AG	Expected Rx for the IOL selected	=(1336*(1.336***AA2**-(4/3-1)***Y2**)-**F2***(**Y2-AE2-W2**)*(1.336***AA2**-(4/3-1)*(**AE2+W2**)))/(1.336*(12*(1.336***AA2**-(4/3-1)***Y2**)+**Y2*AA2**)-0.001***F2***(**Y2-AE2-W2**)*(12*(1.336***AA2**-(4/3-1)*(**AE2+W2**))+(**W2+AE2**)***AA2**))
AH	Predicted ACD	=**W2+AE2**

(continued)

Table 36.10 (continued)

Column	Row 1	Row 2
SRK/T calculations with an optimised IOL constant		
AI	Axial Length	=B2
AJ	Optimized A-Constant	For every case, use the optimized A-Constant value from **Sheet 1, Cell BX4**
AK	ACD Constant	=0.62467***AJ2**-68.747
AL	Mean K	=L2
AM	Radius – SRK/T	=337.5/**AL2**
AN	LCOR	=IF(**AI2**>24.2,-3.446+1.716***AI2**-0.0237***AI2**^2,**AI2**)
AO	Cw	=-5.41+0.58412***AN2**+0.098***AL2**
AP	H	=**AM2**-SQRT(**AM2**^2-**AO2**^2/4)
AQ	ACD estimate	=**AP2**+**AK2**-3.336
AR	Vertex Distance	=12 (twelve mm is the standard vertex distance)
AS	na	=1.336
AT	nc	=1.333
AU	ncm1	=0.333
AV	Retinal Thickness	=0.65696-0.02029***AI2**
AW	LOPT	=**AI2**+**AV2**
AX	Expected RX for IOL selected	=(1336*(**AS2***AM2**-**AU2***AW2**)-F2*(**AW2**-**AQ2**)*(**AS2***AM2**-**AU2***AQ2**))/(**AS2***(12*(**AS2***AM2**-**AU2***AW2**)+**AW2***AM2**)-0.001***F2***(**AW2**-**AQ2**)*(12*(**AS2***AM2**-**AU2***AQ2**)+**AQ2***AM2**))
AY	IOL for Emmetropia	=(1000***AS2***(**AS2***AM2**-**AU2***AW2**))/((**AW2**-**AQ2**)*(**AS2***AM2**-**AU2***AQ2**))
Haigis calculations with an optimised IOL constants		
AZ	a0	For every case, use the optimized a0 value from Sheet 2, Cell M11
BA	a1	For every case, use the optimized a1 value from Sheet 2, Cell M12
BB	a2	For every case, use the optimized a2 value from Sheet 2, Cell M13
BC	Pre op ACD	=E2
BD	Axial Length	=B2
BE	RC1	=((1.3375-1)/**L2**)*1000
BF	Desired Rx	=G2
BG	d	=**AZ2**+**BA2***BC2**+**BB2***BD2**
BH	PC	=(1331.5-1000)/**BE2**
BI	Vertex Distance	=12 (twelve mm is the standard vertex distance)
BJ	Rx for VD	=BF3/(1-**BI3***0.001***BF3**)
BK	T1	=1336*(1336-**BR2***(**BD2**-**BG2**))
BL	T2	=1336*(**BD2**-**BG2**)+**BG2***(1336-**BR2***(**BD2**-**BG2**))
BM	Calculated IOL power	=**BK2**-**BL2**
BN	Z1	=1336*(1336-**BR2***(**BD2**-**BG2**))
BO	Z2	=1336*(**BD2**-**BG2**)+**BG2***(1336-**BR2***(**BD2**-**BG2**))
BP	Z	=**BN2**/**BO2**
BQ	Post op Refraction	=K2
BR	Implanted IOL	=F2
BS	Expected Rx with Implanted IOL	=(**BP2**-**BH2**)/(1+(**BP2**-**BH2**)*(12*0.001))
REFRACTIVE OUTCOME ANALYSIS USING OPTIMISED IOL CONSTANTS		
BT	PE Hoffer	=**K2**-**U2**
BU	PE Holladay 1	=**K2**-**AG2**
BV	PE SRK/T	=**K2**-**AX2**
BW	PE Haigis	=**K2**-**BS2**
BX	Absolute PE Hoffer	=ABS(**K2**-**U2**)

Table 36.10 (continued)

Column	Row 1	Row 2
BY	Absolute PE Holladay 1	=ABS(**K2-AG2**)
BZ	Absolute PE SRK/T	=ABS(**K2-AX2**)
CA	Absolute PE Haigis	=ABS(**K2-BS2**)
CB	Blank	
CC	Labels for CA	CC2: "Hoffer Q" CC3: "Holladay 1" CC4: "SRK/T" CC5: "Haigis"
CD	MNE Values	CD2: =Average(BT:BT) CD3: =Average(BU:BU) CD4: =Average(BV:BV) CD5: =Average(BW:BW)
CE	MAE Values	CE2: =Average(BX:BX) CE3: =Average(BY:BY) CE4: =Average(BZ:BZ) CE5: =Average(CA:CA)

Note: The average MNE values should be very close to 0 if the optimized IOL constants are correct and appropriate for this sample

using the derived IOL constants. This sheet should be named "**Calculation with opt. constants**".

For each formula, there is an optimization and a calculation section. The code is formatted to be used on an excel spreadsheet. It must be stressed that this is a research tool and it must not be used on actual calculations on patients. Also, before using the formulae to optimise constants, one should check for any transcription errors and following that, validate the outcomes against an approved IOL calculator containing the above IOL power formulae.

Each column of the table should be transposed into a row. Entries in the first column of the table are the column letters, starting with A. Entries in the second column of the table are the headers. Entries in the third column represent the formula code. Once the newly transposed first row containing the letters A, B, C is confirmed to identify with the column letters, this first row can be deleted, leaving the headers row as the first row and the code row as the second row. The code can be transferred to the rest of the rows automatically using excel. Data should then be entered for columns A to J. The other columns will automatically calculate various parts of each IOL formula on sheet 1 (Table 36.8).

The columns representing IOL constants are empty. One then uses the Goal Seek function on Microsoft Excel to calculate the IOL constant by iteration for each case so that the calculated IOL power matches the IOL power used to achieve the actual post-operative refraction. This is the IOL constant value for each case that would have resulted in the IOL power that was actually used to reach the observed refractive prediction. Please see the macro code on Table 36.11, which automates the process for any number of eyes. The macro can be activated by a button which can be designed with excel. It is worth noting that the optimization macro is coded to use a sample of 250 cases (rows 2 to 251). If you use a different number, change the last number in the code. Excel allows the insertion of buttons in each sheet, which can be linked to each macro.

First, the "clear calculations" macro should be used. Then, by running the optimization macro, the IOL constant will be calculated for each case to achieve 0 prediction error for the IOL power used. When this is done on 100 or so cases, all the IOL constants can be averaged and this represents the optimised IOL constant, which can be used in Sheet 3 for every new case, as long as the same IOL model and biometer is used.

Table 36.11 Macro codes for IOL constant optimization

Name of macro	Code
| Sheet 1:<br>"Clear Calculations" Macro | ```
Sub ClearCalculations()
Sheets("Constant optimization").Select
    Range("BH2:BH336").Select
    Selection.ClearContents
    Range("AK2:AK336").Select
    Selection.ClearContents
    Range("X2:X336").Select
    Selection.ClearContents
    Range("N2:N336").Select
    Selection.ClearContents
    Sheets("Input Data for Optimisation").Select
End Sub
``` |
| Sheet 1:<br>"Optimization" Macro | ```
Sub Optimization()
Sheets("Constant optimization").Select
    Dim k
    For k = 2 To 251
    Cells(k, "BM").GoalSeek Goal:=Cells(k, "BR"), ChangingCell:=Cells(k, "BG")
    Next k
    Dim q
    For q = 2 To 251
    Cells(q, "V").GoalSeek Goal:=Cells(q, "F"), ChangingCell:=Cells(q, "M")
    Next q
    Dim s
    For s = 2 To 251
    Cells(s, "AF").GoalSeek Goal:=Cells(s, "F"), ChangingCell:=Cells(s, "W")
    Next s
    Dim a
    For a = 2 To 251
    Cells(a, "AX").GoalSeek Goal:=Cells(a, "K"), ChangingCell:=Cells(a, "AJ")
    Next a
End Sub
``` |

Haigis Formula

The code on Table 36.9 contains the mathematical calculations which perform double regression and derive the a0 a1 and a2. For the sheet named "**Haigis optimization**", one copy pastes the values of measured pre op ACD (column E on Sheet 1), measured Axial Length (column B on sheet 1) and optimised "d" (column BG on Sheet 1). The former two are X1 and X2 respectively and "d" is Y. Sheet 2 will automatically perform double regression calculations to derive a0 (intersect), a1 (ACD coefficient) and a2 (AL coefficient). These can then populate the a0 a1 and a2 columns AZ, BA, BB on Sheet 3 "**Calculation with opt.constants**".

B. A Maths-Free Approach for Obtaining and Refining IOL Constants

When starting to use a new IOL model, it is important to find the optimized IOL constants for the biometry machine used. These can be obtained from the biometry machine representative, the IOL manufacturer, or a public database, such as the IOL Con website (iolcon.org). All surgeons carrying out cataract surgery should audit their refractive outcomes, and they should confirm that their mean prediction error is very close to 0. If this is not close to 0, one can use the mathematical approaches described above. Alternatively, for small refinements of an IOL constant, there is a very simple approach, which can be equally effective.

For the formulae Hoffer Q, Holladay 1, Barrett Universal, Holladay 2, the Olsen, and the Haigis (a0), a change of 1 unit of IOL constant translates to 1.3D of prediction change at the spectacle plane [56]. Vice versa, for every 1.0D change in mean prediction error, the IOL constant changes by 0.77 in magnitude for the Hoffer Q pACD, the Holladay 1 sf, the Barrett Surgeon Factor, the Holladay 2 ACD, the Olsen ACD, and the Haigis a0. For the "A constants" for each 1D of change in MPE, the SRKT A constant, the T2 A constant, and the Kane A constant will change by 1.25 units. Table 36.12 below summarises these changes and provides examples. The Haigis should ideally be triple optimized (i.e., modifying a0, a1, and a2 using a double regression approach as discussed later). <u>With this method, only a0 is modified, so this approach is not recommended for optimizing the Haigis formula. Please refer to the section on triple optimization of the Haigis.</u>

C. Optimizing Single-Variable Unpublished IOL Power Formulae

For many of the newer IOL power formulae, the code is not available in order to perform the mathematical approach described above. There is another approach to do that. By having access to an IOL calculator which contains the hidden formula code, one can set up a bot/macro/script to perform repeat IOL power calculations for the IOL power used and vary the IOL constant iteratively for each eye, in order to match its predicted refraction to the post of refraction. By then averaging these values for a sample of eyes, one obtains the optimized IOL constant.

Some members of the IOL power club have offered to help surgeons with optimizing their IOL constants. Dave Cooke can be contacted at dcooke@greateyecare.com. He asks for at least 100 eyes meeting the inclusion/exclusion criteria above. He can send a spreadsheet that can be filled in.

IOL Formulae Requiring a Different Approach to Optimizing Their Constant(s)

A. The Haigis Formula

The Haigis formula uses three IOL constants a0, a1, and a2. It is very important that all three constants are optimized for the IOL used [11]. Compared to the third generation IOL power formulae, the Haigis formula uses a more accurate method for predicting the effective lens position (ELP) by the use of a regression formula that takes into account the pre-op ACD and axial length when predicting the ELP. a0, a1, and a2 are the intersect and the coefficients for the ACD and AL, respectively.

$$ELP = a0 + a1 * ACD + a2 * AL$$

For the optimization, 250 eyes are used and the ELP is back-calculated for each eye to match the IOL power used for the post-op refraction. Then, by performing double linear regression using these theoretical ELPs against ACD and AC, the values for a0 as the intersect, the a1 as the ACD coefficient, and the a2 as the AL coefficient (see Textbox 1 for details on the methodology). Optimising the a1 and the a2, this corrects any systemic bias in estimating the ELP for the specific IOL, across the pre-op ACD and pre-op AL ranges.

In addition, it is important to note that for all thin-lens IOL power formulae, the calculated effective lens position is the theoretical position of an infinitesimally thin lens, which would yield the same effective power as the implanted IOL. The effective lens position is NOT the actual post-operative anterior chamber depth.

B. The Olsen Formula

The Olsen formula is a thick lens formula and has separated the constants into two categories [57]. The first category has to do with the actual dimensions and physical properties of the IOL, which are typically provided by the IOL manufacturer: the refractive index, the anterior and posterior radius of curvature of the optic, the central IOL thickness, and the spherical aberration of the IOL (SA) (the IOL thickness and radii of curvature used are the nominal values for a 21.0D IOL as provided by the manufacturer and not the specific IOL thickness for the particular IOL power to be used). The second category is the *ACD Constant*. What makes this ACD constant

Table 36.12 Guide for changing the IOL constant with respect to the mean prediction error

Mean Prediction Error (D)	−0.50	−0.40	−0.30	−0.20	−0.10	0.00	+0.10	+0.20	+0.30	+0.40	+0.50
Hoffer Q pACD Holladay 1 sf	Decrease constant by 0.39	Decrease constant by 0.31	Decrease constant by 0.23	Decrease constant by 0.15	Decrease constant by 0.08	No Change of the IOL constant	Increase constant by 0.08	Increase constant by 0.15	Increase constant by 0.23	Increase constant by 0.31	Increase constant by 0.39
Barrett UII Surgeon Factor Holladay 2 ACD Olsen ACD Haigis a0 (NOT a1, a2)											
SRK/T A constant T2 A constant Kane A constant	Decrease constant by 0.625	Decrease constant by 0.500	Decrease constant by.375	Decrease constant by 0.250	Decrease constant by 0.125	No Change of the IOL constant	Increase constant by 0.125	Increase constant by 0.250	Increase constant by 0.375	Increase constant by 0.500	Increase constant by 0.625

different from other thin lens formulae is that the *ACD constant* is related to the physical IOL location. It is the average post-op ACD for a specific IOL model, derived from actual measurements of post-op AC, from the corneal epithelium to the anterior surface of the IOL, using a biometer.

To obtain an optimized Olsen ACD value, the surgeon selects a sufficiently large sample of eyes implanted with the same IOL model in the bag. For each eye, the **actual** post-op ACD is measured using optical biometry. Then, the surgeon calculates the average post-op ACD for the entire sample, and this value is entered as the ACD constant for this specific IOL model for the Olsen formula.

When the optimized Olsen ACD value is entered, the software for the Olsen formula then calculates the constant C, which denotes the average anteroposterior position of the center of the IOL within the capsular bag after implantation.

$$\textbf{Predicted } \text{Postop ACD} = \text{Preop ACD} + C * (\text{Lens Thickness}) - \frac{\text{IOL Thickness}}{2}$$

The surgeon does not need to perform any calculations to derive the C constant, all this is done by the software once the average post-op ACD is provided for a sample of eyes.

The geometry of the optic and haptics influences the anteroposterior location of the optic inside the capsular bag, so the C Constant varies from the IOL model to the IOL model in a similar way to other IOL constants, that is 1 mm of change corresponds to 1.4D of change in refraction at the spectacle plane. As the post-op ACD and the C constant are derived from physical data and not from an iterative process, there is a chance that the mean prediction error may not be 0 following optimization. This can be further refined to 0 using the empirical approach summarised in Table 36.12.

Another advantage of the Olsen formula is that one can use the physical location of the IOL for the first eye (by measuring the post-op ACD of that eye) to improve predictions for the second eye by replacing the predicted ACD value with the post-op ACD measured in the fellow eye [58], and this measurement should preferably be performed at least 1- month post-op [59].

C. The Naeser 1 and 2 formulae

The Naeser 1 formula is a thick lens vergence formula, which was first published in 1990 and 1997 [60, 61]. It predicts the post-op IOL position (in this case, the position of the post-op posterior lens capsule) using a double regression formula with respect to pre-op AL, pre-op ACD, and an intercept, similar to the Haigis formula, but in this case, the predicted position of the posterior lens capsule corresponds to the actual physical position and not a theoretical ELP.

Then, an optimized theoretical pre-op axial length value (the theoretical ideal pre-op AL to achieve 0 prediction error) is back calculated using another regression equation with an intercept and the actual pre-op AL with its coefficient. One establishes the value of the AL coefficient and the intercept based on the number of eyes. Once the intercept and the coefficient are determined, all future pre-op axial length measurements are converted to an optimized AL value using the optimized regression formula before entering that value in the equation.

For the first version of the formula (Naeser 1), one needs the actual physical dimensions (anterior and posterior radii for each IOL power and central IOL thickness) for each IOL power across the range of powers for that IOL model. This can be obtained using the manufacturer's cutting cards, but as this is proprietary information, they can be difficult to obtain. For the second version of the formula (Naeser 2) [62], these physical characteristics may be calculated with minimal loss of prediction accuracy.

D. The K6 Formula

This is a thin-lens general vergence formula with a single A-constant that was developed using thick-lens techniques and then modified to work as a thin-lens formula. By measuring the post-op ACD in a number of eyes, one can solve the general vergence equation by back-calculating to find the total corneal power (K) using 6 variables (AL, Ks, ACD, CCT, LT, and HCD). The axial length is from a slightly modified CMAL (using slightly different refractive indices from what CMAL used) [63]. CMAL stands for Cooke's modified Axial Length, which corrects biases related to the proportion of the lens and vitreous optical path in short and long eyes as well as establishing the limit of the axial length at the RPE and not at the ILM as most formulas do. The K6 formula was developed with the Alcon

IOL system. If a markedly different IOL platform is used, some internal adjustments to the formula need to be made, in addition to using a different A-constant (personal communication with the author).

E. The Castrop Formula

This formula uses a Gaussian thick lens formula for the cornea and a thin lens vergence formula for the IOL [64]. The ELP is derived from a regression equation containing the Axial Length (AL), the central corneal thickness (CCT), the Aqueous Depth (AQD), the Mean corneal radius (R_{mean}), and the Lens Thickness (LT).

$$\textbf{ELP} = 0.61 + 0.049 * AL + 0.000729 * CCT + 0.680 * AQD - 0.123 * R_{mean} + \textbf{\textit{C}} * LT$$

For eyes with a pathological cornea or previous refractive surgery, the ELP can be estimated by omitting the mean corneal radius and using

the formula below. In post-refractive eyes, the IOL power calculation needs true corneal power measurements.

$$\textbf{ELP} = -0.09 + 0.037 * AL + 0.000602 * CCT + 0.715 * AQD + C * LT$$

The original version of the formula contains two constants; one called C, which relates to the IOL model, and another called R used for offsetting other systematic errors derived from IOL optic asphericity or offsets related to the biometry method, etc. A new 3-constant version keeps

the C constant as it is but divides the other constant into an "H" offset related to the biometry machine and an "R" related to refractive components (such as the amount of spherical aberration of the IOL), which cannot be dealt with Gaussian optics (personal communication with the author).

$$\textbf{ELP} = 0.045 * AL + 0.761 * ACD - 0.042 * \bar{r}_{ant} + \textbf{\textit{C}} * LT + \textbf{\textit{H}}$$

The Castrop constants should be optimized using post-op refractions and iterative calculations.

Conclusions

When performing IOL power calculations, the optimized IOL constants used should be specific to (1) the model of the IOL to be implanted and (2) the biometry machine that was used. The starting values of these IOL constants should be provided by the biometry machine manufacturers via their representatives. Further optimizing the IOL constant for the individual surgeon is not

expected to offer additional benefits for most surgeons' outcomes.

All cataract surgeons should audit their refractive outcomes to ensure that both their mean prediction error is 0 and their precision is within current standards. For the few surgeons who have an average prediction error significantly different from 0D, the IOL constant can be refined further to achieve a 0 mean prediction error. An important caveat to consider is that when using vision lanes shorter than 6 m for subjective refraction, the post-op refractive outcomes need adjusting to a far point of 6 m before they are used to guide IOL constant optimization.

The impact of using optimized IOL constants on refractive outcomes is often more significant compared to the small differences in outcomes between modern IOL power formulae.

Acknowledgments I thank Dr. Giacomo Savvini for providing the formula code for the Hoffer Q Holladay 1, SRK/T, and Haigis on MS Excel, Dr. Jaime Aramberri, and Dr. David Cooke for performing additional optimization calculations for unpublished IOL power formulae.

References

1. Aristodemou P, Knox Cartwright NE, Sparrow JM, Johnston RL. Intraocular lens formula constant optimization and partial coherence interferometry biometry: refractive outcomes in 8108 eyes after cataract surgery. J Cataract Refract Surg. 2011 Jan;37(1):50–62. https://doi.org/10.1016/j.jcrs.2010.07.037.
2. Dubey R, Birchall W, Grigg J. Improved refractive outcome for ciliary sulcus-implanted intraocular lenses. Ophthalmology. 2012 Feb;119(2):261–5. https://doi.org/10.1016/j.ophtha.2011.07.050.
3. Knox Cartwright NE, Aristodemou P, Sparrow JM, Johnston RL. Adjustment of intraocular lens power for sulcus implantation. JCRS. 2011;37(4):798–9.
4. Eom Y, Song JS, Kim HM. Modified Haigis formula effective lens position equation for ciliary sulcus-implanted intraocular lenses. Am J Ophthalmol. 2016 Jan;161:142–49.e1-2. https://doi.org/10.1016/j.ajo.2015.09.040.
5. Eom Y, Hwang HS, Hwang JY, Song JS, Kim HM. Posterior vault distance of ciliary sulcus-implanted three-piece intraocular lenses according to ciliary sulcus diameter. Am J Ophthalmol. 2017 Mar;175:52–9. https://doi.org/10.1016/j.ajo.2016.11.015.
6. Millar ER, Allen D, Steel DH. Effect of anterior capsulorhexis optic capture of a sulcus-fixated intraocular lens on refractive outcomes. J Cataract Refract Surg. 2013 Jun;39(6):841–4. https://doi.org/10.1016/j.jcrs.2012.12.034.
7. McMillin J, Wang L, Wang MY, Al-Mohtaseb Z, Khandelwal S, Weikert M, Hamill MB. Accuracy of intraocular lens calculation formulas for flanged intrascleral intraocular lens fixation with double-needle technique. J Cataract Refract Surg. 2020 Dec 9. https://doi.org/10.1097/j.jcrs.0000000000000540.
8. Randerson EL, Bogaard JD, Koenig LR, Hwang ES, Warren CC, Koenig SB. Clinical outcomes and lens constant optimization of the Zeiss CT Lucia 602 lens using a modified Yamane technique. Clin Ophthalmol. 2020 Nov 17;14:3903–12. https://doi.org/10.2147/OPTH.S281505.
9. Norrby S. Sources of error in intraocular lens power calculation. J Cataract Refract Surg. 2008 Mar;34(3):368–76.   https://doi.org/10.1016/j.jcrs.2007.10.031.
10. Tehrani M, Krummenauer F, Kumar R, Dick HB. Comparison of biometric measurements using partial coherence interferometry and applanation ultrasound. J Cataract Refract Surg. 2003 Apr;29(4):747–52. https://doi.org/10.1016/s0886-3350(02)01739-x.
11. Haigis W, Lege B, Miller N, Schneider B. Comparison of immersion ultrasound biometry and partial coherence interferometry for intraocular lens calculation according to Haigis. Graefes Arch Clin Exp Ophthalmol. 2000 Sep;238(9):765–73. https://doi.org/10.1007/s004170000188.
12. Hoffer KJ, Shammas HJ, Savini G. Comparison of 2 laser instruments for measuring axial length. J Cataract Refract Surg. 2010 Apr;36(4):644–648. https://doi.org/10.1016/j.jcrs.2009.11.007.   Erratum in: J Cataract Refract Surg. 2010 Jun;36(6):1066.
13. Rabsilber TM, Jepsen C, Auffarth GU, Holzer MP. Intraocular lens power calculation: clinical comparison of 2 optical biometry devices. J Cataract Refract Surg. 2010 Feb;36(2):230–4. https://doi.org/10.1016/j.jcrs.2009.09.016.
14. Huang J, Chen H, Li Y, Chen Z, Gao R, Yu J, Zhao Y, Lu W, McAlinden C, Wang Q. Comprehensive comparison of axial length measurement with three swept-source OCT-based biometers and partial coherence interferometry. J Refract Surg. 2019 Feb 1;35(2):115–20. https://doi.org/10.3928/1081597X-20190109-01.
15. Cooke DL, Cooke TL, Suheimat M, Atchison DA. Standardizing sum-of-segments axial length using refractive index models. Biomed Opt Express. 2020 Sep 25;11(10):5860–70. https://doi.org/10.1364/BOE.400471.
16. Kanclerz P, Hoffer KJ, Przewłócka K, Savini G. Comparison of the upgraded Revo NX with the IOLMaster 700 and the Lenstar. J Cataract Refract Surg 2020 Dec 14. https://doi.org/10.1097/j.jcrs.0000000000000541.
17. Li J, Chen H, Savini G, Lu W, Yu X, Bao F, Wang Q, Huang J. Measurement agreement between a new biometer based on partial coherence interferometry and a validated biometer based on optical low-coherence reflectometry. J Cataract Refract Surg. 2016 Jan;42(1):68–75. https://doi.org/10.1016/j.jcrs.2015.05.042.
18. Yang JY, Kim HK, Kim SS. Axial length measurements: comparison of a new swept-source optical coherence tomography-based biometer and partial coherence interferometry in myopia. J Cataract Refract Surg. 2017 Mar;43(3):328–32. https://doi.org/10.1016/j.jcrs.2016.12.023.
19. Yang CM, Lim DH, Kim HJ, Chung TY. Comparison of two swept-source optical coherence tomography biometers and a partial coherence interferometer. PLoS One. 2019 Oct 11;14(10):e0223114. https://doi.org/10.1371/journal.pone.0223114.
20. Tañá-Rivero P, Aguilar-Córcoles S, Tello-Elordi C, Pastor-Pascual F, Montés-Micó R. Agreement between two swept-source OCT biometers and a Scheimpflug partial coherence interferometer. J Cataract Refract Surg. 2020 Nov 23. https://doi.org/10.1097/j.jcrs.0000000000000483.

21. Oh R, Oh JY, Choi HJ, Kim MK, Yoon CH. Comparison of ocular biometric measurements in patients with cataract using three swept-source optical coherence tomography devices. BMC Ophthalmol. 2021 Jan 27;21(1):62. https://doi.org/10.1186/s12886-021-01826-5.

22. Fişuş AD, Hirnschall ND, Findl O. Comparison of two swept-source optical coherence tomography-based biometry devices. J Cataract Refract Surg. 2020 Aug 5. https://doi.org/10.1097/j.jcrs.0000000000000373.

23. Haddad JS, Barnwell E, Rocha KM, Ambrosio R Jr, Waring Iv GO. Comparison of biometry measurements using standard partial coherence interferometry versus new Scheimpflug tomography with integrated axial length capability. Clin Ophthalmol. 2020 Feb 4;14:353–8. https://doi.org/10.2147/OPTH.S238112.

24. Ortiz A, Galvis V, Tello A, Viaña V, Corrales MI, Ochoa M, Rodriguez CJ. Comparison of three optical biometers: IOLMaster 500, Lenstar LS 900 and Aladdin. Int Ophthalmol. 2019 Aug;39(8):1809–18. https://doi.org/10.1007/s10792-018-1006-z.

25. Huang J, McAlinden C, Huang Y, Wen D, Savini G, Tu R, Wang Q. Meta-analysis of optical low-coherence reflectometry versus partial coherence interferometry biometry. Sci Rep. 2017 Feb 24;7:43414. https://doi.org/10.1038/srep43414.

26. Shetty N, Kaweri L, Koshy A, Shetty R, Nuijts RMMA, Roy AS. Repeatability of biometry measured by IOLMaster 700, Lenstar LS 900 and Anterion, and its impact on predicted intraocular lens power. J Cataract Refract Surg. 2020 Nov 23. https://doi.org/10.1097/j.jcrs.0000000000000494.

27. Savini G, Taroni L, Schiano-Lomoriello D, Hoffer KJ. Repeatability of total Keratometry and standard Keratometry by the IOLMaster 700 and comparison to total corneal astigmatism by Scheimpflug imaging. Eye (Lond). 2021 Jan;35(1):307–15. https://doi.org/10.1038/s41433-020-01245-8.

28. Calvo-Sanz JA, Portero-Benito A, Arias-Puente A. Efficiency and measurements agreement between swept-source OCT and low-coherence interferometry biometry systems. Graefes Arch Clin Exp Ophthalmol. 2018 Mar;256(3):559–66. https://doi.org/10.1007/s00417-018-3909-9.

29. Pereira JMM, Neves A, Alfaiate P, Santos M, Aragão H, Sousa JC. Lenstar® LS 900 vs Pentacam®-AXL: comparative study of ocular biometric measurements and intraocular lens power calculation. Eur J Ophthalmol. 2018 Nov;28(6):645–51. https://doi.org/10.1177/1120672118771844.

30. Ruiz-Mesa R, Abengózar-Vela A, Ruiz-Santos M. Comparison of a new Scheimpflug imaging combined with partial coherence interferometry biometer and a low-coherence reflectometry biometer. J Cataract Refract Surg. 2017 Nov;43(11):1406–12. https://doi.org/10.1016/j.jcrs.2017.08.016.

31. Tu R, Yu J, Savini G, Ye J, Ning R, Xiong J, Chen S, Huang J. Agreement between two optical biometers based on large coherence length SS-OCT and Scheimpflug imaging/partial coherence interferometry. J Refract Surg. 2020 Jul 1;36(7):459–65. https://doi.org/10.3928/1081597X-20200420-02.

32. Srivannaboon S, Chirapapaisan C, Chonpimai P, Loket S. Clinical comparison of a new swept-source optical coherence tomography-based optical biometer and a time-domain optical coherence tomography-based optical biometer. J Cataract Refract Surg. 2015 Oct;41(10):2224–32. https://doi.org/10.1016/j.jcrs.2015.03.019.

33. Hoffer KJ, Hoffmann PC, Savini G. Comparison of a new optical biometer using swept-source optical coherence tomography and a biometer using optical low-coherence reflectometry. J Cataract Refract Surg. 2016 Aug;42(8):1165–72. https://doi.org/10.1016/j.jcrs.2016.07.013.

34. Cheng H, Li J, Cheng B, Wu M. Refractive predictability using two optical biometers and refraction types for intraocular lens power calculation in cataract surgery. Int Ophthalmol. 2020 Jul;40(7):1849–56. https://doi.org/10.1007/s10792-020-01355-y.

35. Rohrer K, Frueh BE, Wälti R, Clemetson IA, Tappeiner C, Goldblum D. Comparison and evaluation of ocular biometry using a new noncontact optical low-coherence reflectometer. Ophthalmology. 2009 Nov;116(11):2087–92. https://doi.org/10.1016/j.ophtha.2009.04.019.

36. Omoto MK, Torii H, Masui S, Ayaki M, Tsubota K, Negishi K. Ocular biometry and refractive outcomes using two swept-source optical coherence tomography-based biometers with segmental or equivalent refractive indices. Sci Rep. 2019 Apr 25;9(1):6557. https://doi.org/10.1038/s41598-019-42968-3. Erratum in: Sci Rep. 2020 Jul 31;10(1):13181.

37. Shammas HJ, Ortiz S, Shammas MC, Kim SH, Chong C. Biometry measurements using a new large-coherence-length swept-source optical coherence tomographer. J Cataract Refract Surg. 2016 Jan;42(1):50–61. https://doi.org/10.1016/j.jcrs.2015.07.042.

38. Huang J, Savini G, Li J, Lu W, Wu F, Wang J, Li Y, Feng Y, Wang Q. Evaluation of a new optical biometry device for measurements of ocular components and its comparison with IOLMaster. Br J Ophthalmol. 2014 Sep;98(9):1277–81. https://doi.org/10.1136/bjophthalmol-2014-305150.

39. Nemeth G, Modis L Jr. Ocular measurements of a swept-source biometer: repeatability data and comparison with an optical low-coherence interferometry biometer. J Cataract Refract Surg. 2019 Jun;45(6):789–97. https://doi.org/10.1016/j.jcrs.2018.12.018.

40. Mandal P, Berrow EJ, Naroo SA, Wolffsohn JS, Uthoff D, Holland D, Shah S. Validity and repeatability of the Aladdin ocular biometer. Br J Ophthalmol.

2014 Feb;98(2):256–8. https://doi.org/10.1136/bjophthalmol-2013-304002. Erratum in: Br J Ophthalmol. 2015 Dec;99(12):1746.

41. Reitblat O, Levy A, Kleinmann G, Assia EI. Accuracy of intraocular lens power calculation using three optical biometry measurement devices: the OA-2000, Lenstar-LS900 and IOLMaster-500. Eye (Lond). 2018 Jul;32(7):1244–52. https://doi.org/10.1038/s41433-018-0063-x.

42. Kongsap P. Comparison of a new optical biometer and a standard biometer in cataract patients. Eye Vis (Lond). 2016 Oct 17;3:27. https://doi.org/10.1186/s40662-016-0059-1.

43. Hua Y, Qiu W, Xiao Q, Wu Q. Precision (repeatability and reproducibility) of ocular parameters obtained by the Tomey OA-2000 biometer compared to the IOLMaster in healthy eyes. PLoS One. 2018 Feb 27;13(2):e0193023. https://doi.org/10.1371/journal.pone.0193023.

44. Haigis W. Matrix-optical representation of currently used intraocular lens power formulas. J Refract Surg. 2009 Feb;25(2):229–34. https://doi.org/10.3928/1081597X-20090201-09.

45. Holladay JT. Standardizing constants for ultrasonic biometry, keratometry, and intraocular lens power calculations. J Cataract Refract Surg. 1997 Nov;23(9):1356–70. https://doi.org/10.1016/s0886-3350(97)80115-0.

46. Bucher PJ. Anterior chamber depth with sulcus and capsular bag placed IOGEL lenses. J Cataract Refract Surg. 1990 Nov;16(6):737–40. https://doi.org/10.1016/s0886-3350(13)81017-6.

47. Gimbel HV. Evolving techniques of cataract surgery: continuous curvilinear Capsulorhexis, down-slope sculpting, and nucleofractis. Semin Ophthalmol. 1992 Dec;7(4):193–207. https://doi.org/10.3109/08820539209065108.

48. Armstrong TA. Refractive effect of capsular bag lens placement with the capsulorhexis technique. J Cataract Refract Surg. 1992 Mar;18(2):121–4. https://doi.org/10.1016/s0886-3350(13)80916-9.

49. Hughes RA, Aristodemou P, Sparrow JM, Kaye S. Multilevel multivariate modelling of the effect of gender and patient co-morbidity on spherocylindrical refractive outcome following cataract surgery – submitted for publication late 2020 – scientific reports.

50. Simpson MJ, Charman WN. The effect of testing distance on intraocular lens power calculation. J Refract Surg. 2014 Nov;30(11):726. https://doi.org/10.3928/1081597X-20141021-01.

51. Hoffer KJ. The Hoffer Q formula: A comparison of theoretic and regression formulas. J Cataract Refract Surg. 1993;19(11):700–12. Errata: 1994;20(6):677 and 2007;33(1):2–3

52. Holladay JT, Prager TC, Chandler TY, Musgrove KH, Lewis JW, Ruiz RS. A three-part system for refining intraocular lens power calculations. J Cataract Refract Surg. 1988 Jan;14(1):17–24. https://doi.org/10.1016/s0886-3350(88)80059-2.

53. Retzlaff JA, Sanders DR, Kraff MC. Development of the SRK/T intraocular lens implant power calculation formula. J Cataract Refract Surg. 1990;16:333–40. Errata: 1990;16:528 and 1993;19(5):444–446

54. Hoffer KJ. Errata in printed Hoffer Q formula. J Cataract Refract Surg. 2007;33:2–3.

55. Retzlaff JA, Sanders DR, Kraff MC. Erratum in. J Cataract Refract Surg. 1990 Jul;16(4):528.

56. Cooke DL, Cooke TL. Effect of altering lens constants. J Cataract Refract Surg. 2017 Jun;43(6):853. https://doi.org/10.1016/j.jcrs.2017.05.001.

57. Olsen T. Calculation of intraocular lens power: a review. Acta Ophthalmol Scand. 2007 Aug;85(5):472–85. https://doi.org/10.1111/j.1600-0420.2007.00879.x.

58. Olsen T. Use of fellow eye data in the calculation of intraocular lens power for the second eye. Ophthalmology. 2011 Sep;118(9):1710–5. https://doi.org/10.1016/j.ophtha.2011.04.030.

59. Muthappan V, Paskowitz D, Kazimierczak A, Jun AS, Ladas J, Kuo IC. Measurement and use of postoperative anterior chamber depth of fellow eye in refractive outcomes. J Cataract Refract Surg. 2015 Apr;41(4):778–84. https://doi.org/10.1016/j.jcrs.2014.08.034.

60. Naeser K, Boberg-Ans J, Bargum R. Biometry of the posterior lens capsule: a new method to predict pseudophakic anterior chamber depth. J Cataract Refract Surg. 1990 Mar;16(2):202–6. https://doi.org/10.1016/s0886-3350(13)80731-6.

61. Naeser K. Intraocular lens power formula based on vergence calculation and lens design. J Cataract Refract Surg. 1997 Oct;23(8):1200–7. https://doi.org/10.1016/s0886-3350(97)80316-1.

62. Næser K, Savini G. Accuracy of thick-lens intraocular lens power calculation based on cutting-card or calculated data for lens architecture. J Cataract Refract Surg. 2019 Oct;45(10):1422–9. https://doi.org/10.1016/j.jcrs.2019.05.021.

63. Cooke DL, Cooke TL. Approximating sum-of-segments axial length from a traditional optical low-coherence reflectometry measurement. J Cataract Refract Surg. 2019 Mar;45(3):351–4. https://doi.org/10.1016/j.jcrs.2018.12.026.

64. Wendelstein J, Hoffmann P, Hirnschall N, Fischinger IR, Mariacher S, Wingert T, Langenbucher A, Bolz M. Project hyperopic power prediction: accuracy of 13 different concepts for intraocular lens calculation in short eyes. Br J Ophthalmol. 2021 Jan 27. https://doi.org/10.1136/bjophthalmol-2020-318272.

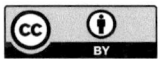

Graham D. Barrett

The search for improvements for more accurate methods to improve refractive outcomes began after Harold Ridley's implantation of the first intraocular lens implant (IOL) in 1949 [1]. There were many aspects of Ridley's intraocular lens that were appropriate, including the choice of polymethylmethacrylate (PMMA) as a lens material, placement in the posterior chamber, and even the method of storage with 10% sodium hydroxide for sterilization neutralized prior to implantation. The post-op refraction, however, was $-24.00/+6.00 \times 30^0$ as the calculation of the required IOL power based on the curvature of the implant did not fully consider the refractive index of the IOL and needed significant refinement.

Biometry at this stage was also rudimentary. The corneal curvature could be measured by keratometers based on the Javal–Schiotz keratometer introduced in 1880 [2], but measurement of the axial length (AL) by A scan ultrasound was only introduced commercially in 1970 (Kretztechnik AG) [3]. Optical biometry greatly enhanced the ability to measure AL with greater precision with partial coherence interferometry (PCI) available with the first IOLMaster introduced in 1999 [4].

Automated keratometers based on LEDs were integrated with optical biometers so that the measurement of corneal curvature was now less dependent on the skill of the user and more repeatable. Optical biometers based on swept-source ocular coherence tomography (SS-OCT) [5] such as the IOLMaster 700 introduced in 2014 further improved the accuracy of AL measurements with a reduction in the standard deviation from 25μm to 8 μm. Modern biometers can measure additional parameters such as central corneal thickness (CCT), lens thickness (LT), and corneal diameter (CD) measurements of the corneal limbus more accurately, in addition to the anterior chamber depth (ACD), available with earlier technology.

Improvements in technology have played a key role, but equally important to refractive outcomes, are the formulas required to predict the required IOL for individual patients with the available information from modern biometers.

It was not common in the early decades of IOL implantation to use a standard IOL power, e.g., 18.0 D, or adjust this power by adding the preop refraction multiplied by a factor of 1.25D. The first formula was derived by Fyodorov [6] in 1967 based on Gaussian optics/vergence calculation and was followed by formulas developed by CD Binkhorst (1972) [7], Colenbrander (1973) [8], Hoffer (1974, publ 1981) [9], Thijssen (1975) [10], Van der Heijde (1975) [11], and the regression-based SRK (1981) [12], which introduced the A-constant. These are considered first-generation formulas where the calculated ACD in

G. D. Barrett (✉)
Lions Eye Institute, Sir Charles Gairdner Hospital, University of Western Australia, Perth, WA, Australia
e-mail: graham.barrett@uwa.edu.au

© The Author(s) 2024
J. Aramberri et al. (eds.), *Intraocular Lens Calculations*, Essentials in Ophthalmology,
https://doi.org/10.1007/978-3-031-50666-6_37

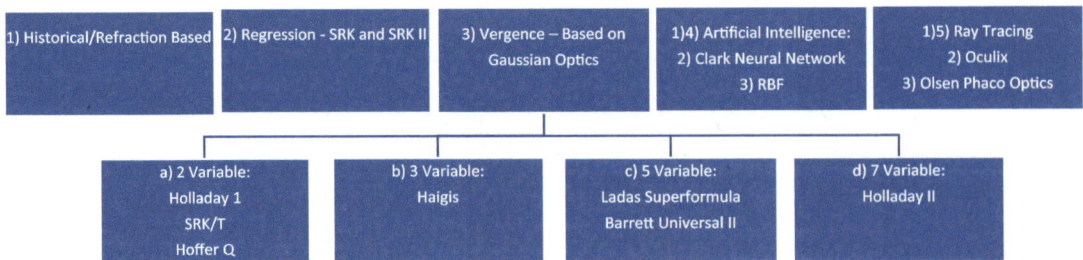

Fig. 37.1 Chart to display the classification of formulas based on the method of prediction

the vergence calculation was not adjusted by any other parameter.

Second-generation formulas were introduced by Hoffer (1982) using the AL to predict the ACD, which was soon followed by R Binkhorst and the SRK II [13] formula. Soon these were followed by the third-generation theoretical formulas using the Al and the K for ACD prediction; the Hoffer Q [14] (1993), Holladay I [15] (1988), and SRK/T [16] (1990).

These formulas were the mainstay of formula prediction for about 25 years until recently when fourth-generation formulas that considered additional parameters such as pre-op ACD and LT were introduced including Barrett Universal (1987) [17, 18], Olsen (1987) [19], Haigis (1990) [20], and Holladay II (1996) [21].

More recent formulas could be considered fifth-generation formulas as they incorporate additional calculation methods including ray tracing and artificial intelligence. These included formulas such as Okulix (2005) [22], Barrett Universal II (2014) [23], Olsen C (2014) [24], Evo (2016), Hill RBF (2016) [25], Pearl DGS (2020) [26], Kane (2019) [27], and Hoffer QST (2020) [28]. The latter list is not exhaustive, and many new formulas have been published in recent years.

Classifying formulas into generations is always controversial as the distinction is somewhat arbitrary, and the date of introduction and grouping is not always sequential. A more logical classification was suggested by an editorial in the *Journal of Cataract and Refractive Surgery* in June 2017 based on the method of prediction [29]. The formulas classified according to the method of prediction are displayed in a chart in Fig. 37.1.

Unfortunately, even this classification has limitations as formulae based on vergence calculations or even ray tracing require a data-driven element to refine the effective lens position (ELP). This component can incorporate artificial intelligence as a strategy to refine the ELP and are therefore, hybrid in nature.

Furthermore, a formula, such as Barrett Universal II, which is a theoretical formula incorporating paraxial ray tracing for the cornea and IOL, uses third-order polynomial regression to refine data-driven refinement of the ELP. The essence of AI whether based on neural networks or similar algorithms relies on the ability of computers to recognize patterns or dependencies, which are not always evident to the individual observer. Some authorities, however, believe that the outcome of AI analysis of large datasets is not distinctive from this statistical method using smaller datasets [30].

Barrett Universal II (BUII)

The reason that the Barrett Universal formula is based on paraxial ray tracing is that this allows the input of custom parameters for refractive index and radii of curvature. This allowed me to calculate the required IOL power for the hydrophilic acrylic IOL I first implanted in August 1983, which was a one-piece foldable lens with an asymmetrical optic and different radii of curvature to conventional PMMA IOLs available at the time [31]. The prediction of the lens position is based on a theoretical model eye I conceived where the ciliary plane is determined as the intersection of an anterior sphere—related to the radius of the cornea—and a posterior sphere—related to the radius of the globe. The lens factor (LF) is the lens constant that indicates the distance from the ciliary plane to the location of the IOL and varies with the lens model characteristics. A relationship between the LF and an equivalent a constant was derived as surgeons are more familiar with the latter value for different IOLs. The radius of the globe (RG) is a difficult parameter to measure, and initially, this was determined empirically and later from actual clinical data using polynomial regression in BUII.

The Barrett Universal II is the core of the Barrett toric calculator [32–34], which incorporates a theoretical model to explain the observed behavior of the posterior cornea based on the ellipticity of the corneal limbus. As such, it differs from a population-based method to derive the posterior cornea, and a unique posterior cornea is calculated for each eye according to the measured parameters.

Similarly, the Barrett True K is based on the BUII with an additional theoretical model to account for the disrupted relationship of the anterior and posterior cornea in eyes that had undergone myopic [35] or hyperopic [36] refractive surgery including RK [37]. Keratoconus is another example where the relationship of the posterior and anterior radii is altered, and more recently, a solution for this condition has been added to the online True K available at apacrs.org [38].

A formula based on paraxial ray tracing treats the IOL as a thick lens, unlike many formulas where the optic is regarded as a thin lens. The BUII calculates the first and second principal planes for the predicted IOL power for an individual eye, which requires relatively complex calculations and iterative solutions. Traditional formulas can typically be condensed to a single line in a spreadsheet, but the BUII requires 750 lines of code in its simplest form and up to 3000 lines of code in the more complex formulas incorporating toric and post-refractive predictions.

Several published studies have compared the BUII to other formulas, and it has been shown to perform well and be equivalent to other top-ranking formulas [39, 40] when targeting emmetropia as well as ametropia in the context of modest monovision [41].

Future strategies to improve IOL power prediction that is worthy of consideration include modifications to biometry, measurements, and the inclusion of additional parameters with existing formulas.

Classical vs. Segmental AL

Traditional pathways to improve ELP power prediction include collecting large datasets and different methods of interpreting the relationship within them. In addition, using the outcome of the first eye undergoing cataract surgery has also proved helpful in refining the outcome of the second eye undergoing cataract surgery [42].

Recent papers have demonstrated that using different refractive indices for each ocular segment as opposed to using a single refractive index can improve the accuracy of traditional formulas such as Holladay 1 or SRK/T. Traditional formulas tend to have a myopic prediction error for short eyes and a hyperopic prediction error for long eyes [43, 44]..

An optical biometer provides an optical path length (OPL) which needs to be transformed into a geometrical path length (GPL) for use in formulas. The average refractive index was derived from the refractive indices of the different segments and then weighted in proportion to the segmented ALs in the Gullstrand model eye.

$$GPL = OPL / 1.3549$$

The Classical Axial Length (CAL), as listed in the Partial Coherence Interferometer (PCI) IOLMaster, is adjusted from the GPL calculated with the group refractive index such that it remains compatible with immersion ultrasound.

$$CAL = GPL - 1.3033 / 0.957$$

The measured optical path length was transformed by Haigis [45] by the regression equation to be compatible with the AL measured by immersion ultrasound. As the latter is in essence a segmental calculation, the derived geometrical path length (Classical Axial Length) can also be regarded as segmental in nature despite using a group refractive index to measure the optical path length.

The Segmented Axial Length (SAL) is the sum of the GPL of the individual segments calculated using their respective refractive indices:

$$SAL = CCT_{GPL} + AQD_{GPL} + LT_{GPL} + VD_{GPL}$$

Where CCT = Central Corneal Thickness, AQD = Aqueous Depth, LT = Lens Thickness, and VD = Vitreous Depth.

A geometrical path length whether derived from optical biometry in the fashion described above by Haigis for the original IOLMaster and subsequent biometers (CAL), or by considering the individual refractive indices (SAL), relies on assumptions. An empirical adjustment will be impacted by the nature of the original dataset used for this purpose, and the individual refractive indices of the media are assumed values and may vary with the density of a cataract as well as the wavelength of a biometer. Despite these limitations, however, it appears logical for a formula to be optimized according to the method used to derive the AL from the measured optical path length.

The Argos biometer uses segmented AL. Arthur Cummings (Dublin, Ireland) collected a dataset with AL measured by the Lenstar (CAL) and the Argos Biometer (SAL). Using these data, I determined a linear relationship between the two methods of AL measurement:

$$AL_{SAL} = AL_{CAL}{}^{*}0.96 - LT^{*}0.014 + 1.04$$

This is similar but not identical to the modified AL determined by Cooke—CMAL.

$$CMAL = 1.23853 + 0.95855^{*} Traditional\,AL - 0.05467^{*} LT$$

The refractive indices used by the Lenstar are not identical to those utilized by the Argos device, which could explain the differences. Unlike the Lenstar, the Argos biometer uses Gullstrand refractive indices, developed for white light (~550 nm), and does not scale the refractive indices to the wavelength of the instrument (1060 nm).

The AL calculated using a global refractive index (CAL) is similar to that calculated with segmental AL (SAL) for average eyes but tends to be longer for short eyes and shorter for long eyes [32].

I used the regression formula I derived from Arthur Cummings' data to transform the AL measured by the Lenstar in a series of 5000 eyes to compare the prediction accuracy using CAL or SAL with Holladay 1 representing traditional formulas and BUII. The lens constant was first optimized for both formulas such that the mean error (ME) was zero.

CAL vs. SAL Holladay 1

The MAE for Holladay 1 using CAL was 0.37, and MedAE was 0.287. The percentage of cases predicted within ±0.50 D was 74.8%.

A trend line in a scatter plot graph of the prediction error versus AL showed a left-leaning downward slope with a myopic prediction error for short eyes and a hyperopic error for long eyes.

Using SAL, the MAE and MedAE reduced to 0.35 and 0.276, respectively, and the prediction error within ±0.50 D improved to 75.9%. The trend line in the scatter plot graph of prediction error versus AL was now quite flat.

CAL vs. SAL BUII

The MAE for BUII using CAL was 0.32, and MedAE was 0.25. The percentage of cases predicted within ±0.50 D was 80.2%.

A trend line in a scatter plot graph of the prediction error versus AL showed a relatively flat curve. Using SAL, the MAE was not altered (remaining 0.32) but the MedAE increased slightly to 0.26. The prediction error within ±0.50 D declined to 78.9%. The trend line in the scatter plot graph of prediction error versus AL sloped downward to the right indicating a trend to hyperopic outcomes for short eyes and myopic outcomes for long eyes.

The comparison confirmed, the previously published data by Cooke et al. and Li Wang et al., that while the use of SAL improved the prediction error and removed AL prediction bias for traditional formulas, it actually diminished the prediction accuracy for more modern formulas such as BUII and Olsen This is because the modern formula that performs well has been optimized for CAL and the algorithms correct for AL bias.

This poses a quandary for a surgeon's selection of formulas when using a biometer such as Argos, which utilizes SAL. I, therefore, derived a version of BUII optimized for this Sum of Segments method.

The EyeSuite software on the Lenstar OLCR machine has research export file capabilities, which can provide the optical path length for the segments as an "air" value. The formula was derived from 17,000 eyes with this data, and the segmented AL was calculated from the optical path length using the same refractive indices as the Argos device. In order to maintain consistency with conventional IOL constants, the SAL AL was offset so the average SAL and CAL were equal—the difference in short and long ALs between SAL and CAL was preserved by this strategy. The optimization was derived using the actual radii of the single model SN60WF IOL, but the derived formula is intended to be used with the default biconvex model used in the existing BUII formula.

Validation of BUII SAL (Barrett True AL Formula)

The new formula based on SAL (Barrett True AL) was validated in a dataset of 595 eyes who had biometry performed with the Argos biometer shared by John Shammas. The Shammas validation dataset was not used in any fashion in the derivation or optimization of the Barrett True AL formula.

1. The standard BUII formula based on CAL was compared to four traditional formulas—Haigis, Hoffer Q, Holladay 1, and SRK/T.

2. The standard BUII formula based on CAL was then compared to the new Barrett True AL Formula based on SAL including subgroup analysis of short (<= 22.5 mm) and long eyes (> = 25.5 mm).

The IOL implanted in all cases was the Alcon SN60WF. An optimized constant was calculated for each formula such that the ME was 0.00 D. IOL constants for all formulas were optimized in this analysis. The constant for this dataset is somewhat higher for all formulas, e.g., the optimized a constant for SRK/T was 119.24. This may indicate a shorter refracting lane than 6.0 m, which is not common in the USA, but the refraction was not adjusted in this analysis.

The error in prediction for each formula was calculated, and the ME, SD, MAE, MedAE, as well as the percentage of cases within ±0.25 D, ±0.50 D, ±0.75 D, and ± 1.00 D determined using an excel spreadsheet. The results are listed in Tables 37.1, 37.2, 37.3, 37.4, and 37.5 for BUII (CAL), Haigis, Hoffer Q, Holladay 1, and SRK/T formulas, respectively.

A scatter plot of prediction error vs. AL was constructed for each formula with a linear trend line to evaluate whether significant bias existed

Table 37.1 ME = mean error, SD = standard deviation, MAE = mean absolute error, MedAE = median absolute error, and percentage of cases within intervals for BUII (CAL) formula

BUII (CAL)	% within D	ME	SD	MAE	MedAE
<±0.25 D	47.90%	0.0	0.376	0.310	0.260
<±0.50 D	80.54%				
<±0.75 D	96.98%				
<±1.00 D	99.50%				

Table 37.2 ME = mean error, SD = standard deviation, MAE = mean absolute error, MedAE = median absolute error, and percentage of cases within intervals for Haigis formula

Haigis (CAL)	% within D	ME	SD	MAE	MedAE
<±0.25 D	42.86%	0.0	0.408	0.330	0.298
<±0.50 D	77.82%				
<±0.75 D	93.45%				
<±1.00 D	99.16%				

Table 37.3 ME = mean error, SD = standard deviation, MAE = mean absolute error, MedAE = median absolute error, and percentage of cases within intervals for Hoffer Q formula

Hoffer Q (CAL)	% within D	ME	SD	MAE	MedAE
<±0.25 D	46.05%	0.0	0.410	0.333	0.287
<±0.50 D	74.79%				
<±0.75 D	93.11%				
<±1.00 D	99.33%				

Table 37.4 ME = mean error, SD = standard deviation, MAE = mean absolute error, MedAE = median absolute error, and percentage of cases within intervals for Holladay 1 formula

Holladay 1 (CAL)	% within D	ME	SD	MAE	MedAE
<±0.25 D	45.04%	0.0	0.388	0.322	0.281
<±0.50 D	77.98%				
<±0.75 D	96.30%				
<±1.00 D	99.83%				

Table 37.5 ME = mean error, SD = standard deviation, MAE = mean absolute error, MedAE = median absolute error, and percentage of cases within intervals for SRK/T formula

SRK/T (CAL)	% within D	ME	SD	MAE	MedAE
<±0.25 D	43.03%	0.0	±0.408	0.337	0.297
<±0.50 D	75.13%				
<±0.75 D	94.79%				
<±1.00 D	99.66%				

between these parameters The graphs are displayed in Figs. 37.2, 37.3, 37.4, 37.5, and 37.6 for BUII (CAL), Haigis, Hoffer Q, Holladay 1, and SRK/T formulas, respectively.

Comparison of Standard BUII Formula Based on CAL to Haigis, Hoffer Q, Holladay 1, and SRK/T

BUII has the lowest error in prediction in terms of MAE and MedAE as well as the percentage of cases with a prediction error within ±0.50 D. The trend line, however, for the scatter plot graph of prediction error versus AK slopes downwards to the right indicating a significant relationship

which is atypical for this formula when analyzing datasets based on CAL.

The scatter plot is similar to the Haigis formula. The trend line for prediction error vs. AL is typically flatter with the Haigis formula than Hoffer Q, Holladay, and SRK/T formulas when comparing formulas in a dataset based on CAL.

Comparison of Standard BUII Formula Based on CAL to the New Barrett True AL Formula Based on SAL

The prediction accuracy for BUII (SAL) listed in Tables 37.6 and 37.7 is maintained for long eyes and improves for short eyes compared to BUII (CAL) in Tables 37.6 and 37.7—the most impressive feature is the flat trend line in Fig. 37.7, which suggests the potential for improved accuracy with larger datasets.

Classical formulas with only basic optimization such as Holladay 1 improved their prediction with SAL as compared to CAL as demonstrated previously with flattening of the curve in prediction error vs. AL with SAL.

Using a biometer based on SAL, however, could potentially have an adverse impact on more sophisticated formulas as they already have a relatively flat curve of prediction error vs. AL over the range of ALs encountered clinically.

This is evident in a comparison of the outcomes in the Shammas dataset comprising eyes measured with the Argos device. The formulas can be refined in the future with actual Argos data, but the present derivation appears to resolve the issues of using formulas optimized for classical ALs with a sum of segments-based AL such as the Argos device.

The trend line of the Barrett True AL formula based on SAL (Fig. 37.7) is flat unlike the bias evident using the BUII formula based on CAL (fig. 37.2).

The optimized constant for the true AL formula (SAL) was LF = 1.972 versus LF = 1.99 for the standard BUII (CAL), indicating that no change in the IOL constant is required when using the new formula.

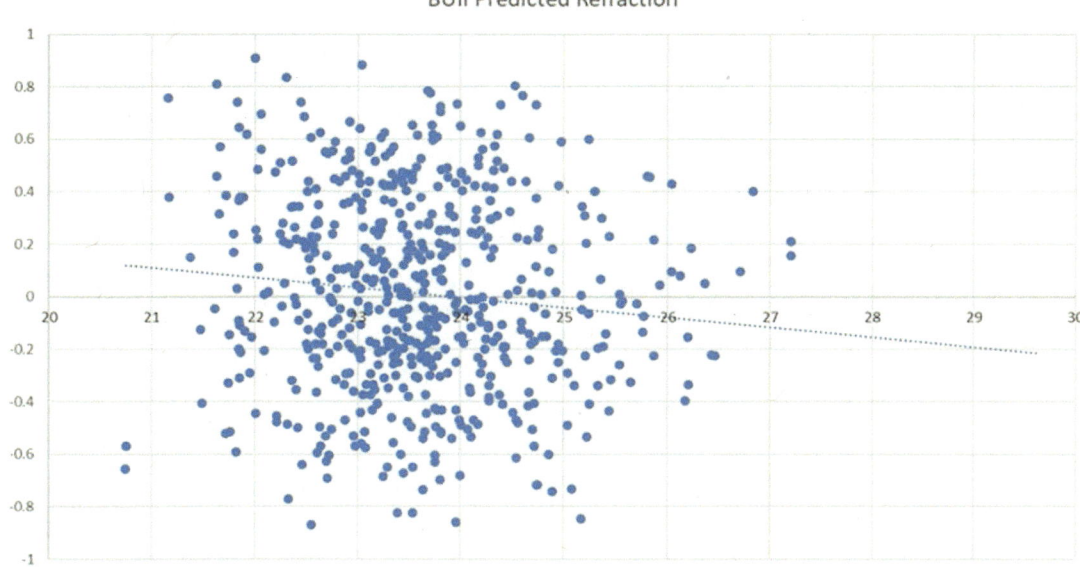

Fig. 37.2 Scatter plot of prediction error vs. AL for BUII (CAL) formula

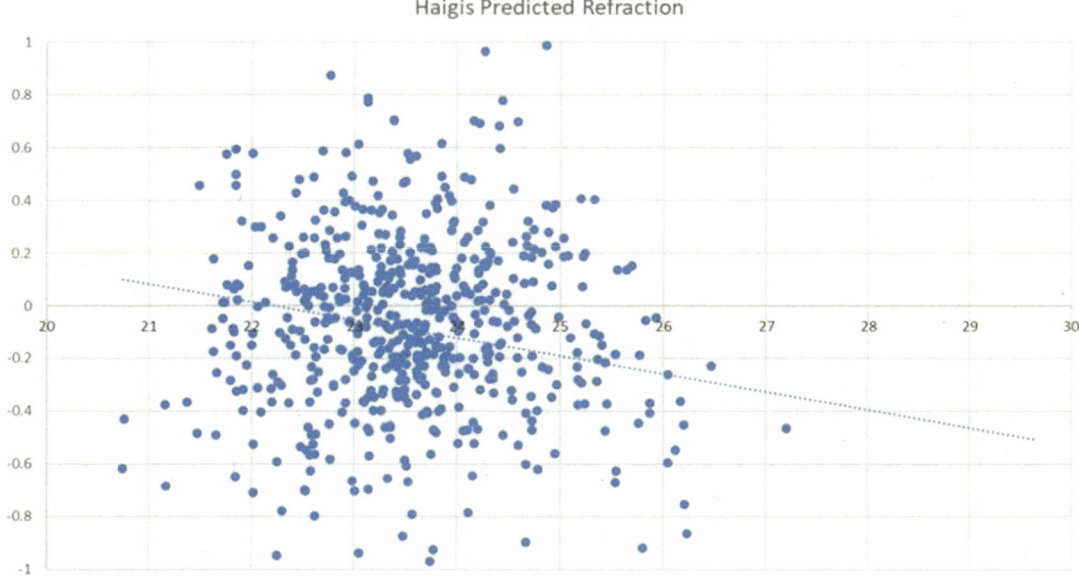

Fig. 37.3 Scatter plot of prediction error vs. AL for Haigis formula

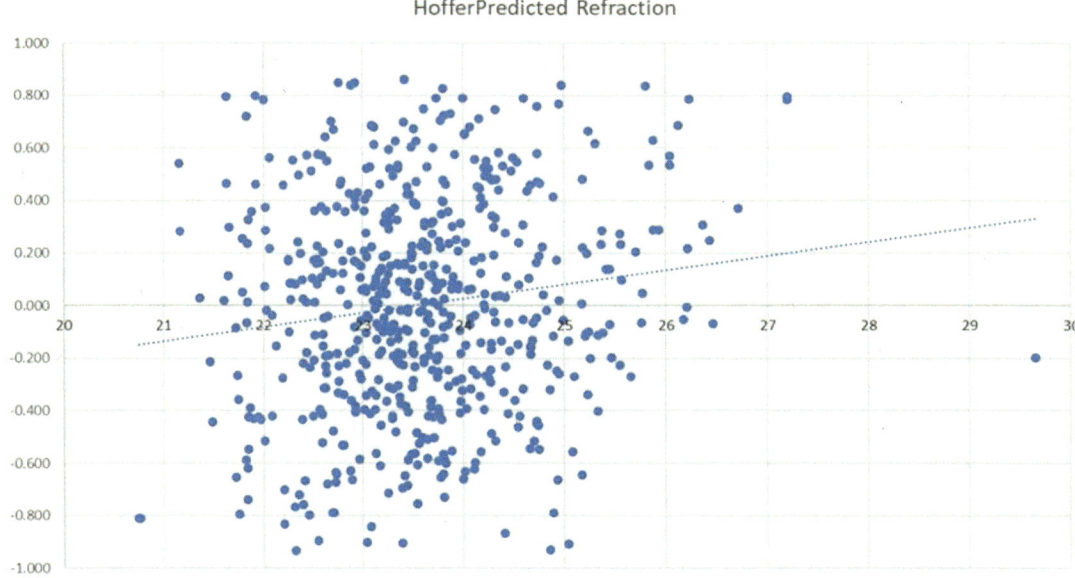

Fig. 37.4 Scatter plot of prediction error vs. AL for Hoffer Q formula

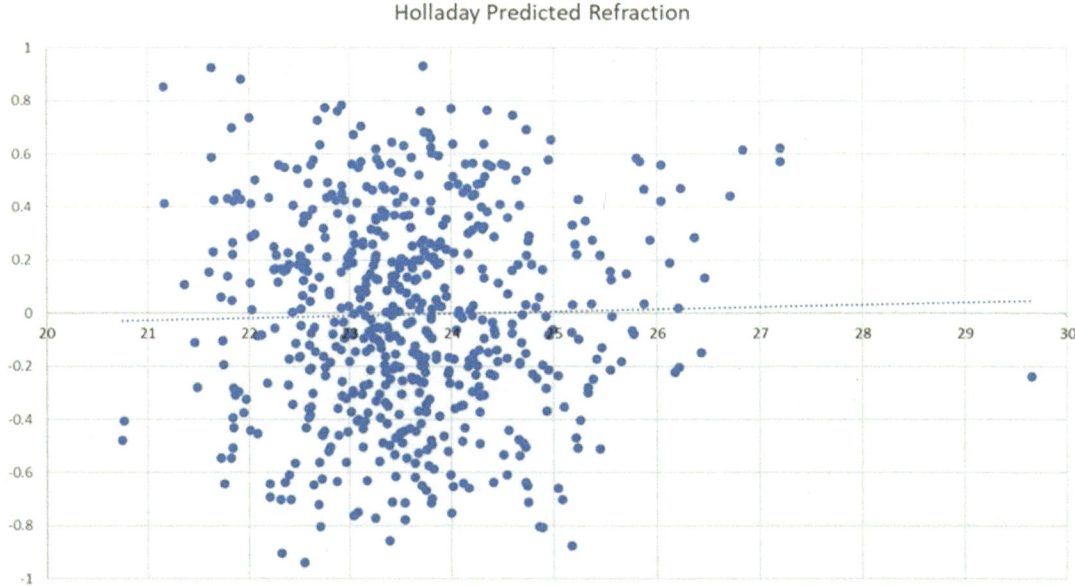

Fig. 37.5 Scatter plot of prediction error vs. AL for Holladay 1 formula

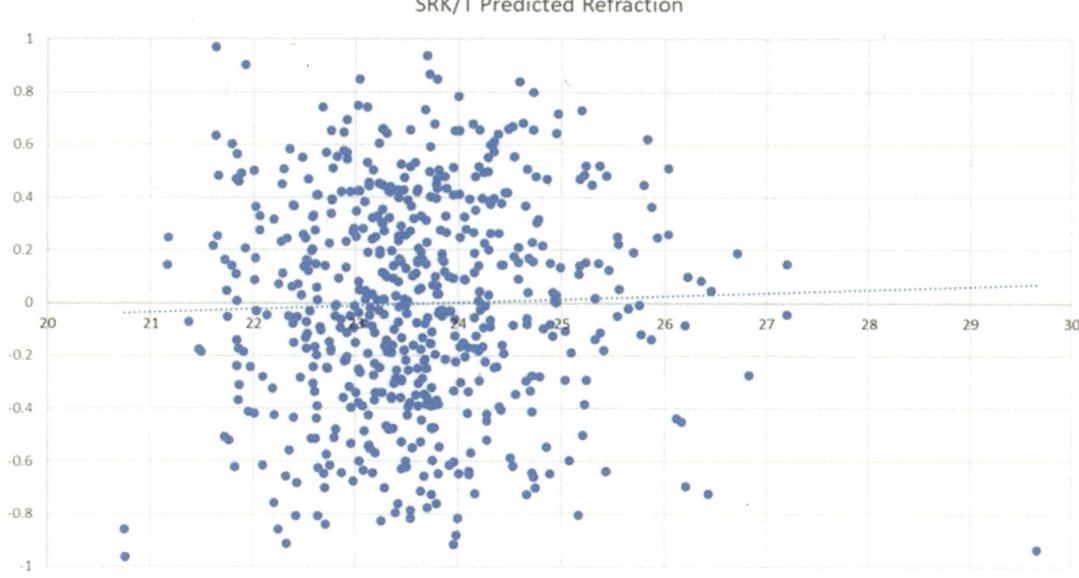

Fig. 37.6 Scatter plot of prediction error vs. AL for SRK/T formula

Table 37.6 ME, SD, MAE, Med.AE, and percentage of cases within intervals for BUII (CAL) formula grouped according to axial length

BUII (CAL) No of eyes 595 Lens factor = 1.972	All eyes (*n* = 595)	Short eyes <= 22 mm (*n* = 43)	Average eyes > = 22 mm < = 25 mm (*n* = 495)	Long eyes > 25 mm (*n* = 57)
Mean prediction error	0.01	0.12	0.01	−0.067
Standard deviation	0.380	0.440	0.371	0.341
Mean absolute prediction error	0.310	0.391	0.306	0.275
Median absolute error	0.260	0.380	0.255	0.225
Maximum absolute error	1.135	1.040	1.135	1.090
% < =0.25 D	47.90%	34.88%	48.08%	56.14%
% < =0.50 D	80.50%	67.44%	80.61%	89.47%
% < =0.75 D	96.98%	90.70%	97.58%	96.49%
% < =1.00 D	99.50%	97.64%	99.80%	98.25%

Table 37.7 ME, SD, MAE, Med.AE, and percentage of cases within intervals for BUII (SAL) formula grouped according to axial length

Barrett true axial length (SAL) No. of eyes 595 Lens factor = 1.972	All eyes (*n* = 595)	Short eyes <= 22 mm (*n* = 43)	Average eyes > = 22 mm < = 25 mm (*n* = 495)	Long eyes > 25 mm (*n* = 57)
Mean prediction error	−0.008	−0.077	0.002	−0.048
Standard deviation	0.37	0.41	0.37	0.32
Mean absolute prediction error	0.305	0.361	0.305	0.264
Median absolute error	0.264	0.317	0.261	0.224
Maximum absolute error	0.996	0.863	0.996	0.857
% < =0.25 D	48.40%	37.21%	48.89%	52.63%
% < =0.50 D	80.34%	72.09%	80.00%	89.47%
% < =0.75 D	96.97%	95.35%	97.17%	96.49%
% < =1.00 D	100.0%	100.0%	100.0%	100.0%

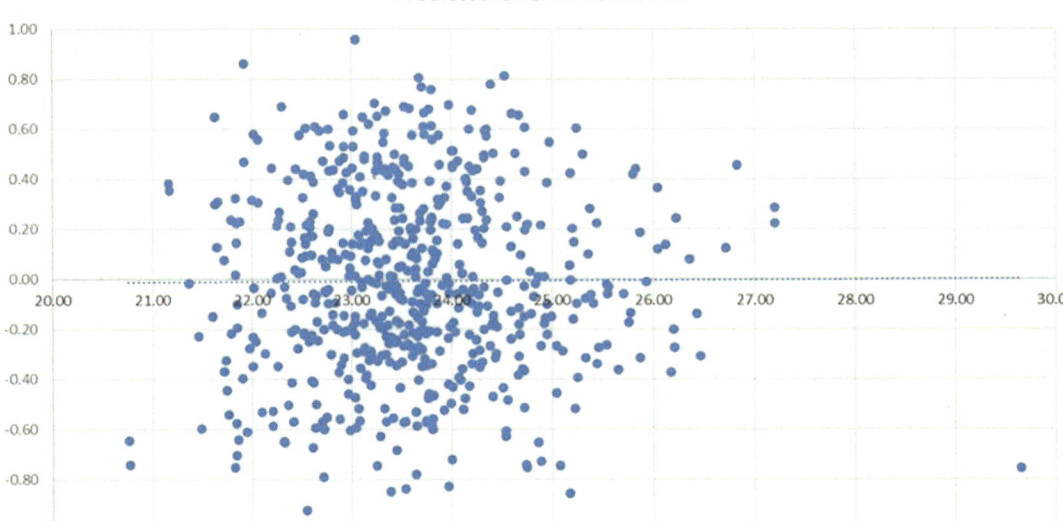

Fig. 37.7 Scatter plot of prediction error vs. AL for BUII (CAL) formula

Summary

The prediction accuracy is maintained for long eyes and improves for short—the most impressive feature is the flat trend line, which suggests improved accuracy with larger datasets.

Classical formulas with only basic optimization such as Holladay improved their prediction with SAL as compared to CAL as demonstrated previously with flattening of the curve in prediction error vs. AL with SAL.

Using a biometer based on SAL, however, could potentially have an adverse impact on more sophisticated formulas as they already have a relatively flat curve of prediction error vs. AL over the range of ALs encountered clinically.

This is evident in a comparison of the outcomes in the Shammas dataset comprising eyes measured with the Argos device. The formulas can be refined in the future with actual Argos data but the present derivation appears to resolve the issues of using formulas optimized for classical ALs with a sum of segments-based AL such as the Argos device.

Measurements

In 2008, Sverker Norrby [46] identified postoperative intraocular lens (IOL) position, postoperative refraction determination, and preoperative AL as the major sources of error contributing to errors in prediction after cataract surgery.

Improvements in the accuracy of optical biometry more recently with swept-source OCT and improved formulas have reduced the impact of these factors although subjective postoperative refraction remains a confounding factor in comparing outcomes. Variability in keratometry remains an important source of error in predicting spherical outcomes, particularly astigmatism, following cataract surgery, and arguably now should be listed as the most important factor.

I compared the repeatability of measuring AL, corneal power, and astigmatism on two separate biometers on the same visit in 144 consecutive eyes during routine pre-op biometry on the same day.

The axial difference in mm was converted to diopters by multiplying by 2.5 to facilitate a comparison of the impact compared to keratometry measured in diopters. The mean difference in AL between the two devices was −0.02 D with a SD of ±0.05 while the MAE was 0.038 and MedAE was 0.025 D. A scatter radar plot superimposed on a target is a useful method to demonstrate the repeatability of measurements and shows how consistent AL measurements have become when measured by two different modern biometers.

The mean difference in keratometry between the two devices was −0.01 D with an SD of ±0.15 while the MAE was 0.10 and MedAE was 0.07 D. The standard deviation of the measurements is greater than AL measurements, but the radar scatter graph demonstrates that the difference in mean Ks is within ±0.25 D for the majority of eyes.

The mean vector difference in magnitude of the cylinder between the two devices was −0.56 D with an SD of ±0.57 while the MAE difference magnitude of the cylinder was 0.55 D and MedAE was 0.41 D. The centroid difference in the measured astigmatism between the two devices was −0.10 D @ 79.2°. The difference between the x and y values of each vector displayed in a double-angle plot demonstrates that the differences in corneal astigmatism vary more widely than the mean K or AL between different devices.

Measures such as using Warren Hill's validation criteria are helpful and are optimizing the corneal surface, but measuring corneal astigmatism is not always repeatable. I have developed a K calculator, which is an integral part of the online Barrett toric calculator for deriving a vector mean or median K when measuring corneal astigmatism from different devices for toric IOL calculations. In a study of 128 patients, the median K of three devices provided the most accurate prediction as it de-emphasizes outliers. The improvement for spherical prediction was modest but the improvement in predicting post-op residual astigmatism was up to 10% and clinically significant [47, 48]. This is why I use the K calculator within the online Barrett toric calculator using three different devices, IOLMaster, Lenstar, and Pentacam to select the sphere and toric cylinder recommendation in all cases.

Additional Parameters

Originally formulas utilized AL and K as the primary measured ocular parameters to predict intraocular lens power. These remain the most important parameters whether the formula is based on vergence calculations, data-driven regression, or artificial intelligence. Pre-op phakic ACD measured from the corneal vertex (epithelium) to the anterior surface of the lens is also correlated to determine the effective lens position of an IOL and was included in the Haigis formulas and most recent formulas. The so-called aqueous depth (AQD) does not include the corneal thickness and is equally useful as a measured parameter to improve outcome prediction. The contribution of different factors can be identified using statistical correlation and pre-operative LT, horizontal CD, and CCT all show a relationship to prediction error. These parameters can be included in a formula and the Holladay II uses up to 7 parameters. The BUII can utilize up to 5 parameters including pre-op ACD, LT, and horizontal CD but can also be used with only AL and K [49].

The utility of the additional parameters is evident in the analysis of 287 consecutive eyes by considering the MAE and MedAE as well as the percentage of eyes with a predicted outcome within ±0.50 D.

The error in prediction reduces with the inclusion of additional parameters. A graph of the percentage of eyes with a prediction error within ±0.50 D vs. the number of parameters demonstrates improved prediction accuracy with ACD and LT as additional parameters but the trend line plateaus indicate less impact with the addition of horizontal CD.

Gender, ethnicity, age, and pre-op refraction are other demographic factors that are correlated with the prediction of refractive outcomes that can be considered for inclusion to improve the prediction of formulas. Gender appears to be the most relevant as female eyes tend to have a more myopic prediction error than male eyes for short ALs and a hyperopic outcome for long eyes compared to male eyes is evident in the analysis of large datasets [50]. Even if the data used for formula refinement is not considered separately, a gender bias may still be evident as the representation of gender is unequal in the age group undergoing cataract surgery due to factors such as the longevity of females over males. Deriving separate data-driven algorithms for male and female eyes is likely to improve outcomes.

Many formulas use a thin lens model and do not take into account the change in the principle plane that occurs with different IOL powers. Ray tracing including paraxial ray tracing such as BUII uses a thick lens model and allows the lens parameters to be calculated for each lens power predicted. Ideally, this calculation could include the actual lens parameters such as the radii of curvature or asphericity as these vary with different manufacturers. The impact of individual IOL parameters will have a greater impact on shorter eyes and using actual radii should improve prediction accuracy in this context. Specific IOL parameters are proprietary and are not generally known so assumptions such as an equi-biconvex model can be utilized. In addition, IOL-specific regression such as the Haigis triple optimization is another route to address this aspect of IOL prediction.

New Parameters

Improvements in technology have enabled us to measure anatomical parameters that were not feasible with earlier optical biometers and ultrasound. Scheimpflug tomographers have been able to measure the posterior cornea as have more recent optical biometers based on a swept-source OCT. Direct measurement of the posterior cornea rather than using an estimate based on an assumed value of the keratometer index or even the Gullstrand ratio in the paraxial equation for corneal power may potentially improve spherical and astigmatic refractive outcomes following cataract surgery.

Typically, a new total corneal power is provided by devices or biometers that measure the corneal power such as "True Net Corneal Power" or "Total Keratometry." These measurements

may not be equivalent as there is no standard with regard to values such as the refractive index of the cornea or aqueous that may be used in these equations. Furthermore, unless the measurement is adjusted to be compatible with the traditional Gullstrand ratio, the lens constants that users have been accustomed may not be appropriate. Formulas utilize corneal power in a variety of ways including the actual vergence calculation as well as the prediction of the actual IOL position. A customized formula is required to utilize the new parameter, and the issue is accounted for within the online Barrett formulas in that it allows the user to enter the measured posterior cornea rather than the total corneal power. The formula is incorporated into biometers such as the IOLMaster 700 where it is referred to as the Barrett TK. If the measured PCA option is selected, then the posterior cornea values PK1 and PK2 from the IOLMaster or the equivalent posterior cornea values from the Pentacam can be entered. The measured posterior corneal power will then be used for the sphere and toric prediction, which is equivalent to the Barrett TK on the IOLMaster 700. The online formulas require a user to select the instrument by which the posterior cornea has been measured, and the algorithm is adjusted accordingly. In addition, the formulas recognize that not all unexplained astigmatism after cataract surgery is due to the posterior cornea and contains additional algorithms to compensate for factors such as lens tilt. For unusual corneas such as keratoconus or post-refractive cases, the improvement in prediction is significant.

Post-Refractive Formulas

I developed the True K formula, which is based on BUII in order to improve outcome prediction in eyes that have had previous refractive surgery. The formula utilizes the history of the refractive change due to the procedure but can also be used if this information is not available. Compensation for the double K issue where a different K is required for the vergence calculation than that for the prediction of the IOL position is incorporated within the formula. An algorithm for the change in corneal thickness that may occur in certain refractive procedures is also included within the formula. The True K has proved to be effective for patients who have undergone myopic LASIK when the refractive history is known and when no history is available as published in 2016. In a publication in the JCRS in 2018, the True K formula proved to be accurate for patients who had undergone laser correction for hyperopia, and the True K has been shown to be accurate when compared to other methods for RK as published in ophthalmology in 2019. The online True K has a distinctive feature that allows the user to enter the most recent pre-cataract surgery refraction, which has not been impacted by nuclear sclerosis-induced myopia without the preop refraction. This is different than PRK or LASIK where both the pre- and post-refractive procedure refraction is required for the entered refractive history to be taken into consideration. This improves the accuracy in prediction for post-RK eyes as the progressive hyperopia, which may be considerable, is taken into account in the prediction of the IOL power required post-RK.

More recently in version 2.5, a solution for keratoconus is provided within the True K of the online True K formula on the APACRS website. The cornea is steep and irregular within the keratoconus, which is one of the reasons for imprecise measurements particularly in relation to the pupil and visual axis. The most important reason for poor prediction in keratoconus, however, is the altered relationship between the posterior and anterior cornea not dissimilar to post-refractive surgery but in its own unique fashion. This latter relationship is addressed in the True K option for keratoconus by a predictive algorithm or direct measurements of the posterior cornea.

The most accurate method of prediction within the True K formula appears to be a recent modification that allows the True K to incorporate the measured posterior cornea, the so-called True K TK. Similar to the toric, when the measured posterior cornea option is selected, a new page appears where you select the device used and enter the measured posterior cornea values listed within the IOLMaster 700 as the PK1 and

PK2 values or corresponding values from other devices such as Scheimpflug devices that are also able to measure the posterior corneal power or radius.

Lawless and co-workers published a relatively large series of their patients consisting of 72 eyes that had undergone previous myopic or hyperopic refractive surgery. Their results confirmed that the True K with the inclusion of the posterior cornea provided the most accurate and repeatable option in both myopic and hyperopic patients undergoing cataract surgery without prior refractive information [51].

An important issue that is not widely appreciated is the need for a custom toric calculator when selecting a Toric IOL in an eye that has undergone previous refractive surgery. The theoretical assumptions within standard toric calculators to predict the posterior cornea or population-based regression methods are no longer valid in the context of toric IOL prediction after cataract surgery.

The True K Toric Calculator was designed specifically for toric prediction post-refractive surgery and, in version 2.0, can now be used with the predicted posterior cornea or a measured option for posterior corneal astigmatism (PCA). In addition, the True K Toric calculator now includes the K calculator, which allows the user to enter up to three different values for the anterior cornea and then calculates a new integrated K or median vector, which is used for the calculation. This is particularly helpful when the Ks of different devices vary, which is not unusual in eyes that have undergone refractive surgery.

The default mode for the True K Toric is the theoretical PCA but I have found that utilizing the measured posterior cornea from SS-OCT provides greater accuracy not only for spherical prediction as previously mentioned but also for toric prediction particularly when no refractive history is available.

In a small series of 28 eyes from my own patients, the method that provided the greatest percentage predicted within ±0.50 D was the True K Toric calculator utilizing the measured posterior cornea from an SS-OCT device.

Formula for Unexpected Refractive Outcome

Managing an unexpected refractive outcome after cataract surgery can be daunting. Corneal refractive surgery or a lens-based solution can be considered whether by exchanging the implanted lens, adding a piggyback, or rotating an existing toric IOL. There are several formulas that can provide some of the required calculations such as the rule of thumb for spherical power, Holladay R for Lens exchange, Astigmatism Fix or Assort for lens rotation, and the vergence formula for the required piggyback IOL but sourcing these different formulas can be confusing.

I, therefore, developed the Barrett Rx (Asia-Pacific Association of Cataract and Refractive Surgeons (APACRS)), which can be used to provide a solution for each of these scenarios in a single formula. The default mode for the Rx is the ELP mode. Here, the actual effective lens position or ELP is calculated from the post-op refraction and used as the basis for the vergence calculation. Alternatively, the IOL mode can be selected, and here, the IOL constant for the implanted lens model is used to determine the ELP. The latter is preferred when the problem is not the ELP prediction but rather due to an abnormal cornea, for example, post-refractive surgery, or a suspected case of lens power mislabeling.

The implanted IOL power and post-op refractions need to be entered including the actual alignment if this is a toric IOL. The lens constant of the implanted lens and that of the planned IOL exchange are also required. It is important to note that the optical ACD and lens thickness are the phakic preop parameters and not the post-op measurements.

Once the data are entered, select calculate and then Rx exchange IOL to display the recommended spherical IOL, toric cylinder, and alignment required for an IOL exchange targeting the desired post-op refraction.

Selecting Rx piggyback on the top menu to display the alternative piggyback IOL, once again both spherical, toric power, and alignment.

Finally look at either the bottom of the IOL exchange or piggyback page, and the Rx formula will display a graph and let you know where to rotate the existing lens for the minimum residual astigmatism.

The Rx is a comprehensive formula that provides the required calculations to manage an unexpected refractive outcome in terms of IOL Exchange, piggyback lens implantation, or toric IOL rotation with both an ELP and IOL option to determine the expected ELP [52].

There are many studies comparing the prediction accuracy of different formulas. One of the most recent comparing 13 formulas was published by Savini et al.,

this year in the BJO [53]. All the modern formulas performed well, and the standard deviation was lowest with BUII. There was certainly no discernible difference in the accuracy of formulas and the method of derivation whether by Gaussian optics or artificial intelligence.

Isaac Newton in his famous book on natural philosophy and mathematics noted that what we know is a drop and what we do not know is an ocean. I would add that when it comes to modern IOL calculations, we should use every drop of knowledge available.

References

1. Ridley NHL. Intraocular acrylic lenses. Trans Ophthalmol Soc UK. 1951;71:617–21. Oxford Ophthalmological Congress, 1951.
2. Javal LE, Schiotz H. Un Opthalmometre Pratique. Annales d'Oculistique. 1881;86:5–21.
3. Ossoinig KC. Proceedings of the 3rd meeting of the International Society for Ultrasonic Diagnosis in Ophthalmology (SIDUO), Vienna, Austria, 1969.
4. Fercher AF, Mengedoht K, Werner W. Eye-length measurement by interferometry with partially coherent light. Opt Lett. 1988;13(3):186–8.
5. Fercher AF, Drexler W, Hitzenberge CK, Lasser T. Optical coherence tomography—principles and applications. Rep. Prog. Phys. 2010;66:239.
6. Fyodorov SN, Galin MA, Linksz A. Calculation of the optical power of intraocular lenses. Investig Ophthalmol. 1975;14:625–8.
7. Binkhorst CD. Power of the prepupillary pseudophakos. Br J Ophthalmol. 1972;56(4):332–7.

8. Colenbrander MC. Calculation of the power of an iris clip lens for distant vision. Br J Ophthalmol. 1973;57(10):735–40.

9. Hoffer KJ. Lens power calculation and the problem of the short eye. Ophthalmic Surg. 1982;13(11):962.

10. Thijssen JM. The emmetropic and the iseikonic implant lens: computer calculation of the refractive power and its accuracy. Ophthalmologica. 1975;171(6):467–86.

11. Van der Heijde GL. A nomogram for calculating the power of the prepupillary lens in the aphakic eye. Bibl Ophthalmol. 1975;83:273–5.

12. Sanders DR, Kraff MC. Improvement of intraocular lens power calculation using empirical data. J Amer Intra-Ocular Implant Soc. 1980;6(3):263–7.

13. Sanders DR, Retzlaff J, Kraff MC. Comparison of the SRK II formula and other second generation formulas. J Cataract Refract Surg. 1988;14(2):136–41.

14. Hoffer KJ. The Hoffer Q formula: A comparison of theoretic and regression formulas. J Cataract Refract Surg. 1993;19(11):700–12. Errata: 1994;20(6):677 and 2007;33(1):2–3.

15. Holladay JT, Prager TC, Chandler TY, Musgrove KH, Lewis JW, Ruiz RS. A three-part system for refining intraocular lens power calculations. J Cataract Refract Surg. 1988;14(1):17–24.

16. Sanders DR, Retzlaff JA, Kraff MC, Gimbel HV, Raanan MG. Comparison of the SRK/T formula and other theoretical and regression formulas. J Cataract Refract Surg. 1990;16(3):341–6. Erratum 1990;16(4):528.

17. Barrett GD. Intraocular lens calculation formulas for new intraocular lens implants. J Cataract Refract Surg. 1987;13(4):389–96.

18. Barrett GD. An improved universal theoretical formula for intraocular lens power prediction. J Cataract Refract Surg. 1993;19(6):713–20.

19. Olsen T. Theoretical approach to intraocular lens calculation using Gaussian optics. J Cataract Refract Surg. 1987;13(2):141–5.

20. Haigis W. Strahldurchrechnung in Gauß'scher Optik zur Beschreibung des Systems Brille-Kontaktlinse-Hornhaut-Augenlinse (IOL). 4. Kongreß d. Deutschen Ges. f. Intraokularlinsen Implant., Essen, Germany 1990, hrsg.v. K Schott, KW Jacobi, H Freyler, Springer Berlin, 1991: 233–246.

21. Holladay JT, Holladay IOL. Consultant computer program. TX, Holladay IOL Consultant: Houston; 1996.

22. Preussner PR, Wahl J, Weitzel D. Topography-based intraocular lens power selection. J Cataract Refract Surg. 2005;31(3):525–33.

23. Barrett GD. A formula for all seasons. Supplement to cataract and refractive surgery Today/Europe. 2014.

24. Olsen T, Hoffmann P. C constant: new concept for ray tracing-assisted intraocular lens power calculation. J Cataract Refract Surg. 2014;40(5):764–73.

25. IOL Power Calculator for Cataract Surgery|Hill-RBF Calculator. https://rbfcalculator.com/.

26. Debellemanière G, Dubois M, Gauvin M, Wallerstein A, Brenner LF, Rampat R, Saad A, Gatinel D. The PEARL-DGS formula: the development of an open-source machine learning-based thick IOL calculation formula. Am J Ophthalmol. 2021;232:58–69.

27. Connell BJ, Kane JX. Comparison of the Kane formula with existing formulas for intraocular lens power selection. BMJ Open Ophthalmol. 2019;4(1):e000251.

28. Shammas HJ, Taroni L, Pellegrini M, Shammas MC, Jivrajka RV. Accuracy of newer IOL power formulas in short and long eyes using sum-of-segments biometry. J Cataract Refract Surg. 2022; https://doi.org/10.1097/j.jcrs.0000000000000958.

29. Koch DD, Hill W, Abulafia A, Wang L. Pursuing perfection in intraocular lens calculations: I. Logical approach for classifying IOL calculation formulas. J Cataract Refract Surg. 2017 Jun;43(6):717–8.

30. Cheng X, Davis D, Matloff N, Davis D, Mohanty P. Polynomial regression as an alternative to neural nets. arXiv. 2019:1806.06850v3.

31. Barrett GD. A new hydrogel intraocular lens design. J Cataract Refract Surg. 1994;20(1):18–25.

32. Barrett GD. Flight of the arrow - Toric IOL prediction. Boston, MA: Film Festival, American Society of Cataract & Refractive Surgeons; 2014.

33. Abulafia BGD, Kleinmann G, Ofir S, Levy A, Marcovich AL, Michaeli A, Koch DD, Wang L, Assia E. Prediction of refractive outcomes with toric intraocular lens implantation. J Cataract Refract Surg. 2015;41(5):936–44.

34. Ferreira TB, Ribeiro P, Ribeiro FJ, O'Neill JG. Comparison of astigmatic prediction errors associated with new calculation methods for toric intraocular lenses. J Cataract Refract Surg. 2017;43(3):340–7.

35. Abulafia A, Hill WE, Koch DD, Wang L, Barrett GD. Accuracy of the Barrett true-K formula for intraocular lens power prediction after laser in situ keratomileusis or photorefractive keratectomy for myopia. J Cataract Refract Surg. 2016;42(3):363–9.

36. Vrijman V, Abulafia A, van der Linden JW, van der Meulen IJE, Mourits MP, Lapid-Gortzak R. ASCRS calculator formula accuracy in multifocal intraocular lens implantation in hyperopic corneal refractive laser surgery eyes. J Cataract Refract Surg. 2019;45(5):582–6.

37. Turnbull AMJ, Crawford GJ, Barrett GD. Methods for intraocular lens power calculation in cataract surgery after radial keratotomy. Ophthalmology. 2020;127(1):45–51.

38. Ton Y, Barrett GD, Kleinmann G, Levy A, Assia EI. Toric intraocular lens power calculation in cataract patients with keratoconus. J Cataract Refract Surg. 2021;47(11):1389–97.

39. Melles RB, Holladay JT, Chang WJ. Accuracy of intraocular lens calculation formulas. Ophthalmology. 2018;125(2):169–78.

40. Roberts TV, Hodge C, Sutton G. Lawless M; contributors to the vision eye institute IOL outcomes registry. Comparison of Hill-radial basis function, Barrett universal and current third generation formulas for the

calculation of intraocular lens power during cataract surgery. Clin Exp Ophthalmol. 2018;46(3):240–6.

41. Turnbull AMJ, Hill WE, Barrett GD. Accuracy of intraocular lens power calculation methods when targeting low myopia in monovision. J Cataract Refract Surg. 2020;46(6):862–6.

42. Wang L, Cao D, Weikert MP, Koch DD. Calculation of axial length using a single group refractive index versus using different refractive indices for each ocular segment: theoretical study and refractive outcomes. Ophthalmol. 2019;126(5):663–70.

43. Cooke DL, Cooke TL. A comparison of two methods to calculate axial length. J Cataract Refract Surg. 2019;45(3):284–92. https://doi.org/10.1016/j.jcrs.2018.10.039.

44. Shammas HJ, Shammas MC, Jivrajka RV, Cooke DL, Potvin R. Effects on IOL power calculation and expected clinical outcomes of axial length measurements based on multiple vs. single refractive indices. Clin Ophthalmol. 2020;14(6):1511–9.

45. Haigis W, Lege B, Miller N, Schneider B. Comparison of immersion ultrasound biometry and partial coherence interferometry for intraocular lens calculation according to Haigis. Graefe's Archive for Clin and Exp Ophthalmol. 2000;238:765–73.

46. Norrby S. Sources of error in intraocular lens power calculation. J Cataract Refract Surg. 2008;34(3):368–76.

47. Barrett GD, Lipsky L. Integrated K to improve toric IOL prediction. Washington, D.C.: Presented American Society of Cataract & Refractive Surgeons; April 2018.

48. Graham B. Plotting the right course. Vienna, Austria: European Society of Cataract and refractive surgeons film festival; 2018.

49. Vega Y, Gershoni A, Achiron A, Tuuminen R, Weinberger Y, Livny E, Nahum Y, Bahar I, Elbaz U. High agreement between Barrett universal II calculations with and without utilization of optional biometry parameters. J Clin Med. 2021;10(3):542.

50. Zhang Y, Li T, Reddy A, Nallasamy N. Gender differences in refraction prediction error of five formulas for cataract surgery. BMC Ophthalmol. 2021;21(1):183. https://doi.org/10.1186/s12886-021-01950-2.

51. Lawless M, Jiang JY, Hodge C, Sutton G, Roberts TV, Barrett G. Total keratometry in intraocular lens power calculations in eyes with previous laser refractive surgery. Clin Exp Ophthalmol. 2020;48(6):749–56.

52. Savini G, Di Maita M, Hoffer KJ, Næser K, Schiano-Lomoriello D, Vagge A, Di Cello L, Traverso CE. Comparison of 13 formulas for IOL power calculation with measurements from partial coherence interferometry. Br J Ophthalmol. 2021;105(4):484–9.

53. Barrett GD. The Barrett Rx formula: predicting IOL power based on refraction after cataract surgery. Barcelona. Spain: European Society of Cataract & Refractive Surgeons; 2015. https://escrs.conference-2web.com/#!contentsessions/12537.

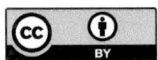

The Castrop IOL Formula

Peter Hoffmann and Achim Langenbucher

The basic IOL power formula is quite old; to our knowledge, it was first described by Fyodorov [1] and by Gernet and Ostholt [2]. This paraxial vergence formula considers three refractive surfaces, a spectacle correction (or target refraction) located at d_{vertex} in front of the cornea, a thin lens cornea with P_{cornea}, and an intraocular lens implant with refractive power P_{IOL} located at ELP behind the cornea:

$$P_{IOL} = \frac{n_{vitreous}}{AL - ELP} - \cfrac{1}{\cfrac{1}{\cfrac{1}{\cfrac{1}{P_{spectacle}} - d_{vertex}} + P_{cornea}} - \cfrac{ELP}{n_{aqueous}}}$$

All distances in [m].

$n_{cornea} = 1.376$.

$n_{air} = 1.000$ (rounded).

$n_{aqueous} = 1.336$.

All classical Gaussian optics IOL formulae date back to this approach. Many derivates exist. They differ mostly in how "ELP" (effective lens position) is dealt with. We used this equation as the basis for our IOL calculation. In daily practice, it makes sense to solve the equation for $P_{spectacle}$ instead of P_{IOL}.

In recent years, many formulae have emerged that are neither published nor disclosed or documented. Some of them provide great results, and some provide less convincing results under specific conditions. We feel it is crucial to understand how the formula acts, and how it processes the input data. Therefore, we would like to document our own approach in detail.

In classical formulae, we identified four typical sources of error that can be cured quite easily.

1. Most conventional formulae consider the cornea as a thin lens model and use a fictitious refractive index of either 1.3375 or 1.332 to convert the mean front surface radius measured paracentrally to "corneal power" K. As this approach tends to overestimate the corneal power by 0.4 to 1.1 D, the IOL power is underestimated accordingly. To compensate for this,

P. Hoffmann (✉)
Augen- und Laserklinik Castrop-Rauxel, Castrop-Rauxel, Germany

A. Langenbucher
Experimentelle Opthalmologie, Universität des Saarlandes, Homburg/Saar, Germany
e-mail: Achim.Langenbucher@uks.eu

© The Author(s) 2024
J. Aramberri et al. (eds.), *Intraocular Lens Calculations*, Essentials in Ophthalmology,
https://doi.org/10.1007/978-3-031-50666-6_38

the fictitious lens position ELP is moved to a position located behind the biconvex lens. This will lead to the next problem. To avoid this, corneal power is calculated using a thick lens model and the measured radii as "equivalent power" (distances in mm). If no data on the posterior curvature is available, we assume a ratio of 0.84 that was derived from very large ssOCT data sets and which is very close to the accepted Liou & Brennan ratio [3]

$$r_{post} = 0.84 \cdot r_{ant}$$

for an untreated cornea. To avoid confusion with the traditional "K," we will call this P_{cornea}.

$$P_{cornea} = \frac{n_{cornea} - n_{air}}{r_{ant}} + \frac{n_{aqueous} - n_{cornea}}{r_{post}} - \frac{CCT}{n_{cornea}} \cdot \frac{n_{cornea} - n_{air}}{r_{ant}} \cdot \frac{n_{aqueous} - n_{cornea}}{r_{post}}$$

P_{cornea} is referenced to the principal plane. From a physical point of view, it would be correct to reference the front vertex. As we want to keep "compatibility" with manufacturer's indications like Tomey's ACCP or Heidelberg's TCRP, we kept the principal plane as a reference. This will become important when it comes to odd cornea, e.g., post LASIK when we can simply replace the whole P_{cornea} term with a power value derived by the manufacturer's software. The difference between the principal plane and front vertex will be ≈ 50 μm in an average cornea, so the systematic deviation will be quite small.

2. As the corneal power is overestimated, a given lens power with a realistic ELP (ELP matches the physical or anatomical position of the IOL) would lead to an underestimation of the lens power and therefore to a hyperopic error. When ELP is assumed to be located behind the physical IOL position, the resulting IOL power will increase, and the error is compensated on average. However, in eyes with unusual combinations of axial length and corneal radii, this will lead to systematic errors. This can be avoided when the ELP is very close to its real position inside the eye. In all biconvex IOL designs, the principal plane of the IOL will be located between the front and back IOL vertex, and in most IOL models on the market, the position is close to the center plane of the lens (see below). A very simple equation according to Olsen [4] had been used in an early version of the Castrop formula (distances in mm):

$$ELP = -0.18 + ACD + C \cdot LT$$

"C" describes the fraction of crystalline lens thickness where the ELP will be presumed. It can vary with haptic and optic design as well as step vault at the edge. Typical values will be between 0.35 and 0.42.

However, IOL position prediction can be further improved when axial length and corneal radii are included in the regression. In contrast, corneal diameter does not reduce the variance in the prediction significantly; therefore, it was omitted. The following equations were derived from a large set of eyes where crystalline lens thickness and position and IOL position were measured optically (distances in mm).

$$ELP = 0.610 + 0.049 \cdot AL + 0.729 \cdot CCT + 0.680 \cdot AQD - 0.123 \cdot r1_{ant} + C \cdot LT + H$$

(historical version used in Wendelstein's paper)

$$ELP = 0.045 \cdot AL + 0.761 \cdot ACD - 0.042 \cdot \bar{r}_{ant} + C \cdot LT + H$$

(recent version)

where r1$_{ant}$ (flat r) as well as $\bar{r}_{ant}$ refers to the base curve of the corneal front surface. In eyes with prior corneal refractive surgery or corneal pathology, corneal radii should be left out and the following equation without corneal radii used instead.

$$ELP = -0.09 + 0.037 \cdot AL + 0.602 \cdot CCT + 0.715 \cdot AQD + C \cdot LT + H$$

(historical version used in Wendelstein's paper)

$$ELP = 0.036 \cdot AL + 0.753 \cdot ACD + C \cdot LT + H$$

(recent version)

Alternate multiple regressions using AS-OCT data like lens diameter, lens curvatures, and lens equator position have also been successfully tested and can reduce prediction error even further. However, these data will not be available to most users and are, therefore, not included in the current version of the formula.

IOLs with planar haptics and steeper anterior radii will have a smaller C than IOLs with posteriorly angulated or stepped haptics and/or designs where the main power is located on the posterior curvature. It is important that "C" optimization does not yield a significant skewness (the median is significantly different from the arithmetic mean). The remaining small offsets can be compensated for by adding an offset to the presumed refraction ("R" for "Rauxel"). This avoids systematic errors. The version of the formula that was used in Wendelstein's paper [5] used only C and R and worked quite well. However, Langenbucher showed H as a designated offset to be beneficial, so it is recommended to use it in conjunction with the new ELP regressions from now on.

3. Axial length is measured optically. This means that the optical path length has to be converted into a *geometrical* path by dividing it by the refractive index. However, the refractive index of the eye is not constant. For the average eye, the group refractive index will be assumed as 1.3549 according to the first IOLMaster versions [6]. In very long eyes, the fraction of vitreous will be larger, and consequently, the group refractive index will be smaller leading to hyperopic error. The opposite is true for short eyes. To overcome this problem, the best solution would be to replace the group refractive index with a sum-of-segments approach with different indices for each segment of the eye instead. There will still be some imprecision as the index of the cataractous lens material is unknown, but systematic errors will be significantly reduced. Unfortunately, none of the biometers able to *measure* sum-of-segments will *indicate* "new" AL but use the "old" value instead (FDA, compatibility issues). We have to thank Cooke [7] for publishing a regression formula that provides a linear regression for a correction of the axial length derived from a LenStar LS900 biometer, which mimics the sum-of-segments.

4. We used Cooke's regression to transform traditional optical AL to "AL$_{new}$."

$$AL_{new} = 1.23854 + 0.95855 \cdot AL_{old} - 0.05467 \cdot LT$$

5. Some small systematic error will remain due to lens properties, and surgical and optometric technique and needs to be adjusted. In conventional formulae, several influencing variables are squeezed into the ELP (e.g., A constant). The most important ones will be the lane distance for refractometry, ambient light, haptic design, asphericity of surfaces (or spherical aberration of the pseudophakic eye), decentration (the more aspheric, the more hyperopic error), or tilt of the lens and capsulotomy properties. This will unavoidably lead to trend errors. In our opinion, it is

better to compensate for systematic refractive deviation by an additional simple offset instead of fudging the ELP.

It is important to understand that "ELP" in the context of the Castrop formula consists of two parts. First, the Lens Equator position (LEQ) will be derived from preoperative input variables (AL, ACD, LT, and [r]) by a multiple linear regression. This resembles an *anatomical* position that can actually be measured by an Anterior Segment OCT. In the future, deep learning algorithms may replace the multiple regression leading to even better results [8]. In this regression, "C" acts as a coefficient (see equations).

Depending on the IOL design, the relevant principal plane H′ will differ from the lens equator plane (LEQ). This is handled by an offset in the linear regression that we call "H" ("Homburg") as its use as a third degree of freedom was suggested by Langenbucher. In an equiconvex IOL, H′ will be located posterior to LEQ, in a typical modern IOL with a steeper anterior curvature, H′ will move anteriorly. When the exact design data of the IOL is known for all power values (Coddington factor), H could be adjusted systematically for any power step. In daily practice, a single "H" would represent the IOL model. It is well known that discrete steps in shape factors (e.g., Alcon SA60AT 25.0–29.5) may lead to systematic deviations.

We feel that every surgeon should do subsequent work on his refractive outcomes. We also think it is more appropriate to add a third constant (besides C and H) instead of fudging the ELP. We call this constant "R" for "Rauxel." In recent studies, we defined "emmetropia" for a lane distance of 6 m = 20 ft. If emmetropia shall be defined for infinity, R should be changed accordingly (decrease R by $\frac{1}{6}$).

At the moment, optimization of 2 formula constants (C and R) or 3 formula constants (C, H, and R) is performed sequentially starting with C and H based on a multivariable linear regression and in a second step by adjusting R to nullify the mean signed formula prediction error for a set of clinical data. Langenbucher developed an algorithm to optimize all three degrees of freedom simultaneously using nonlinear optimization strategies. With a Levenberg–Marquardt algorithm [9], all 3 constants of the Castrop formula can be optimized *en bloc* for minimization of root mean squared refraction error as the target criterion. This will soon be integrated into the IOLcon. org Website.

To summarize, the core of our formula is identical to the basic IOL power formula. Corneal power will be derived from radii using thick-lens Gaussian optics; if posterior radii and/or CCT are not available, they will be modeled according to Liou & Brennan. ELP is predicted from a multiple regression developed from true anatomical data enhancing Olsen's C concept ("Castrop" constant with or without "Homburg" offset). If the cornea has been tampered with or is difficult to measure, a simpler regression omitting corneal radius is recommended. Axial length is transformed according to Cooke. The remaining systematic offsets are accounted for by adding an offset R ("Rauxel").

The formula attempts to eliminate systematic errors (axial length, cornea, and chamber depth) as much as reasonable. It can also be used in post-LASIK eyes with great success if the "true corneal power" can be measured and calculated separately, e.g., CASIA2 ACCP or Anterion TCRP. The derived corneal power can be used to overwrite P_{cornea}. Alternatively, P_{cornea} can also be used, but it must be kept in mind that our simple Gaussian formula cannot deal with aspheric surfaces appropriately. It can be used in minus power cases as well as IOL powers up to and even beyond 40 D without further adjustments and good precision [5].

However, the limits of Gaussian optics still apply. Asphericity, decentration, and tilt of optical elements cannot be dealt with directly. The finer details of the Liou and Brennan eye model cannot be used to the fullest advantage. To break the chains, Gaussian optics would have to be replaced by geometric optics ("raytracing"). Unfortunately, as the design properties of the specific IOLs are not disclosed, and the local corneal power and height data might be unreliable

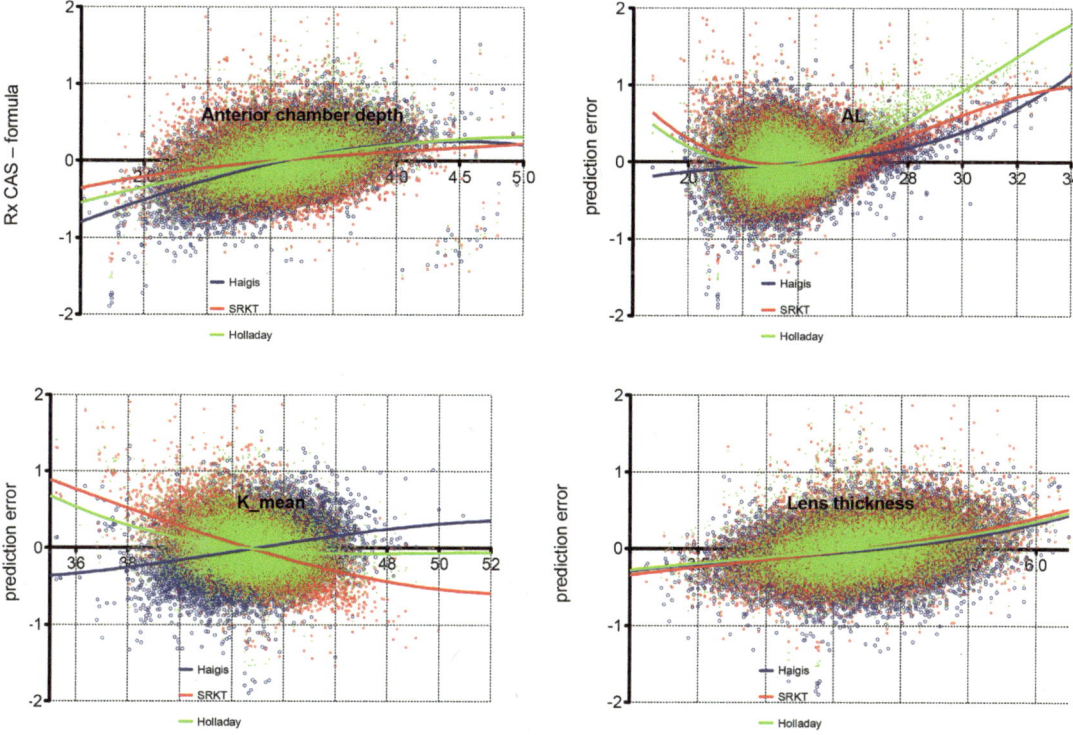

Fig. 38.1 Trend errors of Haigis, Holladay, and SRK/T with ACD, axial length, corneal power, and crystalline lens thickness

due to limitations in the respective measurement techniques such as anterior segment OCT or even more Scheimpflug imaging, this is not applicable in clinical routine, and the Gaussian approach would still make sense.

We believe that trend errors immanent to classical IOL formulae ([10–12] should be avoided whenever possible. This would specifically improve IOL calculation in any eye that is far away from statistical "normality," the especially short axis in combination with flat radii. It would also get you rid of the ritual of choosing from different formulae depending on the biometry data. As mentioned above, the way to achieve this is to avoid skewed outdated eye models and mixing up properties that do not belong together.

In a data set of 904 consecutive eyes, the Castrop formula achieved a standard deviation of the prediction error of 0.35 D (mean absolute error MAE = 0.28 D), compared to 0.39–0.42 D (MAE 0.31–0.34 D) for the classical formulae

Haigis, Hoffer Q, Holladay, and SRK/T – still very good values when compared to the literature (Fig. 38.1). Threefold optimization with the new ELP regression will improve results slightly but will yield more robust results for certain IOL such as B&L EnVista MX60.

When spherical IOLs are excluded (n = 365), the standard deviation will decrease to 0.31 D for the Castrop formula and 0.37–0.41 D for the classical formulae. In aspheric IOL, refraction will be more precise due to less pseudo accommodation; hence, the relative difference between formulae will increase as one of the major sources of stochastic error is decreased.

In very short eyes, the relative advantage will be even greater. The performance in these difficult eyes will be better than any classical formula and on par with Okulix raytracing, Pearl DGS, and Kane formula [5]. It compares very favorably to other modern formulae in normal and short eyes [13–15] (Fig. 38.2).

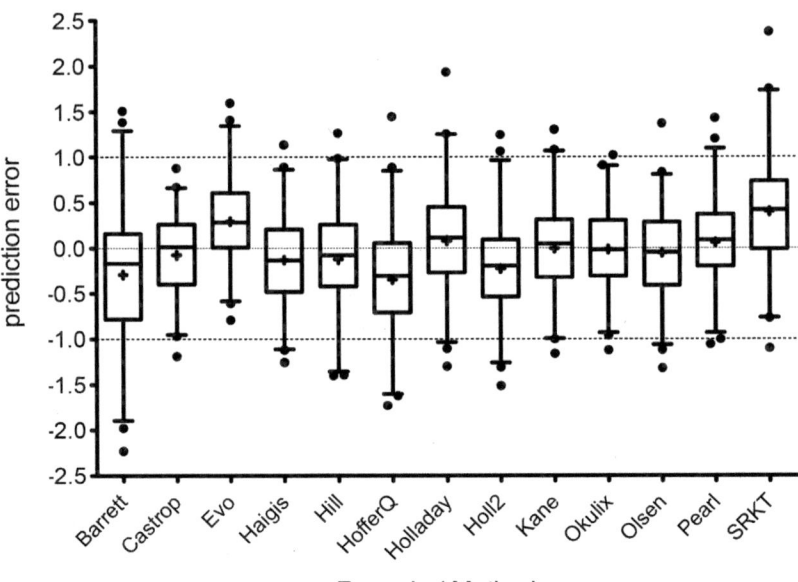

Fig. 38.2 Prediction error as box plot for 13 classical and new formulae. This is a data set of 95 very short eyes implanted with IOL powers of 30 D or more. This can be directly compared to [13]. The box plot was chosen to visualize the mean as well as the standard deviation/spread

The formula is available as an Excel spreadsheet. The screenshot will give you an impression (Fig. 38.3). Optimized constants for six different acrylic IOLs used in our clinic have been derived, see Table below (Tables 38.1 and 38.2). As more postoperative data are coming in, 2- or 3-way optimization can be carried out fully automatically using Langenbucher's software. We now recommend using the web-based version that includes a batch processing option: https://iolcon.org/lpcm.php

A stand-alone version in executable code will soon be available, see Screenshot (Fig. 38.4). This software tool is capable of calculating toric (or stigmatic) intraocular lenses for any spherocylindrical target refraction as well as predicting spherocylindrical refraction at the spectacle plane. For calculation of the IOL power, the following parameters are required: target refraction, vertex distance, flat and steep front surface radii, central corneal thickness (optional), flat and steep corneal back surface radii (optional), phakic anterior chamber depth and lens thickness, axial length, as well as formula constants C, H, and R. For prediction of the postoperative spherocylindrical refraction, the following parameters are required: equivalent power and torus (optional) of the lens implant, vertex distance for spectacle correction, flat and steep front surface radii, central corneal thickness (optional), flat and steep corneal back surface radii (optional), phakic anterior chamber depth and lens thickness, axial length, as well as formula constants C, H, and R. In addition, this software is able to batch-process data from an Excel table if available in a special template format ("Browse"). In this batch processing lens, power is calculated, refraction is predicted en bloc from a data set, and the respective results are added with new columns in the Excel sheet. With a sufficient number of data, the Castrop formula constants are derived using nonlinear optimization for the root mean squared prediction error of equivalent refraction. These optimized constant data are also added to the excel table. A web-based version of the formula is available at https://iolcon.org/lpcm.php

It is our concern that every detail of this IOL calculation approach is transparent and public domain. We believe this is the best way to guarantee scientific integrity and improve clinical outcomes without barriers or paywalls. Further improvements in measuring hardware can easily be adopted. It does make sense to merge the formula with an IOL database like IOLcon.org as all other modern formulae are not disclosed and can, therefore, not be optimized with user-generated data in an automated way.

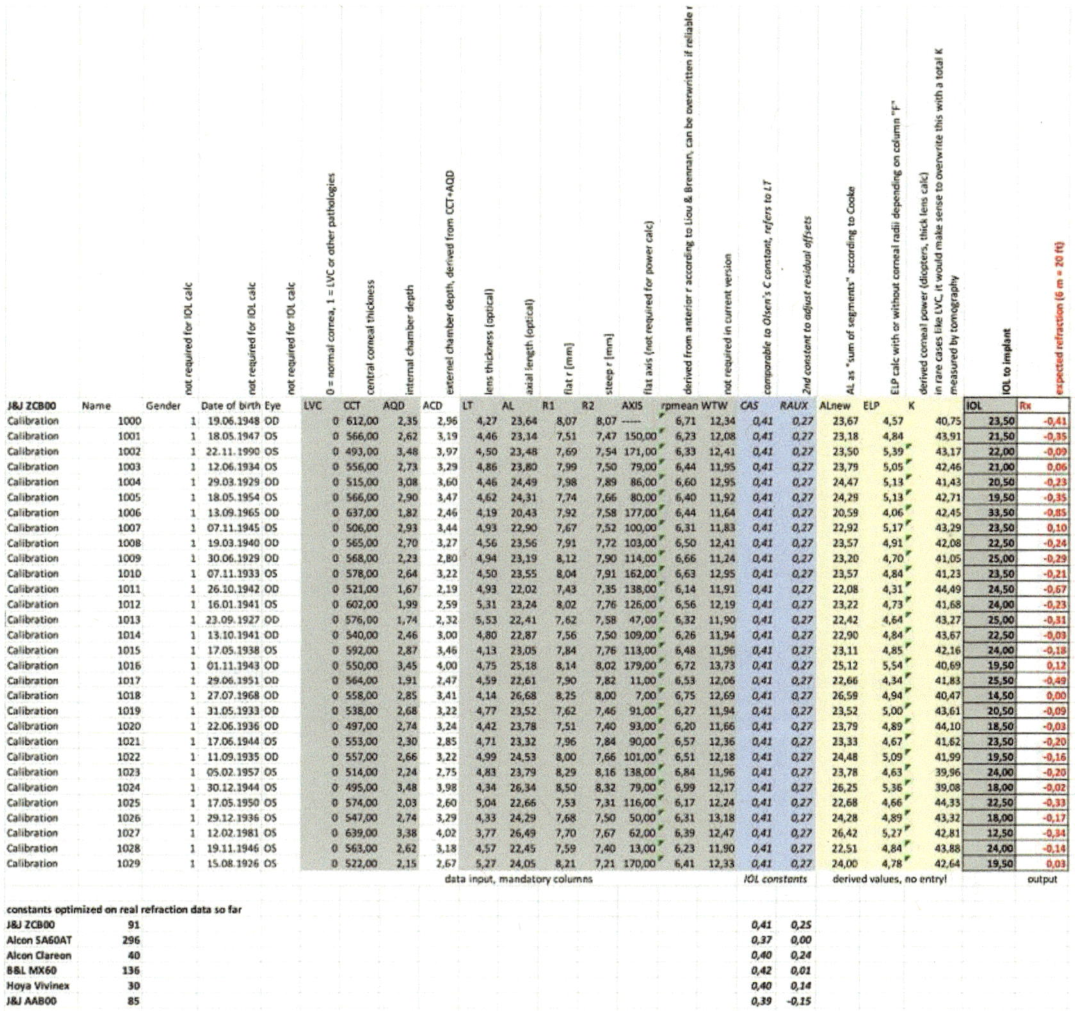

Fig. 38.3 Screenshot of Excel spreadsheet used for IOL studies. It is self-explaining and can be used to process large data sets for clinical studies

The spreadsheet contains the following data (data input, mandatory columns; IOL constants; derived values, no entry!; output):

J&J ZCB00	Name	Gender	Date of birth	Eye	LVC	CCT	AQD	ACD	LT	AL	R1	R2	AXIS	rpmean	WTW	CAS	RAUX	ALnew	ELP	K	IOL	Rx
Calibration	1000	1	19.06.1948	OD	0	612,00	2,35	2,96	4,27	23,64	8,07	8,07 -----		6,71	12,34	0,41	0,27	23,67	4,57	40,75	23,50	-0,41
Calibration	1001	1	18.05.1947	OS	0	566,00	2,62	3,19	4,46	23,14	7,51	7,47	150,00	6,23	12,08	0,41	0,27	23,18	4,84	43,91	21,50	-0,35
Calibration	1002	1	22.11.1990	OS	0	493,00	3,48	3,97	4,50	23,48	7,69	7,54	171,00	6,33	12,41	0,41	0,27	23,50	5,39	43,17	22,00	-0,09
Calibration	1003	1	12.06.1934	OS	0	556,00	2,73	3,29	4,86	23,80	7,99	7,50	79,00	6,44	11,95	0,41	0,27	23,79	5,05	42,46	21,00	0,06
Calibration	1004	1	29.03.1929	OD	0	515,00	3,08	3,60	4,46	24,49	7,98	7,89	86,00	6,60	12,95	0,41	0,27	24,47	5,13	41,43	20,50	-0,23
Calibration	1005	1	18.05.1954	OS	0	566,00	2,90	3,47	4,62	24,31	7,74	7,66	80,00	6,40	11,92	0,41	0,27	24,29	5,13	42,71	19,50	-0,35
Calibration	1006	1	13.09.1965	OD	0	637,00	1,82	2,46	4,19	20,43	7,92	7,58	177,00	6,44	11,64	0,41	0,27	20,59	4,06	42,45	33,50	-0,85
Calibration	1007	1	07.11.1945	OS	0	506,00	2,93	3,44	4,93	22,90	7,67	7,52	100,00	6,31	11,83	0,41	0,27	22,92	5,17	43,29	23,50	0,10
Calibration	1008	1	19.03.1940	OD	0	565,00	2,70	3,27	4,56	23,56	7,91	7,72	103,00	6,50	12,41	0,41	0,27	23,57	4,91	42,08	22,50	-0,24
Calibration	1009	1	30.06.1929	OD	0	568,00	2,23	2,80	4,94	23,19	8,12	7,90	114,00	6,66	11,24	0,41	0,27	23,20	4,70	41,05	25,00	-0,29
Calibration	1010	1	07.11.1933	OS	0	578,00	2,64	3,22	4,50	23,55	8,04	7,91	162,00	6,63	12,95	0,41	0,27	23,57	4,84	41,23	23,50	-0,21
Calibration	1011	1	26.10.1942	OD	0	521,00	1,67	2,19	4,93	22,02	7,43	7,35	138,00	6,14	11,91	0,41	0,27	22,08	4,31	44,49	24,50	-0,67
Calibration	1012	1	16.01.1941	OS	0	602,00	1,99	2,59	5,31	23,24	8,02	7,76	126,00	6,56	12,19	0,41	0,27	23,22	4,73	41,68	24,00	-0,23
Calibration	1013	1	23.09.1927	OD	0	576,00	1,74	2,32	5,53	22,41	7,62	7,58	47,00	6,32	11,90	0,41	0,27	22,42	4,64	43,27	25,00	-0,31
Calibration	1014	1	13.10.1941	OD	0	540,00	2,46	3,00	4,80	22,87	7,56	7,50	109,00	6,26	11,94	0,41	0,27	22,90	4,84	43,67	22,50	-0,03
Calibration	1015	1	17.05.1938	OS	0	592,00	2,87	3,46	4,13	23,05	7,84	7,76	113,00	6,48	11,96	0,41	0,27	23,11	4,85	42,16	24,00	-0,18
Calibration	1016	1	01.11.1943	OD	0	550,00	3,45	4,00	4,75	25,18	8,14	8,02	179,00	6,72	13,73	0,41	0,27	25,12	5,54	40,69	19,50	0,12
Calibration	1017	1	29.06.1951	OD	0	564,00	1,91	2,47	4,59	22,61	7,90	7,82	11,00	6,53	12,06	0,41	0,27	22,66	4,34	41,83	25,50	-0,49
Calibration	1018	1	27.07.1968	OD	0	558,00	2,85	3,41	4,14	26,68	8,25	8,00	7,00	6,75	12,69	0,41	0,27	26,59	4,94	40,47	14,50	0,00
Calibration	1019	1	31.05.1933	OD	0	538,00	2,68	3,22	4,77	23,52	7,62	7,46	91,00	6,27	11,94	0,41	0,27	23,52	5,00	43,61	20,50	-0,09
Calibration	1020	1	22.06.1936	OD	0	497,00	2,74	3,24	4,42	23,78	7,51	7,40	93,00	6,20	11,66	0,41	0,27	23,79	4,49	44,10	18,50	-0,03
Calibration	1021	1	17.06.1944	OS	0	553,00	2,30	2,85	4,71	23,32	7,96	7,84	90,00	6,57	12,36	0,41	0,27	23,33	4,67	41,62	23,50	-0,20
Calibration	1022	1	11.09.1935	OD	0	557,00	2,66	3,22	4,99	24,53	8,00	7,66	101,00	6,51	12,18	0,41	0,27	24,48	5,09	41,99	19,50	-0,16
Calibration	1023	1	05.02.1957	OS	0	514,00	2,24	2,75	4,83	23,79	8,29	8,16	138,00	6,84	11,96	0,41	0,27	23,78	4,63	39,96	24,00	-0,20
Calibration	1024	1	30.12.1944	OS	0	495,00	3,48	3,98	4,34	26,34	8,50	8,32	79,00	6,99	12,17	0,41	0,27	26,25	5,36	39,08	18,00	-0,02
Calibration	1025	1	17.05.1950	OS	0	574,00	2,03	2,60	5,04	22,66	7,53	7,31	116,00	6,17	12,24	0,41	0,27	22,68	4,66	44,33	22,50	-0,33
Calibration	1026	1	29.12.1936	OS	0	547,00	2,74	3,29	4,33	24,29	7,68	7,50	50,00	6,31	13,18	0,41	0,27	24,28	4,89	43,32	18,00	-0,17
Calibration	1027	1	12.02.1981	OS	0	639,00	3,38	4,02	3,77	26,49	7,70	7,67	62,00	6,39	12,47	0,41	0,27	26,42	5,27	42,81	12,50	-0,34
Calibration	1028	1	19.11.1946	OS	0	563,00	2,62	3,18	4,57	22,45	7,59	7,40	13,00	6,23	11,90	0,41	0,27	22,51	4,84	43,88	24,00	-0,14
Calibration	1029	1	15.08.1926	OS	0	522,00	2,15	2,67	5,27	24,05	8,21	7,21	170,00	6,41	12,33	0,41	0,27	24,00	4,78	42,64	19,50	0,03

constants optimized on real refraction data so far

J&J ZCB00	91		0,41	0,25
Alcon SA60AT	296		0,37	0,00
Alcon Clareon	40		0,40	0,24
B&L MX60	136		0,42	0,01
Hoya Vivinex	30		0,40	0,14
J&J AAB00	85		0,39	-0,15

Table 38.1 Optimized constants C and R as used in the BJO paper (old ELP regression)

IOL	Optic	Haptic	C	R	Sample size
Alcon Clareon	Aspheric	1 piece planar C	0.40	0.24	40
Alcon Acrysof SA60AT/SN60AT	Spheric	1 piece planar C	0.37	0.00	296
B&L EnVista MX60	Aspheric neutral	1 piece planar C	0.42	−0.02	243
Hoya Vivinex	Aspheric	1 piece planar C	0.40	0.14	30
J&J AAB00	Spheric	1 piece stepped C	0.39	−0.15	85
J&J ZCB00	Aspheric	1 piece stepped C	0.41	0.24	91

Table 38.2 Optimized with two/three constants C, (H), and R using the new ELP regression. 3-way optimization for $n < 50$ is not sensible. Any result with $n < 50$ should be used with caution. In parenthesis: improvement of variance of 3-way vs. 2-way optimization

IOL	Optic	Haptic	C	H	R	Sample size
Alcon Acrysof SA60AT/ SN60AT	Spheric	1 piece planar C	0.34 0.34	0.00 0.01	0.07 0.05	296 (< 0.1%)
Alcon Clareon	Aspheric	1 piece planar C	0.35 –	0.00 –	0.40 –	40
B&L EnVista MX60	Aspheric neutral	1 piece planar C	0.41 0.36	0.00 0.50	−0.01 −0.45	243 (5.6%)
Hoya Vivinex	Aspheric	1 piece planar C	0.40	0.00	0.00	30
J&J AAB00	Spheric	1 piece stepped C	0.390 0.42	0.00 −0.20	−0.28 −0.22	85 (1.7%)
J&J ZCB00	Aspheric	1 piece stepped C	0.43 0.42	0.00 0.10	−0.07 −0.14	91 (0.8%)

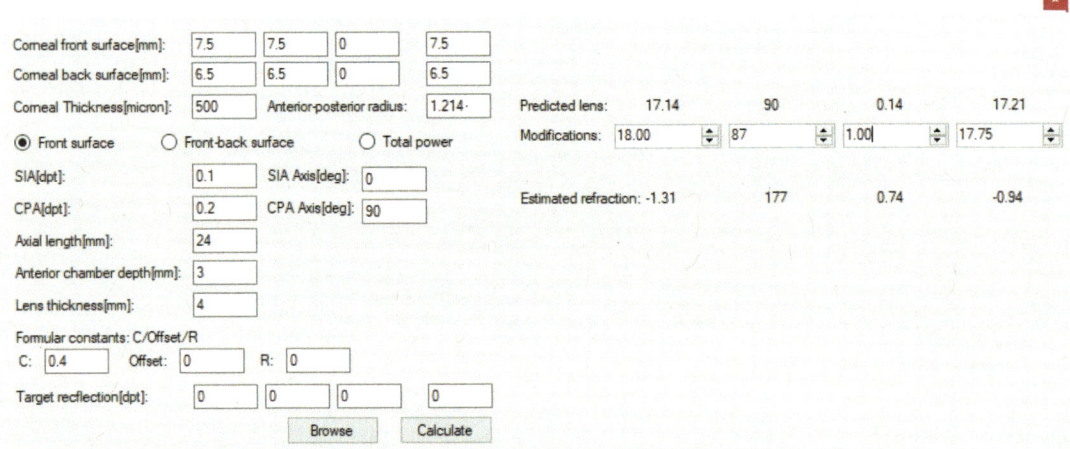

Fig. 38.4 Screenshot of stand-alone software written by Langenbucher. It is possible to import spreadsheets for batch processing

References

1. Fyodorov SN, Kolinko AI. Estimation of optical power of the intraocular lens. Vestn Oftalmol. 1967;4:27.
2. Gernet H, Ostholt H, Werner H. Die präoperative Berechnung intraocularer Binkhorst-Linsen. In: 122. Versammlung des Vereins Rheinisch-Westfälischer Augenärzte. Balve: Zimmermann; 1970. p. 54–5.
3. Liou HL, Brennan NA. Anatomically accurate, finite model eye for optical modeling. J Opt Soc Am A Opt Image Sci Vis. 1997;14(8):1684–95.
4. Olsen T, Hoffmann PC. C constant: new concept for ray tracing-assisted intraocular lens power calculation. J Cataract Refract Surg. 2014;40(5):764–73.
5. Wendelstein J, Hoffmann PC, Hirnschall N, Fischinger IR, Mariacher S, Wingert T, et al. Project hyperopic power prediction: accuracy of 13 different concepts for intraocular lens calculation in short eyes. Br J Ophthalmol. 2021;106(6):795–801.
6. Haigis W, Lege B, Miller N, Schneider B. Comparison of immersion ultrasound biometry and partial coherence interferometry for intraocular lens calculation according to Haigis. Graefes Arch Clin Exp Ophthalmol. 2000;238(9):765–73.
7. Cooke DL, Cooke TL. Approximating sum-of-segments axial length from a traditional optical low-coherence reflectometry measurement. J Cataract Refract Surg. 2019;45(3):351–4.
8. Langenbucher A, Szentmáry N, Wendelstein J, Hoffmann PC. Artificial intelligence, machine learn-

ing and calculation of intraocular lens power. Klin Monatsbl Augenheilkd. 2020;237(12):1430–7.

9. Langenbucher A, Szentmáry N, Cayless A, Müller M, Eppig T, Schröder S, et al. IOL formula constants - strategies for optimization and defining standards for presenting data. Ophthalmic Res. 2021;64(6):1055–67.

10. Haigis W. IOL calculation according to Haigis [Internet]. 1996 [cited 2012 Jan 25]. http://www.augenklinik.uni-wuerzburg.de/uslab/ioltxt/haie.htm.

11. Holladay JT, Prager TC, Chandler TY, Musgrove KH, Lewis JW, Ruiz RS. A three-part system for refining intraocular lens power calculations. J Cataract Refract Surg. 1988;14(1):17–24.

12. Retzlaff JA, Sanders DR, Kraff MC. Development of the SRK/T intraocular lens power calculation formula. J Cataract Refract Surg. 1990;16:333–40. Errata: 1990;16:528 and 1993;19(5):444–446.

13. Kane JX, Melles RB. Intraocular lens formula comparison in axial hyperopia with a high-power intraocular lens of 30 or more diopters. J Cataract Refract Surg. 2020;46(9):1236–9.

14. Melles RB, Kane JX, Olsen T, Chang WJ. Update on intraocular lens calculation formulas. Ophthalmology. 2019;126(9):1334–5.

15. Hipólito-Fernandes D, Elisa Luís M, Gil P, Maduro V, Feijão J, Yeo TK, et al. VRF-G, a new intraocular lens power calculation formula: a 13-formulas comparison study. Clin Ophthalmol. 2020;14:4395–402.

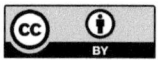

CSO IOL Calculation Module

39

Gabriele Vestri, Francesco Versaci,
Giacomo Savini, and Jaime Aramberri

Historically, the refining process of IOL (Intraocular Lens) calculation has passed through classes of formulas, which more and more accurately have determined the spherical power of an intraocular lens, but, at the same time, have lost adherence to the physical laws, which rule the behaviour of light. As an extreme consequence of this trend, a new family of IOL calculation formulas completely based on deep learning has been recently proposed: in this outermost case, the deterministic optical approach is completely neglected and the IOL power is the output of a neural network.

In a parallel pathway during the latest decades, ray-tracing methods have taken hold in physics and engineering for optical design and analysis. This approach calculates the path of rays of light through a sequence of regions with different refractive indices [1]. Simple problems can be analysed by propagating a few rays, while a more detailed analysis requires a computer to simulate many rays. This approach allows at the same time a return to the physics of light propagation and, if accurate input data are available, to customize the IOL calculation for each patient.

The most famous IOL calculation formulas are mainly modified versions of the Gaussian formulas for a diopter followed by a thin lens. The eye is simply modelled as a spherical diopter with power equal to the average keratometry, which is calculated using only the anterior corneal radius and a refractive index that is not the stromal one, but a weighted version of that of the stroma and of the aqueous. This is a trick to include the effect of the posterior corneal radius when this measurement is not available, but this is a valid approximation only if the ratio between the anterior and the posterior corneal radii (Gullstrand's ratio) is that of the average eye (i.e. 1.22). Therefore, most of the IOL formulas neglect the measurement of the posterior corneal surface. This was surely necessary when tomographers were not available on the market. Moreover, they consider the intraocular lens as a thin lens with zero thickness characterized by a certain value of power.

Basic Concepts

CSO's (Costruzione Strumenti Oftalmici) approach to IOL calculation is an attempt to apply the most advanced engineering calculation method to this problem. The IOL module was made avail-

G. Vestri (✉) · F. Versaci
CSO s.r.l., Florence, Italy
e-mail: g.vestri@csoitalia.it; f.versaci@csoitalia.it

G. Savini
IRCCS Bietti Foundation, Rome, Italy

Studio Oculistico d'Azeglio, Bologna, Italy
e-mail: giacomo.savini@startmail.com

J. Aramberri
Clínica Miranza Begitek, San Sebastian, Spain

Clínica Miranza Ókular, Vitoria, Spain
e-mail: jaimearamberri@telefonica.it

© The Author(s) 2024

J. Aramberri et al. (eds.), *Intraocular Lens Calculations*, Essentials in Ophthalmology,
https://doi.org/10.1007/978-3-031-50666-6_39

able first in 2011 for Sirius, CSO's anterior segment tomographer, which combines Placido disc and Scheimpflug camera and, then, in 2017 for MS-39, CSO's anterior segment tomographer, which integrates Placido disc with optical coherence tomography (OCT) technology.

The measured data of the ocular anterior segment, i.e. the altimetric data of the anterior and posterior corneal surfaces and of the iris, are used in combination with the altimetric data of the intraocular lens to build a three-dimensional model of the eye. In this way, the corneal surfaces are considered with their possible asymmetry, tilt, decentration and irregularities. The intraocular lenses are modelled using the nominal parameters provided by the manufacturers, their thickness is no longer neglected and possible aspherical profiles can be taken into account as well as possible toric shapes.

For each simulated ray entering the pupil of the eye, the software calculates its intersection with the first corneal surface (Fig. 39.1). At this point, it applies Snell's refraction law to get the direction of the refracted ray by knowing the incident ray, the normal of the first corneal surface at their intersection point and the refractive indices of air and stroma. The refracted ray is traced towards the posterior corneal surface and their intersection is calculated. At this point, Snell's refraction law is newly applied to get the direction of the refracted ray in the aqueous towards the intraocular lens. This procedure is applied to every other optical interface between cornea and retina, i.e. to the surfaces of the intraocular lens.

Once the path of a bundle of rays from the outside of the eye to its retina is known, it is possible to determine the wavefront error of the examined eye by subtracting the optical path length of the whole bundle of rays from that of an ideal aberration-free optical system.

In addition to defocus and astigmatism or, in other words, refraction (sphere, cylinder, axis and spherical equivalent), a great amount of optical information of the analysed eye can be extracted from the wavefront error:

- *Refractive map*: this map shows the refractive error for any ray passing through the pupil. This is useful to evaluate the presence of possible defocus, astigmatism and asymmetries in the optical ocular system.
- *Point spread function (PSF)*: the PSF is the impulse response of an optical system (in this case the eye after the IOL implant) to a luminous infinitesimal spot at an infinite distance. It provides the clinician with a visual method to understand the effect of aberrations on the ocular system. Ideally, the PSF should be a tiny circular point for an aberration-free optical system. Its shape is distorted and its dimen-

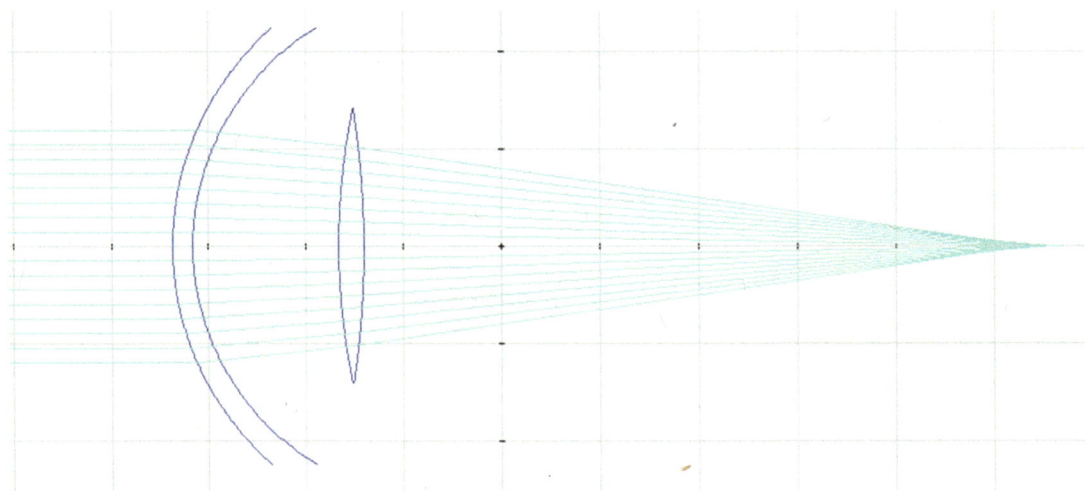

Fig. 39.1 Ray tracing: two-dimensional simplified model of cornea and IOL

sions are enlarged by the presence of aberrations. For example, astigmatism tends to make the PSF a line whose orientation is the direction of the astigmatism; coma gives it the aspect of a comet. Just to keep in mind a numerical reference, the size of the PSF should be less than 1′ for getting a visual acuity of 1.0 or less than 0.5′ for getting a visual acuity of 2.0.

- *Focusing chart:* this chart contains, for the selected intraocular lens, the curve for the merit figure of visual acuity obtained with various corrections of the sphere (Fig. 39.2). From a different point of view, the focusing chart shows how the visual acuity varies at the various distances of the observed object. This chart is therefore useful to evaluate the depth of field for the pseudo-phakic eye. The wider the curve, the wider the interval where visual acuity is kept near its best-corrected value. The higher the curve, the higher the best-corrected visual acuity. The dotted curve shows the diffraction-limited case, i.e. the ideal limit of an aberration-free system. This constitutes a superior limit, which cannot be reached by real eyes. Of course, the simulation does not consider the neurological component of vision, but only the optical one.

The ray-tracing calculation is done by the software for each available power of the selected IOL model. The previous results are shown for the lens, which best satisfies the requirement of the target equivalent sphere chosen by the surgeon. They can also be consulted by the user for the lenses whose powers are included in an interval centred on the power of the best lens. If the IOL model is toric, the software also makes the results available for each of the available IOL cylinders. The software proposes the axis of the astigmatic component of the WFE (wavefront error) as the default option for the IOL orientation. The user can manually change this axis if necessary.

Ignoring the complexity of the whole wavefront, paraxial IOL formulas can only provide the predicted spherical equivalent or, at most, a predicted cylinder applying the same method to two ocular meridians. It is obvious that this prediction is reliable only if the ocular surfaces (anterior corneal surface, posterior corneal surface and IOL) are regular toric surfaces, aligned on the same axis, with no tilt, with the same orientation of their principal axes or, at least, there are no significant deviations from the previous ideal conditions.

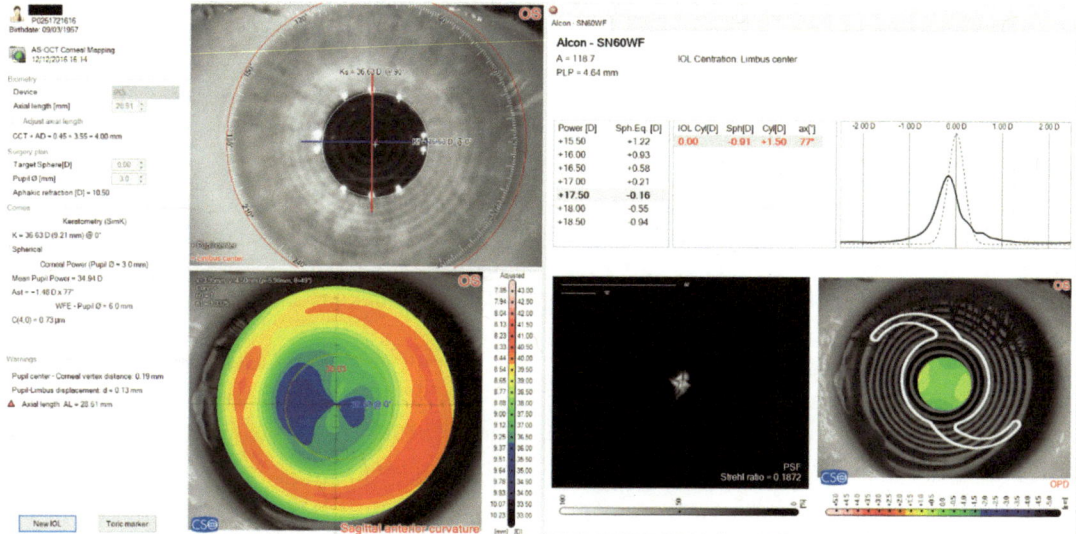

Fig. 39.2 IOL calculation screen. Left column: relevant indices. Central column: iris frontal view with SimK values and sagittal curvature map. Right column with four different sections: IOL power and expected spherical equivalent and refraction data (top left); focusing chart (top right); PSF (bottom left); OPD or refractive error map (bottom right)

Prediction of the IOL Position

One of the most important sources of the refractive error in the selection of the IOL power is certainly the prediction error of the IOL postoperative position.

Third- and fourth-generation formulas generally try to predict this value by multiple regression analysis based on parameters such as the preoperative axial length, corneal curvature radius, anterior chamber depth, crystalline lens thickness and so on. Their predicted value ELP (Effective Lens Position) is not a real geometric distance between two ocular optical interfaces, but is a fictitious distance of the thin lens from the corneal vertex and serves only to make the calculation effective. Because of its nature, it cannot even be checked by a measurement in the postoperative tomographic examination.

On the contrary, when a ray-tracing approach or paraxial thick lens formulas are adopted, it is necessary to predict the real position of the implanted lens. CSO's software makes this prediction by considering some iris points on the external perimeter of the iris, which are used to calculate a best-fit plane whose tilt and position are used as an estimation of the plane where the IOL will lie after the implant. In the case of Sirius, the fitted points are the vertices of the iridocorneal angles, i.e. the intersection points between the posterior corneal surface and the anterior surface of the iris. In the case of MS-39, the fitted points are the intersection points between the anterior surface of the iris and the line passing through the scleral spur and perpendicular to the posterior corneal surface. The position of the best-fit plane is then adjusted by the A-constant, which is an indicator of the "position trend" of a certain IOL model. The predicted value PLP (which stands for Predicted Lens Position) is a real geometric distance, i.e. the distance between the posterior corneal surface and the anterior surface of the IOL.

Performing the IOL Power Calculation

The IOL calculation module is launched from the IOL icon in the main menu display. The screen is divided into three sections (Fig. 39.2). The left one contains the main indices involved in IOL power calculation: biometry figures, where the user has to input manually the axial length and choose the type of biometer (partial coherence interferometry or immersion/applanation ultrasound); surgical plan, where target refraction and pupil size are selected; corneal powers, both keratometry and raytraced total values. The central column contains two graphic representations: the SimK indices over the iris frontal image and a selectable corneal map, either the keratometry or the total refractive power. The right column is the space where the results of the optical calculation are shown.

Once the axial length is input and target refraction and pupil size are accepted, the software allows to choose the IOL model. In this window, the IOL constant is checked and the predicted lens position (PLP) is calculated. Sometimes, the software cannot satisfactorily identify the angle structures (scleral spur and iris root in the case of MS-39 or iridocorneal angles in the case of Sirius) and requires manual editing to give way to the PLP calculation (Fig. 39.3). After that, the above-mentioned results show up in the right column of the screen distributed in four panels:

- The selected IOL and the predicted refractive result, both in spherical equivalent and sphere-cylinder notation;
- The PSF display with the calculated Strehl ratio;
- The OPD (optical path difference) or WFE (wavefront error) map (or the refractive error map) calculated for the measured pupil;
- The focusing chart.

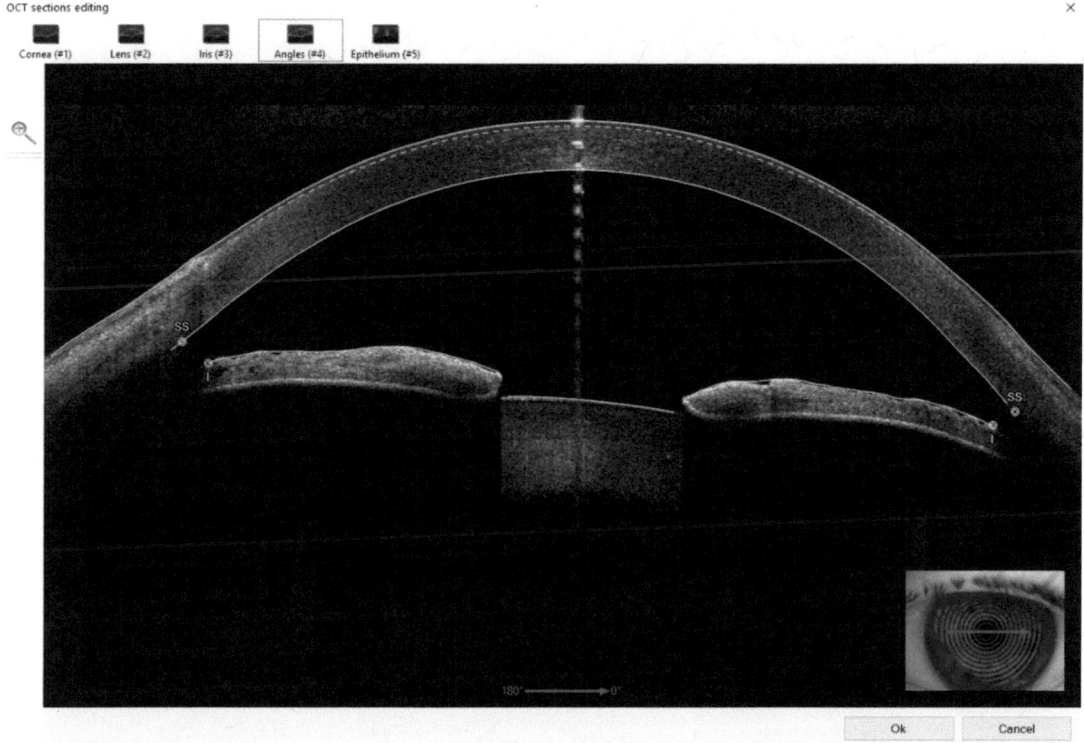

Fig. 39.3 Scleral spur (SS) and iris root (I) manual identification

Examples of Application

CSO's IOL module was created to manage a wide range of eyes, in particular those that underwent corneal refractive surgery [2] and highly astigmatic and/or irregular corneas.

In post-refractive surgery cases, the traditional IOL formulas are affected by three main sources of errors. First, inaccurate estimation of corneal power from the keratometry of anterior corneal surface occurs when the classical keratometric index of 1.3375 is adopted ("keratometric index error"). Second, if the chosen keratometry is SimK, corneal power is extracted from the values of the axial curvature map in a paracentral ring-shaped zone, which may partially overlap with the surgical transition zone in cases where the optical zone is small or decentred ("radius error"). Third, incorrect estimation of the ELP by thin-lens IOL power calculation formulas occurs when the post-refractive surgery anterior corneal radius is used as a predictive factor, such as in the

case of the Hoffer Q, Holladay 1, Holladay 2 and SRK/T formulas ("formula error"). This leads to an underestimation of the ELP and thus of IOL power, which results in postoperative hyperopia. To overcome these problems, several methods have been proposed. For example, the Double-K method [3] uses the anterior corneal radius before refractive surgery to estimate the ELP and its value after refractive surgery for the IOL power calculation by the vergence formula. Although it is a reliable method, it requires the knowledge of historical data and, if those are unavailable, the method cannot be applied. Conversely, CSO's method is not influenced by the keratometric index error, because it applies ray tracing to the measured three-dimensional height data of corneal surfaces with the proper refractive index for each ocular medium. In addition, the prediction for IOL position is not impaired by previous refractive surgery, because it does not consider the anterior corneal curvature, but it is based on iris reference points, which are not modified by

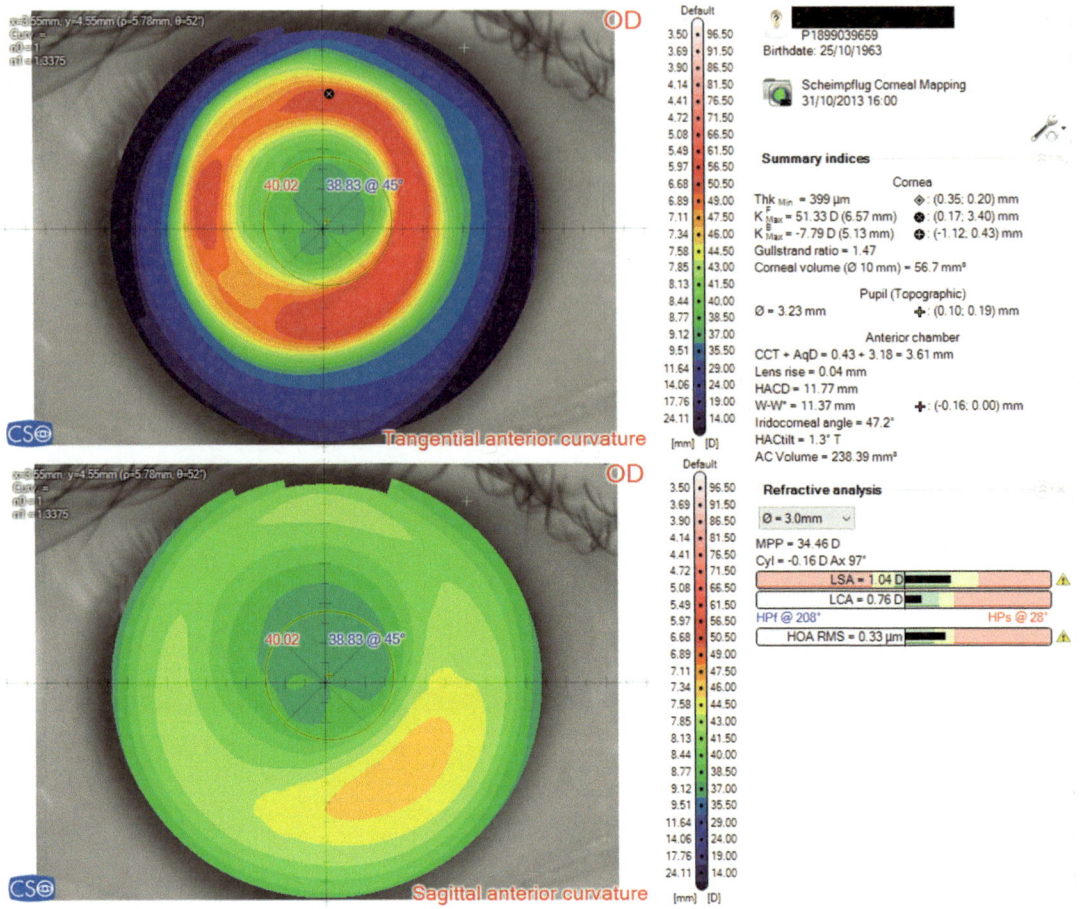

Fig. 39.4 Post-LASIK surgery case

this kind of surgery. The prediction error of the IOL position is therefore theoretically the same in all kinds of eyes.

In Fig. 39.4, the case of a myopic eye, which underwent LASIK surgery, is shown. The tangential curvature maps clearly show that the optical zone is neither very well centred with respect to the corneal vertex nor to the pupil vertex. The average value for the SimK is 39.42 D; the mean pupil power, which is the total corneal power calculated through ray tracing within the pupil diameter of 3 mm, is 34.46 D. This big difference is due to the calculation zone for the SimK, which is an annulus centred on the corneal vertex with internal and external radii of about 1 and 1.8 mm, respectively, on an average cornea (Fig. 39.5). In this case, as in many other cases, the calculation zone includes a portion of the surgical transition zone where the curvatures are steep, and this portion is not in the pupillary zone when the pupil is in photopic conditions. This is a further reason, in addition to the invalid hypothesis beyond the keratometry index (Gullstrand ratio is here 1.47), which makes the SimK value a wrong choice for the IOL calculation in this case and similar ones.

CSO's software considers the portion of the cornea within the actual pupil of the patient to perform ray tracing. The axial length of this eye was 30.28 mm and it was chosen to implant an Alcon SN60WF with a power of 17 D. The PLP was 4.31 mm while the real position turned out to be 4.41 mm. This denotes good behaviour of the predictive algorithm for the IOL position. The predicted refraction was $-2.59 + 0.21 \times 180$,

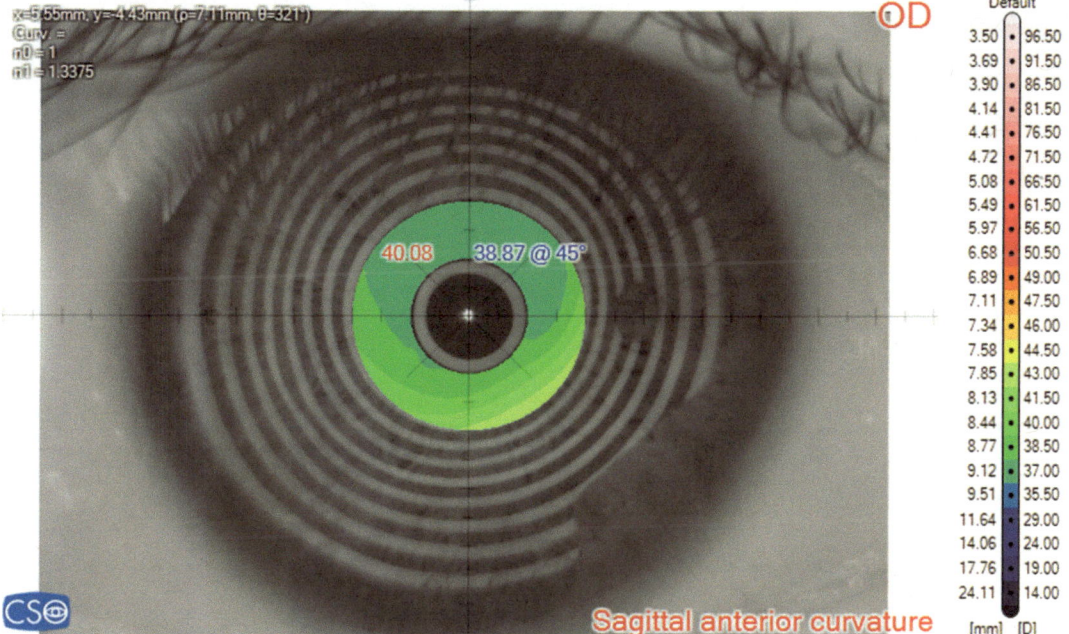

Fig. 39.5 Annular region of sagittal (axial) curvature map used to calculate the values of SimK. The annulus, centred on the corneal vertex with internal and external radii of about 1 and 1.8 mm on an average cornea, includes a portion of the surgical transition zone where the curvatures are steep. The values of SimK are not a proper choice for IOL calculation also because they include the effect of the surgical transition zone, which is external to the pupil region in photopic conditions

which is rather similar to the measured subjective refraction $-2.75 + 0.5 \times 5$.

Another typical case where the IOL module can be useful is shown in Fig. 39.6. This is the case of an eye, which underwent PRK (photorefractive keratectomy) to correct a hyperopic defect of about 3 D. The Gullstrand ratio is here 1.11, quite lower than the mean normal value. Even in this case, the calculation assumptions of keratometry, in particular the value of the keratometric index, lose their validity. Furthermore, the value of curvature modified by PRK leads many formulas to a wrong prediction of the IOL position. CSO's predicted position (3.57 mm), which is based on anatomical structures not altered by surgery, was close to the actual one (3.69 mm). The predicted refraction was $-1.82 + 0.93 \times 106$ (Fig. 39.7), while the subjective refraction was $-1.50 + 0.75 \times 90$. The equivalent spherical error was -0.23 D and could be almost zeroed if we would input the actual position in the software. In this case, it appears that the residual error on

refraction can be fully ascribed to the error on the estimated IOL position.

As regards astigmatic corneas, CSO's method is able to manage correctly both anterior and posterior corneal surfaces, which may be not coaxial, have a different orientation of the astigmatism and a pupil position relatively displaced from the corneal vertex.

The case shown in Fig. 39.8 is an eye with a toric cornea. The total corneal astigmatism calculated through the WFE over a pupil diameter of 3 mm is with-the-rule $+3.36 \times 114$ and derives from the contributions of the anterior and posterior components, respectively, $+3.78 \times 113$ and $+0.44 \times 16$.

The implant of a non-toric intraocular lens would leave a cylinder too high to be borne by the patient without the help of spectacles or contact lenses. This is clear from the refraction table and, for an expert eye, from the OPD/WFE map. The use of a toric IOL would allow cancelling almost totally the cylinder. The predicted

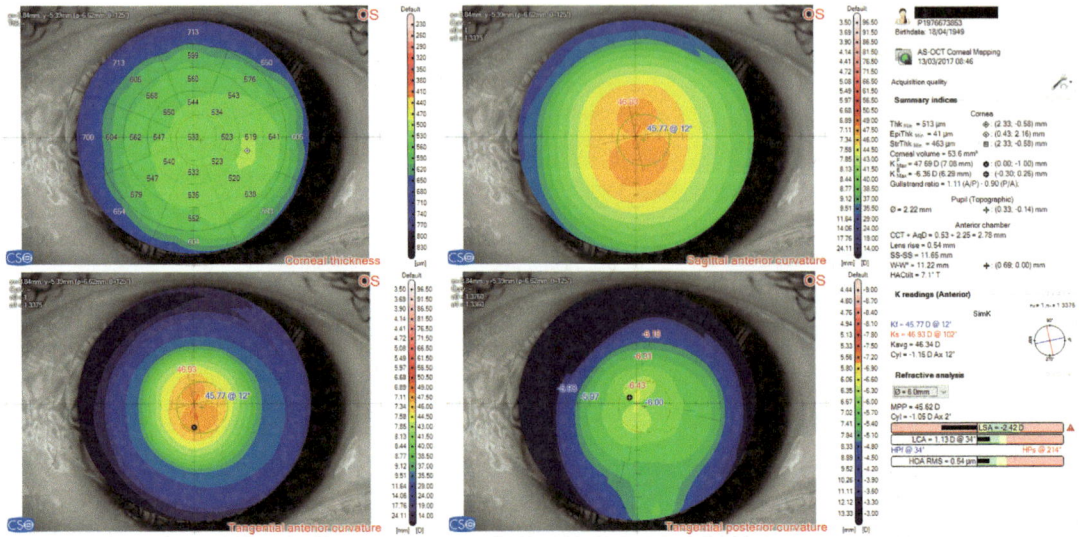

Fig. 39.6 Overview of the topographic maps for an eye, which underwent PRK in order to correct a hyperopic defect

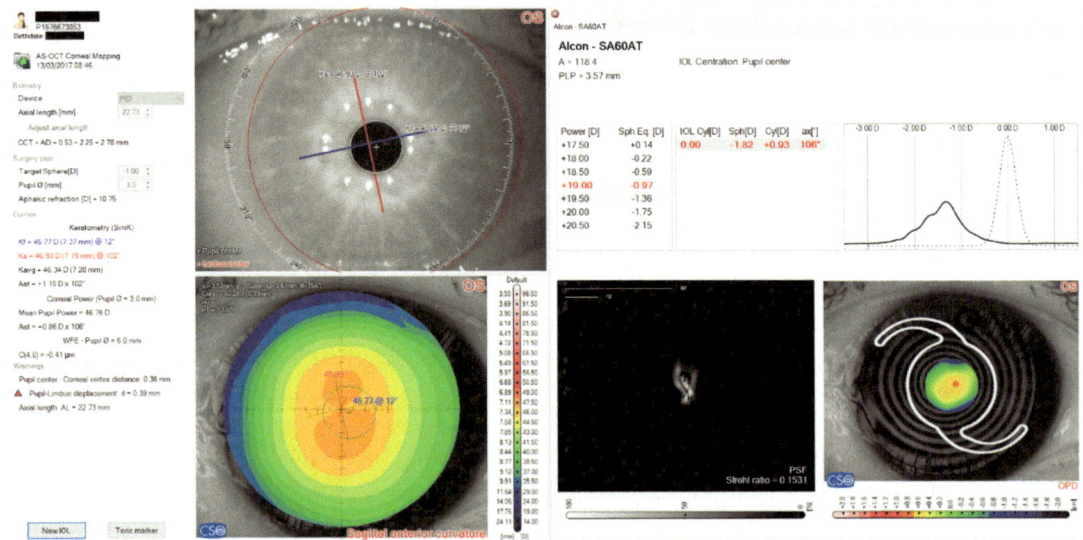

Fig. 39.7 IOL calculation for the eye, which underwent PRK in order to correct a hyperopic defect

refraction is −1.05 + 0.37 × 110 with an IOL cylinder of 4.5 D (Fig. 39.9). Unfortunately, the clinician chose to implant a cylinder (−3.75 D) inferior to the one suggested by this software and the patient showed a residual cylinder of 1 D after the IOL implant (−1 + 1 × 125). This case shows a very good agreement between the actual subjective refraction and the one predicted by the software, as it appears in the residual cylinder of +0.88 x 112 calculated for the

IOL with a cylinder equal to the implanted value.

CSO's IOL module is also theoretically designed to manage correctly even more irregular corneas like the keratoconic or post-graft ones. Eyes after DMEK (Descemet Membrane Endothelial Keratoplasty) or DSAEK (Descemet's Stripping Automated Endothelial Keratoplasty) are likely to suffer problems similar to those of post-refractive surgery eyes when

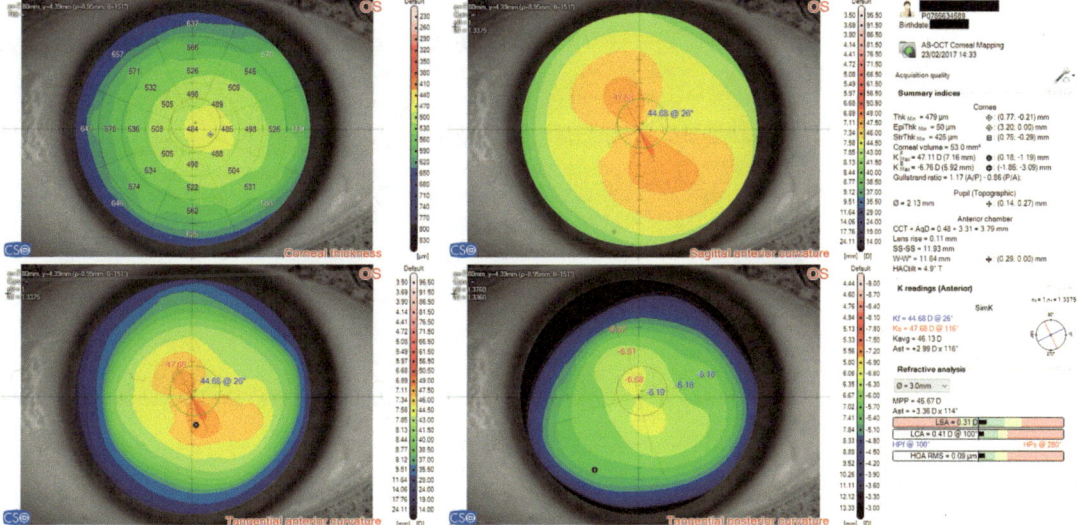

Fig. 39.8 Overview of the topographic maps for a toric cornea

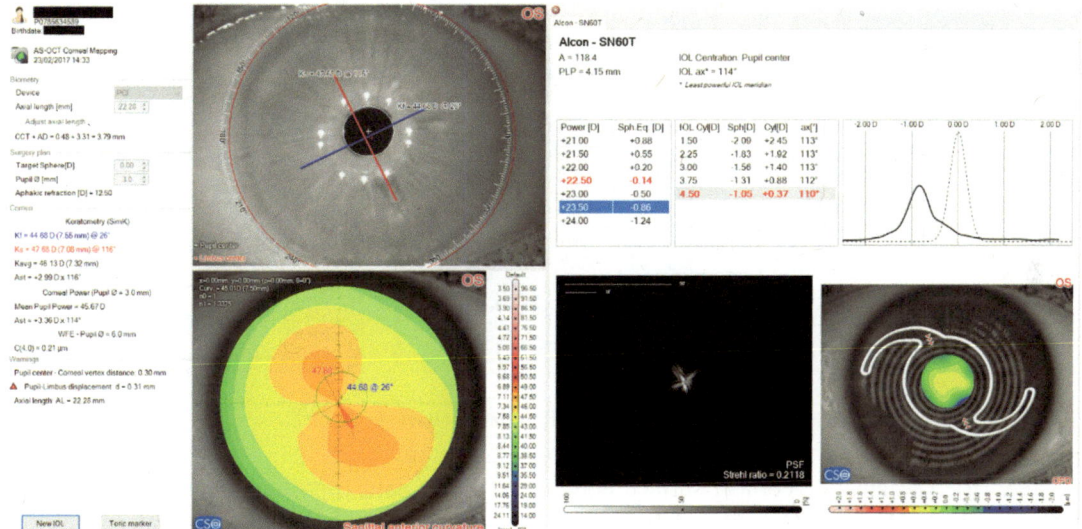

Fig. 39.9 IOL calculation for a toric cornea where a toric model was chosen for the implant. The table at the centre of the screen contains the predicted spherical equivalent for the various IOL powers; the table at its right contains the predicted refraction for each cylinder of the selected IOL power

keratometry values are adopted as corneal power. Of course, in these cases, the measurements may be affected by more severe measurement errors, which decrease the reliability of the calculations. Nonetheless, it is to be noticed that in all these cases, the aberrations are so high that we cannot hope to reach a good visual acuity by simply correcting the sphere and cylinder through an IOL. The software is able to highlight these cases by showing an irregular wavefront error and a flat focusing chart, which can be a useful indication for the surgeon of poor expectations for the visual acuity of the patient.

The next case we present in this chapter is an eye, which underwent an endothelial transplantation (DSAEK) before the cataract surgery

Fig. 39.10 OCT section of the eye, which underwent DSAEK before cataract surgery. The donor tissue is clearly visible below the patient's posterior corneal surface

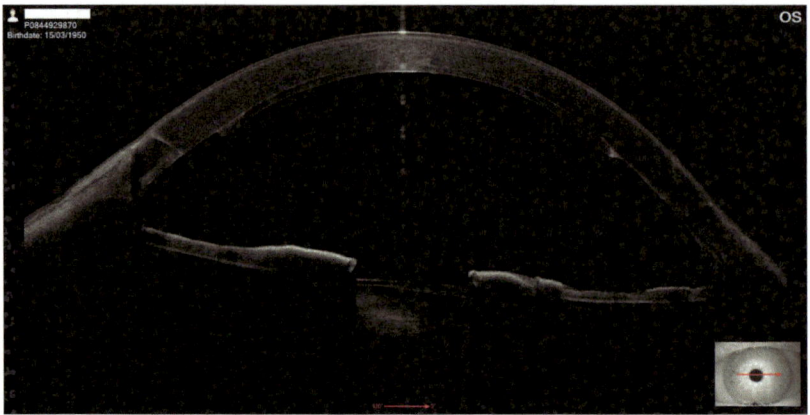

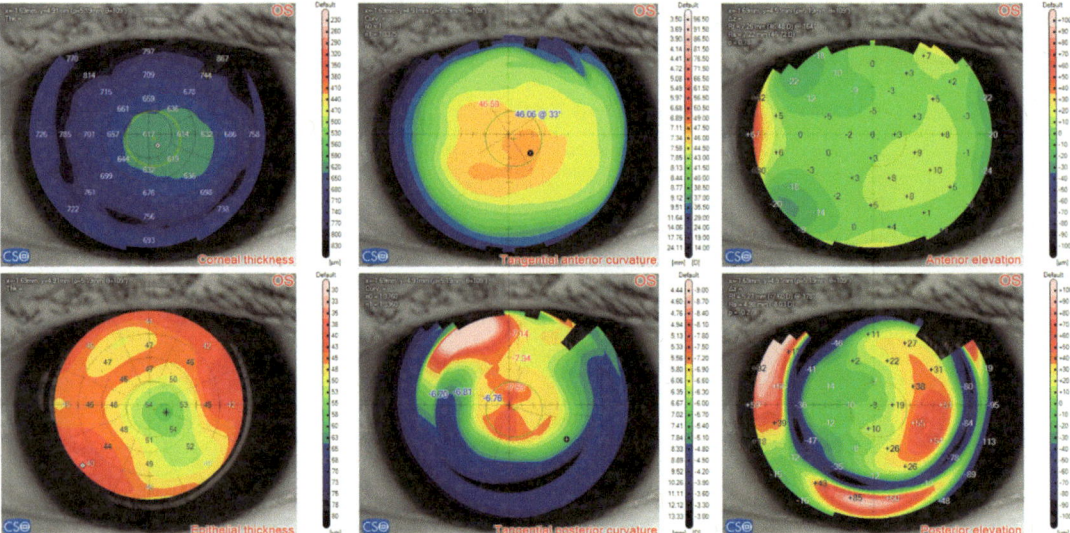

Fig. 39.11 Overview of the eye, which underwent DSAEK before cataract surgery

(Fig. 39.10). The anterior corneal surface does not exhibit particular anomalies. It is a bit steeper than the average cornea and has a certain degree of asymmetry along the vertical direction (Fig. 39.11). The posterior corneal surface has a rather high degree of toricity, which translates into a not negligible astigmatic component of the wavefront error + 0.81 × 4 (Fig. 39.12). The anterior astigmatic component is +1.06 × 74. The two astigmatic components out of phase of 70° produce a total corneal astigmatism of +0.67 × 50. The Gullstrand ratio between the anterior and the posterior curvature is 1.29. The implanted IOL was an AMO Tecnis1 ZCB00 with a power of 23 D. The predicted IOL position was 4.68 mm while the actual position was verified to be 4.49 mm after the implant. The refraction predicted by the software was −0.52 + 0.67 × 50 (Fig. 39.13) in good agreement with the subjective refraction after the surgery, which was 0 + 0.50 × 60. Even though the transplant altered the posterior corneal surface and introduced new aberrations (astigmatism in particular), greater than those of a normal unoperated eye, the software was not misled in the correct choice of the IOL.

The next example is the eye of an airplane pilot, who underwent RK (radial keratotomy) in 1989. He had a good visual quality until 2017, when he began to see the peripheral cuts of the

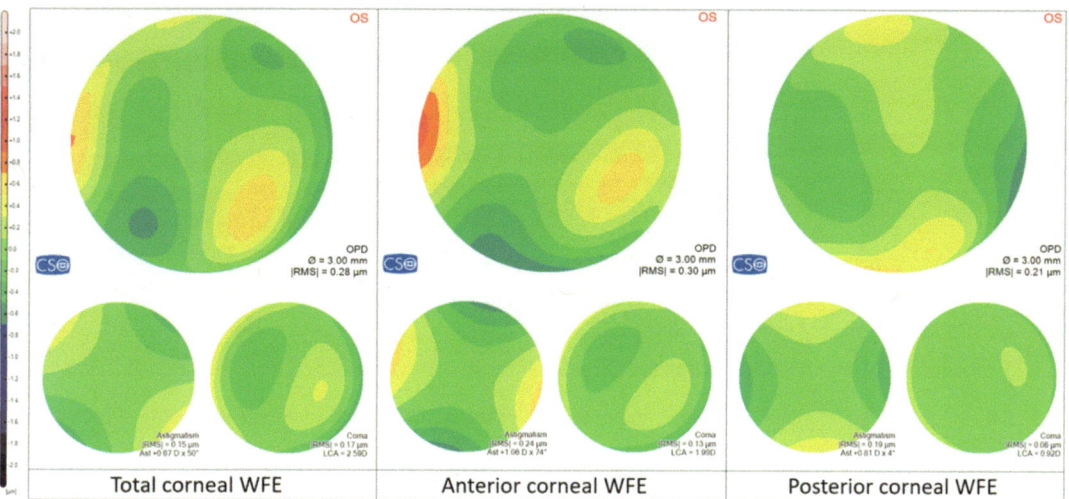

Fig. 39.12 DSAEK case: total corneal wavefront error and its contributions from anterior and posterior corneal surfaces. The smaller maps at the bottom of the image show the components of astigmatism and coma for each of the WFEs shown at the top of the image

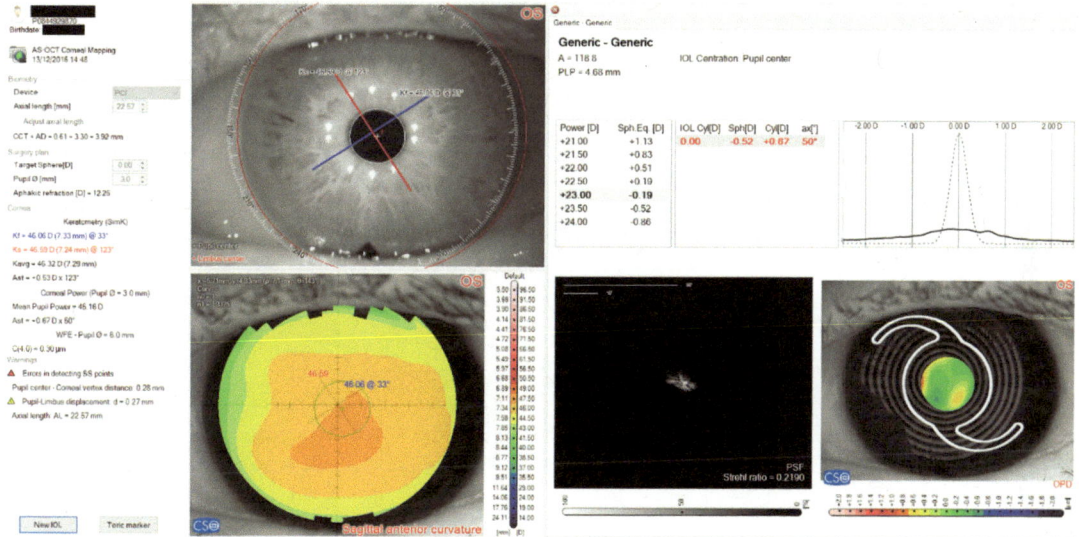

Fig. 39.13 IOL calculation for the eye, which underwent DSAEK surgery before cataract surgery

previous surgery and some central halos, due to an incipient cataract (Fig. 39.14). An improvement of visual quality was possible by administrating pilocarpine, but the vision was too dark. This condition prevented him from doing his job.

The scotopic pupil diameter was about twice the optical zone diameter (Fig. 39.15).

The preoperative evaluation led to lensectomy with the implantation of an IC-8 (AcuFocus Inc.,

California, USA). This is a single-piece hydrophobic acrylic posterior chamber IOL, which combines small aperture optics with a monofocal IOL to achieve extended depth of focus and reduce the influence of corneal aberrations. The calculation was performed with the IOL module adopting the nominal value 120.5 for the A-constant. An IOL with a power of 18 D was chosen (Fig. 39.16).

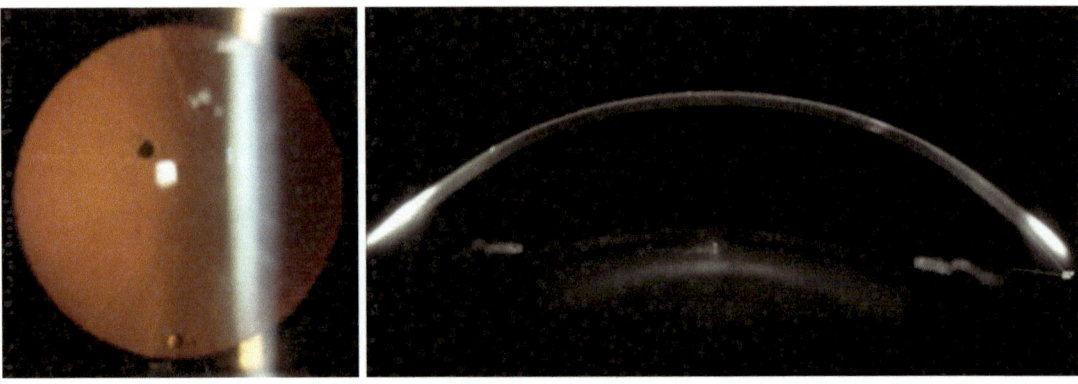

Fig. 39.14 Slit lamp frontal image and Scheimpflug section of the post-RK case: incipient cataract is only visible in the second image

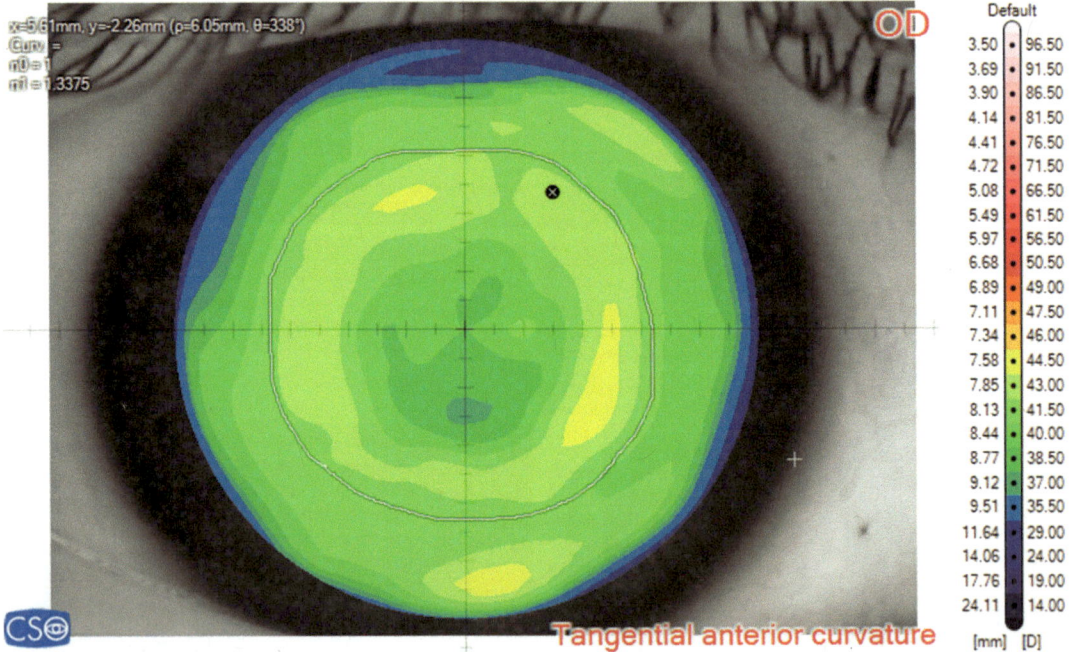

Fig. 39.15 Tangential anterior map for the post-RK case: the scotopic pupil diameter is about twice the optical zone diameter

The predicted refraction was $-0.27 + 0.43 \times 52$ and the postoperative outcome was emmetropy; moreover, the pinhole enabled the patient good uncorrected near vision. Halos disappeared and peripheral cuts were excluded from the optical zone by the IOL small aperture. The patient could resume his job.

The next case is an eye, which underwent PRK in 1999 for a correction of 9 D myopia. In 2019, it was necessary to recur to cataract surgery (Fig. 39.17). A monofocal IOL was implanted but the result was fairly far from the expected one: the patient complained of monocular diplopia, uncorrected visual acuity (UCVA) was 0.3

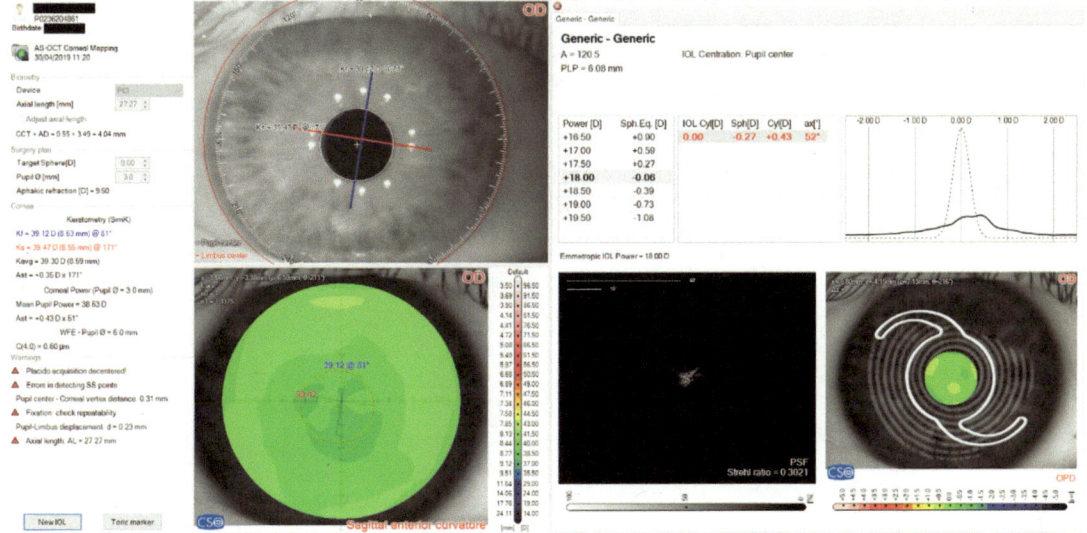

Fig. 39.16 IOL calculation for the post-RK case

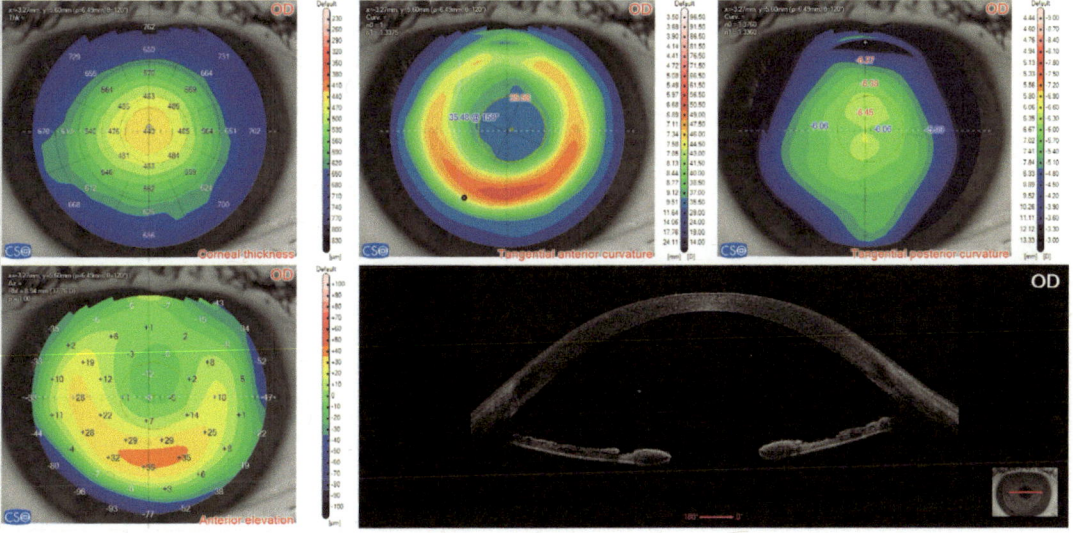

Fig. 39.17 Topographic maps and OCT section for the post-PRK eye, where the removal of the first implanted IOL was necessary

and corrected distance visual acuity (CDVA) was 0.8 with a residual hyperopic refraction (+1.75 + 0.50 × 30). The surgeon thought that the poor visual outcome was due to the combination of wrong IOL power and laser-induced corneal aberrations and proposed an IOL exchange with the implantation of an IC-8. This time the IOL power (24 D) for a target spherical equivalent of −0.5 D was calculated by the IOL module. The predicted refraction was −0.62 + 0.15 × 36 (Fig. 39.18). The postoperative result was emmetropia with UCVA equal to 1.

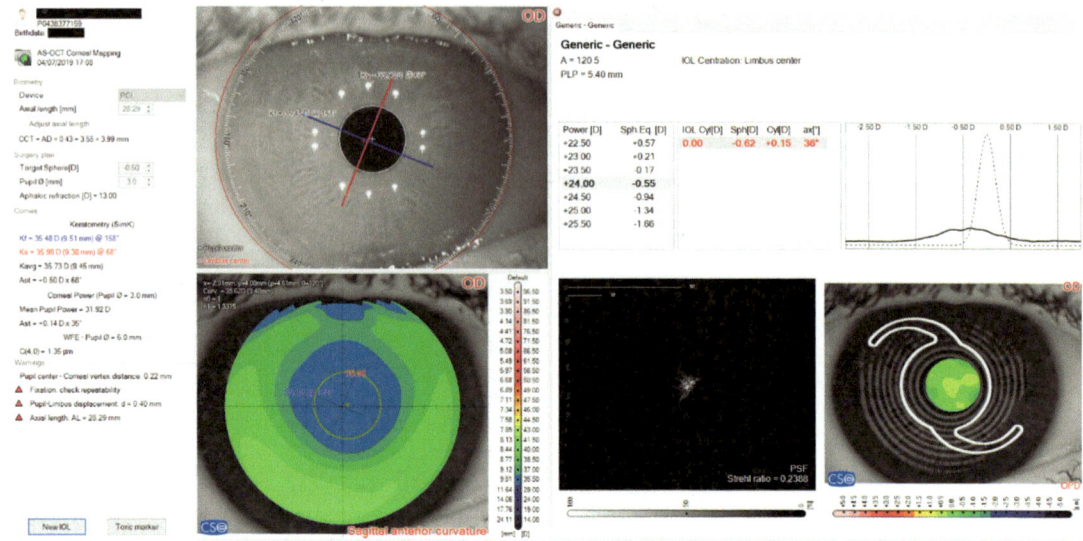

Fig. 39.18 Post-PRK case: IOL calculation for the new IOL implant

References

1. Born M, Wolf E, Bhatia A, et al. Principles of optics: electromagnetic theory of propagation, interference and diffraction of light. 7th ed. Cambridge: Cambridge University Press; 1999.

2. Savini G, Hoffer KJ, Ribeiro FJ, Mendanha Dias J, Coutinho CP, Barboni P, Schiano-Lomoriello D. Intraocular lens power calculation with ray tracing based on AS-OCT and adjusted axial length after myopic excimer laser surgery. J Cataract Refract Surg. 2022;48(8):947–53.

3. Aramberri J. Double-K method to calculate IOL power after refractive surgery. Journal of Cataract & Refractive Surgery. 2005;31(2):255–6.

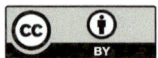

Emmetropia Verifying Optical (EVO) Formula

Tun Kuan Yeo

The Emmetropia Verifying Optical (EVO) formula, currently in version 2.0, consists of a suite of algorithms for intraocular lens (IOL) power and toric prediction, as well as post-myopic laser vision correction IOL power and toric prediction. The formula is based on the theory of emmetropization, hence its name, and is freely available online [1].

History

In the middle of 2015, while researching toric IOL calculations, a theoretical method for the prediction of posterior corneal astigmatism was discovered and created. While this posterior corneal astigmatism algorithm could be applied directly and successfully to existing third-generation IOL formulas for toric predictions, there was a desire to create a new IOL formula that could fully utilize it. The aim subsequently was to develop a formula of high accuracy that could leverage the advances in measurements using optical biometry, be devoid of any axial length or corneal power bias and combine with the new posterior corneal astigmatism algorithm. In June 2016, the EVO formula (version 1.0) for IOL power was therefore completed together with its toric counterpart,

the EVO toric formula. This version of the formula utilized axial length, corneal power (K), anterior chamber depth (ACD), lens thickness (LT) and horizontal Corneal Diameter (CD) measurements as its input parameters, with the latter two being optional. The formula was first presented at the European Society of Cataract and Refractive Surgeons Meeting in 2016 in a comparative study of 817 eyes and showed that it had the lowest mean absolute error (MAE) and median absolute error (MedAE) when compared to the Barrett Universal II, Haigis, Hill-RBF v1.0, Hoffer Q, Holladay I and SRK/T formulas, with no significant bias against axial length and K (Fig. 40.1) [2].

In June 2019, the formula underwent an update to version 2.0, with improved accuracy and added several additional functionalities including prediction for post-myopic laser vision correction eyes with or without clinical history, or Total Keratometry measurements from the IOLMaster 700 (Zeiss, Jena, Germany), in addition to an option for the Argos (Movu, Santa Clara, USA) biometer. The input parameters were changed to axial length, K, ACD, LT and central corneal thickness (CCT), with the latter two being optional. However, it was also recognized that there are cases where only the axial length and K measurements could be used, such as patients with aphakia or eyes with subluxated cataracts where the ACD would have deviated from its physiological value. Therefore, the for-

T. K. Yeo (✉)
Department of Ophthalmology, Tan Tock Seng Hospital, Singapore, Singapore

J. Aramberri et al. (eds.), *Intraocular Lens Calculations*, Essentials in Ophthalmology,
https://doi.org/10.1007/978-3-031-50666-6_40

Fig. 40.1 Graphs of the prediction error of the EVO formula against axial length (top) and K (bottom) with corresponding trend lines show no significant bias in a study of 817 eyes

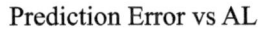

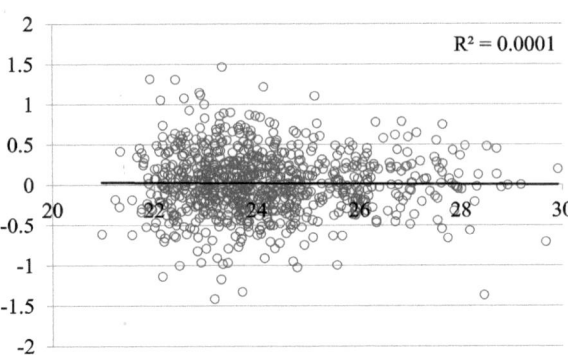

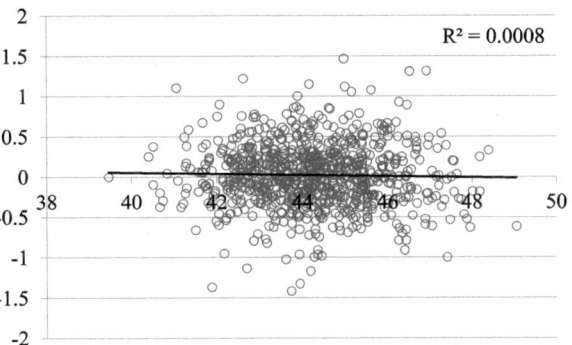

mula was designed to be capable of calculations with just two parameters, axial length and K, as well.

Description

The EVO formula is a thick lens formula based on Gaussian optics principles and therefore takes into account the anterior and posterior corneal curvatures, central corneal thickness, as well as the geometry of the IOL. The decision to base the formula on thick lens optics rather than thin lens optics was to improve accuracy by modelling the formula in close approximation to the optics of the actual physical eye, allowing flexibility in changing the geometry of the IOL for different lenses and enabling easy scalability in future updates of the formula. This is because new mea-

surement parameters can be more readily incorporated into a thick lens formula compared to a thin lens formula. An example would be the posterior corneal radius from either optical coherence tomography (OCT) or Scheimpflug machines. The basic equation for a thick lens formula is

$$P = \frac{n}{L - d2} - \frac{n}{\dfrac{n}{K} - d1}$$

P = IOL power.

n = 1336.

L = axial length.

K = corneal power.

$d1$ = distance from the anterior corneal vertex to the first principal plane of IOL.

$d2$ = distance from the anterior corneal vertex to the second principal plane of IOL.

Axial Length

From the equation above, we can see that axial length is one of the most important variables in IOL power calculations. In the past, axial length was measured using ultrasound A-scan, which is the distance from the anterior cornea to the internal limiting membrane (ILM) of the retina. With the introduction of optical biometry in 1999, it was then possible to measure the retinal pigment epithelium (RPE) with higher resolution and repeatability. However, at that time, it was not possible to measure lens thickness, and difficult to ascertain the actual refractive indices of the different media of the eye relative to the wavelength of the optical biometer. Furthermore, IOL formulas then were ultrasound based. Therefore, Dr. Wolfgang Haigis derived a regression equation to convert the optical path length obtained in the IOLMaster (Zeiss, Jena, Germany) to an immersion ultrasound equivalent. For EVO v2.0, its axial length is derived using Cooke's modified axial length (CMAL) [3] with further adjustments to suit the model of the formula and account for retinal thickness. The resulting axial length therefore represents an optical axial length to the RPE. CMAL is an elegant solution that adds variability to the axial length as a function of lens thickness change, which cannot be attained using the Haigis regression.

$$CMAL = 1.23853 + 0.95855 * AL - 0.05467 * LT$$

CMAL = Cooke's modified axial length.
AL = traditional axial length.
LT = lens thickness.

Corneal Power

Another important factor in IOL calculations is of course corneal power. The corneal power for the EVO formula is derived using Gaussian thick lens equations. The anterior corneal radius is utilized to derive a predicted posterior corneal radius with the Gullstrand ratio of 0.883. A fixed corneal thickness of 540 μm is assumed when a CCT value is not available, otherwise, the measured CCT value is used. The fixed corneal thickness is the average central corneal thickness obtained from the EVO development dataset. With the information above, the total corneal power and the corneal principal planes can then be calculated with the equations below:

$$Ant\,K = \frac{376}{r}$$

$$Pos\,K = -\frac{40}{0.883 * r}$$

$$Total\,K = Ant\,K + Pos\,K - \left(\frac{CCT}{1000}\right) * Ant\,K * Pos$$

$$C1 = \left(\frac{CCT}{1376}\right) * \left(\frac{Pos\,K}{Total\,K}\right) * 1000$$

$$C2 = -\left(\frac{1.336 * \left(\frac{CCT}{1000}\right)}{1.376}\right) * \left(\frac{Ant\,K}{Total\,K}\right) * 1000$$

r = anterior corneal radius.
Ant K = anterior corneal power.
Pos K = posterior corneal power.
CCT = central corneal thickness.
Total K = total corneal power.
$C1$ = first principal plane of the cornea.
$C2$ = second principal plane of the cornea.

Lens Geometry

Another benefit of thick lens optics is the ability to model different IOLs. Not all IOLs are the same and the lens geometry of certain models can differ significantly. The EVO formula provides four options to represent four commonly used IOL models of different lens geometry on its website, namely 'Standard', 'Tecnis', 'AR40e/E/M' and 'MA60MA'. The 'Standard' option represents the majority of IOLs such as SN60WF (Alcon, Texas, USA). With this model, the formula assumes a biconvex lens configuration with a 1:1 anterior-to-posterior ratio. The formula also predicts the anterior and posterior lens radii and

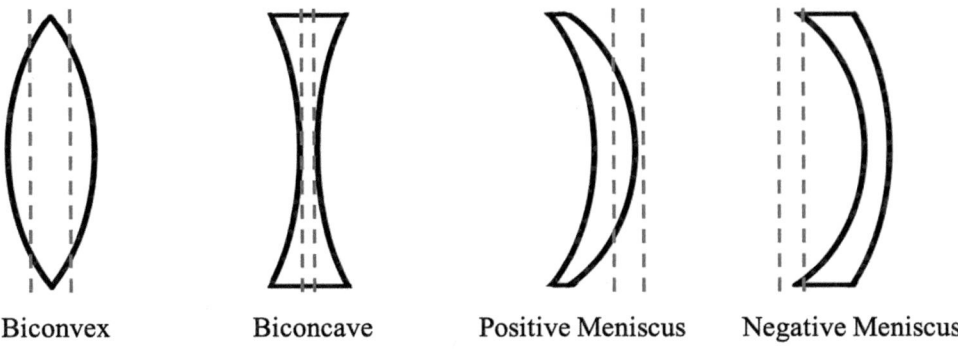

| Biconvex | Biconcave | Positive Meniscus | Negative Meniscus |

Fig. 40.2 Different lens shapes and their respective principal planes

the change in IOL thickness as the power of the IOL changes. The principal planes of the IOL can then be calculated and combined with the predicted pseudophakic lens position to be applied to the basic thick lens formula shown above in deriving the predicted lens power. The 'Tecnis' option is modelled for IOLs of the Tecnis platform such as ZCB00 (Johnson & Johnson, Florida, USA). I believe that the IOLs of the Tecnis platform differ from most standard IOLs, based on back-calculated clinical results and physical evaluation of the IOL. The 'AR40e/E/M' and 'MA60MA' options represent the IOL models AR40e, AR40E and AR40M (Johnson & Johnson, Florida, USA), and MA60MA and MA60MN (Alcon, Texas, USA), respectively. Although usually grouped with having the same lens constants for each version of the IOL, these are in fact different IOLs of different lens geometry. While the AR40e and MA60MA have a biconvex structure, the AR40M and MA60MN are instead meniscus. The latter are low or minus diopter IOLs and contribute to some of the hyperopic errors seen in traditional thin lens formulas in long eyes. This is mainly due to the significant change in the principal planes of the IOL when transitioning from a biconvex to meniscus structure. The EVO formula, however, models this change in lens geometry and principal planes for these IOLs, to avoid similar issues (Fig. 40.2). It is important to note that not all low or minus diopter IOLs are in a meniscus structure. An example would be the 409 M IOL (Zeiss, Jena, Germany), where the 'Standard' option should be used.

Effective Lens Position

We often use the term effective lens position (ELP) to describe the predicted position of the IOL for a formula. However, ELP is probably more suited to describe thin lens formulas, and I prefer the term pseudophakic lens position for thick lens formulas. This is because the ELP in a thin lens formula roughly equates to the second principal plane of the IOL. However, the structure of the EVO formula is such that it predicts the pseudophakic lens position and then derives the principal planes of the IOL, rather than predicting the second principal plane directly. Anatomically and functionally, this appears to be more logical. Predicting where the IOL sits within the eye is the core of any IOL formula. The EVO formula is based on the theory of emmetropization, to predict its pseudophakic lens position. It is postulated that the main driver for the process of emmetropization is the cornea, and the shape of the cornea does not change significantly after infancy, as opposed to the axial length. Therefore, the formula uses the corneal power as a reference and suggests that for any particular corneal power, there is a fixed lens position and axial length to attain emmetropia. Not all eyes attain emmetropia in adulthood, either due to genetic or environmental factors. If for a particular corneal power, the axial length differs from the emmetropic axial length, then there should be a corresponding change in the lens position in relation to the axial length. With this, an 'emmetropia factor' could be derived to describe every eye. Since we are unable to obtain the actual crystalline lens power or shape of an eye before cataract development, the predicted pseudophakic lens position is also adjusted using ACD and LT. LT serves mainly to correct the ACD measurement as the lens changes in thickness with cataract development, which would impact the ACD parameter. Hipolito-Fernandes et al. in their paper systematically illustrated the importance of the LT parameter, in determining what is the actual physiological ACD as opposed to a value altered by the cataract [4]. The addition of CCT as a variable has an impact in changing the calculated corneal power but also the predicted pseudophakic lens position since EVO uses corneal power in its prediction. The use of all five parameters then gives the formula multi-dimensional capability in predicting the pseudophakic lens position, which is derived through a combination of regression and iterative techniques.

Performance

Version 1.0 of the EVO formula was first compared in a large study of 13,301 eyes by Melles et al. in 2019, which showed that it outperformed Hill-RBF 2.0, Holladay 2, Haigis, Holladay 1, Hoffer Q and SKR/T [5]. Savini et al. then showed in their subsequent study of 150 eyes, using a swept-source optical coherence tomography (OCT) biometer and comparing 15 formulas, the EVO v1.0 formula achieved the lowest mean absolute error (MAE) and standard deviation of error, and the highest percentage of eyes within 0.50 D [6].

Further independent studies later revealed the performance of the updated EVO v2.0 formula. Cheng et al. in 2020 compared 12 formulas and concluded that the most accurate prediction of post-operative refraction can be achieved with the Barrett, EVO v2.0, Kane and Olsen formulas, with an improvement of the EVO v2.0 over its earlier version [7]. A paper by Hipolito-Fernandes et al. in 2020 looked at 13 formulas in 828 eyes and noted that the most accurate formulas were EVO v2.0, Kane and VRF-G overall and for all

axial length subgroups, indicating that the EVO v2.0 did not have any bias against axial length [8]. For short eyes, another paper by Kane in 2020 looked at extremely short eyes with an IOL power of 30 or more diopters and reported that Kane and EVO v2.0 were the most accurate [9]. As for long eyes, Zhang et al. [10] and Tan et al. [11] both showed in separate papers that EVO v2.0 had the lowest MAE and median absolute error (MedAE), and highest percentages of eyes within 0.50 D in this group of eyes. In addition, Hipolito-Fernandes et al. in another paper reported that EVO v2.0 was reliable and stable in eyes with extreme ACD and LT combinations [4]. This was in contrast to the Haigis and Hill-RBF 2.0 formulas which had a bias against LT. Finally, an interesting paper that looked at eyes that underwent combined silicone oil removal and cataract surgery showed EVO v2.0 as having the highest prediction accuracy in this special population [12]. Therefore, there is good evidence that EVO v2.0 performs well for all axial length subgroups and in eyes with different ACD and LT combinations.

Toric Prediction

The EVO toric formula utilizes the EVO formula as its core, to predict its pseudophakic lens position. It is therefore an ELP-based toric formula rather than a fixed ratio toric formula. This means that it does not assume a fixed position of the IOL in all eyes but predicts the IOL position depending on the parameters of the eye and considers this in its calculation of a toric IOL. The EVO toric formula also predicts posterior corneal astigmatism and models different toric IOL designs in its calculations. The toric models on the formula website are 'Anterior', 'Posterior' or 'Bitoric', representing the location of the toric surface on the IOL. I believe that the principal planes of a toric IOL differ from that of a non-toric IOL of the same power, and also change depending on the location of the toric surface. All the above are taken into consideration in the calculations for a toric IOL within the formula. In addition, on the formula website, the different toric steps of different companies are also taken into account, with the calculations adjusted depending on the model of toric IOL selected. For example, the toric steps for SN6AT (Alcon, Texas, USA) are completely different from MX60T (Bausch and Lomb, Quebec, Canada).

The performance of the EVO toric formula was first presented at ASCRS in 2019, and the study looked at 117 eyes implanted with SN6AT IOLs [13]. The EVO toric formula performed similarly to the Barrett toric formula, and was statistically better than the Abulafia-Koch regression formula, the Johnson & Johnson online toric calculator and the Holladay 1 toric formula. Pantanelli et al. in 2020 further reported that the EVO toric formula outperformed the legacy enVista toric calculator (Bausch and Lomb, Quebec, Canada) with regard to eyes with low astigmatism [14]. Furthermore, Kane et al. in 2020 reported the EVO toric formula performed similarly to the Barrett toric formula and Abulafia-Koch regression formula and had better performance than the Naeser-Savini and Holladay 2 toric formulas [15].

Post-Myopic Laser Vision Correction

Version 2.0 of the EVO formula included the ability to predict post-myopic laser vision correction eyes such as photorefractive keratectomy (PRK), laser-assisted in situ keratomileusis (LASIK) and SMILE (small incision lenticule extraction). This can be used for both toric and non-toric IOL predictions. The calculations can be performed with or without clinical history, and the clinical history required are the refractions before and after laser vision correction. In addition, with the introduction of the new parameter called 'Total Keratometry' (TK) on the IOLMaster 700 (Zeiss, Jena, Germany) optical biometer, the formula is also able to predict post-myopic LVC eyes using the PK (posterior K) value from the machine. Prediction using PK is based on a novel 'reverse double-K method' as published in 2020 [16]. [1] PK is first converted to the posterior corneal radius [2].

Assuming the posterior corneal radius was not significantly altered by previous LVC, the pre-refractive surgery anterior corneal radius can then be calculated by dividing the measured posterior radius with the Gullstrand ratio of 0.883. This presumed pre-refractive surgery anterior radius is used to generate the pseudo-phakic lens position of the formula [3]. The measured TK value is used to generate the actual corneal power in the formula. EVO using TK was shown in a study of 64 eyes with previous LVC to have the lowest MAE, MedAE and standard deviation of the error, and the highest percentage of eyes within 0.50 D when compared to the Barrett True-K, Barrett True-K with TK, Haigis-L, Haigis with TK and Shammas-PL formulas [16].

Conclusion

The EVO v2.0 formula is one of the new modern IOL formulas available today. It has been shown to be of high accuracy in a wide range of biometric measurements (axial length, K, ACD and LT). There is also good evidence showing its good performance for both toric predictions and in eyes with previous myopic laser refractive surgery. However, it is understood that the quest for accuracy never ends, and as its name implies, the EVO formula will continue to be updated and evolve, to achieve higher accuracy and attain further capabilities.

References

1. Emmetropia Verifying Optical Formula v2.0. https://www.evoiolcalculator.com.
2. Yeo TK. EVO: A new intraocular lens formula. European Society of Cataract and Refractive Surgeons Meeting 2017, Lisbon, Portugal.
3. Cooke DL, Cooke TL. Approximating sum-of-segments axial length from a traditional optical low-coherence reflectometry measurement. J Cataract Refract Surg. 2019;45(3):351–4.
4. Hipólito-Fernandes D, Luís ME, Serras-Pereira R, Gil P, Maduro V, Feijão J, Alves N. Anterior chamber depth, lens thickness and intraocular lens calculation formula accuracy: nine formulas comparison. Br J Ophthalmol. 2020;106(3):349–55.

5. Melles RB, Kane JX, Olsen T, Chang WJ. Update on intraocular lens calculation formulas. Ophthalmology. 2019;126(9):1334–5.

6. Savini G, Hoffer KJ, Balducci N, Barboni P, Schiano-Lomoriello D. Comparison of formula accuracy for intraocular lens power calculation based on measurements by a swept-source optical coherence tomography optical biometer. J Cataract Refract Surg. 2020;46(1):27–33.

7. Cheng H, Kane JX, Liu L, Li J, Cheng B, Wu M. Refractive predictability using the IOLMaster 700 and artificial intelligence-based IOL power formulas compared to standard formulas. J Refract Surg. 2020;36(7):466–72.

8. Hipólito-Fernandes D, Elisa Luís M, Gil P, Maduro V, Feijão J, Yeo TK, Voytsekhivskyy O, Alves N. VRF-G, a new intraocular lens power calculation formula: a 13-formulas comparison study. Clin Ophthalmol. 2020;14:4395–402.

9. Kane JX, Melles RB. Intraocular lens formula comparison in axial hyperopia with a high-power intraocular lens of 30 or more diopters. J Cataract Refract Surg. 2020;46(9):1236–9.

10. Zhang J, Tan X, Wang W, Yang G, Xu J, Ruan X, Gu X, Luo L. Effect of axial length adjustment methods on intraocular lens power calculation in highly myopic eyes. Am J Ophthalmol. 2020;214:110–8.

11. Tan X, Zhang J, Zhu Y, Xu J, Qiu X, Yang G, Liu Z, Luo L, Liu Y. Accuracy of new generation intraocular lens calculation formulas in Vitrectomized eyes. Am J Ophthalmol. 2020;217:81–90.

12. Zhang J, Wang W, Liu Z, Yang G, Qiu X, Xu J, Jin G, Li Y, Zhang S, Tan X, Luo L, Liu Y. Accuracy of new generation intraocular lens calculation formulas in eyes undergoing combined silicone oil removal and cataract surgery. J Cataract Refract Surg. 2020;47(5):593–8.

13. Yeo TK, Barrett GD. A comparison of new and existing toric formulas. San Diego, USA: American Society of Cataract and Refractive Surgeons Meeting; 2019.

14. Pantanelli SM, Kansara N, Smits G. Predictability of residual postoperative astigmatism after implantation of a Toric intraocular lens using two different calculators. Clin Ophthalmol. 2020;14:3627–34.

15. Kane JX, Connell B. A comparison of the accuracy of 6 modern Toric intraocular lens formulas. Ophthalmology. 2020;127(11):1472–86.

16. Yeo TK, Heng WJ, Pek D, Wong J, Fam HB. Accuracy of intraocular lens formulas using total keratometry in eyes with previous myopic laser refractive surgery. Eye (Lond). 2020;35(6):1705–11.

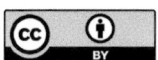

The Haigis Formula

Wolfgang Haigis and Kenneth J. Hoffer

The Thin Lens Formula

Popular formulas for intraocular lens (IOL) power calculation like the Hoffer Q [1], the Holladay 1 [2], and the SRK/T [3] are based on the optics of thin lenses. In thin lens optics, cornea and lens (crystalline or IOL) are replaced by infinitely thin lenses (Fig. 41.1) with refractive powers K (corneal power) and P (IOL power), separated by a distance d. This fictional distance is sometimes referred to as optical anterior chamber depth (ACD, measured from epithelium to IOL principle plane), which has no measurable counterpart, in contrast to the acoustical or optical ACD measured by biometers (from epithelium to lens). In 1997, Holladay [4] proposed the term effective lens position (ELP) for d.

where D_L dioptric power of the lens (or IOL), L axial length (AL), R corneal radius of curvature, $n = 1.336$, $d =$ ACD, $R_X =$ refraction (desired or actual), $d_x =$ vertex distance (=12 mm), D_C dioptric power of the cornea, and n_C index of refraction of the cornea.

Thus, all theoretical formulas may be reduced to the elementary thin lens formula:

$$D_L = \frac{n}{L-d} - \frac{n}{\dfrac{n}{z}-d} \text{ where } z = D_C + \frac{R_x}{1-R_x \cdot d_x} \text{ and } D_C = \frac{n_c-1}{R} \tag{41.1}$$

Wolfgang Haigis was deceased at the time of publication.

W. Haigis (Deceased)
Würzburg University Eye Department, Würzburg, Germany

K. J. Hoffer (✉)
St. Mary's Eye Center, Santa Monica, CA, USA

Stein Eye Institute, UCLA, Los Angeles, CA, USA
e-mail: KHofferMD@StartMail.com

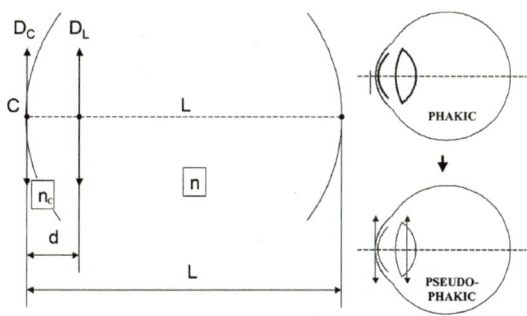

Fig. 41.1 Thin lens model: emmetropic eye where the cornea and lens are reduced to infinitely thin lenses

© The Author(s) 2024
J. Aramberri et al. (eds.), *Intraocular Lens Calculations*, Essentials in Ophthalmology,
https://doi.org/10.1007/978-3-031-50666-6_41

The theoretical formulas differ in how measurement values from a patient are translated into the variables L, d, and D_C of Eq. 41.1. Table 41.1 gives an overview of how different formulas handle this conversion. Included is the calculation according to Haigis [5],[A,B] which is dealt with in more detail later. The individual recipes for data translation reflect of course the different working set-ups of the formula authors.

The main differences between the theoretical formulas lie in the prediction functions for the optical ACD or d, i.e., in the terms for d for each of their formulas. These functions depend, among others, on the AL; they are necessarily based on the author's experience with one or more IOL types in the form of individual constants like Hoffer's "personalized ACD" (pACD), Holladay's Surgeon Factor (SF), or the A constant (SRK/T). All of these constants may readily be transformed into each other [6, 7]. For example, if the A constant = 118.0, then the SF = 1.223 and pACD = 4.97. Figure 41.2 shows such prediction curves (optical ACD d vs AL) for the

Hoffer Q, Holladay 1, and SRK/T formulas, all based on an A constant of 118.0.

Since all IOL constants may be calculated from each other, there is basically just one constant, i.e., one number characterizing a given lens for all available powers, irrespective of IOL shape factor, lens material, index of refraction, diameter, etc. This, in the author's opinion, is insufficient for a meaningful lens characterization, as will be illustrated below.

Effect of Lens Geometry on IOL Position

Following the concept of Norrby [8] and taking the capsular bag equator position (EP) as a measure for the IOL position and considering small, medium, and long eyes, the schematic AL dependence is shown in Fig. 41.3. Small eyes have a shallower ACD with the capsular bag equator lying more anteriorly, while in long eyes, the lens lies deeper in the eye with the bag equator position more posteriorly.

This behavior is backed up by clinical findings on 15,123 eyes [9] (unpublished data) in Fig. 41.4. From preoperative high precision immersion ultrasound measurements of ACD (AC) and lens thickness (LT) as shown, the AL dependence of EP was deduced under the assumption EP = AC + 0.4*LT.

Figure 41.5 gives a schematic representation of the positions of the image principal planes of IOLs with different shape factors and geometry (here e.g., plano-convex and asymmetric biconvex) in eyes with different ALs. It is this posi-

Table 41.1 Differences in theoretical IOL formulas: all are based on thin lens optics (Eq. 41.1)

Formula	n_C	L	IOL constant
SRK/T	1.3330	AL + fx (AL)	A constant
Holladay 1	4/3	AL + 0.2	SF
Hoffer Q	1.3360	AL	pACD
Haigis	1.3315	AL	a_0, a_1, a_2

where n_C index of refraction of the cornea, *fx* function of, *SF* surgeon factor, *pACD* personalized ACD. AL in these formulas is the ultrasound measurement from the cornea epithelium to the anterior surface of the retina, whereas the optical biometry AL measurement is to the pigment epithelium

Fig. 41.2 Prediction curves for the optical ACD (d) in Eq. 41.1 for different theoretical formulas and an A constant of 118.0 (for SRK/T), equivalent to SF = 1.223 (for Holladay 1), and pACD = 4.97 (for Hoffer Q)

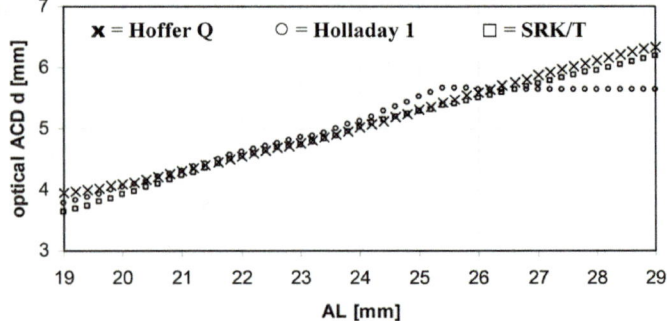

Fig. 41.3 Schematic of the dependence of the EP position of the capsular bag equator on the AL of the eye

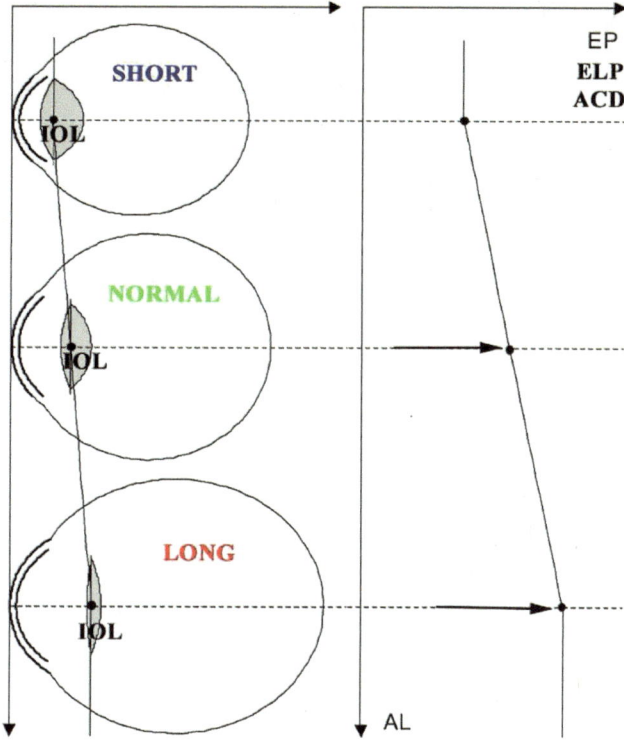

Fig. 41.4 Anterior chamber (AC), lens thickness (LT), and assumed position of the capsular bag equator position (EP) vs AL for 15,123 eyes. Data points: running means and assumption for EP: EP = AC + 0.4*LT

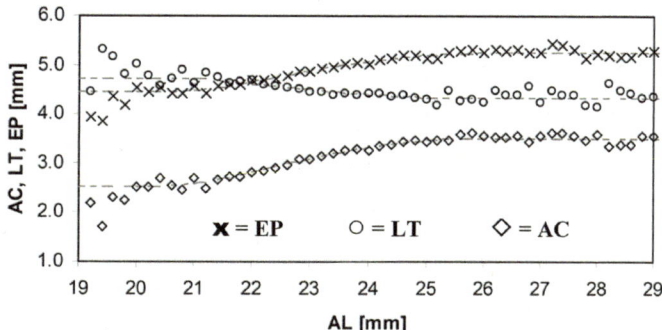

tion (of the image principal plane) that essentially determines d in Eq. 41.1. It is clearly evident from this that different IOLs are characterized by different AL dependencies of their optical ACDs. Thus, a curve (e.g., prediction of d vs AL) rather than a number (IOL constant) seems more useful for the characterization of an IOL.

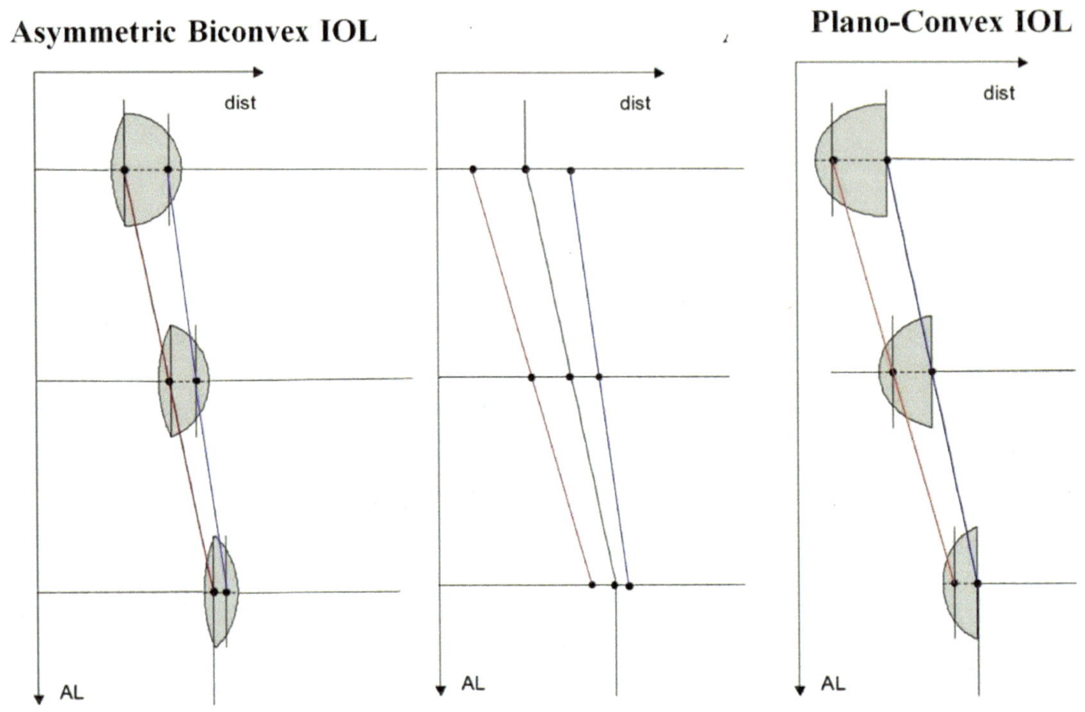

Asymmetric Biconvex IOL

Plano-Convex IOL

Fig. 41.5 Schematic representation of IOLs of different shape factors in eyes with different ALs (from short at the top to long at the bottom). The **red** lines near the **anterior vertex** and the **blue** near the **posterior vertex** of both the plano-convex and the biconvex IOL denote the positions of the image anterior and posterior principal planes, respectively, for the 2 IOL types

Calculations According to Haigis

Using the thick lens algorithm [10] for IOL calculation in the 1980s, we (like many others [11–13]) were looking for ways to predict the PO IOL position by means of multiple regression analysis performed on preoperative data [14]. We found the main contributions to the predictability of PO AC (ACpost) to stem from the AL and the preoperative ACD (AC) as shown in Table 41.2. Therefore, we predicted the (acoustically or optically) measurable PO ACD (ACpost) according to:

$$ACpost = c_0 + c_1{}^* AC + c_2{}^* AL \qquad (41.2)$$

The constants c_0, c_1, and c_2 were followed by a double linear regression analysis. Since the thick lens formula requires lens design data (e.g., radii of curvature, central thickness, and precise refractive indices) for every individual IOL power, which manufacturers are hesitant to release, we turned back again to the thin lens formalism of Eq. 41.1. This time, however, we applied the regression prediction to the optical ACD[A].

$$d(\text{Haigis}) = d = a0 + a1{}^* AC + a2{}^* AL \qquad (41.3)$$

The constants a0, a1, and a2 were found to be quite typical for a given IOL [15]. This led to the idea of using this set of numbers for the characterization of different IOLs.

$$ACpost = a0 + a1{}^* AC + a2{}^* LT + a3{}^* AL + a4{}^* CC \qquad (41.4)$$

Table 41.2 Correlation coefficient for the prediction of the measurable PO ACD using the formula

Parameter used for regression	AC	LT	AL	CC	AC, LT	AC, AL	AC,LT,AL	AC,LT,AL,CC
Correlation coefficient	68%	36%	44%	6%	68%	70%	70%	71%

Fig. 41.6 AL dependence of the optical ACD d in Eq. 41.1 for IOL types 90D, 755 U, and SI40 for the Haigis formula with optimized lens constants. Note that the curves are different not only in the vertical position but also in the form

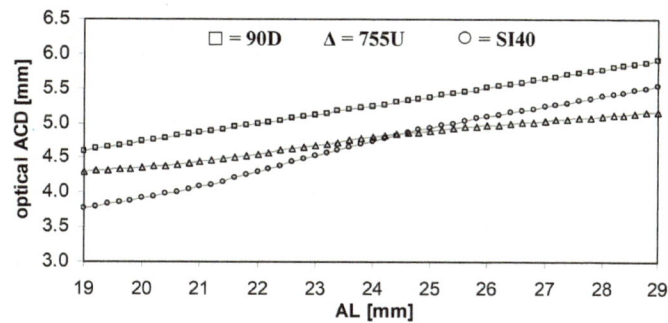

for plano-convex IOL type CILCO KR2U, where *AC* preoperative ACD, *LT* lens thickness, *AL* axial length, and *CC* corneal radius of curvature [14].

Olsen [12, 13] uses a similar regression approach with even more variables to predict PO IOL positions. However, apart from being characterized by their classical ACD constants, no further differentiation is made between different IOLs. Likewise, Holladay's IOL calculation program does not use more than one lens constant to characterize a given IOL.

An essential aspect of Eq. 41.3 lies in the fact that with three constants (a0, a1, and a2), it is possible to model the AL dependence of the optical ACD of a given lens, thus characterizing the IOL by a curve rather than a number. Since the preoperative ACD is dependent on AL (Fig. 41.4),

d(Haigis), as defined by Eq. 41.3, is a function of the AL. The specific form of the resulting curve is determined by the specific values of a0, a1, and a2 (Fig. 41.6).

Generally, for a given lens, the numerical values of the three constants (a0, a1, and a2) are derived from a double regression analysis of d vs AC and AL, where d is the optical ACD producing the true PO refraction (see below). However, for this purpose, the PO data must be available. Prior to knowing this, an alternate method to determine a0, a1, and a2 is necessary.

It was found [16] that quite a number of IOLs could well be described by a fixed value of a1 = 0.4 and a2 = 0.1. Therefore, in "standard mode," we set a1 = 0.4 and a2 = 0.1 and derive a0 from the manufacturer ACD constant ACDconst according to:

$$a0 = ACDconst - 0.40^* meanAC - 0.10^* meanAL \qquad (41.5)$$

where mean AC = 3.37 and mean AL = 23.39 [14].

Using the standard conversion between ACDconst and the A constant [6, 7] Eq. 41.5 is equivalent to:

$$\mathbf{a0 = 0.62467^* A - const - 72.434} \qquad (41.6)$$

Thus, the Haigis formula takes the form of Eq. 41.1, with *d* = d(Haigis) given by Eq. 41.3

and the additional substitutions n_C = 1.3315 and *L* = AL (from ultrasound or optical biometry).

Optimization of Constants

As long as PO results are not available to derive the three constants (a0, a1, and a2), the Haigis formula has to be used in the standard

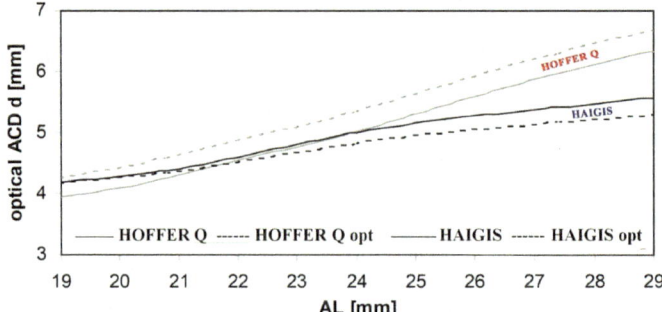

Fig. 41.7 AL dependence of the optical ACD d in Eq. 41.1 for IOL type 755 U and Haigis and Hoffer Q formulas using standard (solid lines) as well as optimized (dashed lines) lens constants. Note that optimization of the Hoffer Q constant results simply in a vertical curve shift, whereas in the Haigis algorithm, the curve *shape* is changed

mode, in which two of the three constants in formula 41.2 are set to the default values (a1 = 0.4 and a2 = 0.1) and the third constant (a0) is calculated from one of the classical lens constants (e.g., a pACD, SF or A constant) as given by the IOL manufacturer (see Eq. 41.5 or Eq. 41.6).

If, however, stable PO refraction results are at hand, it is possible to optimize the formula performance by personalizing all three Haigis lens constants. This may be done in two ways:

1. Only one constant is personalized, namely a0 or.
2. All three constants (a0, a1, and a2) are optimized.

Single Optimization (Optimization of a_0 Only)

If only a0 is optimized, then the situation is comparable to optimizing constants for other IOL formulas: there is only one number. In this case, a0 is iteratively adjusted until the mean prediction error (MPE) for a given set of patient records becomes zero, i.e.,

$$\text{MPE} = \text{Rx}_{\text{true}} - \text{Rx}_{\text{calc}} = 0 \qquad (41.7)$$

Here, Rx_{true} denotes the spherical equivalent of the stable PO refraction at best corrected visual acuity (BCVA), and Rx_{calc} is the calculated refraction according to:

$$R_x = \frac{q - D_C}{1 + d_x \cdot (q - D_C)} \qquad (41.8)$$

$$\text{where } q \text{ is } q = \frac{n^* \left[n - D_L^* (L - d) \right]}{n^* (L - d) + d^* \left[n - D_L^* (L - d) \right]}$$

Optimizing (personalizing) the a0 is equivalent to shifting the curve, which describes the AL dependence of the optical ACD (d), up and down until a mean zero prediction error (Eq. 41.7) is reached (Fig. 41.7). This is very much like adjusting the pACD constant, the SF or the A constant in the other theoretical formulas. It has to be noted that in this case, one and the same d vs AL curve is used for all IOLs. After personalization (as just described), the theoretical formulas differ in the way a given IOL is represented by the formula-inherent d vs AL curve. However, one must remain aware that what may serve well for one type of IOL may not work for another IOL type (e.g., may differ in shape factor).

With the three constants approach, it is possible not only to adjust the position of the d vs AL curve but also to modify its shape. Thus, different IOLs may be characterized by different curves. The lens geometry is no longer built into the formula but is defined externally instead.

Triple Optimization (optimization of a_0, a_1, and a_2)

The optimization process, as has already been described, goes back to the time when Hoffer

[17, 18] correlated the ultrasound PO (pseudo-phakic) ACD with his preoperative ACD as well as when the AL was corrected by means of a double linear regression analysis. However, instead of using the ultrasonically determined acoustic ACD, the optical biometer ACD is now used for the regression analysis.

As a first step, for every patient record, the d value of the optical biometer ACD is calculated, which caused the measured PO refraction for the implanted IOL power. For this purpose, a quadratic equation for d is easily derived from the thin lens formula Eq. 41.1 by elementary algebraic transformations:

$$D_L^* d^2 - D_L^* (L + n/z) * d + n^* (L - n/z) + D_L^* L^* n / z = 0 \tag{41.9}$$

with a quadratic equation solution:

$$d = \frac{1}{2 \cdot a} \cdot \left(-b - \sqrt{b^2 - 4 \cdot a \cdot c} \right)$$

where $a = D_L$, $b = -D_L^*(L + n/z)$ and

$$c = \left[n^* \left(L - \frac{n}{z} \right) + D_L^* L^* \frac{n}{z} \right] \tag{41.10}$$

Having calculated d for every patient record, a double linear regression analysis is performed with d being the dependent variable and AC and AL the independent variables. As a result, the constants a0, a1, and a2 are obtained such that equation $d = a0 + a1*AC + a2*AL$ is fulfilled.

Being aware that the optimization procedure determines the d vs AL curve, it is clear that the range of ALs for this analysis must be as broad as possible. It is of special importance to include ALs <21 mm and > 25 mm to cover the total range of available IOL powers. This implies that the analysis has to be based on a sufficiently large number of patients (a minimum >50). If only a small AL range would serve as a basis for optimization, good results naturally can only be expected for this very range while out-of-range ALs could lead to less accurate results.

Clinical Measurements

Methods

For an illustration of the formula performance and comparison with current power calculation algorithms, we retrospectively reviewed 990 patients implanted in the capsular bag with either:

1. A biconvex silicone plate lens [Chiron Adatomed 90D] $n = 118$,
2. A biconvex PMMA lens [Rayner 755 U] $n = 101$ or,
3. A biconvex silicone lens [Allergan SI40NB] $n = 771$.

Expected refraction was calculated using the formulas Haigis, Hoffer Q, Holladay 1, SRK II, and SRK/T and compared to the actually achieved stable PO refractions.

Results

First, the lens constants (as published by the manufacturers) were used for IOL power calculation; the results of which are shown in Table 41.3. The Haigis formula operating in non-optimized standard mode can be seen to produce slightly myopic results, whereas all other formulas end up on the hyperopic side. Clinically, it is always better to err on the slight myopic side than the hyperopic. The amount of deviation from target refraction differs from lens to lens. The SRK II results differ significantly from those of the theoretical formulas with respect to standard deviation as well as prediction percentages.

For each formula and IOL, individualized constants were subsequently calculated so as to produce a mean zero prediction error between actual and calculated refraction. Table 41.4 shows the results. Again, SRK II performs worse than the theoretic formulas, which produce good results. It is not possible to decide from this data which one of these actually is the

Table 41.3 Mean error (ME) between actual and calculated refraction (REF true-calc) using three IOL styles and percentages of refraction predictions within ±1.00 D and ± 2.00 D of error using manufacturer lens constants with each formula. The Haigis formula is used in "standard mode"

Standard	Rayner 755 U (n = 101)			Chiron 90D (n = 118)			Allergan SI40 (n = 771)		
Formula	ME [D]	% ± 2D	% ± 1D	ME [D]	% ± 2D	% ± 1D	ME [D]	% ± 2D	% ± 1D
SRK II	0.68 ± 0.74	95.0	71.3	0.82 ± 1.07	89.0	54.2	0.42 ± 0.73	96.8	82.9
SRK/T	0.53 ± 0.68	96.0	81.2	0.55 ± 0.82	94.9	70.3	0.29 ± 0.64	98.2	90.4
Holladay 1	0.46 ± 0.65	97.0	82.2	0.53 ± 0.77	95.8	72.0	0.24 ± 0.60	98.4	91.4
Hoffer Q	0.48 ± 0.65	97.0	84.2	0.56 ± 0.74	95.8	76.3	0.29 ± 0.60	98.7	91.2
Haigis	−0.21 ± 0.67	100	87.1	−0.28 ± 0.75	97.5	78.0	−0.38 ± 0.60	98.2	87.3

Table 41.4 Mean error (ME) between actual and calculated refraction (REF_true-calc) and percentages of refraction predictions within ±1.00 D and ± 2.00 D, if optimized constants were used with each formula. Haigis*1: single optimization (only a0 optimized); Haigis*3: triple optimization (all 3 constants optimized)

Optimized	Rayner 755 U (n = 101)			Chiron 90D (n = 118)			Allergan SI40 (n = 771)	
Formula	ME [D]	% ± 2D	% ± 1D	ME [D]	% ± 2D	% ± 1D	% ± 2D	% ± 1D
SRK II	0.00 ± 0.75	98.0	85.1	0.00 ± 1.07	94.1	66.9	97.8	86.4
SRK/T	0.00 ± 0.64	100.0	88.1	0.00 ± 0.77	97.5	83.9	98.3	90.7
Holladay 1	0.00 ± 0.63	100.0	86.1	0.00 ± 0.73	98.3	86.4	98.8	92.6
Hoffer Q	0.00 ± 0.65	100.0	88.1	0.00 ± 0.72	99.2	83.9	99.1	91.4
Haigis*1	0.00 ± 0.66	99.0	87.1	0.00 ± 0.76	98.3	81.4	98.7	92.5
Haigis*3	−0.04 ± 0.63	100.0	87.1	−0.01 ± 0.72	99.2	83.9	99.1	93.0

Table 41.5 Mean absolute error (MAE) between actual and calculated refraction (REF_true-calc) before and after optimization of constants for each formula in three IOL groups

MAE	Rayner 755 U (n = 101)		Chiron 90D (n = 118)		Allergan SI40 (n = 771)	
Formula	MAE ± SD Pre Opt	MAE ± SD Post Opt	MAE ± SD Pre Opt	MAE ± SD Post Opt	MAE ± SD Pre Opt	MAE ± SD Post Opt
SRK II	0.81 ± 0.59	0.56 ± 0.49	0.82 ± 1.07	0.83 ± 0.67	0.63 ± 0.56	0.52 ± 0.52
SRK/T	0.66 ± 0.55	0.50 ± 0.41	0.77 ± 0.61	0.60 ± 0.48	0.51 ± 0.48	0.44 ± 0.44
Holladay 1	0.61 ± 0.51	0.48 ± 0.41	0.72 ± 0.59	0.56 ± 0.47	0.48 ± 0.44	0.42 ± 0.42
Hoffer Q	0.62 ± 0.51	0.50 ± 0.41	0.72 ± 0.58	0.54 ± 0.47	0.50 ± 0.44	0.43 ± 0.42
Haigis*1	0.56 ± 0.41	0.52 ± 0.41	0.65 ± 0.46	0.58 ± 0.49	0.54 ± 0.47	0.42 ± 0.42
Haigis*3	------	0.49 ± 0.40	------	0.54 ± 0.48	------	0.42 ± 0.42

"best" formula since a possible ranking would change from IOL to IOL. The Haigis opt3 (with all three constants optimized) obviously performs better than Haigis opt1 (with only a0 optimized) and compares favorably to the other formulas. In general, it is evident from Tables 41.3 and 41.4 that individualization of lens constants results in a better performance of all formulas.

When comparing different algorithms, it is essential to consider not only the mean prediction error (ME) but also the mean absolute error (MAE)[1]. Table 41.5 shows the MAE before and after optimization of constants. For all formulas, the MAEs are also reduced by constant personalization while, again, the SRK II ranks last, and Haigis opt3 can be found in the top group.

For IOL 755 U, optimization yielded values between 117.68 and 118.84; for IOL 90D, optimization values were between 118.31 and 119.73, and for IOL SI40NB, values were from 117.55 to 118.52. Thus, in terms of A constants, optimization led to changes in them of the order of ~1.20 D for the 755 U, ~1.40 D for the 90D, and ~ 1.00 D for the SI40NB. The slopes (m) will be discussed below.

Fig. 41.8 AL dependence of the prediction error ΔRx (= $Rx_{true}-Rx_{calc}$) between actual and calculated PO refraction with IOL type 755 U for the Holladay 1 and SRK II formulas with optimized lens constants

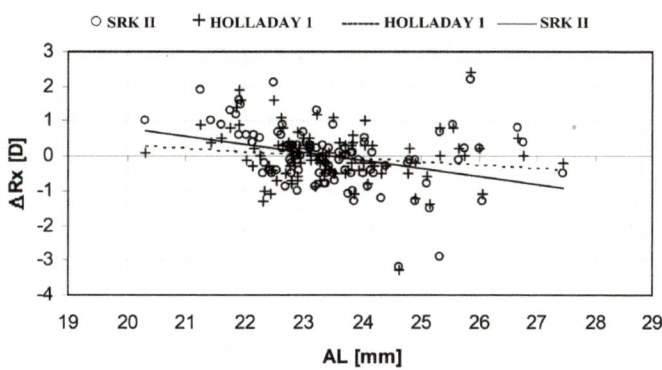

Fig. 41.9 AL dependence of the prediction error ΔRx (= $Rx_{true}-Rx_{calc}$) between actual and calculated PO refraction with IOL type 755 U for the Haigis and Hoffer Q formulas with optimized lens constants

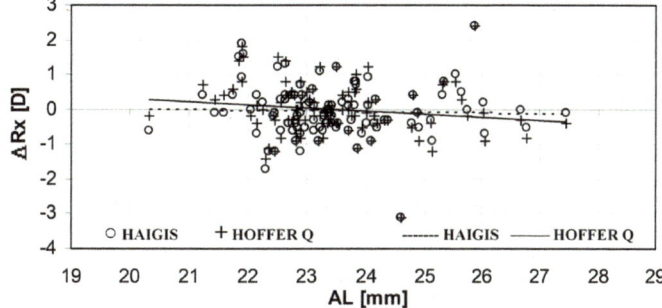

Table 41.6 Summary of the optimized lens constants found and translated into A constants for ease of comparison and slopes of the regression line y = m x + t describing the AL dependence of the prediction error $\Delta REF_{true-calc}$ between actual and calculated PO refraction for different IOL formulas. The smaller the slope (m): the smaller the AL dependent error of refraction prediction

Optimized Formula	Rayner 755 U (*n* = 101)		Chiron 90D (*n* = 118)		Allergan SI40 (*n* = 771)	
	opt A-con	Slope	opt A-con	Slope	opt A-con	Slope
SRK II	118.84	−0.29	119.73	−0.56	118.52	−0.20
SRK/T	118.61	−0.16	119.29	−0.15	118.33	−0.05
Holladay 1	118.59	−0.13	119.33	−0.14	118.31	−0.01
Hoffer Q	118.59	−0.11	119.35	−0.06	118.36	+0.05
Haigis*1	117.76	−0.09	118.40	−0.06	117.57	+0.03
Haigis*3	117.68	0.00	118.31	−0.01	117.55	0.00

where *opt A-con* optimized A constant. A constants used: 755 U (118.0), 90D (118.7), and SI40 (118.0)

Minimizing refraction errors should not only produce a mean error of zero but ideally a zero prediction error for all ALs. It may well be that equal errors of opposite signs for long and short eyes cancel each other out, thus still producing an average of zero. Therefore, it is important to check the AL dependence of the prediction error ΔRx (= $Rx_{true}-Rx_{calc}$ = ME). The slopes of the respective regression lines should be as close to zero as possible to indicate an AL-independent behavior. For lens 755 U, Fig. 41.8 shows the prediction error ΔRx between actual and calculated PO refraction vs AL with optimized constants for SRK II and Holladay 1 and Fig. 41.9 for the Hoffer Q and Haigis formulas. The respective slopes (m) for all formulas and all IOLs are also summarized in Table 41.6. It clearly follows from these findings that the "single-constant-formulas" (Hoffer Q, Holladay 1, SRK II and SRK/T) "pay a price" for a mean zero error with

Table 41.7 Mean absolute prediction errors (MAEs) in different AL ranges for 2 IOLs (Alcon MA60BM and SA60AT) using current IOL power formulas

AL	Haigis	Hoffer Q	Holladay 1	Holladay 2	SRK/T
20–21.99	0.25	0.25	0.25–0.50,	0.25	**0.51–1.00.**
22–24.49	0.25	0.25	0.25	0.25	0.25
24.50–25.99	0.25	0.25	0.25	0.25	0.25
26–28	0.25	0.25–0.50,	0.25	0.25	0.25
28–30	0.25	0.25–0.50,	0.25	0.25	0.25–0.50,
Minus power IOLs	0.25	**Not recommended**	0.25–0.50,	0.25	**0.51–1.00.**

non-zero prediction errors in short and long eyes. The largest is for the SRK II and the least is for the Hoffer Q. The better performance of the Haigis algorithm as indicated in the zero slopes stems from using three IOL constants instead of just one as pointed out earlier.

We see here the AL dependence of the optical ACD (d) for the Hoffer Q and Haigis formulas in standard and optimized modes (for lens 755 U). These graphs may be compared to Fig. 41.2 (which is based on the respective standard constants). For the plot characterizing the Haigis calculation, which makes use of AC in addition to AL (see Eq. 41.5), the model dependence of Fig. 41.4 was used. Optimization causes a vertical translation of the standard Hoffer Q curve, whereas, in the Haigis algorithm, the shape of the curve is altered. Thus, it is possible to create an individual curve shape for a given lens as opposed to the standard shape used in the other formulas.

Accordingly, different IOLs represented by different sets of constants a0, a1, and a2 will have different d vs AL curves, as is shown in Fig. 41.6 for our 3 IOLs: each one is individually positioned, with individual shape.

Once properly optimized (over a large range of ALs), the three constants approach allows good results irrespective of AL. This has also been observed by others, as Table 41.7 shows.

In Summary

The Haigis formula is based on thin lens optics just as does the Hoffer Q, Holladay 1, and SRK/T. In this respect, it makes use of the ele- mentary basic thin lens formula. It does not compare to SRK I/II, which are purely empirical. However, while all other formulas use only one constant (the pACD constant, the SF, or the A constant) for a given IOL, the Haigis formula uses three (a0, a1, and a2). In addition, apart from the AL, the ACD is taken to serve as a predictor for the PO IOL position. By this approach, it is possible to represent an IOL by a curve (optical ACD vs AL) rather than just a single number. The three constants can be derived from a statistical analysis of PO results for a sufficient number of patients (minimum >50) supplied for a given IOL.

In the standard mode, i.e., as long as this optimization process has not been carried out yet, two of the three constants of the Haigis formula are set to default values (a1 = 0.4 and a2 = 0.1), whereas the third constant (a0) is derived from one of the classical lens constants. (e.g., A constant) given by the IOL manufacturer. Therefore, in default mode, the Haigis formula is "just another theoretical formula," which, in general, has a slightly better performance for long and short eyes due to the fact that the clinical experience in the formula-inherent prediction curves stems from more recent IOLs as compared to other IOL formulas.

The power of the Haigis formula evolves after optimization, i.e., individualization of constants, as it allows a mean zero prediction error for the PO refractions irrespective of AL. There are two optimization modes:

1. Classical optimization on the basis of 1 constant, which is inherent in other theoretical

formulas: to individualize the constant of a specific IOL. The constant under question is iteratively changed to achieve a mean zero prediction error for the postop refraction. However, a mean zero error might be due to balanced errors in short and long eyes. Generally, the smallest AL-dependent errors were found with the Haigis formula.

2. Optimization of three constants: in this case, the constants a0, a1, and a2 are derived from a statistical analysis of PO results. The range of ALs for this analysis should be as broad as possible. Thus, for every IOL, an individual curve is defined for optimum prediction of the PO IOL position allowing a mean zero prediction error for all ALs.

Performance of the Haigis formula with no personalization (optimization) is as good or bad as the other theoretical formulas, and with optimization of 1 constant, it is often better for short and long eyes. When all three constants are optimized, performance is better for all ALs and all IOL types.

Acknowledgments The authors wish to thank the surgeons Z. Duzanec (University Eye Clinic, Würzburg, Germany) and J. Brändle (Füssen, Germany) for providing the patient IOL data.

References

1. Hoffer KJ. The Hoffer Q formula: A comparison of theoretic and regression formulas. J Cataract Refract Surg. 1993;19(11):700–12. Errata: 1994;20(6):677 and 2007;33(1):2–3.
2. Holladay JT, Musgrove KH, Prager TC, Lewis JW, Chandler TY, Ruiz RS. A three-part system for refining intraocular lens power calculations. J Cataract Refract Surg. 1988;14:17–24.
3. Retzlaff JA, Sanders DR, Kraff MC. Development of the SRK/T intraocular lens power calculation formula. J Cataract Refract Surg. 1990;16:333–40. Errata: 1990;16:528 and 1993;19(5):444–446.
4. Holladay JT. Standardizing constants for ultrasonic biometry, keratometry, and intraocular lens power calculation. J Cataract Refract Surg. 1997;23:1356–70.
5. Haigis W, Lege B, Miller N, Schneider B. Comparison of immersion ultrasound biometry and partial coherence interferometry for IOL calculation according to Haigis. Graefes Arch Clin Exp Ophthalmol. 2000;238:765–73.
6. Holladay JT. International intraocular lens & implant registry 2000. J Cataract Refract Surg. 2000;26:118–34.
7. Retzlaff J, Sanders DR, Kraff MC. Lens implant power calculation - a manual for ophthalmologists & biometrists. 3rd ed. Thorofare NJ, USA: Slack Inc.; 1990.
8. Norrby NE, Korany G. Prediction of intraocular lens power using the lens haptic plane concept. J Cataract Refract Surg. 1997;23(2):254–9.
9. Haigis W, Gross A: Modellrechnungen zur Vorhersage von IOL-Konstanten. In: Vörösmarthy D, Duncker G, Hartmann CH 10. Kongress der Deutschen Gesellschaft für Intraokularlinsen-Implantation und Refraktive Chirurgie, Budapest 1996, Springer-Verlag, Berlin, Heidelberg, New York, pp. 288-294, 1997.
10. Haigis W: Strahldurchrechnung in Gauß'scher Optik zur Beschreibung des Systems Brille-Kontaktlinse-Hornhaut-Augenlinse (IOL), 4. Kongreß d. Deutschen Ges. f. Intraokularlinsen Implant., Essen 1990 , hrsg.v. K Schott, KW Jacobi, H Freyler, Springer Berlin, pp. 233–246, 1991.
11. Lepper RD, Trier HG. Refraction after intraocular lens implantation: results with a computerized system for ultrasonic biometry and for implant lens power calculation. In: Ophthalmic Ultrasonography: Proceedings of the 9th SIDUO Congress, Leeds, UK July 20–23, 1982 1983 Dec 31. Dordrecht: Springer Netherlands; 1983. p. 243–8.
12. Olsen T. Prediction of intraocular lens position after cataract extraction. J Cataract Refract Surg. 1986;12:376–9.
13. Olsen T, Corydon L, Gimbel H. Intraocular lens power calculation with an improved anterior chamber depth prediction algorithm. J Cataract Refract Surg. 1995;21:313–9.
14. Haigis W, Waller W, Duzanec Z, Voeske W. Postoperative biometry and keratometry after posterior chamber lens implantation. Eur J Implant Ref Surg. 1990;2:191–202.
15. Haigis W. Einfluß der Optikform auf die individuelle Anpassung von Linsenkonstanten zur IOL-Berechnung. In: Rochels R, GIW D, Hartmann CH, editors. 9. Kongress d. Deutsch. Ges. f. Intraokularlinsen Implant., Kiel 1995. Berlin, Heidelberg, New York: Springer-Verlag; 1996. p. 183–9.
16. Haigis W, Kammann J, Dornbach G, Schüttrumpf R. Vorhersage der postoperativen Vorderkammertiefe bei Implantation von PMMA- und Silikonlinsen im Kapselsack. In: 7. Kongr. d. Deutsch. Ges. f. Intraokularlinsen Implant., Zürich 1993. Berlin, Heidelberg, New York: Springer-Verlag; 1993a. p. 505–10.

17. Hoffer KJ. Biometry of the posterior capsule: a new formula for anterior chamber depth of posterior chamber lenses. (Chapter 21) Current Concepts in Cataract Surgery (Eighth Congress). In: Emery JC, Jacobson AC, editors. Appleton-century crofts. New York, NY; 1983. p. 56–62.

18. Hoffer KJ. The effect of axial length on posterior chamber lenses and posterior capsule position. Curr Concepts Ophthalmic Surg. 1984;1(1):20–2.

Additional Sources

Haigis W: IOL calculation according to Haigis: http://ocusoft.de/ulib/czm/index.htm. Accessed Mar 22, 2023.

Haigis W, Duzanec Z, Kammann J, Grehn F: Benefits of using three constants in IOL calculation. Poster. 1999 Joint Meeting, American Academy of Ophthalmology, Pan-American Association of Ophthalmology , Orlando, FL, 1999.

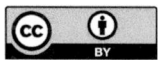

Warren E. Hill and Jonas Haehnle

The nineteenth-century American author Mark Twain once observed that change occurs at the edges and works its way in. Rather than instantly being thrust upon us, a fundamental shift in how we work gradually arises from areas outside things familiar.

In 1962, Everett Rodgers outlined how individuals are likely to adopt new technology in his book *The Diffusion of Innovations* [1]. Most are unfamiliar with this seminal work, but almost everyone knows the vocabulary originating from it.

Rodgers observed that 16% of any group presented with a new technology consists of what he refers to as "laggards" who will change what they do only if no other option is available. Another 34% consists of a "late majority" who borders on cynical and only follows established norms. Thirty-four percent are the "early majority" who will try something new only after someone else tries it first. 13.5% are "early adopters" who quickly see the value of a new idea and incorporate it. 2.5% could be termed "innovators." The adoption of new technology is never universal, regardless of how transformative it may be.

It is a little appreciated fact that much of the technology used in ophthalmology comes to us from other areas. We all know the story of Charles Kelman. His idea of phacoemulsification for cataract surgery arose from a form of tooth-cleaning technology in the 1950s. The first American physicist to receive the Nobel Prize, Albert Michelson, developed the nineteenth-century principle of interferometry. Adolf Fercher at Carl Zeiss in Germany and Wolfgang Haigis at the University of Würzburg used this principle to measure the axial length of the human eye with a previously unknown accuracy and reproducibility [2–5].

There are many examples of ophthalmology, in general, and eye surgeons, in particular, freely borrowing technologies from other fields. The adoption of artificial intelligence for intraocular lens (IOL) power selection is no different.

Accuracy

The evolution of intraocular lens power calculation accuracy, and the technology driving it, is often one step behind the demands of each new and more sophisticated generation of intraocular lenses. For more than 40 years, ophthalmologists have been pursuing perfection, only to face a variety of obstacles at multiple levels.

A significant limitation of all vergence-based intraocular lens power selection methods is

W. E. Hill (✉)
East Valley Ophthalmology, Mesa, AZ, USA
e-mail: hill@doctor-hill.com

J. Haehnle
Haag-Streit AG, Köniz, Switzerland
e-mail: Jonas.Haehnle@haag-streit.com

© The Author(s) 2024
J. Aramberri et al. (eds.), *Intraocular Lens Calculations*, Essentials in Ophthalmology,
https://doi.org/10.1007/978-3-031-50666-6_42

estimating the effective lens position (ELP), which can account for as much as 30% of the calculation accuracy [6, 7]. Even though more modern methods tend to do better than older ones, an exact plan for determining the ELP remains elusive.

The Haigis formula optimization database of more than 300,000 cases shows that most cataract surgeons have a ± 0.50 D accuracy of 78%. Only 6% of surgeons have an 84% ±0.50 D accuracy, while less than 1% of surgeons have a ± 0.50 D accuracy of 92% or better [8]. As cataract surgeons, we all are being judged by patients and peers by our refractive outcomes. There remains much room for improvement.

While traditional and more modern formulas each have benefits, it is becoming evident that IOL power selection based solely on Gaussian optics may have reached an expiration date. Given this seemingly insurmountable limitation, why not move in an entirely different direction? [9] In other words, fundamentally change the conditions of the exercise. Exploring how an artificial intelligence model might be used to solve this problem seemed to be the obvious next step in today's world of increasingly sophisticated development software.

Artificial Intelligence for IOL Power Selection

The first attempt at using artificial intelligence for IOL power selection was by the American ophthalmologist Gerald Clarke, MD, assisted by Jeannie Burmeister, RN, in 1997 [10]. The authors used a neural network and compared the accuracy of these predictions to the first version of the Holladay formula published in 1988 [11].

In this study, using conventional 10-MHz ultrasound to measure axial length, the Holladay formula had a ± 0.50 D accuracy of 38%. In comparison, the neural network had an accuracy of 62.5%. While not consistent with today's accuracy standards, the use of artificial intelligence resulted in an enormous improvement. However,

such an approach did not gain traction due to rudimentary computing power, software that was challenging to set up and refine, and a tendency to overfit the data. Like many groundbreaking ideas, it was years ahead of its time. Artificial intelligence for this purpose would not be tried again in a meaningful way until more than a decade later.

The way a neural network works is by mimicking the human neuron. It has inputs similar to neuronal dendrites and a system of summation and recalculation, very much like a cell body. It transfers the output in a way similar to a neural axon. During the evaluation phase, inputs merge into a final prediction through the network containing mathematical weights. These weights are adjusted and then readjusted throughout training by repeatedly moving prediction errors through the network via a process known as backpropagation.

In 2012, a core group of ophthalmologists and Peter Maloney, an engineer working at the American company MathWorks, began to investigate IOL power selection using artificial intelligence, employing radial basis functions [12]. The original investigators included Li Wang, MD PhD, and Doug Koch, MD, both from Baylor University in Houston, Texas; Sheridan Lamb, MD, a private practitioner in Du Page, Illinois; Johnny Guyton, MD, a private practitioner in Warner-Robins, Georgia; Adi Abulafia, MD, a hospital-based ophthalmologist in Israel and Warren Hill, MD, as the project leader. Later, Jonas Haehnle, PhD, a mathematician working at Haag-Streit AG in König, Switzerland, was added. This group has since expanded to a total of 44 investigators in 22 countries.

The project's stated objective was to increase patient safety and physician confidence and reduce the many burdens associated with an unanticipated refractive outcome. The final goal was to create a self-validating IOL power selection method as simple to use as the iPhone, independent of vergence calculations and without reliance on the effective lens position [8].

Making the Most of What's Available

A significant benefit of artificial intelligence is that it can bypass some shortcomings of current measurement technologies and make the most of what's available. This approach is also well-suited to solve real-world problems where ideal models are unavailable or less accurate than desired. IOL power selection is the poster child for the lack of a perfect, real-world model.

Physical models based on Gaussian optics assume that the measurements correctly represent the physical reality, which is rarely the case. Some of these measurements have systematic biases that must be identified and, if possible, corrected. There are also varying levels of measurement uncertainty. For example, the combination of directly measured anterior and posterior keratometry for virgin eyes is generally less accurate than anterior keratometry and a theoretical mathematical model for the posterior cornea. Significant challenges also arise with measurements that use the summation of segmental axial length. The lens thickness measurement has systematic errors and a high uncertainty level due to the cataractous lens's unknown refractive index.

Physical models also need to make assumptions about certain aspects that cannot be measured. As previously mentioned, the effective lens position is an essential aspect of IOL power selection based on a Gaussian model. There are times when the physical model amplifies a given prediction error. This is more of a problem for advanced physical models than simpler ones. These ultimately must be solved using data-driven approaches.

Artificial intelligence model-based approaches avoid such errors. For example, ELP prediction errors are no longer amplified with high IOL powers. Therefore, even the first version of Hill-RBF achieved accuracies in short eyes that were better than the more traditional IOL calculations of that time.

And not least of all, purely data-driven approaches using artificial intelligence are also free of an implicit bias of the researcher. Our method learns from the data how good the measurements can be.

Developing a Real-World Artificial Intelligence Calculator

The first problem our team faced was determining which preoperative measurements we should evaluate. Initially, 13 parameters were considered, including nontraditional metrics such as the spherical aberration of the anterior cornea, pupil size, patient gender, patient age, as well as the more traditional preoperative measurements of axial length, central corneal power, anterior chamber depth, lens thickness, the IOL power implanted, the postoperative spherical equivalent, and the horizontal corneal diameter. A genetic algorithm was used to help sort this out.

Essentially, a genetic algorithm is an evolutionary, iterative factor selection process. A basic model is created, followed by multiple iterations. Subsequent iterations are then modified in a semi-random manner, creating a series of new models. During the optimization process, the best-performing candidate models are identified, retained, and then ranked. This exercise is repeated, and those factors that produce the best-performing models are identified over time.

This approach has similarities to the process of natural selection as described by Darwin but would be more correctly termed artificial selection. It has been shown to outperform manual optimization methods [13–17].

The preoperative measurements resulting in the highest overall prediction accuracy were 1. axial length, 2. mean keratometry, 3. anterior chamber depth, 4. the observed postoperative spherical equivalent, and 5. the IOL power implanted.

Using 681 eyes implanted with the Alcon SN60WF intraocular lens, we fit this data to a 97.8% ±0.50 D accuracy for the artifical intelli-

Table 42.1 Genetic algorithm factor selection

Number of factors selected	3	4	5	6	7	8
	PostOpSE	PostOpSE	PostOpSE	PostOpSE	PostOpSE	PostOpSE
	Axial length	Axial length	Axial length	Axial length	Axial length	Axial length
Calculation factors	Kmean	Kmean	Kmean	Kmean	Kmean	Kmean
		ACD	ACD	ACD	ACD	ACD
			PreOpSE	PreOpSE	PreOpSE	PreOpSE
				Age	Age	Age
					CCT	CCT
						CD
Fitting dataset (within ±0.50 D)	91.2%	97.8%	93.1%	94.6%	95.1%	94.8%
Validation dataset (within ±0.50 D)	82.6%	90.2%	89.3%	92.2%	91.9%	92.7%
Number of out-of-bounds points	9	15	35	57	73	92
Overall ranking	6	1	5	2	3	4

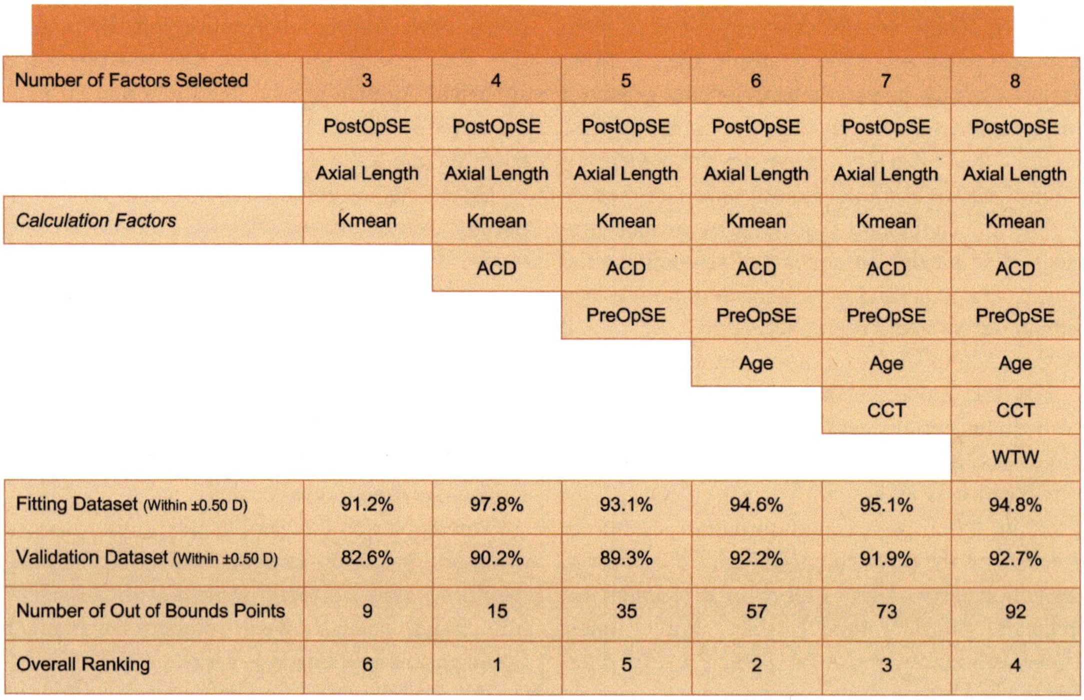

Number of Factors Selected	3	4	5	6	7	8
	PostOpSE	PostOpSE	PostOpSE	PostOpSE	PostOpSE	PostOpSE
	Axial Length	Axial Length	Axial Length	Axial Length	Axial Length	Axial Length
Calculation Factors	Kmean	Kmean	Kmean	Kmean	Kmean	Kmean
		ACD	ACD	ACD	ACD	ACD
			PreOpSE	PreOpSE	PreOpSE	PreOpSE
				Age	Age	Age
					CCT	CCT
						WTW
Fitting Dataset (Within ±0.50 D)	91.2%	97.8%	93.1%	94.6%	95.1%	94.8%
Validation Dataset (Within ±0.50 D)	82.6%	90.2%	89.3%	92.2%	91.9%	92.7%
Number of Out of Bounds Points	9	15	35	57	73	92
Overall Ranking	6	1	5	2	3	4

Fig. 42.1 Genetic algorithm factor selection

gence model. 20% of this database had been held out for independent validation. The resulting ±0.50 D accuracy for this independent validation dataset was 90.2%. These outcomes were very encouraging, suggesting that we were on a solid footing (Table 42.1) (Fig. 42.1).

Confident in the preoperative factors selected, this data was then fit to an artificial intelligence model. For the activation function, a radial basis function was used in the hidden layer. The difference between the output layer and the fitting dataset was calculated. This process was then recalculated using a backward

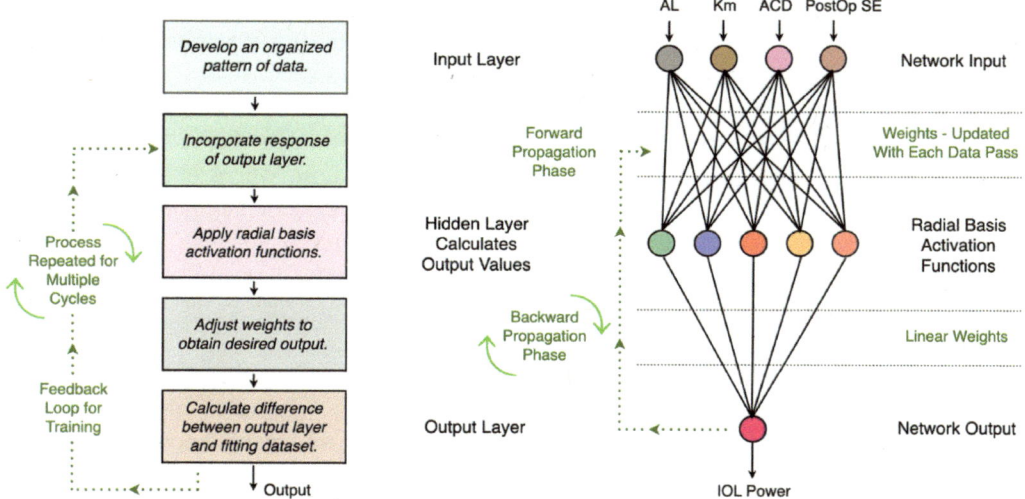

Fig. 42.2 The basic organization of a radial basis function neural network used for IOL power selection

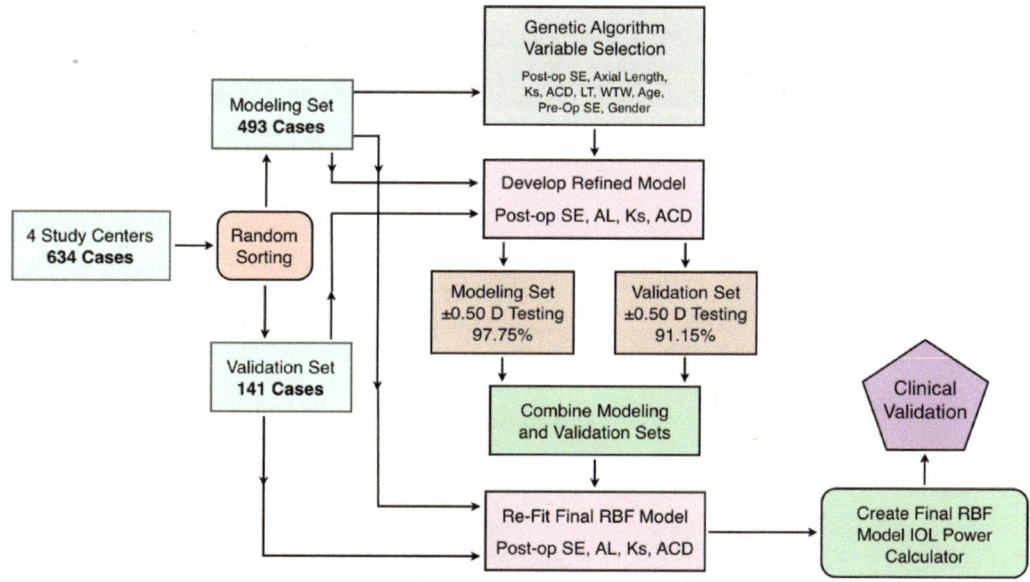

Fig. 42.3 The initial design for the creation of the Hill-RBF IOL power selection method

propagation cycle, and the output was adjusted until a maximum accuracy was obtained [11] (Fig. 42.2).

Our first experience showed several unanticipated features. First, we were able to take a cloud of data and reduce it to a straight line. Second, the calculation method showed no bias, indicating that the accuracy would be limited only by the quality and quantity of data. Whether this was a long eye, a short eye, or an eye with an unusual anterior segment, only the breadth and depth of the patient database mattered. The initial design for the creation of the Hill-RBF IOL power selection method is outlined in Fig. 42.3.

Boundary Models

One standard tool in engineering is the concept of a boundary model. The idea behind this is to identify a data range outer boundary edge, inside which will still result in a specific level of calculation accuracy.

Artificial intelligence-based predictions for many different applications routinely have such meta-models that make predictions about prediction accuracy. Far from being a restriction with the erroneous assumption that all out-of-bounds calculations are useless, a boundary model instead makes transparent the approach's limitations that other methods typically hide.

The boundary model for the Hill-RBF method was created by developing a surface in a four-dimensional space that separates the region where the training data guarantees a 90% prediction ±0.50 D accuracy from the area where no such guarantee exists. The four dimensions are 1. axial length, 2. anterior chamber depth, 3. mean keratometry, and 4. the predicted postoperative

spherical equivalent. This surface can be visualized in the form of six pairwise boundaries, as shown in Fig. 42.4.

Those cases where all data points fall within all boundary models are identified as "in-bounds," and those where one or more of the data points fall outside any boundary model are identified as "out-of-bounds." The user is notified as to the boundary status of each calculation (Fig. 42.5).

Our initial experience showed Hill-RBF to be no worse when calculating out-of-bounds cases than other IOL calculation methods. Globally, the boundary model makes known the limitations of all technologies and can be used as an additional tool to manage patient expectations.

As the breadth and depth of the patient database increases, the surface of the four-dimensional space also increases, with a resulting decrease in the number of out-of-bounds indications. By the time version 3 was completed, enough patient data was available that even highly unusual eyes would give an in-bounds indication (Fig. 42.6).

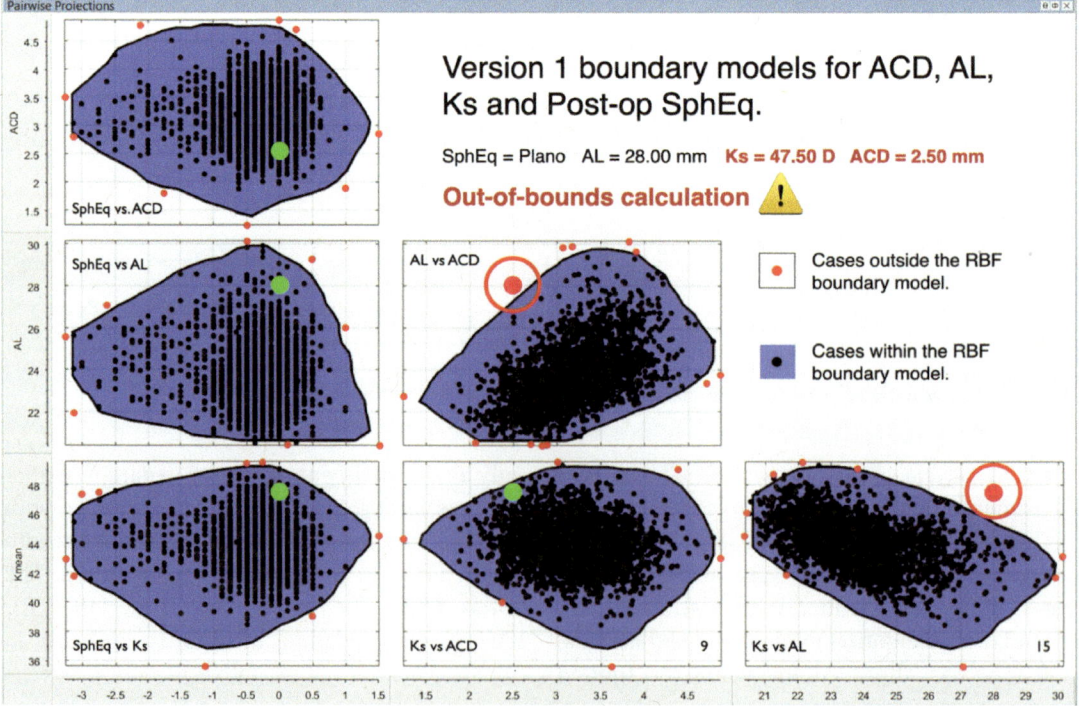

Fig. 42.4 The six pairwise boundary models used for version 1 of the Hill-RBF artificial intelligence IOL power selection method

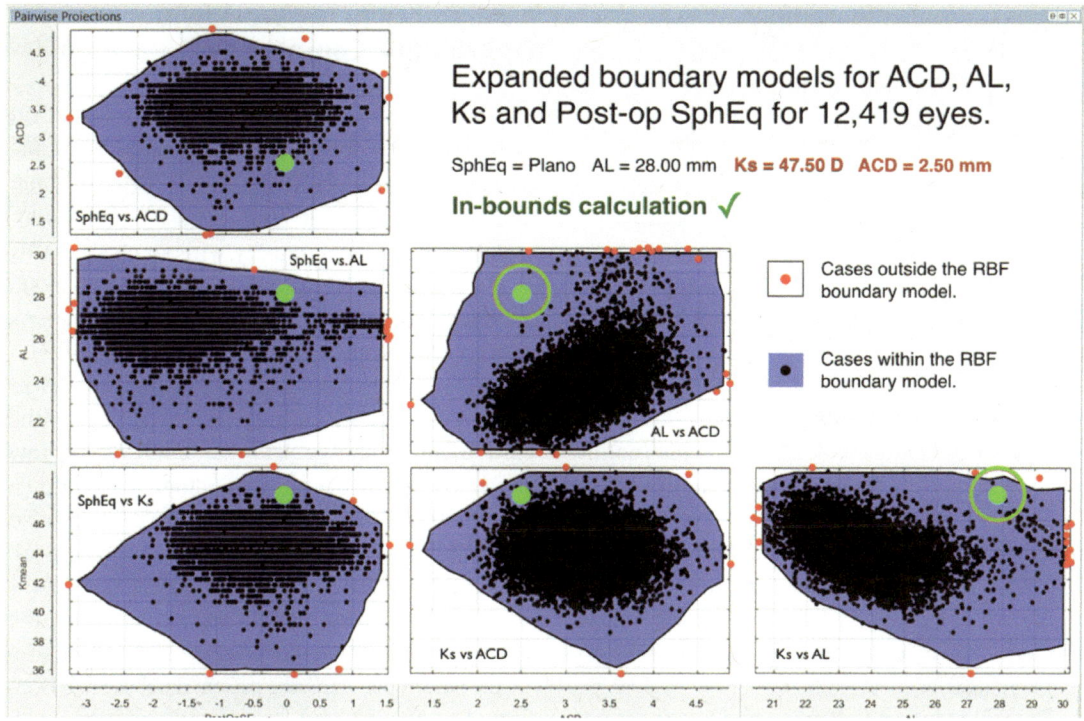

Fig. 42.5 Boundary model of version 2 of the Hill-RBF artificial intelligence IOL power selection method. Note how preoperative measurements that were out-of-bounds for version 1 are now in-bounds measurements for version 2

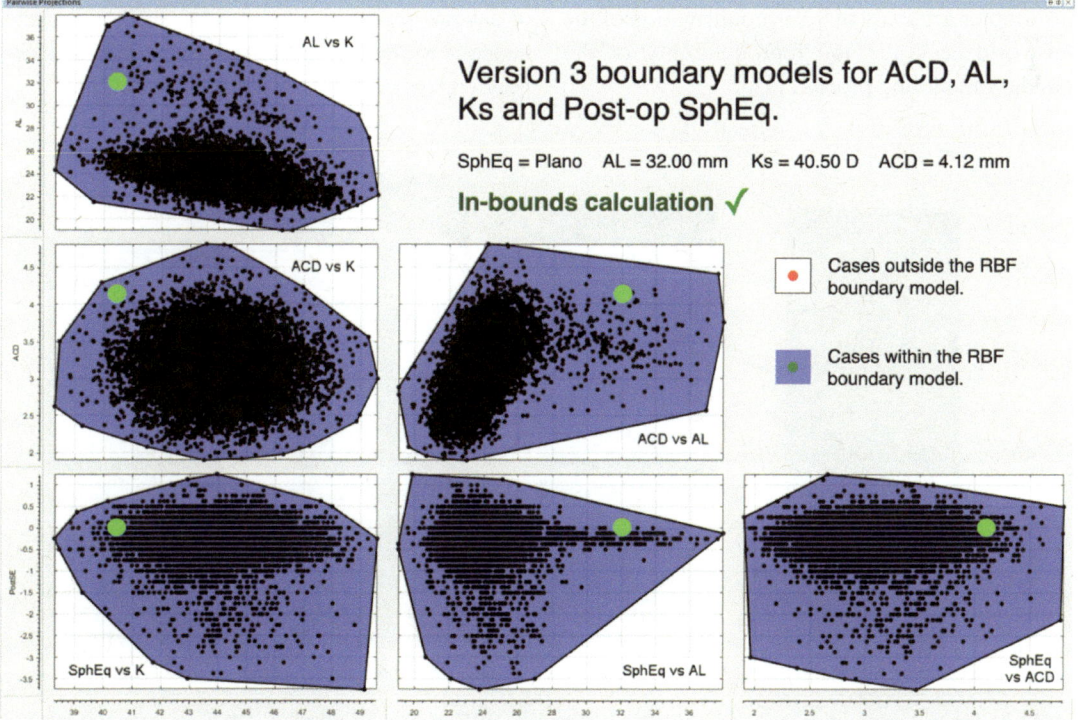

Fig. 42.6 The six pairwise boundary models for version 3 of the Hill-RBF artificial intelligence IOL power selection method. Note that for all preoperative measurements, a highly unusual eye still falls within the borders of each boundary model

A curious feature of the Hill-RBF method was that the in-bounds and the out-of-bounds accuracies were often similar for a wide range of surgeon datasets for the moderate to high axial hyperope.

First Prospective Study

By 2016, there was enough data to successfully create a useable artificial intelligence model and conduct a prospective study. This study consisted of 459 consecutive cases carried out at three independent study centers with an IOL power ranging from +7.50 D to +30.00 D, axial lengths ranging from 20.97 mm to 29.10 mm, a preoperative anterior chamber depth ranging from 2.13 mm to 4.59 mm, and a mean central corneal power ranging from 39.59 D to 48.06 D. The overall ±0.50 D accuracy for all cases in this study was 91.0% [17] (Fig. 42.7).

The following year, Roman and his group presented a study at the Los Angeles meeting of the American Society of Cataract and Refractive Surgery showing that the Hill-RBF method had a half-diopter accuracy of 92%, confirmation of the real-world accuracy and reproducibility of the boundary modeling process [18].

Availability to the Worldwide Ophthalmic Community

The initial success of this calculation method led to its inclusion within the Haag-Streit EyeSuite software. There was also created an online calculator at www.rbfcalculator.com for use by the worldwide ophthalmic community without charge [19].

By March 2018, a total of more than 12,000 eyes had been collected from our study centers around the world. This expanded dataset was refitted to a new artificial intelligence model as version 2, focusing on improved accuracy for the high axial hyperope and the addition of low power meniscus design intraocular lenses down to −5.00 diopters. This additional data also allowed for a greatly expanded boundary model. By 2023, approximately 15,000 caluclations were being performed on a weekly basis for the online version of the calculator.

By December 2020, the patient database had been further expanded and significantly refined, with improved accuracy for high axial hyperopes with IOL powers up to +34.00 diopters. There was also improved accuracy for eyes with odd combinations of anterior segment measurements such as unusual keratometry, horizontal corneal diameter, lens thickness, and the central corneal thickness (CCT).

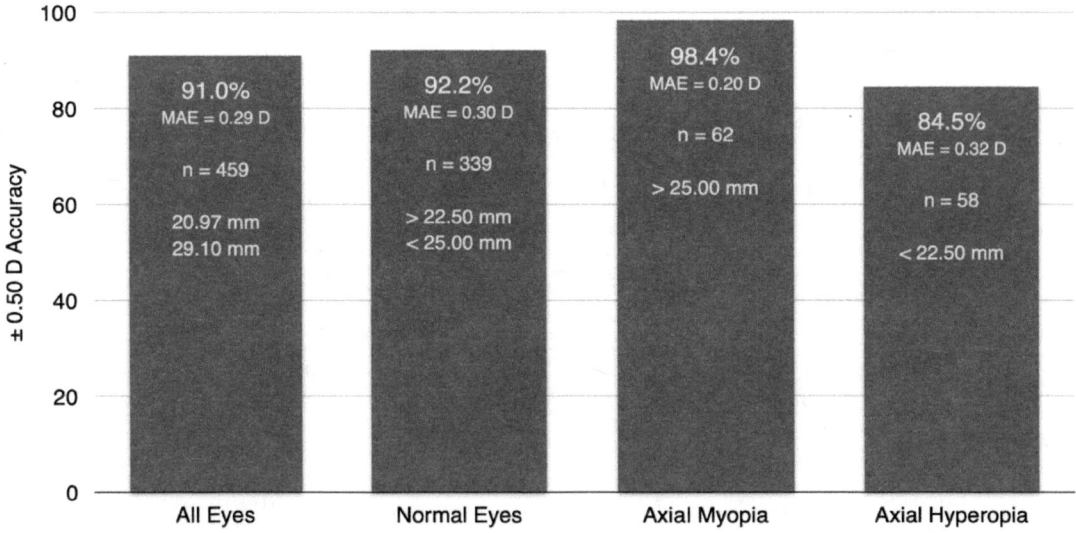

Fig. 42.7 The first prospective study using version 1 of the Hill-RBF artificial intelligence IOL power selection method

IOL	Cases	RBF 3	RBF 2	Barrett	Holladay I	SRK/T
SN60WF	301	89.6	89.5	89.1	86.6	82.0
SN60WF	668	88.7	88.6	88.1	86.4	84.9
Hoya 230	576	98.0	97.9	97.0	96.7	92.0
SN60WF	385	87.7	86.3	85.7	83.7	83.1
SN60WF	187	85.6	84.0	84.3	81.3	78.7
SN60WF	428	92.3	91.3	91.9	89.1	86.5
ZCB00	157	96.5	95.3	93.0	82.6	82.6
SN60WF	3,445	92.0	91.6	90.8	89.4	87.7
SN60WF	88	89.1	87.1	84.8	76.6	80.9
SN60WF	214	93.1	92.8	92.7	90.0	90.0
SN60WF	440	92.2	92.5	90.9	93.3	90.3
SN60WF	300	87.5	87.5	87.1	83.9	82.9
SN60WF	2,751	86.5	84.2	84.5	83.8	81.5
	9,940	**91.2%**	89.3%	87.3%	87.4%	85.3%

±0.50 D Weighted
Averages

Fig. 42.8 Unpublished prerelease validation study of version 3 of the Hill-RBF artificial intelligence IOL power selection method

It should also be noted that artificial intelligence is capable of uncovering previously unappreciated relationships. The discovery that gender can exert an influence on IOL power is an example. Gender was also added as a calculation factor for version 3.

Currently, version 3 is available on the Haag-Streit Lenstar LS-900 and the online calculator at rbfcalculator.com. This most recent version has almost no out-of-bounds indications for normal eyes undergoing cataract surgery and a significantly reduced number of out-of-bounds presentations for unusual eyes.

During the validation process for version 3, a study was carried out of 9940 eyes not used to create the artificial intelligence model. Version 3 showed a weighted ±0.50 D accuracy of 91.2%. This level of accuracy is expected, given a 90% accuracy boundary model. Using this same database, version 2 of the RBF model had a ± 0.50 D accuracy of 89.3% (Fig. 42.8).

Current Accuracy

A study in the *Journal of Cataract and Refractive Surgery* concluded that version 3 of the Hill-RBF method has the lowest standard deviation and best overall ±0.50 D accuracy of the available

Formula	≤ 0.25 D			≤ 0.50 D			≤ 0.75 D			≤ 1.00 D		
	SS-OST (K)	SS-OST (TK)	OLCR (K)	SS-OST (K)	SS-OST (TK)	OLCR (K)	SS-OST (K)	SS-OST (TK)	OLCR (K)	SS-OST (K)	SS-OST (TK)	OLCR (K)
BUII	59%	57%	58%	92%	92%	91%	100%	99%	98%	100%	100%	100%
EVO 2.0	65%	62%	63%	92%	91%	91%	99%	99%	98%	100%	100%	100%
Haigis	65%	59%	54%	87%	88%	90%	98%	98%	99%	100%	100%	100%
HILL-RBF 2.0	62%	58%	56%	92%	90%	94%	99%	99%	96%	100%	100%	100%
HILL-RBF 3.0	68%	62%	62%	93%	95%	93%	100%	99%	99%	100%	100%	100%
Hoffer Q	54%	46%	48%	80%	81%	80%	93%	91%	95%	99%	99%	99%
Holladay 1	53%	53%	58%	80%	80%	81%	95%	93%	94%	100%	98%	98%
Holladay 2	48%	44%	·	79%	78%	·	96%	95%	·	99%	99%	·
Kane	66%	63%	53%	90%	91%	87%	99%	99%	98%	100%	99%	100%
SRK/T	54%	51%	54%	80%	81%	81%	95%	95%	92%	97%	99%	99%
Olsen	·	·	56%	·	·	84%	·	·	97%	·	·	99%

Fig. 42.9 The refractive accuracy of IOL power selection methods currently in use in 2021. (Tessler M, Cohen S, Wang L, et al. *J Cataract Refract Surg*. 2021 May 18 Published ahead of print. Used with permission)

Formula	SD	Hill-RBF 3.0	BUII	EVO 2.0	Kane	Hill-RBF 2.0	Haigis	Holladay 1	SRK/T	Holladay 2	Hoffer Q
Hill-RBF 3.0	0.266	1.000									
BUII	0.282	0.980	1.000								
EVO 2.0	0.285	0.980	0.980	1.000							
Kane	0.287	0.980	0.980	0.980	1.000						
Hill-RBF 2.0	0.290	0.031	0.980	0.980	0.980	1.000					
Haigis	0.311	0.080	0.980	0.980	0.980	0.980	1.000				
Holladay 1	0.367	0.000	0.000	0.002	0.001	0.000	0.142	1.000			
SRK/T	0.377	0.000	0.000	0.000	0.002	0.000	0.405	0.980	1.000		
Holladay 2	0.386	0.000	0.000	0.000	0.000	0.000	0.015	0.980	0.980	1.000	
Hoffer Q	0.387	0.000	0.000	0.002	0.000	0.000	0.000	0.980	0.980	0.980	1.000

Fig. 42.10 Comparison of a heteroscedastic standard deviation and the corresponding p-value of IOL power selection methods currently in use in 2021. (Tessler M, Cohen S, Wang L, et al. *J Cataract Refract Surg*. 2021 May 18 Published ahead of print. Used with permission)

calculation methods currently in use [20] (Figs. 42.9 and 42.10).

New Applications for Increased Sensitivity and Accuracy

During travels to Taiwan, Hong Kong, and mainland China, our Chinese colleagues told us that they were not happy with the accuracy of traditional vergence formulas developed using databases based mostly on Caucasian eyes.

Unpublished work by our teams has shown that the Chinese and Caucasian eyes appear to have subtle anatomic differences that influence IOL power selection. Mathematical tools with adequate sensitivity to detect subtle differences between Caucasian and Han Chinese eyes are now available.

Presently, a multicenter study is underway to develop an artificial intelligence model to improve IOL power selection accuracy for the Han Chinese eye [21, 22]. We now have study centers in the cities of Hangzhou, Guangzhou, Singapore, Hong Kong, and Taipei.

Challenges

An undeniable challenge is that any data-driven approach is only as good as the data used for its creation. We are grateful beyond words to the many surgeons who helped make Hill-RBF a success by contributing patient data.

Summary

The renowned Austrian American pianist Arthur Schnabel once said Mozart's piano sonatas are "too easy for children and too difficult for professionals." [23] For surgeons, the highly accurate outcomes of an artificial intelligence solution may seem simple. However, the complexity can push us to the edge of our abilities to develop these solutions.

As previously stated, a 78% ±0.50 D accuracy is typical using standard technology. With careful attention to preoperative measurement quality, ocular surface optimization, and more modern vergence formulas, this accuracy can improve to 84% or better. However, with the same attention to preoperative measurements, plus the addition of IOL power selection by artificial intelligence, the possibility of ±0.50 D accuracy of 90% is readily achievable.

We believe that the future of ophthalmology is bright. Incremental improvements in IOL power selection accuracy will eventually take us toward the goal of a 100% ±0.50 D accuracy.

Disclosures

Dr. Hill licenses the Hill-RBF method to Haag-Streit AG Switzerland for use on the Lenstar LS900.
Dr. Haehnle is an employee of Haag-Streit AG, Köniz, Switzerland.
The services of MathWorks were supported, in part, by an unrestricted grant from Haag-Streit AG, Switzerland.
The online Hill-RBF IOL power calculator at *https://rbfcalculator.com* is provided without charge to the global ophthalmic community.

References

1. Rogers EM. Diffusion of innovations. 5th ed. New York: Free Press; 2003.
2. Fercher AF, Roth E. Ophthalmic laser interferometer Proc SPIE. 1986;658:48–51.
3. Fercher AF. Optical coherence tomography. J Biomed Opt. 1996;1:157–73.
4. Haigis W. Optical coherence biometry in Kohnen T. (ed): modern cataract surgery. Dev Ophthalmol. Basel Karger. 2002;34:119–30.
5. Hill WE. The IOLMaster. Tech Ophthalmol. 2003;1(1):62–7.
6. Olsen T. Calculation of intraocular lens power: a review. Acta Ophthalmol Scand. 2007;85:472–85.
7. Norrby S. Sources of error in intraocular lens power calculations. J Cataract Refract Surg. 2008;34:368–76.
8. Hill WE. Something borrowed, something new. The Charles Kelman Innovator's lecture of the American Society of Cataract and Refractive Surgery, Boston, MA, 2014.
9. Hill WE. Intraocular lens power calculations: are we stuck in the past? Clin Exp Ophthalmol. 2009;37:761–2.
10. Clarke G, Burmeister J. Comparison of intraocular lens computations using a neural network versus the Holladay formula. J Cataract Refract Surg. 1997;23:1585–9.
11. Holladay JT, Musgrove KH, Prager TC, Lewis JW, Chandler TY, Ruiz RS. A three-part system for refining intraocular lens power calculations J Cataract Refract Surg 14(1):17–24, January 1988.
12. Broomhead DS, Lowe D. Royal Signals and radar establishment memorandum 4148, 1988.
13. Broadhurst D, Goodacre R, Jones A, Rowland JJ, Kell DB. Genetic algorithms as a method for variable selection in multiple linear regression and partial least squares regression, with applications to pyrolysis mass spectrometry. Anal Chim Acta. 1997;348:71–86.
14. Borrás E, Ferre J, Boqué R, Mestres M, Aceña L, Busto O. Data fusion methodologies for food and beverage authentication and quality assessment. – a review. Anal Chim Acta. 2015;891:1–4.
15. MathWorks Documentation Center. How the genetic algorithm works? https://www.mathworks.com/help/gads/how-the-genetic-algorithm-works.html
16. Depczynski U, Frost VJ, Molt K. Genetic algorithms applied to the selection of factors in principal component regression. Anal Chim Acta. 2000;420(2):217–27.
17. Akaike H. A new look at the statistical model identification. IEEE Trans Autom Control. 1974;19(6):716–23.

18. Roman JM, et al. Comparison of Intraoperative Aberrometry, Hill-RBF, Holladay II, Haigis, Barrett Universal II and Olsen formulas for IOL Power Calculations. Presented at the 2017 Annual Meeting of the American Society of Cataract and Refractive Surgery.

19. The Hill-RBF online calculator at RBFCalculator.com Accessed 15 Aug 2021.

20. Tessler M, Cohen S, Wang L, Koch DD, Zadok D, Abulafia A. Evaluating the prediction accuracy of the Hill-RBF 3.0 formula using a heteroscedastic statistical method. J Cataract Refract Surg. 2021;48(1):37–

43. May 18 Electronically published ahead of print. https://doi.org/10.1097/j.jcrs.0000000000000702.

21. Hill WE, Improving IOL, Power selection. The Helen Keller lecture of the University of Alabama Department of ophthalmology and visual sciences. Birmingham, AL; 2018.

22. Hill WE, Improving IOL, Selection P. The 40th anniversary Rayner medal lecture of the United Kingdom and Ireland Society of Cataract and Refractive Surgeons. London, England; 2016.

23. An Encyclopedia of Quotations About Music. Shapiro N. 1st ed. New York, NY: Doubleday; 1978.

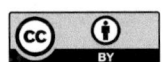

Hoffer Formulas

43

Kenneth J. Hoffer

Introduction

This is a personal history of my intraocular lens (IOL) power formula developments since 1974. I had always been fairly good at math and physics in high school and college, and I was driven by the competition I faced starting a new practice in Santa Monica, CA, which had a more than adequate supply of cataract surgeons. My goal was to get the best possible postoperative refraction results to compete in that environment.

In the Spring of 1974, I was planning to do my first IOL and to use a new Kretz 7200MA A-scan immersion ultrasound unit recommended to me by Karl Ossoinig [1] (Iowa City, IA) to measure the axial length (AL) so I could calculate the IOL power (P) that I would need to make the patient emmetropic. To begin, I needed a formula.

The Hoffer-Colenbrander Formula [First Generation]

For advice on a formula to use, I contacted Dr. Cornelius Binkhorst (Terneuzen, Holland) (famous for the Binkhorst 4-loop IOL and leading us to extracapsular implantation with his

2-loop iridocapsular lens). He recommended what he was using, a formula by Prof. MC Colenbrander (Leyden, Holland), which had just been published in the 1973 British Journal of Ophthalmology [2].

When first trying to use his formula, I found it very cumbersome and I needed to convert the formula in three important ways. First, I redefined the parameters of the formula to A = axial length (in mm), K = average corneal power (in diopters (D)), C = anterior chamber depth (in mm), and P = IOL power (in D). Secondly, I had to change parts of the formula so that it would be able to accept the axial length (AL) and anterior chamber depth (ACD) in millimeters rather than meters. In the early 70s, we all used a standard 3.5 mm for the ACD for the prepupillary IOLs and 2.95 for all anterior chamber (AC) lenses.

Finally, and most importantly, I added a factor R to the corneal power (K) in the formula; R being the postoperative (PO) spherical equivalent (SE) refractive error in diopters (D) at the corneal plane. I considered that the refractive error could be treated as a contact lens on the cornea, and its value could be algebraically added to the power of the cornea. I then recognized the need to correct R from a vertex distance of 12 mm (in the spectacle plane) to the plane of the cornea (0 mm). Now, the formula could calculate the IOL power for any desired postoperative refractive error instead of just for emmetropia (R = 0) (Table 43.1). This became

K. J. Hoffer (✉)
St. Mary's Eye Center, Santa Monica, CA, USA

Stein Eye Institute, UCLA, Los Angeles, CA, USA
e-mail: KHofferMD@StartMail.com

© The Author(s) 2024
J. Aramberri et al. (eds.), *Intraocular Lens Calculations*, Essentials in Ophthalmology,
https://doi.org/10.1007/978-3-031-50666-6_43

Table 43.1 Formulas developed by the author (1974–2020)

1974: Hoffer Emmetropia/Ametropia formula
P = (1336/(AL-ACD-0.05))−(1.336/((1.336/(K + R))−((pACD +0.05/1000)))
Where R = Rx/(1−0.012*Rx)

$$P = \frac{1336}{A-C-.05} - \frac{1.336}{\dfrac{1.336}{K+R} - \dfrac{C+.05}{1000}}$$

Where P = IOL power (D), AL = axial length (mm), ACD = anterior chamber depth (epithelium to the lens, mm), K = average K (D), Rx = desired or PO refractive error in glasses (vertex 12 mm), and R = refractive error at the corneal plane (both D).

1974: Hoffer Refractive Error formula

$$R = \frac{1.336}{\dfrac{1.336}{\dfrac{1336}{A-C-.05} - P} + \dfrac{c+.05}{1000}} - K$$

R = (1.336/(1.336/(1336/(AL−ACD−0.05)−P) + (ACD + 0.05)/1000))−K
Where Rx = R/(1 + 0.012*R)

1974: Hoffer Axial Length formula
AL = 1336/(P + (1.336/((1.336/(K + R))−((ACD + 0.05)/1000)))) + ACD + 0.05
Where R = Rx/(1−0.012*Rx)

1974: Hoffer Iseikonia

$$I = \frac{1336}{L-C-.05} - \frac{1.336}{\dfrac{1.336}{K+S} - \dfrac{C+.05}{1000}}$$

I = (1336/(L-ACD-0.05))−(1.336/((1.336/(K + S))−((ACD + 0.05)/1000)))
Where I = iseikonic IOL power, A = axial length, L = axial length of the other eye (L-0.657 only if eye is phakic), K = corneal power, ACD = anterior chamber depth, P = IOL power, Rx = refractive error, S = refractive error of other eye.

1978: Hoffer + Axial Length-dependent ELP
Hoffer formula using ACD = 2.92*AL−2.93

1993: Hoffer Q formula [Hoffer Formula using an ELP prediction formula (Q formula) based on AL and Tangent of K]
Hoffer formula but ELP is calculated by the Q formula for ELP below:
ELP = pACD +0.3(AL−23.5) + (tan K)^2 + (0.1 M*(23.5−AL)^2 * (tan(0.1(G-AL)^2))−0.99166
Where M and G are limiters for AL values in the Q formula ONLY.
If AL ≤ 23, M = 1 and G = 28. If AL > 23, M = −1 and G = 23.5. If AL > 31, AL = 31. If AL < 18.5, AL = 18.5
MOST IMPORTANT: The above limits *only* apply to the Q formula.
Solving for pACD by back calculation requires a quadratic equation:

$$pACD = \left[\frac{A+N - \sqrt{(A-N)^2 + 4\left[\dfrac{N-A}{\dfrac{P}{1336}}\right]}}{2} \right] - .05$$

pACD = ((AL + N−SQRT[(AL−N)2 + 4((N−A)/(P/1336))])/2−0.05
where N = 1336/(K + R) and R = Rx(1−0.12*Rx)

Table 43.1 (continued)

2004: Hoffer H [Holladay 2 formula simplified]
In the Holladay 2 formula, an estimated scaling factor (ESF) multiplies the ELP.
$\text{Log}(ESF_p) = +1.18 \log(AL_p/23.45) - 0.89 \log(43.81/K_p)^2 + 0.28 \log(CD_p/11.7)^2 - 0.18 \log((ACD + LT)/(ACD_p + LT_p)) + 0.21 \log((1-Rx*[Rx])/400)$
If LT is unknown use: $LT_p = 4 + Age_p/100$.
$ELP_p = SF*ESF_p$.
The above is the reason for entering the age of the patient.
ESF_p = inverse log of $[\log(ESF_p)]$ where $_p$ = patient's value.
In the Hoffer H formula, we replaced his standard biometric values with ours and deleted the entry of the patient's preoperative Rx.
$\text{Log}(ESF_p) = +1.18 \log(AL_p/23.65) - 0.89 \log(43.81/K_p)^2 + 0.28 \log(CD_p/11.52)^2 - 0.18 \log((3.24 + 4.63)/(ACD_p + LT_p))$
Final $ELP = ELP*ESF$

2015: Hoffer H-5 [Hoffer H formula using gender and race of patient]
We replace the standard biometry values (AL, K, ACD, and LT) in the Hoffer H formula (above) with the averages for the gender and race of the individual patient using the biometric race and gender values of our published study [3].

2020: Hoffer QST
See text

what I called the "Hoffer-Colenbrander" formula for several years until Dr. Robert Drews (then President of ASCRS) recommended that I call it simply the Hoffer formula because it really was no longer the Colenbrander formula.

Because of the R factor, the Hoffer formula could now, by back calculation, be used to calculate the PO refractive error resulting from any given IOL power. I also wrote an iseikonic (equal image size in both eyes) formula based on the written recommendations made by Colenbrander in his article (Table 43.1). I tried to publish these formulas but were rejected by all the journals I submitted them so I gave up. At that point in time, respected journals were not interested in publishing anything to do with IOLs. The fact that I was completely unknown did not help either. So, in 1975, I had to start a journal (JCRS) to publish my first paper on lens calculation [4]. Unfortunately, the formulas I had written were not published [5] until 1981, 7 years after they were written, in a less prominent journal that no longer exists (Ophthalmic Surgery).

Adding the First AL-Dependent ACD [Second Generation]

We obtained reasonably good results with the formula for that era, but in 1978, I performed an analysis of the relationship between the AL and the 3-month PO ACD measured by a Haag-Streit optical pachymeter. It was published later in 1983 in a textbook by Jared Emery [6] and in 1984 [7], in a short-lived publication submitted only at the plea of the Chairman of my residency program, Dr. Robert Jampel (the Editor). The results showed a direct relationship ($r = 0.67$) between the AL and ACD (Fig. 43.1). A regression formula resulted such that the PO ACD could be estimated by first multiplying the AL by 0.292 and then subtracting 2.93 (Table 43.1).

The problem was that this regression formula was only good for that one IOL style I was using. I (or others) would have to repeat this for every other IOL model making it not universally useful for others. This AL-dependent prediction of the ACD was later defined by Holladay as the first second-generation formula. Later, Richard Binkhorst (New York, NY) also took this into

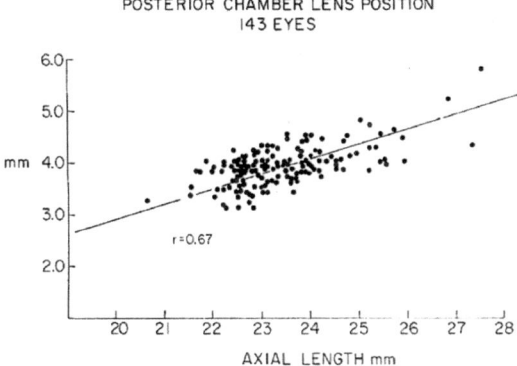

Fig. 43.1 Measurement of the anterior surface of the cornea to the anterior surface of the posterior chamber lens implant (ACD) in relation to the axial length of 143 eyes with a one-piece PMMA posterior chamber lens fixated in the bag, from 1978

consideration but used a different formulation to accomplish it. In 1988, Sanders did the same with the SRK regression formula, calling it the SRK II [8], but by that time it was a little too late for regression formulas.

The Hoffer Q Formula [Third Generation]

In 1988, Holladay [9] introduced the first third-generation formula, which made the predicted ACD dependent on the AL and the K. It made sense to me, as the cornea became steeper (higher K reading) the ACD was deeper. Unfortunately, he used R. Binkhorst's formula for his base instead of the Colenbrander. He used a Fyodorov formula to calculate a predicted corneal height (distance from anterior cornea to iris plane). To get an ACD (or estimated lens position (ELP)), he had to determine the remaining distance from the iris plane to the principle plane of the IOL, a distance he called the surgeon factor (SF). Since this distance could not be measured preoperatively, he calculated it from a series of PO patients and used the average value for future calculations. This required him to solve the quadratic formula for ACD and SF.

After analyzing my results comparing the Hoffer-AL and Holladay formulas, I found the Holladay to be more accurate in a series of 153 eyes (unpublished). I thus planned on using only his formula in the future, but Holladay strongly urged me to update my formula and make it so it could be personalized, for which I have since been incredibly grateful.

So, with a Casio programmable calculator in hand, I worked on an ACD prediction algorithm using the AL and K during our family vacation in Florida. The calculator has memory banks labeled from A to Z, and I started by placing my first iteration of a trial formula in memory bank A. After many iterations [10], it was the memory bank Q that I used to store the final successful ACD trial formula using the tangent of K. I became so accustomed to going to the Q memory bank, I decided to call this ACD prediction method the Q formula, and thus, it became the Hoffer Q formula [11] (Table 43.1). Holladay recommended I call it the Hoffer 2 and come up with a new variable termed the Hoffer ACD factor that would be akin but not equal to his SF. I decided against that for three reasons. First, the base Hoffer formula had not changed since 1974 and therefore should not be referred to as a "Hoffer 2." Secondly, I had changed the calculation of ACD input 10 years earlier (ACD = 2.92AL−2.93) and now was simply changing it again by using the new Q formula. Thirdly, I did not want to create a new IOL-dependent lens constant that would be as alien to most ophthalmologists as the SF was when it was first introduced. The world had three lens constants (ACD, A-con, and SF) and that was enough. I wanted to use a value everyone was familiar with, the ACD, calling it the personalized ACD (or pACD). To solve for ACD and enable personalization, I too had to solve for it using the original base Hoffer formula. This required solving a quadratic equation (Table 43.1). After weeks of frustration trying to do it myself, I finally gave up and it was done for me by Lincoln Chase PhD of the mathematics department at UCLA. Years later, Holladay admitted to me that he had to get a Baylor University math professor to do it for him also. Math is not always easy.

For the Q formula, I did not use the Fyodorov corneal height calculation; instead, I used a tangent of the K. Before publishing the Hoffer Q formula, I needed to perform a study to show that it was superior to the Holladay and SRK/T [12]. I input the surgical data and biometry of 450 eyes in which I had implanted a Jaffe 6-mm one-piece PMMA lens in the capsular bag. This would be the largest uniform series of eyes operated on by one surgeon, using one lens style and the same biometry instruments and surgical technique. The results revealed that the Hoffer Q was statistically equal to the Holladay, but not better. It was statistically superior to the SRK I and II but not the SRK/T even though it appeared to be clinically more accurate.

I decided to analyze the effect of AL on the three theoretic formulas. I started by defining AL ranges as short (<22 mm), normal (22–24.5 mm), medium long (24.5–26 mm), and very long (>26 mm), which are now used by most researchers. My results showed that the Hoffer Q was more accurate than the other two in eyes shorter than 22.0 mm, but because of the small number of short eyes in that range (36), I could not show statistical superiority (which was often noted by Holladay in his presentations). To further verify this result, I asked Dr. James Gills to provide me with biometric data on short eyes and his staff (Myra Cherchio) was able to provide me with

data on 830 eyes shorter than 22 mm and a repeat analysis on this series showed Hoffer Q to be statistically more accurate ($p < 0.0001$) than the Holladay and SRK/T formulas in short eyes, which unfortunately I never had time to publish. In 2011, Aristodemou [13] finally published the statistical superiority of the Hoffer Q, but in eyes shorter than 21.0 mm, in his landmark 8,000 eye large study from the UK.

In response to this, in 1996, Holladay developed the Holladay 2 formula (never published), which calculates a scaling factor (ESF) for the estimated lens position (ELP) by using the logarithms of the preoperative AL, K, the corneal diameter (CD), the anterior segment length (ASL) (composed of lens thickness (LT) and ACD), and preoperative refractive error using mean values for those parameters to better predict the postoperative IOL position. I had taken a photograph of the structure of the formula during an ASCRS course he gave where he first described it and stated it would soon be published. Thomas Olsen (Aarhus, Denmark) had proposed the use of most of these same parameters in his Olsen formula [14, 15] a decade earlier. I did not pursue these concepts because I felt it would be difficult to get ophthalmologists to obtain a measurement of ACD, LT, and CD on every routine cataract. Of course, all this changed in 2009, with the introduction of newer optical biometers that are readily able to provide all these parameters.

Interested in comparing this new Holladay 2 formula, in 2000 I published a study [16] using the Holladay IOL Consultant computer program, to compare the Holladay 2 with the Hoffer Q, Holladay 1, and SRK/T formulas in 317 silicone plate-haptic lens cases operated on by me. The results showed the Holladay 2 (H-2) to be equal to but not better than both the Hoffer Q in short eyes and the SRK/T in long eyes. It also showed the Holladay 2 to be far inferior to the Holladay 1 in eyes with ALs between 22 and 26 mm and especially eyes 24.5–26 mm, where the Holladay 1 has always been the absolute best. Thus, the extremes of AL were improved with the H-2, but it sacrificed the accuracy in the middle range, the majority of eyes. In 2019, Holladay 1 and Holladay 2 were upgraded by improvements in the Wang/Koch AL adjustment formulas [17], which have improved their accuracy quite a bit.

I cannot leave out the unfortunate history of the typographical errors that occurred in the original publication of the Hoffer Q formula by the journal. A crucial minus sign was left out, and the example calculation answers were switched. In the erratum that was published later, I made changes to the formula whereby the limitations on ACD were replaced by limitations on the AL but only in the Q part of the formula. Readers thought that the AL limitation was an addition to the ACD limits and used both of them (in the Q formula and the vergence formula). These problems were due to journal typesetting and me. All errors were made clear in a 2007 letter to the editor in JCRS. The worst example of the errors caused was that by Tomey (Japan) in their A-scan ultrasound instrument. They programmed it without a license or contacting me. In 2001, a publication by Oshika et al. [18] (Table 43.2) showed the Hoffer Q to be the worst formula (mean error of +11.44 D) in a small series of microphthalmic eyes where in actuality it was the most accurate (mean error of +2.80 D). Tomey corrected this, issued an erratum, and apologized for the error. Due to the harm it could cause patients, I now ask to have a license signed for commercial use of my trademarked name whereby I can assure it is programmed correctly.

Table 43.2 (a) Results found by Oshika, et al. [18] on microphthalmic eyes using the Hoffer Q, Holladay 1, SRK/T, and SRK II formulas (Note: Hoffer Q the worst). (b) The corrected real results later produced by Tomey[16Erratum] (after they corrected their mistake) showing the Hoffer Q the best

Formula	ME ± SD	Range
Hoffer Q	**+11.44 ± 0.49**	**+4.08 to +21.70**
Holladay 1	+2.74 ± 4.47	−0.60 to +10.20
SRK II	+11.94 ± 7.07	+4.22 to +21.60
SRK/T	+4.40 ± 4.34	+0.40 to +11.17

Formula	ME ± SD	Range
Hoffer Q	**+2.80 ± 1.83**	**−4.02 to +5.00**
Holladay 1	+3.03 ± 4.23	−0.56 to +10.20
SRK II	+11.94 ± 7.07	+4.22 to +21.60
SRK/T	+4.40 ± 4.34	+0.40 to +11.17

where *ME* mean error, *SD* standard deviation

There have been many new IOL formulas and many studies comparing them over the years, such as the Barrett Universal II, the EVO 2.0, Haigis, Kane, Ladas, Olsen C-factor, Panacea, Pearl GPS, and RBF, all showing improvements over the standard old Hoffer Q/Holladay 1/ SRK/T formulas. The Hoffer Q in short eyes has stood the test of time for almost 30 years and most all studies prove the results I first published; the Hoffer Q is not superior in all AL ranges.

The Hoffer H Formula [Fourth Generation]

In 2004, to attempt to improve the Holladay 2 formula, I replaced Holladay's mean biometry values with my previously published ones from 1980 [10, 19] for the average AL, K, ACD, CD, and LT in the algorithms used for the Holladay 2 ESF calculation and omitted the preoperative refraction which I thought could be very error-prone due to changes brought about by the cataract. I called it the Hoffer H formula (H for Holladay) and after testing it against the Hoffer Q/Holladay 1/SRK/T formulas on a large series of eyes, I found that its singular benefit was a real statistical increase in the percentage of eyes within a prediction error of ±0.13 D (21%), ±0.25 D (38%) and ± 0.50 D (64%), but the other parameters were basically the same or less. The results were presented as a poster at the American Academy of Ophthalmology Meeting in 1994 but based on a lack of enthusiasm from colleagues, I never published it or did much more with it.

The Hoffer H-5 Formula [Fifth Generation]

Eleven years later, in 2015, waking up in the middle of the night on a cross-country Amtrak train trip, I came up with an idea that, since there were differences in biometry between genders and various races, it might be better to change those parameters in the Holladay 2 and Hoffer H formulas suited to the gender and race of the individual patient. I made a note and fell back asleep. It was

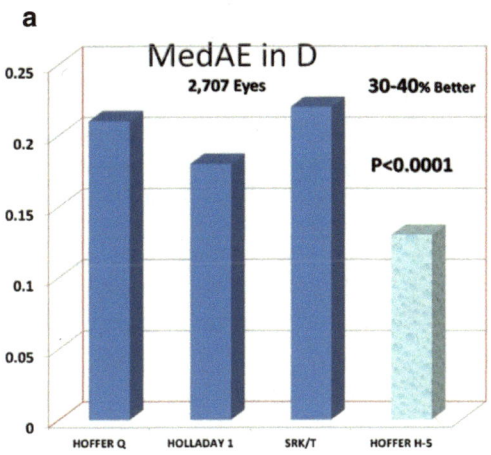
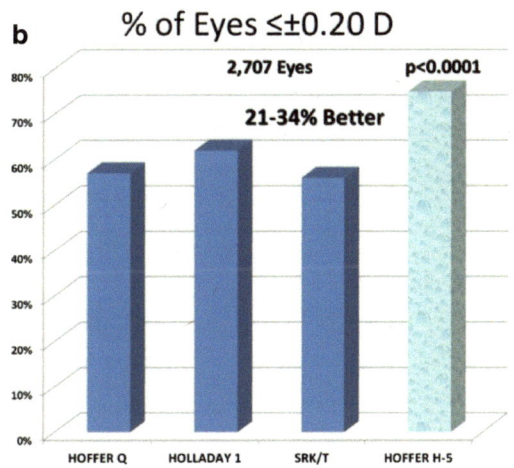

Fig. 43.2 (**a**) Results of MedAEs of the Hoffer H-5 compared to the Hoffer Q, Holladay 1, and SRK/T formulas showing it to be 30–40% statistically better in 2,700 multiracial eyes in 2017. (**b**) A similar comparison of the percentage of eyes within ±0.20 D showing the Hoffer H-5 with 21–34% statistically better in 2,700 eyes

many months later when I discovered the note and set about, with Giacomo Savini (Bologna, Italy), to follow up on it. We first performed a thorough review of the literature regarding the gender and racial differences in biometry and came up with the proper values for them, which were published in 2017 [3]. After an analysis using a large series of 2,700 multiracial eyes from around the world, we found definite statistically significant improvements in accuracy (Figs. 43.2) over the standard Hoffer Q/Holladay 1/SRK/T formulas [20] but were unable to test it against the newer formulas because of the massive task of entering 2,700 eyes individually into each formula's website or program. Not much interest was developed for the new formula by colleagues or industry.

The Hoffer QST Formula 2020 [Using Artificial Intelligence]

After years of frustration that the Hoffer Q formula was limited to reasonable accuracy in normal eyes and better accuracy only in short AL eyes and considering ways to address it, it took the evidence of studies such as by Eom et al. [21] and Melles et al. [22] to point out the effect that the lack of preoperative ACD had on its poor performance in some eyes, but it was the stimulus of

a suggestion to improve the Hoffer Q by Tun Kuan Yeo of Singapore, at an IOL Power Club (IPC) annual meeting in St. Pete Beach, FL, in 2018 that stimulated us to finally do something about it. He suggested making alterations to the index of refraction or adding preoperative ACD, which the Haigis formula [23] had made prominent. It was even considered during the formulation of the Q formula but seemed too cumbersome for clinicians to measure ACD in 1993.

With those aims, Dr. Savini and I began a series of alterations to the basic Q formula using those ideas. We were getting remarkably close (but never better) to the accuracy of the newer more accurate formulas. But then, in collaboration with Dr. Leonardo Taroni (Bologna, Italy), we set about investigating the limitations of the Hoffer Q and finding a way to overcome them.

The first limitation that came to our attention was the correlation between the prediction error (PE) and the preoperative ACD. The Hoffer Q tends to overestimate the IOL power in eyes with shallow ACDs (leading to myopic errors) and underestimate it in eyes with deep ACDs (leading to hyperopic errors) (Fig. 43.3). This finding confirms the results of previous studies [21, 22]. The second limitation is the weak performance in eyes longer than 26.0 mm, where the Hoffer Q tends to provide hyperopic outcomes.

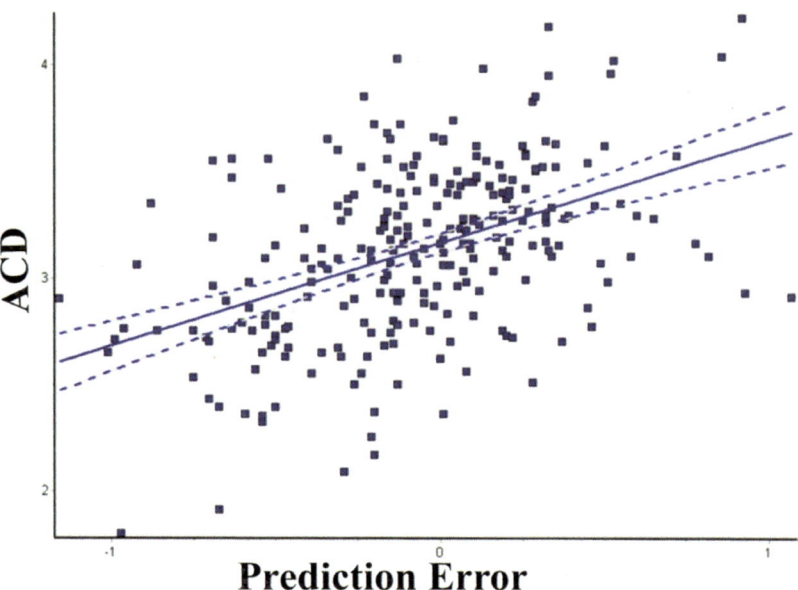

Fig. 43.3 Linear regression ($p < 0.0001$, $r = 0.4552$, r2 = 0.2072) shows that the prediction error (PE) of the Hoffer Q is related to the anterior chamber depth (ACD). Data from 253 eyes implanted with the same IOL after constant optimization. Line: regression; dotted lines: 95% confidence

We started our project of improving the Hoffer Q by using classical statistics such as linear regression and were able to achieve better results than the original formula, but it was not yet possible to reach the accuracy of the newest formulas. We found that the solution was in machine learning, an artificial intelligence that provides us with a nonlinear regression model. The next step was to decide which elements of the original Hoffer Q may deserve updating and we first focused on the effective lens position (ELP), as this is one of the main contributors to errors in IOL power calculation using modern biometry [24, 25]. We collected 537 highly accurately-measured eyes with the same monofocal IOL and zeroed their PE by optimizing the ELP. We subtracted the original Hoffer Q lens constant (pACD) from the optimized ELP giving us a new ELP correcting factor (we called a T-factor) for each eye. Maintaining the same pACD value of the Hoffer Q formula allows us to calculate the new ELP equation using an easily available constant for every single IOL, such as those published on the User Group for Laser Interference Biometry (ULIB, http://ocusoft.de/ulib/c1.htm) or IOLCON (https://iolcon.org) websites. At this point, using machine learning, we created a new model that uses gender and biometric data as input (e.g., AL, ACD, and corneal radius) to calculate the T-factor. Preliminary analyses revealed that other biometric parameters (LT and CD) do not improve ELP prediction, so they were not included in our model.

As a second step, we developed a customized AL adjustment for long eyes following the same method adopted for the T-factor. Briefly, we zeroed the PE of around 200 long eyes (AL > 25.0 mm) optimizing the AL. After determining the AL adjustment from the difference in the original AL and the optimized one, we developed a nonlinear model to estimate it.

Thus, the Hoffer QST has an AL adjustment similar to the Wang-Koch, but superior because (1) it is not dependent only on AL but also uses the input of our model gender and several biometric data (AL, Kavg, ACD, and R) and (2) we use a nonlinear regression model. The Hoffer QST accuracy is maintained over the entire spectrum of ALs and in all IOL models we have tested so far. John Shammas et al. showed its

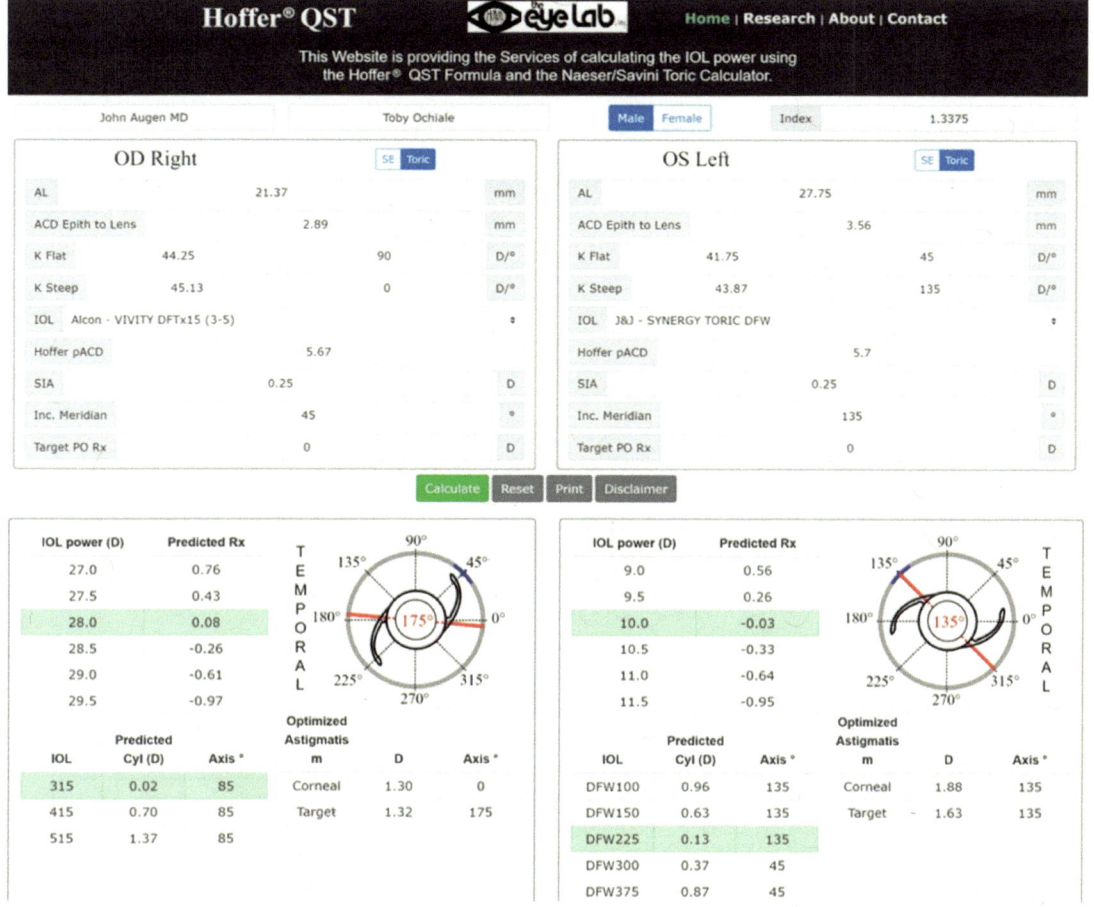

Fig. 43.4 The Hoffer QST website with Naeser/Savini Toric calculation for a short OD and a long OS

accuracy using the Argos biometer [24], which uses a "Sum of Segments" method to measure AL using a specific speed for each part of the eye as developed by David Cooke [26]. This results in an AL slightly different from all the other biometers.

In conclusion, we updated the Hoffer Q formula by means of new algorithms and machine learning generating the new Hoffer QST (Hoffer Q/Savini/Taroni) formula [27].

The Hoffer QST formula calculator is available to be used for free on our website (Figs. 43.4) at www.HofferQST.com (or www. EyeLab.com and www.IOLPower.com), and it

includes the accurate Naeser/Savini Toric calculator with a complete printout (Fig. 43.5) for the chart or electronic medical record. It is also available on the new (September 2022) ESCRS IOL Calculator [https://iolcalculator.escrs.org] and will be available on the new Optopol REVO NX Spectral Domain OCT biometer and the Heidelberg Anterion biometer.

We have added a "Research" section (Fig. 43.6) at the top of the home page that allows the user to download specified Excel spreadsheets to be populated with your data, uploaded to the site, and receive multiple simultaneous calculations or Hoffer QST lens constant (pACD)

OD Right Eye

Calculation: Toric
AL: 24.92 mm
ACD Epith to Lens: 3.02 mm
K Flat: 41.99 D
K Flat Axis: 5 °
K Steep: 44.39 D
K Steep Axis: 95 °
IOL: Alcon - VIVITY DFTx15 (3-5)
Hoffer pACD: 5.67
SIA: 0.2 D
Inc. Meridian: 0 °
Target PO Rx: 0

IOL power (D)	Predicted Rx
16.0	0.70
16.5	0.39
17.0	0.06
17.5	-0.26
18.0	-0.59
18.5	-0.92

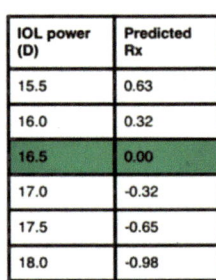

IOL	Predicted Cyl (D)	Axis °
315	0.75	94
415	0.20	94
515	0.35	4

Optimized Astigmatism	D	Axis °
Corneal	1.66	95
Target	1.86	94

OS Left Eye

Calculation: Toric
AL: 24.97 mm
ACD Epith to Lens: 3.08 mm
K Flat: 42.5 D
K Flat Axis: 174 °
K Steep: 44.54 D
K Steep Axis: 84 °
IOL: Alcon - VIVITY DFTx15 (3-5)
Hoffer pACD: 5.67
SIA: 0.2 D
Inc. Meridian: 0 °
Target PO Rx: 0

IOL power (D)	Predicted Rx
15.5	0.63
16.0	0.32
16.5	0.00
17.0	-0.32
17.5	-0.65
18.0	-0.98

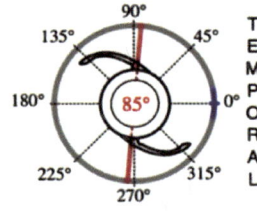

IOL	Predicted Cyl (D)	Axis °
315	0.47	85
415	0.08	175
515	0.62	175

Optimized Astigmatism	D	Axis °
Corneal	1.36	84
Target	1.56	85

Fig. 43.5 Hoffer QST website calculation printout sheet for Toric IOLs

optimization. We are hoping this may stimulate other formula authors to add this to their websites.

Our results show the Hoffer QST to be equal to or better (depending on the parameter measured) than all the latest most accurate formulas available today. Our published clinical results with the formula [27] show that this new version is a definite improvement over the Hoffer Q and will help define its role in today's cataract surgery.

From 1974 to 2024 has been an enjoyable 50 years involved in IOL power formula creation.

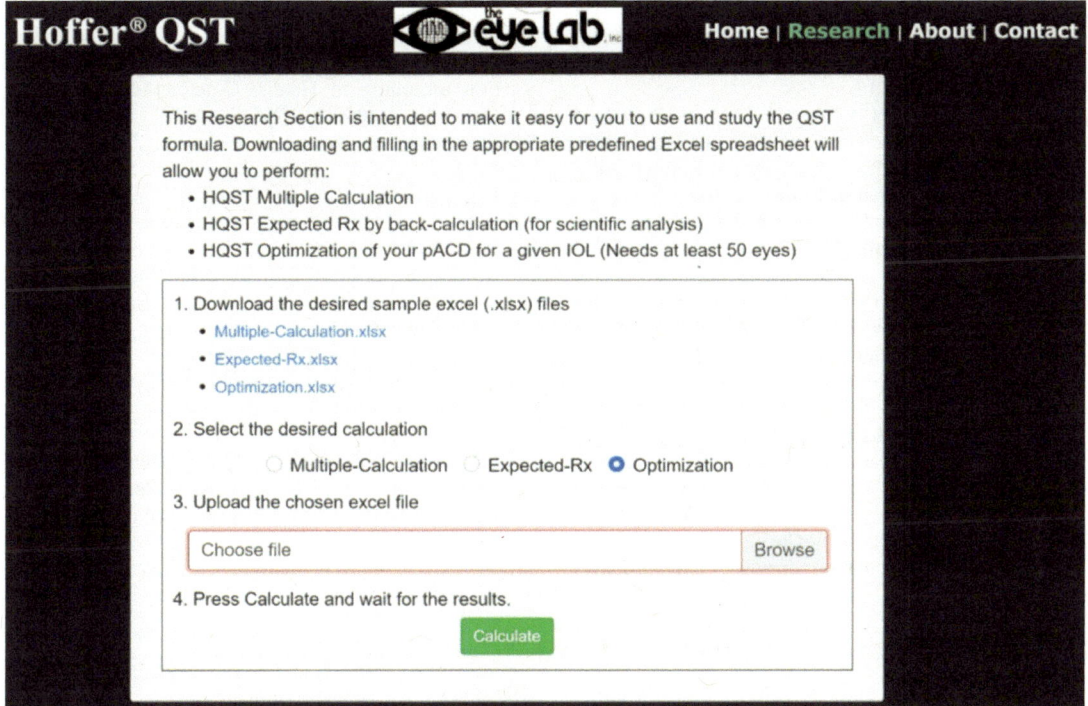

Fig. 43.6 Hoffer QST Research Page for pACD lens constant optimization and multiple calculations for analyses and formula comparison studies by researchers

References

1. Ossoinig KC. Standardized echography: basic principles, clinical applications and results. Int Ophthalmol Clin. 1979;19:127–210.
2. Colenbrander MC. Calculation of the power of an iris-clip lens for distance vision. Br J Ophthalmol. 1973;57:735–40.
3. Hoffer KJ, Savini G. Effect of gender and race on ocular biometry. Int Ophthalmol Clin. 2017;57(3):137–42.
4. Hoffer KJ. Mathematics and computers in intraocular lens calculation. J Cataract Refract Surg. 1975;1(1):3.
5. Hoffer KJ. Intraocular lens calculation: the problem of the short eye. Ophthalmic Surg. 1981;12:269–72.
6. Hoffer KJ. Biometry of the posterior capsule: a new formula for anterior chamber depth of posterior chamber lenses. (Chapter 21) Current Concepts in Cataract Surgery (8th Congress), Emery, JC, Jacobson, AC (Eds). New York: Appleton-Century Crofts; 1983. p. 56–62.
7. Hoffer KJ. The effect of axial length on posterior chamber lenses and posterior capsule position. Curr Concepts Ophthalmic Surg. 1984;1:20–2.
8. Sanders DR, Retzlaff J, Kraff MC. Comparison of the SRK II formula and the other second generation formulas. J Cataract Refract Surg. 1988;14:136–41.
9. Holladay JT, Praeger TC, Chandler TY, Musgrove KH. A three-part system for refining intraocular lens power calculations. J Cataract Refract Surg. 1988;14:17–24.
10. Hoffer KJ. Biometry of 7,500 Cataractous eyes. Am J Ophthalmol. 1980;90:360–8.
11. Hoffer KJ. The Hoffer Q formula: a comparison of theoretic and regression formulas. J Cataract Refract Surg. 1993;19:700–12. Errata 1994;20(6):677 and 2007;33(1):2–3.
12. Retzlaff J, Sanders DR, Kraff MC. Development of the SRK/T intraocular lens implant power calculation formula. J Cataract Refract Surg. 1990;16:333–40. erratum 1990;16(4):528.
13. Aristodemou P, Knox Cartwright NE, Sparrow JM, Johnston RL. Formula choice: Hoffer Q, Holladay 1, or SRK/T and refractive outcomes in 8108 eyes after cataract surgery with biometry by partial coherence interferometry. J Cataract Refract Surg. 2011;37(1):63–71.
14. Olsen T. Prediction of intraocular lens position after cataract extraction. J Cataract Refract Surg. 1986;12:376–9.
15. Olsen T. Theoretical approach to IOL calculation using Gaussian optics. J Cataract Refract Surg. 1987;13:141–5.
16. Hoffer KJ. Clinical results using the Holladay 2 intraocular lens power formula. J Cataract Refract Surg. 2000;26:1232–7.

17. Wang L, Holladay JT, Koch DD. Wang/Koch axial length adjustment for the Holladay 2 formula in long eyes. J Cataract Refract Surg. 2018;44(10):1291–2. Erratum: 2019;45:117.

18. Oshika T, Imamura A, Amano S, et al. Piggyback foldable intraocular lens implantation in patients with microphthalmos. J Cataract Refract Surg. 2001;27:841–4. Erratum 2001;27:1536.

19. Hoffer KJ. Axial dimension of the human cataractous lens. Arch Ophthalmol. 1993;111:914–8. Erratum 1993;111:1626.

20. Hoffer KJ, Savini G. Clinical results of the Hoffer H-5 formula in 2,707 eyes: first 5th generation formula based on gender and race. Int Ophthalmol Clin. 2017;57(4):213–9.

21. Eom Y, Kang SY, Song JS, et al. Comparison of Hoffer Q and Haigis formulae for intraocular lens power calculation according to the anterior chamber depth in short eyes. Am J Ophthalmol. 2014;157:818–24.

22. Melles RB, Holladay JT, Chang WJ. Accuracy of intraocular lens calculation formulas. Ophthalmology. 2018;125:169–78.

23. Haigis W, Lege B, Miller N, Schneider B. Comparison of immersion ultrasound biometry and partial coherence interferometry for intraocular lens calculation according to Haigis. Graefes Arch Clin Exp Ophthalmol. 2000;238:765–73.

24. Shammas HJ, Taroni L, Pellegrini M, Shammas MC, Jivrajka RV. Accuracy of newer intraocular lens power formulas in short and long eyes using sum-of-segments biometry. J Cataract Refract Surg. 2022;48(10):1113–20.

25. Norrby S. Sources of error in intraocular lens power calculation. J Cataract Refract Surg. 2008;34(3):368–76.

26. Cooke DL, Cooke TL. A comparison of two methods to calculate axial length. J Cataract Refract Surg. 2019;45(3):284–92.

27. Taroni L, Hoffer KJ, Pellegrini M, Enrico L, Schiavi C, Savini G. Comparison of the new Hoffer QST with 4 modern accurate formulas. J Cataract Refract Surg. 2023;49(4):378–84. https://doi.org/10.1097/j.jcrs.0000000000001126.

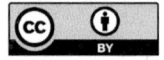

David L. Cooke and Jaime Aramberri

Introduction

Jack Holladay has authored over a hundred articles from how to calculate visual acuity to piggyback IOLs to negative dysphotopsia. He has authored numerous book chapters and books. He has been perhaps most tireless in the several hundred scientific presentations he has made, often staying after the lecture to help teach someone with lingering questions. Fortunately, he survived a type 1 aortic aneurysm repair in February 2010 [1]. Unfortunately, as a result, he has retired from clinical practice. Though he is still active in consulting, he has had to limit his involvement in additional projects, such as writing this chapter.

This chapter intends to focus on the two IOL power formulas that bear his name: Holladay 1 and Holladay 2 formulas. The second formula is closely linked to his software, Holladay IOL Consultant (HIC); several of its main features will be mentioned at the end. This chapter will begin with a basic math and science section, followed by a brief history of IOL power formulas until the time of the Holladay 1 formula.

Basic Math and Science

Holladay 1 is a thin-lens vergence formula. This was necessary when IOL power formulas started because the posterior curvature of the cornea could not be clinically measured and IOL companies did not provide any information about IOL physical features. Vergence of light is calculated from the object to image plane by means of well-defined analytical formulas that operate paraxially. Lens thicknessLens thickness is neglected in thin-lens formulas.

The main advantage of a thin-lens formula is simplicity. Both the powers of the cornea and of the IOL are defined by a single number (in diopters, D). A single lens constant can be used to change from one IOL type to another. In regular eyes, these formulas can perform with similar accuracy to more complex models, avoiding some disadvantages: Thick-lens raytracing models require the measurement of the posterior corneal curvature and the front and back radii of the IOL (usually not available). Artificial intelligence formulas require huge amounts of data; they tend to treat unusual eyes as "out-of-bounds," eyes because the algorithm has not yet been exposed to such eyes. In addition, artificial intelligence creates complex "black-box" mathematical formulas that are difficult to comprehend and impossible to write or compute simply.

D. L. Cooke (✉)
Department of Neurology and Ophthalmology,
Michigan State University, College of Osteopathic
Medicine, East Lansing, MI, USA

Great Lakes Eye Care, St. Joseph, Michigan, USA

J. Aramberri
Clínica Miranza BEGITEK San Sebastián/Clínica
ÓKULAR Vitoria, Vitoria-Gasteiz, Spain

© The Author(s) 2024

J. Aramberri et al. (eds.), *Intraocular Lens Calculations*, Essentials in Ophthalmology,
https://doi.org/10.1007/978-3-031-50666-6_44

A thin-lens formula is one that uses the general vergence formula. This can be calculated from the relationships between the vergence of light on the IOL, the power of the IOL, and the vergence of light on the retina (Fig. 44.1). These are all derived from the definition of vergence, where vergence (diopters) = n/d, where d is the focal distance between the lens and the focal plane, and n is the refractive index for that space.

Basic General Vergence Formula

$$IOL = \frac{1336}{AL - ELP} - \frac{1336}{\dfrac{1336}{TCP} - ELP} \quad (44.1)$$

If an IOL power is being determined for refraction other than for emmetropia, the following refraction component is added to TCP:

$$\frac{1000}{\dfrac{1000}{Ref} - Vertex} \quad (44.2)$$

AL is the axial length of the eye (mm). ELP is the effective lens position or location of the principal plane of IOL power (mm). IOL is the optical power of the implanted IOL (D). Ref is the postoperative refraction at the spectacle plane (D). Vertex is the spectacle back vertex distance (mm), and TCP is the total corneal power (D). Note that total corneal power does not refer to any specific company's calculation for corneal power.

A thin-lens formula is not necessarily inferior to a thick-lens formula, as long as all variables are correctly defined and the eye fulfills the conditions of paraxial optics. Unfortunately, assumptions and fudge factors have been used in all formulas because physiological accuracy has not yet been realized: Keratometry K value assumes a certain anterior-to-posterior curvature ratio when an arbitrary corneal index of refraction is used to take into account the posterior corneal power (like the corneal standard index of refraction 1.375), and the exact AL is still uncertain (see axial length chapter of this book). Because of these non-physiologic components in the thin-lens formula, the ELP is best considered an imaginary location in space that makes the formula predictions work.

The general vergence formula (GVF) needs only five variables (for the rest of this chapter, vertex distance will be considered a constant, such as 12 mm and not a variable): AL, ELP, IOL, TCP, and ref. The GVF can be manipulated to solve for any one of its five variables. Because ELP is in the denominator twice, some of the calculations can be complex. For simplicity, a box will be used instead of the actual calculations. Box 44.1 solves for the ideal IOL power, given a desired post-op refraction, and Box 44.2 solves for the desired refraction, given an IOL power.

Incorporated into the ELP is a lens constant that moves the ELP anteriorly or posteriorly, depending on the value. Every thin-lens formula works this way. When a desired post-op refraction is entered into most IOL calculators, they first use box 1 to determine the ideal IOL. They then choose a few adjacent available IOL powers, plug them into box 2, and give the predicted refraction for several IOL options.

Hoffer Q, Haigis, SRK/T, T2, and Holladay 1 and Holladay 2 all use the same box. The only

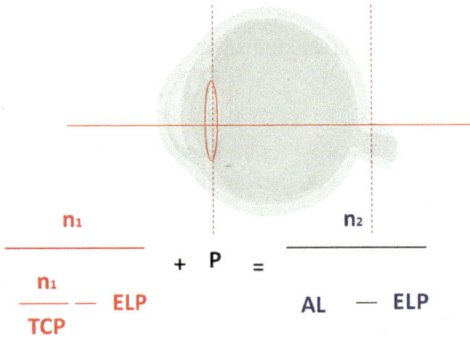

Fig. 44.1 Vergence of light on the retina is equal to the vergence on the IOL plus the IOL power (P). Effective lens position (ELP) is the distance from the cornea to the IOL, TCP is the total corneal power (diopters); AL is the axial length; and n1 and n2 are the indices of refraction of aqueous and vitreous, respectively. From this equation, IOL power can be easily calculated

Box 44.1

$$\boxed{IOL} = \boxed{\; \boxed{AL} \quad \boxed{TCP} \quad \boxed{ELP} \quad \boxed{Ref} \;}$$

Box 44.2

$$\boxed{Ref} = \boxed{\; \boxed{AL} \quad \boxed{TCP} \quad \boxed{ELP} \quad \boxed{IOL} \;}$$

differences are created by changes in TCP, AL, and ELP.

Brief History of IOL Power Formulas

Initially, there were no IOL power formulas. An 18-diopter IOL was placed (anterior to the iris) in every patient after cataract surgery. In 1967, Fyodorov published a method to choose individualized IOLs in the Russian literature [2]. In 1973, Colenbrander [3] published this ELP to go in the basic GVF:

$$ELP = (ACD - 0.05) \qquad (44.3)$$

In 1975, Fyodorov submitted this concept to the English literature [4].

$$ELP = r - \sqrt{\left(r^2 - \frac{(HWTW+1)^2}{4} \right)} \qquad (44.4)$$

where r is the corneal radius and HCD is the horizontal CD or corneal diameter.

In 1981, Binkhorst 2 introduced axial length into the ELP calculations.

$$ELP = \left(\frac{Minimum\ of\ 26\ or\ AL}{23.45} \right) \times ACD \qquad (44.5)$$

To determine ELP, Colenbrander used an unadjusted measurement of the ACD, Fyodorov used corneal measurements, and Binkhorst 2 modified ELP based on AL [5]. In 1988, Holladay published the first of his two formulas giving way to the third generation of vergence thin-lens formulas [6] being the first to use both axial length and Ks to compute the ELP. Two years later, the SRK/T [7] [8] came out, also using both axial length and Ks in Fyodorov's square root ELP function.

Holladay 1 Formula

It is important to acknowledge that this formula was completely disclosed in Holladay's paper because it has allowed readers to understand the details of the whole process. The main innovation of the Holladay 1 formula was the ELP calculating algorithm based on two predicting variables: AL and K. His formula can be decomposed as the sum of three values (Fig. 44.2):

$$ELP = Corneal\ thickness + Corneal\ height\,(H) + Surgeon\ factor\,(sf)$$

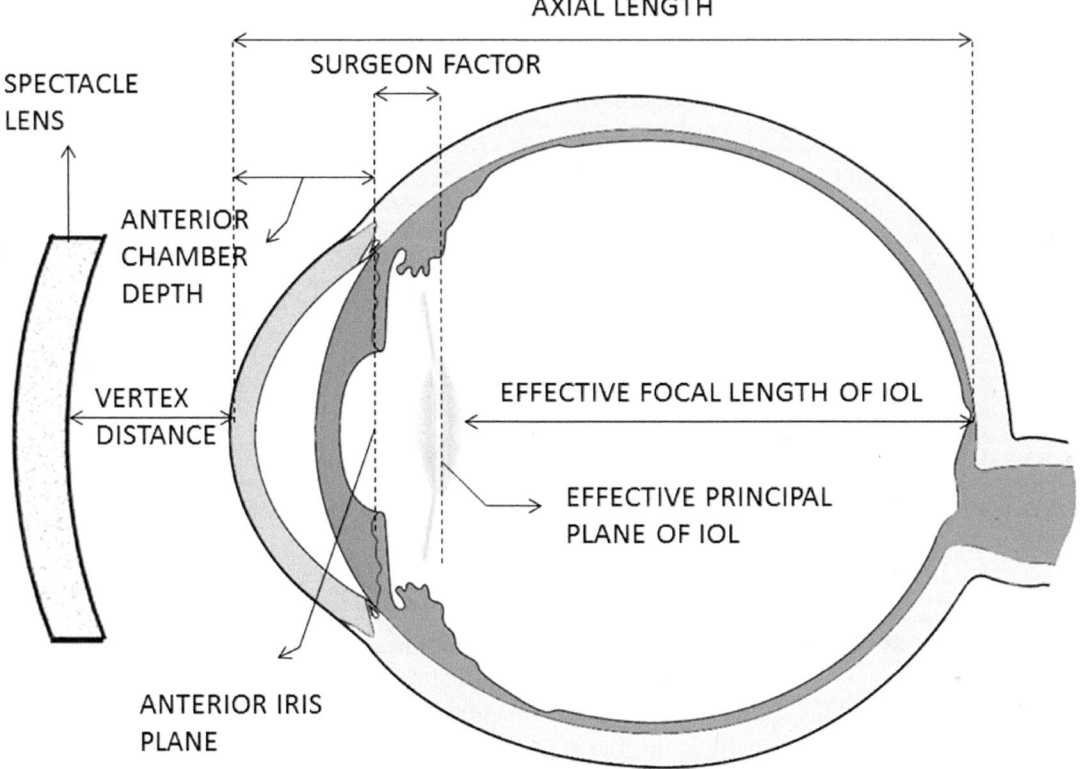

Fig. 44.2 Significant distances for IOL power calculation. Adapted from Holladay's paper [6]

Corneal thickness is a constant: 0.56 mm.

Corneal height (H) is the distance from the endothelium to the iris plane. It was calculated using the equation that calculates the height of a dome previously used for the same task by Fyodorov.

$$H = r - \sqrt{\left(r^2 - \frac{A^2}{4} \right)} \qquad (44.6)$$

where r is the radius of curvature of the cornea and A is the corneal diameter. One clever consideration was to limit the values under the square root so that the value could never be negative value. This was achieved by limiting functions both for r and A, which will become rag and AG:

$$rag = r, if \ r < 7, then \ rag = 7 \qquad (44.7)$$

$$AG = \frac{12.5 \times AL}{23.45}, if \ AG > 13.5,$$
$$then \ AG = 13.5 \qquad (44.8)$$

where AL is the measured axial length of the eye. As a consequence of these functions, the rag will never be lower than 7 mm and the corneal diameter will never be higher than 13.5 mm. With these modifications, the corneal height equation becomes

$$H = rag - \sqrt{\left(rag^2 - \frac{AG^2}{4} \right)} \qquad (44.9)$$

The sum of corneal thickness and corneal height yields the anterior chamber depth (ACD), defined by Holladay as the distance from the corneal vertex to the anterior iris plane.

The surgeon factor (sf) is the distance from the iris plane to the principal plane of IOL. However, even if this value represents that physical magnitude, Holladay proposed that it should be used as an adjustment factor to take account of any bias of the calculation process: biometer, keratometer, refraction accuracy, surgical technique, etc. In his paper, he also proposed a set of

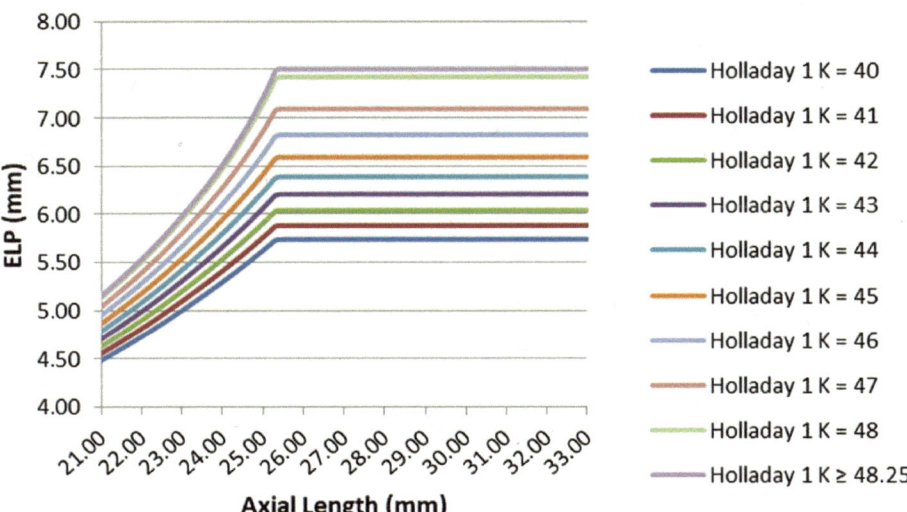

Holladay 1 ELP Prediction (sf = 1.8)

Legend:
- Holladay 1 K = 40
- Holladay 1 K = 41
- Holladay 1 K = 42
- Holladay 1 K = 43
- Holladay 1 K = 44
- Holladay 1 K = 45
- Holladay 1 K = 46
- Holladay 1 K = 47
- Holladay 1 K = 48
- Holladay 1 K ≥ 48.25

Fig. 44.3 ELP prediction as a function of AL for different average K values. It can be seen that for each K value, the ELP increase stops once the AL = 25.32 mm. In addition, all average Ks steeper than 48.5 D have identical ELP curve. *ELP* effective lens position

equations to back-calculate sf from the refractive results in order to personalize this factor for each surgeon in the article's appendix.

The final ELP equation becomes

$$ELP = 0.56 + rag - \sqrt{\left(rag^2 - \frac{ag^2}{4} \right)} + sf \quad (44.10)$$

It is interesting to graph this ELP function to better understand its behavior with different combinations of AL and K: For any K value, ELP arrives at a maximum value at AL = 25.32 mm; this maximum will increase as K increases until a threshold value of 48.25 D is reached. From then on, the ELP is at its maximum value. Figure 44.3 represents one such plot, where sf = 1.8.

As has been explained, capping of the ELP is the result of limiting the values of A and r in the corneal height (H) equation (Eq. 44.6) to avoid a negative number under the square root, but this can lead to some incorrect predictions in the real world: large anterior segments (e.g., megalocornea) where the IOL could settle very deep in the eye, probably would not predict correctly with this algorithm. In some keratoconus eyes, high K values create this ELP limit, while, in contrast,

the SRK/T tends to overestimate ELP, which fortuitously compensates for the abnormal anterior/posterior ratio of these eyes minimizing the hyperopic refraction trend of the Holladay 1.

Beyond the ELP equation, the Holladay 1 formula included a modification for AL and total corneal power (TCP): AL = al + 0.2. A retinal thickness constant value of 0.2 mm is added to the measured AL: TCP = 1000/(3 × r). This equation means that TCP is recalculated from the K measured by the keratometer, which is based on the standard keratometric index of refraction, 1.3375, to a value where the corneal index of refraction is the same value proposed by Binkhorst: 4/3.

Holladay 2 Formula

The Holladay 2 is identical to the Holladay 1 formula except for the ELP calculations [9]. The Holladay 2 ELP algorithm uses more predictors than AL and Ks. It also uses anatomic anterior chamber depth (ACD), lens thickness (LT), corneal diameter or horizontal CD (HCD), pre-op refraction, and age. Surgeons were initially asked to use a metal gauge device to measure HCD for the Holladay 2 formula. It was about half the size of a credit card and had various half-circles drawn on an edge. The surgeon was to match the half-circle to the circle of the cornea. Obviously, when the IOLMaster was able to also measure HCD along with ACD, LT, and AL, this was a welcomed improvement by surgeons who used the Holladay 2 formula.

This formula has not been published and is only available within the software Holladay IOL Consultant® and in different biometry and corneal topography devices. It is adapted to perform calculations in particular situations such as eyes that have undergone previous corneal refractive surgery where an alternative K value can be calculated with different methods. Afterward, the Holladay 2 formula will be used in a double-K manner to avoid the ELP estimation error (see the dedicated chapter in this book). In eyes filled with silicone oil or with a scleral buckle, the calculation is automatically adjusted. The toricity of the IOL is also calculated as described by Holladay in 2019. It is the difference between the postoperative refractive astigmatism in the corneal plane and the preoperative keratometric astigmatism [10]. This will empirically compensate for any of the following involved factors: posterior corneal astigmatism, IOL tilt and decentration, and any unknowns. The toric conversion from the corneal plane to IOL will be a function of ELP and IOL power as calculated by the formula.

Axial Length Adjustment

Holladay 1 was designed with ultrasound. It has suffered prediction accuracy at extreme axial lengths. Recently, it has been suggested that perhaps the switch from immersion, segmental ultrasound to optical biometry was at least partially responsible [11]. When optical biometry was modified to produce sum-of-segments axial length, these ultrasound-derived formulas did much better, for both long and short eyes, than when conventional optical biometric axial lengths were used. A modified sum-of-segments axial length, CMAL, was shown in one paper to improve both Holladay 1 and Holladay 2 at extreme axial lengths [12].

After co-authoring a paper that studied formula predictions with two large databases developed by Kaiser Permanente [13], Jack Holladay used those eyes to re-calibrate optical biometry AL for long eyes. He regressed to the ideal back-calculated axial lengths, which made the Holladay 1 and Holladay 2 formulas improve. Rather than a simple linear regression, he used a polynomial nonlinear regression [14]. The advantage of this over CMAL is that it does not require lens thickness.

These are the formulas proposed by Holladay to adjust the AL when its value is >24 mm:

$$AL \left(Holladay\, 1\, formula \right) = 0.0000462655^* A2 \wedge 5 - 0.0070852534^* A2 \wedge 4 + 0.4320542309^* A2 \wedge 3$$
$$- 13.1162616532^* A2 \wedge 2 + 199.1238629431^* A2 - 1190.3984759734$$

$$AL \left(Holladay\, 2\, formula \right) = -0.0001154786^* A2 \wedge 3 + 0.0032939472^* A2 \wedge 2$$
$$+ 1.001040305^* A2 - 0.3270056564$$

where A2 is the AL measured by the optical biometer (non-segmented measurement).

Formula Performance

Holladay 1 has performed well through the years. Being a mainstay for standard-length eyes since a paper in 1993 [15] where Hoffer found that Hoffer Q was ideal in short eyes, SRK/T was ideal in long eyes, and Holladay 1 was ideal for the bulk of the eyes in the middle.

Though results are similar, Holladay 1 tends to outperform Holladay 2 for normal-length eyes. The value of Holladay 2 improves greatly for longer eyes, especially when AL is adjusted. Perhaps hundreds of studies have compared these formulas. A few of the larger ones were selected to highlight the results.

Aristodemou et al. [16] studied Hoffer Q, Holladay 1, or SRK/T in 8108 eyes after cataract surgery, evaluating more than one IOL model. His group found that Holladay 1 had the best mean absolute error for eyes from 23.50 mm to 25.99 mm.

Another study of 1079 eyes, of 1079 patients, compared results of eyes measured with (Lenstar data) and without (IOLMaster 500 data) lens thickness [17]. Holladay 1 was better than Holladay 2, SRK/T, and Hoffer Q. However, when LT was added as a variable in these same eyes, Holladay 2 became the best of these formulas.

A paper by Kane et al [18] compared 3241 patients. Following the general rule, for medium (AL > 22.0 mm to <24.5 mm) and medium long (AL ≥ 24.5 to <26.0 mm) eyes, Holladay 1 was once again the best of these four formulas, but the Holladay 2 was better for the long eyes (> 26 mm). Note that the actual differences among these formulas were quite small. The maximum difference in mean absolute error between Barrett and T2, SRKT, and Haigis was about 0.08 diopter (Fig. 44.4).

In the previously mentioned Kaiser Permanente study [13], Melles studied two IOL models in 18,501 eyes from 18,501 patients. The Holladay 2 had the lowest standard deviation of these four formulas, but only slightly better than Holladay 1. When the original Wang-Koch long-eye adjuster was applied to Holladay 1, it became the best of all these formulas.

In an update of this study [19], a subgroup analysis of 13,301 eyes with SN60WF implants showed that in all breakdowns of eyes with axial lengths over 22.5. Holladay 2 was better than Holladay 1, Hoffer Q, and SRK/T. For eyes between 22.5 and 25.5, Holladay 1 was better than Hoffer Q and SRK/T, but for eyes longer than 25.5, SRK/T was the best of these three formulas.

None of the prior studies used the Holladay 1 or 2 formulas with the updated nonlinear regression AL. In 2019, a study of 10,930 eyes from the UK National Health Services evaluated Holladay 2 using the updated formula with nonlinear regression AL [20]. It compared 9 IOL power formulas, ranking them by mean absolute error. The authors found the Holladay 2 to be the second-best formula for short eyes (≤ 22.00 mm) and for long eyes (≥ 26.00 mm).

In Tables 44.1 and 44.2, the outcomes of Holladay 1 and Holladay 2 published in the last 5 years are presented.

Holladay IOL Consultant Software.

The Holladay HIC program has several helpful additions beyond merely containing the

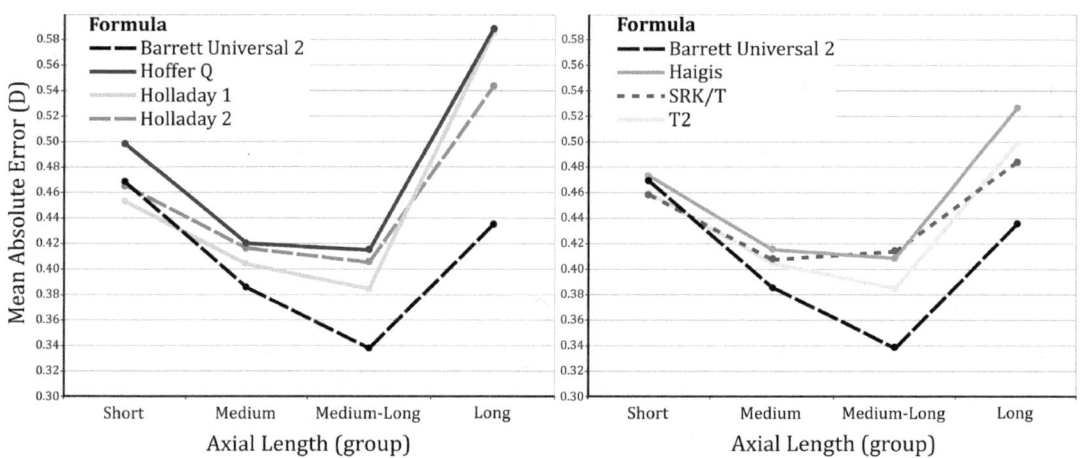

Fig. 44.4 (From Kane paper [18]) Mean absolute error plotted against AL groups for the Barrett Universal II, Hoffer Q, Holladay 1, Holladay 2, Haigis, SRK/T, and T2 formulas. Formulas were grouped to allow easier visualization

Table 44.1 Holladay 1 formula outcomes in recently published papers. IOLM: IOLMaster. SD: standard deviation

First author	Year	Mean	SD	MAE	MEDAE	% in ±0.50 D	% in ±1.00 D	N
Cooke [17] (Lenstar)	2016	0.00	0.408	0.320	0.268	79.1	98.6	1079
Cooke [17] (IOLM 500)	2016	0.00	0.414	0.326	0.270	79.5	98.4	1079
Kane [18]	2016	0.00	n.a.	0.408	0.326	69.4	99.6	3241
Kane [21]	2017	−0.01	n.a.	0.398	0.321	70.1	94.3	3122
Næser [22]	2019	−0.06	0.36	0.290	0.250	85.0	100.0	151
Melles [13]	2018	0.00	0.453	0.351	0.287	75.0	96.8	18,501
Melles [13] (W-K)	2018	0.00	0.439	0.340	0.275	76.6	97.2	18,501
Darcy [20]	2020	0.00	0.512	0.397	0.321	69.6	94.4	10,930
Taroni [23]	2020	0.00	0.382	0.298	0.257	82.4	98.9	101
Hipolito-Fernandes [24]	2020	0.00	0.461	0.361	0.299	74.3	96.1	828
Tsessler [25] (Lenstar)	2021	0.02	0.38	0.29	0.21	81.0	98.0	153
Tsessler [25] (IOLM 700)	2021	−0.05	0.37	0.29	0.24	80.0	100.0	153
Tsessler [25] (IOLM 700 + TK)	2021	0.02	0.38	0.29	0.24	80.0	98.0	153

MAE mean absolute error, *MEDAE* median absolute error, *W-K* Wang-Koch AL correction, *TK* total keratometry by IOL Master 700, *n.a.* not available

Table 44.2 Holladay 2 formula outcomes in recently published papers

First author	Year	Mean	SD	MAE	MEDAE	% in ±0.50 D	% in ±1.00 D	N
Cooke [17] (Lenstar) Presurg ref	2016	0.00	0.423	0.336	0.288	76.6	98.4	557
Cooke [17] (IOLM 500) Presurg ref	2016	0.00	0.432	0.346	0.297	75.2	98.1	557
Cooke [17] (Lenstar) no ref	2016	0.00	0.404	0.318	0.261	79	98.1	557
Cooke [17] (IOLM 500) no ref	2016	0.00	0.417	0.331	0.287	79.3	97.7	1079
Kane [18]	2016	0.00	n.a.	0.420	0.341	67.4	99.7	3241
Kane [21]	2017	−0.01	n.a.	0.410	0.337	68.2	94.4	3122
Melles [13]	2018	0.00	0.450	0.350	0.285	75.4	97.0	18,501
Darcy [20]	2020	0.00	0.503	0.390	0.312	71.0	94.9	10,930
Taroni [23]	2020	0.00	0.411	0.322	0.285	82.4	97.8	101
Tsessler [25] (IOLM 700)	2021	−0.18	0.39	0.34	0.28	79	99	153
Tsessler [25] (IOLM 700 + TK)	2021	0.10	0.40	0.33	0.29	78	99	153

IOLM IOLMaster, *SD* standard deviation, *MAE* mean absolute error, *MEDAE* median absolute error, *AL* axial length correction, *TK* total keratometry by IOL Master 700, *n.a.* not available, *Presurg ref.* pre-surgery refraction used in the calculation, *No ref.* pre-surgery refraction not used in the calculation

Holladay 2 formula. There is a complete set of options to address most of the situations found in the clinical practice: post-LASIK and post-RK eyes, silicone-filled eyes, scleral buckle, keratoconus, etc. Calculation of the IOL power can be adjusted for sulcus implantation. The HIC program can use a refractive formula, thereby not needing an AL, for these calculations in either aphakic or pseudophakic eyes: secondary implants, and phakic IOL calculations.

There is a toric pre-op planner menu to perform toric IOL calculations where the IOL placement axis and the expected refraction for the selected lens are clearly displayed (Fig. 44.5a) and a postoperative toric analysis module that

calculates the total SIA and the rotation needed to achieve the best possible refraction (Fig. 44.5b). The latter is done by two methods, from postoperative Ks and refraction and from the observed IOL meridian and postoperative refraction, which allows double-checking to detect any incorrect data. These toric calculations are done taking into account the effect of ELP and IOL power by the Holladay 2 formula.

After surgery, two software modules allow the surgeon to study postoperative results: One calculates the postoperative surgically induced refractive change (SIRC) both for refraction values and for keratometry values (Fig. 44.6). The other back-calculates five variables individually from the actual values. These are AL, K, post-op

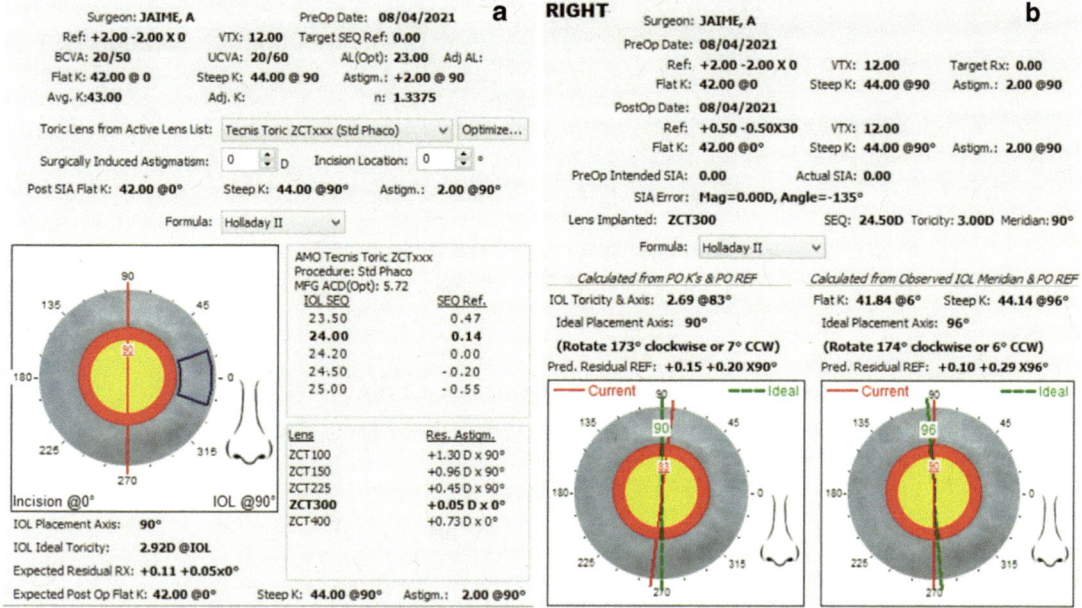

Fig. 44.5 (**a** and **b**)On the left is the toric IOL planner where the toric IOL and the predicted refraction are displayed. On the right is the toric IOL postoperative back calculator where the rotation of the implanted IOL that will yield the minimum astigmatism is calculated by two methods

Rx, IOL power, and IOL constant (Fig. 44.6b). These can be useful to look for the reason for a postoperative refractive surprise as four of these variables can be checked again.

There is a powerful aggregate data analysis tool called surgical outcomes assessment program (SOAP) that offers prediction error analysis allowing for different selection criteria, a complete induced astigmatism study, and IOL constant optimization for SRK/T, Hoffer Q, Holladay 1, and Holladay 2 formulas.

Acknowledgments Many of the references and much understanding of the early formulas were enhanced from this manual: Retzlaff JA, Sanders DR, and Kraff M. Lens Implant Power Calculation A manual for ophthalmologists and biometrists Ed 3. 1990 Slack.

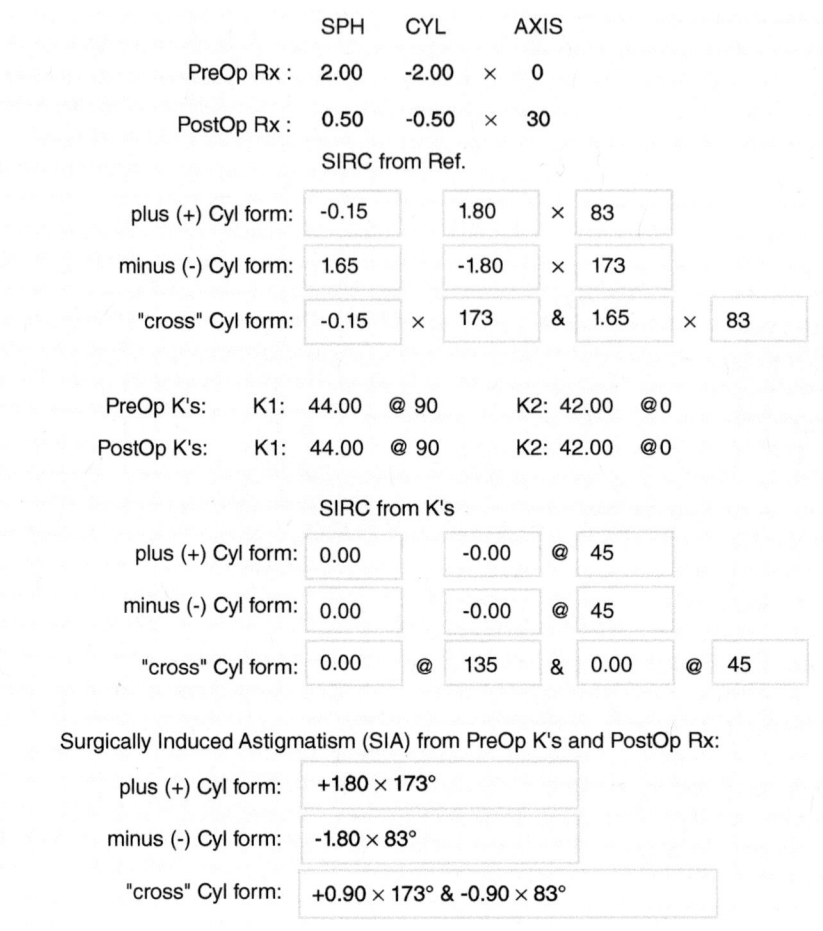

a

	SPH	CYL		AXIS
PreOp Rx :	2.00	-2.00	×	0
PostOp Rx :	0.50	-0.50	×	30

SIRC from Ref.

plus (+) Cyl form:	-0.15	1.80	×	83
minus (-) Cyl form:	1.65	-1.80	×	173
"cross" Cyl form:	-0.15	× 173	& 1.65	× 83

PreOp K's: K1: 44.00 @ 90   K2: 42.00 @0
PostOp K's: K1: 44.00 @ 90   K2: 42.00 @0

SIRC from K's

plus (+) Cyl form:	0.00	-0.00	@	45
minus (-) Cyl form:	0.00	-0.00	@	45
"cross" Cyl form:	0.00	@ 135	& 0.00	@ 45

Surgically Induced Astigmatism (SIA) from PreOp K's and PostOp Rx:

plus (+) Cyl form:	+1.80 × 173°
minus (-) Cyl form:	-1.80 × 83°
"cross" Cyl form:	+0.90 × 173° & -0.90 × 83°

Fig. 44.6 (**a** and **b**)On the left is the surgically induced refractive change (SIRC) calculator. On the right is the postoperative back calculator that is useful to analyze unexpected postoperative refractions

b   Actual Values:

Implanted IOL Power SEQ: 24.50

PostOp SEQ Ref: 0.250   VTX: 12.0

PreOp Adj AL: 23.00

PreOp Avg K: 43.00

Lens Constant(LC): 5.724   MFG

BackCalculated Values (Calculated from 4 measured values)

                                                                From:

IOL Power SEQ: 23.830   D.   (K, AL, LC, Ref)

SEQ Ref: -0.203   D.   (K, AL, LC, IOL)

Adj AL: 22.808   mm   (K, LC, IOL, Ref)

Avg. K: 42.405   D.   (AL, LC, IOL, Ref)

LC: 6.019   (K, AL, IOL, Ref)

Prediction Error: -0.453   D.   (Pred Ref - PO Ref)

Fig. 44.6 (continued)

References

1. http://www.hicsoap.com/biography.php.
2. Fyodorov SN, Kolonko AI. Estimation of optical power of the intraocular lens. Vestnik Oftalmologic (Moscow). 1967;4:27.
3. Colenbrander MC. Calculation of the power of an iris clip lens for distant vision. Br J Ophthalmol. 1973;57(10):735–40.
4. Fyodorov SN, Galin MA, Linksz A. Calculation of the optical power of intraocular lenses. Investig Ophthalmol. 1975;14(8):625–8.
5. Binkhorst RD. Intraocular lens power calculation manual: a guide to the Author's TI 58/59 IOL power module. Ed 2 ed. New York: Binkhorst RD; 1981.
6. Holladay JT, Prager TC, Chandler TY, Musgrove KH, Lewis JW, Ruiz RS. A three-part system for refining intraocular lens power calculations. J Cataract Refract Surg. 1988;14:17–24.
7. Retzlaff JA, Sanders DR, Kraff MC. Development of the SRK/T intraocular lens implant power calculation formula. J Cataract Refract Surg. 1990;16:333–40. erratum, 528
8. Retzlaff JA, Sanders DR, Kraff MC. Comparison of the SRK/T formula and other theoretical and regression formulas. J Cataract Refract Surg. 1990;16:341–6.
9. It can be shown that only ELPs differ between Holladay 1 and Holladay 2 programs from the following: The HIC program back-calculates ideal ELP for Holladay 2 formula. Taking this back-calculated Holladay 2 ELP and inserting it as the ELP in the Holladay 1 program gives identical predictions as the Holladay 2 program.
10. Holladay JT, Pettit G. Improving toric intraocular lens calculations using total surgically induced astigmatism for a 2.5 mm temporal incision. J Cataract Refract Surg. 2019;45:272–83.
11. Cooke DL, Cooke TL. A comparison of two methods to calculate axial length. J Cataract Refract Surg. 2019;45(3):284–92.
12. Cooke DL, Cooke TL. Approximating sum-of-segments axial length from a traditional optical low-coherence reflectometry measurement. J Cataract Refract Surg. 2019;45(3):351–4.
13. Melles RB, Holladay JT, Chang WJ. Accuracy of intraocular lens calculation formulas. Ophthalmology. 2018;125(2):169–78.
14. Wang L, Holladay JT, Koch DD. Wang-Koch axial length adjustment for the Holladay 2 formula in long eyes. J Cataract Refract Surg. 2018;44(10):1291–2. Erratum J Cataract Refract Surg. 2019 Jan;45(1):117.

15. Hoffer KJ. The Hoffer Q formula: a comparison of theoretic and regression formulas. J Cataract Refract Surg. 1993;19:700–12. (Zuberbuhler B, Morrell AJ. Errata in printed Hoffer Q formula. J Cataract Refract Surg. 2007;33(1):2; author reply 2–3. https://doi.org/10.1016/j.jcrs.2006.08.054.)

16. Aristodemou P, Knox Cartwright NE, Sparrow JM, Johnston RL. Formula choice: Hoffer Q, Holladay 1, or SRK/T and refractive outcomes in 8108 eyes after cataract surgery with biometry by partial coherence interferometry. J Cataract Refract Surg. 2011;37(1):63–71.

17. Cooke DL, Cooke TL. Comparison of 9 intraocular lens power calculation formulas. J Cataract Refract Surg. 2016;42(8):1157–64.

18. Kane JX, Van Heerden A, Atik A, Petsoglou C. Intraocular lens power formula accuracy: comparison of 7 formulas. J Cataract Refract Surg. 2016;42(10):1490–500.

19. Melles RB, Kane JX, Olsen T, Chang WJ. Update on intraocular lens calculation formulas. Ophthalmology. 2019;126(9):1334–5.

20. Darcy K, Gunn D, Tavassoli S, Sparrow J, Kane JX. Assessment of the accuracy of new and updated intraocular lens power calculation formulas in 10930 eyes from the UK National Health Service. J Cataract Refract Surg. 2020;46(1):2–7. https://doi.org/10.1016/j.jcrs.2019.08.014. PMID: 32050225

21. Kane J, van Heerden A, Atik A, Petsoglou C. (2017). Accuracy of 3 new methods for intraocular lens power selection. J Cataract Refract Surg. 2017;43:333–9.

22. Næser K, Savini G. Accuracy of thick-lens intraocular lens power calculation based on cutting-card or calculated data for lens architecture. J Cataract Refract Surg. 2019;45:1422–9.

23. Taroni L, Hoffer KJ, Barboni P, Schiano-Lomoriello D, Savini G. Outcomes of IOL power calculation using measurements by a rotating Scheimpflug camera combined with partial coherence interferometry. J Cataract Refract Surg. 2020;46(12):1618–23.

24. Hipolito-Fernandes D, Luis M, Gil P, Maduro V, Fejiao J, Yeo T, Alves N. VRF-G, a new intraocular lens power calculation formula: a 13 formulas comparison study. Clin Ophthalmol. 2020;14:4395–402.

25. Tsessler M, Cohen S, Wang L, Koch DD, Zadok D, Abulafia A. Evaluating the prediction accuracy of the hill-RBF 3.0 formula using a heteroscedastic statistical method. J Cataract Refract Surg. 2022;48(1):37–43.

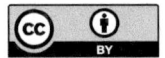

Intraoperative Aberrometry

Sean Ianchulev

Over the last decade, the growing adoption of presbyopia-correcting IOLs has created a growing need for high-precision cataract surgical outcomes driving an unprecedented clinical interest and research in IOL power calculation and biometry. In fact, the number of IOL power estimation studies increased dramatically over the last decade: from an average of 3 per year from 2010 through 2014 to an average of more than 17 per year from 2018 through 2020, with at least 36 formulas and biometric methodologies identified in 2010–2020. [1].

Precision has continued to increase as a result of these innovative approaches, and we see more than 70–75% of eyes within 0.5D of target refractive outcomes [2]. Thanks to advancements in IOL calculators, postoperative mean absolute prediction errors (MAEs) have continued to improve—a further 25% decrease in less than 10 years from 0.4 to 0.3 MAE between 2008 and 2018. [3, 4] On the instrumentation front, biometric precision has accounted for a significant part of that progress as newer technologies seem to have closed the precision gaps in keratometry and axial length measurement variability. Today, instruments such as the IOLMaster and Lenstar allow more accurate IOL power calculations to

be performed with a high level of biometric resolution of less than 20 microns [5].

Nevertheless, challenges remain. Effective lens position (ELP) estimation remains a significant source of formulaic predictive uncertainty, despite the fact that newer formulas have been developed and older ones have been optimized with the goal of improving the accuracy of IOL power calculations. Conventional intraocular lens power formulas generally fall into several categories: vergence (Hoffer Q, Holladay 1 and 2, and SRK/T), artificial intelligence (RBF AI), ray tracing (Olsen), or a combination approach (Kane). All of these biometry methods are accurate in normal and long axial length eyes but less so in short axial length eyes, mainly because errors in axial length measurement or ELP estimation are magnified by the higher dioptric power of the IOL. While Hoffer Q and Haigis seem to perform better in that category, there is still a significant need for a more precise estimation. In addition, all of the conventional predictive models have shortcomings when it comes to eyes that have had prior refractive surgery where the postoperative refractive errors are larger than what the conventional models predict in normal eyes.

Despite significant differences across the various IOL formulas, they mostly share the same basic principle deriving from Fyodorov's original equation—they are based on preoperative anatomic parameters, such as axial length and

S. Ianchulev (✉)
Department of Ophthalmology, New York Eye and Ear of Mount Sinai, New York, NY, USA

J. Aramberri et al. (eds.), *Intraocular Lens Calculations*, Essentials in Ophthalmology,
https://doi.org/10.1007/978-3-031-50666-6_45

corneal curvature, which they use to derive an optical variable—IOL power. The improved second-, third-, and fourth-generation formulas have pushed the predictive efficacy of the preoperative methodology higher, but most of the formulas now operate on the plateau part of their efficacy curve. As surgeons and patients continue to reach for the emmetropic nirvana and postoperative spectacle independence, new approaches and technologies are needed, which can inflect the efficacy curve or put us on a different one altogether.

Intraoperative Refractive Biometry: Aphakic Method

One novel approach that dramatically departs from conventional preoperative methodologies was first introduced by Ianchulev et al. in 2003. Intraoperative refractive biometry was one of the first technologies to deliver automated, on-demand surgical biometry in the operating room more than a decade before intraoperative OCT, imaging, and sensing technologies started to enter the surgical paradigm. In its first embodiment and original implementation, intraoperative refractive biometry used a near-infrared autorefractor to obtain an "optical biopsy" of the eye after the extraction of the cataractous lens. During this unique transiently aphakic state, the surgeon can measure the aphakic spherical equivalent of the eye. Assuming minimal distortion of ocular optics during surgery (as is typical of today's minimally invasive phaco techniques) and high accuracy of auto-refracting devices, the aphakic spherical equivalent informs us about the optical deficit of the aphakic eye at the vertex distance of measurement. Converting and correlating this to the power at the intraocular plane of the final lens position are the basis of the original Ianchulev formulaic method of estimating the emmetropic IOL power biometrically in the OR. The Ianchulev formula was empirically derived as a correlation between the aphakic spherical equivalent and the emmetropic IOL power. It added further validation to earlier theoretical constructs based on Bennett-Rabbetts 1 schematic eye vari-

ants, which demonstrate that the expected ratio between the aphakic spherical equivalent and the final emmetropic power is in the range of 1.75–2.01.

This new aphakic methodology positioned the science of IOL power estimation on a new curve of innovation, which was not limited to preoperative assessments but introduced a biometric methodology to the intraoperative surgical paradigm. Because of its purely refractive approach, which is less dependent on anatomic corneal curvature and axial length (which are inherently factored in optically into the aphakic autorefraction), one would expect less confounding by the effect of prior refractive surgery. In fact, preoperative anatomic measurement could be eliminated altogether in this purely aphakic refractive paradigm where diagnostic optical biometry is done "on the table" at the point of cataract surgery. In addition, any optical effect of the surgical incision on the cornea could also be captured in this intraoperative setting.

While the portable intraoperative autorefractor was initially used for this aphakic method, applying the technique intraoperatively was not trivial. Initial clinical experience has shown that in order to achieve the full potential of this method, control over and experience with a number of variables are important. A reliable autorefractor such as the portable Retinomax (Nikon Optical, NJ, USA) or the Nidek AR-20 device (Nidek, Co. Ltd., Japan) should be used because many autorefractors were not optimized to the refractive range of the aphakic setting. Vertex distance, visual axis centration, and parallax are important, as are post-phaco corneal status, intraocular pressure (over/under-filled AC), and type of viscoelastic used for chamber maintenance (Fig. 45.1).

Early clinical work by Ianchulev, Leccisotti, and Wong demonstrated the clinical utility of intraoperative refractive biometry for IOL power estimation. The first formula for intraoperative autorefraction was derived in 2003 and later reported by Ianchulev et al. in a series of 38 eyes, six of which were post-prior LASIK patients. [6] The range of the axial length was 21.4–25.2 mm with a range of IOL power implanted from 12.0

to 28.5 D. Autorefraction vertex distance was 13.1, and A constant of the IOL used was 118.40. A strong linear correlation was found in a series of 38 eyes across a wide range of emmetropic IOL powers (Fig. 45.2).

Using linear regression, the following empiric formula was derived based on a strong "linear fit" between aphakic spherical equivalent and emmetropic IOL:

$$\text{Ianchulev formula}: P = 2.01 \times ASE$$

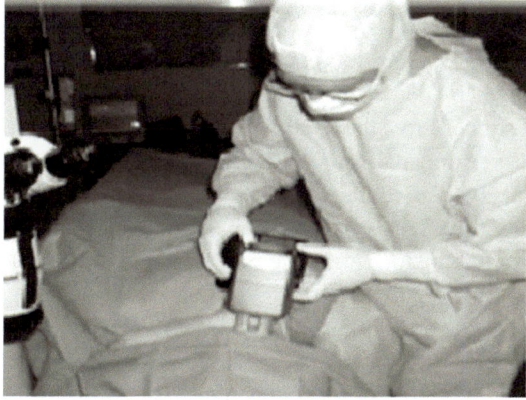

Fig. 45.1 An intraoperative refractometry after cataract removal and prior to IOL implantation: a portable autorefractor used during cataract surgery

where P = emmetropic IOL power, ASE aphakic spherical equivalent.

In the published series, more than 93% of the variability of the final emmetropic power is accounted for by the linear relationship with aphakic spherical equivalent—in standard eyes, the conventional formulas and the optical refractive model showed equivalent predictive efficacy with a correlation coefficient of 0.96. In addition, 83% of the LASIK eyes and 100% of the normal eyes were within ±1 D of the final IOL power when aphakic autorefraction was used, compared with 67% of LASIK eyes and 100% of the normal eyes using the conventional method.

Several other studies provided additional validation of the original technique and formula described by Ianchulev et al. In a prospective, non-comparative consecutive case series of 82 myopic eyes with a mean preoperative spherical equivalent of −12.80 D [range − 3 D to −27 D], Leccisotti et al. derived a modification of Ianchulev's formula for the myopic population: [7].

$$\text{Leccisotti formula}: P = 1.3 \times ASE + 1.45$$

where P = emmetropic IOL power and ASE aphakic spherical equivalent.

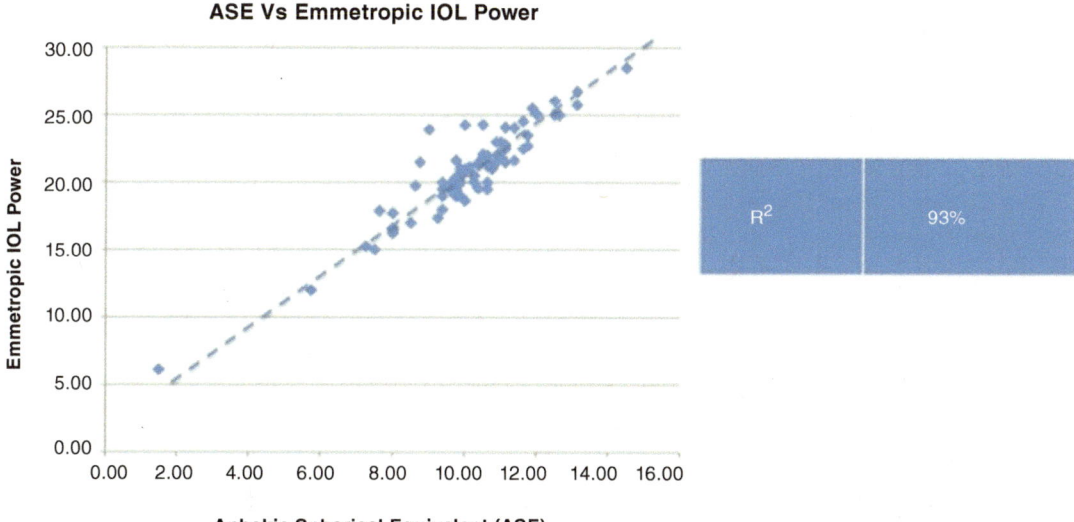

Fig. 45.2 Linear regression of the original Ianchulev et al. series between emmetropic IOL power and aphakic spherical equivalent (ASE)

A more definitive study by Wong et al. compared the Ianchulev formula with and without a Leccisotti modification in a series of 182 eyes and demonstrated that while the Ianchulev formula holds across the wide spectrum of IOL powers, the Leccisotti modification performs

slightly better in myopic eyes (AL >25) [8]. In addition, another set of intraoperative aphakic refractive formulas was derived from this series as follows:

$$\text{For AL} < 25.5\,\text{mm} : P = 1.97 \times \text{SE}$$

$$\text{For AXL} \geq 25.5\,\text{mm} : P = 0.015 \times \text{SE2} + 1.5 \times \text{SE} + 1.5$$

where P = emmetropic IOL power and ASE aphakic spherical equivalent.

Ultimately, the original methodology by Ianchulev et al. demonstrated that one can develop a purely refractive intraoperative paradigm for IOL calculation, which helps solve important aspects of IOL estimation in post-Lasik eyes. It can also be applicable to the standard cataract case where refractive biometry can refine and verify the final IOL calculation. With the development of new integrated equipment that streamlines automated refraction at the point of surgery, significantly higher accuracy can be achieved from measurement standardization, better centration of autorefraction, and incorporation of additional intraoperative parameters in optical analysis such as keratometry. Intraoperative refractive biometry for IOL calculation may ultimately represent another important tangential point along the expanding interface between cataract and refractive surgery.

While these early efforts with intraoperative aphakic biometry set the stage for subsequent progress and introduced a new technological curve of development for IOL power estimation, there were challenges with the intraoperative refractive technique. Similar to conventional methods, it did not address the perennial problem of effective lens position (ELP). It was dependent on suboptimal biometric instrumentation (autorefractors), which was not specifically designed for the aphakic range nor the intraoperative setting. While simple and effective as a one-step purely refractive measurement, which eliminated the need for preoperative assessments, there was more to be desired for standardization and improved efficacy.

Intraoperative Aberrometry

The original clinical efforts on intraoperative aphakic autorefraction in early 2000 were bolstered by better refractive technology specifically designed for the intraoperative setting. Using wavefront analysis to characterize the entire optical system of the eye, both lower and higher order aberrations, was a natural evolution for high-precision refractive biometry. Previously, in optimizing treatment algorithms for laser keratorefractive surgery, wavefront analysis was introduced to the cataract surgical paradigm as a guidance system for intraocular lens power selection and astigmatic correction with LRIs and toric IOLs.

Technologies

The Hartmann-Shack interferometer system was the most common wavefront aberrometry technology in clinical use. Mechanistically, it works by projecting a ray of infrared light onto the retina and analyzing its reflection as it travels back through the pupil, after being focused by an array of lenslets [9]. The array of spot images is captured by a video sensor, and these spot images are computationally compared to their presumed locations in an aberration-free system while in the process generating a wavefront aberration map.

While a number of Hartmann-Shack systems were in clinical use (LADARWave, WaveScan, and Zywave) for laser refractive surgery, these systems were not suited for intraoperative use in cataract surgery. They needed to be adapted in order to attach to the surgical microscope and further optimized for aphakic measurements.

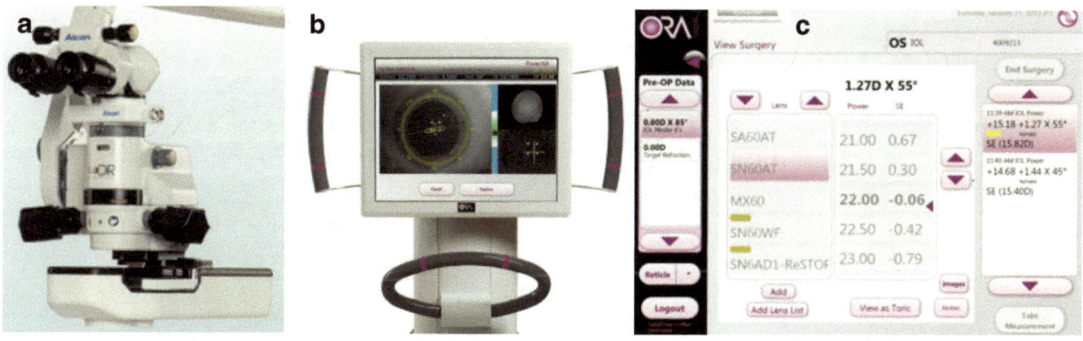

Figs. 45.3 ORA system™ (Alcon): (**a**) Aberrometer adjusted to the operating microscope. (**b**) Centration and alignment screen. (**c**) User interface

The ORA (formerly Orange) intraoperative wavefront aberrometer, manufactured by WaveTec (Alcon), is the first intraoperative aberrometry system designed for use during cataract surgery (Fig. 45.3). ORA may also be one of the first automated biometry systems for intraoperative diagnostic use in ophthalmology. In addition, it incorporated one of the first cloud-based surgical data collection tools with the help of WaveTec AnalyzOR, which accumulates data from all ORA users. The global surgical dataset of outcomes allowed for software updates, formula optimizations, and surgeon factor adjustments—in a continuous effort to increase the system's predictive accuracy.

The ORA uses a Talbot-Moiré interferometry [10]. In Talbot-Moiré technology, the device processes the optical wavefront through a pair of gratings set a particular distance and angle apart. The grating pair diffracts the transiting wavefront and that diffraction produces a fringe pattern whereby a subsequent analysis of the fringe pattern aberrations produces a refractive value. The Talbot-Moiré interferometry is different from the Hartman Schack device—it has increased speed and is small enough to be coupled with the surgical microscope for intraoperative use. The ORA device was optimized for both aphakic and pseudophakic biometry so that it can guide and inform IOL power selection, toric IOL power and axis, and both length and axis of limbal relaxing incisions [11].

Intraoperative aberrometry with the ORA is technically seamless and well integrated into the

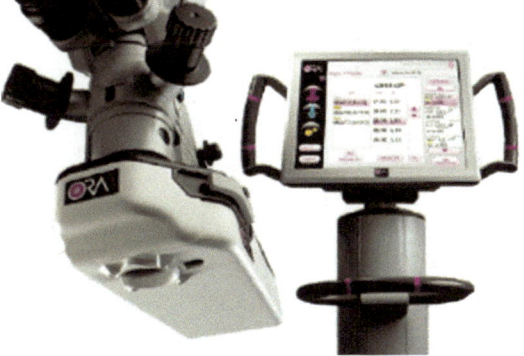

Fig. 45.4 ORA system

cataract surgical flow process. The aberrometer is attached to the surgical microscope and is small enough that it does not interfere with the surgeon's view (Fig. 45.4).

Measurement

While it takes less than thirty seconds to obtain a refractive measurement, there are essential steps to ensure precise results (Figs. 45.5, 45.6, 45.7, and 45.8). For testing the aphakic refraction, it is important to have a sealed incision and avoid overhydration. The central cornea needs to be kept clear and free of distortion. IOP should be at physiologic levels, ideally between 18 and 30 mmHg. Minimize any external pressure and interferences from the speculum and drapes. An important question is whether to have the anterior chamber filled with BSS or viscoelastic and whether the type of viscoelastic and its specific refractive index affect the predictive accuracy of

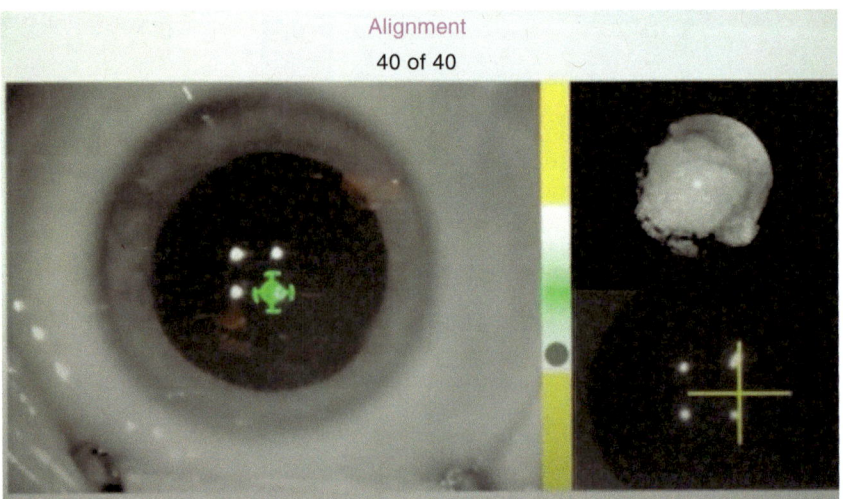

Fig. 45.5 Centration screen

Fig. 45.6 Measurement
and IOL power
calculation

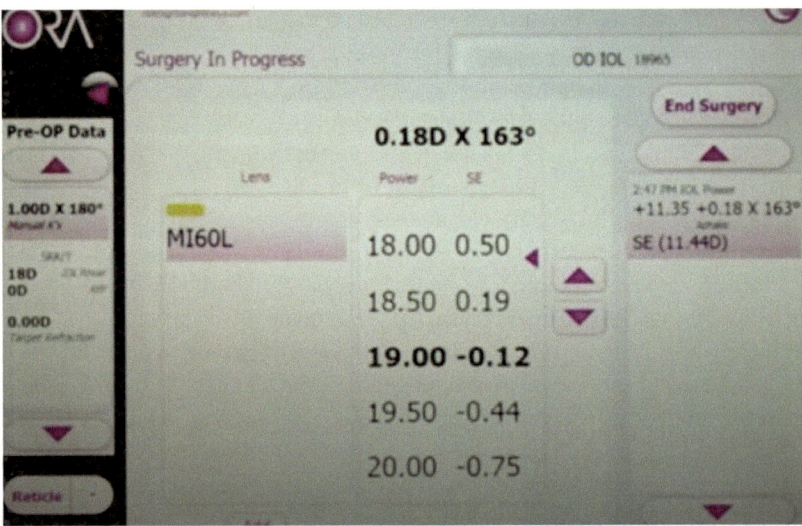

intraoperative aberrometry. That question was answered in a study of 120 eyes, which investigated the correlation between predicted power error (based on an index of refraction disparity between balanced salt solution (BSS) and ophthalmic viscosurgical device (OVD)) and actual aphakic power error. The IOL power determination was lower with OVD filling the chamber—mostly a result of the differences in the index of refraction between BSS and the OVDs used. The results for DisCoVisc and Amvisc Plus suggested an IOL power approximately 0.50 D lower than readings taken with BSS, while the difference for the other agents was less than 0.25 D. In addition, the MAE outcomes were lower with BSS than with OVD, with the exception of Amvisc, for which the results were identical. The differences were statistically significant with DisCoVisc ($P < 0.001$) and Amvisc Plus.

Another aspect of clinical investigation is whether the type of speculum/blepharostat used may impact the biometry. A controlled prospective study examined several speculum configurations and their refractive impact [12]. It concluded that the speculum with the least impact on the IA reading is the open-blade threaded blepharostat.

Fig. 45.7 In vivo calculation of residual astigmatism

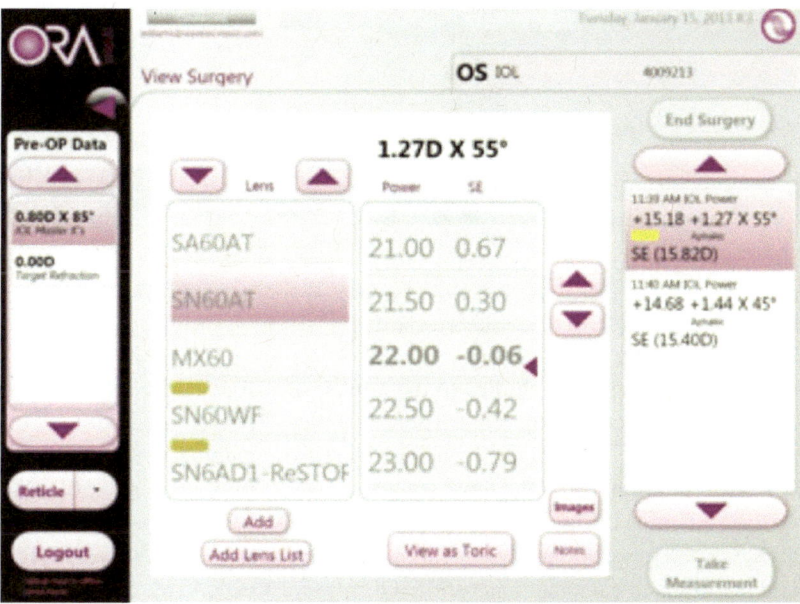

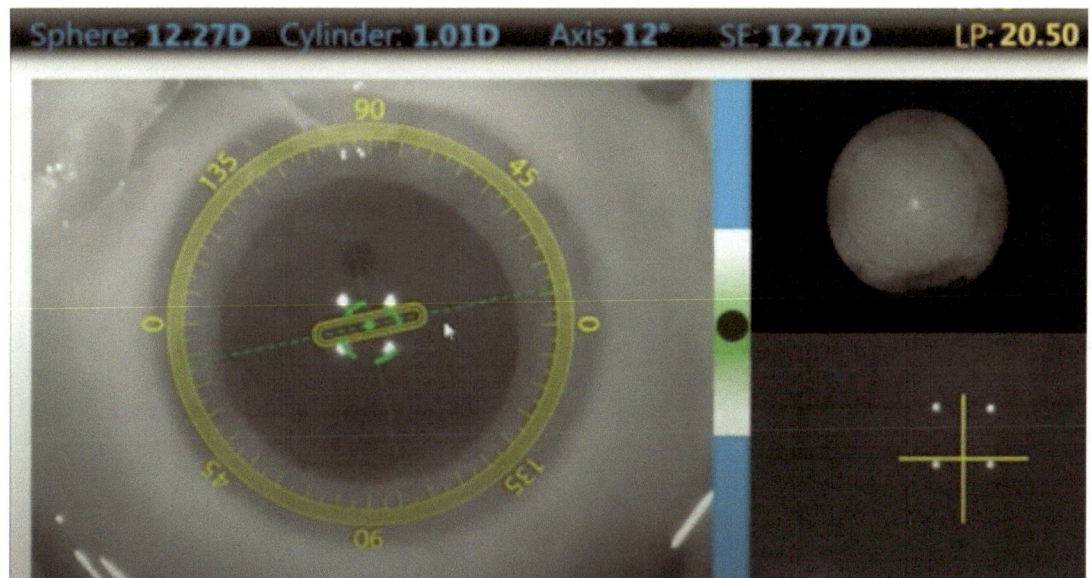

Fig. 45.8 IOL alignment during surgery

Intraoperative Aberrometry for IOL Power Calculation

The first-generation ORange device demonstrated only moderate utility—the correlation between the pseudophakic wavefront refraction from the first-generation ORange device with the 1 week postoperative autorefraction in 32 eyes showed a modest Pearson correlation coefficient of $r = +0.56$, $P < 0.001$ [13].

Over time as the technology and its predictive algorithms improved, so did its clinical utility. With increased adoption and clinical use, the number of studies has shown a dramatic increase

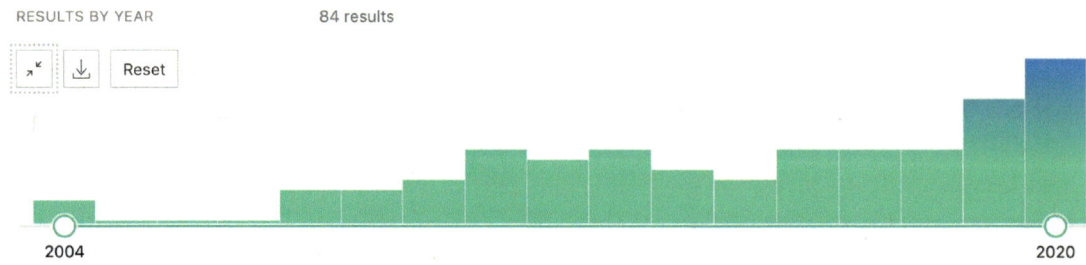

RESULTS BY YEAR   84 results

2004   2020

Fig. 45.9 Clinical studies about intraoperative aberrometry: 2004–2020

as well, with close to 90 studies to date, most of which in the last couple of years. There is a race to the emmetropic nirvana as physicians increase their use of premium IOLs and try to deliver superior outcomes (Fig. 45.9).

One of the main applications of intraoperative aberrometry is to calculate and refine IOL power. The other is for astigmatism management. While intraoperative aberrometry ushered in a new on-demand, on-the-table intraoperative paradigm for high-precision biometry and guided IOL implantation, the last decade has also seen parallel improvements of conventional preoperative biometry, driven by higher-fidelity biometric instrumentation for AL and keratometry and by incremental gains in predictive accuracy of our formulaic calculators. Let us examine the latest clinical evidence on intraoperative aberrometry and how it compares to the preoperative paradigm.

Normal Eyes

In virgin eyes, intraoperative aberrometry demonstrates high predictive efficacy. Cionni et al. reported one of the largest milestone studies on intraoperative aberrometry with 24,375 subjects and 32,189 eyes in 2018 [4]. This study used real-world retrospective de-identified data from the ORA cloud analytical aggregator across multiple surgeons. Because the database comprised real-world data from a variety of surgical centers, the preoperative formulas used by surgeons were not standardized or necessarily optimized. Interoperative aberrometry (IA) using the ORA System and preoperative biometry were per-

formed for all cases. The key endpoints were IOL power prediction error with IA vs. preoperative calculation and percentage of cases with prediction error $\leq 0.50D$. When examining all 32,189 IOL implants, mean and median absolute prediction errors were significantly lower with IA (ORATM System) vs. preoperative calculation ($P < 0.001$). This was also observed for the subset of eyes in which the power of the implanted IOL differed from the preoperatively calculated IOL power ($P < 0.0001$). Absolute prediction error ≤ 0.50 D was achieved significantly more frequently with IA: 81.9% vs. 75.9% of eyes, $P < 0.0001$, for all IOLs and 81.3% vs. 68.8%, $P < 0.0001$, for the subset of eyes in which the power of the implanted IOL differed from the preoperatively calculated IOL power. Given the large dataset, many additional findings and analyses were informative. Mean and median absolute prediction errors for non-toric and toric IOLs were consistent with the full dataset. For non-toric IOLs, the absolute prediction error with IA was $\leq 0.50D$ in 82.4% of eyes (vs. 76.8% with the preoperative calculation). For toric IOLs, the absolute prediction error with IA was $\leq 0.50D$ in 80.8% of eyes (vs. 74.3% with the preoperative calculation). In 8850 (26.7%) of eyes overall, the IOL power recommended by IA differed from the preoperatively planned IOL, and the surgeon implanted the IA-recommended IOL power.

Smaller clinical reports provide further support to the clinical utility of ORA with most of them demonstrating superior fidelity and predictive accuracy of the intraoperative biometric approach.

A further study by Zhang et al. [14] in 295 eyes reported similar benefits. This is a nonrandomized, consecutive retrospective study to compare the outcomes of IA using the ORATM System versus optical biometry alone for IOL power calculation in eyes undergoing cataract surgery with monofocal IOLs. Subjects fell into four subgroups: (1) pre-ORA group: 61 eyes (20.7%) had cataract surgery with IOLMaster measurements, but without IA using the ORATM System; (2) BOTH group: 107 eyes (36.3%) had the same IOL power recommendation from IOLMaster and IA; (3) ORATM group: For 95 eyes (32.2%), the final IOL power implanted was chosen from ORA recommendations rather than IOLMaster. (4) IOLMaster group: For 26 eyes (8.8%), the final IOL power implanted was based on surgeon's best choice from IOLMaster measurements rather than IA. The percentage of eyes within an error range less than ±0.5D of *target refraction* was 65.3%, 80.4%, 73.1%, and 63.9% for ORA, BOTH, IOLMaster, and pre-ORA groups, respectively. The percentage of eyes within an error range less than ±0.5D of *predicted refraction* was 66.3%, 79.4%, and 69.2% for ORA, BOTH, and IOLMaster groups, respectively. Absolute error was significantly reduced in eyes where IA and IOLMaster recommended the same IOL power based on preoperative target refraction compared with IOL selection based on IA (ORATM System) or IOLMaster alone. Overall, IA using the ORA System provided postoperative refractive results comparable to conventional biometry for monofocal IOL selection.

Not every study showed superior efficacy of intraoperative aberrometry. Davison et al. [15] reported on a single clinic, 112 subjects with a retrospective chart review using the ORATM System in determining the IOL sphere power in eyes with no previous ocular surgery. IOL power calculation results from IA with the ORATM System, and the preoperative calculation was similar in nearly half of the cases (47%, 73/155). For toric and multifocal IOLs, there was a statistically significant bias toward lower-powered lenses with IA with the ORATM System ($P < 0.01$). There were only three instances in which preoperative and IA (ORATM System) calculations differed by 1.5 D; in all instances, an adjustment of the preoperative lens power by 0.5 D toward the IA calculation showed a positive effect. In 35% (22/63) of cases in which IOL power differed by at least 0.5 D between IA with the ORATM System and preoperative calculation, the surgeon chose (for nonspecific reasons) the non-optimal method.

Long Eyes

A study by Hill et al. [16] in 51 consecutive eyes aimed to compare the accuracy of IA and the Hill-radial basis function (RBF) formula with other formulas based on preoperative biometry in predicting residual refractive error. Cataract surgery was performed in eyes with axial myopia (axial length [AL] >25 mm) using standard preoperative measurements, IA and Hill-RBF formula for IOL power calculation. IA with the ORATM System was better than all formulas based on preoperative biometry and as effective as the AL-optimized Holladay 1 formula in predicting residual refractive error and reducing hyperopic outcomes.

- The proportion of patients within ±0.5 D of the predicted error was 74.5%, 62.8%, 82.4%, 79.1%, 73.9%, 76.7%, and 80.4% for SRK/T, Holladay 1, AL-optimized Holladay 1, Holladay 2, Barrett Universal II, and Hill-RBF formulas and IA groups, respectively ($P = 0.09$).
- There was a statistically significant difference between AL-optimized Holladay 1 and IA.
- The groups differed significantly with respect to hyperopic outcomes ($P < 0.007$), occurring in 70.6%, 76.5%, 49.0%, 74.4%, 76.1%, 74.4%, and 45.1% of eyes in the SRK/T, Holladay 1, AL-optimized Holladay 1, Holladay 2, Barrett Universal II, Hill-RBF formulas, and IA groups, respectively. The difference was not statistically significant between AL-optimized Holladay 1 and IA.

These data also suggest that patients with axial myopia can benefit from the use of IA.

Short Eyes

As we mentioned earlier, conventional preoperative formulas were less efficacious in the setting of short eyes, with the Hoffer Q offering the highest predictive efficacy for that subgroup. What is the utility of intraoperative aberrometry in this setting? In a single-center retrospective consecutive case series, Sudhakar et al. compared the accuracy of preoperative biometry-based formulas to intraoperative aberrometry (IA) using the ORA System, with respect to predicting refractive outcomes after cataract surgery in 51 short eyes. [17] Cataract surgery with monofocal, multifocal, and/or toric IOL implantation in short eyes, where standard preoperative measurements and IA were performed. Key outcomes of interest were the difference between predicted and actual postoperative spherical equivalent (SE) (numerical error) and the proportion of eyes within ±0.5 D and ± 1.0 D of their target SE refraction.

- Without optimizing the formulas for the study population (i.e., not using n lens constants and surgeon factors that were specifically optimized for short eyes), the mean numerical errors (MNEs) associated with Hoffer Q, Holladay 2, Haigis, Barrett Universal II, Hill-RBF, and IA (ORATM System) were − 0.08 (95% confidence interval [CI], −0.30 to 0.13), −0.14 (95% CI, −0.35 to 0.07), +0.26 (95% CI, 0.05 to 0.47), +0.11 (95% CI, −0.10 to 0.32), +0.07 (95% CI, −0.14 to 0.28), and + 0.00 (95% CI, −0.21 to 0.21), respectively ($P < 0.001$). The proportion of eyes within ±0.5 diopter (D) of the predicted SE with Hoffer Q, Holladay 2, Haigis, Barrett Universal II, Hill-RBF, and IA (ORATM System) were 49.0%, 43.1%, 52.9%, 52.9%, 60.8%, and 58.8%, respectively ($P = 0.06$). A Bonferroni analysis showed that Hoffer Q, Holladay 2, and IA (ORATM System) had the lowest MNEs and were not significantly different from one another; there was no statistically significant difference with regard to the proportion of eyes within ±0.5 D and ± 1.0 D of the target SE.

- Optimizing for the study population (in those patients receiving one of the monofocal IOLs) changed the performance of many of the formulas with regard to the proportion of eyes within ±0.5 D and ± 1.0 D of the target SE; however, these differences were small and not significant. IA using the ORATM System remained one of the best-performing methods, but its performance was not statistically different from the other methods. When a formula and IA predictions differed by 0.5 D or more, IA's ability to recommend a more emmetropic outcome was no better than chance (50%). For example, when there were disagreements greater than 0.5 D, the Barrett Universal II would have outperformed IA 13.7% of the time, and IA would have outperformed Barrett Universal II 13.6% of the time.

Eyes with Previous Corneal Refractive Surgery

Similar to the clinical setting with short eyes, this is where conventional biometry plateaus in its efficacy. There have been a plethora of formulas and calculators designed specifically for this with adjustments and fudge factors trying to improve our ability to estimate the emmetropic IOL power after prior refractive surgery, and this ends up being one of the most taxing aspects of preparing the patient and the surgeon for the cataract surgery, particularly with premium cases where the expectations are so high.

One of the larger studies on this was reported by Ianchulev et al. in 2014 [18]. It is a retrospective consecutive case series from 66 surgeons and 246 eyes, which was designed to evaluate intraoperative aberrometry using the ORA System for IOL power calculation. Cataract surgery after prior myopic LASIK or photorefractive keratectomy, where standard preoperative measurements and IA using ORA were performed. Key outcomes of interest were the median absolute error of prediction and percentage of eyes within ±0.50 diopters D and ± 1.00 D of refractive prediction error. With IA, 67% of eyes were within ±0.5 D,

85% were within ±0.75 D, and 94% were within ±1.0 D of the predicted outcome. This was significantly more accurate than the other preoperative methods: prediction with IA was almost 45% more accurate than the surgeon's best choice (46% within ±0.5 D) and 34% more than the Shammas method, which came in second (50% within 0.5 D. These outcomes were consistent across all endpoints for 0.75 D and 1.0 D postoperative refractive thresholds. In 246 eyes (215 first eyes and 31 second eyes), IA achieved the greatest predictive accuracy, with a median absolute error of 0.35 D (95% confidence interval, 0.35–0.43 D; $P < 0.0001$) and mean absolute error of 0.42 D. All other methods demonstrated at least a 45% higher error than IA, which in the case of surgeon best choice was 70% higher at 0.60 D (95% confidence interval, 0.58–0.73 D).

Another study by Fram et al. [19] is a retrospective consecutive case series (two surgeons) designed to evaluate intraoperative aberrometry using the ORA system and compare it to preoperative IOL power calculation in 59 eyes with prior LASIK surgery. Patients with historical data ($n = 20$ eyes) were compared using the Masket regression formula, Haigis-L, IA, and Optovue. In the groups with historical data, 35–70% of eyes were within ±0.25 D, 60–85% were within ±0.50 D, 80–95% were within ±0.75 D, and 90–95% were within ±1.00 D of targeted refractive IOL power prediction error. The MedAE was 0.21 D for the Masket regression formula, 0.22 D for the Haigis-L formula, 0.25 D for IA, and 0.39 for Optovue. The MAE was 0.28 D for the Masket regression formula, 0.31 D for the Haigis-L formula, 0.37 D for IA, and 0.44 D for Optovue. There was no statistically significant difference among the methods.

Patients without historical data ($n = 39$ eyes) were compared using Haigis-L, IA (ORA System), and Optovue. In the group without historical data, 49% of eyes were within ±0.25 D, 69–74% were within ±0.50 D, 87–97% were within ±0.75 D, and 92–97% were within ±1.00 D of targeted refractive IOL power prediction error. The MedAE was 0.26 D for Haigis-L, 0.29 D for IA (ORATM System), and 0.28 D for Optovue. The MAE was 0.37 D for Haigis-L,

0.34 D for IA (ORATM System), and 0.39 D for Optovue. There was no statistically significant difference among the methods. Overall, IA aberrometry and Fourier-domain OCT-based formula showed promising results when compared with established methods. The findings of improved benefit with IA and Fourier-domain OCT-based IOL formula were particularly meaningful in patients for whom prior data are not available.

Not all clinical evaluations showed positive results of IA in the post-refractive setting. There are a number of smaller studies that did not report convincing benefits of IA. Some used the first-generation technology, ORange, which lacked in predictive accuracy [20]. Furthermore, in the setting of prior RK, biometric challenges continue to overwhelm both conventional formulas and intraoperative aberrometry. Fortunately, in these modern times, there are not many patients left with RK, but a case report by Zhang et al. [21] illustrates the difficulties in that population. After cataract surgery and IOL power calculations using IA (ORA System), a patient with a history of RK showed hyperopic refraction. This was the experience of the author as well when we used IA in our practice in subjects with RK. The corneal distortion is so pronounced in these patients that small decentration from the visual axis can dramatically change the refractive result.

Intraoperative Aberrometry for Astigmatism Correction

Of recent, cataract surgery has become a growing platform for the simultaneous management of astigmatism using LRIs or toric IOLs, intraoperative guidance with the wavefront aberrometry system could not have been a more timely development. On-the-table instantaneous biometric guidance for toric IOLs in particular has been an essential ancillary tool given that small misalignments of the toric IOL can negate its efficacy and ability to correct the astigmatic axis. For every degree of misalignment, about 3% of the lens cylinder power is lost [22]. It is not impossible to end up with misalignments greater than 20°-30° where the effect of the toric correction will be null. Also, the astigmatic axis and power can change based on the intraoperative surgical approach due to the effect of the corneal incision. It certainly seems advantageous to evaluate and confirm the refractive parameters of the eye with respect to astigmatic after eliminating the refractive interference of the cataractous lens and factoring in the intraoperative effect of the corneal incision. The ORA features a large dynamic range of −5 to +20 D, using Talbot moiré interferometry to determine the refractive state of the eye. Because of this, ORA can measure phakic, aphakic, and pseudophakic refraction of the eye, both cylinder and sphere. The aberrometer calculates and confirms IOL power after cataract removal and IOL implantation and determines the magnitude and axis of astigmatism after cataract removal and limbal relaxing incisions. It provides continuous, real-time refractive feedback for astigmatic correction when the surgeon is rotating toric IOLs, titrating limbal relaxing incisions or peripheral corneal relaxing incisions, and performing arcuate incisions with a femtosecond laser.

Another consideration with regard to astigmatism correction is posterior astigmatism. ORA can play an important role by uncovering the impact of the posterior cornea following lens removal. Dr. Koch confirmed that the posterior cornea can have, on average, 0.3 D of astigmatism. This can be significant particularly for multifocal patients, who are extremely sensitive to small degrees of astigmatism.

Regular Astigmatism

Multiple studies provide growing evidence and clinical validation for the advantages of intraoperative aberrometry for astigmatic correction. By far, the largest series comes from the Ora aggregate clinical database. Cionni et al. reported one of the largest milestone studies on intraoperative aberrometry with 24,375 subjects and 32,189 eyes in 2018 [4]. This study used real-world retrospective de-identified data from the ORA cloud analytical aggregator across multiple surgeons. While the study did not specifically address toric

axis alignment, it provides important assurance that patients with toric IOL implantation demonstrate similar high fidelity of refractive correction as non-toric IOLs. Mean and median absolute prediction errors for non-toric and toric IOLs were consistent with the full dataset. For non-toric IOLs, the absolute prediction error with IA was ≤0.50D in 82.4% of eyes (vs. 76.8% with the preoperative calculation). For toric IOLs, the absolute prediction error with IA was ≤0.50D in 80.8% of eyes (vs. 74.3% with the preoperative calculation).

Several studies are informative with respect to the use of intraoperative aberrometry in the setting of LRIs. Packer et al. [23] conducted a retrospective, case-control chart review to assess whether the use of intraoperative aberrometry reduces the frequency of postoperative laser enhancements compared with cases in which aberrometry was not used in 67 eyes of 48 subjects. Mean postoperative follow-up was 3 months in the IA group and 6 months in the control group. Overall, laser enhancements were performed in seven eyes of five patients, for a rate of 10.4%. The excimer laser enhancement rate was 3.3% (one patient) in the IA group and 16.2% (six patients) in the control group. The odds ratio of a laser enhancement without intraoperative aberrometry was 5.71 ($P = 0.21$) although statistical significance was not reached in this small sample size.

With respect to toric IOL application of intraoperative aberrometry, a large retrospective review investigated factors associated with residual refractive astigmatism after toric IOL implantation in more than 3000 cases [24]. Higher measured surgically induced astigmatism (calculated as the vector difference between the preoperative and postoperative keratometry) was most associated with higher levels of reported residual astigmatism. While there were no differences in the residual refractive astigmatism values associated with use or non-use of a femtosecond laser system, the use of intraoperative aberrometry was associated with significantly lower refractive cylinder values (approximately 0.20 D, $P < 0.01$); the odds ratio indicates a 29% higher likelihood of needing a new IOL rather than being able to successfully rotate the current IOL. Overall, higher levels of residual refractive astigmatism when present after cataract surgery were most associated with large measured differences in preoperative to postoperative keratometry and intraoperative guidance by aberrometry was associated with lower levels of residual refractive astigmatism.

Another study by Waisbren et al. compared intraoperative aberrometry versus conventional methods and took another look at the toric setting. [25] This is a retrospective case series from two surgeons designed to compare intraoperative refractive biometry to conventional methods for intraocular lens (IOL) power calculation in patients receiving toric IOLs with a sample size of 104 eyes. Patients in the intraoperative aberrometry cohort achieved a statistically significant lower MAE (0.25 ± 0.22) compared to those in the conventional calculations cohort (0.34 ± 0.29) ($P = 0.05$). In the IA group, 45/52 (87%) of eyes were within 0.5 D of the targeted refraction, compared to 41/52 (79%) in the conventional preoperative calculation group ($P = 0.437$). With the help of IA, surgeons were able to reduce astigmatism to <1 D in 45/52 (87%) of patients compared to only 36/52 (69%) of patients who underwent conventional planning ($P = 0.059$). In the IA (ORA System) group, 14/52 (27%) had no postoperative residual astigmatism vs. 18/52 (35%) of the conventional group. Absolute error was significantly improved in patients using IA, while other variables tested, such as proximity to the targeted axis, were also improved but did not achieve statistical significance.

Similar findings are evident from the study reported by Woodcock et al. [26]. This is a multicenter prospective cohort study comparing astigmatic outcomes in patients having toric IOL implantation with intraoperative aberrometry measurements in one eye and standard power calculation in the contralateral eye. The study enrolled 248 eyes of 124 patients. The percentage of eyes with astigmatism of 0.50 D or less at 1 month was higher in the IA group than in the standard group (89.2% versus 76.6%) ($P = 0.006$). The number of patients (14 [53.8%]) falling outside the intended astigmatic target (<0.50 D) was lower in the IA group than in the standard group. The proportions of eyes with postoperative refractive astigmatism of 0.25 D or less, 0.75 D or less, and 1.00 D or less were also higher in the IA group. Similarly, mean postoperative astigmatism was lower in the IA group than in the standard group (0.29 ± 0.28 D versus 0.36 ± 0.35 D; $P = 0.041$). Overall, compared with standard methods, the use of IA increased the proportion of eyes with postoperative refractive astigmatism of 0.50 D or less and reduced the mean postoperative refractive astigmatism at 1 month.

The number of patients falling outside the intended astigmatic target was reduced by more than half in the IA cohort when compared with the group in which the toric calculator was used.

Salomon et al. conducted a toric study, which further informs of the high efficacy of intraoperative guidance for astigmatic correction during IOL implantation [27]. It is a prospective randomized case series to compare refractive outcomes of intraoperative computer-assisted registration and intraoperative aberrometry (IA) using the ORA system for the reduction in cylinder during toric IOL placement in 104 eyes. Toric IOL implantation after phacoemulsification was assisted by intraoperative computer-assisted registration in one group and intraoperative aberrometry in a separate group (contralateral eye). The mean postoperative remaining refractive astigmatism was below 0.5D: -0.29 ± 0.22 D and -0.46 ± 0.25D with intraoperative computer-assisted registration and IA, respectively. In the computer-assisted registration group, more than 25% of the cases had no postoperative astigmatism, compared with 8% of cases in the IA group. Overall, 92.2% of cases in the computer-assisted registration group had remaining refractive astigmatism of 0.50 D or less, compared with 76.5% in the IA group. The median absolute error in predicting cylindrical correction by IOL was similar for both guidance systems: 0.35 D in the intraoperative computer-assisted registration group and 0.39 D in the IA group, irrespective of the axis ($P = 0.91$). While it appears that the computer-assisted registration group may have a slightly better corrective impact for the astigmatic aberration, it is validating to see such a high degree of precision for intraoperative surgical guidance systems. Another more recent study by Salomon et al. [28] appears to indicate that further advancements in digital alignment technologies may provide outcomes that are as good or even better than those seen with intraoperative aberrometry.

Astigmatism After Corneal Refractive Surgery

This seems to be a clinical setting in the sweet spot for intraoperative aberrometry. A study by Yesilirmak et al. [29] informs to this exact population. It is a retrospective case review of intraoperative aberrometry for toric IOL power selection in eyes with a history of refractive surgery and significant residual astigmatism following refractive surgery—fifteen eyes; 12 eyes had a history of myopic LASIK and three of hyperopic LASIK. Mean residual astigmatic prediction using IA was 0.64 ± 0.61 D, and the mean postoperative manifest astigmatism was 0.74 ± 0.63 D. Twenty-seven percent of the eyes had 0.25 D or less of astigmatism postoperatively, 47% had 0.50 D or less, 60% had 0.75 D or less, and 73% had 1.00 D. Mean IA prediction error was 0.43 ± 0.33 D, compared to a mean prediction error of 0.77 ± 0.56 D for the calculated preoperative lens choice using the IOLMaster ($P = 0.03$) and 0.61 ± 0.34 D using the online ASCRS calculator ($P = 0.08$). 80% of the treated eyes ended up with a spherical equivalent of 0.75 D or less, whereas only 53% of them would have achieved this if the calculated preoperative lens per IOLMaster had been implanted instead.

Conclusion

Intraoperative aberrometry was a timely answer to a major clinical need at the turn of the century when millions of post-LASIK patients were entering the cataract age and the general population started to demand high-fidelity refractive outcomes more suitable to their active lifestyle. Intraoperative aberrometry broke off from the 50-year-old

Fyodorov paradigm of preoperative IOL power estimation, inflected the conventional biometry curve of preoperative formulas away from its deepening plateau, and ushered ophthalmic surgery into the new age of intraoperative guidance and biometry as the first such technology to enter the operating room. It was also one of the first cloud-based analytics platforms for any ophthalmic diagnostic and imaging technology, which used aggregate population data to improve software, algorithms, and, ultimately, patient outcomes.

References

1. Pubmed search on IOL power estimation performed 03.04.2021
2. Liu J, Wang L, Chai F, Han Y, Qian S, Koch DD, Weikert MP. Comparison of intraocular lens power calculation formulas in Chinese eyes with axial myopia. J Cataract Refract Surg. 2019;45(6):725–31.
3. Behndig A, Montan P, Stenevi U, Kugelberg M, Zetterström C, Lundström M. Aiming for emmetropia after cataract surgery: Swedish National Cataract Register study. J Cataract Refract Surg. 2012;38(7):1181–6.
4. Cionni RJ, Dimalanta R, Breen M, Hamilton C. A large retrospective database analysis comparing outcomes of intraoperative aberrometry with conventional preoperative planning. J Cataract Refract Surg. 2018;44(10):1230–5.
5. Eleftheriadis H. IOLMaster biometry: refractive results of 100 consecutive cases. Br J Ophthalmol. 2003;87(8):960–3.
6. Ianchulev T, Salz J, Hoffer K, Albini T, Hsu H, Labree L. Intraoperative optical refractive biometry for intraocular lens power estimation without axial length and keratometry measurements. J Cataract Refract Surg. 2005;31(8):1530–6.
7. Leccisotti A. Intraocular lens calculation by intraoperative autorefraction in myopic eyes. Graefes Arch Clin Exp Ophthalmol. 2008;246(5):729–33.
8. Wong AC, Mak ST, Tse RK. Clinical evaluation of the intraoperative refraction technique for intraocular lens power calculation. Ophthalmology. 2010;117(4):711–6.
9. Ríos S, López D. Modified shack-Hartmann wavefront sensor using an array of superresolution pupil filters. Opt Express. 2009;17(12):9669–79.
10. Sarver EJ, Van Heugten TY, Padrick TD, Hall MT. Astigmatic refraction using peaks of the interferogram Fourier transform for a Talbot Moiré interferometer. J Refract Surg. 2007;23(9):972–7.
11. Wiley WF, Bafna S. Intra-operative aberrometry guided cataract surgery. Int Ophthalmol Clin. 2011;51(2):119–29.

12. Lafetá Queiroz RF, Kniggendorf DV, de Medeiros AL, Hida WT, Nakano CT, Carricondo PC, Nosé W, Rolim AG, Motta AFP. Clinical comparison of speculum's influence on intraoperative aberrometry reading. Clin Ophthalmol. 2019;13:953–8.

13. Chen M. Correlation between ORange (gen 1, pseudophakic) intraoperative refraction and 1-week post-cataract surgery autorefraction. Clin Ophthalmol. 2011;5:197–9.

14. Zhang Z, Thomas LW, Leu SY, Carter S, Garg S. Refractive outcomes of intraoperative wavefront aberrometry versus optical biometry alone for intraocular lens power calculation. Indian J Ophthalmol. 2017;65(9):813–7.

15. Davison JA, Potvin R. Preoperative measurement vs intraoperative aberrometry for the selection of intraocular lens sphere power in normal eyes. Clin Ophthalmol. 2017;11:923–9.

16. Hill DC, Sudhakar S, Hill CS, King TS, Scott IU, Ernst BB, Pantanelli SM. Intraoperative aberrometry versus preoperative biometry for intraocular lens power selection in axial myopia. J Cataract Refract Surg. 2017;43(4):505–10.

17. Sudhakar S, Hill DC, King TS, Scott IU, Mishra G, Ernst BB, Pantanelli SM. Intraoperative aberrometry versus preoperative biometry for intraocular lens power selection in short eyes. J Cataract Refract Surg. 2019;45(6):719–24.

18. Ianchulev T, Hoffer KJ, Yoo SH, Chang DF, Breen M, Padrick T, Tran DB. Intraoperative refractive biometry for predicting intraocular lens power calculation after prior myopic refractive surgery. Ophthalmology. 2014;121(1):56–60.

19. Fram NR, Masket S, Wang L. Comparison of intraoperative Aberrometry, OCT-based IOL formula, Haigis-L, and Masket formulae for IOL power calculation after laser vision correction. Ophthalmology. 2015;122(6):1096–101.

20. Canto AP, Chhadva P, Cabot F, Galor A, Yoo SH, Vaddavalli PK, Culbertson WW. Comparison of IOL power calculation methods and intraoperative wavefront aberrometer in eyes after refractive surgery. J Refract Surg. 2013;29(7):484–9.

21. Zhang F. Optiwave refractive analysis may not work well in patients with previous history of radial keratotomy. Am J Ophthalmol Case Rep. 2018;10:163–4.

22. Browne AW, Osher RH. Optimizing precision in toric lens selection by combining keratometry techniques. J Refract Surg. 2014;30(1):67–72.

23. Packer M. Effect of intraoperative aberrometry on the rate of postoperative enhancement: retrospective study. J Cataract Refract Surg. 2010;36(5):747–55.

24. Potvin R, Kramer BA, Hardten DR, Berdahl JP. Factors associated with residual astigmatism after Toric intraocular lens implantation reported in an online Toric intraocular lens Back-calculator. J Refract Surg. 2018;34(6):366–71.

25. Waisbren E, Ritterband D, Wang L, Trief D, Koplin R, et al. Intraoperative biometry versus conventional methods for predicting intraocular lens power: a closer look at patients undergoing Toric lens implantation for astigmatic correction. J Eye Cataract Surg. 2017;3:27. https://doi.org/10.21767/2471-8300.100027.

26. Woodcock MG, Lehmann R, Cionni RJ, Breen M, Scott MC. Intraoperative aberrometry versus standard preoperative biometry and a toric IOL calculator for bilateral toric IOL implantation with a femtosecond laser: one-month results. J Cataract Refract Surg. 2016;42(6):817–25.

27. Solomon JD, Ladas J. Toric outcomes: computer-assisted registration versus intraoperative aberrometry. J Cataract Refract Surg. 2017;43(4):498–504.

28. Solomon KD, Sandoval HP, Potvin R. Evaluating the relative value of intraoperative aberrometry versus current formulas for toric IOL sphere, cylinder, and orientation planning. J Cataract Refract Surg. 2019;45(10):1430–5.

29. Yesilirmak N, Palioura S, Culbertson W, Yoo SH, Donaldson K. Intraoperative Wavefront Aberrometry for Toric intraocular lens placement in eyes with a history of refractive surgery. J Refract Surg. 2016;32(1):69–70.

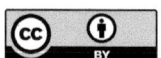

Kane Formula

Jack X Kane

The Kane formula was created in 2017 using a large database of cases (~30,000) to develop the underlying algorithm. The formula is based on theoretical optics and incorporates both regression and artificial intelligence components to further refine its predictions. The formula was created using high-performance cloud-based computing (a way to leverage the power of the cloud to create a virtual supercomputer capable of performing many decades worth of calculations in a few days). Variables used in the formula are axial length, keratometry, anterior chamber depth, lens thickness, central corneal thickness, and patient biological sex. Lens thickness and central corneal thickness are optional variables as these are not available on all biometry platforms. The formula is available for use free of charge at www.iolformula.com.

Since its inception, the formula has consistently been shown to be the most accurate in a variety of studies and subgroups of eyes. The first paper to assess the formula was a single-surgeon study of 846 patients using a single IOL type, which demonstrated that it was more accurate than the Hill-RBF 2.0, Barrett Universal 2, Olsen, Holladay 2, Haigis, Hoffer Q, Holladay 1, and SRK/T formulas [1].

The improved accuracy compared to other modern formulas was further established in an update to the landmark paper by Melles et al. in *Ophthalmology* [2]. This paper—the largest to date on IOL power calculation—studied 18,501 eyes of 18,501 patients assessing the performance of the Barrett Universal 2, Olsen, Haigis, Holladay 2, Holladay 1, and Hoffer Q and found that the Barrett Universal 2 formula was the most accurate. The update to this paper [3] included four additional formulas that were not available for the original study (Kane, Olsen 4-factor, EVO, and Hill-RBF 2.0) and assessed their accuracy using the same dataset as the original paper. This update showed a new leader, with the Kane formula, demonstrating the highest percentage of eyes within ± 0.25, ± 0.50,± 0.75, and± 1.00 D and the lowest standard deviation, mean absolute error, and median absolute error for both the SN60WF and SA60AT IOLs. It was the most accurate formula for short, medium, medium long, and extremely long axial length eyes. In this study, the formula outperformed the long-established best formula for short eyes—with 34.2% reduction in the mean absolute error compared with the Hoffer Q—and the best formula for long eyes—with a 33.3% reduction in the mean absolute error compared to the SRK/T. Compared with the Barrett, which was the best performing in the original study, the reduction in mean absolute error was 12.5% in the short axial

J. X. Kane (✉)
Northern Health Ophthalmology Unit,
Melbourne, Australia

© The Author(s) 2024

J. Aramberri et al. (eds.), *Intraocular Lens Calculations*, Essentials in Ophthalmology,
https://doi.org/10.1007/978-3-031-50666-6_46

length group and 7.4% in the long axial length group.

Another major study from the NHS of 10,930 patients published in the *Journal of Cataract and Refractive Surgery* also demonstrated the improved accuracy of the Kane formula compared to the Hill-RBF 2.0, Olsen, Barrett, Haigis, Hoffer Q, Holladay 1, Holladay 2, and SRK/T. This study also showed the formula to be the most accurate in both short and long axial length eyes and for each IOL type included in the study [4]. This confirmed the finding of the Melles et al. study [3] with the superior performance of the formula across the entire axial length spectrum. These two studies are the largest published to date by a significant margin, and their findings were unequivocally in favor of using the Kane formula.

A review article [5] was published in *Ophthalmology* in 2020 looking at every IOL power formula study over the past 10 years. This study assessed 68 papers on IOL power calculation identifying 36 unique formulas that had been studied (not including obsolete formulas such as SRKII) over the preceding 10 years. The paper

showed that despite only being created in 2017, the overall weight of evidence over the previous 10 years demonstrated that the Kane formula (see Fig. 46.1) was the most accurate over the entire axial length and in both the short eye (≤22.0 mm) and long eye (≥26.0 mm) subgroups. The study demonstrated the tendency of new formulas to have a single paper that shows their excellent results, which were either never studied again or failed to replicate their success with subsequent independent papers, which highlights the need to proceed with caution before adapting a new IOL formula.

Since this review paper, many additional studies have continued to demonstrate the excellent performance of the Kane formula in a variety of different subgroups including short axial length and long axial length, in a variety of anterior chamber depth (ACD) and lens thickness (LT) subgroups and with a variety of different devices.

Short axial length eyes are the most difficult to predict because the high IOL powers inserted lead to the exquisite sensitivity of the effective lens position to any errors in prediction. A JCRS paper [6] of 182 patients having an IOL power of

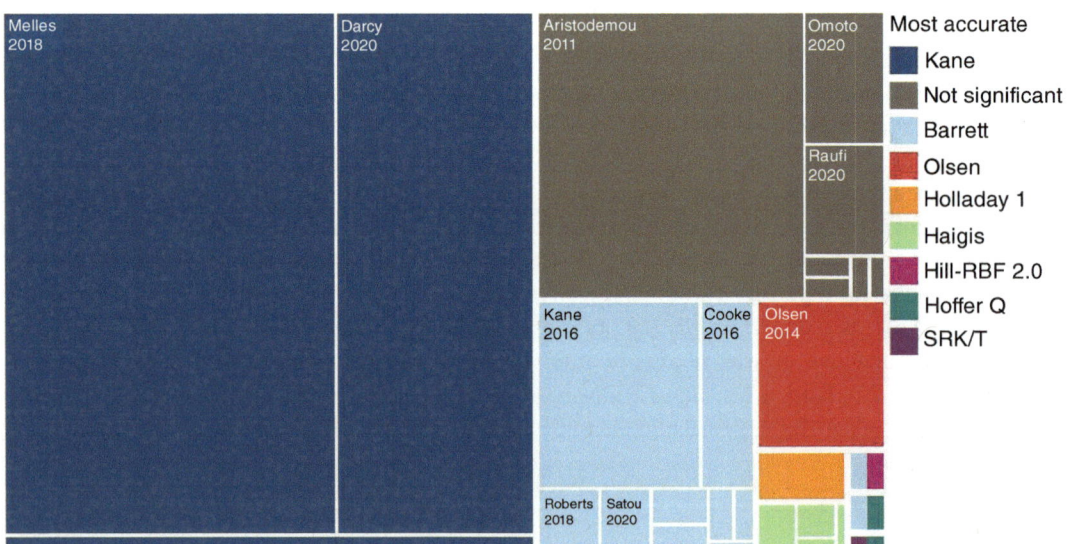

Fig. 46.1 Treemap of studies that assessed the entire axial length spectrum summarizing the most accurate formula. Each separate box represents a different study, the color of the box represents the most accurate formula for

that study, and the relative size of the box represents the size of the study. (Adapted from Kane and Chang [5] with permission)

≥30 diopters inserted (utilizing a database of 28,349 eyes) demonstrated that the Kane formula had the highest percentage of eyes within ± 0.50 D compared to the other studied formulas (EVO 2.0, Barrett, Hill-RBF 2.0, Olsen, and conventional formulas). The improvement was an additional 22.0% of eyes within ± 0.50 D compared to the Barrett formula. Other studies have confirmed these findings with a study of 150 short eyes (axial length ≤ 21.5 mm or IOL power ≥ 28.5) demonstrating that the Kane formula was the equal most accurate formula [7] and another paper with 241 eyes with an axial length ≤ 22.0 mm showed again that it was the equal most accurate formula [8].

In long axial length eyes, the findings of the review have been further confirmed by two additional papers [9, 10], which both demonstrated that the Kane formula had the most accurate results compared to all other studied formulas including the Barrett, EVO, and Hill-RBF 2.0 in eyes with axial length ≥ 26.0 mm. In extreme myopia (axial length ≥ 30.0 mm), the benefit of the Kane formula over the others was even more significant.

An interesting study [11] looking at the performance of formulas based on ACD and LT subgroups demonstrated no significant bias of the formula in any of the nine ACD and LT subgroups. In this study of 628 patients, the Kane formula had the highest percentage of patients within ± 0.50 D. Another study [12], on a new formula (the VRF-G) by the creator of the VRF-G, demonstrated that the Kane formula had the lowest mean absolute error and standard deviation of the prediction error compared with all 12 other formulas in the 828 patients studied.

The findings of the review have been replicated with multiple different devices including ANTERION [13] (Heidelberg) where the formula had the highest percentage of eyes within ± 0.50 D, on the Lenstar (Haag-Streit) where it had the highest percentage of eyes within ± 0.50 D, [14] and on the IOLMaster 700 (Zeiss) where

in 410 patients it had the highest percentage of eyes within ± 0.50 D and the lowest mean absolute error and standard deviation of the prediction error [15].

Additionally, it has been shown to be accurate in other specific populations including post-vitrectomy eyes where it was the only formula to not have a systematic bias [16] and in the aged population where it had the equal highest percentage of eyes within ± 0.50 D [17].

The formula performs well across the entire axial length range, in short and long eyes, in all combinations of anterior chamber depth and lens thickness, and in other studied populations. The use of the formula may free ophthalmologists from the outdated practice of using a variety of formulas depending on the axial length of the patient.

Toric Formula

The Kane toric formula uses an algorithm incorporating regression, theoretical optics, and artificial intelligence techniques to calculate the total corneal astigmatism. It then applies an ELP-based approach to calculate the residual astigmatism for a particular eye and IOL power combination.

In the largest study on toric IOL formula accuracy published in *Ophthalmology* [18], the Kane toric formula was shown to be more accurate than all currently available toric formulas (Barrett, Abulafia-Koch, Holladay 2 with total SIA, EVO 2.0, and Næser-Savini). The formula resulted in a higher percentage of eyes within ± 0.50 D of the astigmatic prediction error with 5.7% more compared to the next best-performing formula (the Barrett toric formula) and 12.7% compared to the worst-performing formula in the study (the Holladay 2 toric formula with total SIA). The Kane toric formula performed the best for with-the-rule, against-the-rule, and oblique astigmatism cases (Fig. 46.2).

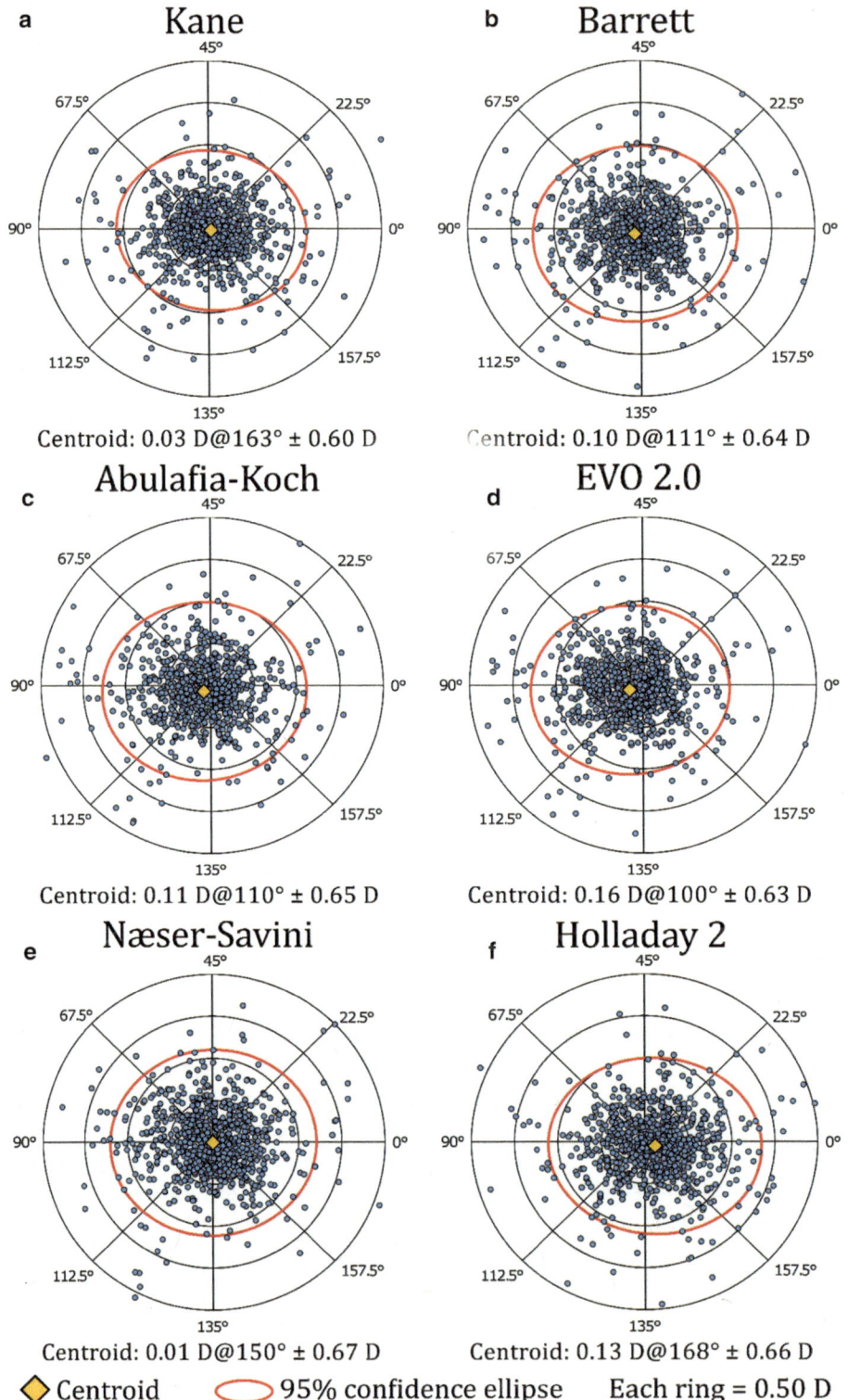

a Kane
Centroid: 0.03 D@163° ± 0.60 D

b Barrett
Centroid: 0.10 D@111° ± 0.64 D

c Abulafia-Koch
Centroid: 0.11 D@110° ± 0.65 D

d EVO 2.0
Centroid: 0.16 D@100° ± 0.63 D

e Næser-Savini
Centroid: 0.01 D@150° ± 0.67 D

f Holladay 2
Centroid: 0.13 D@168° ± 0.66 D

◆ Centroid   ⬭ 95% confidence ellipse   Each ring = 0.50 D

Fig. 46.2 Double-angle plots of the prediction error for each of the formulas assessed (A-F) using the postoperative keratometry and the actual measured IOL axis. The centroids and SDs for each formula are also shown. Adapted from Kane and Connell [18] with permission

Keratoconus Formula

The Kane keratoconus formula is a purely theoretical modification of the original Kane formula. It uses a modified corneal power, derived from anterior corneal radii of curvature, that better represents the true anterior/posterior ratio in keratoconic eyes. The formula also minimizes the effect of corneal power on the ELP calculation to enable more accurate predictions. The variables used in the formula are identical to those in the original formula, and the formula works with standard biometric devices. The same A-constant that is used for a particular IOL for non-keratoconic patients should be used.

This formula was first presented at the 15th IPC meeting in Napa with an article in *Ophthalmology* in 2020 [19]. This article described the largest study of keratoconus patients. In 146 eyes of 146 patients who had IOLMaster biometry, it was found that the Kane keratoconus formula had the best results. It achieved 8.3% more patients within ± 0.50 D than the SRK/T and 7.1% more within ± 0.50 D than the Barrett in mild keratoconus. In moderate keratoconus, it demonstrated an additional 5.4% within ± 0.50 D compared to the Barrett and 13.5% compared to the SRK/T. In severe keratoconus (where average keratometry was ≥53 D), it achieved 20% more within ± 0.50 D compared with the Barrett and 12% more than the SRK/T and had 32% more within ± 1.00 D compared with the Barrett and 28% more than the SRK/T. Another study [20] that included eight eyes with an average keratometry reading over 48 D showed the improved performance of the Kane keratoconus formula compared with the original Kane formula. Comparing the Kane versus the Kane keratoconus formula in these eyes showed a reduction in the mean absolute error from 1.54 D for the original Kane formula to 0.54 D for the Kane keratoconus formula and change from a high hyperopic prediction error + 1.11 D to a low myopic prediction error − 0.15 D.

References

1. Connell BJ, Kane JX. Comparison of the Kane formula with existing formulas for intraocular lens power selection. BMJ Open Ophthalmol. 2019;4(1):e000251. https://doi.org/10.1136/bmjophth-2018-000251.
2. Melles RB, Holladay JT, Chang WJ. Accuracy of intraocular lens calculation formulas. Ophthalmology. 2018;125(2):169–78. https://doi.org/10.1016/j.ophtha.2017.08.027.
3. Melles RB, Kane JX, Olsen T, Chang WJ. Update on intraocular lens calculation formulas. Ophthalmology. 2019;126(9):1334–5. https://doi.org/10.1016/j.ophtha.2019.04.011.
4. Darcy K, Gunn D, Tavassoli S, Sparrow J, Kane JX. Assessment of the accuracy of new and updated intraocular lens power calculation formulas in 10930 eyes from the UK National Health Service. J Cataract Refract Surg. 2020;46(1):2–7. https://doi.org/10.1016/j.jcrs.2019.08.014.
5. Kane JX, Chang DF. Intraocular lens power formulas, biometry, and intraoperative aberrometry. Ophthalmology. 2020;128(11):e94–e114. https://doi.org/10.1016/j.ophtha.2020.08.010.
6. Kane JX, Melles RB. Intraocular lens formula comparison in axial hyperopia with a high-power intraocular lens of 30 or more diopter. J Cataract Refract Surg. 2020;46(9):1236–9. https://doi.org/10.1097/j.jcrs.0000000000000235.
7. Wendelstein J, Hoffmann P, Hirnschall N, et al. Project hyperopic power prediction: accuracy of 13 different concepts for intraocular lens calculation in short eyes. Br J Ophthalmol. 2021;106(6):795–801. https://doi.org/10.1136/bjophthalmol-2020-318272.
8. Voytsekhivskyy OV, Hoffer KJ, Savini G, Tutchenko LP, Fernandes D. Clinical accuracy of 18 IOL power formulas in 241 short eyes. Curr Eye Res. 2021;46(12):1832–43. https://doi.org/10.1080/02713683.2021.1933056.
9. Cheng H, Wang L, Kane JX, Li J, Liu L, Wu M. Accuracy of artificial intelligence formulas and axial length adjustments for highly myopic eyes. Am J Ophthalmol. 2021;223:100–7. https://doi.org/10.1016/j.ajo.2020.09.019.
10. Ang RT, Rapista AB, Remo JM, Tan-Daclan MT, Cruz E. Clinical outcomes and comparison of intraocular lens calculation formulas in eyes with long axial myopia. Taiwan J Ophthalmol. 2021;12(3):305–11. https://doi.org/10.4103/tjo.tjo_7_21.
11. Hipólito-Fernandes D, Luís ME, Serras-Pereira R, et al. Anterior chamber depth, lens thickness and intraocular lens calculation formula accuracy: nine formulas comparison. Br J Ophthalmol.

2020;106(3):349–55. https://doi.org/10.1136/bjophthalmol-2020-317822.

12. Hipólito-Fernandes D, Elisa Luís M, Gil P, et al. VRF-G, a new intraocular lens power calculation formula: a 13-formulas comparison study. Clin Ophthalmol. 2020;14:4395–402. https://doi.org/10.2147/OPTH.S290125.

13. Szalai E, Toth N, Kolkedi Z, Varga C, Csutak A. Comparison of various intraocular lens formulas using a new high-resolution swept-source optical coherence tomographer. J Cataract Refract Surg. 2020;46(8):1138–41. https://doi.org/10.1097/j.jcrs.0000000000000329.

14. Cheng H, Li J, Cheng B, Wu M. Refractive predictability using two optical biometers and refraction types for intraocular lens power calculation in cataract surgery. Int Ophthalmol. 2020;40(7):1849–56. https://doi.org/10.1007/s10792-020-01355-y.

15. Cheng H, Kane JX, Liu L, Li J, Cheng B, Wu M. Refractive predictability using the IOLMaster 700 and artificial intelligence–based iol power formulas compared to standard formulas. J Refract Surg. 2020;36(7):466–72. https://doi.org/10.3928/1081597X-20200514-02.

16. Tan X, Zhang J, Zhu Y, et al. Accuracy of new generation intraocular lens calculation formulas in Vitrectomized eyes. Am J Ophthalmol. 2020;217:81–90. https://doi.org/10.1016/j.ajo.2020.04.035.

17. Reitblat O, Gali HE, Chou L, et al. Intraocular lens power calculation in the elderly population using the Kane formula in comparison with existing methods. J Cataract Refract Surg. 2020;46(11):1501–7. https://doi.org/10.1097/j.jcrs.0000000000000308.

18. Kane JX, Connell B. A comparison of the accuracy of six modern toric IOL formulas. Ophthalmology. 2020;127(11):1472–86. https://doi.org/10.1016/j.ophtha.2020.04.039.

19. Kane JX, Connell B, Yip H, et al. Accuracy of intraocular lens power formulas modified for patients with Keratoconus. Ophthalmology. 2020;127(8):1037–42. https://doi.org/10.1016/j.ophtha.2020.02.008.

20. Ton Y, Barrett GD, Kleinmann G, Levy A, Assia EI. Toric intraocular lens power calculation in cataract patients with keratoconus. J Cataract Refract Surg. 2021;47(11):1389–97. https://doi.org/10.1097/j.jcrs.0000000000000638.

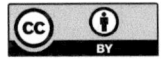

Ladas Super Formula: Origin and Evolution with AI

47

John Ladas, Uday Devgan, Albert Jun, and Aazim Siddiqui

Introduction

The first formulas to determine the power of an IOL to achieve a specific refractive outcome were introduced in the 1970s by Colenbrander, Fyodorov, and Binkhorst. [1–3] Over the ensuing 50 years, many significant advances have been made to improve outcomes. Reasons for this have been more precise measurements of the structural variables of the eye in addition to improved theoretical analysis of these variables. Further, "adjustments" to these formulas were made when the formulas appeared to underperform. Our interest and contribution are the way we visualize formulas, compare them, combine them, and ultimately adjust them using artificial intelligence. Our ability to achieve this has occurred because computing power and modeling advancements have made this much more viable.

J. Ladas (✉)
Maryland Eye Consultants and Surgeons, Silver Spring, MD, USA

Wilmer Eye Institute, Devgan Eye, Los Angeles, CA, USA

U. Devgan
Wilmer Eye Institute, Devgan Eye, Los Angeles, CA, USA

A. Jun
Wilmer Eye Institute, Baltimore, MD, USA
e-mail: aljun@jhmi.edu

A. Siddiqui
Solomon Eye Associates, Bowie, MD, USA

Formulas throughout the years have been described in multiple ways, one of which is by "generations." [4] However, some formulas do not uniquely fit into a specific category. The SRK I was a regression-based formula characterized as the first generation and used actual outcome data for its development. [5, 6] This first empiric formula was further modified by axial length. [7] Perhaps, this was the first attempt at "adjusting" a formula.

The next generation of formulas was theoretical in that they used the measurement of axial length and corneal power to predict the effective lens position of the implanted IOL. These formulas included the Hoffer Q, Holladay 1, and SRK/T. [8–10] Further, important to our work is that particular formulas have been proven to work best with specific eyes. For instance, it was generally accepted that the Hoffer Q worked particularly well with short eyes, Holladay 1 with average eyes, and SRK/T with longer eyes. This was likely related to the way that the effective lens position was calculated by each formula.

There has also been much interest and work over the last 25 years to determine the variables beyond axial length and corneal power that may lead to improved outcomes. Additional variables have been shown to improve outcomes when accounted for individually. For instance, the Wang-Koch adjustment for axial length has been applied to eyes greater than 25 mm. [11, 12] It is doubtful that any axial length adjustment should

© The Author(s) 2024

J. Aramberri et al. (eds.), *Intraocular Lens Calculations*, Essentials in Ophthalmology, https://doi.org/10.1007/978-3-031-50666-6_47

start and stop at exactly 25 mm. Others have proposed incorporating additional variables to account for a multitude of factors. The Holladay 2 formula released in 1996 includes additional variables of lens thickness, corneal diameter distance, preoperative refraction, and age [13]. Other potential variables that have been suggested to have an effect on IOL prediction include equatorial lens position, age, race, gender, aphakic refraction, relative ratio of various eye segments, C-factor, posterior corneal power, corneal thickness, specific lens design, and exact power of the IOL [4, 14–19]. These variables do not occur in a vacuum and are likely intimately related to other variables such as ACD.

So, with the following assumptions we started to work on and continue to modify our formula. These assumptions include that specific formulas perform better in certain eyes, targeted "adjustments" can improve outcomes, and there are multiple variables that can be used with these adjustments. If now one takes into consideration the computing power that is available, there seems to be a path forward that uses all of these ideas to optimize outcomes.

LSF 1.0

The first step for our group in developing and working with formulas was to start thinking about them differently. Although various theoretical formulas seemed to use different constants and variables, their mathematical structure was very similar. This "visual" interpretation of formulas has been used in other mathematical disciplines. Using the best "peer-reviewed" literature, we created a formula that used multiple parts of various formulas and added adjustments. Figure 47.1 shows what the formula looked like graphically when it was first published. [20] This initial iteration that we described in the article included parts of the Hoffer Q, the Holladay 1, and the SRK/T. Further, the Wang-Koch adjustment was

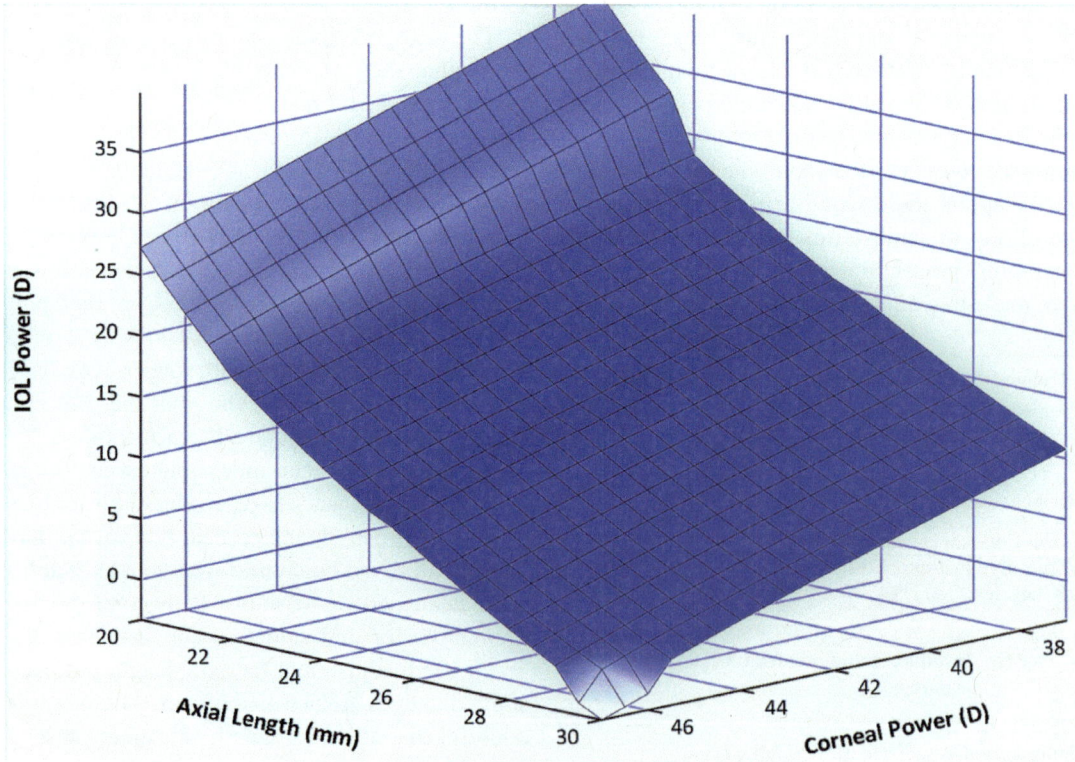

Fig. 47.1 Original Super Formula LSF 1.0 with adjustments

used where appropriate. We certainly could have chosen more formulas and adjustments to include but decided upon this for our initial iteration. Further, as mentioned in our original article, we felt that this approach leads to a better conceptual understanding of formulas and becomes a framework for further improvements.

One additional but important facet of thinking about these formulas differently is that specific formulas and specific variables within them can be compared. For instance, Fig. 47.2 demonstrates a graphical analysis of where formulas diverge in their prediction by more than one diopter. The green areas demonstrate when formulas, given a set of variables, are similar. The red areas show when the predictions diverge. Resolving these areas of greatest discrepancy is of clinical relevance as we try to understand and improve formulas in these particular regions.

Analyzing the differences between formulas can allow for better allocation of resources to determine where advances will likely come from and what variables will lead to them. Also, we are able to observe subtle differences in how a particular variable such as ELP calculation can affect a particular formula [21].

The use of multiple formulas leads to better outcomes by selecting the most accurate formula for a particular eye and has been demonstrated in the literature throughout the years. Data presented from our group at ASCRS also demonstrated superior results when compared against modern formulas with this approach reaching 85% of eyes within 0.5 diopters of predicted refraction, which was the best of all formulas tested [22].

To our knowledge, only one other study has attempted to analyze the original iteration. Cooke

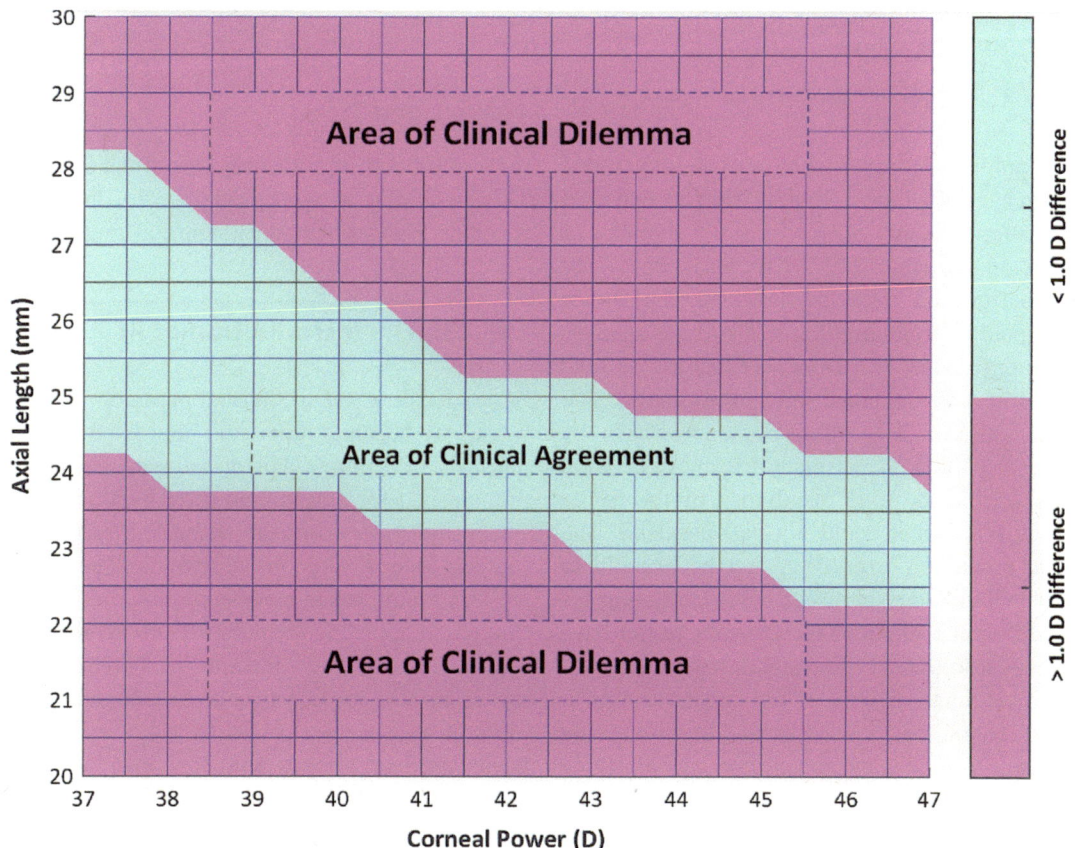

Fig. 47.2 Ladas-Siddiqui plot showing areas of agreement and divergence among formulae

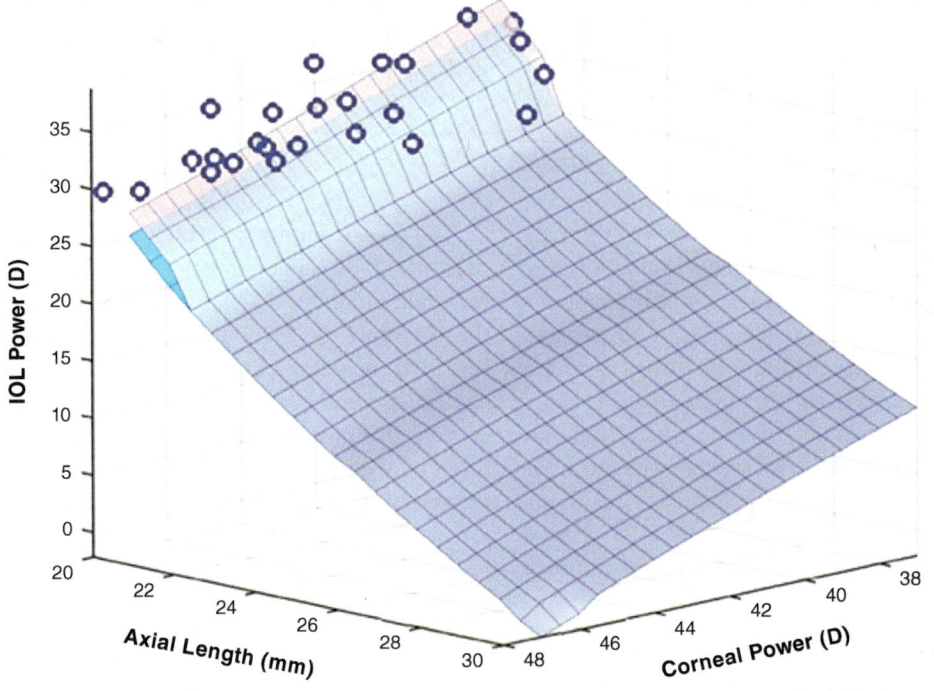

Fig. 47.3 Schematic of "targeted" adjustments

IMAGE COURTESY UDAY DEVGAN, MD

et al. published a paper where they demonstrated that in eyes of all axial lengths, it performed well with approximately 80% within 0.5 diopters of predicted refraction [23]. This was one of the best-performing formulas; however, the author attempted to program it himself without contacting our group so we are not sure that it was done correctly and included all adjustments. The authors also made an interesting comment in the manuscript that is pertinent to our discussion here. He noted, "one peculiarity of the Super Formula is that it could not be optimized. The mean prediction error could not be brought to zero." Optimizing it correctly by accounting for the different regions of the formula would have perhaps resulted in even better performance.

The ultimate benefit of the super formula is that it is a framework to adjust and improve going forward. With this approach, one can adjust or target short eyes rather than move an A-constant up or down across a range of eyes. For instance, Fig. 47.3 is a schematic of how a particular region (short axial length) can be targeted and adjusted without influencing other regions of the formula. This is similar to what is done with the well-accepted Wang-Koch adjustment for long eyes.

LSF 2.0. The Introduction of AI

After deciding on a starting point or "framework," we began to refine and improve the original LSF 1.0 formula. Historically, as mentioned previously, a formula was adjusted by moving the A-constant up or down across the entire spectrum of eyes. Indeed, surgeons were told to "personalize" a formula based on twenty or so cases. The thought of adjusting formulas based on relatively few outcomes is not uncommon. For example, instances of a specific formula recommendation or "adjustment" to a particular set of eyes have been based on studies with less than 100 outcomes [8, 11, 24, 25]. These thought leaders had less resources and outcome data to work with. Further, as new IOLs came on the market, the Users Group for Interferometry (ULIB) was

Fig. 47.4 Schematic of our AI algorithm used to adjust a formula

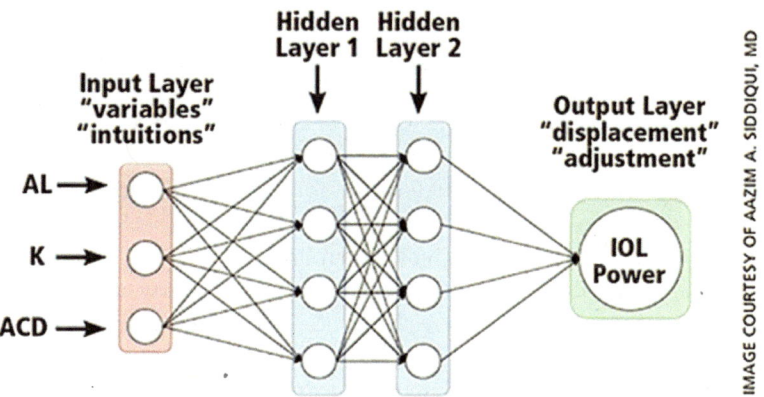

IMAGE COURTESY OF AAZIM A. SIDDIQUI, MD

developed to hone A-constants for large groups of surgeons. While all of this was certainly helpful and improved outcomes, it seemed to us that outcome analysis could be improved upon by treating "adjustments" differently.

Thus, further advancements and adjustments are unlikely to be conceived as single variables or discrete formulas, and progress using such approaches likely would be inefficient compared to machine learning methods. Artificial intelligence and deep learning seem particularly suited for this task and have the ability to "weigh" the effect of multiple variables on reaching a desired outcome.

There are two categories of machine learning, and both could be applicable to cataract surgery and IOL calculations. These include unsupervised and supervised learning. Unsupervised learning uses input data to discover similarities among datasets. Unsupervised learning has been used by our group to predict which eyes are particularly susceptible to poor refractive outcomes, for instance, predicting eyes that are likely to have an outcome of greater than one diopter of targeted refraction.

Supervised learning, which is more pertinent to our discussion here, is the other branch of machine learning that utilizes outcome data, in addition to the input variables, to develop a predictive model. This is the type of learning that we primarily use to improve formulas. Regression-based supervised learning uses specific algorithms to establish the relationship between the input variables it is given and the outcome.

Cataract surgery and IOL calculations are particularly suited to this task in medicine. This is because cataract surgery is precise, its inputs and outcomes are mathematical, and the outcome is known within a matter of weeks. Methods of supervised nonlinear regression machine learning models that we use include support vector regression, extreme gradient boost, and neural networks.

As mentioned earlier, our approach to AI differs from others in that it starts with a "blueprint" or framework formula (the original LSF) and uses outcome data to "adjust" each eye individually. The approach described in this paper is contrasted with forms of deep learning such as the Hill-RBF (radial basis function) that "back calculate" an algorithm from a fixed dataset. With our approach, there are no instances where a calculation is "out of bounds" because of paucity of data [26]. A schematic of our methodology is demonstrated in Fig. 47.4. As seen in the figure, we use the input variables of axial length, corneal power, and ACD and then develop an algorithm that "predicts" the error. This error would be seamlessly used to adjust an eye with similar input variables. By doing this, we mitigate the potential downsides of AI while maximizing its ability to refine a formula. Also, this particular approach can be used to add additional input variables such as posterior corneal power or total corneal power.

Our initial algorithm to introduce AI used vetted and refined outcome data supplied by in-house data and trusted colleagues. The use of outcome data for AI and its reliability cannot be emphasized enough. We feel that our concept of adjusting a baseline formula is novel and unique. The LSF 2.0 included further adjustments based on outside studies that included 8000 eyes and an in-house library of outcome data that included 3000 eyes. This was used to adjust the formula and was tested on our internal data. We currently have more than 6000 eyes available in our library data and continue to test, refine, and introduce new algorithms.

Our formula has recently been tested and performed well compared to all modern formulas with one of the lowest mean absolute errors [27]. Indeed, the results of this study are shown in the table below. The predicted error demonstrated the lowest standard deviation of all formulas tested as well as superior results for eyes within predicted refraction.

PE ± SD	MedAE	PE ≤ ±0.50 D	PE ≤ ±1.00 D
−0.003 ± 0.366	0.220	85.71%	98.90%

In addition to creating AI-enhanced formulas from our original baseline formula, we are also able to improve existing formulas. Recent work from our group has demonstrated that we can improve multiple generations of formulas with our methodology [28]. Indeed, multiple supervised learning algorithms were used to improve the MAE, MedAE, and eyes within 0.5 diopters of the target with various formulas. Other work presented elsewhere has shown that this can be done with other formulas such as the Barrett Universal II and Haigis. Interestingly, when we enhance a formula with a specific set of variables, we see each formula improve to a similar threshold. From a theoretical standpoint, it is perhaps predictable that each algorithm was able to predict and adjust each of the formula's "errors" individually and for each eye in a way that could never be written in a mathematical formula by a human.

The most recent version of our formula can be found at www.iolcalc.com. The formula is updated as needed and will continue to evolve. The input of the formula is straightforward, and biometer inputs can be uploaded and auto-populated to the interface seen below in Fig. 47.5.

The Ladas Super Formula can also be accessed securely via a smartphone application (Fig. 47.6).

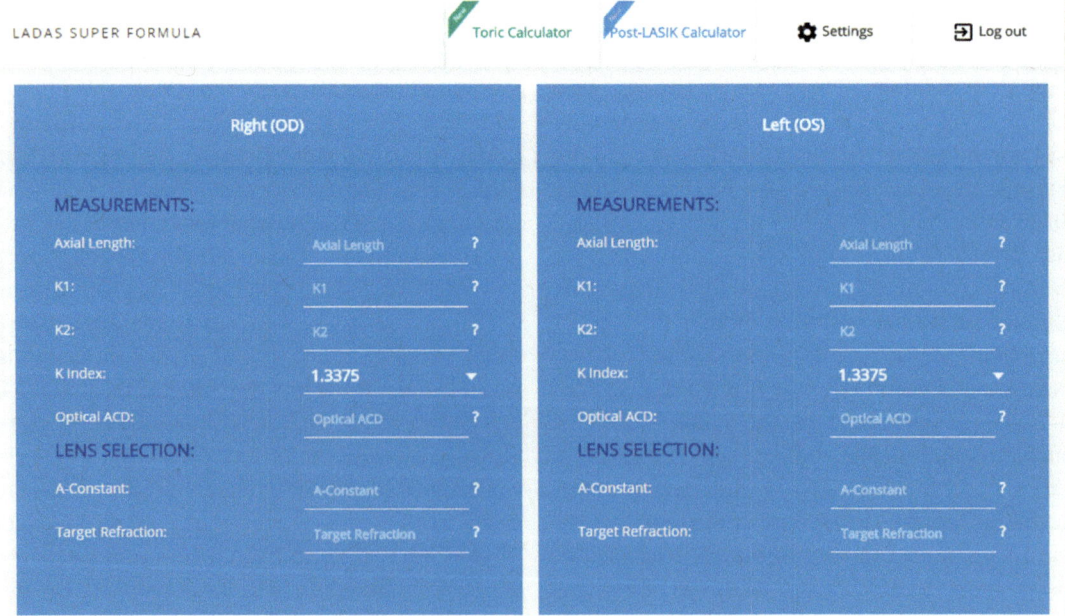

Fig. 47.5 Data input screen on iolcalc.com

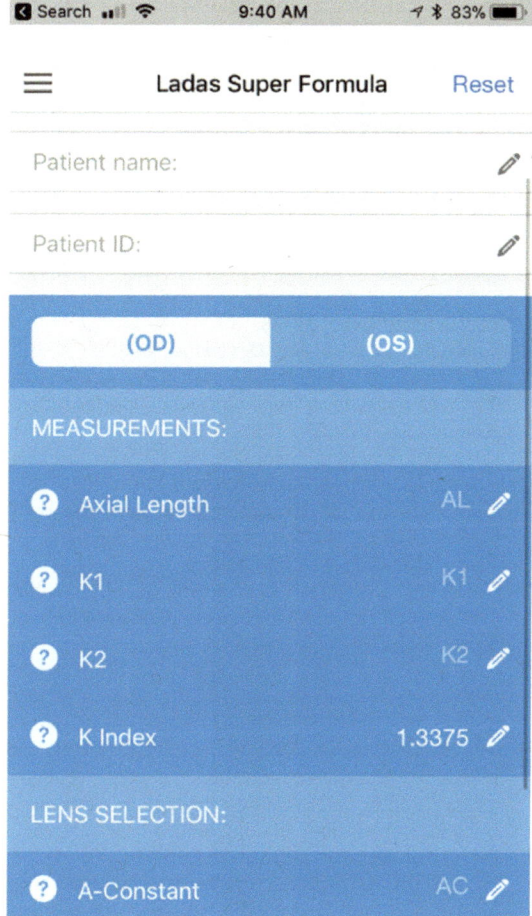

Fig. 47.6 Smart phone app for calculations and input of outcome data

occur with MRx acquisition. However, the correlation between ARx and MRx for the purposes of IOL formula optimization is still unclear and is being currently investigated in ongoing studies. Given a correlation exists between the two modalities for this purpose, then integration of AI in this schema may be useful by allowing the collection of big data and leading to the development of AI-based IOL formulas.

We have presented a pilot study that demonstrated no significant difference between the spherical equivalent of manifest refraction and autorefraction in pseudophakic eyes [29]. Further, we can demonstrate that MRx can be substituted with ARx for basic refinement of formulas.

There are many potential benefits of AI integration in automated refraction. Customized AI-IOL calculation formulas may be developed for a given surgeon using the surgeon's own postoperative data. This could help account for surgeon-to-surgeon variation, which is responsible for a significant portion of error in current IOL calculation methodologies. This could also allow for a system of optimization, which improves upon itself in a recurrent manner. Furthermore, with the "big data" stored within an automated refractor, it will be able to characterize an eye as one with "standard" parameters or one with "unusual" parameters. Thus, AI could preoperatively highlight eyes that are "at risk" for a postoperative refractive surprise.

Automation of the Process and Next Steps

Generally, refining IOL formulas has required the availability of accurate postoperative data. Usually, these data are composed of preoperative biometry and postoperative manifest refraction (MRx) data taken from multiple high-volume surgeons. However, MRx measurements are often suboptimal due to technique variability, room length, patient's subjective participation, and time taken to perform measurements. The use of autorefraction (ARx) or wavefront data can potentially help eliminate most issues that

Conclusion

It takes time for ideas to catch on, but the use of artificial intelligence will definitely be a part of the future of IOL calculations. While better mathematical algorithms will certainly be developed by our group and others in and outside ophthalmology, I believe our approach that uses both deep learning algorithms coupled with the accumulation of massive amounts of objective postoperative data to further refine formulas will eventually become the norm. Only time will tell.

References

1. Colenbrander MC. Calculation of the power of an iris-clip lens for distance vision. Br J Ophthalmol. 1973;57:735–40.
2. Fyodorov SN, Galin MA, Linksz A. Calculation of the optical power of intraocular lenses. Investig Ophthalmol. 1975;14:625–8.
3. Binkhorst RD. Intraocular lens power calculation. Int Ophthalmol Clin. 1979;19:237–52.
4. Olsen T. Calculation of intraocular lens power: a review. Acta Ophtalmologica Scandinavica. 2007;85(5):472–85.
5. Sanders DR, Kraff MC. Improvement of intraocular lens power calculation using empirical data. J Am Intraocul Implant Soc. 1980;6:263–7.
6. Retzlaff J. A new intraocular lens calculation formula. J Am Intraocul Implant Soc. 1980;6(2):148–52.
7. Sanders DR, Retzlaff J, Kraff MC. Comparison of the SRK II formula and other second-generation formulas. J Cataract Refract Surg. 1988;14(2):136–41.
8. Hoffer KJ. The Hoffer Q formula: a comparison of theoretic and regression formulas. J Cataract Refract Surg. 1993;19(6):700–12.
9. Holladay JT, Prager TC, Chandler TY, Musgrove KH, Lewis JW, Ruiz RS. A three-part system for refining intraocular lens power calculations. J Cataract Refract Surg. 1988;14(1):17–24.
10. Retzlaff JA, Sanders DR, Kraff MC. Development of the SRK/T intraocular lens implant power calculation formula. J Cataract Refract Surg. 1990;16(3):333–40.
11. Wang L, Shirayama M, Ma XJ, Kohnen T, Koch DD. Optimizing intraocular lens power calculations in eyes with axial lengths above 25.0 mm. J Cataract Refract Surg. 2011;37(11):2018–27.
12. Wang L, Holladay JT, Koch DD. Wang-Koch axial length adjustment for the Holladay 2 formula in long eyes. J Cataract Refract Surg. 2018;44(10):1291–2.
13. Mahdavi S, Holladay J. IOLMaster 500 and integration of the Holladay 2 formula for intraocular lens calculations. European Ophthalmic Review. 2011;5(2):134–5.
14. Melles RB, Holladay JT, Chang WJ. Accuracy of intraocular lens calculation formulas. Ophthalmology. 2018;125:169–78.
15. Olsen T. Prediction of the effective postoperative (intraocular lens) anterior chamber depth. J Cataract Refract Surg. 2006;32(3):419–24.
16. Cooke DL, Cook TL. Approximating sum-of-segments axial length from a traditional optical low-coherence reflectometry measurement. J Cataract Refract Surg. 2019;45(3):351–4.
17. Olsen T, Corydon L, Gimbel H. Intraocular lens power calculation with an improved anterior chamber depth prediction algorithm. J Cataract Refract Surg. 1995;21(3):313–9.
18. Yoo YS, Whang WJ, Hwang KY. Use of the crystalline lens equatorial plane (LEP) as a new parameter for predicting postoperative IOL position. Am J Ophthalmol. 2019;198:17–24.
19. Olsen T. The Olsen formula. In: Shammas HJ, editor. Intraocular lens power calculations. NJ, Slack: Thorofare; 2004. p. 27–38.
20. Ladas JG, Siddiqui AA, Devgan U, Jun AS. A 3-D "super surface" combining modern intraocular formulas to generate a "super formula" and maximize accuracy. JAMA. 2015;133(12):1431–6.
21. Devgan U. Anterior chamber depth plays critical role in IOL calculations. Ocular Surgery News; 2016.
22. Siddiqui AA, et al. Evaluation of a novel intraocular lens formula that integrates artificial intelligence. Washington, DC: ASCRS; 2018. p. 2018.
23. Cooke DL, Cooke TL. Comparison of 9 intraocular lens power calculation formulas. J Cataract Refract Surg. 2016;42(8):1157–64.
24. Haigis W. Intraocular lens calculation after refractive surgery for myopia: Haigis-L formula. J Cataract Refract Surg. 2008;34:1658–63.
25. Masket S, Masket SE. Simple regression formula for intraocular lens power adjustment in eyes requiring cataract surgery after excimer laser photoablation. J Cataract Refract Surg. 2006;32:430–4.
26. Hill-RBF Method. Released: October 2017/V2.0. Haag-Streit AG Koeniz, Switzerland https://www.haag-streit.com/fileadmin/Haag-Streit_Diagnostics/biometry/EyeSuite_IOL/Brochures_Flyers/White_Paper_Hill-RBF_Method_20160819_2_0.pdf.
27. Taroni L, Hoffer KJ, Barboni P, Schiano-Lomoriello D, Savini G. Outcomes of IOL power calculation using measurements by a rotating Scheimpflug camera combined with partial coherence interferometry. J Cataract Refract Surg. 2020;46:1618–23.
28. Ladas J, Ladas D, Lin SR, Devgan U, Siddiqui AA, Jun AS. Improvement of multiple generations of intraocular lens formulae with a novel approach using artificial intelligence. Transl Vis Sci Tech. 2021;10(3):7.
29. Chang S, Ladas J, Solomon J, Jeng B. Analysis and refinement of intraocular lens formulas with objective data. AAO; 2021.

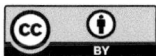

Norrby Formulas for IOL Power Calculation

48

Sverker Norrby

S. Norrby (✉)
Eindhoven, Netherlands

Prologue

My education and experience were in polymer science and technology. One of my first tasks at Pharmacia was to come up with a method to assign A-constants without the need for a clinical study. Although the SRK II formula was dominant at the time, I realized that the A-constant had something to do with the optics of the eye and the depth at which the IOL ended up. Having only high school knowledge in optics, I bought O'Shea's textbook on the subject [1]. It taught me that optical calculations are ideally treated in spreadsheets, which greatly helped me get a grip on the matter.

Next, I turned to the clinical department for studies in which the postoperative IOL position had been measured. My working hypothesis was that the position of the IOL was dependent on the plane where the haptics made contact with eye tissue. I termed it the lens haptic plane (LHP) and postulated that it was common to all IOL models implanted in the bag and that the offset from the plane was determined by the detailed mechanical and optical design of each IOL model. After a lot of calculations, an "average eye" emerged. For a new IOL model, it was "implanted" with the power that made that eye emmetropic. From there, we could back-calculate the A-constant. This procedure was eventually published [2].

In the process of developing the LHP concept, I became aware that biometry instruments could differ systematically from each other. This, rather than a surgical technique, required "personalization" of formula constants. To assess the differences, I asked several friends to measure my own eyes. The data collected resulted in a paper [3] that was accepted by the editor without peer review.

In a subsequent paper [4], differences between ultrasound and optical measurement of anterior chamber depth were studied. In another study [5], systematic differences between two ultrasound devices were investigated, followed by a suggestion [6] as to how to deal with them by transformation of data. With the introduction of the Zeiss IOLMaster in 1999, a new gold standard for axial length (AL) measurement was set. However, while it measures the optical AL to the retinal pigment epithelium and A-scan ultrasound measures to the inner limiting membrane, the output was re-calculated to agree with A-scan ultrasound [7], which in fact introduced systematic bias. This was commercially understandable but is unfortunate.

Systematic differences remain a problem in keratometry. The measured quantity is the corneal radius of curvature, which is transformed to

J. Aramberri et al. (eds.), *Intraocular Lens Calculations*, Essentials in Ophthalmology,
https://doi.org/10.1007/978-3-031-50666-6_48

corneal power by means of the keratometric index. As pointed out by Olsen [8], the index 1.3315 affords the power in the second principal plane (also known as the back principal plane, or the image principal plane), which should be used for thin lens calculations. The value 1.332 puts the power at the anterior surface of the cornea, while the index 1.3375, which is used in many keratometers, gives the power at the posterior vertex. The latter overestimates corneal power by about 0.80 D. In commonly used thin lens IOL power formulas, this is compensated by adjusting the formula constant(s) to result in a virtual IOL position that is posterior to the true one.

When I retired on July 1, 2010, I felt it was time to come up with an IOL power formula of my own. It became three formulas. They were presented at the IOL Power Club meeting on April 27–29, 2012, in Nashville/Memphis, USA. They have not been published until now, a decade later.

Data

The data for this chapter was obtained in conjunction with a study [9] of IOL stability at Moorfields Eye Hospital (London, UK) involving the models Tecnis ZA9003 (3-piece) and Tecnis ZCB00 (1-piece) from AMO, Santa Ana, CA, USA. The company was later acquired by Johnson & Johnson Vision, Jacksonville, FL, USA.

Preoperatively measured AL, anterior chamber depth (ACD, anterior cornea to anterior lens), and corneal radius (CR) obtained with the IOLMaster software V.5 version (Carl Zeiss Meditec AG, Germany) are used. The implanted IOL powers had been calculated by the SRK/T formula. Refraction was determined 1 year postoperatively using a trial frame with the chart at 4 m. There are 44 complete datasets available for each IOL model. The data for ZA9003 were used for the development of the formulas and are summarized in Table 48.1.

Table 48.1 Overview of parameters used for IOL model ZA9003: AL = axial length, ACD = anterior chamber depth (anterior cornea to anterior lens), CR = anterior corneal radius of curvature, and SE = spherical equivalent spectacle lens refraction. There were 44 complete datasets available

Variable	Obtained with	Mean	SD	Range
Pre-op AL (mm)	IOLMaster	23.51	± 0.64	22.02–25.37
Pre-op ACD (mm)	IOLMaster	2.98	± 0.33	2.32–3.83
Pre-op CR (mm)	IOLMaster	7.73	± 0.28	7.28–8.35
Pre-op IOL power (D)	SRK/T	21.75	± 1.71	17.5–26.0
Post-op SE (D)	Trial frame @ 4 m	−0.82	± 0.38	0.00–1.75

Norrby Thick Lens Formula

In 2004, I published a thick lens calculation scheme for IOL power calculation based on the LHP concept [10]. I no longer subscribe to several features in it, hence this new attempt.

The Tecnis lenses are designed to eliminate the average spherical aberration caused by the cornea. In that case, thick lens paraxial ray tracing should be appropriate for IOL power calculation. In a thick lens calculation model, every refracting surface is at its true position. There are no virtual principal planes involved. However, because spectacle lenses are labeled with their back vertex power, they can preferably be treated as thin lenses at the vertex distance from the cornea. In the model, the vertex distance is assumed to be 12 mm.

The anterior corneal surface is the reference for target distance, AL, and IOL position. In a previous paper [11], it was found that the position of the posterior IOL surface could be estimated by the formula.

$$pLP = 3.074 + 0.06524^* AL + 0.2957^* ACD$$

This formula was found to be valid for both ZA9003 and ZCB00. With the anterior capsule mechanically compromised by the capsulorrhexis, it could be argued that the intact posterior capsule becomes a support for the IOL optic for any model. It is open to others to prove or disprove this postulate. It is at least valid for the two models used here.

For the cornea, only the anterior radius is known by measurement. The le Grand eye model [12] is adopted to obtain the posterior radius by multiplication with the ratio 6.5/7.8 = 0.833. The corneal thickness is 0.55 mm. For the refractive indices of the ocular media, the Gullstrand [13] values of 1.376 for the cornea and 1.336 for aqueous and vitreous are chosen. Curvatures, thickness, and refractive index of the IOL must be obtained from the manufacturer. As a former employee, they are available to me, but I am not at liberty to divulge them in detail. A spreadsheet to generate a dummy equi-biconvex IOL for use here is given in Table 48.2.

Finally, for the purpose of optimization a thin refracting surface is introduced in the same plane as the posterior IOL surface. It is initially given zero power.

The ray tracing scheme is given in Table 48.3. The output, t6 in the table, we could call the optical back focal length (OBFL). The vitreous depth (VD) is the distance from the IOL to the inner limiting membrane and can be calculated as AL—pLP. The retinal thickness (RT) is the distance from the inner limiting membrane to the pigment epithelium. Assuming it is the same as the correction applied by the Zeiss IOLMaster to obtain AL from the measured optical path length, it can be calculated [7] as RT = −0.0429*AL + 1.3033 mm. For all cases pooled, RT was found to be (mean 0.29; SD ± 0.03; range 0.21 to 0.36; in mm). For simplicity, the mean value is used. The geometrical back focal length thus becomes GBFL = VD + 0.29 mm. The eye is focused if OBFL and GBFL are equal.

For the 44 cases with ZA9003, OBFL = 18.34 mm and GBFL = 18.31 mm were found without optimization ($N = 0$ D). To assess the agreement on the case level, the refractions that produced identical OBFL and GBFL values were calculated per case. The results are summarized in Table 48.4.

To use the formula, input the desired Rx to aim for and find the le IOL power that results in OBFL being just short of GBFL. Then, calculate the expected resulting Rx. This trial-and-error approach may be somewhat awkward for practical use, but a macro could be written to automate the procedure.

Table 48.2 Spreadsheet formulas to generate input for a dummy equi-biconvex design. The values in column B result in a 20 D IOL

	A	B	C	D
1	IOL radii Ra = −Rp (mm)	13.255	Power of each surface (D)	=(B2-B3)/B1*1000
2	RI of IOL	1.469		
3	RI of aqueous/vitreous	1.336	Central thickness (mm)	=2*(B1-SQRT(B1^2-(B5/2)^2)) + B4
4	IOL edge thickness (mm)	0.3		
5	IOL optic diameter (mm)	6	IOL power	=2*D1−D3/B2*D1^2/1000

Table 48.3 Norrby thick lens formula ray tracing scheme. The tracing calculations involve height and slope. The other rows provide input for the calculations. The trace is opened by setting the slope s0. The value 2.5 is arbitrary to produce convenient height values. Any value would produce the same end result. The trace is closed by the calculation of t6, the distance from the IOL to the focal point, at which the ray has zero height at the image surface. The equation for pLP, the distance from anterior cornea to poste- rior IOL, is given in the text. The refractive error (Rx) can be given as input or calculated as output. Surface 6 is a corrector for use in optimization by adjusting N, initially set to zero. The system is in focus if the optical back focal length (OBFL; t6 in the scheme) is equal to the geometric back focal length (GBFL; defined in the text). If the scheme is set up as an Excel spreadsheet, its Goal Seek utility can be conveniently used to find the Rx by the condition that the difference between OBFL and GBFL be zero

Surface	0 Target	1 Spectacle	2 Anterior cornea	3 Posterior cornea	4 Anterior IOL	5 Posterior IOL	6 Corrector	7 Image
Thickness (mm)	$t0 = 3988$	$t1 = 12$	$t2 = 0.55$	$t3 = pLP-t4-t2$	$t4 = $ IOL thickness	$t5 = 0$	$t6 = -h6/s6$	
Refractive index	$n0 = 1$	$n1 = 1$	$n2 = 1.376$	$n3 = 1.336$	$n4 = $ IOL Refractive index	$n5 = 1.336$	$n6 = 1.336$	
Curvature(mm)			$r2 = $ corneal anterior radius	$r3 = r2*6.8/7.7$	$r4 = $ IOL anterior radius	$r5 = $ IOL posterior radius		
Power (D)		$p1 = Rx$	$p2 = 1000*(n2-n1)/r2$	$p3 = 1000*(n3-n2)/r3$	$p4 = 1000*(n4-n3)/r4$	$p5 = 1000*(n5-n4)/r5$	$p6 = N$	
Height (mm)	$h0 = 0$	$h1 = h0 + s0*t0$	$h2 = h1 + s1*t1$	$h3 = h2 + s2*t2$	$h4 = h3 + s3*t3$	$h5 = h4 + s4*t4$	$h6 = h5 + s5*t5$	$h7 = 0$
Slope	$s0 = 2.5/t0$	$s1 = (n0*s0-h1*p1/1000)/n1$	$s2 = (n1*s1-h2*p2/1000)/n2$	$s3 = (n2*s2-h3*p3/1000)/n3$	$s4 = (n3*s3-h4*p4/1000)/n4$	$s5 = (n4*s4-h5*p5/1000)/n5$	$s6 = (n5*s5-h6*p6/1000)/n6$	

Table 48.4 Results for the Norrby thick lens formula using the 44 cases with the ZA9003 IOL. *SE* spherical equivalent (D); *OBFD* optical back focal length (mm); *GBFD* geometric back focal length (mm). Differences were obtained as calculated minus measured refractions. Unoptimized results

Parameter	OBFD	GBFD	SE measured	SE calculated	SE difference
Unit	mm	mm	D	D	D
Mean	18.34	18.31	−0.82	−0.73	0.09
SD	± 0.62	± 0.58	± 0.38	± 0.23	± 0.32
Range	17.03 to 19.93	17.06 to 19.86	−1.75 to 0.00	−1.16 to −0.18	−0.53 to 0.78

Norrby Thin Lens Formula

Common IOL power formulas are based on thin lens theory, which describes a lens as a plane with an associated power. The power calculation is then reduced to a system of three refracting surfaces: spectacle, cornea, and IOL. This system also lends itself to be set up in a spreadsheet but can be given in closed form. I will first describe the spreadsheet approach.

The spectacle is at a vertex distance of 12 mm from the anterior cornea and is given its labeled power. The cornea is placed at its second principal plane, which is 0.06 mm anterior to the cornea for the le Grand model cornea. The power is calculated as 331.5/CR, where CR is the measured anterior corneal radius of curvature. The posterior IOL surface position, pLP, is computed with the formula given in the previous section. The equivalent plane of the thin lens is at the intersection between an incoming converging ray from the cornea and the outgoing ray. The distance from the posterior plane, IO, was found (mean − 0.35; SD ± 0.05; range − 0.45 to −0.21; unit mm). The negative sign means it is anterior to the posterior IOL surface. The mean is used in the calculations.

Finally, for the purpose of optimization, a thin refracting surface is introduced at the equivalent plane of the IOL. It is initially given zero power. The resulting spreadsheet is given in Table 48.5. The distance from the IOL plane to focus, t4 in the table, is termed optical back focal distance, OBFD, to distinguish it from OBFL used for the thick lens case. The geometrical back focal distance, GBFD, is calculated as.

$$GBFD = AL - pLP + IO + RT$$

using the absolute value of IO. AL is the measured axial length, pLP is the position of the posterior IOL surface, and RT is the retinal thickness given the value of 0.29 mm.

For the 44 cases with ZA9003, OBFD = 18.63 mm and GBFD = 18.66 mm were found without optimization ($N = 0$ D). To assess the agreement on the case level, the refractions that produced identical OBFD and GBFD values were calculated per case. The results are summarized in Table 48.6.

To use the formula, input Rx to aim for and find the le IOL power that makes OBFD equal to GBFD. Choose the next higher available power. Then, calculate the expected resulting Rx.

In closed form, the thin lens formula can be written as

$$P = 1336 \times \left(\cfrac{1}{\cfrac{1.336}{\cfrac{1}{\cfrac{1}{\cfrac{1}{TD-VD} - \cfrac{Rx}{1000}} + (VD - CO)} - \cfrac{0.3315}{CR}} + (CO + (pLP - IO))} + \cfrac{1}{AL - (pLP - IO) + RT} \right)$$

Table 48.5 Norrby thin lens formula ray tracing scheme. The tracing calculations involve height and slope. The other rows provide input for the calculations. The trace is opened by setting the slope s0. The value 2.5 is arbitrary to produce convenient height values. Any value would produce the same end result. The trace is closed by the calculation of t4, the distance from the equivalent plane of the IOL to the focal point, at which the ray has zero height at the image surface. The equation for pLP, the distance from anterior cornea to posterior IOL, is given in the text. CO is the corneal offset, and IO is the IOL offset. They are both negative vectors, but to avoid confusion, their absolute values are used here. CR is the anterior corneal radius of curvature. Rx can be given as input or calculated as output. Surface 4 is a corrector for use in optimization by adjusting N, initially set to zero. The system is in focus if the optical back focal distance (OBFD; t4 in the scheme) is equal to the geometric back focal distance (GBFD; defined in the text). If the scheme is set up as an Excel spreadsheet, its Goal Seek utility can be conveniently used to find Rx by the condition that the difference between OBFD and GBFD be zero

Surface	0 Target	1 Spectacle	2 Corneal plane	3 IOL plane	4 Corrector	5 Image
Thickness (mm)	t0 = 3988	t1 = 12-CO	t2 = CO + pLP-IO	t3 = 0	t4 = -h4/s4	
Refractive index	n0 = 1	n1 = 1	n2 = 1.336	n3 = 1.336	n4 = 1.336	
Curvature(mm)			r2 = CR			
Power(D)		p1 = Rx	p2 = 331.5/r2	p3 = IOL power	p4 = N	
Height(mm)	h0 = 0	h1 = h0 + s0*t0	h2 = h1 + s1*t1	h3 = h2 + s2*t2	h4 = h3 + s3*t3	h5 = 0
Slope	s0 = 2.5/t0	s1 = (n0*s0-h1*p1/1000)/n1	s2 = (n1*s1-h2*p2/1000)/n2	s3 = (n2*s2-h3*p3/1000)/n3	s4 = (n3*s3-h4*p4/1000)/n4	

Table 48.6 Results for the Norrby thin lens formula using the 44 cases with the ZA9003 IOL. SE: spherical equivalent (D); OBFD: optical back focal distance (mm); GBFD: geometric back focal distance (mm). Differences were obtained as calculated minus measured refractions. Unoptimized results

Parameter	OBFD	GBFD	SE measured	SE calculated	SE difference
Unit	Mm	Mm	D	D	D
Mean	18.63	18.66	−0.82	−0.89	−0.07
SD	± 0.60	± 0.58	± 0.38	± 0.27	± 0.33
Range	17.39 to 20.15	17.41 to 20.21	−1.75 to 0.00	−1.33 to −0.23	−0.68 to 0.62

where P is IOL power (D). AL is axial length (mm), Rx is the desired refraction (D), TD is target distance (mm), VD is vertex distance (mm), CR is the corneal radius (mm), pLP is the position of the posterior IOL surface (mm), CO is the corneal offset (mm), IO is the IOL offset (mm), and RT is the retinal thickness (mm). Though CO and IO are negative vectors, their absolute value is used here to avoid confusion. In the present calculations, TD = 4000 mm, VD = 12 mm, CO = 0.06 mm, IO = 0.35 mm, and RT = 0.29 mm have been used as fixed values. pLP is calculated as before.

Norrby Regression Formula

To a physicist, it is obvious that the original SRK formula ($P = A-2.5*AL-0.9*K$) cannot be a correct description of the relation between its parameters, because they do not all have the same dimension. AL has the dimension length, while P and K have the dimension diopter, which is a reciprocal length.

Including also refraction, the following dimensionally correct representation can be set up:

$$0.7 \times P + Rx = C_1 + \frac{C_2}{AL} + \frac{C_3}{CR}$$

The factor 0.7 transforms P to the spectacle plane. The factor varies slightly from eye to eye, but 0.7 is a representative average. The Cs are coefficients found by linear regression to yield

$$0.7 \times P + Rx = -4.262 + \frac{1308}{AL} - \frac{286.0}{CR}$$

for which the statistical R-squared value of 0.93 was found. This means that the relationship accounts for virtually all variance in the data.

Table 48.7 Results for the Norrby regression formula using the 44 cases with the ZA9003 IOL. SE: spherical equivalent (D). Differences were obtained as calculated minus measured refractions

Parameter	SE measured	SE calculated	SE difference
Unit	D	D	D
Mean	−0.82	−0.82	0.00
SD	± 0.38	± 0.16	± 0.33
Range	−1.75 to 0.00	−1.15 to −0.35	−0.77 to 0.73

There is nothing more to be explained. The equation can be re-arranged to solve for either P or Rx. Using the P values implanted and calculating the expected Rx values per case gave the results summarized in Table 48.7 for the 44 cases with ZA9003.

Calculations for Other IOL Models

The three formulas were developed on data from IOL model ZA9003. What about other models? Taking the regression formula as an example, one can proceed as follows for model ZCB00. The labeled A-constant for ZCB00 is 119.3 D and that of ZA9003 is 119.1 D. Powers for ZCB00 are therefore expected to be 0.2 D higher than for ZA9003 on average. This can be calculated by the formula

$$P = \frac{1}{0.7}\left(-Rx - 4.262 + \frac{1308}{AL} - \frac{286.0}{CR}\right) + N$$

where $N = 0.2$ D for ZCB00. Taking the new P, compute the expected refraction with the original equation for ZA9003 (without N) re-arranged to solve for Rx:

$$Rx = -4.262 + \frac{1308}{AL} - \frac{286.0}{CR} - 0.7 \times P$$

Assume you have a patient with AL = 25.37 mm and CR = 8.125 mm. You aim for Rx = −0.25 D. With $N = 0.2$ mm, you find $P = 17.8$ D, which you round up to 18.0 D. With that power, you expect Rx = −0.50 and you find −0.625 as the spherical equivalent. You are probably not bothered by this difference.

Analyzing the 44 cases with ZCB00 in retrospect, $N = 0.2$ D is subtracted from the IOL powers implanted to obtain the corresponding power for ZA9003. Computing the expected refractions yields Rx −0.80 D as the mean, which is −0.25 D more myopic than was found. By adding 0.25/0.7 = 0.36 D, N = 0.56 D is obtained. Rx (D) now becomes (mean − 0.54; SD ± 0.25; range − 0.91to 0.45; unit D), yielding the Rx difference (mean 0.00; SD ± 0.42; range − 1.39 to 1.20; unit D).

The N number approach is general and can be applied to any IOL power formula. If you want to start with a new IOL model, use the formula for your current IOL model, including the formula constant. Add N to the power calculated by your current formula. The starting assumption is that N is equal to the difference between the published A-constants (new A minus old A). Use it for 20 to 40 cases and determine the mean refraction. If you are not happy, you can increase or decrease the N number. Adding 0.36 D to your N number will drive your outcome by a quarter diopter in the myopic direction, subtracting in the hyperopic direction.

Applying the SRK/T formula to the ZA9003 data and optimizing the A-constant to achieve zero mean Rx difference yield the A-constant of 118.6 (D). The discrepancy with the labeled A-constant 119.1 (D) can be explained if the keratometric index of 1.3375 was used in the clinical data underlying the labeled constant. Be sure to use the A-constant of 118.6 (D) when translating results to other models than ZA9003.

Comparisons between the Norrby and SRK/T formulas are given in Table 48.8. First, the Norrby thick and thin formulas were optimized by adjusting N to achieve zero mean difference between calculated and measured refractions. The Norrby regression formula is already optimized by way of its derivation. The results are plotted in Fig. 48.1.

The correction procedure works also for IOL models that do not balance out the corneal spherical aberration. The effect of spherical aberration

Table 48.8 Comparison between optimized results for the Norrby and SRK/T formulas for the 44 cases with the ZA9003 IOL. Results are for calculated minus measured refractions

Parameter	Norrby thick lens formula	Norrby thin lens formula	Norrby regression formula	SRK/T formula
Unit	D	D	D	D
Optimization	$N = 0.14$	$N = -0.09$	$N = 0$	$A = 118.6$
Mean	0.00	0.00	0.00	0.00
SD	± 0.32	± 0.33	± 0.33	± 0.37
Range	−0.63 to 0.69	−0.62 to 0.68	−0.77 to 0.73	−1.01 to 0.64
MeanAE	0.25	0.25	0.27	0.30
MedianAE	0.20	0.18	0.19	0.28

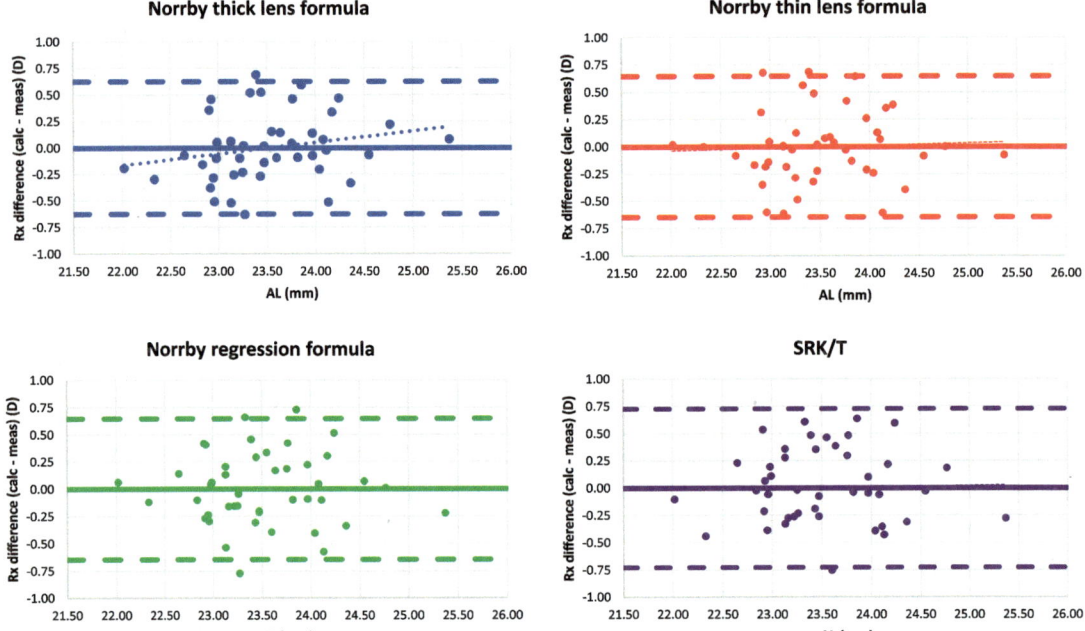

Fig. 48.1 Refraction difference (calculated minus measured) vs. AL for four IOL power calculation formulas for the 44 cases of IOL model ZA9003. The results are optimized for all formulas (see Table 48.8). Dashed lines are 95% limits, and the full line is the mean. Trend lines are dotted and in some cases hidden by the line for the mean. Trend slopes are in all cases not statistically significant: Norrby thick lens formula $F = 0.16$; Norrby thin lens formula $F = 0.77$; Norrby regression formula $F = 0.98$; SRK/T formula $F = 0.87$

is that the best focus is anterior to paraxial focus. This effect is embedded in optimized formula constants. To illustrate the effect of spherical aberration, I used a calculation spreadsheet of mine that can handle aspheric surfaces. For an eye that is emmetropic with a 20 D ZA9003, a spectacle correction of −0.29 D is required if it is replaced by the same power of its spherical predecessor CeeOn 911A, assuming a 3-mm pupil. The effect of the spherical aberration thus gives an apparent increase in IOL power of 0.41 D. Note that the N number correction does not change the position of the IOL, as formulas like SRK/T do.

To challenge the Norrby formulas, prospective studies must be performed. It is then essential that measured AL, CR, and ACD (if used) are consistent with those obtained with the Zeiss IOLMaster software V.5 version that was employed in the data acquisition for their development. Otherwise, data must be corrected by suitable transformation [6] before applying the formulas. It is also important that postoperative refraction is determined with the chart at 4 m, or corrected by the addition of $(1/6–1/4) = 0.08$ D if measured at 6 m.

Toric Calculation with Norrby Formulas

Fam and Lim have published [14] a method to calculate toric IOL sphere and cylinder powers to correct for measured corneal sphere and cylinder powers. It entails calculating the power in the steep and flat meridians separately and by rather elaborate calculations determine the nearest toric IOL power and cylinder combination available and then calculate the expected postoperative refractive outcome in terms of sphere, cylinder, and axis. They illustrate it with the Holladay 1 formula in their paper. I tested the method with other common IOL power formulas, and it works equally well for them. It should work for the Norrby formulas as well.

Another option is to transform the measured corneal cylinder to the IOL plane by dividing it by 0.7. This is how the Alcon toric calculator works (it applies a slightly different value for the transformation). However, as pointed out by Fam and Lim, that is less accurate.

Correction for surgically induced astigmatism in the toric calculation is in my opinion not called for. At least in the data coming from the study used here, no clinically significant surgically induced change was found [15], even though the incision was 3.2 mm. The same observation was made by Hirnschall and colleagues [16].

Future

The Norrby formulas reported here have approximately an MAE of 0.25 D and a MedAE of 0.20 D, which is at least as good as commonly used power calculation formulas. I do not think one can hope to achieve better, considering the uncertainties in the determination of the corneal power [15, 17, 18] required for the power calculation, and the refraction [19, 20] used to assess the outcome. Keratometry has good repeatability [21], but the reproducibility is poor, not due to the

measurement as such, but to fluctuations over time in the curvature of the cornea. Keratometry is thus a larger contributor to outcome error than previously thought [22, 16]. It is plausible that the uncertainty in refraction is correlated with fluctuations in the cornea, but I have not seen any such study. In conclusion, in my opinion, the quest for the ultimate IOL power formula has reached road's end.

For improvement in the predictability of IOL surgery, it is better to concentrate on the consistency of biometry. We are far from a situation where biometry equipment yields the same result for a given measured eye. Take keratometry, where the index used to convert measured curvature to K varies among instruments. The appearance of the IOLMaster may have meant there is a gold standard for AL measurement, but that length is not appropriate for exact optical calculations. Results for ACD and crystalline LT also vary among instruments. Admittedly, they are more difficult and not infrequently impossible to measure. We should aim for a situation where biometry equipment provide a clearly defined output that can be used interchangeably.

Many ophthalmologists believe that inaccuracy in IOL power is a major contributor to outcome error, referring to the international standard for IOL power [23, 24]. For example, a 20 D IOL has a tolerance of ± 0.40 D. Tolerances in industry are ± 3 standard deviations. As responsible for the development of the standard, I have pitifully failed to convince ophthalmologists that the IOL is unlikely to be a main contributor to outcome error. To put it in perspective, fluctuations in keratometry are about ± 0.25 D [15], giving a "specification" of ± 0.75 D for corneal K, with an unknown nominal value. Also, I am not a believer in statistical analysis of large datasets from multiple sources, which are bound to contain measurements obtained by multiple instruments. Likely, the data are also not dimensionally consistent. The result inevitably will be a large blur. What is not significant with 20–40 cases with well-controlled data acquisition is not worth pursuing.

After having advocated IOL calculation by exact ray tracing throughout my career, it came as a sobering revelation that a simple regression formula performed just as well and that AL and corneal curvature are sufficient as input. There is no need to know the ACD, while the estimation of IOL position is crucial for all formulas based on optical calculation, be it based on thin or thick lens theory.

For power calculation in eyes that had corneal refractive surgery, it seems ray tracing is the way to go. However, even in this case I am not wholly convinced any longer. I have ideas to approach it more simply but will not pursue them.

Epilogue

This chapter is the result of ideas, proposals, assumptions, postulates, and opinions that have evolved and matured over the years. It is up to others to pursue, improve, refute, or forget them.

This is my final publication in the field of IOL power calculation. It has been a wonderful journey that has given me many good friends and fond memories.

Acknowledgments I am indebted to many people for this paper. In the first instance, Wolfgang Haigis, PhD, came to Groningen in 1985 to ask for IOL design information for his efforts in power calculation. At that time, he applied thick lens ray tracing [25]. We immediately became friends, and he taught me a lot about optical calculation and biometry during several visits to his laboratory at the Kopfklinikum of the Julius-Maximilians-University Eye Clinic in Würzburg. He sadly passed away on October 15, 2019. Clinical data for my early publications were generated in studies at St. Erik's Eye Hospital, Stockholm, Sweden. I am indebted to Eva Lydahl, MD, PhD, Gabor Koranyi, MD, PhD, and Mikaela Taube, RN, who performed the studies and co-authored the resulting papers. For this chapter, the data were collected at Moorfields Eye Hospital, London, United Kingdom. I owe gratitude to Oliver Findl, MD, MBA, Nino Hirnschall MD, PhD, and Yutaro Nishi, MD. They co-authored several of my later publications. A special thanks is due to Rolf Bergman, PhD. We met at university and were colleagues at Pharmacia and its successors for several years. Rolf made me aware of the shortcomings of conventional statistics (I blush for some of my early papers) and taught me why partial least-squares (PLS) regression is preferable. He performed the analysis for the seminal paper on postoperative IOL position [11]. Finally, I owe gratitude to Kenneth J Hoffer, MD, H John Shammas, MD, Jaime Aramberri, MD, Thomas Olsen, MD, and again Wolfgang Haigis,

PhD. They invited me as a co-founder of the IOL Power Club at its first meeting in 2005, in San Sebastian, Spain. We have had many wonderful meetings, filled with fruitful discussions and joyful events, after that.

References

1. O'Shea DC. Elements of modern optical design. New York: Wiley-Interscience; 1985.
2. Norrby NES. The Lens Haptic Plane (LHP) a fixed reference for IOL implant power calculation. Eur J Implant Ref Surg. 1995;7:202–9.
3. Norrby S. Multicenter biometry study of 1 pair of eyes. Cataract Refract Surg. 2001;27:1656–61.
4. Koranyi G, Lydahl E, Norrby S, Taube M. Anterior chamber depth measurement: a-scan versus optical methods. J Cataract Refract Surg. 2002;28:243–7.
5. Norrby S, Lydahl E, Koranyi G, Taube M. Comparison of 2 A-scans. J Cataract Refract Surg. 2003;29:95–9.
6. Norrby S, Lydahl E, Koranyi G, Taube M. Reduction of trend errors in power calculation by linear transformation of measured axial lengths. J Cataract Refract Surg. 2003;29:100–5.
7. Haigis W, Lege B, Miller N, Schneider B. Comparison of immersion ultrasound biometry and partial coherence interferometry for intraocular lens calculation according to Haigis. Graefe's Arch Clin Exp Ophthalmol. 2000;238:765–73.
8. Olsen T. On the calculation of power from curvature of the cornea. Br J Ophthalmol. 1986;70:152–4.
9. Findl O, Hirnschall N, Nishi Y, Maurino V, Crnej a. Capsular bag performance of a hydrophobic acrylic 1-piece intraocular lens. J Cataract Refract Surg. 2015;41(1):90–7.
10. Norrby S. Using the lens haptic plane concept and thick-lens ray tracing to calculate intraocular lens power. J Cataract Refract Surg. 2004;30:1000–5.
11. Norrby S, Bergman R, Hirnschall N, Nishi Y, Findl O. Prediction of the true IOL position. Br J Ophthalmol. 2017;0:1–7. Erratum: "aLP" in the Formula Quoted Should Be "pLP"
12. LeGrand Y, El Hage SG. Physiological Optics. Berlin: (Springer Verlag; 1980. p. 65–7.
13. Gullstrand A. The dioptrics of the eye. In: Southall JPC, editor. Helmholtz's treatise on physiological optics, vol. 1. (Optical Society of America; 1924. p. 351–2.
14. Bor FH, Ling LK. Meridional nalysis for calculating the expected spherocylindrical refraction in eyes with toric intraocular lenses. J Cataract Refract Surg. 2007;33:2072–6.
15. Norrby S, Hirnschall N, MD, Nishi Y, Findl O. Fluctuations in corneal curvature limit predictability of intraocular lens power calculations. J Cataract Refract Surg. 2013;39:174–9.
16. Hirnschall N, Findl O, Bayer N, et al. Sources of Error in Toric Intraocular Lens Power Calculation. J Refract Surg. 2020;36(10):646–52.

17. Shammas HJ, Chan S. Precision of biometry, keratometry, and refractive measurements with a partial coherence interferometry–keratometry device. J Cataract Refract Surg. 2010;36:1474–8.
18. Shammas HJ, Hoffer KJ. Repeatability and Reproducibility of Biometry and Keratometry Measurements Using a Noncontact Optical Low-Coherence Reflectometer and Keratometer. Am J Ophthalmol. 2012;153:55–61.
19. Bullimore MA, Fusaro RE, Adams CW. The repeatability of automated and clinician refraction. Optom vis Sci. 1998;75:617–22.
20. MacKenzie GE. Reproducibility of Sphero-Cylindrical Prescriptions. Ophthal Physiol Opt. 2008;28:143–50.
21. Shirayama M, Wang L, Weikert MP, Koch DD. Comparison of corneal powers obtained from 4 different devices. Am J Ophthalmol. 2009;148:528–35.
22. Norrby S. Sources of error in intraocular lens power calculation. J Cataract Refract Surg. 2008;34:368–76.
23. International Organization for Standardization. Ophthalmic implants—intraocular lensesdpart 2: optical properties and test methods. Geneva, Switzerland, ISO 2014 (ISO 11979–2).
24. Norrby NES, Grossman LW, Geraghty EP, et al. Accuracy in determining intraocular lens dioptric power assessed by interlaboratory tests. J Cataract Refract Surg. 1996;22:983–93.
25. Haigis W. Strahldurchrechnung in Gaußscher Optik Zur Beschreibung Des LinsensystemsBrille-Kontaktlinse-Hornhaut-Augenlinse (IOL). In: Schott K, et al., editors. 4. Kongreß der Deutschen Gesellschaft für Intraokularlinsen Implantation. Berlin Heidelberg: Springer-Verlag; 1991. p. 233–46.

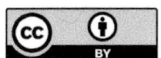

OKULIX Raytracing Software

Paul-Rolf Preußner

Background: Raytracing?

Raytracing sounds like a modern approach. But this impression is wrong. Raytracing was the first calculation method for imaging optics, developed in the beginning of the seventeenth century. The law of refraction of light at a surface that separates two media of different light velocity was first discovered heuristically by Willebrord Snellius (1580–1626). The numerical value of the light velocity in vacuum v_v was not yet known at that time, but the ratio of light velocities in different media was. Therefore, the "index of refraction" $n = v_v / v_m$ was used to optically characterize a specific material with light velocity v_m. Pierre de Fermat (1601–1665) deduced Snell's law a few decades after its invention from a general principle of light propagation. This deduction is often presented to students of physics as an exercise: They have to find out the angular change of light propagation on a surface separating two media of different light velocity under the condition that the total flight time of the light has a minimum. The result of this exercise is Snell's law: $sin\beta_1 \times n_1 = sin\beta_2 \times n_2$ with n_1 and n_2, refractive indices of the two media, and β_1 and β_2, angles of the light ray relative to the normal of the surface at the intersection point.

P.-R. Preußner (✉)
University Eye Hospital Mainz, Mainz, Germany
e-mail: pr.preussner@uni-mainz.de

Nothing more than Snell's law is needed to calculate an imaging optical system, but there is a pitfall: combining expressions of Snell's law for more than one surface generates so-called transcendental equations which are mathematically not solvable. The only way is to apply Snell's law iteratively: Calculate the angle of one ray on one surface, use the result for the next surface, and continue this way for all surfaces and for many rays. This needs the calculation of many sine expressions and of the ray geometry between the surfaces for all rays, altogether called **"raytracing,"** requiring a calculation effort that was not available in the seventeenth century. Thus, despite the availability of the physical know how, optical systems could not be calculated at that time.

About 150 years later Carl Friedrich Gauß (1777–1855) found an approximative solution of the problem. Numerically, the sine can be calculated by a polynomial series: $sin\beta = \beta - \beta^3 / 3! + \beta^5 / 5! - \beta^7 / 7!...$

Gauß abbreviated this series to the first element: $sin\beta \approx \beta$. The accuracy of this approximation is the better the smaller β is. For an optical system consisting of only spherical surfaces and centered to an optical axis, rays with a small angular deviation from this axis could now be calculated in closed formulae, thereby using terms like focal width $f = R / \Delta n$ or power $p = 1 / f$ with R, the radius of the sphere, and Δn, the difference of the refractive indices of both sides of that sphere.

© The Author(s) 2024

J. Aramberri et al. (eds.), *Intraocular Lens Calculations*, Essentials in Ophthalmology,
https://doi.org/10.1007/978-3-031-50666-6_49

The restriction of Gaussian optics to paraxial rays and to spherical surfaces causes inaccuracies which are not tolerable in many applications. Therefore, the seventeenth-century approach of raytracing has meanwhile again replaced Gaussian optics in nearly all optical areas. The main reason to use Gaussian optics, the missing computing power, disappeared with the availability of cheap, powerful computers today.

Also the human eye with its highly vaulted optical surfaces is poorly described by Gaussian optics. The development of a variety of correcting methods for IOL formulas in Gaussian optics was necessary to compensate the bias from a too simplified approach.

IOL Selection in OKULIX

Tracing many rays through a human eye does not yet solve the problem of finding the IOL that fits best to the patient's requirements. This addresses not only the IOL power closest to the target refraction but also higher order optical errors of the pseudophakic eye, in particular, the eye's spherical aberration, and astigmatism.

Generally, patients want to see "sharp," but, other than in a photograph, the major fraction of the light impinging to the optical entrance of the eye does not contribute to the impression of a subjectively sharp image. The human eye can see sharp only in a very small area, the fovea. Outside the fovea, visual acuity steeply decreases to a few percent of the foveal value. This decrease is mostly caused by the neuronal characteristics of the human retina, less by the decrease of optical imaging quality. Therefore, in order not to waist computing power, OKULIX restricts all calculations to the foveal area.

In the unavoidable presence of higher order optical errors of the human eye, the definition of "sharp" is not always unambiguous. Among other influencing parameters, it can even depend on the visual target. A square-edged target may look sharper than a round one with one optics,

but less sharp with another one. Taking into account this ambiguity together with the requirement to obtain IOL calculation results from raytracing which can directly be compared to those of other methods, the following calculation steps are used in OKULIX:

1. Calculation of the paraxial refraction of the eye for each power level of the corresponding IOL model. The results of such paraxial raytracing are identical to those of a thick-lens calculation in Gaussian optics.

2. Calculation of the so-called best focus refraction in a full aperture raytracing, again for all power levels. The best focus of an optical system with spherical aberration is the focal width of the highest flux density. It is the "working" focus used in vision, and it depends on the pupil width. As an example, the refraction difference between paraxial and the best focus refraction of a mean-sized eye implanted with a 21D Alcon SN60AT IOL is $-0.2D$ for a pupil width of 2.5 mm, but $-1.17D$ for 6 mm pupil width. This refraction shift is also responsible for what is commonly called "night myopia." It depends on many parameters, e.g., on the asphericities of all optical surfaces and on the IOL shape factor (see also section "Impact of IOL Shape Factor Variations").

The default pupil width in OKULIX is 2.5 mm in pupil plane, i.e., ≈ 2.9 mm in corneal plane (modifiable by the user). The best focus refraction can be directly compared to the results of all other IOL calculation methods. The difference between the paraxial and the best focus refraction shows the amount of spherical aberration with the chosen IOL model. It is zero in case of zero spherical aberration.

The best focus refractions are indicated for sphere, cylinder, and axis. Thus the user can see from the axis whether the proposed toric IOL power results in an astigmatic under- or overcorrection, see Fig. 49.1.

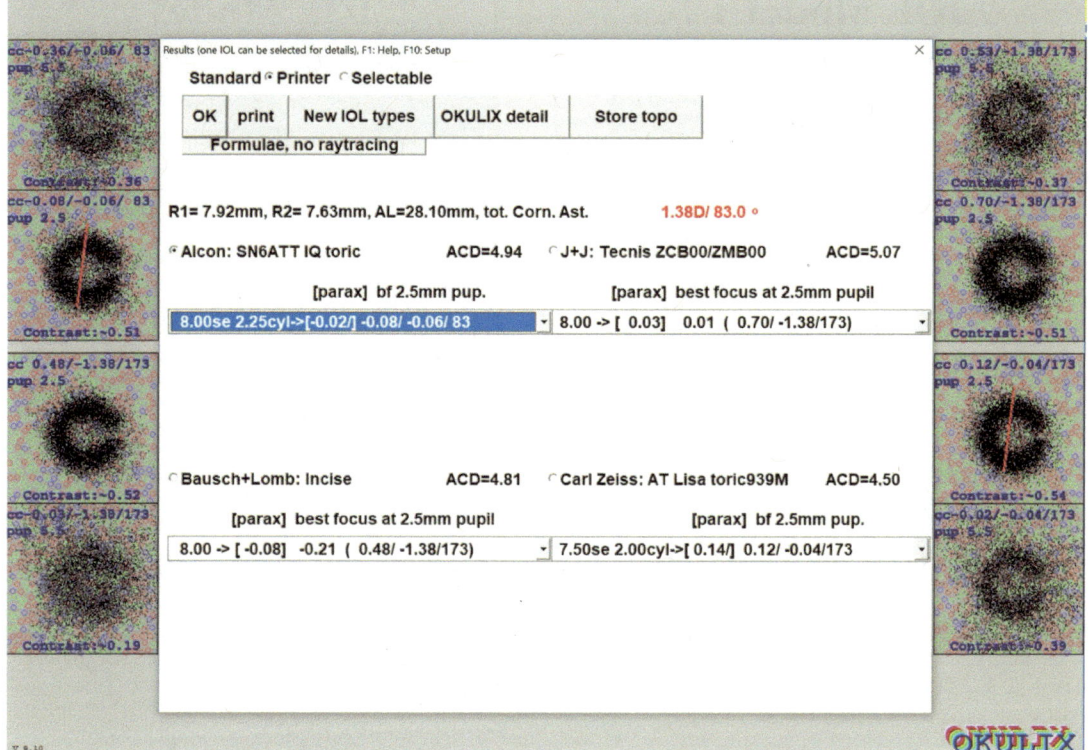

Fig. 49.1 Results of calculation for four IOL models (The predicted refractions are calculated paraxially and for the best focus of the assumed pupil width (default: 2.5 mm) in pupil plane. They are shown for each power level in the sub-windows of the IOL models. Two Landolt rings of visual acuity chart size 1.0 (20/20, 6/6, logMar 0) are simulated for each IOL model and shown above each other, one with normal (e.g., 2.5 mm) and one with large (5.5 mm) pupil size. The simulations are calculated with the best sphero-cylindrical correction which is indicated in blue on top of the subimage. Thus the simulated visual impressions exactly show the impact of all higher order optical aberrations. As a quantitative measure of optical quality the contrast of the Landolt rings is indicated (blue). The total corneal astigmatism, i.e., the combination of anterior and posterior astigmatism, is shown in red. The cylinder axis is additionally plotted in the Landolt ring simulations of toric IOL.)

3. Calculation of simulated Landolt ring images on the retina for the IOL power level closest to the target refraction. These images are calculated for 2.5 mm and 5.5 mm pupil width, thus graphically showing the impact of spherical aberration and other higher order optical errors on image quality, see Fig. 49.1. In both images the sphero-cylindrical refraction errors (in corneal plane) are indicated and the calculation is corrected for them. Without such correction, sphero-cylindrical errors mostly would dominate the image worsening compared to the worsening caused by higher order optical errors.

For toric IOL [6, 20], simulated Landolt rings are additionally calculated not only for the power level closest to the target refraction but also for the neighboring spherical and cylindrical power levels, i.e., altogether nine subimages are produced. This time, calculation is performed for 2.5 mm pupil width only (or for the value chosen by the user) and without correction of residual sphero-cylindrical refraction errors, thus showing the patient's visual impression without glasses, see Fig. 49.2.

IOL Model 1

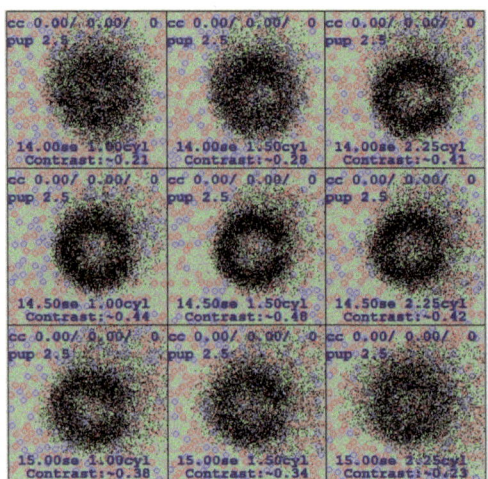

←**Cylindrical Power**→

IOL Model 2

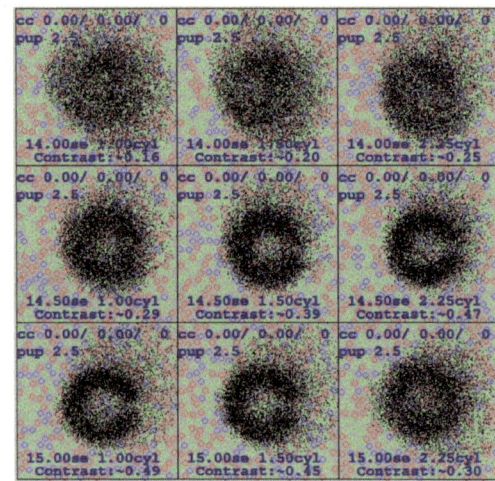

← **Cylindrical Power** →

← **Spherical Power** →

Fig. 49.2 Step 3 of Toric IOL Selection (The central one of the nine Landolt rings corresponds to the "best focus" selection, and the surrounding ones are from the neighboring power steps in sphere (se) and cylinder. The two IOL models differ in design details, in particular, in the asphericity of their surfaces causing different spherical aberrations of the eye. Both IOL models are virtually implanted into the same eye. Note that for IOL model 1 the central subimage corresponds to the best visual impression, but for IOL model 2, the lowest left and the middle right are slightly better, showing the ambiguity of "best optics")

Input Parameters for IOL Calculation

The accuracy of an IOL calculation is always limited by the accuracy of the input data. Many of the current methods are additionally biased from replacing physical input data by assumed parameters. Even if OKULIX tries to avoid this as far as possible, there are unavoidable restrictions:

1. Data that cannot be measured with the available equipment. Corneal asphericity is not measured when only Keratometry is available, and the data of the posterior corneal surface are only measured with instruments providing full tomography: Scheimpflug or OCT devices. In cases of unavailable measurements, OKULIX uses the eye model of Liou and Brennan [9] to complete the missing input data.

2. Data that cannot be measured at all preoperatively: the final IOL position. OKULIX assumes a centered IOL, and however, after the IOL selection the user can define a decentration and simulate the impact on optical quality, e.g., Landolt ring images or wavefront errors.

   OKULIX uses the geometrical IOL position, not a fictitious "effective lens position." The prediction algorithm of IOL position utilizes axial eye length and position and the thickness of the crystalline lens (when measured) and an average IOL position for each IOL model [17]. During the development of OKULIX, this algorithm was refined several times, thereby taking into account postoperative position measurements of different IOL models [15]. In case of a justified assumption (e.g., measurement in the fellow eye), the user can also define the IOL position in OKULIX. In principal, there is no difference of such a prediction algorithm used for ray-tracing compared to the one used for Gaussian optics with respect to accuracy, but an algorithm that predicts "effective" instead of geometrical IOL positions can cause a systematic bias in particular in short eyes.

The measurable input data are described in the following subsections.

Axial Length Data

Axial lengths measured by different devices differ significantly. Even if the IOLMaster (Zeiss, Germany) is de facto established as a worldwide reference, the rational basis to accept this is doubtful as it is based on a relative calibration of the IOLMaster to an ultrasound device [3], making thus this ultrasound device to the universal standard. However, a real "Gold Standard" for axial length measurements does not exist because it is impossible to measure a human eye, e.g., by a mechanical micrometer. To overcome these problems of absolute calibration, during the development of OKULIX, an axial length transformation was developed that was calibrated in a patient collective in which all other parameters were defined with high accuracy. Corneal radii, axial lengths (from IOLMaster), IOL position (from laser interferometry), and refraction were measured in a patient collective of 189 eyes. Together with these data, manufacturer's IOL data (see below) were used for a raytracing calculation. The data set of this pseudophakic sample is mathematically overdetermined, and therefore, we could find a transformation for the axial lengths that made the data consistent [11, 12, 15]. The results of this transformation are used as reference in OKULIX. For other axial length measuring devices, comparing measurements was performed to the IOLMaster in larger patient collectives to establish relative calibrations of all of these devices to one another. Thus each of the devices listed in OKULIX can now be used,

together with an internal transformation procedure, without inducing any systematic differences.

The accuracy of axial length measurements is limited by the unknown properties of the crystalline lens which cannot be measured independently from the thickness in the individual eye: the sound velocity in ultrasound and the refractive index in optical measurements. In order to find out the impact of these parameters on overall accuracy, the axial length was optically measured prior to and after cataract surgery in a large patient collective. In the postoperative measurement, the data (thickness and refractive index of the IOL) were exactly known. The standard deviation of the difference between pre- and postoperative measurements (52 μm, [17]) can be considered as the best measure of the mean error.

In summary, with modern optical axial length measurements, errors are in the order of 50 μm corresponding to ≈0.15D in the refraction prediction. This is valid for all IOL calculation methods.

Corneal Data

Preferably, corneal data should consist of the measured tomography, i.e., anterior topography and spatially resolved thickness. Devices that have a software interface to OKULIX transfer these data automatically. Such devices are Tomey TMS-5 and CASIA, Oculus Pentacam, Ziemer Galilei G6, and Heidelberg Engineering ANTERION. Local posterior corneal radii are calculated from the anterior ones and the local thickness in a straightforward geometrical calculation. Some other devices with an interface to OKULIX only measure anterior topography: Tomey TMS4 and OA2000 and Tracey iTrace. For the latter ones, local posterior radii are calculated according to the Liou and Brennan eye model [9] from the anterior ones: $R_p = 0.83 \times R_a$ with R_p and R_a, local posterior and anterior radii. This calculation should not be performed in eyes after the corneal surgery.

When only keratometric (vertex) radii are measured, they can be used as well for "normal" eyes, again by calculating the posterior vertex radii with the same factor of 0.83 from the anterior ones, and a default value of −0.18 for anterior corneal asphericity. However, in this case, the third step of the IOL selection as described in section "IOL Selection in OKULIX" does not make much sense.

IOL Data

An IOL in OKULIX is defined by anterior and posterior vertex radii, central thickness, refractive index, and asphericity of anterior and posterior surfaces. In toric models, two vertex radii are needed for each anterior or posterior toric surface. These data are different for each power level, whereby "'power" is only used as a label (rather than as a physical parameter). All IOL data in OKULIX come from the IOL manufacturers. To avoid possible data errors, all data are checked for compliance with ISO11979-2 prior to inclusion into the OKULIX database. The notation of toric IOLs also is in compliance with ISO11979-2, for example, 23.5Se2.5Cyl means an IOL with a spherical equivalent of 23.5D and a cylinder power of 2.5D. The meridian of the lowest IOL power which is to be implanted at the axis of highest total corneal power is always indicated by a red line.

Benefits: Applications and Comparisons

IOL Calculation in Eyes After Corneal Surgery

Two significant differences between virgin eyes and eyes after the corneal surgery can cause errors in the IOL calculation:

1. The asphericity of the anterior cornea often changes from a slightly prolate to an oblate asphere after the myopia-correcting corneal surgery. Keratometric measurements assum-

ing a sphere or a prolate asphere then underestimate the vertex radius [13, 14, 16], thus producing a hyperopic outcome of IOL calculations.

2. With changed anterior but more or less unchanged posterior corneal radii after corneal surgery, the ratio between anterior and posterior corneal radii changes as well. When anterior and posterior surfaces are combined to only one surface at the location of the anterior cornea in IOL formulas, thereby defining a so-called fictitious corneal refractive index

$$\hat{n} = n_c + (n_h - n_c) \cdot R_a / R_p - d \cdot (n_c - 1) \cdot (n_h - n_c) / (n_c \cdot R_p)$$

with n_c and n_h, refractive index of cornea and aqueous humor, R_a and R_p, anterior and posterior corneal radii, and d, corneal thickness, this refractive index $\hat{n}$ and the corneal power based thereon are changing as well. After the myopia-correcting corneal surgery, this additionally causes a hyperopic shift.

The said errors do not occur in tomography-based raytracing [2, 21, 23] because all parameters are measured, without making any assumptions, see the following example: In 70 eyes after the myopia-correcting Lasik, Pentacam tomography and IOLMaster Keratometry and axial length measurements were performed prior to the complication-free cataract surgery. Figure 49.3 shows the results together with the impact of the two abovementioned error contributions. In this example, they are both of the

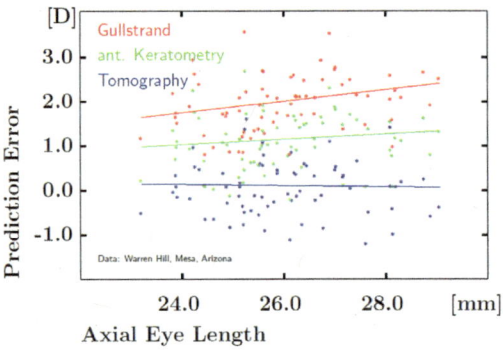

Fig. 49.3 Prediction error in Post-Lasik eyes blue: raytracing based on full tomography green: same posterior radii, but anterior keratometry (IOLMaster) red: anterior keratometry, posterior radii from Gullstrand's eye model

same order of magnitude, but this can differ depending on the details of the Lasik laser protocol.

A more systematic approach of verifying whether the impact of a corneal laser surgery is fully covered by an IOL calculation method is the following: The eyes are measured prior to and after the corneal surgery, and for both measurements, an IOL calculation with the same IOL model and power is performed. The differences of the resulting refractive predictions of the IOL calculations should be identical to the achieved corneal laser refractive corrections. The advantage of this approach is to avoid any error impact of the surgical procedure or of IOL manufacturing errors.

Such an investigation was performed in 204 eyes undergoing SMILE. Pre- and postoperative Pentacam tomography and IOLMaster axial length measurements were performed [8]. The OKULIX results together with those of two other methods using Pentacam anterior vertex radii are shown in Fig. 49.4.

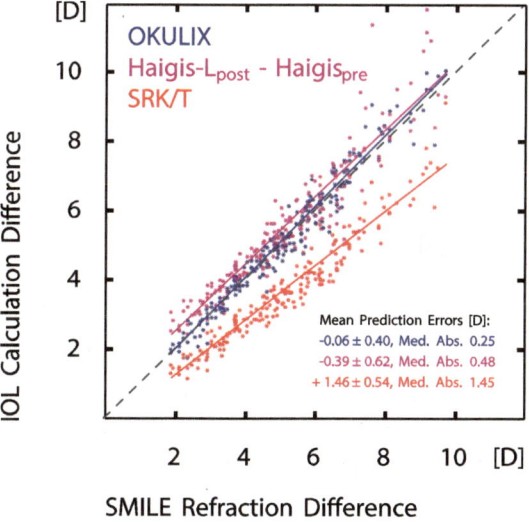

Fig. 49.4 Prediction errors after SMILE (The difference between the refraction prediction of IOL calculation methods prior to and after the SMILE corneal surgery is shown as a function of the achieved refractive correction of the SMILE procedure in 204 eyes)

Very Long Eyes

In very long eyes many IOL formulas produce a hyperopic bias which is not found with OKULIX, see Fig. 49.5. The reason, however, is not the application of raytracing but the use of the appropriate eye model of Liou and Brennan [9]. Replacing the fictitious corneal refractive index $\hat{n}$ of the formulas by the one derived from the Liou and Brennan eye model mostly removes the bias [18, 19]. The wrongly higher $\hat{n}$-value from Gullstrand's eye model is also responsible for the unrealistically high "effective lens position" to compensate the overestimated corneal power in the formulas. This applies also to short eyes.

Impact of IOL Shape Factor Variations

When prediction accuracy was compared to other methods up to the second digit behind the decimal point in a competition, OKULIX was the winner [1]. This, however, is not fully obvious when taking into account the expected error amounts as described in section "Limitations". It can be assumed that the reason is the exact use of the IOL manufacturer's data, in particular, variations of the IOL shape factor with the IOL power level.

The shape factor S of a lens describes the deviation from biconvex or biconcave symmetry: $S = (R_1 + R_2) / (R_1 - R_2)$ with R_1 and R_2, anterior and posterior lens radii. For a symmetric lens, $R_1 = -R_2$ and thus $S = 0$. Many IOL models are symmetric, but the majority of lenses on the market are not. In many of these asymmetric lenses, the shape factor varies between power levels, see Fig. 49.6.

Such shape factor variations also show the occurring inaccuracies when so-called formula constants are adjusted: A correct adjustment would need a separate "constant" for each power level.

Fig. 49.5 Prediction error in very long eyes (The prediction error of 83 eyes measured with IOLMaster (Zeiss) and implanted with Alcon MA60MA IOLs is shown as a function of the axial eye length. Upper image: results of the formulas [3, 4, 7, 22] in the original notation, and lower image: with Liou and Brennan's fictitious corneal refractive index)

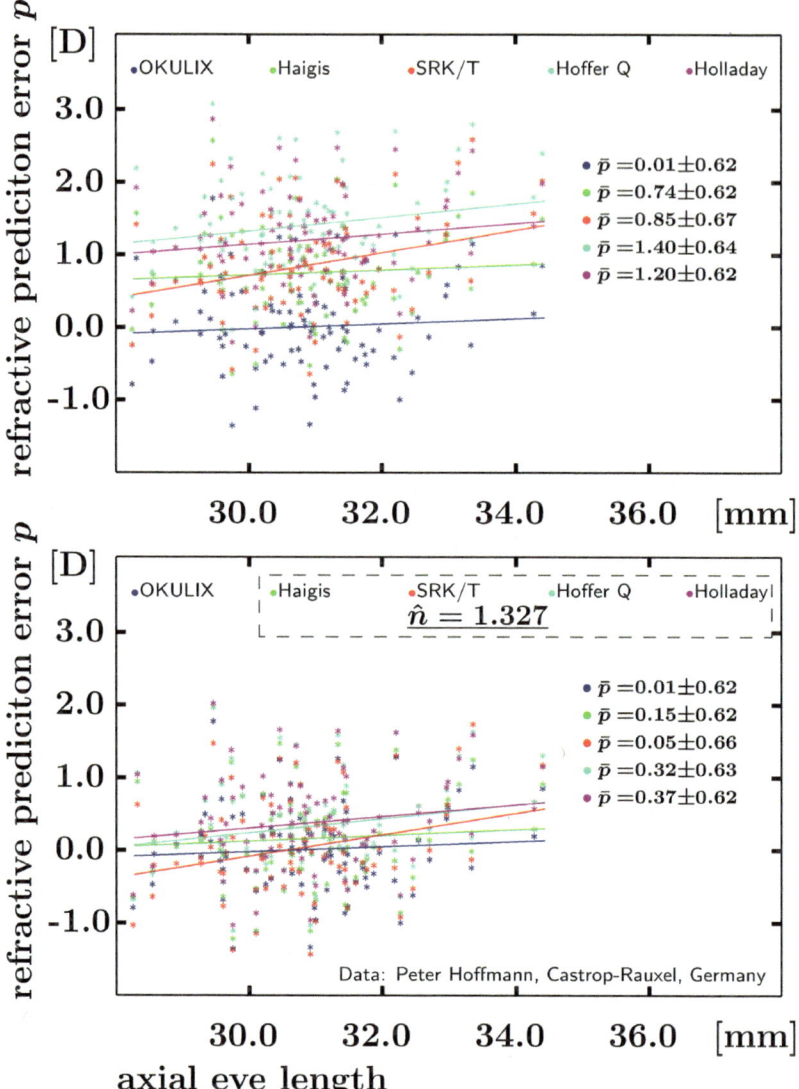

Comparison with the "Big Data" Approach

Systematic deviation patterns of IOL formula predictions from reality can be detected in large collectives implanted with the same IOL model. Moreover, known results from collectives covering the whole range of all input variables can also be used for IOL selections. Such Big Data algorithms do not even need any optical calculation but can predict IOL powers for individual eyes by higher order inter- or extrapolation from the existing refractive outcome of previous IOL implantations. The Hill RBF method uses radial basis functions (RBFs) for such calculations. In a private communication with Warren Hill, Mesa, Arizona, a set of 6004 eyes implanted with Alcon SN60WF IOL was investigated. The refractive prediction differences between four classical formulas in Gaussian optics [3, 4, 7, 22], the RBF

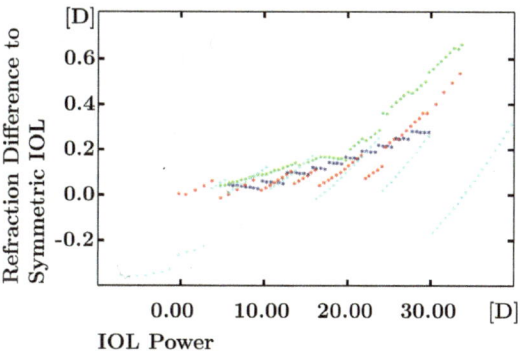

Fig. 49.6 Shape factor variations (For four different IOL models from four manufacturers (four colors), the differences of the predicted refractions between their IOL and a symmetric IOL (shape factor = 0) of the same power, thickness, and refractive index at the same position in the same eye are shown as a function of the IOL power)

method, and OKULIX were calculated. Differences between each of the formulas and OKULIX show a specific pattern, depending on the assumptions (e.g., fictitious corneal refractive index and effective lens position) of the respective formula. Interestingly, these patterns are principally the same for the differences between the formulas and OKULIX on the one hand and for the differences between the formulas and RBF on the other hand, beside some higher noise for RBF, see Fig. 49.7 in which the results of the comparison for the SRK/T- and for the Haigis formula are shown as examples. A systematic difference pattern between RBF and OKULIX is not recognizable. Correspondingly, only mar-

ginal differences were found in the overall accuracy comparison between RBF and OKULIX (e.g., numbers of eyes within a certain prediction error interval, etc.). However, slightly higher prediction accuracy was found for RBF and for OKULIX when compared to the formulas.

The similar results of RBF and OKULIX do not imply that a Big Data approach is equivalent to a raytracing calculation. A Big Data method needs large numbers of previous IOL implantations for each IOL model separately because of the different IOL shape factor patterns of different IOL models (see section "Impact of IOL Shape Factor Variations"). Additionally, in eyes after corneal refractive surgery, a large patient collective would not only be needed for each IOL model but also for the combination of an IOL model and a specific protocol of the corneal laser procedure. This is not feasible. In addition, a Big Data approach would not adequately address rare specific characteristics of an individual eye, e.g., a beginning Keratoconus, which would always be detected by corneal tomography and adequately addressed by a raytracing calculation based thereon. Furthermore, the Big Data approach is restricted to spherical equivalents and cannot predict toric IOL with the same algorithms. Finally, the data set of a Big Data approach is based on data collections from many different locations. The accuracy of these subcollectives is often biased by different refraction habits, see also section "Accuracy of Refraction".

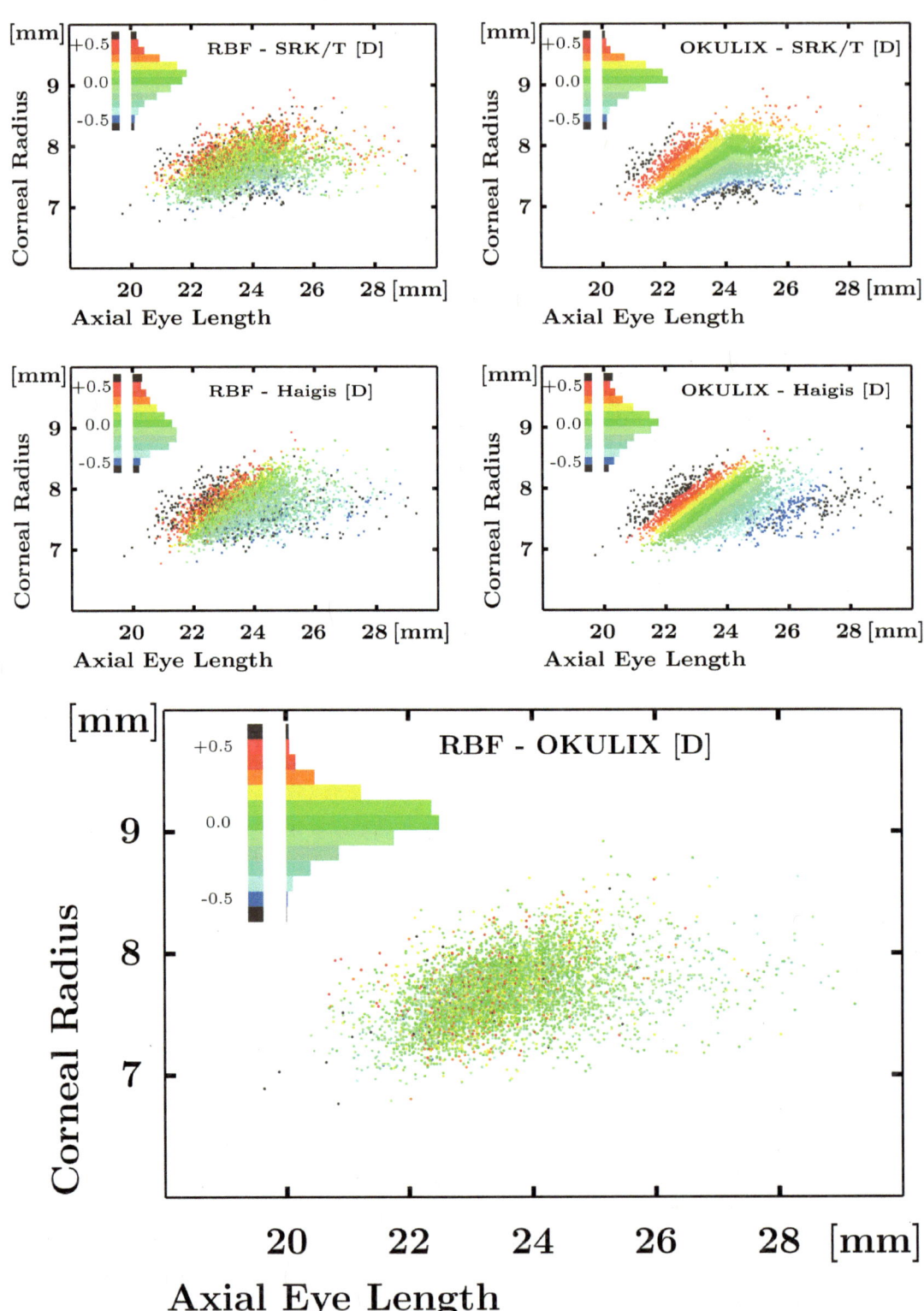

Fig. 49.7 Systematic differences in 6004 eyes (All subimages show the prediction differences (spherical equivalent) of the indicated methods in pseudocolors, as function of axial eye length and mean corneal radius. The pseudocolor definitions (look-up tables) and the histo-gram distributions of the differences are shown in the upper left corners. Differences of more than ±0.5D are indicated in black. Such higher differences are mostly found in the margins of the distribution in the comparisons with the formulas)

Additional Tools

For scientific purposes beyond IOL selection, the corneal module of OKULIX allows additional investigations of the optical properties of the pseudophakic eye. Two-dimensional refraction- or wavefront maps can be calculated and decomposed into Zernike series up to 12th radial order, see Fig. 49.8 for an example.

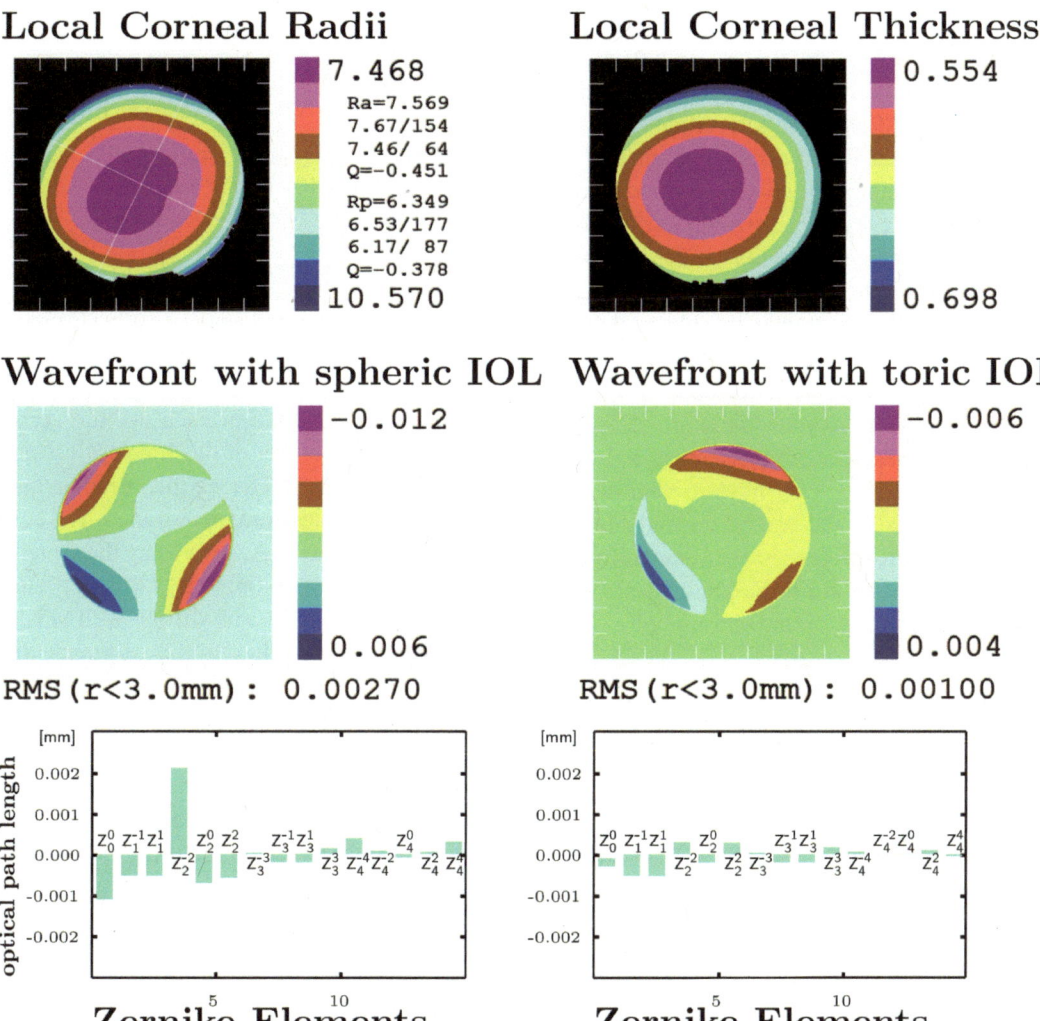

Fig. 49.8 Wavefront analysis with different IOL models (For an eye with an axial length of 25.28 mm and tomography as shown on top, a wavefront analysis is performed with a spheric (left) and a toric (right) IOL. Both IOL models also differ in the asphericities of their surfaces. The root-mean-square error of optical path lengths inside a zone of radius 3 mm is about three times as high for the left compared to the right IOL (0.0027 mm versus 0.001 mm). The first 15 Zernike elements out of the overall 91 are shown on the bottom for both IOL models. All not indicated measures are in millimeters)

Limitations

Accuracy of Refraction

The accuracy of IOL calculations is mostly measured by the prediction error, i.e., the difference between achieved and predicted refraction. But also these achieved refractions are often not well defined. Refraction errors increase with decreasing visual acuity because patients cannot distinguish between different optical situations, the less, the worse their visual acuity, and the higher their pseudoaccommodation width is. In a patient collective of 115 eyes implanted with aberration correcting IOL and visual acuity of 20/20 or better, the mean absolute prediction error was 0.21D, and in 210 eyes implanted with spherical IOL and visual acuity below 20/20, it was two times as high: 0.42D. All eyes were operated complication free by the same surgeon [5].

In addition to such patient-based error sources, also refraction habits can have a significant impact on the results and can be responsible for the major part of differences between different locations which later are to be compensated by so-called constant optimization of IOL calculations.

Accuracy of Placido/Scheimpflug Tomographers

In 83 eyes the measured data of three Placido and Scheimpflug tomographers were compared: Galilei G6, a combined Placido- and Scheimpflug tomographer (Ziemer, Switzerland), Pentacam HR, a pure Scheimpflug device (Oculus, Germany), and TMS-5, again a combined Placido–Scheimpflug device (Tomey, Japan). The recorded data of anterior topography and spatially resolved corneal thickness were transferred to OKULIX, and an IOL calculation was performed for the same IOL in the same position and the same axial length. For each eye the predicted refractions were calculated, together with the mean of the three devices and the differences of the individual values to this mean, see Fig. 49.9

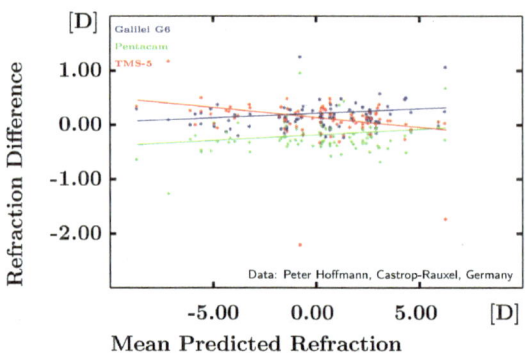

Fig. 49.9 Differences between Placido and Scheimpflug devices (Assuming an IOL (Johnson and Johnson, Sensar AR40e, 21D) at a position of 4.0 mm behind the cornea and an axial length of 23.6 mm, the residual refractions and the differences between the three devices are calculated. The average differences are 0.17 ± 0.24D (Galilei G6), -0.26 ± 0.29 (Pentacam), and 0.08 ± 0.39 (TMS-5))

In addition, the total corneal astigmatism was calculated in OKULIX. For each eye the vector mean of the astigmatisms of the three devices and the vector differences between this mean and the data from each device were determined. The centroids of these differences, describing the systematic deviations, are 0.04D/173° (Galilei G6), 0.14D/93° (Pentacam), and 0.10D/7° (TMS-5). The median absolute values of the astigmatic differences are 0.31D for Galilei G6, 0.33D for Pentacam, and 0.29D for TMS-5.

In summary, the astigmatic differences are small enough to make the three devices exchangeable with respect to the astigmatic error of toric IOL calculations. The spherical differences, however, are just at the limit of acceptability.

Accuracy of OCT Tomographers

In 161 eyes the measured data of three OCT tomographers were compared: ANTERION (Heidelberg Engineering, Germany), CASIA (Tomey, Japan), and IOLMaster700 (Zeiss, Germany). The recorded data of anterior topography and spatially resolved corneal thickness of ANTERION and CASIA were transferred to OKULIX. From these data, anterior and posterior corneal vertex radii and asphericities were

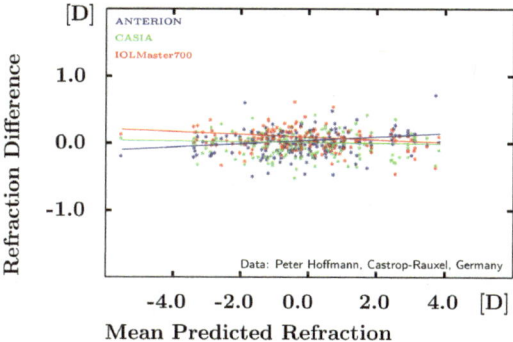

Fig. 49.10 Differences between OCT devices (Assuming the IOL (Johnson and Johnson, Sensar AR40e, 21D) at a position of 4.0 mm behind the cornea and an axial length of 23.6 mm, the average refractions and the differences between the three devices are calculated. The average differences are 0.01 ± 0.21D (ANTERION), -0.03 ± 0.21 (CASIA), and 0.02 ± 0.20 (IOLMaster700))

extracted. For IOLMaster700, anterior and posterior corneal vertex radii were taken from the device because it does not have a software interface to OKULIX. Anterior asphericity was set to -0.18 for the IOLMaster data. An IOL calculation was performed for the same IOL at the same position and the same axial length. For each eye the predicted refractions were calculated, together with the mean of the three devices and the differences of the individual values to this mean, see Fig. 49.10.

In addition the total corneal astigmatism was calculated in OKULIX. For each eye the vector mean of the astigmatisms of the three devices and the vector differences between this mean and the data from each device were determined. The centroids of these differences, describing the systematic deviations, are 0.18D/$120°$ (ANTERION), 0.07D/$70°$ (CASIA), and 0.22D/$4°$ (IOLMaster700). The median absolute values of the astigmatic differences are 0.26D for ANTERION, 0.30D for CASIA, and 0.33D for IOLMaster700.

In summary, the differences between the data of these devices are sufficiently small to make the devices interchangeable with respect to the accuracy of spheric and of toric IOL calculation.

IOL Manufacturing Tolerances

The IOL manufacturing tolerances for an IOL of power P according to ISO11979-2 are ± 0.3D for $|P| < 15$D, ± 0.4D for 15D$\leq P < 25$D, ± 0.5D for 25D$\leq P < 30$D, and ± 1.0D for $P \geq 30$D. Even if many IOL manufacturers claim to produce their IOL with significantly smaller tolerances, it can be assumed that often a major part of systematic power bias of an IOL model is due to an offset in the manufacturing control procedure. OKULIX therefore allows an offset correction of the IOL power of each model which is ultimately comparable to the so-called constant optimizations of IOL formulas.

Conclusions and Future Developments

IOL calculation with OKULIX raytracing can be performed in the same way and with principally the same accuracy in very long eyes, very short eyes [10, 24], postrefractive eyes, and virgin eyes without any knowledge about the eye's history. This advantage on the one hand requires full confidence in the measured data on the other hand, particularly, in corneal tomography. In addition, also reliable measurements of position and the thickness of the crystalline lens are needed for a sufficiently accurate prediction of the IOL position. These requirements on instrumentation are currently not yet generally fulfilled. However, improvements in instrument development and better availability of such reliable instrumentation are to be expected in the near future.

References

1. Cooke DL, Cooke TL. A comparison of two methods to calculate axial length. J Cataract Refract Surg. 2019;45:284–91.
2. Gjerdrum B, Gundersen KG, Lundmark PO, Aakre BM. Refractive precision of ray tracing IOL calculations based on OCT data versus traditional IOL cal-

culation formulas based on reflectometry in patients with a history of laser vision correction for myopia. Clin Ophthalmol. 2021;15:845–57.

3. Haigis W, Lege B, Miller N, Schneider B. Comparison of immersion ultrasound biometry and partial coherence interferometry for intraocular lens calculation according to Haigis. Graefe's Arch Clin Exp Ophthalmol. 2000;238:765–73.

4. Hoffer KJ. The Hoffer Q formula: a comparison of theoretic and regression formulas. J Cataract Refract Surg. 1993;19(11):700–12. Errata: 1994;20(6):677 and 2007;33(1):2–3.

5. Hoffmann P, Wahl J, Preußner PR. Accuracy of intraocular lens calculation with raytracing. J Refract Surg. 2012;28:650–5.

6. Hoffmann P, Wahl J, Hütz W, Preußner PR. A ray tracing approach to calculate toric intraocular lenses. J Refract Surg. 2013;29:402–8.

7. Holladay JT, Musgrove KH, Prager CT, Lewis JW, Chandler TY, Ruiz RS. A three-part system for refining intraocular lens power calculations. J Cataract Refract Surg. 1988;14:17–24.

8. Lazaridis A, Schraml F, Preußner PR, Sekundo W. Predictability of intraocular lens calculation after SMILE for myopia. J Cataract Refract Surg. 2021;47:304–10.

9. Liou HL, Brennan NA. Anatomically accurate, finite model eye for optical modeling. J Opt Soc Am. 1997;14:1684–95.

10. Luo Y, Li H, Gao L, Du J, Chen W, Gao Y, Ye Z, Li Z. Comparing the accuracy of new intraocular lens power calculation formulae in short eyes after cataract surgery: a systematic review and meta-analysis. Int Ophthalmol. 2022. https://doi.org/10.1007/s10792-021-02191-4.

11. Preußner PR, Wahl J, Lahdo H, Findl O. Konsistente IOL-Berechnung. Ophthalmologe. 2000;3:300–4.

12. Preußner PR, Wahl J, Lahdo H, Findl O, Dick B. Ray tracing for IOL calculation. J Cataract Refract Surg. 2002;28:1412–9.

13. Preußner PR, Wahl J, Kramann C. Corneal model. J Cataract Refract Surg. 2003;29:471–7.

14. Preußner PR, Wahl J. Simplified mathematics for customized refractive surgery. J Cataract Refract Surg. 2003;29:462–70.

15. Preußner PR, Wahl J, Weitzel D, Berthold S, Kriechbaum K, Findl O. Predicting postoperative anterior chamber depth and refraction. J Cataract Refract Surg. 2004;30:2077–83.

16. Preußner PR, Wahl J, Weitzel. Topography based IOL power selection. J Cataract Refract Surg. 2005;31:525–33.

17. Preußner PR, Olsen T, Hoffmann P, Findl O. IOL calculation accuracy limits in normal eyes. J Cataract Refract Surg. 2008;34:802–8.

18. Preußner PR, Hoffmann P, Petermeier K. Vergleich zwischen Raytracing und IOL-Formeln der 3. Generation. Klin Monatsbl Augenheilk. 2009;226:83–9.

19. Preußner PR. Intraocular lens calculation in extreme myopia. J Cataract Refract Surg. 2010;36:531–2.

20. Preußner PR, Hoffmann P, Wahl J. Impact of posterior corneal surface on toric intraocular lens (IOL) calculation. Curr Eye Res. 2015;40:809–14.

21. Rabsilber TM, Reuland AJ, Holzer MP, Auffarth GU. Intraocular lens power calculation using ray tracing following excimer laser surgery. Eye. 2007;21:697–701.

22. Retzlaff JA, Sanders DR, Kraff MC. Development of the SRK/T intraocular lens power calculation formula. J Cataract Refract Surg. 1990;16:333–40. Errata: 1990;16:528 and 1993;19(5):444–446

23. Savini G, Hoffer KJ, Schiano-Lomoriello D, Barboni P. Intraocular lens power calculation using Placido disk-Scheimpflug tomographer in eyes that had previous myopic corneal excimer laser surgery. J Cataract Refract Surg. 2018;44:935–41.

24. Wendelstein J, Hoffmann P, Hirnschall N, Fischinger IR, Mariacher S, Wingert T, Langenbucher A, Bolz M. Project hyperopic power prediction: accuracy of 13 different concepts for intraocular lens calculation in short eyes. Br J Ophthalmol. 2020. https://doi.org/10.1136/bjophthalmol-2020-318272.

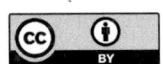

The Olsen Formula

50

Thomas Olsen

The Olsen Formula

The Olsen formula was developed at the time when the Sanders-Retzlaff-Kraff (SRK) method was popular. Although the SRK formula was working all right in the normal range, errors were frequent in the extreme range and the lack of a flexible, optical model was frustrating. So, the ambition was to develop a thick-lens formula based on paraxial ray tracing as assumption-free as possible allowing for the use of real physical dimensions—including the physical position of the IOL— to be used in the formula.

The first step for the author was to realize that the K-reading of the keratometer using the standard index of 1.3375 was wrong (see the "Keratometry" chapter). To avoid confusion, the author has always preferred to input the radius of the K-reading rather than the diopter value. The conversion to corneal power is then done internally by the formula. From the beginning, a fictitious index of 1.3315 based on the Gullstrand ratio of 0.883 was found to give a more realistic value for effective corneal power. This value has later been used by other authors, i.e., Haigis and Barrett, and there seems to be growing consensus among newer formulas that the lower value is a better choice for IOL power calculation.

The paraxial approach allows for thick-lens calculations whereby the cornea and the IOL can be represented as the two-surface optical lenses they are. The advantage is that different optic configurations can be dealt with, and the refractive effect of a, say 1:1 biconvex, 1:2 biconvex, or a meniscus concave-convex IOL, can be calculated independently from the IOL position. All it requires is a knowledge of the shape of the IOL, which must be provided by the IOL manufacturer.

One disadvantage of the paraxial approach is that higher-order aberrations are not taken into account. The most significant aberration is spherical aberration, which plays a role in normal eyes, but can be excessive in abnormal corneas like post-LASIK cases and keratoconus. Hence, from 2012 the Olsen formula was modified to allow exact ray tracing on aspheric surfaces in order to include the effect of spherical aberration in the calculated effective refraction. This meant a change in Gullstrand ratio to 0.83 (which is the value also demonstrated in many Scheimpflug reports) but now in addition using the Q-value of the front and back surface of the cornea for a more detailed calculation of the corneal power. If no Q-values are stated, the program will assume the default normal values. In this way, it was possible to include the effect of the wavefront-corrected spherical aberration of an aspheric IOL.

T. Olsen (✉)
Aros Private Hospital, Aarhus, Denmark

© The Author(s) 2024
J. Aramberri et al. (eds.), *Intraocular Lens Calculations*, Essentials in Ophthalmology,
https://doi.org/10.1007/978-3-031-50666-6_50

A realistic corneal power is required to predict the refractive effect of the IOL using the physical position of the IOL. Once it was found that the position of the IOL could be predicted, the next step was to improve the ELP prediction. Over the years, a number of ELP predictors have been studied by the author: 1) K-reading, ACD and lens thickness (Olsen 1986) [1], 2) K-reading, ACD and axial length, K-reading, ACD, lens thickness, axial length, corneal diameter distance, and refraction [2], and finally 3) ACD and lens thickness measured by laser biometry to arrive at the novel concept called the C-constant approach (Olsen & Hoffmann 2014) [3]. The latter method represented a "heureka" moment in its simple form that proved to be effective and robust without the indirect predictors such as the K-reading, axial length, corneal diameter, refraction, and age with previous methods. The advantage of this approach is that it should work equally effectively in abnormal corneas such as post-LASIK cases, keratoconus, megalocornea, scleral buckling procedure, and horses, if you may.

PhacoOptics® Software

A stand-alone PC software for Microsoft Windows (www.phacooptics.com) was released by the author in 2009. Using paraxial and exact ray tracing, the software package offers a comprehensive system for IOL power calculation and data management.

Because of the ray tracing, the physical data of the IOL need to be stated in more detail than in most formulas. The IOL constants are:

1. Refractive index
2. Anterior and posterior radius of curvature of an average-powered IOL
3. Thickness of an average-powered IOL
4. Wavefront Z(4,0) correction for spherical aberration
5. ACD constant (average value in representative population)

When the physical parameters 1–4 have been entered, it is possible to have item 5, the ACD constant calculated from the SRK/T A-constant, as a first go. However, it is recommended to keep track of the outcome and adjust the ACD constant as more data become available.

Data Entry

Data entry can be made manually or by importing from biometers via a data bridge (xml files or similar). The following biometers are supported for data bridge import:

1. Haag-Streit Lenstar LS900
2. Oculus Pentacam (full cornea analysis)
3. Zeiss IOLMaster 700
4. Topcon Aladdin
5. Tomey OA-2000
6. Ziemer Galilei G6 (full cornea analysis)

The K-readings can be expanded (double-click on the field) to allow entry of posterior curvatures and Q-values if these are available. If no data are input for the posterior surface, the program will assume a default value. In this way, corneal astigmatism can be calculated based on the default posterior cylinder or based on exact measurements. This allows for a full-thickness analysis of the corneal power from tomography data, i.e., captured with the Oculus Pentacam or the Ziemer Galilei G6. This is particularly useful when dealing with post-LASIK cases or other abnormal corneas.

The Olsen formula has also been implemented as a dynamic library into the software of the Haag-Streit Lenstar, the Topcon Aladdin, the Tomey OA-2000, and the Oculus Pentacam.

The IOL power calculation algorithm follows the principles described in this chapter. The prediction of the ELP (rather: the physical IOL position) has been given the flexibility of a 2-factor version and a 4-factor version (selectable by the user). Both versions use the C-constant, which is based on the ACD and the lens thickness, but the 4-factor version uses an additional corrective term based on the K-reading and the axial length. The 4-factor version may have a little more accuracy than the 2-factor version as shown by Cooke and Cooke [4, 5], but is only applicable to normal, virgin eyes. The 2-factor version is independent of the K-reading and the axial length and is therefore more robust in post-LASIK cases and other abnormal cases.

Data Quality Is the Key

All calculations depend on the quality of the input data. Garbage in means garbage out, as everybody knows. To help filter out typing errors or other mistakes, the program will evaluate the plausibility of all data input when in manual entering mode. This plausibility check is performed at three different levels:

1. The out-of-range plausibility of the individual variable
2. The intra-eye plausibility of the input compared to other variables of the same eye (e.g., a flat cornea in a short eye)
3. The inter-eye plausibility of the input compared to existing data of the contralateral eye

The threshold of the plausibility levels can be set in the program settings.

As is the case with any IOL formula, it is important that the K-readings and the axial length are accurate. In addition, the Olsen formula is particularly sensitive to measurement errors of the anterior chamber depth and the lens thickness. This is because the C-constant is entirely dependent on these two variables. It is good clinical practice to check the consistency of the readings, especially for the lens thickness, which may be hard for the biometer software to pick up with good spikes of the anterior and the posterior surface.

Finally, the pupil size should be mentioned. Unlike most other formulas, PhacoOptics does take the pupil size into account as it will play a role when the spherical aberration is high. Care should be taken, however, to check the pupil size if you are importing data from an external biometer, and the patient was dilated at the examination. A safe procedure is to leave the pupil blank, which is the equivalent of a standard pupil size of 3 mm assumed by the program.

Figure 50.1 shows a PhacoOptics screenshot of the preoperative data of a post-LASIK case of the right eye and untouched left eye for comparison. A full-thickness analysis of the right cornea was done by importing the values from the Oculus Pentacam (highlighted fields). The detailed information can be viewed (and edited) by right- or double-clicking the K-reading fields (insert lower right). In this case, the Gullstrand ratio was 0.779 on the post-LASIK right eye and 0.883 (default) on the virgin left eye. An abnormal Q-value for the front surface of the right eye due to the LASIK procedure is noted.

Figure 50.2 shows the IOL power calculation screen of the same post-LASIK case. The IOL type has been selected from a drop-down menu. Both the power, the cylinder, and the axis can be changed by scrolling up and down, and the resulting sphere cylinder and axis are displayed below. By default, the optimum placement axis of the toric has been calculated based on the complete corneal data. The axis can be confirmed by pressing the small button marked? "Cyl axis." Here, a small cylinder was chosen to minimize the astigmatism of the postoperative refraction. The surgically induced astigmatism (SIA) can also be added in a detail window (not shown).

For the post-LASIK case, the ELP prediction was done using a 2-factor algorithm (identical to the C-constant) because the post-LASIK K-reading is unsuited for this purpose. The selection was done after double-clicking the ACD field. Note the nearly identical values for the right and left eye despite the post-LASIK state of the right eye.

Formula Validation

The aim of the Olsen formula was to "divide and conquer" the unknowns of IOL power calculation. On the one side, we have the measurements of corneal power, axial length, and optical properties of the IOL. All measurements must be representative of the physical reality. Also, the physical properties of the IOL must be known so that we can calculate the refractive effect for a given IOL location. On the other side, we have an issue with the prediction of the IOL position for which empirical studies are needed.

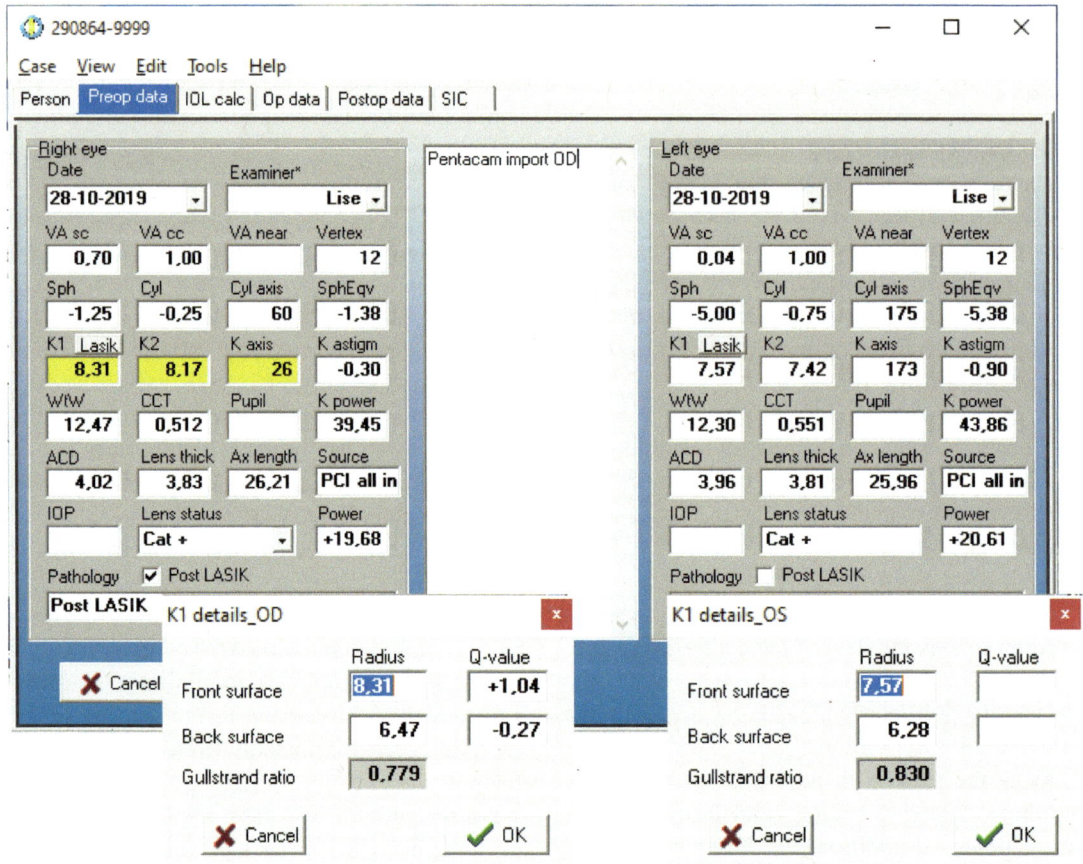

Fig. 50.1 Preoperative data screen of a post-LASIK case on the right eye with untouched left eye. You may note the right-left difference in K-readings. The K-readings of the right eye are highlighted in yellow after Pentacam import, because a full-thickness analysis of the corneal power is wanted. The two inserts at the bottom show the detailed information of the K1-reading (double-click in the K1 field) with complete data on the right eye and default data on the left eye

A critical question is as follows: What if the exact IOL position was known, and would the formula be able to predict the refractive outcome accurately? The question can be answered by recording the actual IOL position after surgery and using this value in the "predictions." This was done by Olsen and Hoffmann [3] in a subset of cases, demonstrating a drop in MAE from 0.39 to 0.36 for a public university series and from 0.30 D to 0.26 D in a private series, respectively, when the actual, measured postoperative IOL position was substituted for the predicted value in retrospect.

For this book chapter, the study concept was repeated with a larger database collected some years ago. The database contained 1622 cases of 1269 university clinic patients with an implanted power ranging from −3.0 to +39.0 D. Ninety percent of the IOLs were of the Alcon Acrysof family (SA60AT, SN60AT, and torics and MA60MA for the low IOL power), and 10% were of the Abbott Tecnis types. The pseudophakic ACD was recorded after surgery with Lenstar laser biometry.

The refractive prediction mean error was found to be −0.13 D ± 0.469 D (SD) with the standard Olsen procedure and −0.019 D ± 0.436 D (SD) when the postoperative, actual ACD was used in the "predictions." The mean error with the postoperative ACD was not significantly

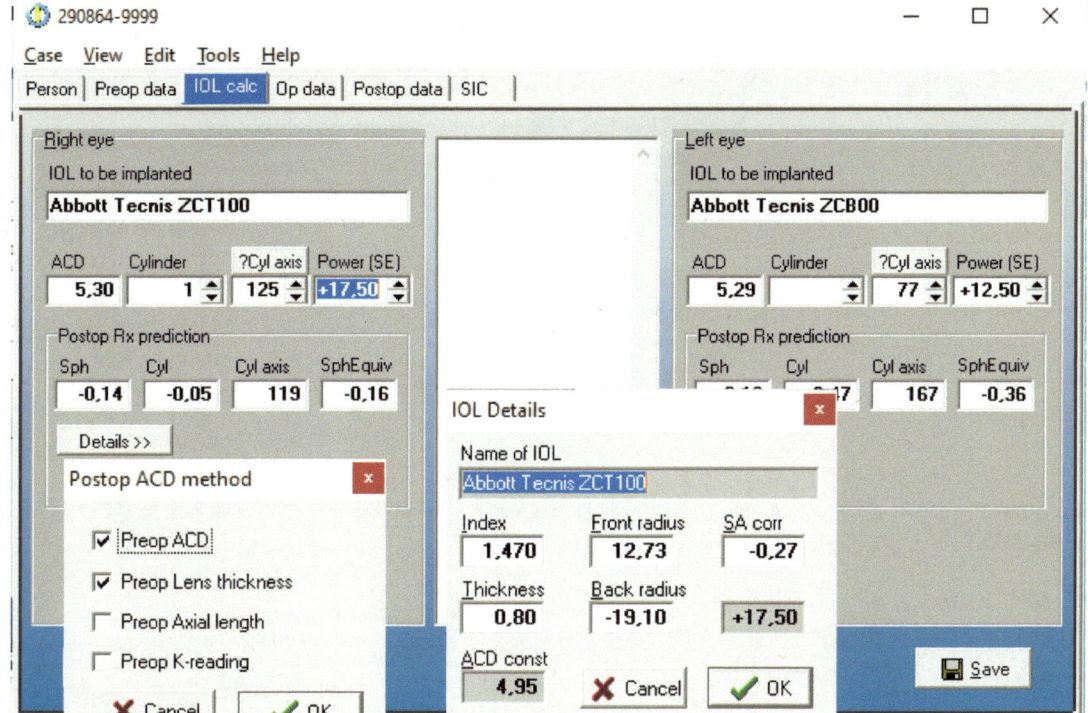

Fig. 50.2 IOL power calculation screen of the right eye post-LASIK case. The ELP prediction was done using a 2-factor algorithm (identical to the C-constant) because the post-LASIK K-reading is unsuited for this purpose. The selection was done after double-clicking the ACD field. An aspheric IOL with a small cylinder has been selected. The IOL details (insert) were called by double-clicking the IOL power field. The program calculates the exact curvatures of the front and back surfaces of the IOL to be used for ray tracing

different from zero. The standard deviation of ±0.436 D corresponded to a mean absolute error (MAE) of 0.35 D, which was significantly lower than that of the normal predictions ($p < 0.01$) (Fig. 50.3). In conclusion, when the IOL position was known, the formula was able to predict the refraction with no bias or offset error (!) and a corresponding improvement in accuracy. This finding means that if the ELP prediction would improve as a result of newer biometry techniques, the Olsen formula can utilize this information and improve the accuracy accordingly.

Another method of verification is to reverse the calculations: From the known postoperative refraction and the IOL position, it is possible to back-solve for the IOL power using ray tracing. This was originally done by Olsen and Funding (2012) [6] who studied 767 eyes with an implanted IOL power of the old Alcon Acrysof type ranging from −2.00 D to +36.0 D. The

actual position of the IOL after surgery was recorded using Haag-Streit Lenstar laser interferometry. Based on the postoperative refraction and the biometric measurements, a ray tracing analysis was performed back-solving for the power of the IOL in situ. The results showed the calculated IOL power to be in good agreement with the labeled power over the entire power range with no offset or bias. This finding was another "heureka" moment for the author showing that the optics of the pseudophakic eye can be described by ray tracing and modern biometry techniques.

For the present book chapter, the study was repeated on the same database as mentioned above. Figure 50.4 shows the correlation between the calculated IOL power in situ and the labeled power for the 1622 cases. The correlation coefficient was 0.99, and the slope of the linear regression equation was not significant from unity. This

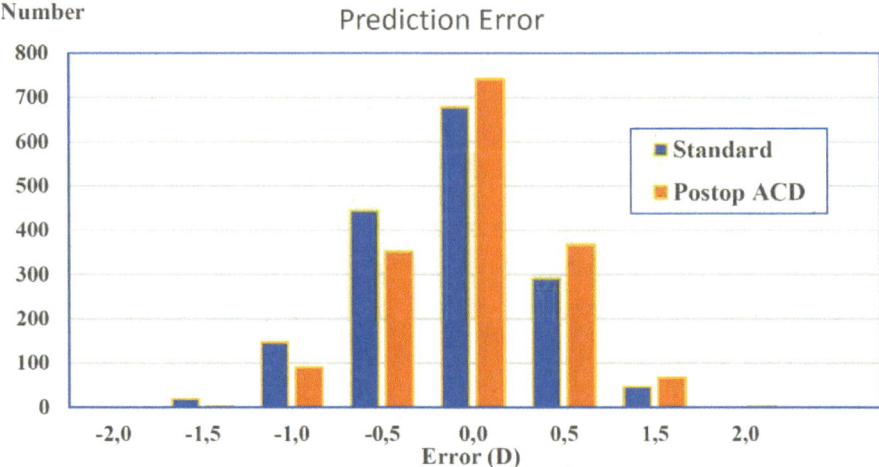

Fig. 50.3 Prediction accuracy of the Olsen formula with and without the usage of the postop ACD in the "predictions"

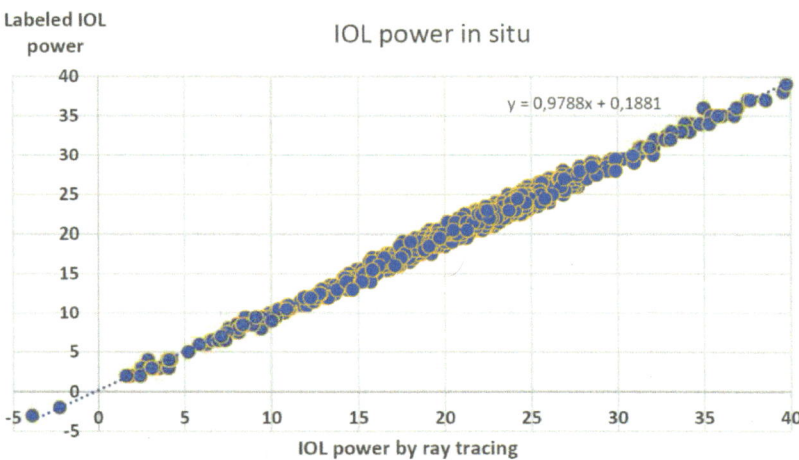

Fig. 50.4 IOL power in situ calculated by exact ray tracing compared to the labeled value

finding can be regarded as a verification of the optical algorithms used in the Olsen formula.

Own History of Calculation Accuracy

The author has over 30 years of experience with IOL power calculation. Looking back, it is amazing how the accuracy has been ever-increasing over time. One reason for the improvement in accuracy has been the unsurpassed accuracy of optical biometry, but other factors such as standardization of surgery and improvement in formula (ELP prediction) have combined to produce

a highly standardized and controlled environment for IOL power calculation.

In Fig. 50.5, the accuracy observed by the author has been tabulated for a period of 30+ years, covering both ultrasound and later optical biometry. The number of cases within 0.5 D accuracy has been computed from the standard deviation of the prediction error observed in each series. Except for the last column (year 2020), all columns have been constructed from the papers published by the author and associates [3, 7–17]. The last column showing 90% of cases within ±0.5 D was the result of an independent study of 469 refractive lens exchange cases using

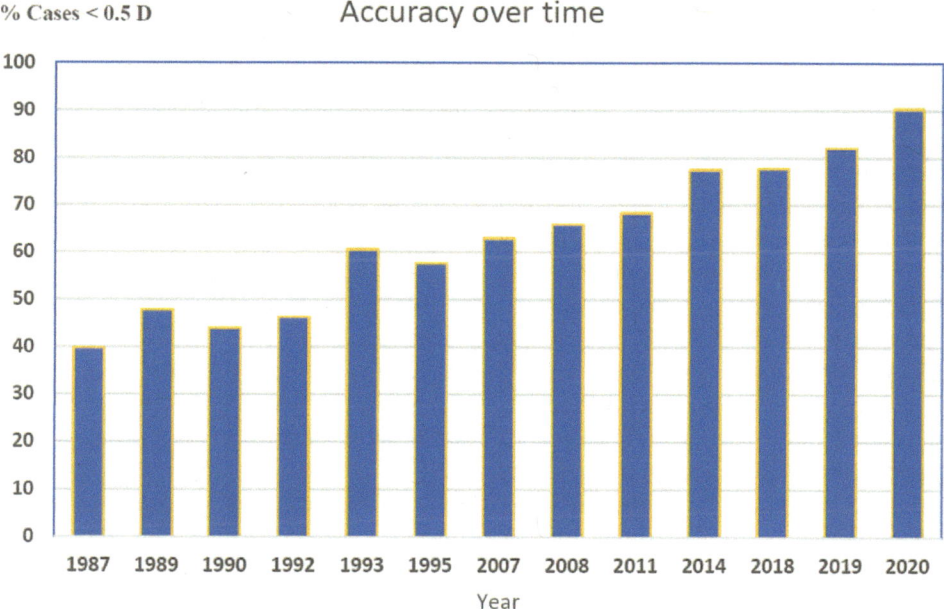

Fig. 50.5 History of IOL calculation accuracy (author's own series)

IOLMaster 700 and the Olsen formula (unpublished).

Recent Clinical Studies

There is a plethora of publications dealing with IOL power calculation, and many new IOL formulas have evolved. The interest comes from the fact that modern lens surgery with a perfect IOL power calculation holds the promise to free the spectacle dependence of the patient. As discussed in the section "The History of IOL Power Calculation Accuracy," the accuracy is approaching 90% of cases within 0.5 D of the target.

As the Olsen formula requires good measurements of the anterior chamber depth and of the lens thickness for the prediction of the IOL position, it is not possible to evaluate the performance of the Olsen formula using the traditional PCI optical biometry (IOLMaster 500) that does not measure the lens thickness. However, more and more studies have emerged using OLCR or swept-source OCT (SS-OCT) that does offer measurements of all intraocular distances by the laser.

One of the largest comparative studies ever was the study by Melles et al. (2018) [15] who investigated the accuracy of seven different formulas in a total of 18,501 cases of AcrySof SN60WF (13,301 cases) and SA60AT (5200 cases) implants using Haag-Streit Lenstar biometry. The lowest prediction error was found with the Barrett Universal II, followed by Olsen, Haigis, Holladay 2, Holladay 1, SRK/T, and Hoffer Q.

The Melles 2018 study was later repeated with updated versions of the Olsen formula (4-factor version rather than the 2-factor version studied in the first paper), the Hill RBF formula (newest version 2), the Holladay 2 (newest version, axial length adjusted for the hyperopic error in long eyes), and 2 newer formulas: the Kane formula and the EVO formula. The most accurate formulas were the Kane, the Olsen, and the Barret formula all achieving more than 80% of the predictions within ±0.50 D of the target, followed by the EVO, the Hill RBF, the Holladay 2, the Haigis, the Holladay 1, the SRK/T, and the Hoffer Q formulas in that order, respectively.

The 2-factor version of the Olsen formula was the version that was originally implemented on the Lenstar biometer. The 2-factor version only takes the anterior chamber depth and lens thickness as parameters and uses the unmodified C-constant concept for the prediction of the IOL position. However, as found by Cooke and Cooke [29, 30] there seems to be a marginal higher accuracy using the 4-factor version that also takes the axial length and the corneal curvature as additional parameters in the prediction of effective lens position. The 4-factor version is the default version of the stand-alone PC software available on the website www.phacooptics.com.

The author has had the opportunity to review the large database of the Melles study and check the prediction accuracy. The database consists of outcome data for many surgeons from many clinics, and therefore, some variation can be found in data quality. Some cases were noted to have recorded highly unlikely values for the lens thickness: for example, a lens thickness of 2.5 in a 76 years old, which is virtually impossible and must be due to a measurement mistake of the Lenstar biometer. Therefore, all cases with lens thickness <3 mm were excluded from the present review. None were excluded because of a high prediction error per se.

Thus, after the exclusion of 92 cases with unlikely lens thickness, the Melles database consisted of 13,209 cases of SA60WF implants suitable for analysis. The standard deviation of the prediction error was found to be ±0.38 D, and the mean absolute error (MAE) was 0.30 D with 81.8% of the cases within ±0.5 D. The material was analyzed for possible bias with the axial length. As shown in Fig. 50.6, no correlation was found between the numerical error and the axial length. This finding is noteworthy as a hyperopic error has been reported for some formulas in the long eyes, giving rise to the Wang-Koch adjustment of the Holladay 1 and the SRK/T formula.

The absolute error showed a trend toward higher error in the short eyes and lower error in the long eyes (Fig. 50.7). The short eyes remain the group of eyes with the highest error, first of all because all measurement errors have a relatively higher impact on a short eye and also because the error of the ELP estimation has a much higher impact on the short eyes (see Fig. 50.8).

When analyzing for bias with the K-reading, no correlation was found between the prediction error and the K-reading (Fig. 50.8). Hence, whether the eye is long, short, or has a steep or flat cornea did not appear to have a significant bias on the formula performance.

Finally, a note on the gender bias would be appropriate since some formulas use gender as a co-predictor. For example, gender was taken as a parameter by the Hoffer H formula [18] and is also included as a parameter in the newer Kane formula [19]. The rationale behind this is that female eyes tend to be a little shorter, have a

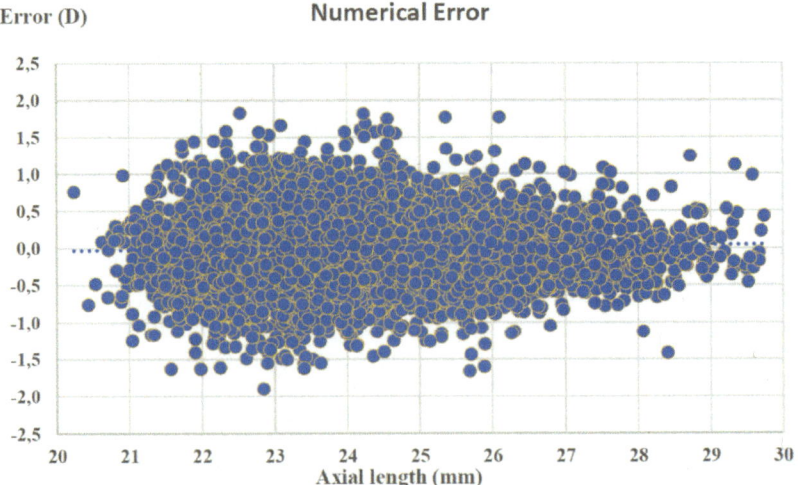

Fig. 50.6 Numerical error vs axial length in 13,209 cases

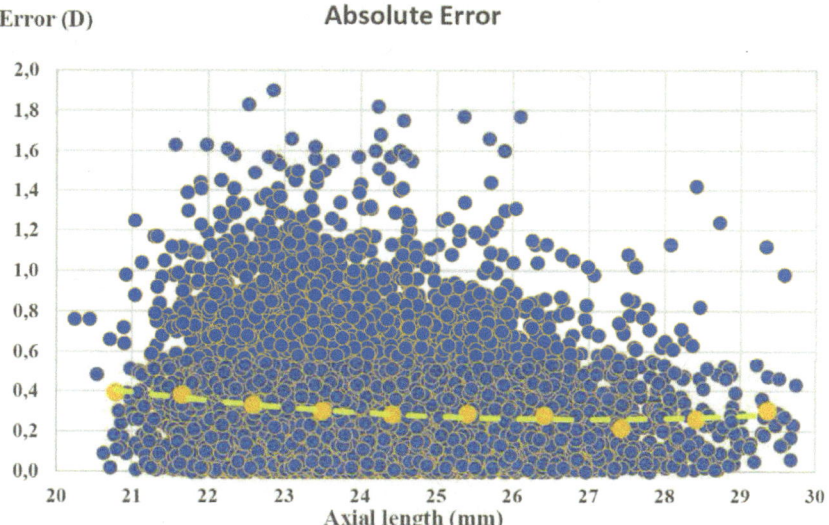

Fig. 50.7 Absolute error vs axial length in 13,209 cases

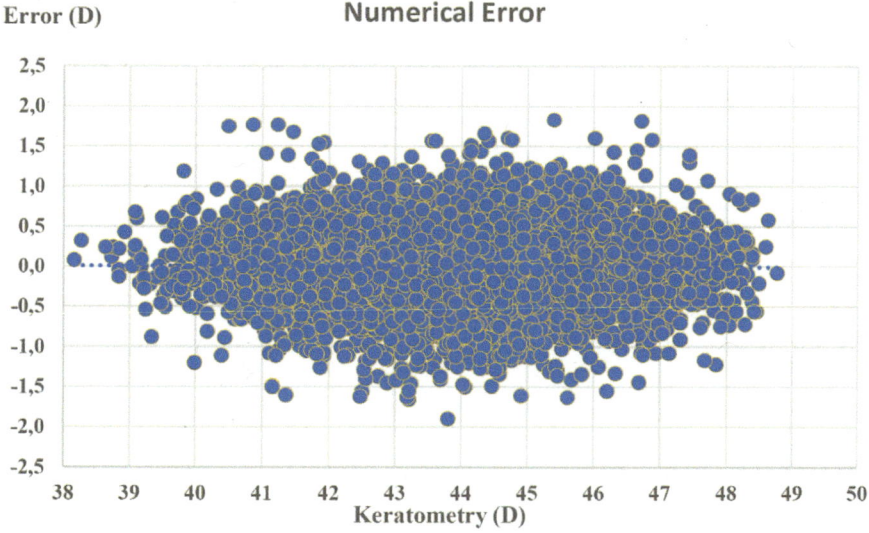

Fig. 50.8 Numerical error vs keratometry reading in 13,209 cases

steeper K-reading, and have a shallower anterior chamber than men. Therefore, one might suspect different behavior with respect to IOL constants and possibly introducing a bias in the IOL power prediction.

Table 50.1 shows the accuracy of the Olsen formula according to gender. The mean numerical error (± SD) was found to be +0.034 D (± 0.387) in males and − 0.029 D (± 0.392) in females. The mean difference was 0.06 D between males and females. Although statistically significant ($p < 0.01$), the difference is not clinically relevant. The lack of systematic bias may be due to the use of the C-constant, which is based on the position and thickness of the crystalline lens and works independently of the K-reading, the axial length, and anterior chamber depth.

Table 50.1 Influence of gender on the prediction accuracy of the Olsen formula

Gender	Error (± SD)	MAE	Range
Males (n = 5409)	+0.034 (± 0.387)	0.307	−1.66 to +1.82
Females (n = 7800)	−0.029 (± 0.392)	0.311	−1.93 to +1.80

References

1. Olsen T. Prediction of intraocular lens position after cataract extraction. J Cataract Refract Surg. 1986;12:376–9.
2. Olsen T. Prediction of the effective postoperative (intraocular lens) anterior chamber depth. J Cataract Refract Surg. 2006;22:419–24.
3. Olsen T, Hoffmann P. C constant: New concept for ray tracing–assisted. intraocular lens power calculation. J Cataract Refract Surg. 2014;40:764–773.
4. Cooke DL, Cooke TL. Prediction accuracy of pre-installed formulas on 2 optical biometers. J Cataract Refract Surg. 2016;42:358–62.
5. Cooke DL, Cooke TL. Comparison of 9 intraocular lens power calculation formulas. J Cataract Refract Surg. 2016;42:1157–64.
6. Olsen T, Funding M. Ray-tracing analysis of intraocular lens power in situ. J Cataract Refract Surg. 2012;38:641–7.
7. Olsen T. Theoretical, computer-assisted prediction versus SRK prediction of postoperative refraction after intraocular lens implantation. J Cataract Refract Surg. 1987;13:146–50.
8. Olsen T, et al. Computerised intraocular lens calculation: clinical results and predictability. Br J Ophthalmol. 1989;73:220–4.
9. Olsen T, et al. Theoretical versus SRK I and SRK II calculation of intraocular lens power. J Cataract Refract Surg. 1990;16:217–25.
10. Olsen T, Gimbel H. Phacoemulsification, capsulorhexis, and intraocular lens power prediction accuracy. J Cataract Refract Surg. 1993;19:695–9.
11. Olsen T, et al. Intraocular lens power calculation with an improved anterior chamber depth prediction algorithm. J Cataract Refract Surg. 1995;21:313–9.
12. Olsen T. Improved accuracy of intraocular lens power calculation with the Zeiss IOLMaster. Acta Ophthalmol Scand. 2007;85:84–7.
13. Preussner P-R, Olsen T, et al. Intraocular lens calculation accuracy limits in normal eyes. J Cataract Refract Surg. 2008;34:802–8.
14. Olsen T. Use of fellow eye data in the calculation of intraocular lens power for the second eye. Ophthalmology. 2011;118:1710–5.
15. Melles RB, Holladay JT, Chang WJ. Accuracy of intraocular lens calculation formulas. Ophthalmology. 2018;125:169–78.
16. Melles, et al. Update on IOL calculation. Ophthalmology. 2019;126:1334–6.
17. Olsen T et al. IOL prediction accuracy with the IOL Master 700. 2020; (data on file).
18. Hoffer KJ, Savini G. Clinical results of the Hoffer H-5 formula in 2707 eyes: first 5th-generation formula based on gender and race. Int Ophthalmol Clin. 2017;57(4):213–9.
19. Darcy K, Gunn D, Tavassoli S, et al. Assessment of the accuracy of new and updated intraocular lens power calculation formulas in 10 930 eyes from the UK National Health Service. J Cataract Refract Surg. 2020;46:2–7.

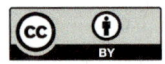

Panacea IOL Calculator

51

David Flikier

Introduction

Ocular biometry and intraocular lens (IOL) power calculations have evolved the last 70 years in the ophthalmology field, and there is still a search for the ideal method of the calculation of the IOL. During the past two decades, the obtained outcomes have improved [1], making it possible to find isolated studies in the literature, with very low absolute median errors (MAE), 0.26–0.28, and cases within a predictive error of ±0.50 D from 86.3 to 89.04% [2], great advances in biometry undoubtedly. However, these outcomes are insufficient if we take into account the current requirements on behalf of the patients and the technology with premium lenses.

When we study groups with a very large number of patients, we still find regular outcomes with median absolute errors superior to 0.310 and with percentages of eyes within the predictive error of ±0.50 D, relatively low for all studied formulas (Melles and cols. [3], Cooke and cols. [4], Kane and cols. [5], and Darcy and cols. [6] finding a MAE for different formulas studied of 0.311–0.383 (Melles) [3], 0.306–0.348 (Cooke) [4], 0.381–0.417 (Kane) [5] and 0.377–0.410 (Darcy) [6] achieving percentages that oscillate between 71.0 to 80.8% (Melles) [3], 75.1–80.6% (Cooke) [4], 66.6–72.8% (Kane) [5], and 68.1–

72.0% (Darcy) [6] of cases between ±0.50 D. In other investigations, with a very representative number of eyes studied, a high percentage of patients was observed (19.4–33.4%) outside the ±0.50 D of residual error [10–12]. In the case of extreme eyes, both greater than 26 mm and smaller than 22 mm, inferior outcomes were found [3, 4].

IOL Panacea Formula and Toric Calculator

Panacea is a formula that begins its development in the year 1997, due to the difficulty experienced during the second half of the 1990s decade, in order to determine the IOL power in eyes after refractive surgery, especially after myopic refractive corrections where a growing number of hyperopic outcomes was found.

It is a theoretical vergence formula with thin lens assumption, where the position of the IOL is estimated through a trigonometric mathematical and multivariable regression method, using predictive anatomical variables, and with an emphasis on optimizing the real corneal power with several factors in order to include eyes and corneas which fall outside the norm.

To come up with the result of the power of the IOL, the method of the calculation program will require mainly three factors:

D. Flikier (✉)
Instituto de Cirugía Ocular, San José, Costa Rica

© The Author(s) 2024
J. Aramberri et al. (eds.), *Intraocular Lens Calculations*, Essentials in Ophthalmology,
https://doi.org/10.1007/978-3-031-50666-6_51

1. The axial length (LAX).
2. The effective lens position (ELPo) estimated through multiple variables: axial length, corneal curvature, anterior chamber depth (ACD), lens thickness (LT), corneal distance (CD), and age.
3. The total corneal power (TCP), or the optimized calculation of the K, is based on the asphericity/spherical aberration, the corneal thickness, the radius of the anterior corneal curvature, the radius of the posterior corneal curvature, and the ratio between the posterior and anterior corneal curvature (P/A).

Axial Length

The LAX has undergone an optimization since the end of the 90 s, thanks to the onset of optical biometry, which led to the reduction of the standard deviation (SD) in 0.1 mm in the case of ultrasound biometry, to <0.01 mm with optical biometry [7, 8] due to its better resolution.

During the last years, this biometric factor has been improved, mainly from three points: Spike Finder or spike detection programs incorporated in the equipment in order to improve the detection of the different internal structures and allow the use of the crystalline thickness and the retina, as reliable variables in biometrical calculations. The optical biometric calculation method by the sum of its segments, (from the sum of segments) [9–12], consisting in assigning an appropriate value for the refraction index to each ocular segment, instead of using a common value for the whole eye, thus improving the measurement of each segment separately [10–12]. This may improve the refractive outcomes in large and short eyes, in some third-generation formulas such as Hoffer Q, SRK/T, and Holladay 1 and 2, but for more modern formulas such as Haigis and Okulix, it will require the modification and optimization of the intraocular lens constants or they would not improve them [10–13]. Finally, the introduction in biometric calculation, of the real measurement of the total retinal thickness, with the use of optical coherence tomography equipment (OCT). Currently, this factor is used as a

fixed value, or corrected with a factor associated with the axial length [14–16], in an indirect form by third-generation formulas, and directly (within their formulas) in many of the fourth-generation formulas. The **Panacea** program includes internal correction modules for axial length and the sum of segments, through optical and regression formulas, as well as including correction factors for extreme biometrics, both for large and short eyes.

Effective Lens Position

The estimation of the effective lens position has been one of the main factors for the improvement of the outcomes in the calculation of the intraocular lens, beginning during the mid-90 s, with the onset of fourth generation formulas, and the increase of variables such as the anterior chamber depth (ACD), the crystalline lens thickness (LT), the corneal distance (CD), age, and others.

The **Panacea** platform uses the axial length, keratometry, ACD and LT variables, as predictive factors for the estimation of the effective lens position, and adds a fifth variable, the relation between the radius of the curvature of the posterior and the anterior surface of the cornea, **the P/A ratio**, to recalculate the keratometry variable in the prediction of the effective lens position. This will be applied in corneas where the P/A ratio is abnormal, in which the anterior surface has suffered a modification mainly after refractive surgery, and the P/A ratio is used to recalculate a previous simulated K, allowing for the correction of the error described by Aramberri (Double K method [17]). Using this variable allows the height of the corneal dome to keep its value as predictive factor of the effective lens position, even in abnormal corneas, automatically (Fig. 51.1).

Total Corneal Power

Besides the two factors previously described, it is imperative to highlight the importance of the third factor, the **total corneal power** in an objec-

Fig. 51.1 Comparison of the variables used by different programs for the prediction of ELPo. Additional use in Panacea of the corneal asphericity and the Gullstrand ratio in order to determine the total corneal power

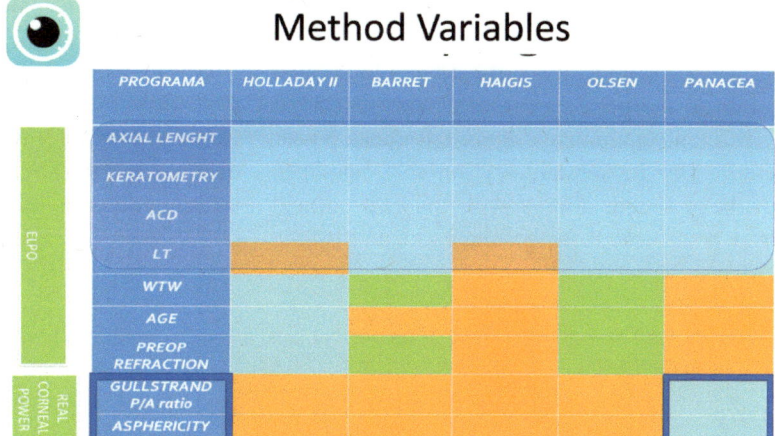

tive manner for the effective calculation of the IOL power, integrating two new variables to the equation, corneal asphericity and the relation between the posterior and the anterior surface of the cornea. All of this with the intent to increase the percentage of emmetropia both for cases of patients with normal corneas and for abnormal corneas (post-refractive laser, post refractive keratotomy, post-keratoplasty, keratoconus and ectasias).

This factor, the total corneal power of the cornea, and the importance of its posterior surface, has taken special relevance in the last 5 years [18, 19], mainly due to the emergence of equipment's offering approximate calculations of the total corneal power in an automatic fashion such as the total keratometry (TK) of the IOL Master 700, by ray tracing and equivalents according to Chao Pan and cols. [20] (dependents of the measured diameter) total corneal refractive power (TCRP) of the Pentacam, Mean Pupil Power (MPP) from Sirius, Total Corneal Power (TCP) from Galilei, etc.; that have been the source of study in recent investigations [21], proving its usefulness in complex cases such as Post photorefractive keratectomy-TCRP [22], Post refractive— [23–25], in Keratoconus [26–28], and in normal eyes—TK [29]. In the study of Fabian and cols. [13], it was demonstrated that both for the Haigis formula as well as for the Barrett's, using TK (Total Keratometry for IOL Master 700), increased the percentage of patients within the +/− 0.50 D in approximately 2%.

There are three corneal factors, complexes of optic mechanisms which interact among themselves, and should be understood and analyzed:

(a) The relation between the posterior and the anterior surface of the cornea.
(b) The corneal asphericity and the spherical aberration.
(c) The corneal multifocality.

Posterior-Anterior Relation/Gullstrand Ratio

For more than a century, the optical physicists, including Gullstrand, designed a strategy in order to estimate the total corneal power (due to the fact that there was only the ability to measure the anterior surface of the cornea, and with that factor alone the whole corneal power had to be calculated), they estimated a "refraction index" for the whole cornea (1.3375) [30, 31], understanding that this presupposed a fixed relation between the radius of the posterior and anterior faces of the cornea at 88%. These calculations induce an estimation error of approximately 0.68 D, due to the fact that the relation for the radius of the posterior and anterior surface (P/A rel.) for the real average cornea is 82.3%, where the estimated refraction index is more adequate at 1.3315–1.3320 [32]. This difference in the keratometry power, is corrected in the lens calculation formulas by correction factors, in some cases such as the A constant, which is why the 1.3375 index is currently being used in keratometry, presumably without any problem.

In studies with patients, it has been found that by comparing the real corneal power (measured by different equipment) against corneal power measured by the keratometry, variable outcomes have been found, always with the real corneal power being less than the one estimated by the keratometry, whose difference oscillates between 0.39 and 0.8 D [19, 27, 33–42], (see Table 51.1).

The use of values in keratometry equivalence tomographers, such as EKR (Equivalent Keratometry Reading, Pentacam equivalent keratometry), make reference to the conversion of the corneal power to a value equivalent to using a fictitious refractory index of 1.3375 on the corneal surface (Fig. 51.2).

Table 51.1 Studies showing keratometry powers vs. total corneal powers by ray tracing and comparative differences among equipment's and studied optic zones [19, 27, 33–42]

Previous studies	Year	Eyes	Km/SimK (instruments)	Total corneal power (instruments)	Difference compared with Km/SimK D (Mean ± SD)
Shirayama and associates	2010	75	43.87 ± 1.22 (IOLMasler) 43.85 ± 1.24 (atlas)	43.37 ± 1.28 (Galilei, 4.0 mm)	−0.50 −0.48
Savini and associates	2011	43	44.04 ± 1.69 (Keraton) 43.83 ± 1.66 (Galilei)	43.44 ± 1.70 (Galilei, 4.0 mm)	−0.60 −0.39
Savini and associates	2012	38	43.67 ± 1.45 (Keraton) 43.46 ± 1.45 (Sirius)	42.87 ± 1.54 (Sirius, 3.0 mm)	−0.80 −0.59
Savini and associates	2013	41	43.88 ± 1.56 (Keraton) 43.85 ± 1.59 (Pentacam)	43.22 ± 1.58 (Pentacam, 3.0 mm)	−0.68 −0.63
Saad and associates	2013	50	43 68 ± 1 68 (IOLMaster) 43.77 ± 1.33 (Pentacam)	43.21 ± 1.32 (Pentacam, 4.0 mm)	−0.47 ± 0.34 −0.56
Seo and associates	2014	100	N/A (Petacam)	N/A (Pentacam, 4.0 mm)	0.7 ± 0.3
Oh and associates	2014	49	43.47 ± 1.02 (Pentacam)	42.76 ± 1.05 (Pentacam, 3.0 mm)	0.71
				43.13 ± 1.12 (Pentacam, 4.0 mm)	0.37
Naeser and associates	2015	951	43.42 ± 1.49 (Pentacam)	42.79 ± 1.50 (Pentacam, 3.0 mm)	0.63
				42.91 ± 1.51 (Pentacam. 4.0 mm)	0.51
Savini and associates	2017	114	43.64 ± 1.44 (Sirius)	43.07 ± 1.41 (Sirius, 3.0 mm)	−0.56 ± 0.23
Savini and associates	2018	68	43.63 ± 1.27 (Galilei)	43.08 ± 1.21 (Galilei, TCP1)	0.55
				41.841 ± 1.18 (Galilei, TCP2)	1.79
		50	43.88 ± 1.57 (Galilei)	43.18 ± 1.53 (Galilei, TCP1)	0.70
				41.92 ± 1.46 (Galilei, TCP2)	1.96
Kimiya and associates	2018	25	43.78 ± 1.89 (Pentacam HR)	43.29 ± 1.91 (Pentacam HR, 3.0 mm)	0.49
Pan and associates	2020	74	43.06 ± 1.33 (allegro Topolyzer)	42.55 ± 1.35 (TRCP Pentacam, 4.0 mm)	−0.52 (0.26)
				42.58 ± 1.38 (MMP Sirius, 4.5 mm)	−0.48 (0.22)
				42.68 ± 0.38 (TCP Galilei, 4.0 mm)	−0.38 (0.24)

Km = Mean Keratometry; Sim K = Simulated Keratometry; TCP = Galilei, Calculated Total Corneal Power; TCRP = Pentacam, Total Corneal Refractive Power; MMP = Sirius Mean Pupillary Power at 4.5 mm

However, "the problem" is magnified in two situations.

1. In the normal population, the standard deviation of the relation between the radius of the curvature on the posterior and anterior faces of the cornea (P/A) is important (there are significant differences within the normal population) and achieves 2.4%. This means that, at 2 standard deviations, the P/A ratio oscillates between 77.5 and 87.1%, and it translates into the measure offered by the keratometry, when using the estimated index at 1.3375, could be mistaken up to 0.40 D, which would induce an error in the calculation of the lens up to 0.65 D (Fig. 51.3).

2. In abnormal corneas, such as the ones after refractive surgery, radial keratotomy, postkeratoplasty, keratoconus, and other corneal ectasias where the P/A ratio can vary even further, reaching values of up to 65% in the case

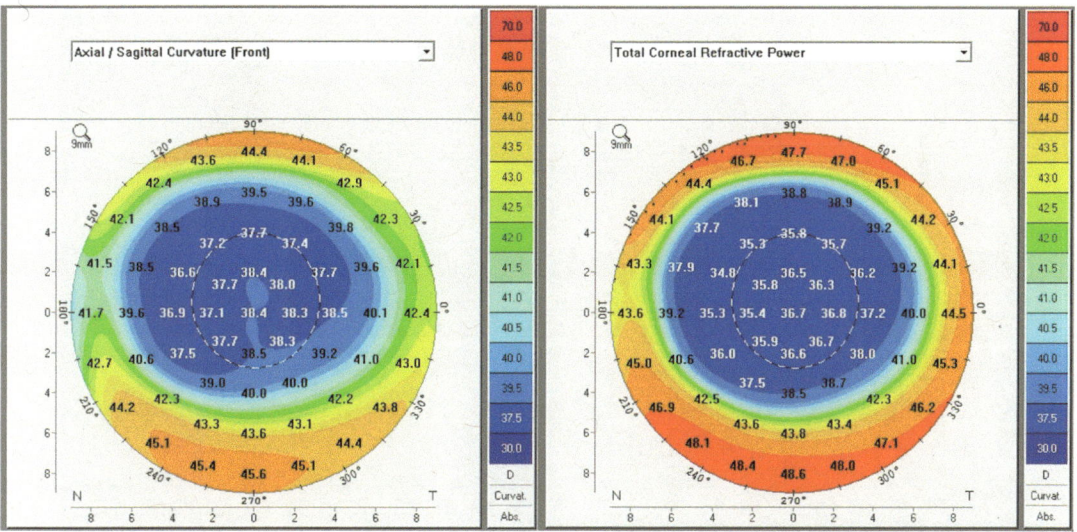

Fig. 51.2 Comparison of the corneal power measured according to the refraction index (RI) of 1.3375 (EKR) similar to keratometry and the total corneal potency

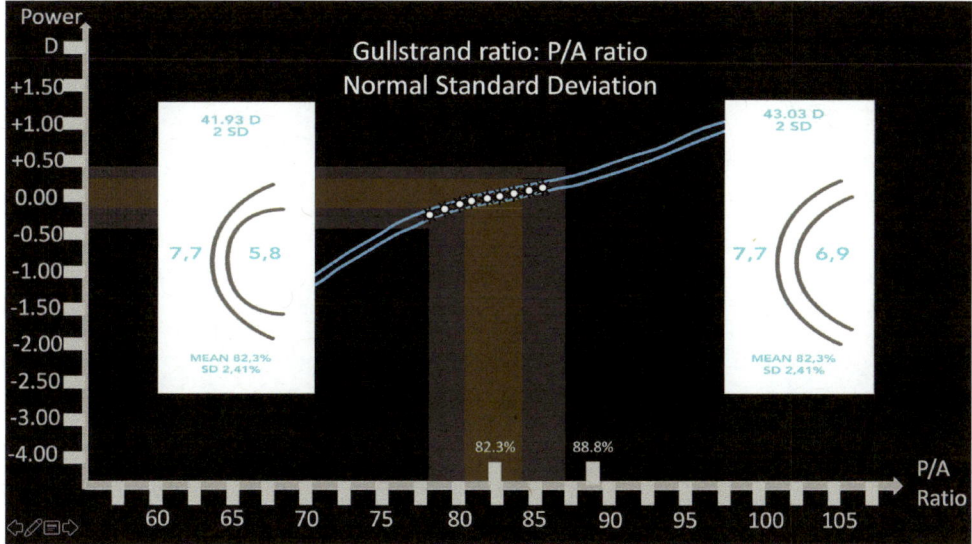

Fig. 51.3 Graph Gullstrand ratio, posterior/anterior ratio vs. gain-loss corneal power. Standard Deviation

of post-myopic, and up to 115% in the post-hyperopic refractive patient, leading into great errors in the measurement of the corneal power (that could total up to errors in the range of several diopters), on behalf of the keratometry or biometers that fail to take into account the posterior surface of the cornea (see Fig. 51.4).

When the reduction of the posterior-anterior ratio is less than 81%, as it happens after a myopic refractive surgery, induces a false over-estimation of the corneal power by the keratometry, and therefore, IOL calculation with less power, and results in a residual hyperopia. To adequately estimate the real power of these corneas, it is required to measure both radii of curvature, anterior and posterior, with a tomographer [43], in order to estimate the real diminished corneal power (Fig. 51.5).

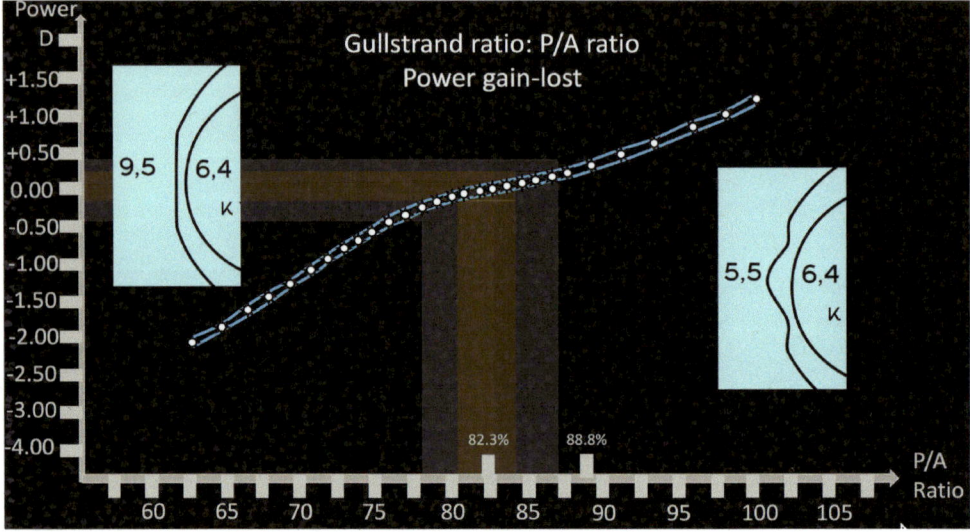

Fig. 51.4 Graph Gullstrand ratio, posterior/anterior ratio vs. gain-loss corneal power. Post-myopic, Post-hyperopic case

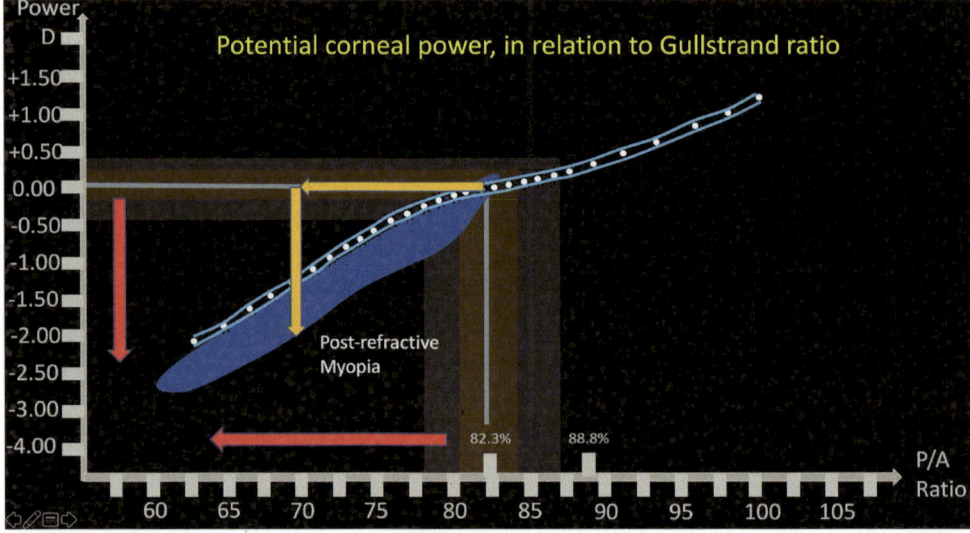

Fig. 51.5 Graph Gullstrand ratio, posterior/anterior ratio vs. gain-loss corneal power in post-myopic refractory surgery. In blue the effect induced by the asphericity, on the power measured by keratometry

Corneal Asphericity and Spherical Aberration

When we are faced with an abnormal corneal asphericity and the induction of the corneal spherical aberration, several aspects should be considered in order to understand how they can affect the estimation of the corneal power and the calculation of the IOL power.

In order to simplify the understanding of the corneal asphericity, if we use the Q term, we need to remember that a sphere has a Q value of 0. In a prolate cornea there is a peripheral flattening and Q will be negative. The human average cornea has a Q value of −0.27. In an oblate cornea the periphery will be steeper than the center and Q will be positive. In this case, as we previously stated, the keratometry which measures a more mid peripheral area, obtains a higher keratometry power than the real flatter central apical one.

Regarding the induction of spherical aberration [44], the light incidence angle in the zones that separate from the optic axis, suffers from greater refraction, making the rays focused on a more proximal point (positive spherical aberration). In a sphere, positive spherical aberration is induced. In order to avoid the induction of positive spherical aberration, a prolate aspheric lens is required (flattening towards the periphery) with a −0.58 asphericity. Since the normal cornea has a lower prolaticity than −0.27, a positive spherical aberration is induced by 0.25 μm (see Fig. 51.6).

On the contrary, in hyperopic refractive surgery, there is a trend to obtain myopic outcomes, due to the steepening of the central anterior surface, the anterior curvature radius (mm) is reduced, and therefore the P/A ratio increases in a significant manner, producing a cornea with greater relative power, than the one measured using the 1.3375 index (the keratometry underestimates the corneal power). The asphericity becomes negative, making the cornea more prolate, and there is a steepening in the center, while flattening indirectly to the periphery. This produces a measure offered by the keratometry, in its mid periphery, which is falsely flatter than the real one on its apical portion (see Fig. 51.7). Keratometry under-estimates the corneal power, and there is a tendency for myopic results.

There are two interesting cases, keratoconus cornea and corneal rings segments, where hyperopic outcomes are frequently observed after performing cataract surgeries and intraocular lens calculations with the majority of formulas, due to

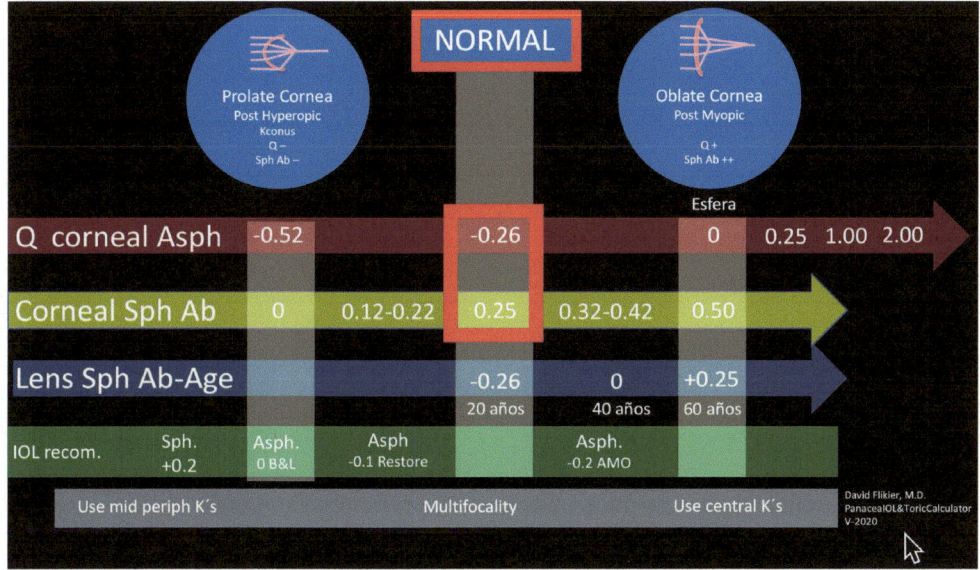

Fig. 51.6 Diagram showing the relation between the corneal asphericity (Q value), the induced aspherical aberration, and the recommended asphericity in the intraocular lens

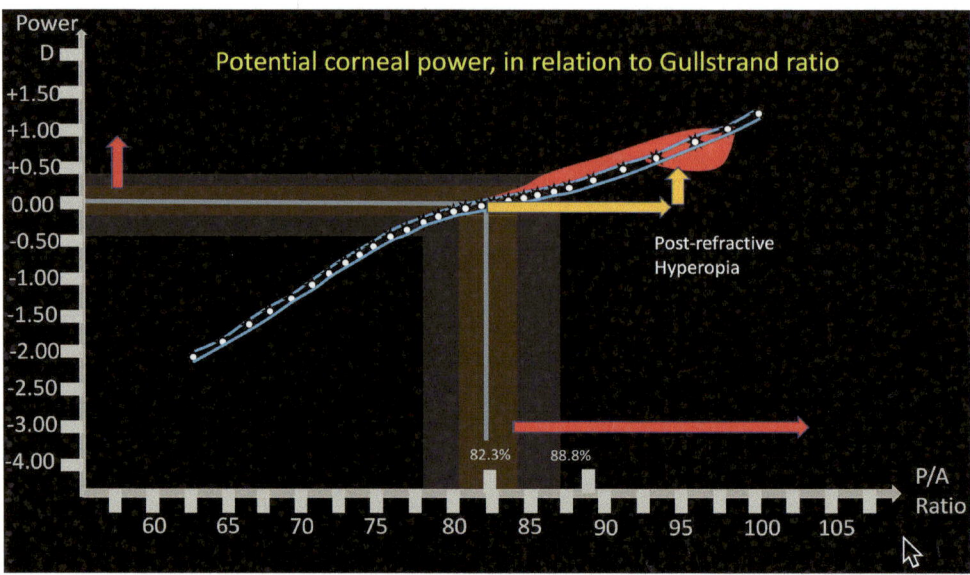

Fig. 51.7 Graph Gullstrand ratio, posterior/anterior ratio vs. gain-loss corneal power in cases of hyperopic refractive surgery

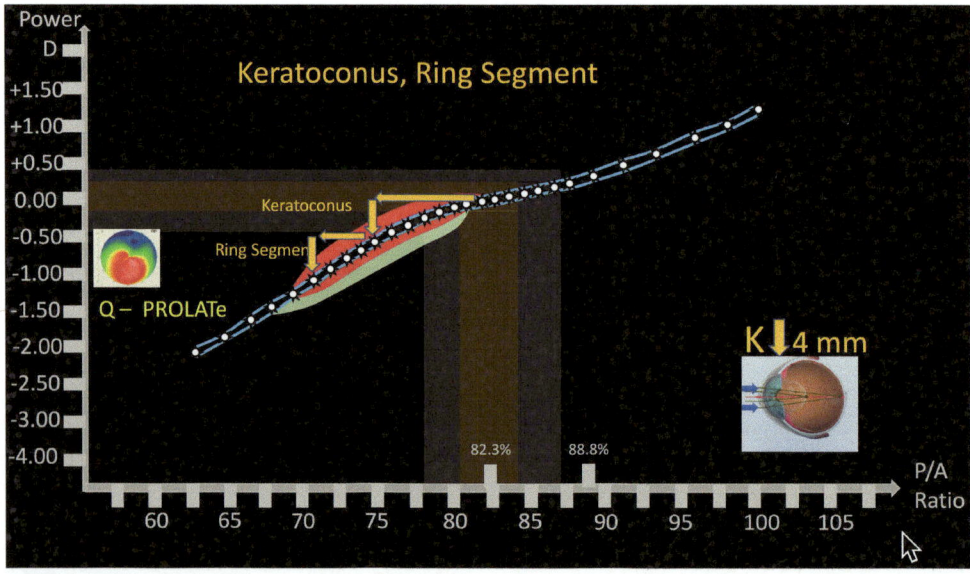

Fig. 51.8 Graph Gullstrand ratio, posterior/anterior ratio vs. gain-loss corneal power in cases with keratoconus and post corneal rings segments

the fact that these corneas present low P/A ratios, a similar effect in the total power of the cornea that appears in the post-myopic refractive surgery, but with high negative asphericities, reducing the effect of the loss of relative corneal power when measuring it with indexes of 1.3375 (see Fig. 51.8).

The last interesting case is found in corneas with marked apical flattening due to keratotomy and post-keratoplasty. In the case of keratotomies, both surfaces of the cornea have suffered flattening, with marked changes on the posterior surface, therefore the P/A relation tends to become markedly positive (differing from the laser myopic surgery). The loss of parallelism varies with penetrating and lamellar keratoplasties, according to the difference in central and peripheral thickness for the different donor discs or receptors, hence the behavior of the P/A ratio and the asphericity of each transplant, and the variability of the reports and their results (see Fig. 51.9).

Observing the relation between the posterior and anterior corneal surface and the asphericity of its anterior surface, it is possible to define the type of cornea we are facing and define the degree of diopter power gains or losses they currently have.

We need to add a fundamental factor, the one from the multifocality influence in the corneas, where the asphericity increases both towards prolaticity, such as in the oblate corneas. If we want to take advantage and maintain multifocality, by implanting the intraocular lens, we must define the power of keratometry which we will use for the calculation of the lens to be placed, so that it will allow the largest percentage of desirable near and far vision.

Corneal Multifocality

We should always consider the multifocality factor in high spherical aberrations. In multifocal corneas there will always be a zone with greater refractive diopter power, if used in an appropriate manner could be programmed for its performance for near vision, and a zone of lower refractive power that would be used for far vision.

In the eye with positive spherical aberration, with an oblate cornea, post myopic refractive surgery, if apical keratometry is used for the IOL calculation, hence for emmetropia, for far vision, the mid peripheric zones and the positive spherical aberration will have a myopization effect, allowing to provide near visual function to multifocality, mainly under mesopic conditions with greater pupillary diameter. If we want to use the multifocality of these corneas, the central apical K's must be used for far vision. This is apical keratometry for the calculations of the intraocular lens, so that the mid peripheral steeper zone would be the one providing the near-close vision. If we were to take the mid peripheral keratometries in order to calculate the intraocular lens, these zones would be the ones who would remain focused for far vision and the central area would remain hyperopic, losing the purpose of the multifocality (see Figs. 51.10, 51.11, and 51.12).

On the contrary, in the prolate cornea, as in apical keratoconus and post-hyperopic refractive

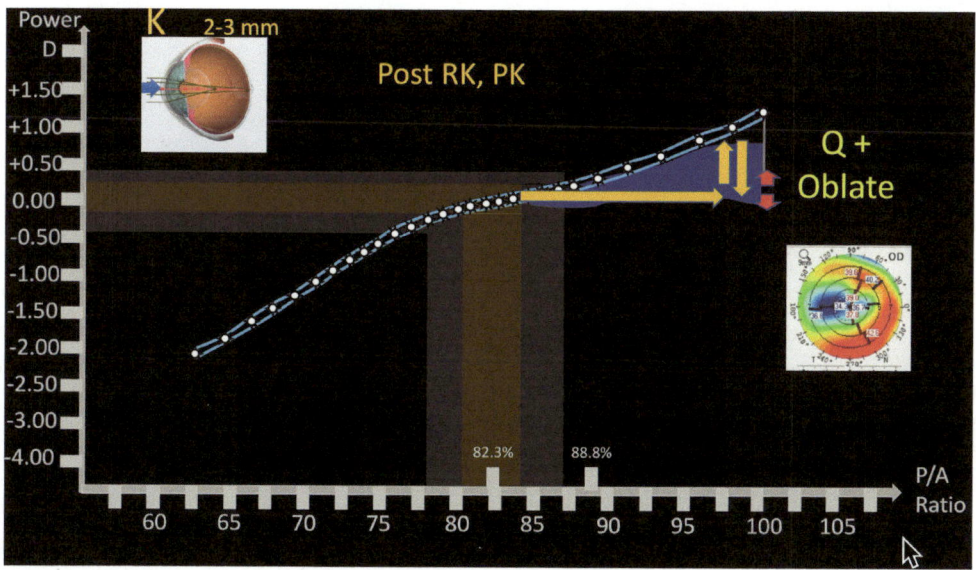

Fig. 51.9 Graph Gullstrand ratio, posterior/anterior ratio vs. gain-loss corneal power in patients with radial keratotomies and keratoplasty

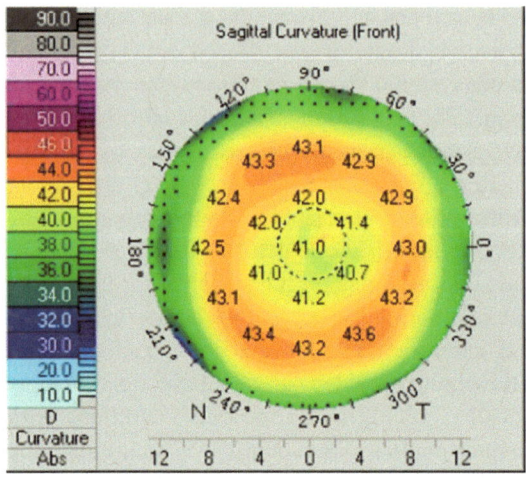

Fig. 51.10 Topographic image of the anterior surface, making corneal oblate asphericity evident, with a lower corneal apical power, in comparison with the higher power in the mid periphery

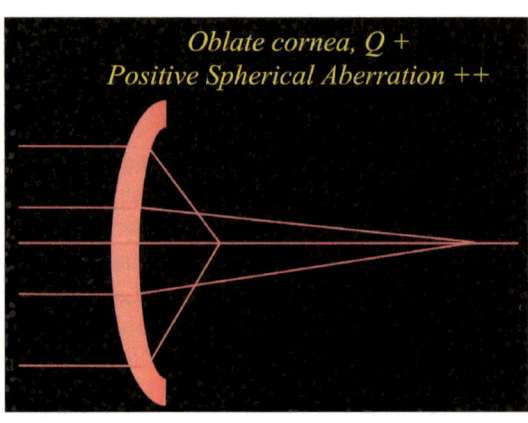

Fig. 51.11 Diagram for positive spherical aberration, the peripheral rays are focused in a point in front of the paraxial rays

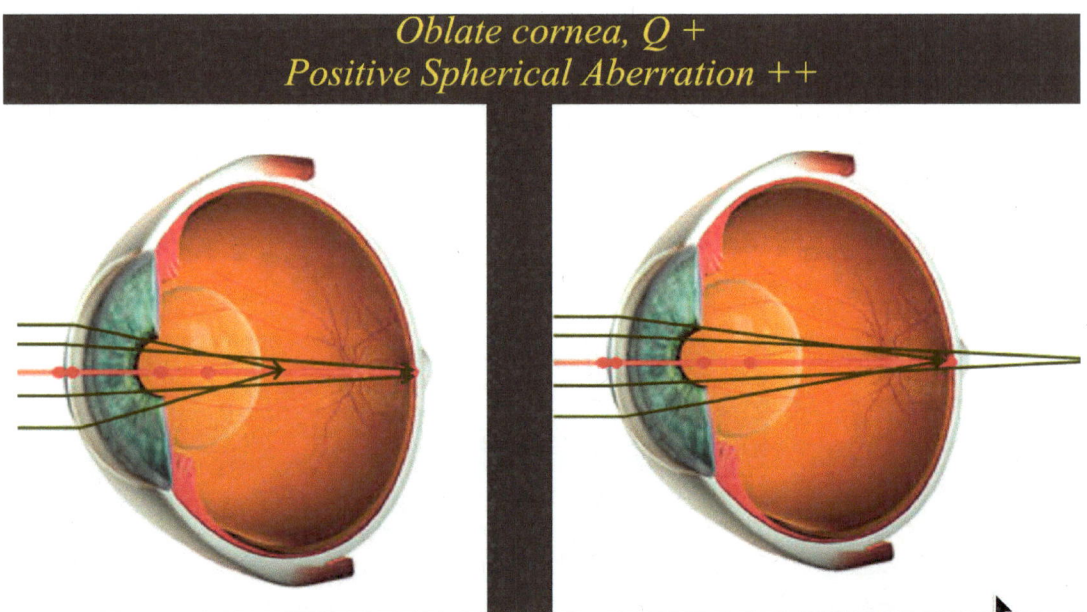

Fig. 51.12 Diagram for the change in spherical aberration in an oblate cornea, by central apical flattening (e.g., Post-Myopic refractive), producing a multifocality, where the paracentral rays are focused on a more posterior point, and the mid peripheral, in a more anterior point

cases, if you wish to use the multifocality, the corneal zones which should be measured are the mid peripheral at 2–4 mm, for far vision, in order to leave the apical K's, which are steeper for near-close vision and thus maintain multifocality, specially under photopic conditions, with miosis, where the rays will go through more apical areas. In these cases, if apical keratometries are used for the lens calculation, the center will lean towards emmetropia, but the mid peripheral cornea to hyperopia and the multifocality idea will be lost (see Figs. 51.13 and 51.14).

In conclusion, if we are to reduce the standard deviation of our results and obtain a greater number of patients close to the expected refractive outcome, we must consider the real corneal power, including the three variables discussed in

our calculation programs: **the corneal P/A ratio, the corneal asphericity and its effect in multifocality** (see Fig. 51.15). This will allow us to improve the results not only in normal corneas, where we understand that the standard deviation of these variables exist and may be significant in some patients, but specially in cases of abnormal pathological corneas such as keratoconus and corneal rings segments, or in corneas altered by surgical procedures such as laser refractive surgery, radial keratotomy or penetrating or lamellar keratoplasties.

From the measured keratometry value captured by the Lenstar or IOL Master 700, in optic zones between 1.6 and 2.8 mm, the Panacea program compensates the total corneal power as a function of the relation between the radius of the corneal curvature, at the posterior and the anterior corneal surfaces (P/A), taking into account the Q corneal asphericity of the anterior corneal surface, and the effect on the rest of the more central cornea, in those cases where a more apical measure is needed in order to take advantage of the multifocality (see Fig. 51.16).

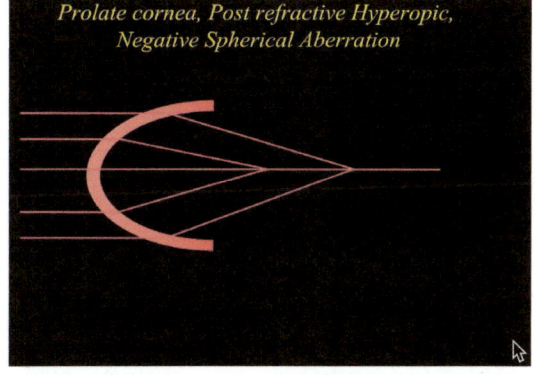

Fig. 51.13 Diagram of the negative spherical aberration, the peripheral rays focused in a point posterior to the paraxials

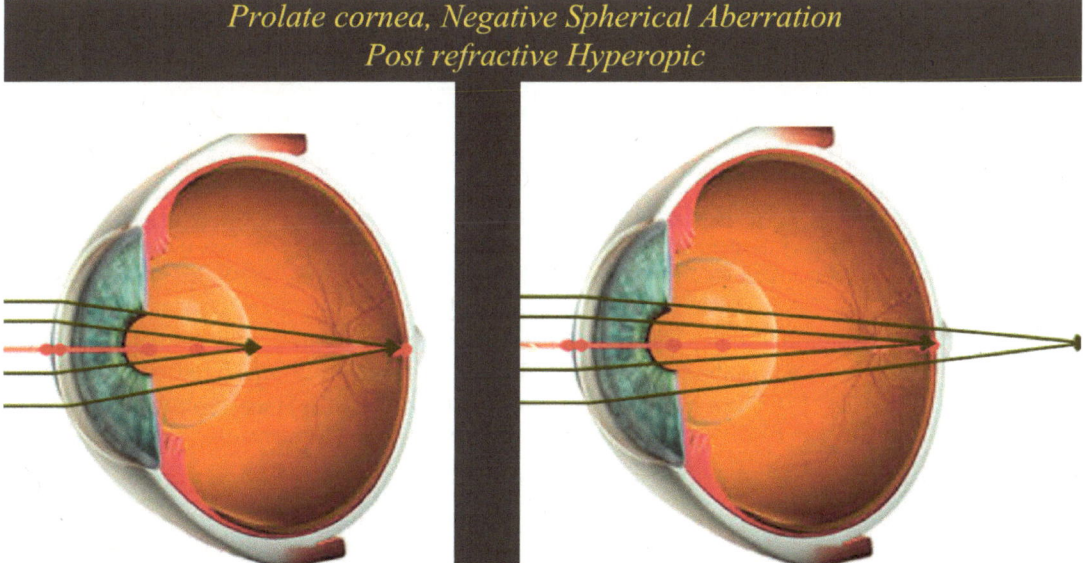

Fig. 51.14 Diagram Spherical aberration in a cornea with high prolaticity, by central apical Steepening (e.g., Post hyperopic refractive), producing a multifocality, where the apical rays are focused in a more anterior point and those at the mid periphery, in a more posterior point

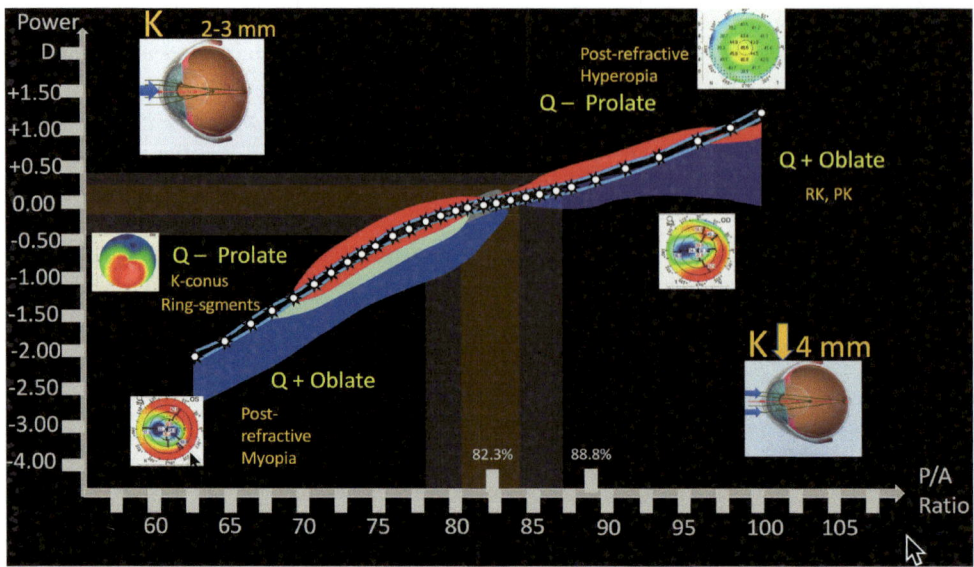

Fig. 51.15 Graph with the relation of the posterior/anterior radius, corneal potency gains or loss in diopters, according to the type of cornea and multifocality

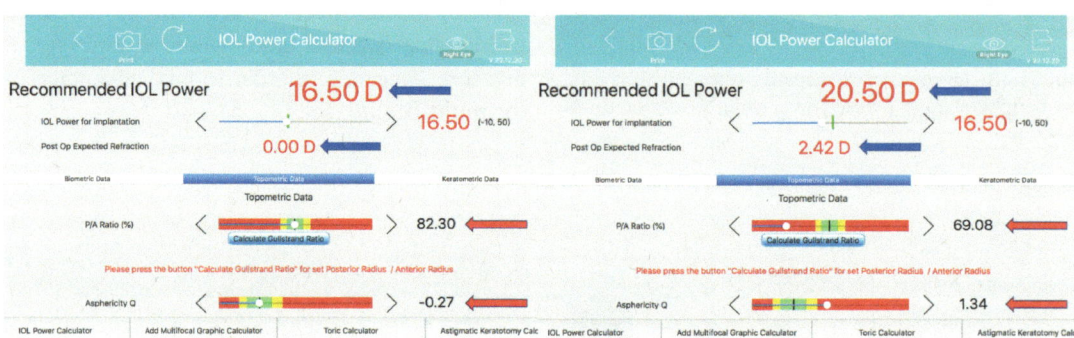

Fig. 51.16 Panacea software images calculating the potency of the IOL according to the P/A ratio in a post-op patient with refractive surgery. 3a: In the first image, the calculations were made assuming the normal PA ratio, as required by any calculator (including the fourth genera-tion formulas). The IOL power calculated is used to provide the patient with emmetrope. 3b: In the second image, the calculation is based on the Real P/A ratio, with a lower P/A, which means that the necessary IOL power is higher, preventing a hyperopic surprise of 2.42 D

The Rocha-de-Lossada and cols. study [45], showed promising results with a better medium absolute error (MedAE 0.178 D) in median axial length, when compared with other 11 formulas, and the results in the groups for ±0.25 D (60.66%) and ±0.75 D (95.08%) (see Table 51.2).

Table 51.2 Comparison of outcomes comparing 12 formulas, in median axial length eyes, axial lengths >22.5 mm and <25 mm (23.44 ± 0.56) (*n* = 122) [45]

| Formula | Refractive prediction error | | | ±0.25 D (%)[a] | ±0.50 D (%)[a] | ±0.75 D (%)[a] | ±1.00 D (%)[a] |
	Opt. ME ± SD (D)	MAE ± SD (D)	Med AE (D)				
Barrett	0.00 ± 0.330	0.263 ± 0.197	0.237	54.92	89.34	98.36	100.00
Pearl	−0.01 ± 0.339	0.263 ± 0.214	0.210	57.38	86.89	95.90	100.00
Holladay	0.00 ± 0.352	0.275 ± 0.219	0.219	54.10	86.89	96.72	98.36
EVO	0.00 ± 0.350	0.271 ± 0.219	0.203	60.66	86.07	95.90	100.00
Hill RBF	0.00 ± 0.354	0.276 ± 0.221	0.240	56.56	86.07	97.54	98.36
Panacea	0.00 ± 0.355	0.266 ± 0.234	0.178	60.66	84.43	95.08	99.18
Olsen	0.00 ± 0.365	0.287 ± 0.224	0.225	55.74	84.43	95.08	99.18
Kane	0.00 ± 0.363	0.280 ± 0.230	0.238	53.28	84.43	95.08	100.00
Haigis	0.00 ± 0.379	0.292 ± 0.240	0.225	56.56	82.79	95.90	98.36
SRK/T	0.00 ± 0.373	0.287 ± 0.237	0.240	53.28	82.79	95.90	98.36
Hoffer Q	0.00 ± 0.359	0.284 ± 0.218	0.233	57.38	81.97	96.72	99.18
Ladas	0.00 ± 0.401	0.313 ± 0.250	0.266	48.36	81.15	92.62	99.18

Opt. ME optimized mean error; *SD* standard deviation; *MAE* mean absolute error; *Med AE* median absolute error; *RBF* radial basis function

[a] Eyes with predictive error between ±0.25D, ±0.50D. ±0.75D and ±1.00D

Availability

Panacea IOL & Toric Calculator may be obtained in an open and free manner, for the following platforms:

Web Panacea: www.panaceaiolandtoriccalculator.com

Mac IPAD: https://apps.apple.com/app/id975426922?ign-mpt=uo%3D4

MacDesktop: https://itunes.apple.com/cr/app/panaceaioltoriccalcd/id1107308495?l=en&mt=12

PC Desktop: www.panaceaioltoriccalc.com

Conclusion

A modern formula must have every available tool in order to increase its good results, including improvements in biometry, such as correction factors in the axial length and its segments, as well as in the real retinal thickness, the estimation of the effective lens position, with the inclusion of new variables if needed, such as the P/A ratio in the optimization of the corneal curvature value used in the estimation of the ELPo.

The total corneal power, and the P/A ratio in particular, are not only important for those "naive" normal corneas, whose standard deviation may induce a significant error in some cases, but it is also of particular importance, in eyes with abnormal corneas, affected after refractive surgeries, lamellar or penetrating keratoplasties, and corneal ectasias.

A formula which considers the relation of both corneal curvatures, the corneal asphericity and the multifocality, can perform the calculations with the objective data taken from a tomograph and a biometer, avoiding the need of formulas that depend on the eye or cornea characteristics.

References

1. Kane JX, Chang DF. Intraocular lens power formulas, biometry, and intraoperative aberrometry: a review. Ophthalmology. 2021;128(11):e94–e114.
2. Savini G, et al. Accuracy of optical biometry combined with Placido disc corneal topography for intraocular lens power calculation. PLoS One. 2017;12(2):e0172634.
3. Melles RB, Holladay JT, Chang WJ. Accuracy of intraocular lens calculation formulas. Ophthalmology. 2018;125(2):169–78.
4. Cooke DL, Cooke TL. Comparison of 9 intraocular lens power calculation formulas. J Cataract Refract Surg. 2016;42(8):1157–64.

5. Kane JX, et al. Accuracy of 3 new methods for intraocular lens power selection. J Cataract Refract Surg. 2017;43(3):333–9.

6. Darcy K, et al. Assessment of the accuracy of new and updated intraocular lens power calculation formulas in 10 930 eyes from the UK National Health Service. J Cataract Refract Surg. 2020;46(1):2–7.

7. Drexler W, et al. Partial coherence interferometry: a novel approach to biometry in cataract surgery. Am J Ophthalmol. 1998;126(4):524–34.

8. Findl O, et al. High precision biometry of pseudophakic eyes using partial coherence interferometry. J Cataract Refract Surg. 1998;24(8):1087–93.

9. Haigis W, et al. Comparison of immersion ultrasound biometry and partial coherence interferometry for intraocular lens calculation according to Haigis. Graefes Arch Clin Exp Ophthalmol. 2000;238(9):765–73.

10. Cooke DL, Cooke TL. A comparison of two methods to calculate axial length. J Cataract Refract Surg. 2019;45(3):284–92.

11. Cooke DL, Cooke TL. Approximating sum-of-segments axial length from a traditional optical low-coherence reflectometry measurement. J Cataract Refract Surg. 2019;45(3):351–4.

12. Wang L, et al. Calculation of axial length using a single group refractive index versus using different refractive indices for each ocular segment: theoretical study and refractive outcomes. Ophthalmology. 2019;126(5):663–70.

13. Cooke DL, et al. Standardizing sum-of-segments axial length using refractive index models. Biomed Opt Express. 2020;11(10):5860–70.

14. Wang L, et al. Optimizing intraocular lens power calculations in eyes with axial lengths above 25.0 mm. J Cataract Refract Surg. 2011;37(11):2018–27.

15. Wang L, Holladay JT, Koch DD. Wang-Koch axial length adjustment for the Holladay 2 formula in long eyes. J Cataract Refract Surg. 2018;44(10):1291–2.

16. Wang L, Koch DD. Modified axial length adjustment formulas in long eyes. J Cataract Refract Surg. 2018;44(11):1396–7.

17. Aramberri J. Intraocular lens power calculation after corneal refractive surgery: double-K method. J Cataract Refract Surg. 2003;29(11):2063–8.

18. Fabian E, Wehner W. Prediction accuracy of Total Keratometry compared to standard Keratometry using different intraocular lens power formulas. J Refract Surg. 2019;35(6):362–8.

19. Savini G, et al. Simulated Keratometry versus Total corneal power by ray tracing: a comparison in prediction accuracy of intraocular lens power. Cornea. 2017;36(11):1368–72.

20. Pan C, et al. A comparative study of Total corneal power using a ray tracing method obtained from 3 different Scheimpflug camera devices. Am J Ophthalmol. 2020;216:90–8.

21. Sandoval HP, et al. Cataract surgery after myopic LASIK: objective analysis to determine best formula and keratometry to use. J Cataract Refract Surg. 2020;47:465.

22. Yoneyama R, et al. Predictability of intraocular lens power calculation in eyes after phototherapeutic keratectomy. Jpn J Ophthalmol. 2020;64(1):62–7.

23. Lawless M, et al. Total keratometry in intraocular lens power calculations in eyes with previous laser refractive surgery. Clin Exp Ophthalmol. 2020;48(6):749–56.

24. Cho K, et al. New method for intraocular lens power calculation using a rotating Scheimpflug camera in eyes with corneal refractive surgery. Sci Rep. 2020;10(1):8992.

25. Wang L, et al. Evaluation of total keratometry and its accuracy for intraocular lens power calculation in eyes after corneal refractive surgery. J Cataract Refract Surg. 2019;45(10):1416–21.

26. Pirhadi S, Maghooli K, Jadidi K. An innovative approach for determining the customized refractive index of ectatic corneas in cataractous patients. Sci Rep. 2020;10(1):16681.

27. Kamiya K, et al. Comparison of simulated Keratometry and Total refractive power for keratoconus according to the stage of Amsler-Krumeich classification. Sci Rep. 2018;8(1):12436.

28. Kamiya K, et al. Predictability of intraocular lens power calculation for cataract with keratoconus: a multicenter study. Sci Rep. 2018;8(1):1312.

29. Srivannaboon S, Chirapapaisan C. Comparison of refractive outcomes using conventional keratometry or total keratometry for IOL power calculation in cataract surgery. Graefes Arch Clin Exp Ophthalmol. 2019;257(12):2677–82.

30. Ho JD, et al. Validity of the keratometric index: evaluation by the Pentacam rotating Scheimpflug camera. J Cataract Refract Surg. 2008;34(1):137–45.

31. Shirayama M, et al. Comparison of corneal powers obtained from 4 different devices. Am J Ophthalmol. 2009;148(4):528–35. e1.

32. Haigis W. Challenges and approaches in modern biometry and IOL calculation. Saudi J Ophthalmol. 2012;26(1):7–12.

33. Naeser K, Savini G, Bregnhoj JF. Corneal powers measured with a rotating Scheimpflug camera. Br J Ophthalmol. 2016;100(9):1196–200.

34. Oh JH, et al. Evaluation of the Pentacam ray tracing method for the measurement of central corneal power after myopic photorefractive keratectomy. Cornea. 2014;33(3):261–5.

35. Saad E, Shammas MC, Shammas HJ. Scheimpflug corneal power measurements for intraocular lens power calculation in cataract surgery. Am J Ophthalmol. 2013;156(3):460–467 e2.

36. Savini G, et al. Accuracy of a dual Scheimpflug analyzer and a corneal topography system for intraocular lens power calculation in unoperated eyes. J Cataract Refract Surg. 2011;37(1):72–6.

37. Savini G, et al. Comparison of methods to measure corneal power for intraocular lens power calcula-

tion using a rotating Scheimpflug camera. J Cataract Refract Surg. 2013;39(4):598–604.

38. Savini G, et al. Repeatability of automatic measurements performed by a dual Scheimpflug analyzer in unoperated and post-refractive surgery eyes. J Cataract Refract Surg. 2011;37(2):302–9.

39. Savini G, et al. Refractive outcomes of intraocular lens power calculation using different corneal power measurements with a new optical biometer. J Cataract Refract Surg. 2018;44(6):701–8.

40. Savini G, Schiano-Lomoriello D, Hoffer KJ. Repeatability of automatic measurements by a new anterior segment optical coherence tomographer combined with Placido topography and agreement with 2 Scheimpflug cameras. J Cataract Refract Surg. 2018;44(4):471–8.

41. Savini G, Taroni L, Hoffer KJ. Recent developments in intraocular lens power calculation methods-update 2020. Ann Transl Med. 2020;8(22):1553.

42. Seo KY, et al. New equivalent keratometry reading calculation with a rotating Scheimpflug camera for intraocular lens power calculation after myopic corneal surgery. J Cataract Refract Surg. 2014;40(11):1834–42.

43. Holladay JT. Accuracy of Scheimpflug Holladay equivalent keratometry readings after corneal refractive surgery. J Cataract Refract Surg. 2010;36(1):182–3. author reply 183-4

44. Wang L, Hill WE, Koch DD. Evaluation of intraocular lens power prediction methods using the American Society of Cataract and Refractive Surgeons Post-Keratorefractive Intraocular Lens Power Calculator. J Cataract Refract Surg. 2010;36(9):1466–73.

45. Rocha-de-Lossada C, et al. Intraocular lens power calculation formula accuracy: comparison of 12 formulas for a trifocal hydrophilic intraocular lens. Eur J Ophthalmol. 2020;31(6):2981–8.

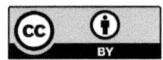

The PEARL-DGS Formula

52

Guillaume Debellemanière, Alain Saad,
and Damien Gatinel

History of the PEARL-DGS Formula

The Postoperative spherical Equivalent prediction using ARtificial Intelligence and Linear algorithms (PEARL) project aims to assess the potential of artificial intelligence (AI) techniques in the IOL calculation field, to determine the optimal architecture of those formulas, and to encourage open research in this field by publishing the experiments and the related code under an open-source license. It was initiated in 2017 in the Anterior Segment and Refractive Surgery Department at Rothschild Foundation by the authors of this chapter. It resulted in a succession of IOL calculation formulas known under the name "PEARL-DGS," DGS representing the initials of the last names of the authors.

Description of the Current PEARL-DGS Formula

General Principles

The PEARL-DGS formula is a thick lens formula that uses AI techniques to predict the distance between the posterior corneal surface and

G. Debellemanière (✉) · A. Saad · D. Gatinel
Foundation Adolphe de Rothschild Hospital,
Paris, France

the anterior IOL surface ("theoretical internal lens position," TILP) [1] (Fig. 52.1). The TILP is an anatomical distance, independent of both the lens principal plane positions and the corneal thickness. The reference TILP (the target to predict) corresponds to the value leading to the real postoperative SE when entered in thick lens equations along with the other optical parameters of the eye and IOL. The formula uses various machine learning algorithms and ensemble methods to predict this value. The refractive index values used in the formula are those of the Atchison eye model [2], except for the corneal index, which was determined empirically during the formula development process. The sum-of-segments AL, approximated by the Cooke-modified AL (CMAL), replaces the AL in the formula. As the thin lens approximation is not used, the real geometric parameters of the considered IOL are ideally used during the development process; otherwise, the formula can be developed using theoretical IOL parameters (for example, biconvex symmetric geometry) and a study of the mean TILP prediction error along the IOL power range is proposed.

Sum-of-Segments AL Calculation

Sum-of-segments AL is obtained by computing the geometric length of each ocular segment [3]

J. Aramberri et al. (eds.), *Intraocular Lens Calculations*, Essentials in Ophthalmology,
https://doi.org/10.1007/978-3-031-50666-6_52

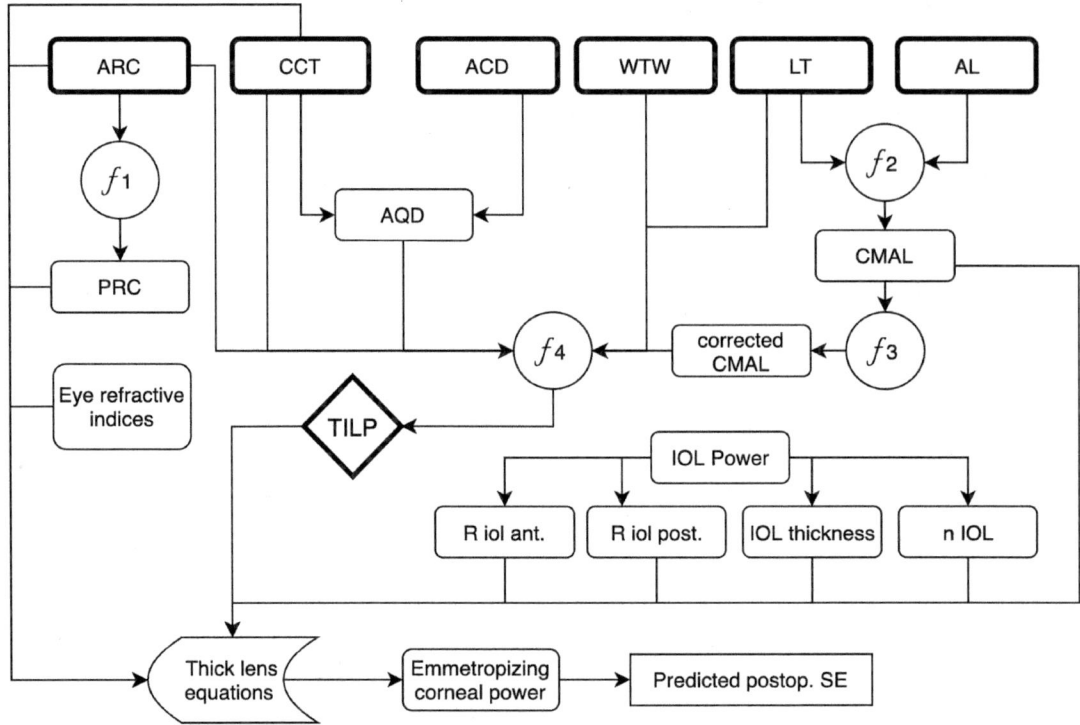

Fig. 52.1 General outline of the PEARL-DGS formula prediction process. The PRC is deduced from the ARC (f1). AL and LT are used to calculate the CMAL (f2). The CMAL is corrected before being used as an input to predict the TILP (f3). The raw CMAL value is used in the optical part of the formula. The ARC and CCT are used in the optical part of the formula and also used as an input to predict the TILP. CD, AQD, and LT are only used to predict the TILP. The TILP is then predicted using 6 biometric parameters (f4). From Debellemanière et al.: The PEARL-DGS Formula: The Development of an Open-source Machine Learning-based Thick IOL Calculation Formula. Am J Ophthalmol. 2021 Dec;232:58–69

(calculated by dividing their optical path length by their own refractive index), rather than using the weighted-average refractive index of the whole eye as described by Haigis [4].

CMAL calculation allows to approximate the sum-of-segments AL in the absence of vitreous thickness value delivered by the biometer [5], which is the case in most clinical settings. CMAL is calculated using the equation $CMAL = (1.23853 + 958.55 \times AL - 54.67 \times LT)/1000$ (AL and LT in meters). Two hundred micrometers was added to this value to account for the retinal thickness, as suggested by Dr. David Cooke (personal communication, February 4, 2021).

In the formula, CMAL is calculated and replaces traditional AL; it is also calculated during the formula development process and the reference TILP is back-calculated using this value as the reference AL.

Optical Principles

The refractive index values of the Atchison eye model are used: n_{aqueous} is set to 1.3374, n_{vitreous} to 1.336, and n_{IOL} is equal to the real refractive of the IOL used in the formula development process. n_{cornea} was set to 1.363. The process that led to the choice of this value is described later in this chapter. The formula is entirely based on thick lens equations (Eqs. 52.1–52.7) (Table 52.1).

Posterior Corneal Radius Prediction

The PRC is inferred from the ARC using two linear regressions. Those regressions were determined using ARC and PRC values from 2052 rotating Scheimpflug camera system measurements (Pentacam, Oculus Optikgerate, Wetzlar, Germany) obtained on eyes with no his-

Table 52.1 Fundamental paraxial optics equations. Signs in the equation respect the Cartesian sign convention: Distances to the left are negative, and distances to the right are positive

	Formula	Explanation
(52.1)	$P = \left(\dfrac{n_{\text{right}} - n_{\text{left}}}{r} \right)$	Surface power for a given radius r and surrounding refractive index n_{right} and n_{left}
(52.2)	$P_{\text{both}} = P_{\text{left}} + P_{\text{right}} - (P_{\text{left}} \times P_{\text{right}} \times d/n)$	Gullstrand formula: Equivalent power of a thick lens. P_{left} and P_{right} are the power of each lens surface. d is the distance between the lenses, and n is the lens refractive index
(52.3)	$f = -n_{\text{left}}/P$	Front focal length of a lens*
(52.4)	$f' = n_{\text{right}}/P$	Back focal length of a lens**
(52.5)	$H = d \times f_{\text{both}}/f_{\text{right}}$	Distance from the left vertex to the first principal plane of a two-lens system. d is the distance between the lenses***
(52.6)	$H' = -d \times f'_{\text{both}}/f'_{\text{left}}$	Distance from the right vertex to the second principal plane of a two-lens system. d is the distance between the lenses***
(52.7)	$d_{\text{o}} = d - H'_{\text{left}} + H_{\text{right}}$	Optical distance between two-lens systems

From Debellemanière et al.: The PEARL-DGS Formula: The Development of an Open-source Machine Learning-based Thick IOL Calculation Formula. Am J Ophthalmol. 2021 Dec;232:58–69

Signs in the equation respect the cartesian sign convention: distances to the left are negative, and distances to the right are positive
* The front focal length of a thick lens is expressed from its first principal plane
** The back focal length of a thick lens is expressed from its second principal plane
*** If the system is itself composed of a lens system, d must be calculated according to the appropriate principal plane positions using Eq. 52.7

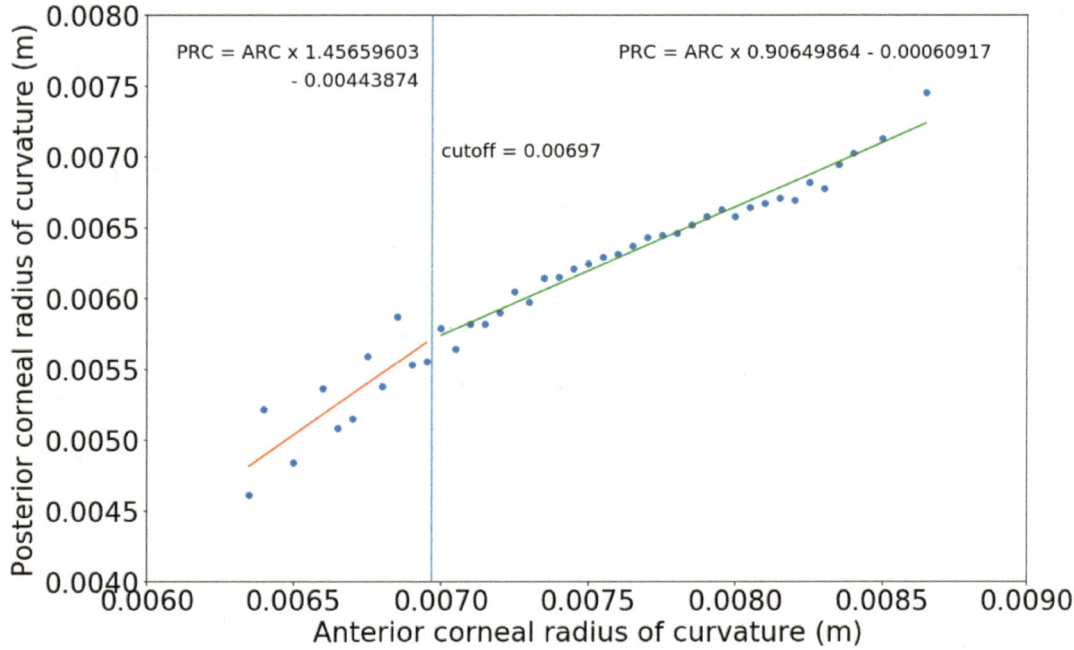

Fig. 52.2 Mean PRC for each ARC step (ARC values are rounded up to 0.05 mm). A cut-off at 7.00 mm was visually defined, and two linear regressions were fitted. The cut-off was then refined to 6.97 mm. From Debellemanière et al.: The PEARL-DGS Formula: The Development of an Open-source Machine Learning-based Thick IOL Calculation Formula. Am J Ophthalmol. 2021 Dec;232:58–69

tory of corneal surgery. The mean PRC was calculated for each step of ARC values rounded to 0.05 mm. A threshold at 7.00 mm ARC was visually identified. Two linear regression algorithms were fitted on both sides of this threshold, which was then slightly modified to 6.97 mm to allow a perfect transition between the PRC values obtained around the threshold.

The linear regressions are presented in Fig. 52.2.

TILP Back-Calculation

The formula is based on the prediction of the TILP value, defined as the theoretical distance between the posterior corneal surface and the anterior IOL surface that leads to the real postoperative SE when entered in thick lens equations along with the other optical parameters of the eye and IOL. The calculation of the TILP must be performed for each eye of the training set, to obtain the reference value that will be used as the target to predict in the algorithms.

The formula allowing this back-calculation is described in Eq. (52.10). If the eye is not emmetropic, the postoperative refraction is added to the total corneal power, and the anterior corneal radius is re-calculated to fit the new total corneal power value (Eqs. 52.8 and 52.9). Equation (52.10) can then be applied (Table 52.2).

TILP Prediction

The PEARL formula takes advantage of various algorithms such as gradient-boosted trees (XGBoost), support vector regression, neural networks (multi-layer perceptron regressor), and standard multiple regression to predict the TILP. The hyperparameters of each model were determined using fivefold cross-validation on the training set.

Predicted SE Calculation

Once the TILP is predicted, it is necessary to calculate the associated refraction at the spectacle plane. This can be done by first calculating the emmetropizing anterior corneal radius, i.e., the theoretical anterior corneal radius leading to emmetropia if the predicted TILP is used in thick lens equations along with the other optical parameters of the eye and IOL, using Eq. (52.11). The emmetropizing total corneal power can then be calculated using this value, using Eq. (52.2). The predicted postoperative SE at the corneal plane is then obtained by subtracting the real total corneal power from the emmetropizing total corneal power (Eq. 52.12). The resulting refraction converted to the spectacle plane is the predicted postoperative SE (Eq. 52.13) (Table 52.3).

Corneal Index Optimization

The refractive index of the cornea varies from 1.337 to 1.432 in the literature [6]. In order to

Table 52.2 Equations used in the formula (lengths are in meters)

(52.8)	$SE_{cornea} = SE_{spectacles}/(1 - d_v \times SE_{spectacles})$	Spectacle plane refraction to corneal plane refraction conversion. d_v is the vertex distance of spectacle lenses
(52.9)	$P_{ant.cornea\ corrected} = \dfrac{P_{cornea\ corrected} \times n_{co} - P_{post.cornea} \times n_{co}}{n_{co} - P_{post.cornea} \times T_{cornea}}$ With $P_{cornea\ corrected} = P_{cornea} + SE_{cornea}$	Calculation of the emmetropizing anterior corneal surface. This equation allows the use of Eq. (52.10) to back-calculate the TILP for the eyes that have a postoperative spherical equivalent different from Plano
(52.10)	$TILP_i = \dfrac{-B \pm \sqrt{C}}{2 \times P_{cornea} \times P_{iol}} + H'_{cornea} - H_{iol}$ with $C = B^2 - 4 \times P_{cornea} \times P_{iol} \times (A \times (n_{aq} \times P_{cornea} + n_{aq} \times P_{iol}) - n_{vit} \times n_{aq})$ and $B = \dfrac{n_{vit} \times n_{aq}}{f'_{cornea}} - n_{aq} \times P_{cornea} - n_{aq} \times P_{iol} - P_{cornea} \times P_{iol} \times A$ and $A = AL - T_{cornea} + H_{iol} - H'_{cornea} - T_{iol} - H'_{iol}$	Back-calculation of the theoretical physical distance between the posterior corneal surface and the anterior IOL surface. The sign of the second term of the numerator in the main equation must be negative for positive IOLs and positive for negative IOLs

From Debellemanière et al.: The PEARL-DGS Formula: The Development of an Open-source Machine Learning-based Thick IOL Calculation Formula. Am J Ophthalmol. 2021 Dec;232:58–69

Table 52.3 Equations used in the formula (lengths are in meters)

(52.11)	$$P_{ant.cornea} = \frac{n_{aq} \times n_{cornea} - P_{post.cornea} \times n_{cornea} \times E}{E \times (n_{cornea} - T_{cornea} \times P_{post.cornea}) + n_{aq} \times T_{cornea}}$$ with $E = TILP + H_{iol} - \dfrac{D \times n_{aq}}{D \times P_{iol} - 1}$ and $D = \dfrac{AL - T_{cornea} - TILP - T_{iol} - H'_{iol}}{n_{vit}}$	Calculation of the emmetropizing anterior corneal surface power using the predicted TILP value and the optical parameters of the eye
(52.12)	$SE_{cornea\ predicted} = P_{cornea\ (emmetropia)} - P_{cornea(real)}$	Calculation of the predicted postoperative refraction (corneal plane)
(52.13)	$SE_{spectacles} = SE_{cornea}/(1 + d_v \times SE_{cornea})$	Corneal plane refraction to spectacle plane refraction conversion. d_v is the vertex distance of spectacle lenses

From Debellemanière et al.: The PEARL-DGS Formula: The Development of an Open-source Machine Learning-based Thick IOL Calculation Formula. Am J Ophthalmol. 2021 Dec;232:58–69

Fig. 52.3 SD of the prediction error as a function of the corneal refractive index value used to develop the formula. From Debellemanière et al.: The PEARL-DGS Formula: The Development of an Open-source Machine Learning-based Thick IOL Calculation Formula. Am J Ophthalmol. 2021 Dec;232:58–69

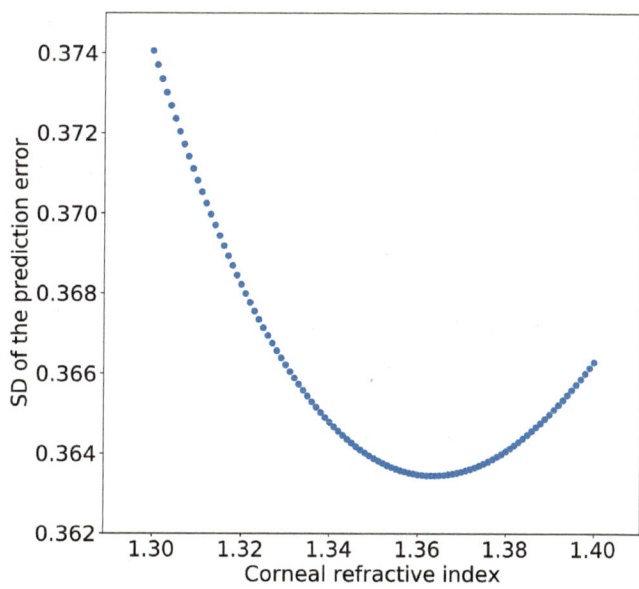

determine the optimal corneal index to use in the formula, a systematic approach was applied, using the eyes of the training set, for a range of corneal refractive index values ranging between 1.30 and 1.40 by 0.001 steps. For each step, reference TILP was back-calculated, a multiple regression was fitted to predict the resulting value from biometric parameters, the predicted TILP was calculated using the regression, the predicted postoperative SE was calculated, the prediction error was calculated, and the standard deviation (SD) of the mean prediction error (PE) was determined. The SD of the mean PE was plotted against the corneal refractive index value, and a concave upward curve was obtained. The refractive index value leading to the lowest SD was selected: in our case, this value was 1.363 (Fig. 52.3).

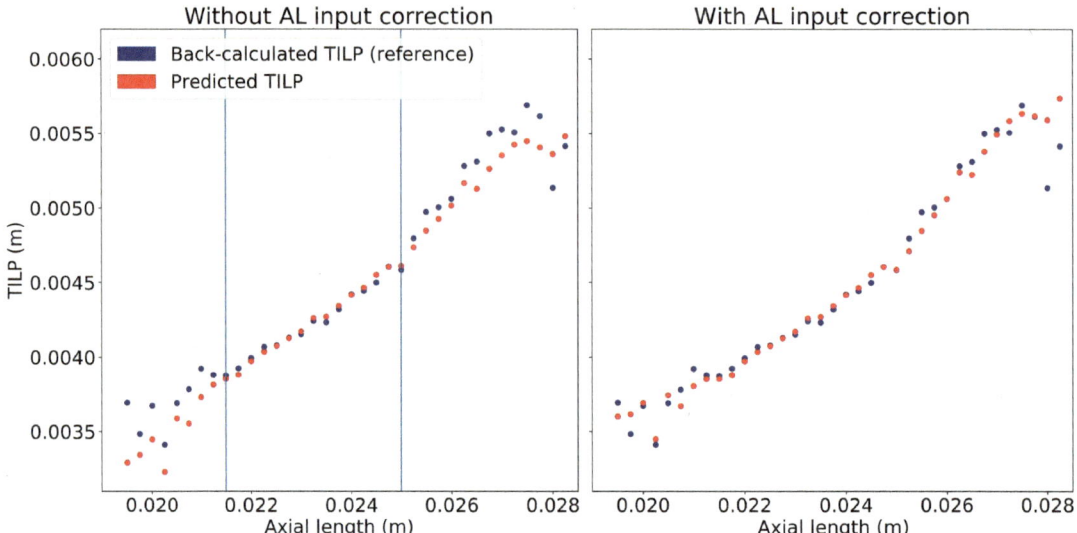

Fig. 52.4 Predicted TILP and back-calculated TILP are plotted against AL, without AL input correction (left) and with input correction (right). AL input correction in multiple regression allows to correct for the TILP prediction error that arises below 21.5 mm and beyond 25 mm. From

Debellemanière et al.: The PEARL-DGS Formula: The Development of an Open-source Machine Learning-based Thick IOL Calculation Formula. Am J Ophthalmol. 2021 Dec;232:58–69

Table 52.4 Modified CMAL calculation, to adapt the CMAL value used as an input in the multiple regression algorithm to the AL

(52.14) $CMAL_{modified} = CMAL + AL\ correction\ factor$ With *AL correction* *factor* $= \mid threshold - AL \mid\ *\ weight$	Corrected CMAL calculation, used as an input in the TILP prediction algorithm. NB: The optical equations use the non-modified CMAL value

From Debellemanière et al.: The PEARL-DGS Formula: The Development of an Open-source Machine Learning-based Thick IOL Calculation Formula. Am J Ophthalmol. 2021 Dec;232:58–69

Extreme AL Adjustment in the Multiple Regression Algorithm

The mean reference TILP values and mean predicted TILP values predicted by the final multiple regression algorithm were calculated for each AL value rounded to the nearest 0.25 mm. The resulting graph is shown in Fig. 52.4. Systematic and increasing errors were identified for very short and very long eyes, after a given threshold, proportional to the distance to this threshold. The error thresholds were visually defined as 21.5 mm and 26 mm, for short and long eyes, respectively.

A correction factor was applied to the CMAL value used as an input in the TILP predicting algorithm. This correction factor was defined as the absolute value of the difference between the

chosen upper/lower threshold and the AL of the considered eye, multiplied by a weight. This correction factor was added to the CMAL value used as an input in the algorithm if its AL was below the lower AL threshold or beyond the upper AL threshold. The optimal weight to apply to short and long eyes was systematically determined for both AL categories. The CMAL value used in the optical part of the equation was never modified (Table 52.4).

Formula Development for IOLs with Unknown Geometry

If a large dataset is available for an IOL of unknown geometry, we propose to apply the following four-step methodology:

- create a theoretical parameter table for the considered IOL, using the real refractive index of the IOL, a refractive index of 1.336 for the medium surrounding the lens (as required by the ISO 11979-2 norm) [7], and a symmetric biconvex shape
- follow the aforementioned formula development process
- calculate the mean TILP prediction error for each IOL power step and look for a pattern of TILP prediction error
- manually account for this error in the TILP prediction function, depending on the IOL power for which the prediction is made.

Prediction for IOLs with Unknown Geometry and No Available Data

To allow a SE prediction for IOLs with no data available, the adjusted SRK/T A constant for each IOL model of a large dataset comprising 28 IOL models was calculated. The predicted TILP was calculated. For each IOL model, this value was shifted by an equal amount for each eye until the mean prediction error was equal to zero for this model. A linear regression was fitted to predict the TILP shift associated with a given SRK/T A constant.

Performances of the PEARL Formula

In the main PEARL-DGS article [1], two test sets of 677 and 262 eyes were analyzed. The PEARL-DGS formula yielded the lowest SD on the first set (± 0.382 D), followed by K6 and Olsen (± 0.394 D), EVO 2.0 (±0.398 D), RBF 3.0, and BUII (± 0.402 D), as well as the lowest SD on the second set (± 0.269 D), followed by Olsen (± 0.272 D), K6 (± 0.276 D), EVO 2.0 (± 0.277 D), and BUII (± 0.301 D).

Independent peer-reviewed studies evaluated and compared the PEARL-DGS formula along with other fourth-generation IOL calculation formulas. In three of seven studies, PEARL-DGS ranked first with a median absolute error (MedAE) varying between 0.190 and 0.310 and

a percentage of eyes with a postoperative refractive error of <0.5 diopter, varying between 74% and 87.1%. In a cohort of short axial eye length, Wendelstein et al. [8] showed that PEARL-DGS, Okulix, Kane, or Castrop formulas had the lowest MAE (0.260, 0.300, 0.300, and 0.270, respectively). Evaluating the refractive result of 171 eyes, Rocha de Lossada [8, 9] found that Barrett and PEARL-DGS performed best for medium eyes (MAE = 0.237 and 0.263, respectively; % eyes <0.5 D = 89.34 and 86.89%, respectively).

Table 52.5 presents and compares the performance of PEARL-DGS and new-generation IOL calculation formulas.

Perspectives

The accuracy of the postoperative refraction calculation depends on the accuracy of the parameters entered in the equation (biometric measurements, IOL geometrical parameters, refractive indices), on the accuracy of the physical lens position prediction, and on how closely the physical model used in the formula approximates the reality. It is therefore interesting to increase the accuracy of the biometric measurements, increase the number of biometric parameters that are measured or known with certainty rather than predicted or assumed, increase the accuracy of the physical models used to perform the calculation, and increase the accuracy of the IOL postoperative physical position.

The PEARL-DGS formula toolbox can be used without modification to back-calculate the TILP value using measured posterior corneal radius and refractive index values, which could increase its performance. Similarly, we advocate for the disclosure of IOL radius of curvatures, thicknesses, and refractive indices by IOL manufacturers.

Our method can also be used without modification to replace the CMAL sum-of-segments AL approximation by an exact, measured sum-of-segments AL value. This more precise way of measuring the AL should logically become the norm. One of the main obstacles for the wide

Table 52.5 Performance comparison of PEARL-DGS and IOL calculation formulas

	Study	First Author	Corresponding Author	Country	Journal	Date	Subgroup
1	Comparison of 13 formulas for IOL power calculation with measurements from partial coherence interferometry	Giacomo Savini	Giacomo Savini	Italy	British Journal of ophthalmology	Jun-20	NA
2	Refractive predictability using the IOLMaster 700 and artificial intelligence–based IOL power formulas compared to standard formulas	Huanhuan Cheng	Mingxing Wu,	China	Journal of refractive surgery	Jul-20	Small groups
3	Outcomes of IOL power calculation using measurements by a rotating camera combined with partial Scheimpflug coherence interferometry	Leonardo Taroni	Leonardo Taroni	Italy	Journal of cataract and refractive surgery	Dec-20	NA
4	Anterior chamber depth, lens thickness and intraocular lens calculation formula accuracy: Nineformulas comparison	Diogo Hipólito-Fernandes	Diogo Hipólito-Fernandes	Portugal	British Journal of ophthalmology	Nov-20	ACD < 3.00 mm / 3.00 < ACD < 3.5 mm / ACD > 3.5 mm
6	VRF-G, a new intraocular lens power calculation formula: A 13-formulas comparison study	Diogo Hipólito-Fernandes	Diogo Hipólito-Fernandes	Portugal	Clinical ophthalmology	Dec-20	
7	Project hyperopic power prediction: Accuracy of 13 different concepts for intraocular lens calculation in short eyes	Jascha Wendelstein	Isaak Raphael Fischinger	Austria	British Journal of ophthalmology	Jan-21	All / SA60AT (n = 111) / ZCB00 (n = 39)

	Study	MedAE (% eyes <0.50D)														
		Barrett Universal II without ACD	Barrett Universal II with ACD	EVO 2.0 without ACD	EVO 2.0 with ACD	Haigis	Hoffer Q	Holladay 1	Holladay 2AL	Kane	Naeser 2	Pearl DGS	RBF 2.0	SRK/T	T2	VRF
1	Comparison of 13 formulas for IOL power calculation with measurements from partial coherence interferometry	0.218 (88%)	0.218 (85.5%)	0.225 (87%)	0.233 (83.5%)	0.240 (82%)	0.229 (84%)	0.232 (88.5%)	0.228 (83%)	0.214 (86.5%)	0.256 (80%)	0.238 (84.5%)	0.215 (85%)	0.223 (86%)	0.228 (88.5%)	0.235 (84.5%)
2	Refractive predictability using the IOLMaster 700 and artificial intelligence–based IOL power formulas compared to standard formulas	NA	0.283	NA	0.293	0.322	0.379	0.376	0.325	0.286	NA	0.305	0.314	0.371	0.317	NA
3	Outcomes of IOL power calculation using measurements by a rotating camera combined with partial Scheimpflug coherence interferometry	NA	0.240 (86.81%)	NA	0.260 (86.81%)	0.244 (78.02%)	0.239 (82.42%)	0.257 (82.42%)	0.285 (82.42%)	0.232 (85.71%)	0.236 (79.12%)	0.190 (86.81%)	0.232 (85.71%)	0.238 (80.22%)	0.245 (85.71%)	0.234 (82.42%)

Table 52.5 (continued)

| Study | MedAE (% eyes <0.50D) | | | | | | | | | | | | | | |
	Barrett Universal II without ACD	Barrett Universal II with ACD	EVO 2.0 without ACD	EVO 2.0 with ACD	Haigis	Hoffer Q	Holladay 1	Holladay 2AL	Kane	Naeser 2	Pearl DGS	RBF 2.0	SRK/T	T2	VRF
4 Anterior chamber depth, lens thickness and intraocular lens calculation formula accuracy: Nineformulas comparison	NA	0.29 (78%)	NA	0.297 (78%)	0.313 (72.7%)	0.295 (71.8%)	0.295 (74.4%)	NA	0.277 (80.2%)	NA	0.270 (81.1%)	0.280 (74.9%)	0.292 (76.7%)	NA	NA
		0.290 (79.6%)		0.297 (80.6%)	0.313 (76.6%)	0.295 (78.6%)	0.288 (79.3%)		0.276 (81.6%)		0.270 (79.9%)	0.280 (77.9%)	0.292 (77.9%)	NA	NA
		0.310 (76.9%)		0.285 (75.7%)	0.319 (75.7%)	0.347 (67.5%)	0.326 (75.7%)		0.286 (76.3%)		0.310 (74%)	0.320 (77.5%)	0.370 (71.6%)	NA	NA
6 VRF-G, a new intraocular lens power calculation formula: A 13-formulas comparison study	NA	0.291 (77.8%)	NA	0.282 (78.5%)	0.309 (74.5%)	0.317 (69.9%)	0.299 (74.3%)	NA	0.274 (79.3%)	0.309 (74.9%)	0.290 (76.9%)	0.291 (76.7%)	0.303 (75.1%)	0.291 (75.5%)	0.293 (76.7%)
7 Project hyperopic power prediction: Accuracy of 13 different concepts for intraocular lens calculation in short eyes	NA	0.330 (62.7%)	NA	0.300 (70%)	0.320 (68%)	0.380 (60.7%)	0.340 (66.7%)	0.380 (66%)	0.300 (78.7%)	NA	0.260 (80%)	0.320 (73.3%)	0.420 (76.9%)	NA	NA
	NA	0.320 (63.1%)	n	0.340 (71.2%)	0.310 (70.3%)	0.380 (62.2%)	0.360 (64%)	0.380 (64.9%)	0.300 (79.3%)	NA	0.270 (77.5%)	0.320 (73%)	0.450 (53.2%)	NA	NA
	NA	0.340 (61.5%)	n	0.260 (66.7%)	0.410 (61.5%)	0.340 (56.4%)	0.250 (74.4%)	0.410 (69.2%)	0.350 (76.9%)	NA	0.260 (87.2%)	0.350 (74.4%)	0.360 (59.3%)	NA	NA

Study	VRF-G	Olsen	Lada SF	Castrop	Okulix	n	IOL	Mean AL +/-SD	Design
1 Comparison of 13 formulas for IOL power calculation with measurements from partial coherence interferometry	NA	NA		NA	NA	200	Hoya Si255	23.66 +/-1.23	Retrospective
2 Refractive predictability using the IOLMaster 700 and artificial intelligence–based IOL power formulas compared to standard formulas	NA	0.283		NA	NA	410	Envista MX60	24.62 +/-2.42	Retrospective
3 Outcomes of IOL power calculation using measurements by a rotating camera combined with partial Scheimpflug coherence interferometry	NA	NA	0.220	NA	NA	91	SN60WF	24.01+/-1.56	Prospective
4 Anterior chamber depth, lens thickness and intraocular lens calculation formula accuracy: Nineformulas comparison	NA	NA	NA	NA	NA	227	SN60WF	22.98 +/-0.66	Retrospective
			NA	NA	NA	299		23.36 +/-0.69	
			NA	NA	NA	169		23.83 +/-0.79	
6 VRF-G, a new intraocular lens power calculation formula: A 13-formulas comparison study	0.273 (79.5%)	NA	NA	NA	NA	828	SN60WF	23.41+/-1.30	Retrospective
7 Project hyperopic power prediction: Accuracy of 13 different concepts for intraocular lens calculation in short eyes	NA	0.330 (70%)	NA	0.270 (74.7%)	0.300 (79.3%)	150	SA60AT or ZCB00	20.98 +/-0.54	Retrospective
	NA	0.330 (68.5%)	NA	0.280 (73.9%)	0.300 (80.2%)	111	SA60 AT		
	NA	0.320 (74.4%)	NA	0.270 (76.9%)	0.280 (76.9%)	39	ZCB00		

adoption of those kinds of innovations is that earlier formulas will perform differently when used with differently measured biometric parameters. Developing a proven, reproducible, and open-source formula-building process could allow researchers to permanently adapt a given formula to new innovations in biometric measurements and newly disclosed IOL parameters.

The advent of OCT in biometry opens new perspectives in the measurement of the anterior segment preoperatively. OCT imaging is unique in its potential ability to both find new biometric parameters (e.g., equatorial lens position [10]) and to directly use anterior segment images in deep learning algorithms, thus opening the door to the use of other powerful AI tools to predict the postoperative lens position.

Acknowledgments The authors would like to sincerely thank Dr Radhika Rampat, Moorfields Eye Hospital, London, UK, for careful proofreading of this chapter.

References

1. Debellemanière G, Dubois M, Gauvin M, Wallerstein A, Brenner LF, Rampat R, Saad A, Gatinel D. The PEARL-DGS Formula: The Development of an Open-source Machine Learning-based Thick IOL Calculation Formula. Am J Ophthalmol. 2021;232: 58–69. https://doi.org/10.1016/j.ajo.2021.05.004.
2. Atchison DA. Optical models for human myopic eyes. Vis Res. 2006;46(14):2236–50.
3. Cooke DL, Cooke TL. A comparison of two methods to calculate axial length. J Cataract Refract Surg. 2019;45(3):284–92.
4. Haigis W, Lege B, Miller N, Schneider B. Comparison of immersion ultrasound biometry and partial coherence interferometry for intraocular lens calculation according to Haigis. Graefes Arch Clin Exp Ophthalmol. 2000;238(9):765–73.
5. Cooke DL, Cooke TL. Approximating sum-of-segments axial length from a traditional optical low-coherence reflectometry measurement. J Cataract Refract Surg. 2019;45(3):351–4.
6. Patel S, Tutchenko L. The refractive index of the human cornea: a review. Cont Lens Anterior Eye. 2019;42(5):575–80.
7. Ophthalmic implants—Intraocular lenses—Part 2: Optical properties and test methods. ISO. 2014. https://www.iso.org/standard/55682.html.
8. Wendelstein J, Hoffmann P, Hirnschall N, Fischinger IR, Mariacher S, Wingert T, et al. Project hyperopic power prediction: accuracy of 13 different concepts for intraocular lens calculation in short eyes. Br J Ophthalmol. 2021;106(6):795–801. https://doi.org/10.1136/bjophthalmol-2020-318272.
9. Rocha-de-Lossada C, Colmenero-Reina E, Flikier D, Castro-Alonso F-J, Rodriguez-Raton A, García-Madrona J-L, et al. Intraocular lens power calculation formula accuracy: comparison of 12 formulas for a tri-focal hydrophilic intraocular lens. Eur J Ophthalmol. 2020;31(6):2981–8.
10. Martinez-Enriquez E, Pérez-Merino P, Durán-Poveda S, Jiménez-Alfaro I, Marcos S. Estimation of intraocular lens position from full crystalline lens geometry: towards a new generation of intraocular lens power calculation formulas. Sci Rep. 2018;8(1):9829.

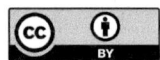

SRK Formula History

53

John Retzlaff and Donald R. Sanders

The seeds that grew into SRK began with the SRK authors, John Retzlaff in Medford Oregon and Manus Kraff and Don Sanders in Chicago, IL, after they independently became discontented with the large number of refractive surprises occurring in their IOL patients. Refractive surprises ocurred despite meticulously measurement of axial length (AL) by applanation, using corneal power (K) and precisely applying the RD Binkhorst formula (as described in his Power Calculation guide) [1].

They studied the IOL power calculation formulas [2–8] which had been published at that time and became familiar with them and their various constants and correction factors. They also noticed that when rearranged, all these formulas were algebraically similar. This is because they are all based on the classical vergence of light formula worked out by Maxwell [9] and others in the 1800s.

Rather than working with the theoretic formula model, Sanders, Retzlaff, and Kraff decided, unknowingly and simultaneously, to pursue the linear regression equation approach, even though they realized biological phenomena are rarely linear.

J. Retzlaff · D. R. Sanders (✉)
Center for Clinical Research, Oak Brook, IL, USA
e-mail: drs@drsmd.com

1977–1980

In 1978, Tom Lloyd, a technician in Jim Gills' office, developed the first linear regression formula for IOL calculation which Gills published in an Editorial [10] in a 1978 Journal of Cataract & Refractive Surgery (JCRS).

Don Sanders met Manus Kraff, while Kraff was the surgical attending during Sanders' last year of residency at Illinois Eye and Ear Infirmary. He finished his residency, accepted a faculty position at the University of Illinois, became the Chief of Ophthalmology at Westside VA Hospital in Chicago, and enrolled in a PhD program at Rush University which gave him access to the University's mainframe computer. While there, he became proficient in the leading statistical software packages of that time (SAS, Statistical Analysis System, and SPSS, Statistical Package for the Social Sciences) and became familiar with programming keypunch cards.

Kraff had the foresight to realize that the best way for him to contribute to ophthalmology would be to analyze clinical data from his extensive and prolific cataract and IOL practice; he was recording data on his cataract/IOL cases on index cards.

It was only natural that they both realized that they could draw on each other's strengths. This resulted in a more than 40-year collaboration with over 40 coauthored peer-reviewed publications, a quarter of which were on IOL power and

© The Author(s) 2024

J. Aramberri et al. (eds.), *Intraocular Lens Calculations*, Essentials in Ophthalmology,
https://doi.org/10.1007/978-3-031-50666-6_53

database computerization. Their first two publications [11, 12] in 1980 were on IOL power calculation. Their first regression formula paper contained an analysis of 923 eyes with six different IOL styles, with each style having at least 120 eyes, a testament to Kraff's data collection skills. Sanders computerized his database, added more variables, and designed protocols. Keypunch cards were ultimately replaced by modem transmission of data for remote analysis as this technology became available.

Meanwhile, in Medford, Oregon, Retzlaff was very busy in his private practice. He had become comfortable with phacoemulsification and was well into IOL implantation. His IOL power calculation research began with his son Steven at Medford High School. This allowed access to the only computer in Southern Oregon powerful enough to do regression analysis.

Fortunately, the district's PhD computer instructor and overseer had John learn enough basic (Gate's and Allen's computer language) to enter data into the system, review the data to weed out entry errors, program the theoretic formulas needed for comparison, and manage the project in general. He procured a regression analysis program robust enough to easily include and test all necessary and available IOL calculation factors (variables) in its hierarchical analysis. He found that picking the brains of his two mathematician duplicate bridge-playing partners was extremely helpful in navigating his way through these unknown waters.

After many months, to his surprise, he found the regression formula he derived to be more accurate than other published formulas available at that time. He presented his positive findings in Portland OR on March 16, 1979, at the 38th Annual Convention of the Oregon Academy of Ophthalmology. By a total coincidence, Kenneth J Hoffer (Chairman of the ASCRS Symposium and Editor of JCRS) was invited to give their Orpha Ellen Reeh Lecture and heard Retzlaff's lecture. He enthusiastically complimented his work and virtually insisted he write up the study and submit it to him for publication in the AIOIS Journal which later became JCRS. Hoffer threatened him that if he did not, he would publish the idea himself. He also told him that his talk would be placed on the program at the next ASCRS Symposium and that if he did not show up, it would be given without him. Retzlaff came and delivered the talk perfectly.

The Journal submitted Retzlaff's paper [13] to Kraff and Sanders to be reviewed. They could have easily killed it. Instead, they wrote a letter to Retzlaff complimenting him on the paper and telling him they were recommending speedy publication. They noted that they themselves were in the midst of a linear regression project and included data, which showed that some of their preliminary regression constants were similar to Retzlaff's regression constants.

A short time later all three were invited individually to each give a presentation of their work at Hoffer's IOL Power Course at the 1979 American Academy of Ophthalmology meeting. They met and an immediate bond formed and intense collaboration began which has continued all these years. There were many phone calls since there was no email and no easy way to exchange data, graphs, and tables. Electronic data exchange was still years away from fruition.

Collaboration Examples

Collaboration 1: One afternoon, Sanders called Retzlaff while he was seeing patients and probably was already half an hour behind schedule. He pointed out the important principle that IOL power data from IOLs of different styles and from different manufacturers must be analyzed separately. Retzlaff quickly and emphatically responded, "Oh, I don't think that's necessary at all." However, Retzlaff quickly realized the irrefutable logic of this principle because, clearly, different IOL styles and manufacturers have different effective powers. He agreed with the principle and adopted it. He had to swallow the bitter fact he had erred by failing to do this in his paper already in publication. It may seem preposterous that John made this error; however, remember that in 1978, some were still, to some extent, in the era of the Standard Lens Method, meaning every patient received the same power IOL (not everyone had an A-scan unit).

Collaboration 2: On another occasion, Retzlaff, referring to the regression equation of the form x = A + By + Cz, told Sanders: "I've started doing regression analysis on different data sets using a fixed 'B' and 'C' constant and allowing only the 'A' constant to vary." After getting an explanation of this peculiar process, Sanders told him, "You can't do that." He responded, "Well, I've done it and it works." This capricious "peculiar process" of doing regression equations with one or more of the constants fixed led to our realization that handling the regression equations in this manner, i.e., calculating an individual A-constant for each style of IOL, provides a single, specific index value for each IOL, a powerful piece of information. Manufacturers could then provide surgeons with the needed A-constants or the surgeons could calculate their own personal A-constants.

Most of our IOL discussions occurred on the weekends. We were doing extensive data analysis. We explored AL and K, preoperative anterior chamber depth (ACD_{PRE}) measured from epithelium to lens, possible correction factors, regression math using multiplicative and exponential terms, and curve fitting. Using regression analysis, we also investigated factors including preoperative refraction (recent and old), cataract type, gender, and age. We did not find that any of these factors improved prediction accuracy.

Preoperative ACD (ACD_{PRE})

During their research into IOL power using regression analysis, Kraff and Sanders measured ACD_{PRE} with the Haag-Streit optical anterior chamber pachymeter to test the predictive value of this variable (ACD_{PRE}) in IOL power calculation. ACD_{PRE}, AL, and K were analyzed in hierarchical steps by the computer program, i.e., the factor most helpful in predicting IOL power was added to the equation first, the factor that was next in importance was added second, and so on. AL was the single most important factor in predicting implant power. K was second in impor-

tance. We found that ACD_{PRE} improved the prediction accuracy by less than 1%. Similarly, using ACD_{PRE} in various mathematical forms (exponents, etc.) was still, in our model, not any more predictive of IOL power than using AL and K alone. Bagan and Brubaker [14] reached the same conclusion in their study of ACD_{PRE}. However, history has shown that this was not true.

1980: SRK Is Born

Determination of the order of the letters in the formula name (what order would the initials be placed: KRS, RKS, SRK) was decided with a coin toss. Kraff contends that the coin toss agreement was, "Retzlaff heads, Sanders tails, and Kraff if the coin lands on its edge and stays there." When that was settled, we developed a logo (Fig. 53.1). We were satisfied that we had thoroughly explored the available variables using multiple mathematical tools. We were delighted we had boiled all this information and all these possibilities down into a truly simple mathematical form:

$$P = A - 2.5^* AL - 0.9^* K$$

This needed only AL, K, and a constant "A" for each IOL. The predictive accuracy of the new formula was compared to previously published formulas, and the SRK was found to be consistently more accurate. Our first two-principle SRK papers were published in 1980, Retzlaff's in April [13] and Sanders and Kraff's in July [12].

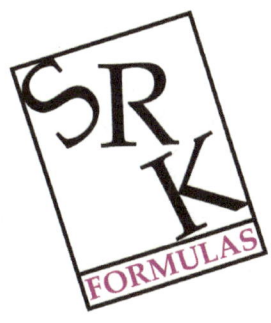

Fig. 53.1 SRK formulas logo

Paper Summary: Retzlaff

"Data from 166 eyes with iridocapsular implants were analyzed and different prediction methods were compared. A new formula was derived which predicted implant power better than any other method. The theoretic formulas and correction factors of Fyodorov, Colenbrander, and others were examined in detail and compared to the more accurate, simpler linear regression formula derived in this study."

Paper Summary: Sanders Kraff

"It can be produced with different constants (A, B, and C) for each type of lens implant and each manufacturer. We have determined the constants for iris-fixated, anterior chamber, and posterior chamber lens implants, based on data from 923 cases. The results have been more accurate than those from presently available theoretical formulas, and the well-known phenomenon of predicting too much dioptric power in eyes with short axial lengths has been avoided. Only 1% of the cases had a predicted lens power more than 3 diopters in error."

The addendum below introduced the exact, first SRK formula.

Addendum: In an attempt to simplify the regression formula even further, in cooperation with Dr. John Retzlaff , we have set the constants B and C the same for all implants and determined the best-fit A-constant. The following formula: Predicted implant power $= A - 2.5 \times AL - 0.9 \times K$ was tested with A = 115.5 (medallion-style lenses, Medical Workshop); A = 114.8 (medallion-style lenses, Intermedics Intraocular); A = 115.7 (Choyce-style lenses, Rayner/Coburn); A = 114.3 (Tennant-style lenses, Precision-Cosmet); and A = 116.0 (single-plane and angulated Shearing-style lenses, IOLAB).

After it was introduced, the simple SRK regression formula was used extensively by ophthalmologists worldwide for many years. During this early period, some ultrasonic AL measuring units did not have built-in IOL power calculation formulas. The most common method of calculation was the use of a Texas Instruments (TI) handheld programmable calculator with the R

Binkhorst formula built into a PROM (programmable read-only) chip. A dedicated thermal printer was attached. This was sold by Sonometrics, the most prominent A-scan manufacturer at the time.

Sanders and Retzlaff decided that to truly gain widespread acceptance of the SRK formula at this early period, they had to make the formula available for the same TI system used by R Binkhorst and Sonometrics. They soon learned that they had to program the PROM chip and purchase a minimum of 1000 chips from TI at a cost of tens of thousands of dollars; any coding errors required scrapping the PROMs.

Fortunately, they tested the step-by-step PROM programming meticulously and repeatedly and our PROM was accurate the first time around. In a short period of time, the SRK team, in conjunction with Sonometrics, sold all of the PROMs and the SRK formula became the most widely used IOL power calculation formula worldwide. Soon thereafter, IOL calculation formulas became more available in A-scan devices further increasing the reach of the SRK formula.

Early 1980s

During the 1980s, the IOL frenzy settled down to a merely exhilarating, challenging, and constantly changing activity. IOL power courses were plentiful. RD Binkhorst, Kenneth J Hoffer and John Shammas, Jack Holladay, Michael Cravy, Bobby Osher, Jim Gills, and Gale Martin, as well as ourselves, were active doing courses. We pounded away on practical issues emphasizing meticulous measurement of AL and K and avoiding mix-ups of data, power calculation reports, and IOLs themselves. During these courses, formulas were not discussed much; the main formulas being used at the time were SRK, R Binkhorst, and less frequently Hoffer; so, there was not much to talk about.

The art of selecting the best IOL power for each individual patient was by considering the patient's previous refraction and spectacle use, then discussing the patient's desires and expectations including monovision, then checking the

IOL power printout for both eyes looking for errors, and finally, selecting the best IOL power for that patient, not necessarily 20/20 distance vision.

Late 1980s SRK II

By the late 1980s, IOL implantation had become an almost universal part of cataract surgery. Patient selection had expanded from only healthy average-length eyes to virtually all cataract surgery eyes. The Holladay 1 formula [15] was published and became available on a TI calculator. It became quite popular, and results showed it superior to the SRK regression. With time, it became increasingly apparent that a pure linear formula was inaccurate in extremely long and short eyes. This led to modifying the original SRK formula by developing the SRK II [16]. The goal was to create a new formula more accurate than existing formulas and to retain simplicity. Extensive modeling and analysis improved the accuracy of the original SRK formula for short (>22 mm) and long (≥25 mm) eyes.

Similar in form to the existing SRK regression formula, power was added to the SRK formula in a stepwise fashion for short eyes and subtracted for long eyes. The SRK II formula was developed from seven data sets: 2068 eyes (which included 167 short eyes, 306 long eyes, and 1595 average eyes). Extensive modeling and analysis improved the accuracy of the original SRK formula and yet retained the simple, do-it-in-your-head characteristic of the original.

Secret Formulas

As a group, the SRK collaborators have always felt that formulas that had hidden or secret relationships between variables were unwise in scientific discourse. They make it more difficult to perform head-to-head comparisons between formulas and methods. Proprietary secret IOL formulas first appeared with the Holladay 2 formula which was marketed in a proprietary software program and later in some biometers. The code

was never published. Since that time, almost all new formulas have been relatively secret. Interestingly, most cataract surgeons are not aware that so many IOL power calculation formulas are secret.

From Fyodorov [2] to SRK/T [18, 19], Hoffer Q [20], and Haigis [21], formulas have all been published in detail so others could test them independently, program and modify them, and learn from them. Having the SRK family of formulas published in detail has certainly not harmed its popularity and commercial success. On the other hand, with the modern use of artificial intelligence (AI) and complex algorithms, it would not be easy for a clinician to duplicate them even if they were published, as has been recently done for the PEARL-DGS formula [17] from France.

1990 SRK/T

In 1987, the SRK II had been completed and was published. Retzlaff was planning retirement from his surgical practice but due to the success of the Holladay 2 formula over the SRK formulas, it was decided to re-evaluate the formula. Retzlaff sets out to (1) create "an empiric formula that uses the nonlinear terms of theoretical formulas" (as so elegantly stated by Rasooly et al. [22]) and (2) compare a new formula to other formulas using an entirely separate independent data set. Thus, two separate data sets were used for the project. Development of the SRK/T formula was done with the first of these data sets (1677 eyes); the comparison of the accuracy of the new formula was done with the second data set (2068 eyes).

SRK/T Development

The project plan was to work with the vergence of light formula [9], which is the basic structure of all theoretic formulas. Early theoretic formulas were restudied. Particular attention was focused on Fyodorov's [2] 1967 corneal height work (which Holladay had used) by utilizing anterior segment measurements. Factors considered in the first SRK publications were tested using regression analysis within the framework of the theoretic formula structure. Extensive optimization efforts including curve fitting and regression using multiplicative and exponential terms were carried out. We presented our development methods and code, in considerable detail, to facilitate continued research into IOL power calculation.

The new IOL power calculation SRK/T formula was developed using the nonlinear terms of the theoretical formulas as its foundation but using empirical regression methodology for optimization. Postoperative anterior chamber depth prediction (ELP), retinal thickness AL correction, and corneal refractive index were systematically and interactively optimized using an interactive process on five data sets consisting of 1677 posterior chamber lens cases. The new SRK/T formula performed slightly better than the Holladay 1, SRK II, R Binkhorst, and Hoffer formulas, which was the expected result as any formula performs superiorly with the data from which it was derived. The comparative accuracy of this formula upon independent data sets is addressed in a follow-up report. The formula derived provides a primary theoretical approach under the SRK umbrella of formulas and has the added advantage of being useable with the SRK A-constants that have been empirically derived over the previous 9 years or using converted anterior chamber depth estimates.

SRK/T Accuracy Comparison: Independent Data Sets

In 1988, Richard Brubaker, chief of ophthalmology at Mayo Clinic, commented to Retzlaff: "You cannot test a formula's prediction accuracy with the data you used to derive the formula." After asking why, Brubaker smiled and said, "You just can't!" The logic of using independent data is so compelling that it should be self-evident but it was not evident to us until it was pointed out by Brubaker. Examination of papers presenting new formulas shows that this principle was also violated by Fyodorov and Galin [4], R Binkhorst [5], Colenbrander [3], Thisson [6],

Holladay [16], and Haigis [20]. Also, how the creators of unpublished formulas handled data set selection to test their formulas' prediction accuracy is impossible to determine because it is secret.

SRK/T Accuracy Comparison 1990

We compared the predictive accuracy of the SRK/T formula to the SRK II, R Binkhorst II, Hoffer, and Holladay 1 formulas in seven series of cases totaling 1050 eyes. In the combined group, the SRK/T and Holladay formulas performed only slightly better than the other formulas. In short eyes (<22 mm), all formulas performed well, with the SRK/T, SRK II, and Holladay formulas performing marginally better (not statistically better). In moderately long eyes (>24.5 and ≤27 mm), the Hoffer and R Binkhorst II formulas had a greater proportion of cases with >2 diopters (D) of error and the SRK/T and Holladay 1 were again marginally better. In the very long eyes (>27 and ≤28.4 mm), there were only 11 cases and all formulas performed well since none had >2.00 D of prediction error. In an extremely long eye data set (>28.4 mm), the SRK II formula clearly gave the poorest result. Eyes of this length occurred in only 0.1% of cases in this unselected series. Results support the contention that the present second- and third-generation formulas give fairly equivalent accuracy. Other factors, such as availability, ease of use, and ability to tailor or individualize them, become major considerations.

SRK/T Errata

It is important to note that, unfortunately, there have been two published errata for the SRK/T 1990 publication (1990;16(3):333–340), one in 1990 and another in 1993.

Immediately after it was first published, Hoffer was attempting to program the formulas of Hoffer, Holladay 1, and the SRK/T into a Casio calculator and discovered a problem with the SRK/T that seemed to be caused by the L_{COR}

(corrected AL formula). He immediately called Retzlaff and luckily reached him right away. Retzlaff knew exactly what the problem was, corrected it, and submitted the erratum to JCRS which was published in the very next issue (JCRS 1990;16(4):528). It specifically corrects two formulas: the first defined the AL correction L_{COR} as $= -3.466 + 1.715*AL-0.237*AL^2$ if the AL was >24.2 and if AL was ≤24.2, then the actual AL was used unaltered. The second was that if the AL was <24.5, then C = 0 but if ≥24.5, then C = −0.50.

The second occurred in 1993 after a published letter to the editor in JCRS by Haigis, who pointed out several issues with the formula leading to a response letter from the authors and a full explanation of the issues raised (1993;19(5):444–446). In the part of the formula for ELP prediction, they left out the limitation on H: "If H < 0, H = 0" creating meaningless results in some cases. The other issue was the sudden drop in results of IOL power when the AL >26 mm.

Since almost all use of the SRK/T formula was through legitimately licensed instruments that were correct and properly programmed, these issues only caused problems for the few who were programming it themselves based only on the original publication.

Closing Remarks and Thoughts

We find it remarkable that a concept and a brand that took shape more than 40 years ago still have relevance and use in clinical ophthalmology today, while the original IOL designs, most of the companies that made them, and the axial length measuring devices upon which SRK formulas were based are no longer used. We feel blessed to be some of the "last men standing" in this field.

References

1. Binkhorst RD. Intraocular lens power calculations manual. New York: Binkhorst RD; 1978.
2. Fyodorov SN, Kolonko AI. Estimation of optical power of the intraocular lens. Vestnik Oftalmologic (Moscow). 1967;4:27.
3. Colenbrander MC. Calculations of the power of an iris-clip lens for distance vision. Br J Ophthalmol. 1973;57:735–40.
4. Fyodorov SN, Galin MA, Linksz A. Calculation of the optical power of an intraocular lens. Invest Ophthal. 1975;14:625–8.
5. Binkhorst RD. Pitfalls in the determination of intraocular lens power without ultrasound. Ophthal Surg. 1976;5:69–82. Ophthal Surg. 1975;6(3):17–31.
6. Thijssen JM. The emmetropic and iseikonic implant lens: computer calculations of the refractive power and its accuracy. Ophthalmologica. 1975;171:467–86.
7. Hoffer KJ. Intraocular lens calculation: the problem of the short eye. Ophthal Surg. 1981;12:269–72.
8. Van Der Heijde GL, Fechner PU, Worst JG. Optical consequences of implantation of a negative intraocular lens in myopic patients [Ger]. Klinische Monatsblatter Fur Augenheilkundle. 1988;193(1):99–102.
9. Maxwell JC. A dynamical theory of the electromagnetic field. Philos Trans R Soc Lond. 1865;155:459–512. Pg 499. [Archived from the original on 28 July 2011].
10. Gills JP. Regression formula (editorial). J Cataract Refract Surg. 1978;4:163. and Minimizing postoperative refractive error. Contact Intraoc Lens Med J. 1980;6:56.
11. Sanders DR, Kraff MC. Computerization of intraocular lens data. J Cataract Refract Surg. 1980;6:156–9.
12. Sanders D, Kraff M. Improvement of intraocular lens power calculation using empirical data. J Cataract Refract Surg. 1980;6(3):263–7. Errata 1981;7(1): 82.
13. Retzlaff J. A new intraocular lens calculation formula. J Cataract Refract Surg. 1980;6:148–52.
14. Bagan SM, Brubaker RF. Prediction of artiphakic anterior chamber depth. Ophthal Surgery. 1980;11(11):768–70.
15. Holladay JT, Praeger TC, Chandler TY, Musgrove KH. A three part system for refining intraocular lens power calculations. J Cataract Refract Surg. 1988;14(17):24.
16. Sanders DR, Retzlaff J, Kraff MC. Comparison of the SRK II formula and the other second generation formulas. J Cataract Refract Surg. 1988;14(3):136–41.
17. Debellemanière G, Dubois M, Gauvin M, Wallerstein A, Brenner LF, Rampat R, et al. The Pearl-DGS formula: the development of an open-source machine learning-based thick IOL calculation formula. Am J Ophthalmol. 2021;232:58–69.
18. Retzlaff J, Sanders DR, Kraff MC. Development of the SRK/T intraocular lens implant power calculations formula. J Cataract Refract Surg. 1990;16(3):333–40. Errata: 1990;16(4):528 and 1993;19(5):444–446.
19. Sanders DR, Retzlaff J, Kraff MC, Gimbell H, Raanan M. Comparison of the SRK/T formula and other theoretical and regression formulas. J Cataract Refract Surg. 1990;16(3):341–6.
20. Hoffer KJ. The Hoffer Q formula: a comparison of theoretic and regression formulas. J Cataract Refract Surg. 1993;19(11):700–12. Errata 1994;20:677 and 2007;33(1):2–3.

21. Haigis W, Lege B, Miller N, Schneider B. Comparison of immersion ultrasound biometry and partial coherence interferometry for intraocular lens calculation according to Haigis. Graefes Arch Clin Exp Ophthalmol. 2000;238:765–73.

22. Rasooly R, Zauberman H. Correlations between ocular optical components, height and head circumference. Ophthalmic Physiol Opt. 1988;8(3):3:51–2.

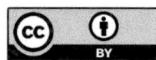

The T2 Formula

54

Richard Sheard, Guy Smith, and David L. Cooke

Introduction

The SRK/T formula was first described in 1990 [1] and has subsequently become one of the most widely used formulas used to predict the intraocular lens (IOL) power for implantation following cataract surgery. The original article contained errors, which were later corrected [2]. In 1993, Haigis reported a further problem with the published version of the SRK/T formula in which, for particular combinations of axial length and corneal power, the formula algorithm may attempt to take the square root of a negative number leading to erroneous results [3]. This is "the imaginary anterior chamber depth (ACD) problem", and in their reply, the SRK/T authors suggested a solution. In the same response, they also discussed that, under certain circumstances, a non-physiological irregularity in the predicted IOL power is observed [3]. The authors called this the "SRK/T cusp" (Fig. 54.1) and invited colleagues to send examples of cases in which this phenomenon was observed to investigate it further.

Our study was the first to investigate the cause of the SRK/T cusp and to systematically evaluate its clinical significance [4]. We then developed a modification of the formula to eliminate the cusp phenomenon and evaluated its performance. We refer to the new formula algorithm as the T2 formula [4].

R. Sheard (✉)
Derwent Eye Specialists, Hobart, Australia
e-mail: richard.sheard@derwenteye.com.au

G. Smith
Great Western Hospital, Wiltshire, UK

Matrix Eye Clinic, Wiltshire, UK
e-mail: guy.smith1@nhs.net

D. L. Cooke
Department of Neurology and Ophthalmology,
Michigan State University, College of Osteopathic
Medicine, East Lansing, MI, USA

Great Lakes Eye Care, St. Joseph, MI, USA

© The Author(s) 2024
J. Aramberri et al. (eds.), *Intraocular Lens Calculations*, Essentials in Ophthalmology,
https://doi.org/10.1007/978-3-031-50666-6_54

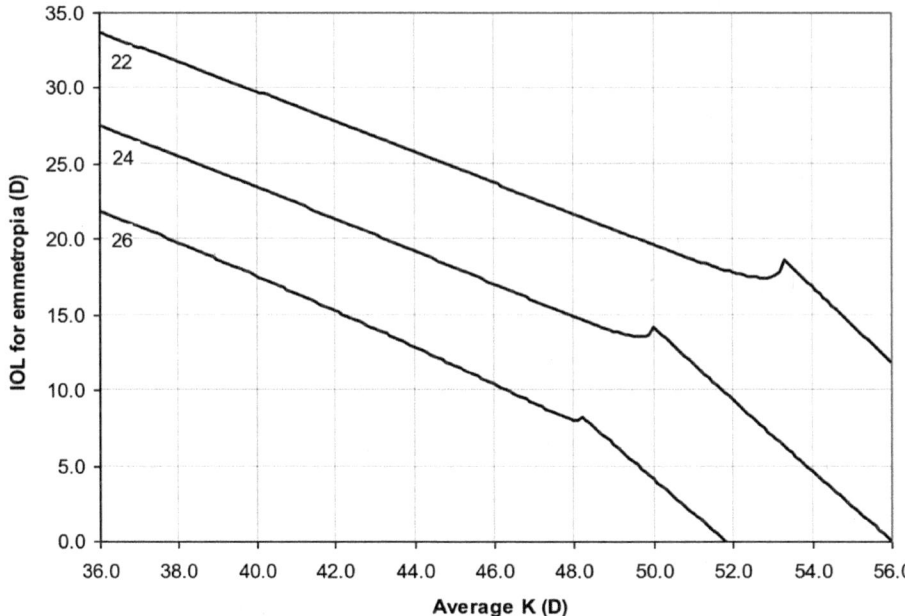

Fig. 54.1 Graph showing non-physiological discontinuity in the IOL power for emmetropia calculated by the SRK/T formula with varying corneal power (K) at three different axial lengths (22, 24 and 26 mm). Reproduced with permission from [4]

Non-physiological Behaviour in the SRK/T Formula

The SRK/T formula determines the required IOL power (in dioptres) for a desired post-operative refraction from the pre-operative average corneal power, K (dioptres), and axial length, L (millimetres).

Our study examined each of the steps of the SRK/T formula algorithm for non-physiological behaviour by varying the input variables and plotting a graph of the output value. For physiological behaviour, one would expect to see a smooth curve over the physiological range of input variables. We defined non-physiological behaviour as an unexpected or illogical discontinuity in the curve, and we observed such non-physiological behaviour in the calculation of corrected axial length and corneal height.

We investigated the possible impact of the non-physiological behaviour of the SRK/T formula with reference to a large cataract surgery database. The reference database records the full biometric data (measured with the IOL Master) and refractive outcome in 11,189 eyes, using ten different models of posterior chamber IOL [4].

Non-physiological Behaviour in the Calculation of Corrected Axial Length

Step 2 of the SRK/T formula algorithm derives the corrected axial length, known as *LCOR*, which for axial lengths greater than 24.2 mm entails a quadratic expression [1–3]. As a result, *LCOR* reaches its maximal value of 27.62 mm at an axial length of 36.20 mm. For axial lengths above this value, *LCOR* progressively decreases, a behaviour which is illogical. We refer to this phenomenon as the "*LCOR* reversal". The LCOR reversal affects only extremely long eyes with axial lengths greater than 36.20 mm. These eyes are very uncommon; in the reference database, we found no such examples [4].

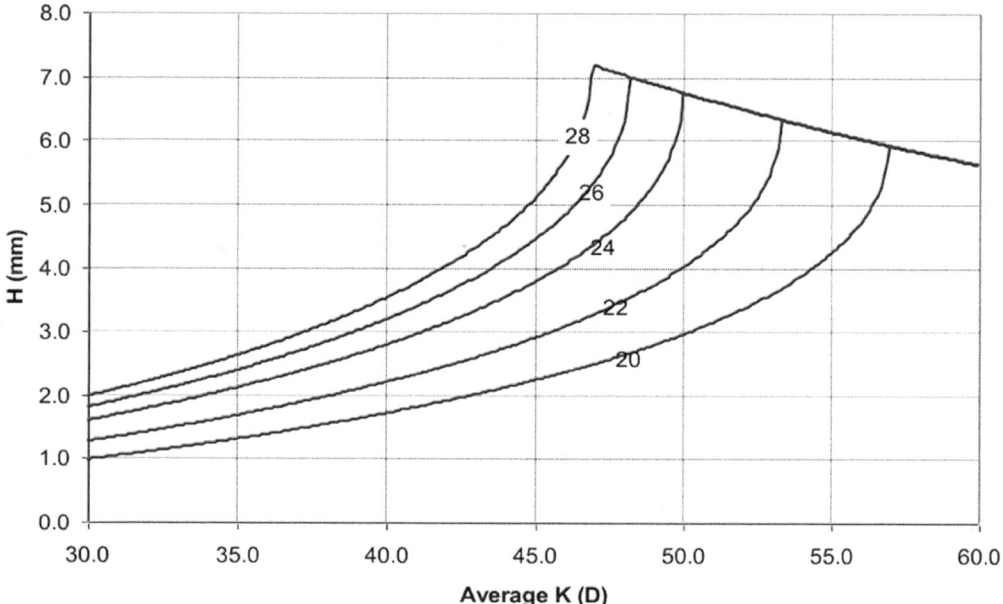

Fig. 54.2 Graph showing the non-physiological variation of the SRK/T calculated corneal height (H) with corneal power (average K) for different axial lengths as indicated (mm). Reproduced with permission from [4]

Non-physiological Behaviour in the Calculation of Corneal Height

Step 4 of the SRK/T formula algorithm calculates the corneal height, H [1–3]. Fig. 54.2 shows the variation of H with various combinations of L and K. The shape of the curve is clearly non-physiological in all cases, with H increasing rapidly to a peak with increasing K, after which the gradient reverses. The shape of the curve resembles the non-physiological irregularity of the SRK/T cusp phenomenon (Fig. 54.1). We therefore refer to the peak of the curve as the corneal height cusp. For a given axial length, L, there is a unique corneal power, K_{cusp}, at which the corneal height, H, is maximal.

Clinical Significance of the Corneal Height Cusp

The shape of the corneal height curves suggests that, in the vicinity of the cusp, the SRK/T formula may over-estimate the corneal height (Fig. 54.2). In consequence, the estimated effec-

tive IOL position will be further from the cornea and closer to the retina, resulting in an overestimate of IOL power. This hypothesis fits empirically with the original observation of the SRK/T cusp (Fig. 54.1) [3].

Figure 54.3 plots the axial length and corneal power of the eyes in the reference database. The figure also plots K_{cusp} against L and, for ease of interpretation, indicates five dioptre-wide bands below the cusp. Two eyes have measured corneal powers greater than K_{cusp} for their axial length ("above the cusp"). 1234 eyes (11.0%) fall into the band within 5 dioptres below the cusp, 9593 (85.7%) are between 5 and 10 dioptres below the cusp and 360 (3.2%) between 10 and 15 dioptres below [4]. The eyes above or close to the cusp may be affected by the SRK/T corneal height error, but it is not possible to determine from these data how many and to what degree.

We applied the SRK/T formula "backwards" to each eye in the reference database to determine the value of H that would be required to give the observed refractive outcome. We refer to this as the back-calculated corneal height, H_{back}. We then calculated the corneal height error, $H - H_{back}$, for

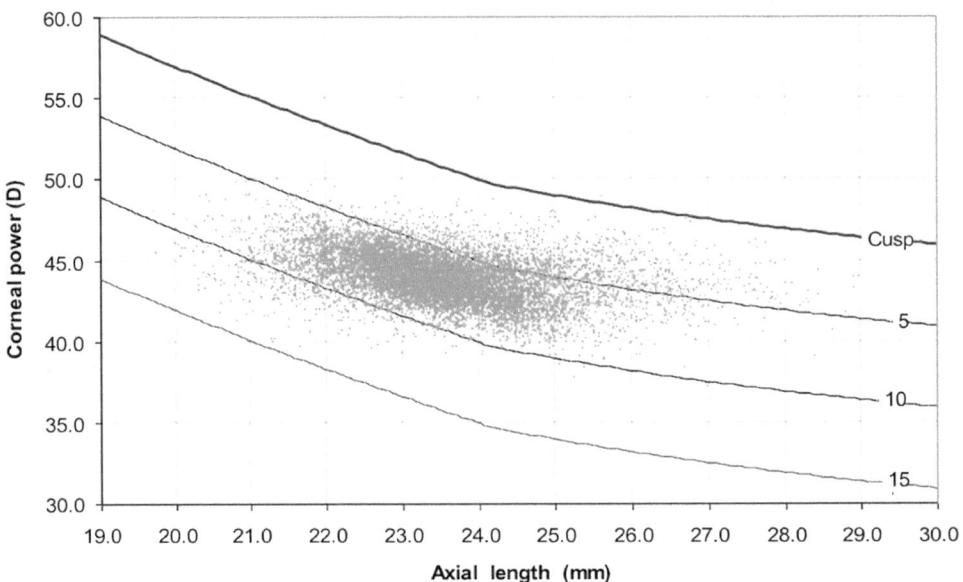

Fig. 54.3 Graph showing the combination of axial length and corneal power at which the SRK/T corneal height cusp occurs (heavy line). The light lines highlight bands 5, 10 and 15 dioptres below the cusp. The points plotted represent the axial length and corneal power combination of the 11,189 eyes from the reference database. Reproduced with permission from [4]

each eye. We segregated eyes from the database into one dioptre bands below the cusp, and Fig. 54.4 shows the mean corneal height error within each band. The graph confirms that the SRK/T formula tends to over-estimate the corneal height as the corneal power approaches the cusp. The SRK/T error in corneal height prediction appears to be systematic, progressively decreasing with increasing distance below the cusp such that, for corneal powers 7 D or more below the cusp, the predicted corneal height tends to be an under-estimate. The differences in corneal height error between the bands were highly statistically significant (one-way ANOVA: $p < 0.0001$) [4].

As we hypothesized, the SRK/T formula tends to over-estimate the corneal height for eyes with a combination of L and K close to the cusp and, as a result, potentially over-estimates the IOL power. However, Fig. 54.4 also shows that SRK/T under-estimates the corneal power for eyes more than 7 D below the cusp with a likely under-estimate of IOL power. These systematic errors, being in opposite directions, will cancel out across a dataset and have therefore not previously been identified. The corneal height error is the most likely explanation for the observation in several studies that the optimized SRK/T A-constant varies with corneal power and, indirectly, axial length [5–8].

The clinical significance of the corneal height error in an individual eye depends on its geometry, but for an average eye (axial length 23 mm and corneal power 44 D) a 0.3 mm error in corneal height prediction results in an IOL power prediction error of 0.25 D. In the reference dataset, 3485 eyes (31.1%) had a corneal height error of more than 0.3 mm [4].

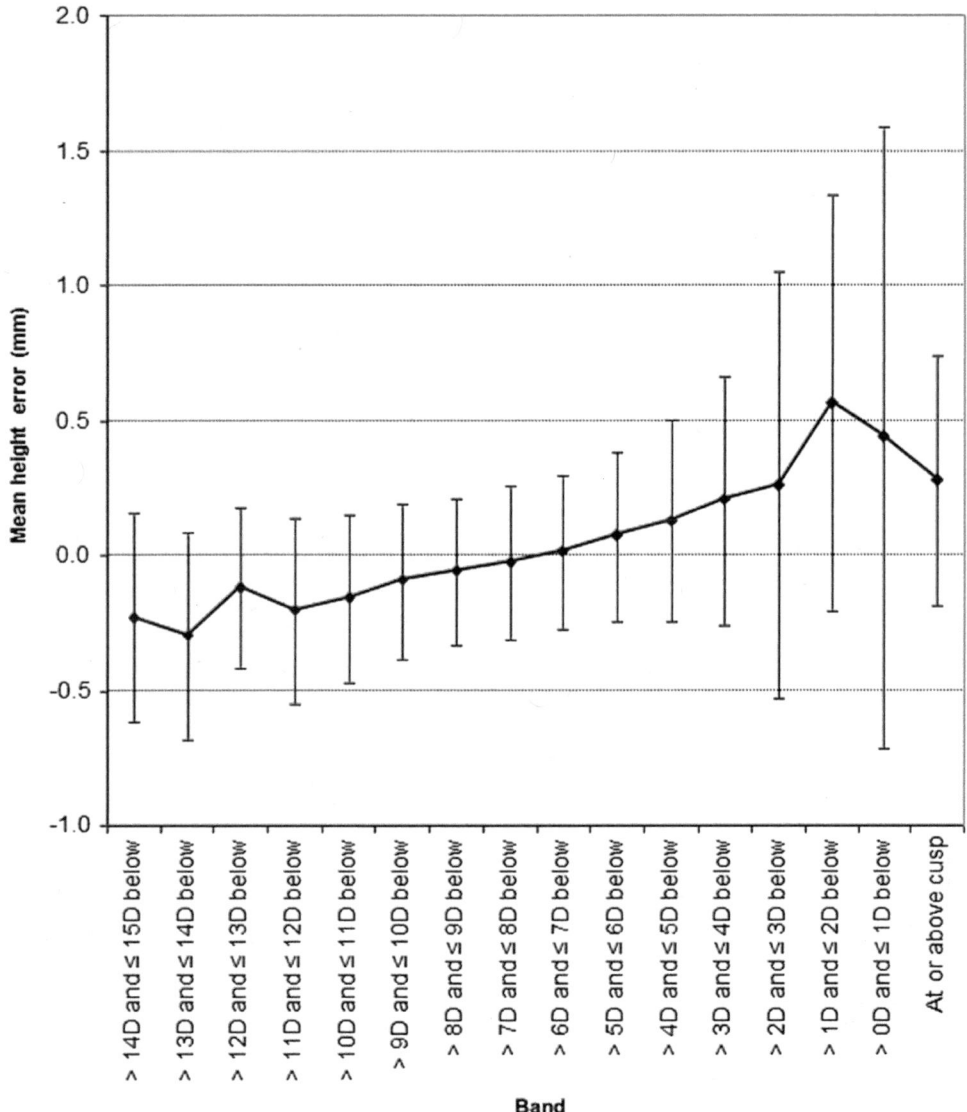

Fig. 54.4 Mean difference between the SRK/T formula's predicted corneal height and the back-calculated corneal height in 11,189 eyes, banded according to their proximity to the cusp (bars indicate standard deviation). Reproduced with permission from [4]

Solution to the SRK/T Cusp: The T2 Formula

The SRK/T cusp arises from the equations employed to predict the corneal height [1–3]. Elimination of the cusp, therefore, requires a new method for corneal height calculation. One solution is to use a regression formula derived from real data, and if a linear regression model is employed, the resulting formula will be free of non-physiological anomalies.

We randomly divided the reference dataset of 11,189 eyes into a development subset used to derive a regression formula for corneal height calculation (5588 eyes), and an evaluation subset to assess its performance in comparison with the standard SRK/T formula (5601 eyes) [4].

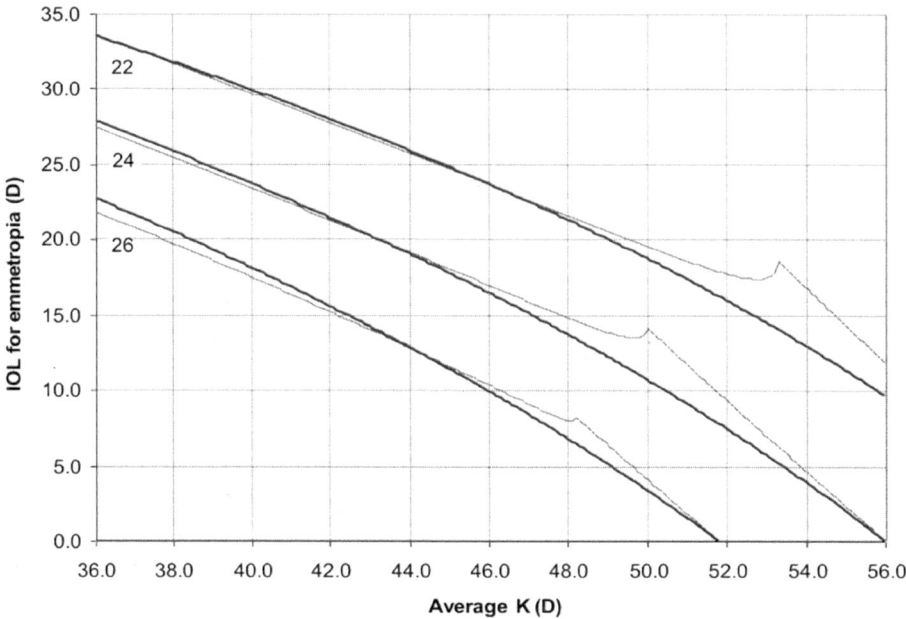

Fig. 54.5 Graph showing IOL power for emmetropia with varying corneal power (K) at three different axial lengths (22, 24 and 26 mm). The heavy lines show the T2 formula and the light lines the SRK/T. Reproduced with permission from [4]

To develop the new corneal height regression formula, we determined H_{back} for each eye in the development subset as described earlier. Multiple linear regression was performed using H_{back} as the dependent variable and corneal power (K) and either axial length (L) or corrected axial length ($LCOR$) as independent variables. Two regression equations were derived for H_2, the estimated corneal height, are as follows:

$$H_2 = -10.326 + 0.32630 \cdot L + 0.13533 \cdot K$$
(54.1)

$$H_2 = -11.980 + 0.38626 \cdot LCOR + 0.14177 \cdot K$$
(54.2)

Equation (54.1) showed a higher correlation coefficient ($R^2 = 0.5566$ vs. 0.5404) and lower standard error (0.3147 vs. 0.3204) and was therefore selected for further investigation. Since the SRK/T formula only uses $LCOR$ as an intermediate step in the corneal height calculation, the use of Eq. (54.1) renders a solution for the $LCOR$ reversal unnecessary. We programmed a new version of the SRK/T formula by simply replacing the corneal height calculation step with Eq. (54.1). We refer to the modified version as the **T2 formula** [4], and Fig. 54.5 confirms the elimination of the SRK/T cusp phenomenon.

Evaluation of the T2 Formula

We compared the clinical performance of the T2 formula with the SRK/T by calculating the spectacle prediction error (PE) of each formula in the evaluation subset of eyes, using separate IOL-specific A-constants optimized for each formula (mean PE: SRK/T 0.0019 D, T2 0.0004 D). When compared to the SRK/T, the T2 formula results demonstrate a significantly lower standard deviation (SD: SRK/T 0.4167 D, T2 0.3960 D; F-test: $p < 0.0001$) and mean absolute error (MAE: SRK/T: 0.3217 D, T2: 0.3052 D; t-test: $p < 0.0001$). Table 54.1 shows the number and proportion of eyes within ±0.25 D, ±0.5 D and ±1 D of prediction for the two formulas; in all cases, the T2 formula shows a statistically significant improvement over the SRK/T.

Table 54.1 Proportion of eyes in the evaluation subset (n = 5601) within ±0.25 D, ±0.5 D and ±1 D of prediction

	SRK/T	T2 formula	McNemar's test
Within ±0.25 D	2710 (48.4%)	2818 (50.3%)	$p = 0.0002$
Within ±0.50 D	4416 (78.7%)	4516 (80.9%)	$p < 0.0001$
Within ±1.00 D	5487 (98.0%)	5510 (98.5%)	$p = 0.0003$

A small number of subsequent studies have evaluated the performance of the T2 formula [9–11]. These confirm that, across the full range of axial lengths, the T2 formula is significantly more accurate than the SRK/T formula and the other third-generation IOL formulas. When analysed according to subgroups of axial length, the T2 formula matches or exceeds the performance of other third-generation formulas for the short-, medium- and medium-long groups [9]. For long eyes (axial length > 26 mm), the results are conflicting. Cooke and Cooke confirmed that the T2 formula is more accurate than the SRK/T in this subgroup also [10], but other series show that the SRK/T formula may be more accurate than the T2 formula [9, 12].

Conclusion

Our study set out to understand the cause of the SRK/T cusp phenomenon and, in doing so, identified a systematic error in corneal height calculation. Our large reference dataset allowed us to evaluate the importance of the corneal height error and to propose a solution. The development of the T2 formula achieved its goal of eliminating the SRK/T cusp and, in consequence, delivered a statistically and clinically significant performance improvement in what was, at the time, the largest independent study to examine the performance of the SRK/T formula. The A-constants required by the T2 formula are almost identical to those of the SRK/T; in our study, they differed by no more than ±0.03 D. The T2 formula can therefore be used as a direct substitute for the SRK/T.

More recent fourth-generation formulas using more ocular measurements (e.g. phakic anterior chamber depth, lens thickness and horizontal corneal diameter in addition to keratometry and axial length) or algorithms employing ray tracing and artificial intelligence paradigms are more accurate than the third-generation formulas, of which the T2 formula is one [13]. It is likely that in routine clinical practice third-generation formulas are now obsolete, but they may retain a role in circumstances where the parameters required by the more modern formulas cannot be measured. For example, phakic anterior chamber depth (ACD) and lens thickness, required by many of the newer formulas, cannot be obtained in aphakic eyes requiring secondary intraocular lens implantation or in pseudophakic eyes requiring IOL exchange, and the measured phakic ACD is likely to be anomalous in eyes with a subluxated crystalline lens. It can be shown that the performance of the fourth-generation formulas is degraded by missing input parameters (personal communication, David Cooke). Li et al. studied refractive outcomes of lens implantation in eyes with insufficient capsular support and demonstrated that the SRK/T formula was the most accurate, including in comparison with the Haigis (requires phakic ACD) and Barrett Universal II formulas (requires phakic ACD and lens thickness) [14]. The authors did not evaluate the T2 formula in their study, but there is no reason to expect that it would not perform better than the SRK/T in this context, similar to the findings in the setting of standard cataract surgery.

References

1. Retzlaff JA, Sanders DR, Kraff MC. Development of the SRK/T intraocular lens implant power calculation formula. J Cataract Refract Surg. 1990;16:333–40.
2. Erratum. J Cataract Refract Surg. 1990;16:528.
3. Haigis W. Occurrence of erroneous anterior chamber depth in the SRK/T formula. J Cataract Refract Surg. 1993;19:442–3. Author reply J Cataract Refract Surg. 1993;19:443–6.
4. Sheard RM, Smith GT, Cooke DL. Improving the prediction accuracy of the SRK/T formula: the T2 formula. J Cataract Refract Surg. 2010;36:1829–34.

5. Petermeier K, Gekeler F, Messias A, et al. Intraocular lens power calculation and optimized constants for highly myopic eyes. J Cataract Refract Surg. 2009;35:1575–81.

6. Aristodemou P, Knox Cartwright NE, Sparrow JM, Johnston RL. Intraocular lens formula constant optimization and partial coherence interferometry biometry: refractive outcomes in 8108 eyes after cataract surgery. J Cataract Refract Surg. 2011;37:50–62.

7. Eom Y, Kang SY, Song JS, Kim HM. Use of corneal power-specific constants to improve the accuracy of the SRK/T formula. Ophthalmology. 2013;120:477–81.

8. Merriam J, Nong E, Zheng L, Stohl M. Optimization of the A constant for the SRK/T formula. Open J Ophthalmol. 2015;5:108–14.

9. Kane JX, Van Heerden A, Atik A, Petsoglou C. Intraocular lens power formula accuracy: comparison of 7 formulas. J Cataract Refract Surg. 2016;42:1490–500.

10. Cooke DL, Cooke TL. Comparison of 9 intraocular lens power calculation formulas. J Cataract Refract Surg. 2016;42:1157–64.

11. Shajari M, Kolb CM, Petermann K, Böhm M, Herzog M, de'Lorenzo N, Schönbrunn S, Kohnen T. Comparison of 9 modern intraocular lens power calculation formulas for a quadrifocal intraocular lens. J Cataract Refract Surg. 2018;44:942–8.

12. Idrobo-Robalino CA, Santaella G, Gutiérrez ÁM. T2 formula in a highly myopic population, comparison with other methods and description of an improved approach for estimating corneal height. BMC Ophthalmol. 2019;19:222.

13. Kane JX, Chang D. Intraocular lens power formulas, biometry, and intraoperative aberrometry. Ophthalmology. 2020;128(11):e94–e114. https://doi.org/10.1016/j.ophtha.2020.08.010.

14. Li Z, Lian Z, Young CA, Zhao J, Jin G, Zheng D. Accuracy of intraocular lens calculation formulas for eyes with insufficient capsular support. Ann Transl Med. 2021;9:324.

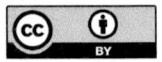

Oleksiy V. Voytsekhivskyy ⓘ

The main method for the calculation of lens power, in most cases, still uses a technique that is based on paraxial optics, which is a simplified version of geometric ray tracing [1–4]. In this case, it is possible to significantly simplify the mathematical calculations and to reduce them to a relatively simple formula in relation to the optical system of the human eye, which can be represented by a system of two thin lenses (IOL and the cornea) as follows [3, 4]:

$$P = \frac{n \times 1000}{AL - C} - \frac{n \times 1000}{V - C}; V = \frac{n \times 1000}{K}; K = \frac{1000 \times (nc - 1)}{r};$$

where P is the optical power of the implanted IOL (D), n is the refraction index of the optical medium (1.336, aqueous humor; 1.000, air), C is the postoperative ELP (mm), AL is the axial length of the eye (mm), K is the refractive corneal power (D), nc is the refractive index of the cornea (1.3375), 1 is the refractive index of air (1.000), and r is the radius of the front surface of the cornea (mm).

The main advantage of this method is its relative simplicity and the need for only one parameter to calculate the IOL power; it is a specific constant determined by the manufacturer of this type of lens. The majority of modern formulas and methods use this formula to calculate the optical power of the intraocular lens with some correction factors; the difference lies only in the

method of predicting the postoperative position of the intraocular lens in the eye [5, 6].

Investigation of Formula

Similar to all currently existing formulas for the calculation of intraocular lens power, this formula can in principle be divided into two main parts: the main formula and the method of predicting the postoperative position of the lens in the eye (ELP). This method uses the so-called classical stigmatic, paraxial optical formula [3, 4], which was proposed more than 150 years ago. Two reference values were used as correction factors: the factor correcting the axial length of the eye and the factor correcting the true refractive power of the cornea. Different authors used different values in their formulas. Binkhorst did a correction for the value of axial length of 0.25 mm and Holladay for 0.20 mm, and Hoffer used no correction factor [6, 7]. The value 0.20 mm for

O. V. Voytsekhivskyy (✉)
Kyiv Clinical Ophthalmology Hospital Eye
Microsurgery Center, Komarov Ave, Medical City,
Kyiv, Ukraine

© The Author(s) 2024
J. Aramberri et al. (eds.), *Intraocular Lens Calculations*, Essentials in Ophthalmology,
https://doi.org/10.1007/978-3-031-50666-6_55

axial length correction was used because it yielded the best result for calculation according to this new method and was similar to that used by other researchers (Binkhorst; Holladay and associates) [3, 4, 6]. For highly myopic eyes was used correction factor obtained empirical way: if

$$AL \geq 26.5\,mm, AL0 = AL + \left(-0.159 \times AL + 4.401\right).$$

The second factor is associated with the conversion of the refractive power of the cornea in true optical power. Recently, many authors [3, 4, 7, 8] have shown the irrationality of using the classic 1.3375 index refraction and the error in the refractive power of the cornea from 0.5 to 1 diopter [3, 4]. The standardized keratometric index of refraction was chosen many years ago, so that an anterior radius of curvature of the cornea of 7.5 mm would yield a power of 45.0 D. The cornea is a thick lens with two surfaces and thicknesses. Using the index of refraction of the corneal stroma of 1.376, a posterior corneal radius that is 1.2 mm steeper, and a corneal thickness of 0.55 mm results in a net corneal power of 44.4 D. This value is approximately 0.56 D less than the standardized keratometric power. As described in detail by Holladay, the value of 4/3 for the net corneal index of refraction is an appropriate value and would have the minimum impact and thus was recommended for use in modern formulas. Olsen recommends using an even lower value of 1.3315 that yielded an appropriate corneal power of 44.20 diopters [3]. Holladay's value of the refraction index was chosen (1.3333) because a more appropriate result was achieved with it than using Olsen value (1.3315) that overestimated the resulting IOL power [3, 5, 9]. Therefore, we used the following correction factor:

$$Ktrue = \frac{\left(4/3 - 1\right)}{\left(1.3375 - 1\right)} = 0.98765431 \times K.$$

Thus, we used a classical stigmatic, paraxial optical formula with an adjusted axial length and a correction of the true optical power of the cornea:

$$P = \frac{1336}{AL_0 - C} - \frac{1336}{\dfrac{1336}{\dfrac{1000}{\dfrac{1000}{tgRef} - Vd} + Ktrue} - C};$$

$$AL_0 = AL + 0.20, \text{if } AL \geq 26.5\,mm, AL_0 = AL + \left(-0.159 \times AL + 4.401\right).$$

P is the optical power of the implanted IOL for emmetropia (D), *n* is the refraction index of aqueous humor and vitreous liquid (1.336) and air (1.000), AL is the axial length of the eye (mm), *C* is the postoperative estimated lens position (ELP) (mm), tgRef is the target postoperative refraction (D), Vd is the spectacle back vertex distance (mm), *K* is the refractive corneal power (D), AL0 is the true axial length (mm), Ktrue is the true refractive corneal power (D), and 0.20 and $(-0.159 \times AL + 4.401)$ are the correction factors of the axial length (mm).

The second and the main part of our formula is a method of predicting the postoperative position of IOL in the eye. Hoffer was one of the first authors who suggested considering this value; for the first time, he applied a factor in changing the ELP values using the axial lengthof the eye. In 1988, Holladay suggested using two variables; namely, he added the value of the refractive power of the cornea to the axial length of the eye and suggested the term "effective lens position." [3, 4] Furthermore, the number of variables used to predict the postoperative position of the lens increased, and some authors suggested considering additional parameters, which are associated with anatomic changes in the anterior segment of the eye [1, 5, 8].

Thus, there are two unknown values in any formula: the optical power of the lens and the postoperative position of the lens in the eye. As we cannot change the first unknown value, the second value is the key in any IOL calculation formula. The main difference between all the formulas used in this study lies in the difference of the algorithms for predicting the postoperative position of lens, which actually determines optical power IOL.

Investigation of Estimated Lens Position

To obtain the regression algorithm of ELP prediction, we used the data group of patients with two different types of lenses, Alcon ReSTOR SN6AD1 (169 eyes) and AMO Tecnis MF ZMB00 (160 eyes). In total, there were 329 eyes.

Based on the data of the preoperative parameters of the eye (AL, K, ACDpre, and CD), the values of the optical power of the two different types of implanted IOLs and the received postoperative manifest refraction empirically based on the multiple regression analysis (SPSS 22.0, IBM) obtained the equation describing the postoperative position of the IOL in the eye, namely the postoperative ELP. To develop the regression formula, multiple linear regression was performed using the ELP as the dependent variable and the axial length (AL), corneal power (K), preoperative anterior chamber depth (epithelium to lens) (ACDpre), and horizontal corneal diameter (CD) as independent variables. For each value of the predicted postoperative ACD, the corresponding regression equation was obtained. More than 700 iterations were performed to obtain the averaged regression equation model. Accordingly, for two different types of lenses (Alcon ReSTOR SN6AD1 and AMO Tecnis MF ZMB00), two regression models were derived as follows:

$$AL \times (CACD \times 0.051 - 0.006) + K \times (CACD \times 0.019 - 0.008) + ACDpre$$
$$\times (CACD \times 0.053 + 0.005) - CD \times (CACD \times 0.013 - 0.003) - (CACD \times 0.959 - 0.013); \quad (55.1)$$

$$AL \times (CACD \times 0.050 - 0.007) + K \times (CACD \times 0.018 - 0.001) + ACDpre$$
$$\times (CACD \times 0.056 + 0.004) - CD \times (CACD \times 0.012 - 0.003) - (CACD \times 0.974 - 0.005); \quad (55.2)$$

where CACD is an ACD constant from the manufacturer, AL is the axial length of the eye (optical method) (mm), K is the refractive power of the cornea (D), $K = (nc - 1)/r$ (D), r is the radius of curvature of the anterior corneal surface (mm), nc is the refractive index of 1.3375, ACDpre is the preoperative anterior chamber depth (epithelium to lens) (mm), and CD is the horizontal corneal diameter (mm).

Equation (55.1) had a higher correlation coefficient ($R^2 = 0.922$ vs. $R^2 = 0.895$) and a lower standard error (0.316 vs. 0.334) than Eq. (55.2) and was therefore selected for further evaluation. A new formula was programmed using Eq. (55.1). The proposed method was called Voytsekhivskyy regression function (VRF). Thus, in the new formula, the ELP is a function of five variables as follows:

$$ELP = f(CACD; AL; K; ACDpre; CD);$$

$$ELP = AL \times (CACD \times D1 - E1) + K \times (CACD \times D2 - E2) + ACDpre$$
$$\times (CACD \times D3 + E3) - CD \times (CACD \times D4 - E4) - offset;$$

where AL is the axial length of the eye (optical method) (mm), K is the refractive power of the cornea (D) and $K = (nc - 1)/r$ (D), r is the radius of curvature of the anterior corneal surface (mm), nc is the refractive index of 1.3375, ACDpre is the preoperative anterior chamber depth (epithelium to lens) (mm), CD is the horizontal corneal diameter (mm), CACD is an ACD constant from the manufacturer, D constants 1–4 and E constants 1–4 are the regression constants obtained empirically by the study, and the offset is the regression equation obtained empirically.

The regression constants are as follows:

$$D1 = 0.051; D2 = 0.019; D3 = 0.053; D4 = 0.013;$$

$$E1 = 0.006; E2 = 0.008; E3 = 0.005; E4 = 0.003.$$

The offset is given by

$$Offset = CACD \times 0.959 - 0.013.$$

CACD Constant of VRF Formula

The main feature of this algorithm is the use of a single IOL constant that is repeated several times and not the use of a number of different constants

[8, 10]. Each of the four preoperative parameters of the eye affects a constant and gives a final value corresponding to the postoperative position of the IOL in the eye. The so-called optical constant of the anterior chamber depth (optical CACD) was used as a constant. The CACD constant was used exclusively as the optical constant due primarily to the fact that the sample was taken from patients whose AL was measured using an optical method (PCI, IOLMaster 500, software version 7.3, Carl Zeiss Meditec AG, Jena, Germany).

There is a method to determine the appropriate optical CACD. The option is to use the regression equation proposed by Haigis [10, 11] for optimized constants to obtain the values of the optical CACD constant from the optical A-constants given by the manufacturer.

$$Optical\ CACD\ constant = (Optical\ A - constant \times 0.62467) - 68.82.$$

where the optical CACD is a constant depth of the anterior chamber for optical measurement techniques, and the optical A-constant is a constant for optical measurement techniques by the manufacturer of the intraocular lens.

Evaluation of VRF Formula

The aim of this study was to develop and compare a new method for predicting the postoperative IOL position and further calculating the optical power of the implanted lens using four parameters: the axial length of the eye (AL), the optical refractive power of the cornea (K), the preoperative anterior chamber depth (epithelium to lens) (ACDpre), and the horizontal corneal diameter (CD). The clinical performance of the VRF formula was compared to that of the other formulas by calculating the spectacle prediction error of each formula in the evaluation subset of eyes using separate IOL-specific constants optimized for each formula. AcrySof IQ SN60WF IOL was used for the evaluation of the second subgroup of patients (494 eyes, Alcon Laboratories, Inc., Fort Worth, TX, USA).

Overall, there was a good correlation between the prediction errors of the seven formulas (best, $r^2 = 0.905$ Haigis; worst, $r^2 = 0.844$ Holladay 2). In general, the VRF formula produced a prediction error similar to that of the Hoffer Q on short eyes, Holladay 1 on medium eyes, T2 on medium-long eyes, and SRK/T on long eyes but of smaller magnitude, as indicated in Fig. 55.1.

The main indicators of formula accuracy were the indices MedAE and MAE [12, 13]. Moreover, the value MedAE was less sensitive to outliers compared to MAE and allowed for a more precise estimate of the refractive error data.

The obtained results were very encouraging. In the first group with short AL (53 eyes), the best result was from the VRF method (MedAE 0.345 D) and the Hoffer Q formula (MedAE 0.350 D) and the worst result was produced by the SRK/T formula (MedAE 0.426 D), which was predictable in short eyes. For the medium AL group (320 eyes), the VRF formula demonstrated the highest accuracy (MedAE 0.302 D) and the least accuracy was demonstrated by the Holladay 2 formula (MedAE 0.338 D). The third group with medium-long AL (70 eyes) showed the best accuracy using the VRF formula (MedAE 0.301 D)

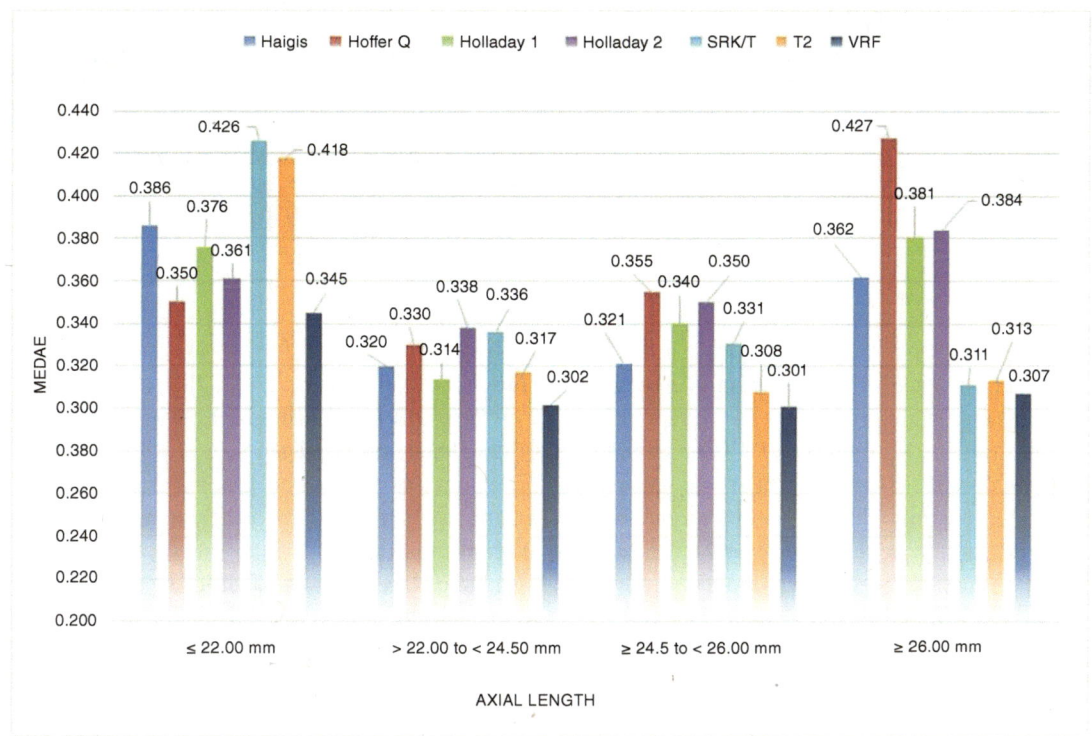

Fig. 55.1 Median absolute error plotted against axial length groups for the Haigis, Hoffer Q, Holladay 1, Holladay 2, SRK/T, T2, and VRF formulas

and the worst using the Hoffer Q formula (MedAE 0.355 D). In the long AL group (51 eyes), the best result was from the VRF (MedAE 0.307 D) and the worst result was from the Hoffer Q formula (MedAE 0.427 D). For the entire AL group, VRF showed better predictability than the other formulas (MedAE 0.305 D). However, there was a very small difference between the corresponding values; most of the formulas were stacked in the value of 0.01 diopters, which indicated the high accuracy of all the presented methods. Overall, 41.3% of the eyes were within ±0.25 D of prediction using the VRF formula and 39.0% using the Haigis formula. The other formulas had lower results of 35.0% for SRK/T and 38.0% for T2 and Hoffer Q. All formulas had prediction errors within ±2 D except T2 at 99.8%. There were no statistically significant differences between the formulas for short eyes, medium eyes (except Holladay 2 and SRK/T, *P* < 0.005, W-test), medium-long eyes, or long eyes (except Holladay 2, *P* < 0.005, W-test). For all axial

length ranges, statistically significant differences were found for Holladay 2 (*P* < 0.005, W-test) and SRK/T (*P* < 0.005, W-test) formulas [14].

Recently, Savini et al. [15] studied the 13 formulas in a sample of 150 average eyes. The lowest MedAE values were achieved with the following formulas: Kane (0.200 D), T2 (0.200 D), Barrett (0.202 D), EVO (0.205 D), RBF (0.205 D), Olsen (standalone) (0.209 D), and VRF (0.215 D). Dunn's posttest analysis showed that only the following paired comparison had statistically significant differences (*P* < 0.005): EVO vs Haigis, EVO vs Hoffer Q, and RBF vs Haigis. The proportion of absolute errors less than ±0.50 D was more than 85% for almost all formulas. The calculation with the EVO and VRF formulas showed the best results on eyes with axial length > 26.00 mm (MedAE 0.168 D and 0.198 D respectively). The results from the current study confirm that the VRF (MedAE 0.210 D) was most accurate than the traditional formulas for average eyes with T2 (MedAE 0.200 D) as an exception (Haigis (MedAE 0.254 D), Hoffer Q (MedAE 0.248 D), Holladay 1 (MedAE 0.249 D), Holladay 2 (MedAE 0.228 D), and SRK/T (MedAE 0.221 D), respectively).

$$\mathrm{Dp} = \frac{n - a\mathrm{Dc}}{(a-k) \times \dfrac{(1 - k\mathrm{Dc})}{n}}; k = r - \sqrt{r^2} - \frac{d2}{4}; \mathrm{Dc} = \frac{1000 \times (\mathrm{nc} - 1)}{r};$$

where "a" represents the axial length (in meters), "k" anterior chamber depth with the pupillary implant in place (in meters), "Dc" the refracting power of cornea (in diopters), "Dp" the refracting power of the intraocular lens (in diopters and assuming a thin lens), and "n" the refractive index of aqueous and vitreous (1.336).

For many years, formulas such as Hoffer Q, Holladay 1, and SRK/T were the gold standard for calculating IOL power, and they remain the standard for many ophthalmologists [3, 7, 17]. The third generation of formulas used two predictors to estimate postoperative lens position, including axial length and cornea power, whereas newer formulas use up to seven predictors (Holladay 2), and some of them even include race and sex (Hoffer H-5) and some just sex (Kane and VRF-G). Recently, more than 30 new methods and formulas for calculating IOL power have appeared (Fig. 55.2) [1, 2, 14, 18–26]. A new generation of IOL power formulas such as Barrett

The VRF-G Formula

The first formula for calculating the optical power of the anterior chamber IOL was suggested by Fyodorov and associates in 1967 [16].

Universal II, Castrop, EVO 2.0, Hoffer QST, Cooke K6, Kane, Karmona, LSF AI, Naeser 2, Olsen, Panacea, Pearl-DGS, and RBF 3.0 have brought a new level of accuracy and allowed cataract surgery to become a refractive procedure. With the existence of many new methods and unsatisfied accuracy of traditional formulas on long eyes, the update of existing classical formulas appeared. The Wang-Koch modification was implemented for Holladay 1, Hoffer Q, and SRK/T formulas [27, 28].

Currently, there are many methods and principles for calculating the optical power of an intraocular lens (IOL). All existing methods can be divided into four groups: methods using the principles of paraxial approximation, or Gaussian optics; methods using the real, exact path of rays in the optical system of the eye, the so-called geometric optics, or ray tracing, models that are based on different algorithms of artificial intelligence (AI) and mixed mathematical algorithms

- - Barrett Universal II
- - Barrett True Axial Length (BTAL)
- - Bayesian Additive Regression Trees (BART)
- - Castrop
- - Emmetropia Verifying Optical 2.0 (EVO)
- - FullMonte IOL (2018)
- - Haigis
- - Hoffer H-5
- - Hoffer Q
- - Hoffer QST (Savini, Taroni)
- - Hoffer Q (Wang-Koch)
- - Holladay 1

- - Holladay 1 (NLR)*
- - Holladay 1 (MWK)□
- - Holladay 1 (Wang-Koch)
- - Holladay 2
- - Holladay 2 (NLR)*
- - Holladay 2 (Wang-Koch)
- - Cooke K6
- - Kane
- - Karmona
- - Ladas Super Formula AI (LSF AI)
- - Naeser 2
- - Nallasamy

- - OKULIX
- - Olsen (OLCR)
- - Olsen (PhacoOptics)
- - Panacea
- - Pearl-DGS
- - Radial Basis Function 3.0 (RBF)
- - SRK/T
- - SRK/T (MWK)□
- - SRK/T (Wang-Koch)
- - T2
- - VRF
- - VRF-G

* Nonlinear Regression　　□ Modified Wang-Koch

Fig. 55.2 IOL power formulas and methods

that featured aforementioned models with a prevalence one of them [1, 2, 14, 18–24]. Interestingly, all recently presented formulas as a rule are mixed models that use artificial intelligence (AI) or ray tracing and are based on traditional vergence formulas.

Today, there is no consensus on the best formula among the available ones. Many researchers have attempted to evaluate the accuracy of these formulas in their investigations. For example, Savini and associates studied the 13 formulas (Barrett Universal II with and without anterior chamber depth (ACD) as a predictor, Emmetropia Verifying Optical 2.0 (EVO), Haigis, Hoffer Q, Holladay 1, Holladay 2, Holladay 2 AL, Kane, Naeser 2, Pearl-DGS, RBF 2.0, SRK/T, T2, and VRF) in 200 eyes with the same IOL model (Si 255; Hoya). The lowest values were achieved with the Kane (0.214 D), RBF 2.0 (0.215 D), BUII with and without ACD (0.218 D), and SRK/T (0.223 D). A percentage ranging from 80% to 88.5% of eyes showed a PE within ±0.50 D, and all formulas achieved more than 50% of eyes with a PE within ±0.25 D. The median absolute error (MedAE) ranged between 0.214 D and 0.256 D, with a statistically significant difference among formulas ($P < 0.0001$) [29]. Cooke and Cooke tested the nine IOL power formulas and found that the formulas yielded different results depending on which machine measurements were used [30]. Taroni and associates compared the 13 IOL power formulas and found that in average eyes with a mean AL 24.01 ± 1.56 mm (range 20.45–28.80 mm), the Pearl-DGS formula was a more accurate predictor of actual postoperative refraction than the other formulas [31].

Investigation of Formulas

The VRF formula is a vergence-based thin-lens formula using four variables: axial length, keratometry, anterior chamber depth, and horizontal corneal diameter. However, it does not consider parameters such as lens thickness and gender, and the published results did not position it as one of the most accurate formulas [29, 31]. This method is a part of the VRF Suite software version 1.3. (V/C/Systems, Kyiv, Ukraine), created and designed specifically for calculating IOL power. This program enables the determination of the optical power of the IOL and planned postoperative refraction for ordinary (VRF and VRF-G formulas) cataract surgery, conditions after corneal refractive surgery (VRF-L and VRF-GL formulas), and cataract surgery in keratoconus (VRF-K) (Fig. 55.3).

The VRF-G (gender) is an unpublished new formula that is based on theoretical optics with regression and ray-tracing components. It uses the optical A-constant for the SRK/T formula and operates eight variables including AL, K, ACDpre (epithelium to lens), LT, horizontal CD (corneal diameter), CCT, preoperative refractive spherical equivalent (SE), and gender. Parameters such as AL, K, ACDpre (epithelium to lens), and gender are mandatory for calculation. It was programmed into IBM PC software and was called VRF Suite V1.3 (Fig. 55.4) [21, 32]. This formula was introduced as a profound modification of the original VRF formula, does not rely on any artificial intelligence (AI) assumption, and showed promising outcome across all axial length range with a special focus on the short eyes [21].

VRF VRF Suite V1.3 (Personal Version)   —   □   ✕

Ordinary Calculation   Corneal Surgery Calculation   Keratoconus Calculation   Documentation   About the Program

VRF FORMULA

The VRF formula was developed in August 2017 using 329 cases with two types of IOLs (Alcon ReSTOR SN6AD1 (169) and J&J Tecnis MF ZMB00 (160)). The formula is based on theoretical optics and incorporates regression components to further refine its predictions. The formula focused on eyes with a long axial length and incorporates a regression algorithm for high-performance accuracy of calculations. An ELP prediction is empirical and takes into account anterior chamber depth that increased accuracy in eyes with unusual anterior segment and drastically reduce the errors seen at the extremes of the various ocular dimensions. Variables used in the formula are an axial length that measured from optical biometry (AL optical), keratometry (K), anterior chamber depth (Ph ACD) and horizontal corneal diameter (WTW).
This study is available in the American Journal of Ophthalmology:
https://www.ajo.com/article/S0002-9394(17)30451-8/fulltext

VRF-G FORMULA

The VRF-G formula uses an algorithm incorporating theoretical Gaussian optics, regression and ray-tracing techniques to calculate the intraocular lens power. This method can be considered a profound modification of the original VRF formula, which was described previously. It uses eight variables to predict IOL power, including mandatory AL, K, ACD (from the epithelium to the lens) and gender, while horizontal CD, LT, CCT and preoperative refractive spherical equivalent (SE) are optional. Recent investigations have shown promising results for this formula, especially in eyes with a short axial length.[1,2] In the large study on IOL formula accuracy on short eyes, the VRF-G formula has been shown to be more accurate (MedAE 0.276 D) than all currently available formulas (Barrett, EVO 2.0, Haigis, Hoffer Q, Holladay 1 and Holladay 2, K6, Kane, LSF AI, Naeser 2, Olsen, Panacea, Pearl-DGS, RBF2.0 SRK/T, T2 and VRF).
This study is available in CURRENT EYE RESEARCH: https://www.tandfonline.com/doi/full/10.1080/02713683.2021.1933056

VRF-L and VRF-GL FORMULAS

The VRF-L and VRF-GL formulas are a profound modification of a classical VRF formula. Both use regression components related to corneal power and axial length estimation in eyes that have been undergone corneal refractive surgery including radial keratotomy (RK) and distinct types of laser surgery (LASIK, LASER, PRK, trans-PRK). The formulas also minimize the errors related to the estimation of the corneal power. There is no requirement for additional variables for the VRF-L and VRF-GL formulas and the formulas work with the same CACD and A-constant used for ordinary patients.

VRF-K FORMULA

The VRF-K (Keratoconus) formula is a theoretical paraxial ray-tracing modification of the original VRF formula. It uses modified linear and nonlinear regression equations for correction of corneal power and anterior chamber depth, which better represents the true corneal power and axial length in keratoconic eyes. The formula also minimizes the errors related to the corneal measurements and estimation of the ELP. There is no requirement for additional variables for the VRF-K formula and the formula works with the same CACD-constant used for non-keratoconic patients. Slightly myopic target refraction is recommended in these patients: -0.25 D.

1. Hipólito-Fernandes D, Luís ME, Gil P, Maduro V, Feijão J, Yeo TK et al. VRF-G, a New Intraocular Lens Power Calculation Formula: A 13-Formulas Comparison Study. Clin Ophthalmol 2020; 14:4395-4402. doi:10.2147/OPTH.S290125.
2. Voytsekhivskyy O, Hoffer KJ, Savini G, Tutchenko L, Hipólito-Fernandes D. Clinical Accuracy of 18 IOL power formulas in 241 short eyes. Curr Eye Res 2021; May 20. doi:10.1080/02713683.2021.1933056. Online ahead of print.

Fig. 55.3 VRF Suite V1.3 with VRF, VRF-G, VRF-L, VRF-GL, and VRF-K formulas

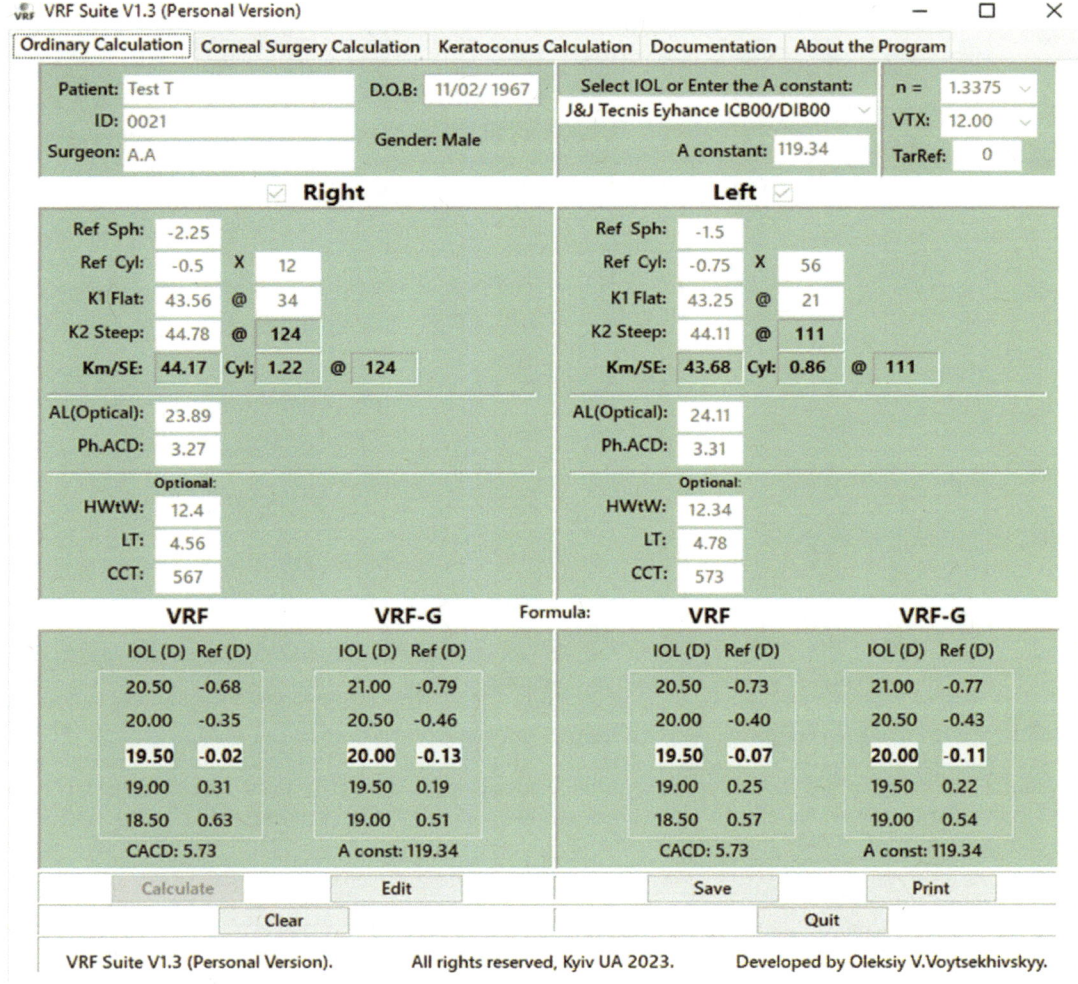

Fig. 55.4 VRF Suite V1.3 with VRF and VRF-G formulas

Evaluation of the Formula

Recently, we investigated the results of 13 formulas for a large database of 828 eyes, with one type of lens (AcrySof SN60WF; Alcon Laboratories, Inc.) [32] Overall, VRF-G showed promising outcomes with the best median absolute error (MedAE 0.273 D) among all methods and was third with the absolute error value (MAE 0.332 D), after Kane (MAE 0.324) and EVO 2.0 (MAE 0.329 D). Additionally, VRF-G produced the highest percentage of eyes within ±0.50 D (79.5%) (Fig. 55.5).

In our other study, we compared 18 IOL power formulas in 241 short eyes [21]. A recently developed new formulas such as K6, Kane, Naeser 2, Olsen, and VRF-G obtained the lowest MedAE compared to other formulas (0.308, 0.300, 0.277, 0.310, and 0.276 D, respectively). Comparison of the absolute prediction errors revealed a statistically significant difference ($P < 0.05$) between some of the newer formulas (K6, Kane, Naeser 2, Olsen, and VRF-G) and the remaining ones. These formulas also yielded the highest percentage of eyes with a PE within ±0.50 D (70.54%,

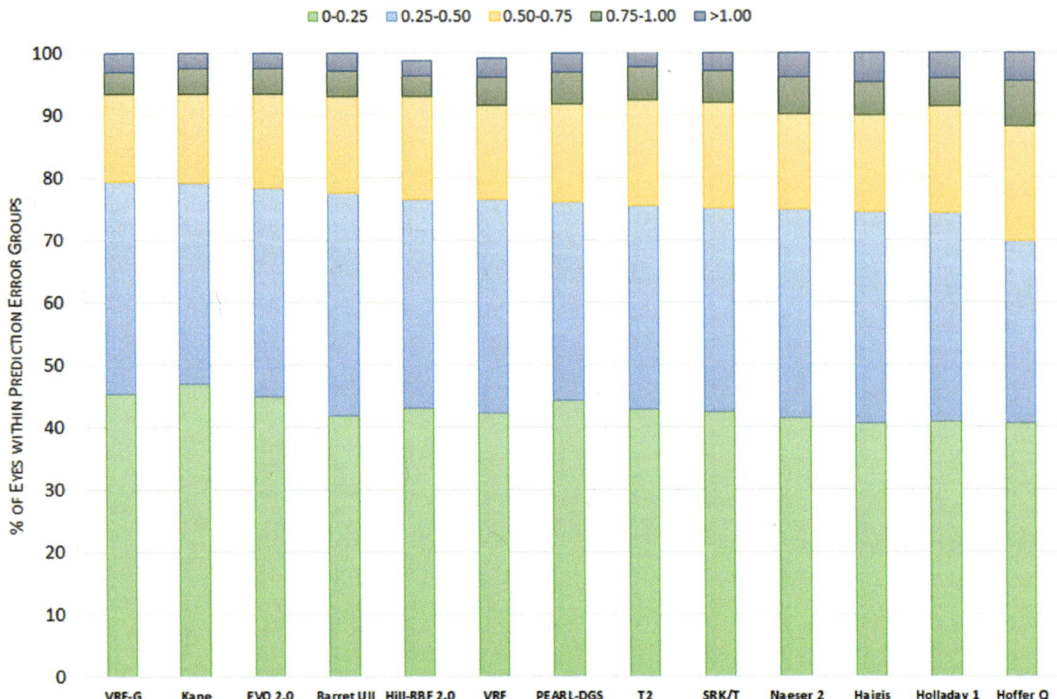

Fig. 55.5 Stacked histogram comparing the percentages of eyes within ±0.25 D, ±0.50 D, ±0.75 D, and ±1.00 D of prediction error. Formulas are ranked according to the higher percentage of eyes within ±0.50 D. In short eyes (n = 82), VRF-G (MAE 0.345 D) produced a smaller absolute error when compared to other formulas. For all AL subgroups, VRF-G had one of the most accurate performances, being slightly worse than Kane and EVO 2.0 formulas (SD and MAE values) [32]

72.20%, 71.37%, 70.95%, and 73.03%, respectively). The VRF-G formula showed the highest percentage of eyes within ±0.50 D (73.03%) and the lowest median absolute error value (MedAE = 0.276 D), with slight superiority over other methods. Overall, it was not worse and equal to existing methods.

Recently, in our investigation, the VRF-G formula (MedAE 0.242 D) had the lowest median absolute error value and outperformed all other formulas [33]. The Haigis (MedAE 0.247 D) and Kane (MedAE 0.263 D) methods demonstrated slightly worse results. The calculation with other formulas was less predictable.

In conclusion, the findings of the present investigations support the idea that the VRF-G formula, as a rule, outperforms the original formulas for short eyes showing promising outcomes on medium and long eyes.

References

1. Olsen T, Hoffmann P. C constant: new concept for ray tracing–assisted intraocular lens power calculation. J Cataract Refract Surg. 2014;40(5):764–73. https://doi.org/10.1016/j.jcrs.2013.10.037.
2. Preussner P-R, Wahl J, Lahdo H, Dick B, Findl O. Ray tracing for intraocular lens calculation. J Cataract Refract Surg. 2002;28(8):1412–9. https://doi.org/10.1016/s0886-3350(01)01346-3.
3. Holladay JT, Prager TC, Chandler TY, Musgrove KH, Lewis JW, Ruiz RS. A three-part system for refining intraocular lens power calculations. J Cataract Refract Surg. 1988;14(1):17–24. https://doi.org/10.1016/s0886-3350(88)80059-2.
4. Holladay JT, Maverick KJ. Relationship of the actual thick intraocular lens optic to the thin lens equivalent. Am J Ophthalmol. 1998;126:339–47. https://doi.org/10.1016/s0002-9394(98)00088-9.
5. Olsen T. Calculation of intraocular lens power: a review. Acta Ophthalmol Scand. 2007;85:472–85. https://doi.org/10.1111/j.1600-0420.2007.00879.x. Epub 2007 Apr 2

6. Binkhorst RD. The optical design of intraocular lens implants. Ophthalmic Surg. 1975;6(3):17–31.
7. Hoffer KJ. The Hoffer Q formula: a comparison of theoretic and regression formulas. J Cataract Refract Surg. 1993;19(6):700–12; Errata 1994; 20:677 and Zuberbuhler B, Morell AJ. Errata in printed Hoffer Q formula [letter]. J Cataract Refract Surg 2007;33(1):2; reply by KJ Hoffer, 2–3. doi: 10.1016/s0886-3350(13)80338-0.
8. Haigis W, Lege B, Miller N, Schneider B. Comparison of immersion ultrasound biometry and partial coherence interferometry for IOL calculation according to Haigis. Graefes Arch Clin Exp Ophthalmol. 2000;238:765–73. https://doi.org/10.1007/s004170000188.
9. Olsen T. On the calculation of power from curvature of the cornea. Br J Ophthalmol. 1986;70:152–4. https://doi.org/10.1136/bjo.70.2.152.
10. Haigis W. The Haigis formula. In: Shammas HJ, editor. Intraocular lens power calculations. Thorofare, NJ: Slack; 2004. p. 41–57.
11. Haigis W. Relations between optimized IOL constants. In: Symposium on cataract, IOL and refractive surgery of the American Society of Cataract and Refractive Surgery (ASCRS), Philadelphia, PA, USA, 1–5 June 2002. Abstracts, p. 112.
12. Hoffer KJ, Aramberri J, Haigis W, Olsen T, Savini G, Shammas HJ, Bentow S. Protocols for studies of intraocular lens formula accuracy [editorial]. Am J Ophthalmol. 2015;160:403–5. https://doi.org/10.1016/j.ajo.2015.05.029. Epub 2015 Jun 25.
13. Murdoch IE, Morris SS, Cousens SN. People and eyes: statistical approaches in ophthalmology. Br J Ophthalmol. 1998;82(8):971–3. https://doi.org/10.1136/bjo.82.8.971.
14. Voytsekhivskyy O. Development and clinical accuracy of a new intraocular lens power formula (VRF) compared to other formulas. Am J Ophthalmol. 2018;185:56–67. https://doi.org/10.1016/j.ajo.2017.10.020.
15. Savini G, Hoffer KJ, Balducci N, Barboni P, Schiano-Lomoriello D. Comparison of formula accuracy for intraocular lens power calculation based on measurements by a swept-source optical coherence tomography optical biometer. J Cataract Refract Surg. 2020;46:27–33. https://doi.org/10.1016/j.jcrs.2019.08.044.
16. Fedorov SN, Kolinko AIKA. [Estimation of optical power of the intraocular lens] [Russian]. Vestn oftalmol. 1967;80:27–31.
17. Retzlaff JA, Sanders DR, Kraff MC. Development of the SRK/T intraocular lens implant power calculation formula. J Cataract Refract Surg. 1990;16(3):333–40. erratum: 528
18. Sheard RM, Smith GT, Cooke DL. Improving the prediction accuracy of the SRK/T formula: the T2 formula. J Cataract Refract Surg. 2010;36(11):1829–34.
19. Barret GD. An improved universal theoretical formula for intraocular lens power prediction. J Cataract Refract Surg. 1993;19(6):713–20.
20. Melles RB, Holladay JT, Chang WJ. Accuracy of intraocular lens calculation formulas. Ophthalmology. 2018;125(2):169–78.
21. Voytsekhivskyy O, Hoffer KJ, Savini G, Tutchenko L, Hipólito-Fernandes D. Clinical accuracy of 18 IOL power formulas in 241 short eyes. Curr Eye Res. 2021;46(12):1832–43.
22. Ladas JG, Siddiqui AA, Devgan U, Jun AS. A 3-D "super surface" combining modern intraocular lens formulas to generate a "super formula" and maximize accuracy. JAMA Ophthalmol. 2015;133(12):1431–6. https://doi.org/10.1001/jamaophthalmol.2015.3832.
23. Melles RB, Kane JX, Olsen T, Chang WJ. Update on intraocular lens power calculation formulas. Ophthalmology. 2019;126(9):1334–5.
24. Kane JX, Melles RB. Intraocular lens formula comparison in axial hyperopia with a high-power intraocular lens of 30 or more diopters. J Cataract Refract Surg. 2020;46(9):1236–9.
25. Næser K, Savini G. Accuracy of thick-lens intraocular lens power calculation based on cutting-card or calculated data for lens architecture. J Cataract Refract Surg. 2019;45(10):1422–9.
26. Cooke DL, Cooke TL. Approximating sum-of-segments axial length from a traditional optical low-coherence reflectometry measurement. J Cataract Refract Surg. 2019;45(3):351–4.
27. Wang L, Holladay JT, Koch DD. Wang-Koch axial length adjustment for the Holladay 2 formula in long eyes. J Cataract Refract Surg. 2018;44(10):1291–2.
28. Wang L, Koch DD. Modified axial length adjustment formulas in long eyes. J Cataract Refract Surg. 2018;44(11):1396–7.
29. Savini G, Di Maita M, Hoffer KJ, Naeser K, Schiano-Lomoriello D, Vagge A, Di Cello L, Traverso CE. Comparison of 13 formulas for IOL power calculation with measurements from partial coherence interferometry. Br J Ophthalmol. 2021;105(4):484–9.
30. Cooke DL, Cooke TL. Comparison of 9 intraocular lens power calculation formulas. J Cataract Refract Surg. 2016;42:1157–64.
31. Taroni L, Hoffer KJ, Barboni P, Schiano-Lomoriello D, Savini G. Outcomes of IOL power calculation using measurements by a rotating Scheimpflug camera combined with partial coherence interferometry. J Cataract Refract Surg. 2020;46(12):1618–23.
32. Hipólito-Fernandes D, Luís ME, Gil P, et al. VRF-G, a new intraocular lens power calculation formula: a 13-formulas comparison study. Clin Ophthalmol. 2020;14:4395–402.
33. Voytsekhivskyy O, Tutchenko L, Hipólito-Fernandes D. Comparison of the Barrett universal II, Kane and VRF-G formulas with existing intraocular lens calculation formulas in eyes with short axial lengths. Eye. 2023;37(1):120–6. https://doi.org/10.1038/s41433-021-01890-7. Epub 2022 Jan 15.

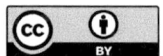

Calculation of Phakic and Pseudophakic Additional Lenses

56

Achim Langenbucher (ORCID), Alan Cayless, and Jens Schrecker

Introduction to Phakic and Pseudophakic Additional Lenses

Traditional methods to compensate for refractive errors are eyeglasses and contact lenses. Especially when correcting higher ametropia, astigmatism, and oblique light incidence, spectacles can themselves create new aberrations, and the frequent use of contact lenses may lead to intolerance, mostly in combination with dry eye syndrome. To overcome these issues, surgical refractive procedures can offer permanent and convenient results. Compared to keratorefractive interventions with excimer and femtosecond laser technologies, additional (implantable) lenses have significant advantages: They allow for a wider range of applications, they do not intensify dry eye syndrome, and the procedure is reversible at any time. Even years after the primary implantation, an exchange or explantation of an additional lens is possible with little surgi-

cal effort and minimal risk to surrounding tissues [1]. Additional IOLs are placed anterior to the crystalline lens (phakic Add-on) or artificial intraocular lens (pseudophakic Add-on). Possible locations are within the anterior eye chamber (haptics at iridocorneal angle or at the front of the iris) or within the posterior chamber in the sulcus ciliaris (Fig. 56.1). Because of potential complications with anterior chamber lenses, these types of IOL are used relatively rarely today. Theoretically, the nodal points of the IOL and eye will become closer together with the increasingly posterior placement of the Add-on, reducing disturbing photic phenomena. Furthermore, the greater distance to the cornea helps to prevent endothelial cell loss. On the other hand, in the case of a phakic eye, such placement increases the risk of triggering cataract development.

In young refractive patients with a clear lens and sufficient accommodation, **phakic Add-on IOLs** are an alternative to keratorefractive procedures, especially in eyes with higher myopia. Despite potential risks of pigment dispersion, pupillary block, and cataract development, modern phakic IOLs are shown to be safe, effective, and stable in many studies [2–5]. The surgical skills for the implantation, exchange, or explantation of these IOL are similar to cataract surgery, and in contrast to corneal laser surgery, the necessary equipment is considerably less expensive. As with all intraocular procedures, there are associated general surgical risks. In addition, a

A. Langenbucher (✉)
Department of Experimental Ophthalmology, Saarland University, Homburg/Saar, Germany
e-mail: achim.langenbucher@uks.eu

A. Cayless
School of Physical Sciences, The Open University, Milton Keynes, UK

J. Schrecker
Department of Ophthalmology, Rudolf-Virchow-Clinics, Glauchau, Germany

© The Author(s) 2024
J. Aramberri et al. (eds.), *Intraocular Lens Calculations*, Essentials in Ophthalmology,
https://doi.org/10.1007/978-3-031-50666-6_56

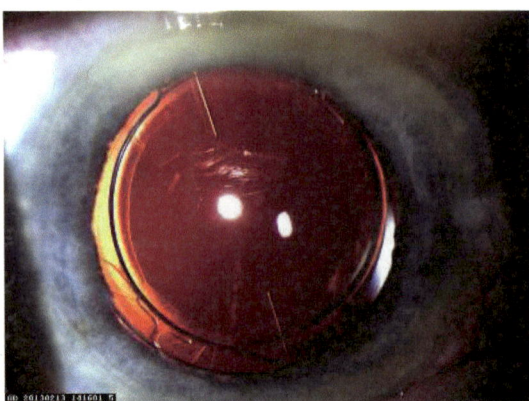 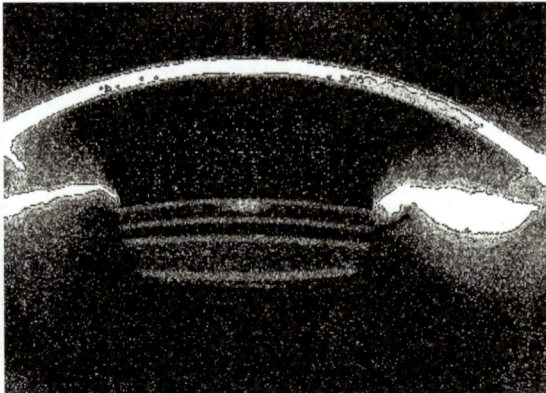

Fig. 56.1 Left: Toric Add-on IOL in front of the primary IOL in the capsular bag. Right: Scheimpflug image of the anterior eye segment with an even gap between the Add-on IOL in the sulcus ciliaris and the IOL in the capsular bag

progressive shallowing of the anterior chamber resulting from increasing lens thickness with age might contribute to the abovementioned issues. A pending issue of toric Add-on models is their potential rotational instability, which could induce crossed cylinders and a deteriorated visual performance even years after surgery [6, 7].

There are four main indications for pseudophakic Add-on IOLs:

1. Within the power calculation of IOLs before cataract or refractive lens surgery, all relevant parameters such as keratometric data, anterior chamber depth, lens thickness, and axial eye length can be measured by modern biometers with high precision. However, despite highly optimized measuring and power calculation methods, postoperative refractive surprises can still occur in some cases. Under such circumstances, pseudophakic Add-on IOLs are a welcome option for fine-tuning [8–13].
2. In situations where the patient decides on the option of pseudo-accommodation only after lens surgery, multifocal Add-ons provide a suitable alternative [8, 14–20] and a persisting deviation from emmetropia can be corrected at the same time.
3. The implantation of an IOL during congenital cataract surgery is another area of application. In the majority of cases, the eye of the child is still growing at the time of surgery and refractive conditions will change significantly.

Because of the limited compliance of a small child, spectacles and contact lenses might not be an optimal solution and the exchange of the IOL in the bag is virtually impossible because of the massive ingrowth. For these reasons, exchangeable additional IOLs can be very helpful within the course of postoperative treatment [21].

4. A fourth indication for Add-ons is after keratoplasty, where the crystalline lens has been replaced before or during this operation [11]. In those cases, the prediction of the appropriate lens power may fail due to the unpredictable or varying corneal power. Here an Add-on IOL can be used to correct any persisting cylindrical and equivalent refraction error [22].

The fundamental **calculation strategy for additional IOLs** was described in 1988 by the so-called Van der Heijde formula [23]. In this paper, a spherical phakic Add-on IOL was calculated for a myopic correction using classical vergence transformation. Langenbucher et al. generalized this formula for the calculation of toric phakic IOLs with spherocylindrical target refraction using a vergence-based formalism by transferring the position of refractive correction from the spectacle plane to the IOL plane [24]. In contrast to intraocular lenses in the capsular bag, the calculation of an additional IOL is based on manifest subjective refraction, axial distance between spectacle back vertex and corneal front vertex, corneal curvature, and the axial position of the Add-on in the eye with respect to the corneal front vertex [22, 24].

Calculation of Additional Lenses

The special situation of calculating additional lenses relates to the transfer, in part or in full, of a preexisting refraction mostly at the spectacle plane, to the plane of the additional lens [2, 3, 15]. This means that there is no change in the optical system posterior to the additional lens plane, and therefore, we have to consider only the anterior eye segment for the calculation of the lens power or for the lateral magnification [24].

There are several options for calculating additional lenses: Calculation could be performed using linear Gaussian optics within the paraxial space, either with formulae based on vergence transform or with matrix algebras, or with ray-tracing strategies based on a ray bundle traced through all refractive surfaces and optical media from the object plane to the plane of the additional lens.

Figure 56.2 displays by way of example the optical model used for calculating the power of an Add-on, for the situation of a phakic lens implantation in the ciliary sulcus. In the upper graph, we have the preoperative situation with a spectacle correction at vertex distance (VD) in front of the cornea, and in the lower graph, the spectacle correction is transferred to the plane of the Add-on, which is located slightly in front of the crystalline lens.

The postoperative position of the Add-on (ELP) can be estimated from the position of the anterior surface of the crystalline lens (CRL for phakic lenses) or the replacement lens (IOL for pseudophakic lenses) and the vault. This vault corresponds to the interspace between the Add-on

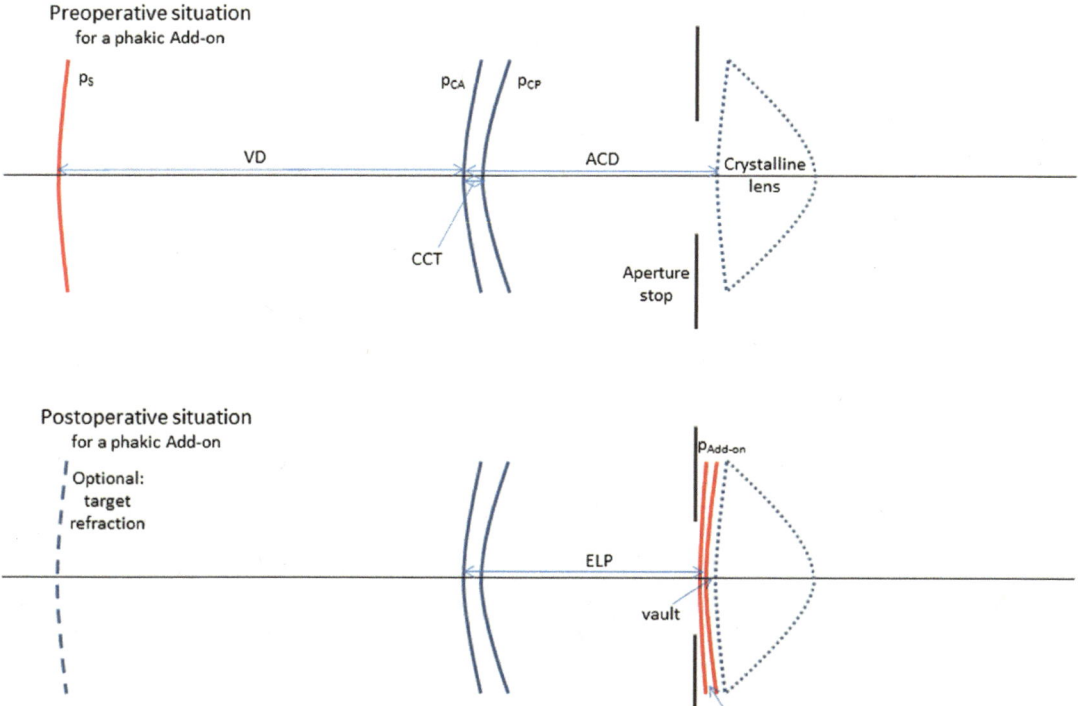

Fig. 56.2 Schematic drawing of the situation before (upper graph) and after (lower graph) implantation of an additional lens (Add-on). The axial position of the Add-on (ELP) is derived from the measured anterior chamber depth (ACD). The aperture stop of the optical system is assumed to be located at the Add-on plane

and the CRL or IOL and ranges between 0.2 and 0.5 mm. Therefore, a biometric measurement prior to Add-on implantation—preferably with optical biometry—is mandatory for the prediction of the estimated Add-on position ELP [24–27].

Our preferred calculation method for the Add-on is using matrix algebra, as the concept directly adds value by predicting the change of lateral magnification (ΔM). Using vergence transform formulae, the estimation of the magnification before and after Add-on implantation requires a separate calculation step. The strategy of matrix calculation is based on a system matrix, which describes and characterizes the paraxial optical properties of the relevant optical part of the eye [28–30]. This system matrix is composed of a product of refraction and translation matrices: A refraction matrix describes the change of ray direction as the ray passes through this surface, and a translation matrix describes the change in lateral ray position as the ray passes through a homogeneous optical medium. For stigmatic (non-toric) situations, the system matrix and all refraction and translation matrices are of dimension 2×2. With an incident ray defined in terms of its slope α_0 and height h_0, the slope α and height h of the ray exiting the optical system described by the system matrix S [28] are defined by

$$\begin{pmatrix} \alpha \\ h \end{pmatrix} = \begin{pmatrix} A & B \\ C & D \end{pmatrix} \begin{pmatrix} \alpha_0 \\ h_0 \end{pmatrix} = S \begin{pmatrix} \alpha_0 \\ h_0 \end{pmatrix}. \quad (56.1)$$

The system matrix S is derived from the product of the respective refraction and translation matrices considered in reverse order (against the ray direction). The refraction and translation matrices P and T are of the form

$$P = \begin{pmatrix} 1 & -p \\ 0 & 1 \end{pmatrix}$$
$$T = \begin{pmatrix} 1 & 0 \\ \dfrac{d}{n} & 1 \end{pmatrix}, \quad (56.2)$$

where p refers to the surface power $p = (n' - n)/r$ (n' and n refer to the refractive indices behind and in front of the refractive surface of radius r),

and d and n refer to the thickness of the refractive index of the homogeneous medium. Both situations of the anterior eye segment, from the spectacle plane to the Add-on plane before and after implantation of the Add-on, are described by system matrices S_{pre} and S_{post}. For example, for a thick lens model of the cornea, both matrices read

$$\begin{aligned} S_{pre} &= T_{iELP} P_{CP} T_{CCT} P_{CA} T_{VD} P_S \\ S_{post} &= P_{Add-on} T_{iELP} P_{CP} T_{CCT} P_{CA} T_{VD} \end{aligned},$$
(56.3)

where T_{iELP}, T_{CCT}, and T_{VD} refer to the translation matrices for the aqueous depth, the cornea, and the vertex distance, and P_{Add-on}, P_{CP}, P_{CA}, and P_S refer to the refraction matrices for the Add-on, the corneal back and front surface, and the refraction correction before Add-on implantation, which is to be transferred (in this case fully) to the Add-on plane.

To obtain the same focus position, the exit vergences of S_{pre} and S_{post} at the Add-on plane must be identical. This means that with

$$S_0 = T_{iELP} P_{CP} T_{CCT} P_{CA} T_{VD} = \begin{pmatrix} A_0 & B_0 \\ C_0 & D_0 \end{pmatrix}$$
(56.4)

for an object located at $-\infty$ (with an entrance vergence of 0 or slope angles $\alpha_0 ' = 0$) and a preoperative refraction at the spectacle plane of p_S, the following condition must be fulfilled:

$$(B_0 - A_0 p_S) D_0 = (D_0 - C_0 p_S)(B_0 - D_0 p_{Add-on})$$
(56.5)

Reformulating Eq. (56.5) yields the refractive power of the Add-on (p_{Add-on}):

$$p_{Add-on} = \frac{B_0}{D_0} - \frac{(B_0 - A_0 p_S)}{(D_0 - C_0 p_S)}. \quad (56.6)$$

The lateral magnification before and after implantation of the Add-on is easily obtained from the respective system matrices S_{pre} and S_{post} [30, 31]. If an optical system S is corrected, either matrix element C or D in Eq. (56.1) equals zero (depending on whether it is corrected for far objects ($D = 0$) or for objects at finite distances ($C = 0$)). Here, our systems S_{pre} and S_{post} are not corrected; therefore, we have to select the chief ray [31] for evaluation of magnification properties. Assuming that the aperture of the system is located at the Add-on plane, this means $h = C\alpha_0 + Dh_0 = 0$, or $h_0 = -C/D\,\alpha_0$. Inserting this into Eq. (56.1) yields a relative lateral magnification $M_{\text{pre/post}}$ of

$$M_{\text{pre/post}} = \frac{\alpha}{\alpha_0} = A - B\frac{C}{D}, \qquad (56.7)$$

A relative change in lateral magnification of ΔM of $M_{\text{post}}/M_{\text{pre}}$.

Clinical Example 1

With a phakic lens, preexisting spectacle correction $p_S = -7$ dpt at a vertex distance VD = 12 mm to be transferred to a correction at ELP = 3.4 mm behind the corneal front apex (e.g., phakic anterior chamber depth: 3.6 mm, vault: 0.2 mm). With a corneal front/back surface radius of 7.77/6.4 mm, a central corneal thickness of 500 μm, and refractive indices of air/cornea/aqueous of 1.0/1.376/1.336, Eq. (56.4) for S_0 becomes

$$S_0 = \begin{pmatrix} 0.4953 & -42.2511 \\ 0.0132 & 0.8907 \end{pmatrix}$$

The power of the Add-on is derived from Eq. (56.6) as $p_{\text{Add-on}} = -7.9925$. Using Eq. (56.3) gives

$$S_{\text{pre}} = \begin{pmatrix} 0.4953 & -38.7843 \\ 0.0132 & 0.9833 \end{pmatrix}$$

$$S_{\text{post}} = \begin{pmatrix} 0.6010 & -35.1322 \\ 0.0132 & 0.8907 \end{pmatrix}$$

According to Eq. (56.7), we calculate a relative magnification of $M_{\text{pre}} = 1.0170$ and $M_{\text{post}} = 1.1227$ and an increase in lateral magnification of 10.4% ($\Delta M = 1.1040$).

Clinical Example 2

In this example, we consider a pseudophakic additional lens, with a post-cataract spectacle correction of $p_S = +3.5$ dpt at a vertex distance

VD = 14 mm to be converted to a correction at an ELP = 4.8 mm behind the corneal front apex (e.g., pseudophakic anterior chamber depth: 5.1 mm, vault: 0.3 mm). Assuming a corneal front/back surface radius of 7.9/6.5 mm, a central corneal thickness of 550 μm, and refractive indices of air/cornea/aqueous of 1.0/1.376/1.336, Eq. (56.4) reads for S_0 becomes

$$S_0 = \begin{pmatrix} 0.4206 & -41.5582 \\ 0.0155 & 0.8488 \end{pmatrix}$$

The power of the Add-on is derived from Eq. (56.6) as $p_{\text{Add-on}} = 5.1894$. Using Eq. (56.3) gives

$$S_{\text{pre}} = \begin{pmatrix} 0.4206 & -43.0304 \\ 0.0155 & 0.7946 \end{pmatrix}$$

$$S_{\text{post}} = \begin{pmatrix} 0.3404 & -45.9628 \\ 0.0155 & 0.8488 \end{pmatrix}$$

According to Eq. (56.7), we calculate a relative magnification of $M_{\text{pre}} = 1.2585$ and $M_{\text{post}} = 1.1782$ and a decrease in lateral magnification of 6.4% ($\Delta M = 0.9362$).

Calculation of Toric Additional Lenses

The matrix scheme as outlined before for stigmatic lenses can easily be generalized for toric additional lenses. Instead of 2 × 2, we have to deal with 4 × 4 matrices for the system matrix [28, 30], the refraction, and the translation matrices, which are composed of 4 2 × 2 sub-matrices A, B, C, and D. The slope angles α_x and α_y and the ray height h_x and h_y of the exiting ray in x-direction and y-direction are calculated from the respective slope angles and height values of the incident ray (α_{x0}, α_{y0}, h_{x0} and h_{y0}) by

$$\begin{pmatrix} \alpha_x \\ \alpha_y \\ h_x \\ h_y \end{pmatrix} = \begin{pmatrix} A_{11} & A_{12} & B_{11} & B_{12} \\ A_{21} & A_{22} & B_{21} & B_{22} \\ C_{11} & C_{12} & D_{11} & D_{12} \\ C_{21} & C_{22} & D_{21} & D_{22} \end{pmatrix} \begin{pmatrix} \alpha_{x0} \\ \alpha_{y0} \\ h_{x0} \\ h_{y0} \end{pmatrix}. \qquad (56.8)$$

The refraction matrix P and the translation matrix T for the astigmatic case are of the form

$$
P = \begin{pmatrix} 1 & 0 & -p_a & -p_d \\ 0 & 1 & -p_d & -p_b \\ 0 & 0 & 1 & 0 \\ 0 & 0 & 0 & 1 \end{pmatrix}
$$

$$
T = \begin{pmatrix} 1 & 0 & 0 & 0 \\ 0 & 1 & 0 & 0 \\ \dfrac{d}{n} & 0 & 1 & 0 \\ 0 & \dfrac{d}{n} & 0 & 1 \end{pmatrix}, \quad (56.9)
$$

where

$$
\begin{aligned}
p_a &= p_1 + (p_2 - p_1)\sin 2(ax) \\
p_b &= p_1 + (p_2 - p_1)\cos 2(ax), \quad (56.10) \\
p_d &= (p_2 - p_1)\sin(ax)\cos(ax)
\end{aligned}
$$

with the refractive power of a surface in meridian 1 (with radius r_1) $p_1 = (n' - n)/r_1$ and meridian 2 (with radius r_2) $p_2 = (n' - n)/r_2$, and with ax as the orientation of meridian 1.

From the refraction and translation matrices, the 4×4 system S_{pre} and S_{post} are calculated according to Eq. (56.3). As S_0 defined in Eq. (56.4) is now a 4×4 matrix and A_0, B_0, C_0, and D_0 are 2×2 matrices instead of scalars, Eq. (56.5) has to be reformulated to ensure that the vergence at the Add-on plane is identical for the preoperative and the postoperative situation:

$$
(B_0 - A_0 P_S) \bullet \text{inv}(D_0 - C_0 P_S) = (B_0 - D_0 p_{\text{Add-on}}) \bullet \text{inv}(D_0). \tag{56.11}
$$

Reformulating Eq. (56.11) yields the refractive power of the Add-on ($p_{\text{Add-on}}$):

$$
p_{\text{Add-on}} = (B_0 - (\text{inv}(D_0))((B_0 - A_0 P_S) \bullet \text{inv}(D_0 - C_0 P_S) \bullet D_0)), \tag{56.12}
$$

where inv. (.) refers to the inverse of the 2×2 matrix (.). Using an eigenvalue decomposition of the 2×2 matrix $p_{\text{Add-on}}$ yields the power in both meridians (eigenvalue 1 and 2), and the orientation of meridian 1 is extracted from eigenvector 1.

According to the stigmatic case, if we select the chief ray, which passes through the center of the aperture stop assumed to be located at the Add-on plane, we obtain

$$
\begin{pmatrix} h_x \\ h_y \end{pmatrix} = C \begin{pmatrix} \alpha_{x0} \\ \alpha_{y0} \end{pmatrix} + D \begin{pmatrix} h_{x0} \\ h_{y0} \end{pmatrix} = \begin{pmatrix} 0 \\ 0 \end{pmatrix}, \tag{56.13}
$$

or

$$
\begin{pmatrix} h_{x0} \\ h_{y0} \end{pmatrix} = -\text{inv}(D) \bullet C \bullet \begin{pmatrix} \alpha_{x0} \\ \alpha_{y0} \end{pmatrix}. \tag{56.14}
$$

Inserting the result of Eq. (56.14) into Eq. (56.8) yields the lateral magnification for the pre-operative or postoperative astigmatic optical system:

$$
M_{\text{pre/post}} = A - B \bullet \text{inv}(D) \bullet C. \tag{56.15}
$$

The situations for lateral magnification [31] in both principal meridians before (blue) and after (red) implantation of a toric Add-on are displayed in a sketch in Fig. 56.3. In this example, the meridian of magnification changes from 70° pre-operatively to 85° postoperatively, whereas the axis of magnification changes from 160 to 175°. The overall magnification as indicated by the dashed lines increases by 25% from preoperative (blue dashed line) to postoperative (red dashed line).

The relative change in magnification is given by

$$
\Delta M = \text{inv}(M_{\text{pre}}) \bullet M_{\text{post}}. \tag{56.16}
$$

Fig. 56.3 Lateral magnification before (blue) and after (red) implantation of a toric Add-on. In this example, the overall magnification gains by 25% (blue and red dashed circles), which indicates that a minus Add-on is implanted. The image distortion (major to minor axis of the ellipse) is typically reduced if the refraction correction is transferred from the spectacle plane to the Add-on plane

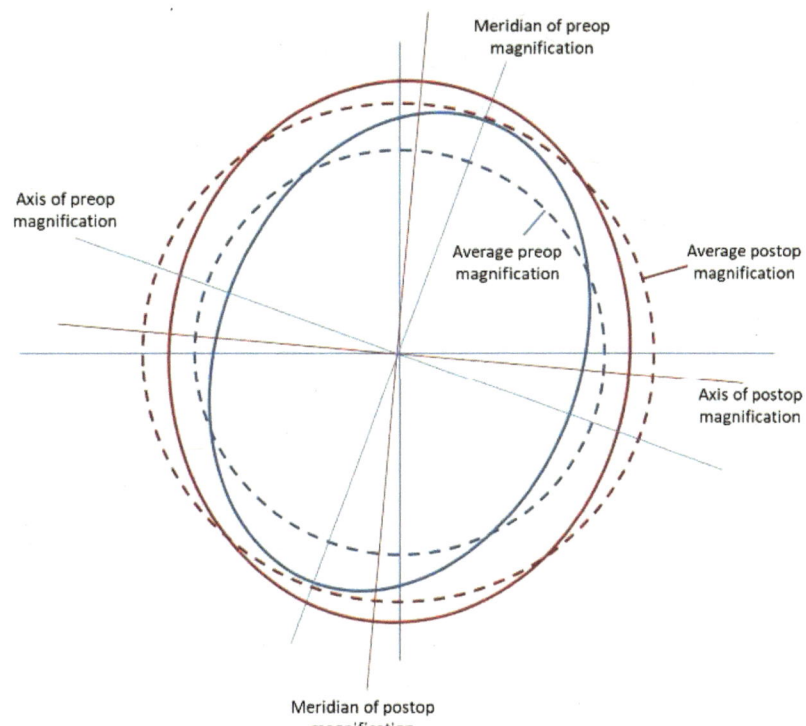

Meridian of preop magnification

Axis of preop magnification

Average preop magnification

Average postop magnification

Axis of postop magnification

Meridian of postop magnification

Again, the principal meridians and the orientation of the principal meridians are extracted from M_{pre}, M_{post}, and ΔM using eigenvalue decomposition.

Clinical Example 3

With a phakic lens, preexisting spectacle correction $p_{S1} = -7$ dpt/A $= 10°$ and $p_{S2} = -10$ dpt/A $= 100°$ at a vertex distance VD = 12 mm to be transferred to a correction at ELP = 3.4 mm behind the corneal front apex. With a corneal front surface shape of 8.0 mm/A $= 20°$ and 7.6 mm/A $= 110°$ and a corneal back surface shape of 6.7 mm/A $= 25°$ and 6.4 mm/A $= 115°$ and a central corneal thickness of 500 μm, and refractive indices of air/cornea/ aqueous of 1.0/1.376/1.336, S_0 according to Eq. (56.4) reads

$$
S_0 = \begin{pmatrix}
0.5057 & 0.0083 & -41.3727 & 0.6915 \\
0.0083 & 0.4851 & 0.6915 & -43.0951 \\
0.0138 & 0.0 & 0.8497 & 0.0025 \\
0.0 & 0.0137 & 0.0025 & 0.8434
\end{pmatrix}
$$

The power of the Add-on is derived from Eq. (56.12) as

$$
p_{Add-on} = \begin{pmatrix}
8.8078 & -0.6138 \\
-0.6138 & 11.9972
\end{pmatrix}.
$$

Converted to standard notation this gives -8.69/A $= 10.53$ and -12.11/A $= 100.53°$, or $-12.11 + 3.42$/A $= 100.53°$. According to Eq. (56.3), S_{pre} and S_{post} read

$$S_{pre} = \begin{pmatrix} 0.5057 & 0.0083 & -37.7912 & 0.5139 \\ 0.0083 & 0.4851 & 0.5012 & -38.2921 \\ 0.0138 & 0.0 & 0.9474 & -0.0043 \\ 0.0 & 0.0137 & -0.0043 & 0.9793 \end{pmatrix}$$

$$S_{post} = \begin{pmatrix} 0.5057 & 0.0083 & -41.3727 & 0.6915 \\ 0.0083 & 0.4851 & 0.6915 & -43.0951 \\ 0.0138 & 0.0 & 0.8497 & 0.0025 \\ 0.0 & 0.0137 & 0.0025 & 0.8434 \end{pmatrix}$$

According to Eq. (56.15), we calculate a relative magnification before (M_{pre}) and after (M_{post}) Add-on implantation, and according to Eq. (56.16), the change in relative magnification as

$$M_{pre} = \begin{pmatrix} 1.0556 & 0.0044 \\ 0.0048 & 1.0212 \end{pmatrix}$$

$$M_{post} = \begin{pmatrix} 1.1770 & -0.0035 \\ -0.0035 & 1.1857 \end{pmatrix},$$

$$\Delta M = \begin{pmatrix} 1.1150 & -0.0082 \\ -0.0086 & 1.1611 \end{pmatrix}$$

and using eigenvalue decomposition gives the principal meridians of magnification preoperatively (1.0562/A = 7.8° and 1.0206/A = 97.8°) and postoperatively (1.1757 A = 19.5° and 1.1869/A = 109.5°) together with the gain in ocular magnification from Add-on implantation (11.35% in 10.3° and 16.26% in 100.3°). Lateral image distortion is reduced from 3.49% preoperatively to 0.94% postoperatively. Example 3 demonstrates that the refractive power of an Add-on is determined mostly by the refraction (sphere, cylinder, and axis) and only to a small amount by the cornea (base curve, astigmatism, and axis).

Simplification for a Thin Lens Model of the Cornea

The calculation strategy for Add-on lenses as shown above can be simplified by considering the cornea as a thin lens with a single refractive surface located at the front apex position of the

meniscus lens. In general, if the corneal front and back surface data are available and the calculation scheme is computerized, there is no need for this simplification to a thin cornea model. Especially after corneal refractive surgery (e.g., LASIK), it is important to consider both corneal surfaces in the calculation concept to avoid refractive surprises, as the ratio of front-to-back surface curvature of the cornea shows some mismatch. Equation (56.3), which describes the situations of the anterior eye segment from the spectacle plane to the Add-on plane before and after implantation of the Add-on, has to be replaced by

$$\begin{aligned} S_{pre} &= T_{ELP} P_{CK} T_{VD} P_S \\ S_{post} &= P_{Add-on} T_{ELP} P_{CK} T_{VD} \end{aligned}, \quad (56.17)$$

where T_{ELP} refers to the translation matrices for the axial position of the Add-on with respect to the anterior front vertex plane of the cornea, and P_{CK} refers to the refraction matrix describing the keratometric power of the cornea. For the stigmatic case (calculation of non-toric Add-on) and the astigmatic case (calculation of toric Add-on), the matrices P_{CK} and T_{ELP} read

$$P_{CK} = \begin{pmatrix} 1 & -\dfrac{n_K - 1}{r} \\ 0 & 1 \end{pmatrix},$$

$$T_{ELP} = \begin{pmatrix} 1 & 0 \\ \dfrac{ELP}{n_{Aqueous}} & 1 \end{pmatrix} \quad (56.18)$$

and

$$P_{CK} = \begin{pmatrix} 1 & 0 & -\left(\frac{n_K-1}{r_1}+\left(\frac{n_K-1}{r_2}-\frac{n_K-1}{r_1}\right)\sin 2(a_1)\right) & -\left(\left(\frac{n_K-1}{r_2}-\frac{n_K-1}{r_1}\right)\sin(a_1)\cos(a_1)\right) \\ 0 & 1 & -\left(\left(\frac{n_K-1}{r_2}-\frac{n_K-1}{r_1}\right)\sin(a_1)\cos(a_1)\right) & -\left(\frac{n_K-1}{r_1}+\left(\frac{n_K-1}{r_2}-\frac{n_K-1}{r_1}\right)\cos 2(a_1)\right) \\ 0 & 0 & 1 & 0 \\ 0 & 0 & 0 & 1 \end{pmatrix},$$

$$T_{ELP} = \begin{pmatrix} 1 & 0 & 0 & 0 \\ 0 & 1 & 0 & 0 \\ \frac{ELP}{n_{Aqueous}} & 0 & 1 & 0 \\ 0 & \frac{ELP}{n_{Aqueous}} & 0 & 1 \end{pmatrix}$$

$$(56.19)$$

Equation (56.4) has to be replaced by

$$S_0 = T_{ELP} P_{CK} T_{VD} = \begin{pmatrix} A_0 & B_0 \\ C_0 & D_0 \end{pmatrix}, \quad (56.20)$$

while all other steps of the calculations remain unchanged.

Simplification Using Linear Modeling

Especially where a computerized calculation scheme is not available in the clinical routine process, the power of a stigmatic Add-on and the change in magnification due to the implantation of an Add-on can easily be estimated using a simple polynomial model. In the case of a toric Add-on, we recommend a calculation instead of such a simplification, as there are some more effect sizes, plus the situation of crossed cylinders which cannot be simplified properly.

As the conversion of refraction from the spectacle plane to the Add-on plane is not linear, we set up a polynomial of third order to describe the effect of p_{Add-on} and a linear function to model ΔM as a function of the spectacle refraction p_S. All of the other parameters such as corneal front and back surface curvature p_{CA} and p_{CP}, corneal thickness CCT, and the axial position of the Add-on ELP were analyzed and can be linearized with a sufficient clinical precision. We derived the coefficients of the polynomial fit function $p_{Add-on} = \text{fit}p_{Add-on}(p_S)$ and ΔM (in %) = $\text{fit}_{\Delta M}(p_S)$ for standard values of $p_{CA} = 7.77$ mm, $p_{CP} = 6.4$ mm, CCT = 500 µm and ELP = 3.4 mm for the phakic Add-on using a least squares optimization process:

$$p_{Add-on} = 2.79\exp{-4} \bullet p_S^3 + 1.88\exp{-2} \bullet p_S^2 + 1.26 \bullet p_S - 2.31\exp{-4}$$
$$\Delta M(\%) = -1.49 \bullet p_S$$

$$(56.21)$$

The effect of all other parameters was analyzed by calculating the gradient of $p_{Add-on} - \text{fit}p_{Add-on}(p_S)$ and ΔM (in %) $- \text{fit}_{\Delta M}(p_S)$.

For the situation of a phakic Add-on, the power of an Add-on and the change in magnification in % due to the implantation of a stigmatic Add-on can be estimated from the following equation:

$$p_{Add-on}(dpt) = 2.79 \bullet exp-4 \bullet p_S(dpt)3 + 1.88 \bullet exp-2 \bullet p_S(dpt)2 + 1.26 \bullet p_S(dpt)$$
$$-2.31 exp-4 - 4.55 \bullet exp-2\big(p_{CA}(mm) - 7.77\big) + 5.99 exp-3 \bullet \big(p_{CP}(mm) - 6.4\big)$$
$$+1.15 exp-5 \bullet \big(CCT(\mu m) - 500\big) + 9.21 exp-2 \bullet \big(ELP(mm) - 3.4\big) \tag{56.22}$$

$$\Delta M(\%) = -1.49 \bullet p_S + 5.06 exp-3\big(p_{CA}(mm) - 7.77\big) - 5.80 exp-4 \bullet \big(p_{CP}(mm) - 6.4\big)$$
$$+2.40 exp-7 \bullet \big(CCT(\mu m) - 500\big) - 9.43 exp-2 \bullet \big(ELP(mm) - 3.4\big). \tag{56.23}$$

For the situation of a pseudophakic Add-on, we derived the coefficients of the polynomial fit function $p_{Add-on} = fit p_{Add-on}(p_S)$ and ΔM (in %) $= fit_{\Delta M}(p_S)$ for standard values of $p_{CA} = 7.77$ mm, $p_{CP} = 6.4$ mm, CCT = 500 μm, and ELP = 4.8 mm using

$$p_{Add-on} = 3.71 exp-4 \bullet p_S^3 + 2.28 exp-2 \bullet p_S^2 + 1.39 \bullet p_S - 3.35 exp-4$$
$$\Delta M(\%) = -1.62 \bullet p_S \tag{56.24}$$

The effect of all other parameters was analyzed by calculating the gradient of $p_{Add-on} - fit p_{Add-on}(p_S)$ and ΔM (in %) $- fit_{\Delta M}(p_S)$.

For the situation of a phakic Add-on, the power of an Add-on and the change in magnification in % due to the implantation of a stigmatic Add-on can be estimated from the following equation:

$$p_{Add-on}(dpt) = 3.71 \bullet exp-4 \bullet p_S(dpt)3 + 2.28 \bullet exp-2 \bullet p_S(dpt)2 + 1.39 \bullet p_S(dpt)$$
$$-3.35 exp-4 - 7.51 \bullet exp-2\big(p_{CA}(mm) - 7.77\big) + 1.04 exp-2 \bullet \big(p_{CP}(mm) - 6.4\big)$$
$$+1.43 exp-4 \bullet \big(CCT(\mu m) - 500\big) + 1.08 exp-1 \bullet \big(ELP(mm) - 4.8\big) \tag{56.25}$$

$$\Delta M(\%) = -1.62 \bullet p_S + 1.12 exp-2\big(p_{CA}(mm) - 7.77\big) - 1.41 exp-3 \bullet \big(p_{CP}(mm) - 6.4\big)$$
$$-1.08 exp-5 \bullet \big(CCT(\mu m) - 500\big) - 1.04 exp-1 \bullet \big(ELP(mm) - 4.8\big). \tag{56.26}$$

Figure 56.4 displays the power of an Add-on and the change in magnification if the refractive correction at spectacle plane is converted to Add-on plane for an example with a vertex distance of 12 mm, a corneal front surface/back surface curvature of 7.77/6.4 mm, a corneal thickness of 500 μm, and a ELP of 3.4 mm (for the phakic Add-on) and 4.8 mm (for the pseudo-phakic Add-on). For a myopic correction ($p_S < 0$), the ratio of p_{Add-on}/p_S yields lower values compared to a hyperopic correction, which is considered with the polynomial fit function of order 3. The change in magnification can be described using a linear fit function as shown in Eqs. (56.21) and (56.22).

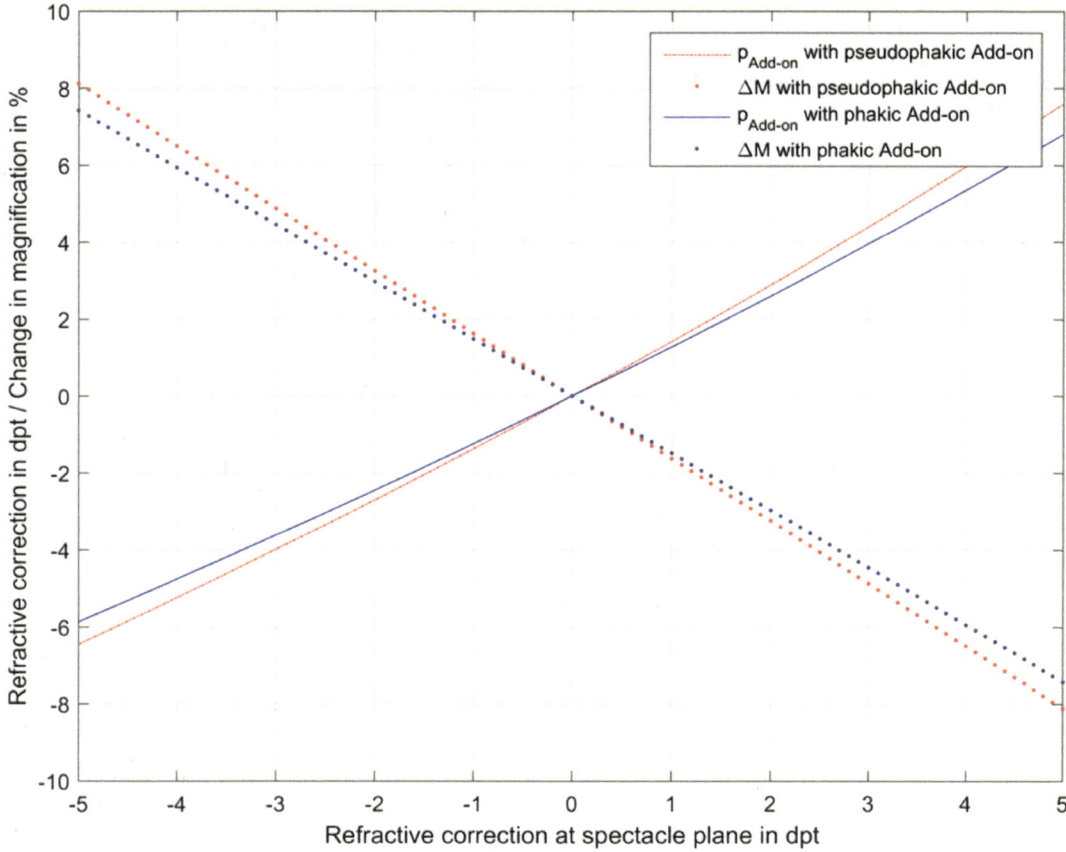

Fig. 56.4 Power of an Add-on and the change in magnification as a function of spectacle refraction to be corrected with the Add-on. This graph depicts an example with a vertex distance of 12 mm, a corneal front surface/ back surface curvature of 7.77/6.4 mm, a corneal thickness of 500 μm, and a ELP of 3.4 mm (for the phakic Add-on) and 4.8 mm (for the pseudophakic Add-on)

References

1. Schrecker J, Feith A, Langenbucher A. Comparison of additional pseudophakic multifocal lenses and multifocal intraocular lenses in the capsular bag. Br J Ophthalmol. 2014;98:915–9. https://doi.org/10.1136/bjophthalmol-2013-304591.

2. Gonvers M, Bornet C, Othenin-Girard P. Implantable contact lens for moderate to high myopia: relationship of vaulting to cataract formation. J Cataract Refract Surg. 2003;29:918–24. https://doi.org/10.1016/s0886-3350(03)00065-8.

3. Kohnen T, Kasper T, Bühren J, Fechner PU. Ten-year follow-up of a ciliary sulcus-fixated silicone phakic posterior chamber intraocular lens. J Cataract Refract Surg. 2004;30:2431–4. https://doi.org/10.1016/j.jcrs.2004.04.066.

4. Tsiklis NS, Kymionis GD, Karp CL, Naoumidi T, Pallikaris AL. Nine-year follow up of a posterior chamber phakic IOL in one eye and LASIK in the fellow eye of the same patient. J Refract Surg. 2007;23:935–7.

5. Lackner B, Pieh S, Schmidinger G, Simader C, Franz C, Dejaco-Ruhswurm I, et al. Long-term results of implantation of phakic posterior chamber intraocular lenses. J Cataract Refract Surg. 2004;30:2269–76. https://doi.org/10.1016/j.jcrs.2004.07.018.

6. Boutillier G, Gueudry J, Aouidid S, Muraine M. Sudden rotation and technique for repositioning Add-On® piggy-back sulcus toric intraocular lenses. J Fr Ophtalmol. 2021;44:e287–90. https://doi.org/10.1016/j.jfo.2020.07.015.

7. Muñoz G, Albarrán-Diego C, Belda L, Rohrweck S. Add-on sulcus-based versus primary in-the-bag multifocal intraocular lens: intraindividual study.

J Refract Surg. 2014;30(5):320–5. https://doi.org/10.3928/1081597X-20140422-02.

8. Sauder G. Sekundäre torische intraokularlinsen-implantation in pseudophake Augen. Das "Add-on"-IOL-system [Secondary toric intraocular lens implantation in pseudophakic eyes. The Add-on IOL system]. Ophthalmologe. 2007;104:1041–5. https://doi.org/10.1007/s00347-007-1660-4.

9. Basarir B, Kaya V, Altan C, Karakus S, Pinarci EY, Demirok A. The use of a supplemental sulcus fixated IOL (HumanOptics Add-On IOL) to correct pseudophakic refractive errors. Eur J Ophthalmol. 2012;22(6):898–903. https://doi.org/10.5301/ejo.5000156.

10. Gundersen KG, Potvin R. Refractive and visual outcomes after implantation of a secondary toric sulcus intraocular lenses. Clin Ophthalmol. 2020;18(14):1337–42. https://doi.org/10.2147/OPTH.S255725.

11. Hassenstein A, Niemeck F, Giannakakis K, Klemm M. Torische AddOn-Intraokularlinsen zur Korrektur hoher Astigmatismen nach pseudophaker Keratoplastik [Toric Add-on intraocular lenses for correction of high astigmatism after pseudophakic keratoplasty]. Ophthalmologe. 2017;114(6):549–55. https://doi.org/10.1007/s00347-016-0386-6.

12. Hengerer FH, Conrad-Hengerer I. Pseudophake additive Intraokularlinsen [Pseudophakic additive lenses]. Klin Monatsbl Augenheilkd. 2017;234(12):e43–55. https://doi.org/10.1055/s-0043-120095.

13. Thomas BC, Auffarth GU, Reiter J, Holzer MP, Rabsilber TM. Implantation of three-piece silicone toric additive IOLs in challenging clinical cases with high astigmatism. J Refract Surg. 2013;29(3):187–93. https://doi.org/10.3928/1081597X-20130212-01.

14. Kohnen T, Klaproth OK. Pseudophake additive Intraokularlinsen [Pseudophakic supplementary intraocular lenses]. Ophthalmologe. 2010;107:766–72. https://doi.org/10.1007/s00347-010-2219-3.

15. Schrecker J, Kroeber S, Eppig T, Langenbucher A. Additional multifocal sulcus-based intraocular lens: alternative to multifocal intraocular lens in the capsular bag. J Cataract Refract Surg. 2013;39:548–55. https://doi.org/10.1016/j.jcrs.2012.10.047.

16. Albayrak S, Comba ÖB, Karakaya M. Visual performance and patient satisfaction following the implantation of a novel trifocal supplementary intraocular lens. Eur J Ophthalmol. 2020;6:1120672120969042. https://doi.org/10.1177/1120672120969042.

17. Gekeler K, Gekeler F. Multifokale und Add-on-Intraokularlinsen [Multifocal and Add-on intraocular lenses]. Klin Monbl Augenheilkd. 2014;231(10):1037, 1039–48; quiz 1049-50. https://doi.org/10.1055/s-0033-1358020.

18. Gerten G, Kermani O, Schmiedt K, Farvili E, Foerster A, Oberheide U. Dual intraocular lens implantation: monofocal lens in the bag and additional diffractive multifocal lens in the sulcus. J Cataract Refract Surg. 2009;35(12):2136–43. https://doi.org/10.1016/j.jcrs.2009.07.014.

19. Palomino-Bautista C, Sánchez-Jean R, Carmona Gonzalez D, Romero Domínguez M, Castillo Gómez A. Spectacle Independence for Pseudophakic patients—experience with a trifocal supplementary add-on intraocular lens. Clin Ophthalmol. 2020;14:1043–54. https://doi.org/10.2147/OPTH.S238553.

20. Schrecker J, Langenbucher A. Visual performance in the long term with secondary Add-on versus primary capsular bag multifocal intraocular lenses. J Refract Surg. 2016;32(11):742–7. https://doi.org/10.3928/1081597X-20160630-02.

21. Amon M, Kahraman G, Schrittwieser H. Primäre (Duett Implantation) und sekundäre Implantation additiver Intraokularlinsen bei kindlicher Katarakt. Spektrum Augenheilkd. 2012;26:21–3.

22. Langenbucher A, Viestenz A, Szentmáry N, Seitz B, Viestenz A. Pseudophake und phake torische Linsen zur Korrektur des kornealen Astigmatismus—theorie und klinische Aspekte [Calculation of pseudophakic and phakic toric lenses for correction of corneal astigmatism—theory and clinical aspects]. Klin Monatsbl Augenheilkd. 2008;225(6):541–7. https://doi.org/10.1055/s-2008-1027502.

23. van der Heijde GL, Fechner PU, Worst JGF. Optische Konsequenzen der implantation einer negativen Intraokularlinse bei myopen Patienten. [Optical consequences of implantation of a negative intraocular lens in myopic patients]. Klin Monatsbl Augenheilkd. 1988;193:99–102. https://doi.org/10.1055/s-2008-1050231.

24. Langenbucher A, Szentmáry N, Seitz B. Calculating the power of toric phakic intraocular lenses. Ophthalmic Physiol Opt. 2007;27(4):373–80. https://doi.org/10.1111/j.1475-1313.2007.00487.x.

25. Eppig T, Gillner M, Walter S, Viestenz A, Langenbucher A. Berechnung phaker Intraokularlinsen [Calculation of phakic intraocular lenses]. Klin Monatsbl Augenheilkd. 2011;228(8):690–7. https://doi.org/10.1055/s-0031-1281598.

26. Eppig T, Viestenz A, Seitz B, Langenbucher A. Berechnung pseudophaker torischer Intraokularlinsen [Calculation of pseudophakic toric intraocular lenses]. Klin Monatsbl Augenheilkd. 2011;228(8):681–9. https://doi.org/10.1055/s-0029-1246046.

27. Holladay JT. Refractive power calculations for intraocular lenses in the phakic eye. Am J Ophthalmol.

1993;116(1):63–6. https://doi.org/10.1016/s0002-9394(14)71745-3.

28. Langenbucher A, Reese S, Sauer T, Seitz B. Matrix-based calculation scheme for toric intraocular lenses. Ophthalmic Physiol Opt. 2004;24(6):511–9. https://doi.org/10.1111/j.1475-1313.2004.00231.x.

29. Langenbucher A, Seitz B. Computerized calculation scheme for bitoric eikonic intraocular lenses. Ophthalmic Physiol Opt. 2003;23(3):213–20. https://doi.org/10.1046/j.1475-1313.2003.00109.x.

30. Langenbucher A, Viestenz A, Szentmáry N, Behrens-Baumann W, Viestenz A. Toric intraocular lenses—theory, matrix calculations, and clinical practice. J Refract Surg. 2009;25(7):611–22. https://doi.org/10.3928/1081597X-20090610-07.

31. Langenbucher A, Viestenz A, Seitz B, Brünner H. Computerized calculation scheme for retinal image size after implantation of toric intraocular lenses. Acta Ophthalmol Scand. 2007;85(1):92–8. https://doi.org/10.1111/j.1600-0420.2006.00721.x.

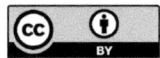

Kenneth J. Hoffer, Filomena Ribeiro,
and Giacomo Savini

Online Calculators for Spherical and Toric IOL Power

ASCRS Post-refractive IOL Calculator

The American Society of Cataract and Refractive Surgery (ASCRS), 15 years ago, developed a free online IOL calculator (https://ascrs.org/tools/post-refractive-iol-calculator) for eyes with previous corneal refractive surgery. The calculator has undergone continuous modifications over time and has three sections.

- **Prior Myopic LASIK/PRK:** Required inputs are axial length (AL), flattest keratometry (K1), steepest keratometry (K2), target refraction (Rx), and the A-constant of a given IOL. If no other parameters are entered, the results of two no-history formulas are shown: the Barrett True-K (see below) and Shammas-PL. Entering anterior chamber depth (ACD, from corneal epithelium to lens) enables the calculation of the Haigis-L formula also. If other parameters are entered (e.g., refractive change induced by the laser), a total of seven formulas with historical data and seven no-history formulas are shown.
- **Prior Hyperopic LASIK/PRK:** Required inputs are the same for myopic LASIK/PRK. A total of four no-history formulas and five formulas with historical data are computed.
- **Prior Radial Keratotomy (RK):** Using the same above mentioned parameters, seven formulas are displayed.

Barrett Formula Website (Fig. 57.1)

The formulas developed by Graham D. Barrett MD are available on the website of the Asia-Pacific Association of Cataract and Refractive Surgery (www.apacrs.org). Under the heading "IOL formulae," it is possible to perform several calculations:

- **For Unoperated Eyes:** The Barrett Universal II formula is available. A dropdown menu enables surgeons to select one of 18 IOL models, each with its own lens factor. Alternatively, if another IOL has to be used, its A-constant is

K. J. Hoffer (✉)
St. Mary's Eye Center, Santa Monica, CA, USA

Stein Eye Institute, UCLA, Los Angeles, CA, USA
e-mail: KHofferMD@StartMail.com

F. Ribeiro
Hospital da Luz Lisboa, Lisbon, Portugal

Lisbon University, Lisbon, Portugal

G. Savini
Studio Oculistico d'Azeglio, Bologna, Italy

G.B. Bietti Foundation I.R.C.C.S., Rome, Italy

© The Author(s) 2024

J. Aramberri et al. (eds.), *Intraocular Lens Calculations*, Essentials in Ophthalmology,
https://doi.org/10.1007/978-3-031-50666-6_57

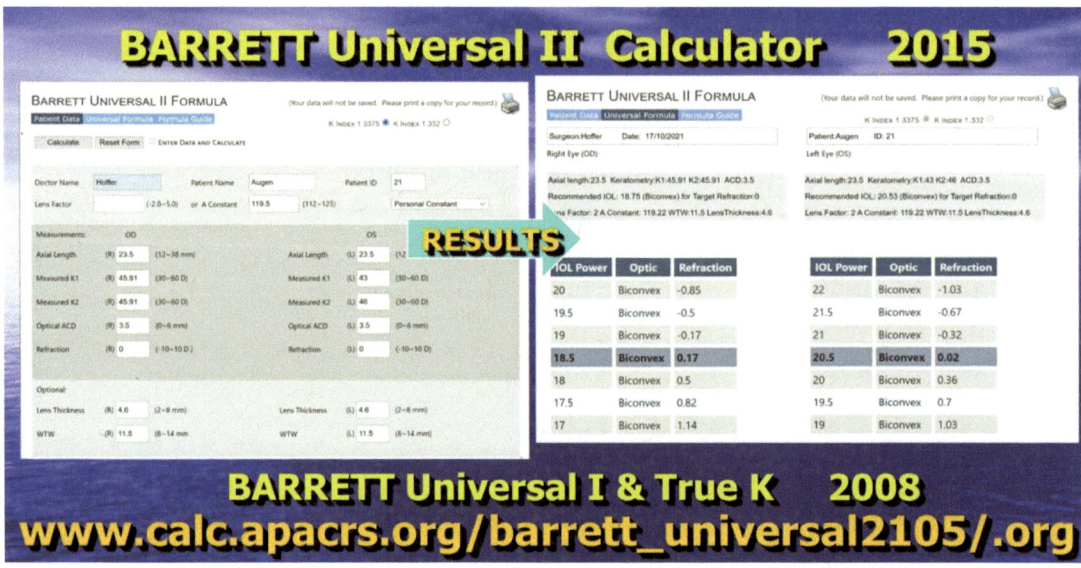

Fig. 57.1 Barrett online calculator

entered and automatically converted into the lens factor. Mandatory entries include AL, K1, K2, and target Rx. The IOL power can also be calculated without entering the ACD, but it is recommended to use this parameter. Optional values are the lens thickness (LT) and horizontal corneal diameter (CD).

- **For Unoperated Eyes Requiring a Toric IOL:** The Barrett Toric calculator is available. The dropdown menu includes 25 IOL models, each with its own lens factor. The A-constant can also be entered for other IOL models. In addition to AL, K1, K2, ACD, and target Rx, the flat axis and steep axis are required. The surgically induced astigmatism (SIA) and the incision location are optional, as well as LT and CD. This calculator offers two interesting opportunities: (1) the possibility to enter the measured posterior corneal astigmatism (PCA), obtained by five different instruments, and (2) the possibility to enter the K1 and K2 of three different devices, whose measurements are averaged. Both options are intended to improve the refractive accuracy. In any case, the keratometric astigmatism (KA) entered by the surgeon is optimized according to an unpublished

method, such that it decreases in eyes with with-the-rule (WTR) astigmatism and increases in eyes with against-the-rule (ATR) astigmatism in order to take the PCA into account. The Barrett toric calculator not only calculates the toric power of the IOL, but also calculates the spherical equivalent (SE) power.

- **For Eyes with Previous Corneal Refractive Surgery and Keratoconus:** (Myopic or Hyperopic LASIK and RK) and for eyes with Keratoconus: The Barrett True-K formula is available and the dropdown menu includes 26 IOL models, each with its own lens factor. The A-constant can be entered for other IOL models. In addition to the parameters needed for the Barrett Universal II formula, users may enter the refractive change induced by LASIK and the measured PCA (either from the IOLMaster 700 or the Pentacam). These parameters have been shown to improve the prediction accuracy in eyes with previous corneal refractive surgery.

- **For Toric IOL Powers in Eyes with Previous Excimer Laser Surgery or RK:** The Barrett True-K toric calculator merges the capabilities of the True-K formula and the standard toric calculator to calculate, but contrary to the True-K formula, it does not offer the keratoconus option.

- **For Special Situations:** The Barrett Rx formula has been developed to calculate the IOL power in situations where a refractive error has occurred after cataract surgery. It enables surgeons to calculate the IOL power of piggyback IOLs or the IOL power when an IOL exchange is preferred. The "patient data" display must be populated with specific values, such as the power of the implanted IOL (SE and, if needed, cylinder) and the postoperative (PO) refraction (sphere, cylinder, and axis). In addition to the PreOp K1 and K2 (with their axes), the PO corresponding values are required. Of course, AL, ACD, and target refraction are mandatory. SIA, LT, and CD are optional. The dropdown menu includes 18 IOL models with their own lens factor. For other IOLs, the A-constant must be entered. With both exchange IOL and piggyback IOL modules, the Rx formula suggests also the best meridian along which the toric IOL should be aligned and predicts the residual astigmatism.

Cooke K6 Formula Website (Fig. 57.2)

The website to access the K6 formula, developed by David L. Cooke, MD, is https://cookeformula.com. This is a thin-lens formula where the effective lens position (ELP) is computed with thick-lens calculations and the AL is internally modified to simulate the sum-of-segment axial length (CMAL, Cooke-modified axial length). The user is provided with the opportunity to select the Argos (Alcon) AL, which eliminates the need for internal AL modification, and can select one out of 5 keratometric indices and 20 IOL models, each with its own A-constant. Required variables are AL (there is an Argos option), central corneal thickness (CCT), ACD, LT, CD, K1 and K2, and target Rx, and these parameters are mandatory for the formula to run.

EVO Formula Website (Fig. 57.3)

The Emmetropia Verifying Optical (EVO) formulas developed by Tun Kuan Yeo, MD, are available at https://www.evoiolcalculator.com/start.aspx. The website includes three calculators.

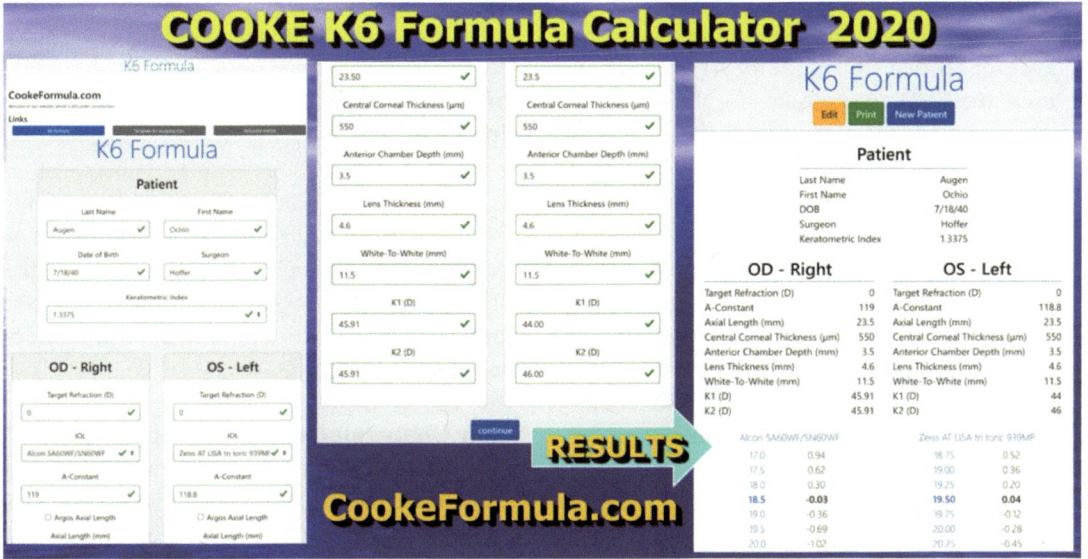

Fig. 57.2 Cooke K6 online calculator

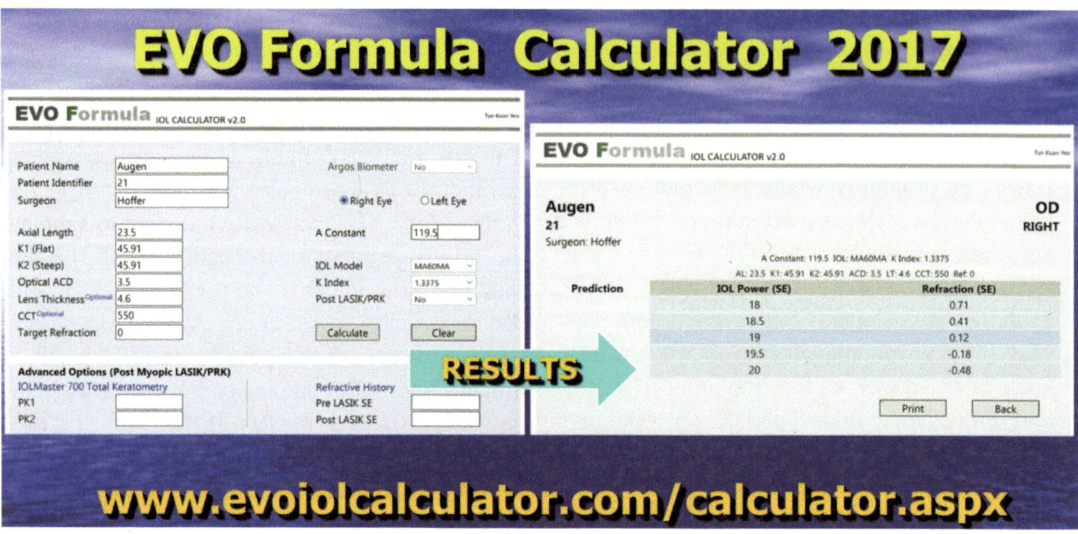

Fig. 57.3 EVO online calculator

- **The EVO (Version 2.0)** (https://www.evoiol-calculator.com/calculator.aspx) is a thick-lens formula and requires five mandatory variables: AL, ACD, K1, K2, and target Rx. LT and CCT are optional. A dropdown menu includes three IOL models. For all other IOL models, it is recommended to enter the www.iolcon.org lens constants. The user has to specify whether the Argos biometer was used or not, as it calculates the AL with the sum-of-segments, which leads to different values in eyes longer than 25 mm. If the Argos has been used, the EVO compensates for the change in AL with respect to traditional optical biometers.
- **The EVO Toric Calculator** (https://www.evoiolcalculator.com/toric.aspx) calculates the cylinder of toric IOLs once the AL, ACD, K1, K2 (with their axes), and target Rx are provided. SIA, LT, and CCT are optional. The dropdown menu offers the choice among four IOL models; for other IOLs, the surgeon has to select whether the toricity is manufactured on the anterior surface of the IOL, on the posterior surface, or both. The results of the toric calculator show the SE power of the IOL, its cylinder, the recommended axis of alignment, and the predicted Rx (sphere, cylinder, and axis).

- **The Post-LASIK EVO Formula Calculator** was developed for eyes that underwent myopic refractive surgery. It can work as a full no-history formula, but it offers the user the opportunity to enter the preoperative (PreOp) and the PO refraction and the posterior corneal curvature (PK1 and PK2) measured by the IOLMaster 700. The post-LASIK option can be selected from both the EVO formula and the EVO toric calculator.

Hoffer QST Formula Website (Fig. 57.4)

The Hoffer QST (Q/Savini/Taroni) is the evolution of the Hoffer Q formula, which has been used for 30 years by ophthalmologists around the world. It can be accessed at https://HofferQST.com and www.EyeLab.com. The calculator offers three options.

- **For Unoperated Eyes:** The improvements of the Hoffer QST over the original Hoffer Q regard the ELP, which is predicted using artificial intelligence (with the average of K1 and K2, anterior corneal radius, Pre-Op ACD, AL, and gender) as inputs of a machine learning algorithm as well as the AL, which is opti-

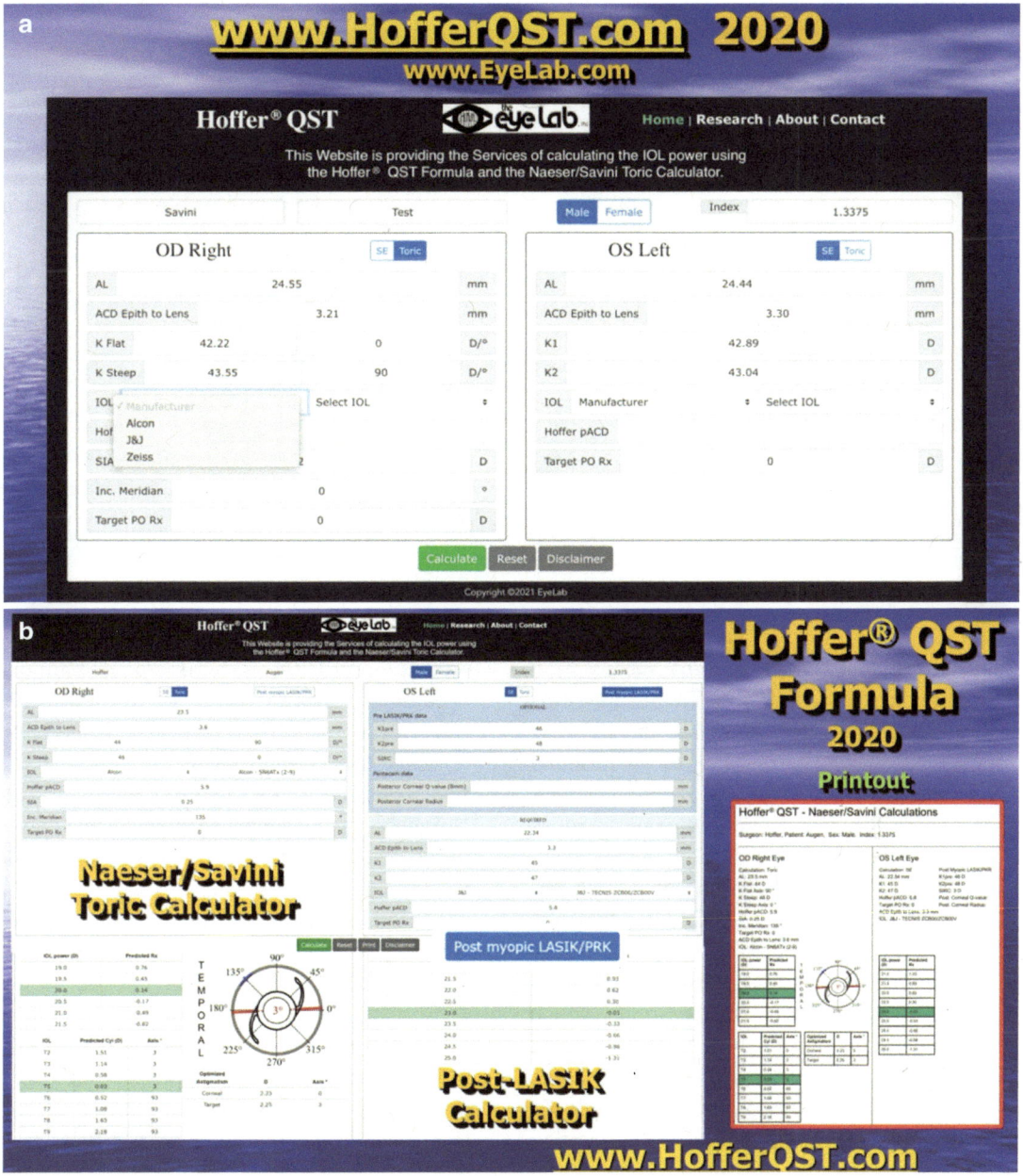

Fig. 57.4 (a) Hoffer QST online calculator: standard calculation page. (b) Hoffer QST online calculator: toric and post-LASIK calculation page with a printout. (c) Hoffer QST online calculator: constant personalization and research

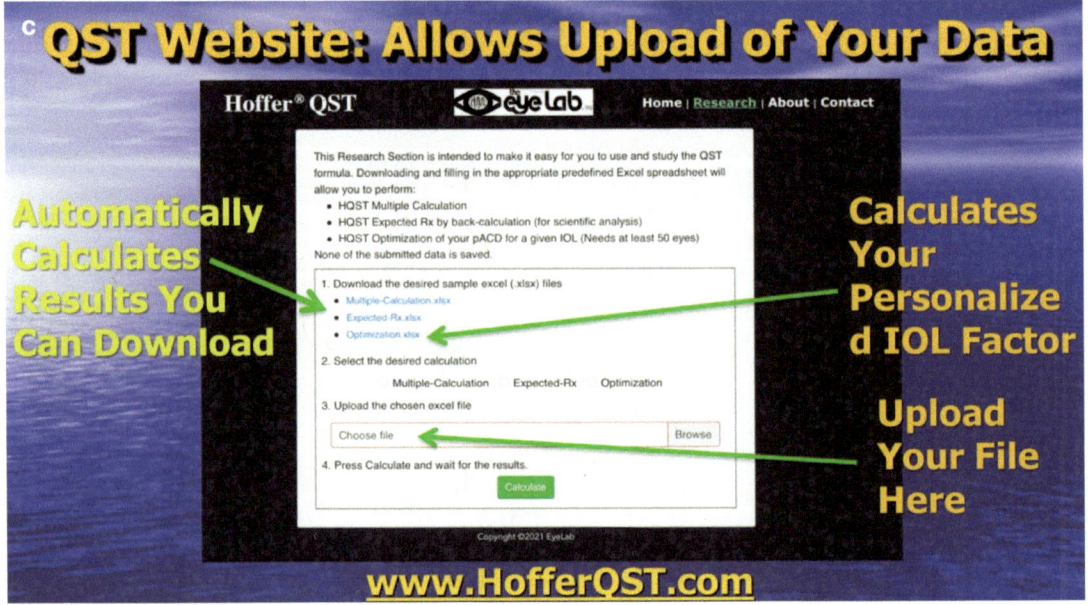

Fig. 57.4 (continued)

mized for long eyes again by means of a machine learning algorithm. The formula was developed in order to maintain the IOLCon pACD constants of the Hoffer Q formula. Required data are AL, ACD, K1, K2, gender, and target Rx. The dropdown menu includes **61 IOL models** from 10 manufacturers.

- **For Toric IOLs:** The Næser/Savini toric calculator is applied to the Hoffer QST formula. In this case, the axes of K1 and K2 and SIA are required. The results are based on the keratometric astigmatism optimization, which reduces the amount of cylinder in eyes with WTR astigmatism and increases it in eyes with ATR astigmatism. The results include the SE power, the cylinder power, and orientation of the IOL, as well as the optimized astigmatism and the predicted refraction.
- **For Post-LASIK Eyes:** This can work as a full no-history method, where AL, ACD, K1 and K2, gender, and target Rx are the only required data. In addition, the refractive change induced by LASIK can be entered. In order to improve the double-K method used to

predict the ELP, the posterior corneal radii or, if Pentacam measurements are available, the posterior corneal curvature and asphericity (Q-value) can be entered.

- **For Research and Constant Optimization:** Uniquely, a research section is available (https://HofferQST.com/research). This was included to help clinicians calculate their personalized lens factor and more importantly for researchers to investigate the outcomes of the Hoffer QST formula in their datasets when comparing the results of various formulas. Five Excel files can be downloaded: (1) a multiple calculation file to calculate the IOL power in large datasets; (2) an expected refraction file to calculate the expected Rx; (3) a multiple calculation file for post-LASIK eyes; (4) an expected refraction for post-LASIK eyes; and (5) an optimization file, which calculates the optimized Hoffer pACD for each dataset. Once these files are filled out with all the data from PO eyes, they can be uploaded and the results are provided to the surgeon anonymously.

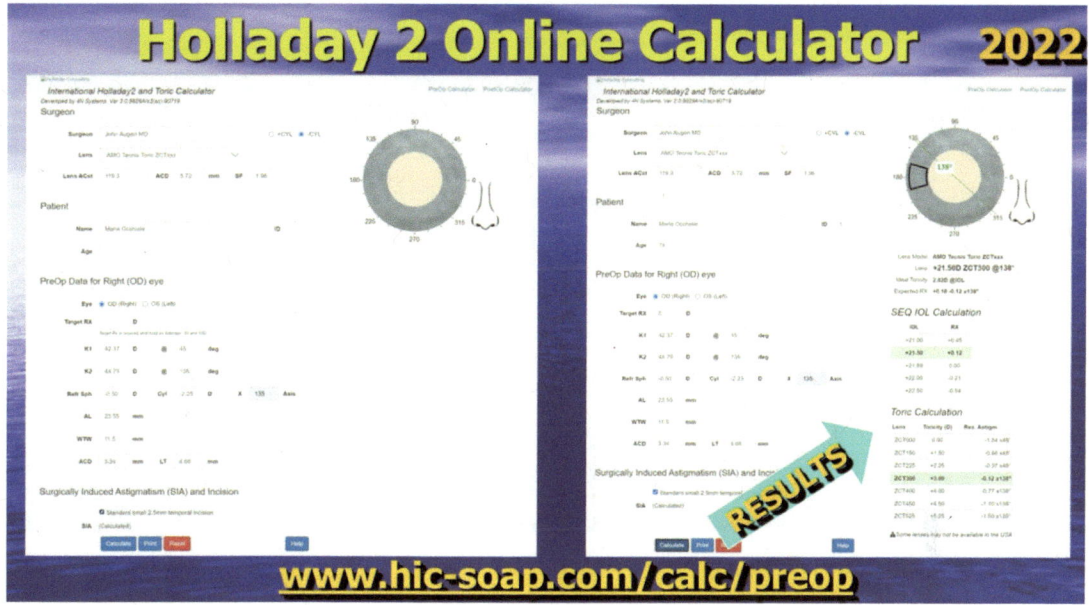

Fig. 57.5 Holladay 2 online calculator

Holladay 2 Formula (Fig. 57.5)

The Holladay 2 and toric calculator can be accessed at https://www.hic-soap.com. The SE power of the IOL is calculated with the Holladay 2 formula and the cylinder with Holladay's toric calculator. Several PreOp variables are necessary: AL, ACD K1 and K2 with their axes, CD, target Rx, and the PreOp Rx. A standard SIA is used, unless the user enters a personalized value. The dropdown menu offers 17 IOL models with their lens constants.

Also, a PO calculator is included to help surgeons rotate the toric IOL if the PO Rx is far from the target. The ideal alignment is calculated from the PO Ks and Rx of the observed IOL alignment and PO Rx.

Kane Formula Website (Fig. 57.6)

The results from the Kane formula, developed by Jack X Kane, MD, can be accessed at https://www.iolformula.com.

- **For Unoperated Eyes:** The Kane formula requires AL, ACD, K1, K2, gender, and target

Rx, while LT and CCT are optional. 14 IOL models are available in the dropdown menu. If another IOL has to be used, its A-constant has to be manually entered. The formula has been developed to have an A-constant similar to the SRK/T A-constant. If the surgeon has an optimized A-constant, then that is recommended for use. Otherwise, the IOLCon SRK/T A-constant for any particular IOL should be used.

- **For Unoperated Eyes with Corneal Astigmatism:** The Kane toric calculator requires the axes of K1 and K2 and SIA to perform the calculation (it is recommended to use an SIA of zero with the Kane toric formula when performing surgery with a temporal incision size of ≤ 2.75 mm). As with other newer generation toric calculators, the keratometric astigmatism is adjusted to take PCA into account. The SE power and cylinder of the toric IOL are provided, as well as the suggested orientation and the predicted refraction.

- **For Unoperated Eyes with Keratoconus:** The Kane formula is specifically adapted. The surgeon must select the "Keratoconus" option, and the same variables as for the standard for-

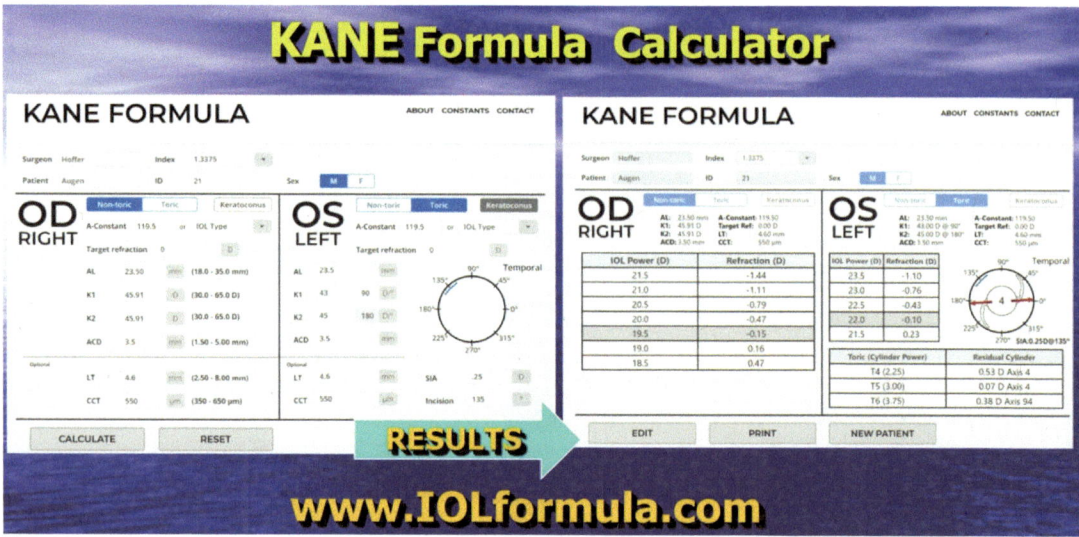

Fig. 57.6 Kane formula online calculator

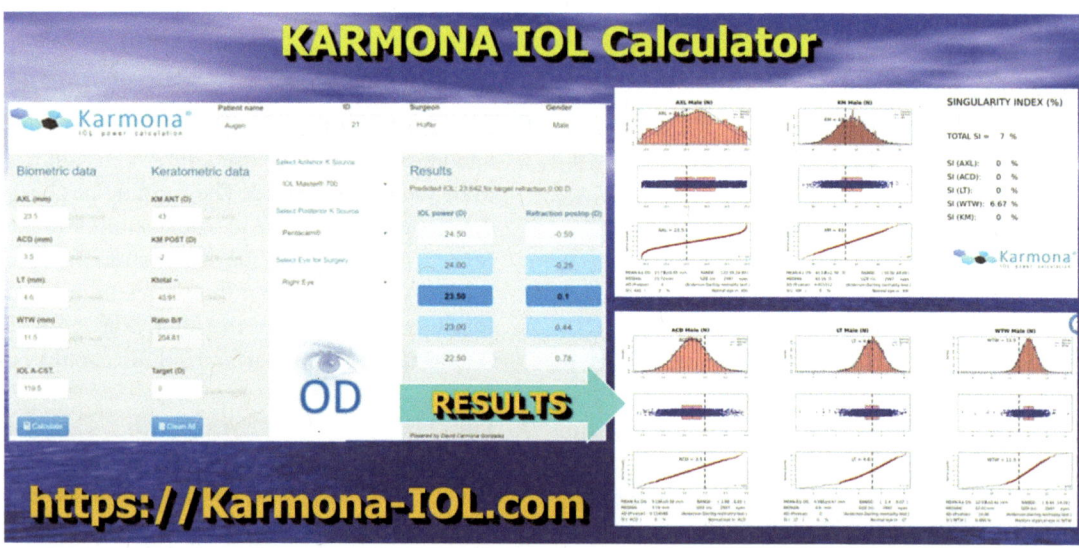

Fig. 57.7 Karmona online calculator

mula are required. The Kane formula for keratoconus is based on a modified corneal power,
derived from the anterior corneal radii of curvature. The formula also reduces the impact of
corneal power on the ELP calculation. A myopic target refraction is recommended in
patients with an average corneal power > 48
D. Between 48 D and 53 D, a target of −0.50
diopter (D) is recommended; between 53 D
and 59 D, a target of −1.00 D is recommended;

and above 59 D, a target of −1.50 to −2.50 D
is recommended.

Karmona Formula Website (Fig. 57.7)

This is another calculation method based on artificial intelligence, available at https://karmona-
iol.com and developed by David Carmona
Gonzales, PhD. Required variables are AL, ACD,

K$_{average}$, CD, and target Rx. LT and posterior K are optional. Standard A-constants have to be entered in order to calculate the IOL power and the expected Rx. Interestingly, a Singularity Index is provided for each eye, with the purpose of alerting the surgeon of unusual combinations of PreOp biometric parameters. The Singularity webpage also features multiple graphs showing the distribution of each parameter compared to the general population. The "Researchers" webpage contains an Excel file that can be downloaded, populated with the biometric data of any surgeon, and uploaded to achieve the results of the Karmona formula for multiple eyes.

Ladas Formula Calculator (Fig. 57.8)

The outcomes of this formula can be obtained at https://www.iolcalc.com. It represents the evolution, based on artificial intelligence and big data methodology, of the original Ladas super formula, which used the best portions of the Haigis, Hoffer Q, Holladay 1, and SRK/T formulas based on AL ranges originally recommended and published by Hoffer [1] in 1993. For unoperated eyes, AL, K1 and K2, and target Rx are sufficient to calculate the SE power of the IOL, whereas PreOp ACD can be entered as an optional input. There are no IOLs to be selected, and the user has to individually enter the A-constant value (default values can be entered in the "Preferences").

The website requires registering with personal information and being approved by them before the calculator can be used. Their toric calculator and a post-LASIK calculator are in development and not yet available.

Nallasamy Formula Website (Fig. 57.9)

This is a method entirely based on artificial intelligence (more specifically, ensemble learning). Calculations can be obtained at https://lenscalc.com. Required data input are AL, ACD, K1, K2, CD, LT, age, and target Rx. CCT is an option. Calculations are available only for one IOL model (AcrySof SN60WF, Alcon).

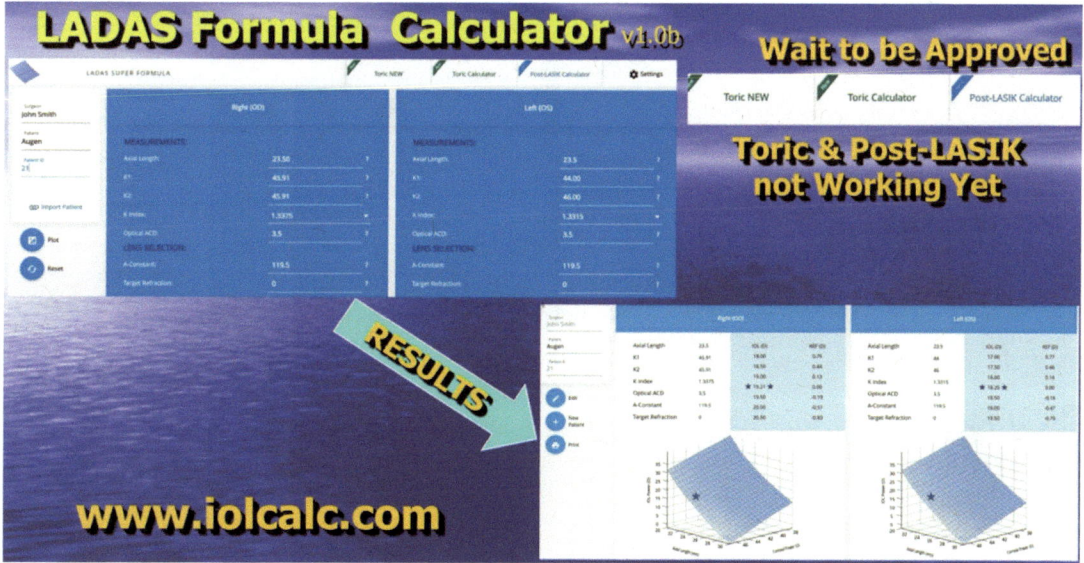

Fig. 57.8 Ladas online calculator

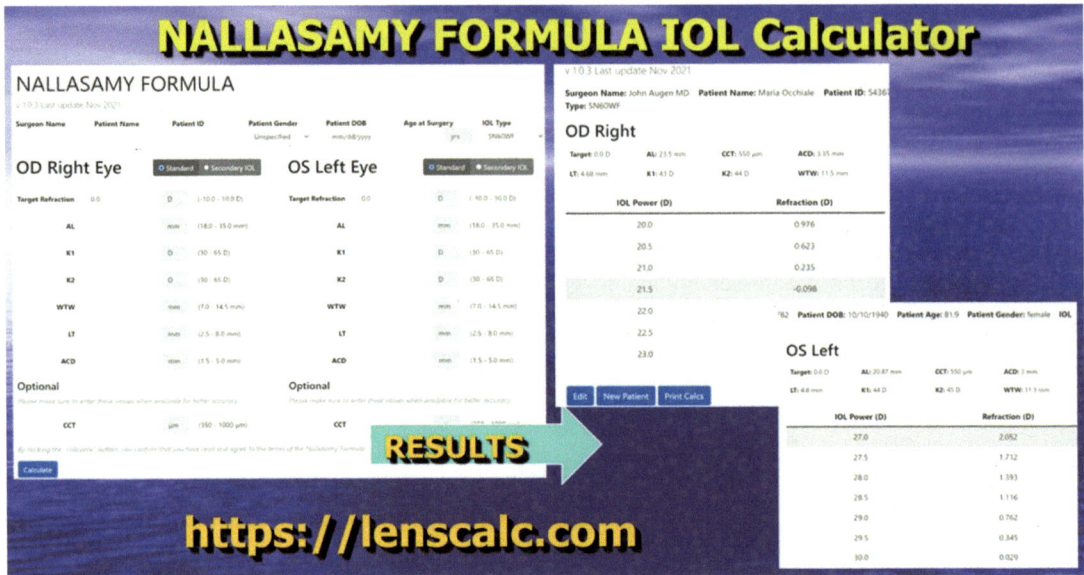

Fig. 57.9 Nallasamy online calculator

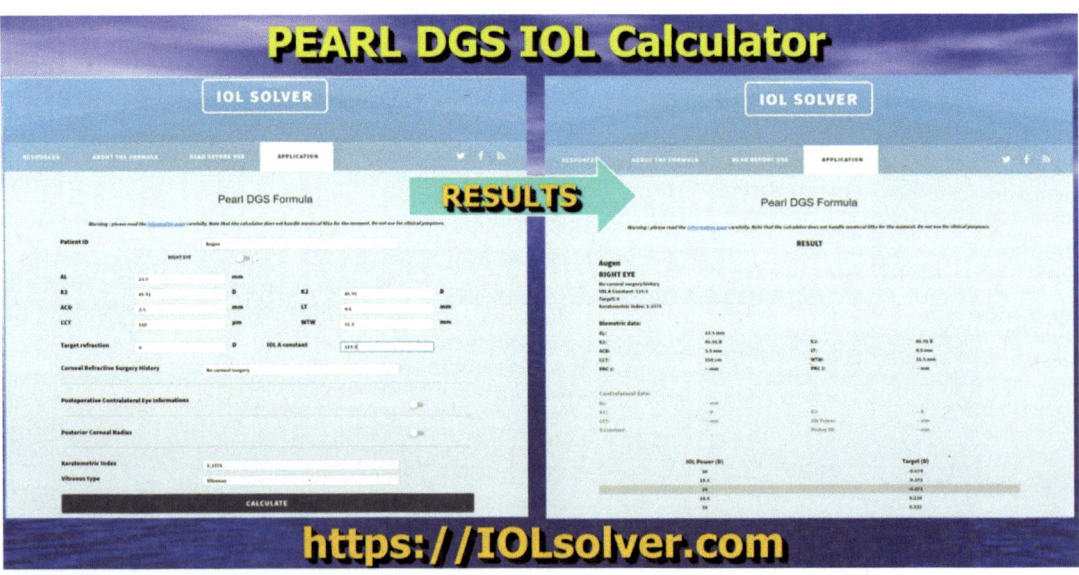

Fig. 57.10 Pearl DGS online calculator

PEARL DGS Formula Website (Fig. 57.10)

Developed by Guillaime Debellemaniere MD, Damien Gatinel MD PhD, Alain Saad MD, the PEARL (PO SE Prediction using ARtificial Intelligence and Linear algorithms), the DGS for-mula is available at **https://iolsolver.com/main**. This is a thick-lens formula considering every radius, thickness, and refractive index. Prediction of the IOL distance from the cornea is based on artificial intelligence. AL is modified according to Cooke (CMAL) to approximate the sum-of-segment AL.

- **For Unoperated Eyes**, AL, ACD, K1, K2, CCT, LT, CD, and target Rx are all mandatory entries. The posterior corneal radii can be entered if measured by any instrument; otherwise, they are predicted from the anterior corneal curvature. The A-constant has to be manually entered. Interestingly, this is the only formula allowing the use of the contralateral eye information if it has had IOL surgery: The user can enter AL, K1, K2, CCT, power of the implanted IOL, and PO Rx to improve the prediction of the IOL power in the second eye.
- **For Eyes with Previous Myopic or Hyperopic Excimer Laser Surgery:** A version of their formula has been developed for these and eyes with previous RK.

RBF 3.0 Calculator Website (Fig. 57.11)

This method, which is available at https://rbfcalculator.com/online/index.html, employs Radial Basis Function, a form of artificial intelligence based on pattern recognition, and has been developed for unoperated eyes. It has been optimized for use with biometry data from the Haag-Streit

Lenstar LS 900 optical biometer in combination with the Alcon SN60WF biconvex IOL for powers from +6.00 D to +30.00 D and IOL powers up to +35.00 D based on a similar biconvex IOL design. For IOL powers from +5.00 D to −5.00 D, it performs best with this combination of biometry devices and the Alcon MA60MA extended range IOL. The RBF calculator may also be used with data from other optical biometers, which provide clinically equivalent biometry data as compared to the Lenstar LS 900 (which is almost all of them except the Argos unit). It may also be used with other biconvex IOL models in the power range of +6.00 D to +35.00 D and other meniscus design IOL models in the power range of +5.00 D to −5.00 D.

Required inputs depend on the optical biometer used. For older instruments, the IOLMaster 500, AL, ACD, K1 and K2, gender, and target Rx are sufficient. For newer instruments, additional optional inputs are LT, CCT, and CD. The "lens constants" section provides users with a list of IOL models and their A-constant to be adopted.

About 1.5% of eyes will be classified as "out of bounds," i.e., cases whose refractive prediction may be less accurate than usual.

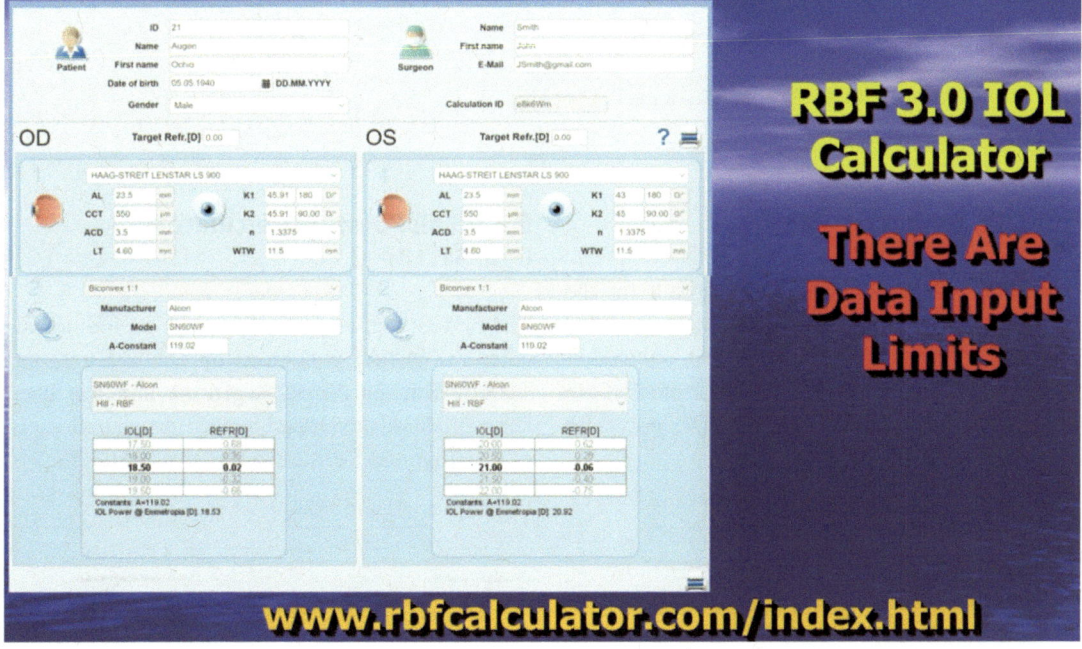

Fig. 57.11 RBF 3.0 online calculator

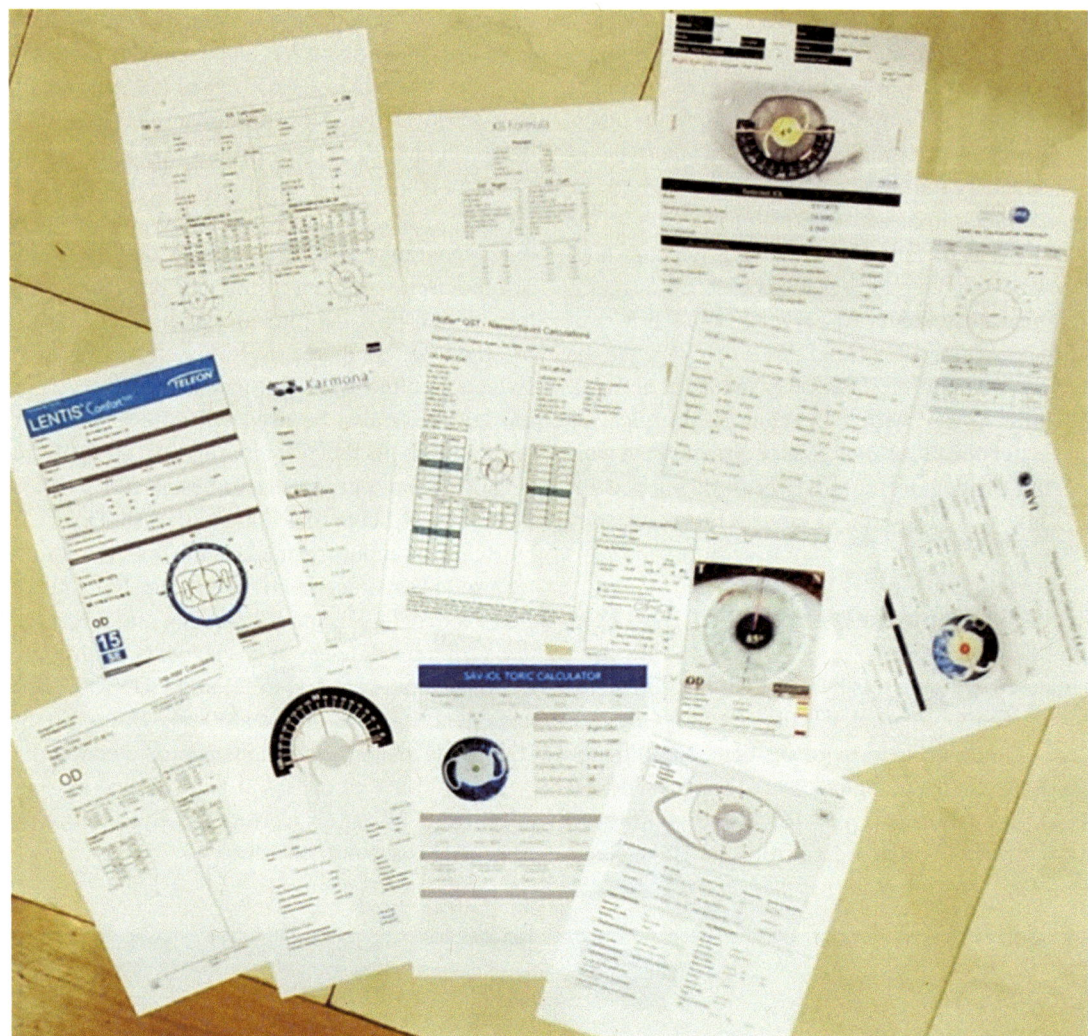

Fig. 57.12 Online website calculator printouts

PRINTOUTS

All formula websites provide a printout for the chart (Fig. 57.12). We are gratified to see that many formulas and websites have added the additional factor of gender which we first pointed out as an important determinant for IOL power in 2017 [2].

ESCRS all Formula Calculator (Fig. 57.13)

The newest and easiest way to use an online calculator was first conceived by Dante Buonsanti MD of Buenos Aires, Argentina and has been sponsored and developed by the European Society of Cataract and Refractive Surgery (ESCRS).

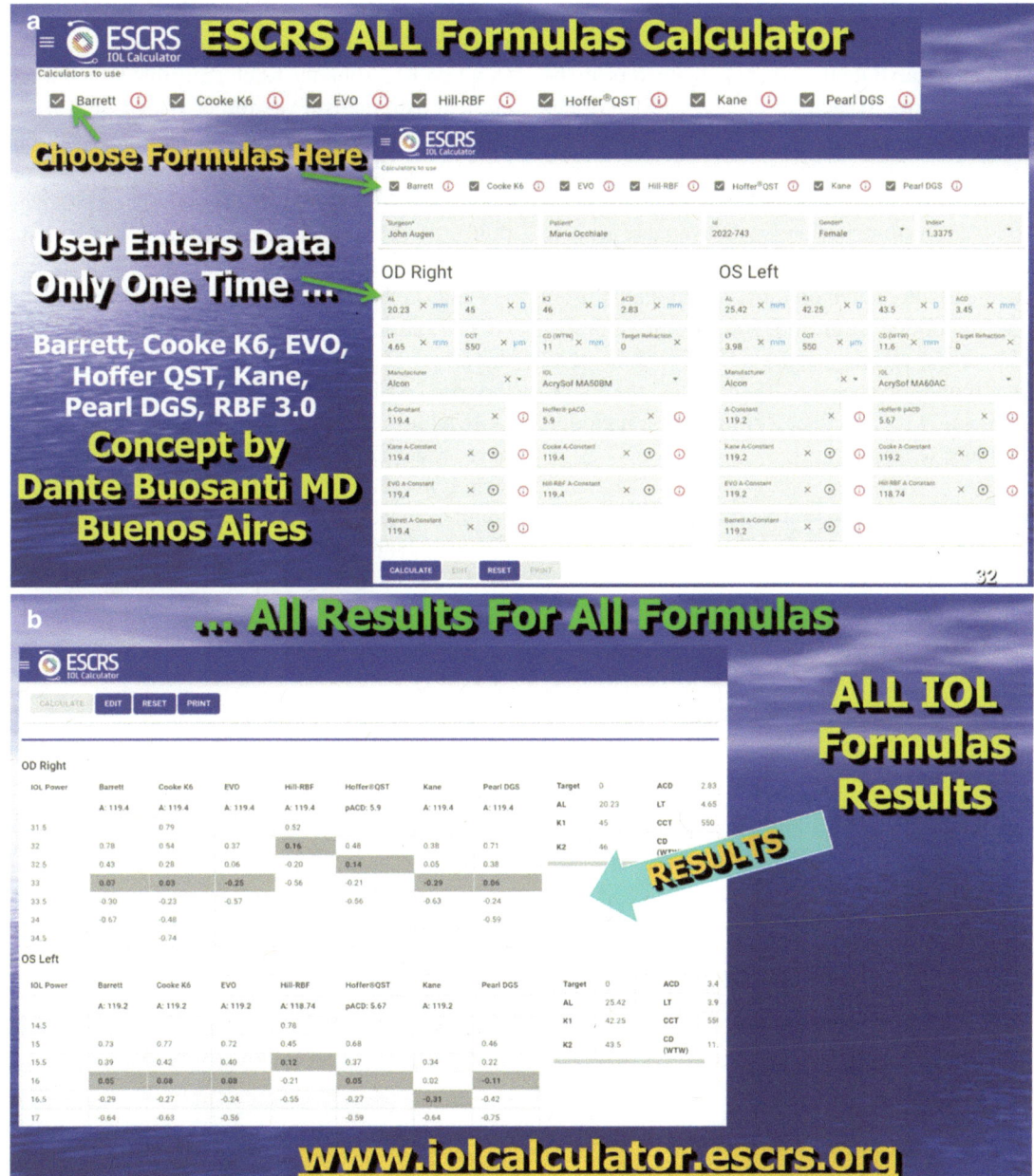

Fig. 57.13 (**a**) ESCRS all formula online calculator: data entry. (**b**) ESCRS all formula online calculator: results when all seven formulas chosen

This calculator (https://iolcalculator.escrs.org/) facilitates the routine effort of ophthalmologists who want to use the latest IOL power formulas for their patients which are not available on their biometer. Users select any or all the formulas they want results for. All they have to do is enter AL, K1, K2, ACD, LT, CCT, CD, gender, and target Rx only one time, and with one click, the results of as many as seven formulas are simultaneously calculated through each formula website: Barrett Universal II, Cooke K6, EVO 2.0, Hoffer QST, Kane, Pearl DGS, and RBF 3.0. This is performed by a Web scraping technology with the permission of all the formula authors. The ESCRS IOL calculator provides recommended lens constants for various IOL models. If a formula specifies a constant for an IOL, the value is obtained from the formula's site. If not, the suggested constants from the IOLCon website are utilized. These constants are optimized if possible, or else those suggested by the manufacturer/ULIB are used. In all cases, an information button is available next to the constant, providing details on where it originated and alternative options. Additionally, users have the option to manually adjust all values. A printout is available that provides the results of all the formulas on one page. There is also the convenient option to use either a comma or a period as a number separator.

Online Calculators for Toric IOL Power

ASSORT Web Calculators

The Alpins Statistical System for Ophthalmic Refractive Surgery Techniques (Assort) has been developed by Noel Alpins MD at www.assort.com. The Web calculators section includes a toric IOL calculator and has two sections: PreOp planning and refractive surprises analysis. The first one requires K1, K2, and steep meridian and provides users with three choices for calculations: standard Ks, Abulafia-Koch adjustment, and total corneal astigmatism (as directly measured by a Scheimpflug camera or an OCT). Once you log in, the calculator is not entirely free, as the use of only four (4) patients is allowed. The spherical power of the IOL is calculated with the Haigis, Hoffer Q, Holladay 1, and SRK/T formula. Formula constants need to be entered by the user.

The refractive surprise analysis can calculate the effect of PO rotation of the toric implant in the case of a refractive surprise.

In addition, a large number of toric calculators have been developed by all manufacturers of toric IOLs (Fig. 57.14). This is a list of the most commonly used:

Alcon: https://www.acrysoftoriccalculator.com

Bausch + Lomb: https://envista.toriccalculator.com

Hanita: https://calc.hanitalenses.com/toric-iol-calculator-v5-01/

Hoya: www.hoyatoric.com

Johnson & Johnson Vision: https://tecnistoric-calc.com

Kowa: https://avanseetoriccalculator.com

Omni: http://www.omnilens.in/portfolio/toric-calculator/

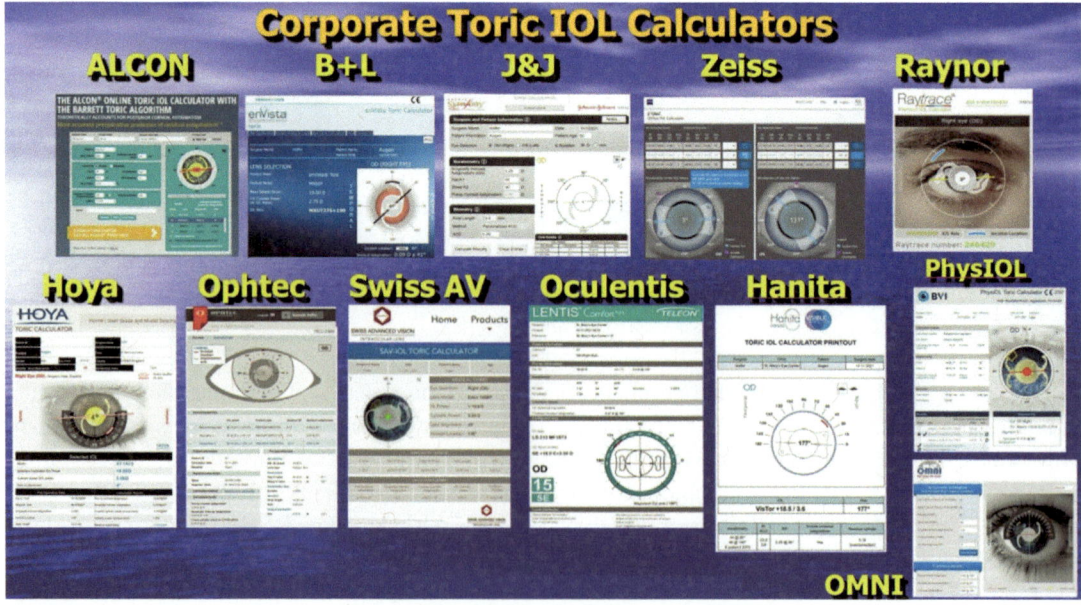

Fig. 57.14 Corporate toric online calculators

Ophtec: https://calculator.ophtec.com/calculator-choice

Physiol: https://www.physioltoric.eu

Rayner: https://www.raytrace.rayner.com

VSY: https://easytoriccalculator.com

Zeiss: https://zcalc.meditec.zeiss.com

Free Downloadable Apps for Spherical and Toric IOL Power

Panacea Formula

This formula, developed by David Flikier MD, of Costa Rica, is not online, but the program can be downloaded at http://www.panaceaiolandtoric-calculator.com/downloads.html. The installed application contains several unique features.

- **The IOL power calculator** is intended for non-toric IOLs to be implanted in unoperated eyes. Required data include AL, ACD, $K_{average}$, and LT. In addition, the ratio of the anterior and posterior corneal radii and the asphericity (Q-value) can be entered to further refine the IOL power calculation. The A-constant of 38 IOL models from five manufacturers is available.
- **The toric calculator** provides the cylinder power of the IOL based on the keratometric astigmatism, calculated from the anterior corneal radii and the flat meridian axis. PCA and SIA can be entered to further improve the predicted outcome.
- **The postop toric calculator** aims to show the ideal toric IOL orientation in eyes that have undergone previous toric IOL implantation but had an unexpected residual astigmatism. After entering the PO Rx (sphere, cylinder, and axis), the AL and K, the cylinder of the

implanted IOL, and its PO alignment, the surgeon can visualize the predicted residual astigmatism. By virtually rotating the IOL from 0 to 180°, it is possible to see the predicted astigmatism for each degree of rotation and select the best IOL orientation. Alternatively, a new toric IOL can be calculated if IOL replacement is planned.

- **The aphakic IOL calculator** is based on the following variables: AL, K, subjective refraction (SE) with vertex distance, A-constant, and anterior-to-posterior corneal radii ratio.

Appendix

In addition to the previously described calculators, it is important to remember two landmark websites. First, the ULIB page (http://ocusoft.de/ulib/c1.htm) was developed by Wolfgang Haigis PhD and was available until 2015. This page contains the optimized constants for hundreds of IOL models. The ULIB website was also the first online calculator, as it enabled individual IOL power calculation with the Haigis, Hoffer Q, and SRK/T formulas. Second, the IOLCon website (https://iolcon.org), developed under the guidance of Prof. Dr. Achim Langenbucher, who continued the work of Haigis, is still collecting and optimizing the constants of newer and older IOL models.

Reference

1. Hoffer KJ. The Hoffer Q formula: a comparison of theoretic and regression formulas. J Cataract Refract Surg 1993;19(11):700–12. Errata 1994;20:677 and 2007;33(1):2-3.
2. Hoffer KJ, Savini G. Effect of gender and race on ocular biometry. Int Ophthalmol Clin. 2017;57(3):137–42.

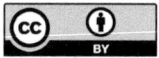

Power Calculations for Spherical and Toric Phakic IOLs

58

Edwin J. Sarver

Introduction

A phakic intraocular lens (PIOL) is implanted into the anterior or posterior chamber of a phakic eye to correct hyperopia or myopia with or without astigmatism. PIOLs are specifically designed to be placed in one of three locations: the angle of the anterior chamber, fixated to the iris, or placed in the sulcus. These lenses are available in high powers and are known to provide highly predictable results [1, 2]. Reporting on ten studies (391 total eyes with sphere range from −6.5 to −33 D), the percentage of eyes with postoperative (PO) refraction within ±1.0 D ranged from 63 to 86% with the median being 75% [2].

Several methods have been developed to accurately calculate the power of a PIOL for a given eye. Both stigmatic and astigmatic power calculation methods are described below. The following is intended to be a sampling of these methods.

Stigmatic PIOL Power Calculations

Russian Method

The Russian method [3] is a particularly simple method that calculates the effective spectacle correction (S) referred to the cornea plane where the back vertex distance (bvd) is assumed to be 12.0 mm and the spectacle lens is translated in air. Equation 58.1 provides the power, P_{PIOL}, of the PIOL as derived via the equation for the effectivity of a lens of power P translated a distance d in a medium of refractive index n and then substituted for the PIOL scenario.

$$P_{PIOL} = \frac{P}{1 - \dfrac{dP}{n}} = \frac{S}{1 - \dfrac{bvd\,S}{1000}} \qquad (58.1)$$

The units employed with the effectivity Eq. (58.1) may be chosen from two sets with either optical powers in diopters (D), distances in meters (m), and index of refraction as a value between 1 and 2, OR optical powers in D, distances in millimeters (mm), and index of refraction multiplied by a factor of 1000. The latter system will be used for all equations in this chapter. Note that for positive translation (light propagation toward the retina) d is positive and for negative translation (light propagation out of the eye) d is negative. For example, if $S = -10$ D, then

E. J. Sarver (✉)
STAAR Surgical Company, Monrovia, CA, USA
e-mail: ejsarver@saavision.com

© The Author(s) 2024
J. Aramberri et al. (eds.), *Intraocular Lens Calculations*, Essentials in Ophthalmology,
https://doi.org/10.1007/978-3-031-50666-6_58

$$P_{PIOL} = \frac{-10.0}{1 - \dfrac{12.0 \times (-10.0)}{1000}} = -8.93\,D$$

van der Heijde's Method

A well-established method for calculating the PIOL power is the van der Heijde equation [3, 4]. This method adds the use of the average keratometry power of the cornea (K) and effective lens position with respect to the anterior cornea (elp). The van der Heijde equation is given in Eq. (58.2).

$$P_{PIOL} = \frac{1336}{\dfrac{1336}{K + S_c} - elp} - \frac{1336}{\dfrac{1336}{K} - elp} \quad (58.2)$$

where S_c is the equivalent power for the spectacle lens of power S for a given bvd as calculated using Eq. (58.1).

Holladay's Method

The vergence formulas of Holladay [5] were derived using a step-along method for the vergence entering the spectacle and eye optical system and stepping along each refracting element (spectacle, cornea, PIOL) and each translation (bvd and elp). Both the preoperative refraction, $PreRx$, and desired PO refraction, $DPostRx$, are considered. Then, given a selected IOL power (IOL), the predicted PO refraction ($PPostRx$) can be calculated. Additionally, a means to optimize the elp was provided so the power calculation could be tuned to a surgeon's data set of eyes. The elp is calculated using Eq. (58.3).

$$elp = 3.74 + sf \quad (58.3)$$

where sf is the surgeon factor optimization parameter and 3.74 is the so-called anatomic anterior chamber depth value [6]. Equation (58.4) calculates the theoretical power for the PIOL.

$$P_{PIOL} = \frac{1336}{\dfrac{1336}{\dfrac{1336}{1000} + K} - elp} - \frac{1336}{\dfrac{1336}{\dfrac{1336}{1000} + K} - elp} \quad (58.4)$$

The predicted PO refraction $PPostRx$ is calculated using Eq. (58.5).

$$PPostRx = \frac{1000}{\dfrac{1000}{\dfrac{1336}{\dfrac{1336}{\dfrac{1336}{\dfrac{1336}{\dfrac{1000}{\dfrac{1000}{PreRx} - bvd} + K} - elp} - IOL} + elp} - K} + bvd} \quad (58.5)$$

The surgeon factor is an optimization parameter that can be used to remove bias in the predicted PO refraction for a given data set. For a given PIOL calculation case, the personalized surgeon factor, psf, can be calculated to arrive at the "perfect" sf value to predict the actual PO refraction (*APostRx*). This is accomplished using Eqs. (58.6)–(58.10).

$$X = \frac{1336}{\dfrac{1000}{\dfrac{1000}{PreRx} - bvd} + K} \quad (58.6)$$

$$Y = \frac{1336}{\dfrac{1000}{\dfrac{1000}{APostRx} - bvd} + K} \quad (58.7)$$

$$A = IOL \quad (58.8a)$$

$$B = -IOL \times (X + Y) \quad (58.8b)$$

$$C = 1336 \times (X - Y) + IOL \times X \times Y \quad (58.8c)$$

$$elp = \frac{-B \pm \sqrt{B^2 - 4AC}}{2A} \quad (58.9)$$

$$psf = elp - 3.74 \quad (58.10)$$

To apply this optimization to a surgeon's data set, Eq. (58.11) is used where M is the number of cases in the surgeon's data set. The *psf* is calculated for each case and then the average is taken to yield the new *sf* to be used in Eq. (58.3) for the *elp* value used in Eqs. (58.4) and (58.5).

$$sf = \frac{1}{M} \sum_{m=1}^{M} psf_m \quad (58.11)$$

Astigmatic PIOL Power Calculations

Sarver's Method

Sarver's method [7] combines the step-along method of Holladay with the use of astigmatic decomposition [8] to yield equations to calculate the ideal toric PIOL (TPIOL) power, to predict the PO refraction for a selected TPIOL, and then calculate a simple optimization parameter to remove bias in the predicted PO refraction error spherical equivalent for a given data set. This method makes use of astigmatic decomposition to generalize vergence from stigmatic to astig-matic in a domain where the components may be linearly combined.

Astigmatic Decomposition

The forward astigmatic decomposition transformation is given in Eq. (58.12).

$$m = s + \frac{c}{2}$$

$$c_0 = c \times \cos(2\theta)$$

$$c_{45} = c \times \sin(2\theta) \quad (58.12)$$

where *s*, *c*, and θ are the standard toric lens parameters; sphere (D), cylinder (D), axis (deg), and m, c_0, and c_{45} are the astigmatic decomposition parameters (all in diopters) where m is the spherical equivalent power.

The axis value θ is the meridian of the toric lens and is limited to the range of 0–180°. For an astigmatic power (in power and axis form) such as keratometric values *steep power @ steep axis + flat power @ flat axis*, the first step is to convert to equivalent s and c axes with negative cylinder values using Eq. (58.13) and then apply Eq. (58.12) to get the equivalent astigmatic decomposition values.

$$s = \text{steep power}$$

$$c = \text{flat power} - \text{steep power}$$

$$\theta = \text{steep axis} \quad (58.13)$$

The inverse astigmatic decomposition transformation for minus cylinder notation is shown in Eq. (58.14).

$$c = -\sqrt{c_0^2 + c_{45}^2}$$

$$s = m - \frac{c}{2}$$

$$\theta = \tan^{-1}\left(\frac{c - c_0}{c_{45}}\right) \quad (58.14)$$

To keep the axis value θ in the range of 0–180, if the calculated value from the arctangent function in Eq. (58.14) is negative, 180 is added to it, and if it is greater than 180, 180 is subtracted from it. Also, note that in programming the astigmatic decomposition equations it is often simpler to use the atan2 function that automatically handles the case where c_{45} is zero.

It is often convenient to denote the forward and inverse astigmatic decomposition transformations of Eqs. (58.12) and (58.14) as shown in Eqs. (58.15) and (58.16), respectively.

$$\begin{bmatrix} m \\ c_0 \\ c_{45} \end{bmatrix} = A \left\{ \begin{bmatrix} s \\ c \\ \theta \end{bmatrix} \right\} \quad (58.15)$$

$$\begin{bmatrix} s \\ c \\ \theta \end{bmatrix} = A^{-1} \left\{ \begin{bmatrix} m \\ c_0 \\ c_{45} \end{bmatrix} \right\} \quad (58.16)$$

Effectivity

In Eq. (58.1), the effectivity equation for a stigmatic lens or vergence is provided. Its equivalent formulation is given in Eq. (58.17).

$$e_{d,n}(P) = \frac{P}{1 - \dfrac{dP}{n}} = \frac{n}{\dfrac{n}{P} - d} \quad (58.17)$$

The left-hand side of Eq. (58.17) is intended to provide a shorthand notation for calculating the effectivity of translating a scalar power P a distance d through a medium of index n. The formulation on the right side of the equation is problematic when the power P is zero, so the center formulation is preferred. The structure of the right side is what leads to the characteristic waterfall structure of Eqs. (58.1), (58.2), and (58.4)–(58.7).

To apply the scalar version of the effectivity equation in 17 to an astigmatic decomposition vector or a sphere, cylinder, and axis vector, it is necessary to find the principal powers, translate each one independently, and then transform the results back to either sphere, cylinder, or axis form or to an astigmatic decomposition vector.

For an astigmatic decomposition vector $\mathbf{V}$, these operations are denoted as shown in Eq. (58.18).

$$E_{d,n}\{\mathbf{V}\} = A\left\{ e_{d,n}\left(A^{-1}\{\mathbf{V}\} \right) \right\} \quad (58.18)$$

Phakic IOL Calculations

The parameters used in the TPIOL calculations are either vectors shown with **bold capital letters** (power or vergence values) or scalars shown with *lowercase italics letters* (distance values). They are listed in Table 58.1.

The *elp* value is the *acd* value offset by the *sf* value and is given in Eq. (58.19).

$$elp = acd + sf \quad (58.19)$$

In this section, calculations are presented for ideal IOL power, predicted refraction, back-calculated surgeon factor, and exchange TPIOL power.

Ideal IOL Power

The combination of the preoperative spectacle correction referred to the cornea, the preoperative

Table 58.1 Parameters for the toric phakic IOL calculations

Symbol	Meaning
bvd	Back vertex distance
elp	Expected lens position
aelp	Actual expected lens position
sf	Surgeon factor
acd	Anterior chamber depth (with respect to anterior cornea)
S	Preoperative spectacle power
CL	Preoperative contact lens
K	Preoperative corneal power
PK	PO corneal power
DS	Desired PO spectacle power
PS	Predicted PO spectacle power
AS	Actual PO spectacle power
IP	Ideal power of the TPIOL
AP	Actual implanted IOL power
CP	Current power = AP at PO axis
EP	Exchange TPIOL power

contact lens (if any), and the corneal power all referred to the IOL plane is denoted $\mathbf{P_1}$ and is given in Eq. (58.20).

$$\mathbf{P_1} = E_{elp,1336} \left\{ \mathbf{K} + \mathbf{CL} + E_{bvd,1000} \left\{ \mathbf{S} \right\} \right\} \tag{58.20}$$

The combination of the desired PO spectacle correction referred to the cornea and the corneal power referred to the IOL plane is denoted $\mathbf{P_2}$ and is given in Eq. (58.21).

$$\mathbf{P_2} = E_{elp,1336} \left\{ \mathbf{K} + E_{bvd,1000} \left\{ \mathbf{DS} \right\} \right\} \tag{58.21}$$

The ideal power of the TPIOL can now be calculated as the difference between the power required at the IOL plane to focus a distant object on the retina $\mathbf{P_1}$ and the power supplied by the desired PO spectacle lens and the cornea referred to the IOL plane $\mathbf{P_2}$. This is specified in Eq. (58.22).

$$\mathbf{IP} = \mathbf{P_1} - \mathbf{P_2} \tag{58.22}$$

Predicted PO Refraction

Usually, the precise TPIOL power calculated in eq. 22 will not be available to the surgeon. TPIOL powers are often quantized in step sizes of 0.50 D. For the actual IOL power, **AP,** selected by the surgeon, the PO refraction **PS** can be predicted using Eq. (58.23).

$$\mathbf{PS} = E_{-bvd,1000} \left\{ E_{-elp,1336} \left\{ \mathbf{P_1} - \mathbf{AP} \right\} - \mathbf{K} \right\} \tag{58.23}$$

Calculating the *elp* Value

Following Holladay's lead, the actual *elp, aelp,* for each case in a surgeon's data set can be calculated and used to optimize future calculations. For this calculation, instead of using astigmatic decomposition values, it is converted to spherical equivalent values. The calculation is performed

by solving a quadratic equation as shown in Eqs. (58.24)–(58.28).

$$a_1 = 1336 \frac{bvd\, S - 1000}{(K + CL)\, bvd\, S - 1000(K + CL + S)} \tag{58.24}$$

$$a_2 = 1336 \frac{bvd\, AS - 1000}{K\, bvd\, AS - 1000(K + AS)} \tag{58.25}$$

$$b = a_1 + a_2 \tag{58.26}$$

$$c = \frac{1336(a_1 - a_2)}{AP} + a_1 a_2 \tag{58.27}$$

$$aelp = \begin{cases} \dfrac{b - \sqrt{b^2 - 4\,c}}{2} & \text{if } b > 0 \\[4mm] \dfrac{b + \sqrt{b^2 - 4\,c}}{2} & \text{otherwise} \end{cases} \tag{58.28}$$

where *S, K, CL, AS,* and *AP* are scalar spherical equivalent values not astigmatic decomposition vectors.

Refractive Surprise Exchange Calculation

Although not presented in [7], the astigmatic decomposition notation can be used to illustrate how to calculate an exchange PIOL power. The need for this calculation can occur when, for example, there is a refractive surprise that requires a lens exchange. In this case, Eqs. (58.29) and (58.30) can be used to calculate the exchange PIOL power (**EP**).

$$\mathbf{P_3} = E_{elp,1336} \left\{ \mathbf{PK} + E_{bvd,1000} \left\{ \mathbf{AS} \right\} \right\} + \mathbf{AP} \tag{58.29}$$

$$\mathbf{EP} = \mathbf{P_3} - E_{elp,1336} \left\{ \mathbf{PK} + E_{bvd,1000} \left\{ \mathbf{DS} \right\} \right\} \tag{58.30}$$

Sample Calculation

A sample TPIOL calculation using eqs. 12 to 30 is presented in this section to make clear how the calculations flow. For this example, the scaler data of back vertex distance *bvd* are 12.0 mm, anterior chamber depth *acd* is 3.55 mm, and surgeon factor *sf* is −0.304 mm. Then, from Eq. (58.18), the expected lens position *elp* is calculated to be 3.25 mm. These scaler parameters are listed in Table 58.2.

The second set of data for this example calculation is the astigmatic powers in normal form and astigmatic decomposition form. These values are given in Table 58.3. In this table, the first column contains the vector parameter symbol, the center column contains the normal astigmatic form values, and the last column contains the equivalent astigmatic decomposition vector elements. For parameters already given by sphere, cylinder, and axis values, Eq. (58.12) is used to calculate the astigmatic decomposition elements. For the corneal power vector **K,** Eq. (58.13) is first used to convert from power and axis format

to sphere, cylinder, and axis, and then Eq. (58.12) is used to compute the astigmatic decomposition elements.

Using the *elp* value from Table 58.2, the astigmatic decomposition elements from Table 58.3, and Eqs. (58.20)–(58.22), the ideal TPIOL power is calculated to be

$$\mathbf{P}_1 = \begin{bmatrix} 39.36 \\ 0.19 \\ 0.52 \end{bmatrix}$$

$$\mathbf{P}_2 = \begin{bmatrix} 47.03 \\ 1.20 \\ -0.30 \end{bmatrix}$$

$$\mathbf{IP} = \begin{bmatrix} -7.66 \\ -1.01 \\ 0.82 \end{bmatrix}$$

Converting this astigmatic decomposition, TPIOL power to sphere, cylinder, and axis components using Eq. (58.14) gives

$$\mathbf{IP} = -7.01 - 1.30 \times 160°$$

If this **IP** value is used for the actual power **AP** of the TPIOL to be implanted, the predicted PO spectacle would be the desired spectacle **DS** value, −0.5 D. If the surgeon instead plans to use the **AP** power of −8.00 − 1.00 × 160, then using Eqs. (58.14), (58.20), and (58.23), the predicted PO spectacle **PS** is calculated as (astigmatic decomposition and sphere, cylinder, and axis forms)

$$\mathbf{PS} = \begin{bmatrix} 0.18 \\ -0.20 \\ 0.15 \end{bmatrix} \rightarrow 0.30 - 0.25 \times 162°$$

Now, suppose the actual PO spectacle power is 0.50–1.25 × 170° and the surgeon would like to consider an exchange lens. Using Eqs. (58.14), (58.29), and (58.30), the exchange lens parameters are computed in astigmatic decomposition and sphere, cylinder, and axis forms.

$$\mathbf{P}_3 = \begin{bmatrix} 39.18 \\ -072 \\ 0.59 \end{bmatrix}$$

Table 58.2 Sample TPIOL calculation scalar parameters

Parameter	Value	Equation
bvd	12.0	
acd	3.55	
sf	−0.304	
elp	3.25	(58.18)

Table 58.3 Sample TPIOL calculation astigmatic parameters in normal and in astigmatic decomposition form

Parameter	Sphere, cylinder, axis	M, C0, C45
S	−6.75 − 1.25 × 160.00	−7.38, −0.96, 0.80
CL	0–0 × 0	0, 0, 0
K	42.20 @ 173.00 + 43.20 @ 83.00	42.70, 0.97, −0.24
DS	−0.5 − 0 × 0	−0.5, 0, 0
AP	−8.00 − 1.00 × 160	−8.50, −0.77, 0.64
AS	0.50–1.25 × 180.00	−0.13, −1.25, −0.00
PK	42.2 @ 169 + 43.5 @ 79	42.85, 1.21, −0.47

$$\mathbf{EP} = \begin{bmatrix} -8.03 \\ -2.22 \\ 1.17 \end{bmatrix} \rightarrow -6.78 - 2.51 \times 166°$$

For available powers near this exchange lens power, the prediction formulas could again be employed to help the surgeon make a selection to yield the best-expected results for the patient.

Next, given the data for this case, the actual *elp* (*aelp*) can be calculated for use in optimizing future results using Eqs. (58.24)–(58.28).

$$a_1 = 37.19$$

$$a_2 = 31.38$$

$$b = 68.58$$

$$c = 254.08$$

$$aelp = 3.93$$

Using this value of 3.93 instead of 3.25 leads to the predicted PO spectacle spherical equivalent equal to the actual PO spectacle spherical equivalent. A data set consisting of historical cases where each one has an *aelp* value could be used to calculate the best constant value *elp* or allow fitting any of a number of machine learning regression models to the data set to improve future results. In the case of using a machine learning regression model, a new *elp* value would be calculated for each future TPIOL case.

Discussion

The set of equations required to support calculations relating to TPIOLs have been provided. This provides the functions of:

1. Calculation of the ideal TPIOL power for a given eye and desired PO spectacle power
2. Prediction of the PO spectacle power for a selected TPIOL power other than the ideal power
3. Calculation of an exchange TPIOL in the event of an unacceptable refractive surprise
4. Back calculation of the *elp* value on a per-case basis to provide a means of building a data set to optimize the predictability of future cases

The same set of equations also supports stigmatic PIOLs, by simply entering 0 for the appropriate cylinder values.

Although not described above, by allowing the surgeon to enter any sphere, cylinder, and axis for the actual TPIOL power **AP**, the effect of axis rotation can readily be calculated using the predicted refraction equations. This analysis would be useful in deciding whether a simple lens rotation would be useful in the event of an unexpected refractive outcome.

MacKenzie [9] and Langenbucher [10] also discuss astigmatic PIOL power calculations using matrix optics and astigmatic decomposition vectors, respectively. The use of matrix optics is numerically equivalent to the astigmatic decomposition approach. However, these references did not present details on how to update the *elp* value to optimize future calculations.

References

1. Wong ACM, Azar DT. Chapter 31: Refractive surgery. In: Phakic IOL power calculations. 2nd ed. Mosby; 2007. p. 401–16.
2. Alio y Sanz JL, Rodriguez-Mier FA. Chapter 39: Refractive surgery. In: Refractive phakic intraocular lens for the correction of myopia and hyperopia (AC and artisan lens). Jaypee Brothers Medical Publishers, LTD; 2000. p. 417–26.
3. Dementiev DD, Hoffer KJ, Sborgia G, Marucchi P, D'Amico A. Chapter 41: Refractive surgery. In: Phakic refractive lens for correction of myopia and hyperopia. Jaypee Brothers Medical Publishers, LTD; 2000. p. 440–61.
4. van der Heijde GL, Fechner PU, Worst JG. [Optical consequences of implantation of a negative intraocular lens in myopic patients]. Klin Monatsbl Augenheilkd. 1988;193:99–102.
5. Holladay JT. Refractive power calculations for intraocular lenses in the phakic eye. Am J Ophthalmol. 1993;116:63–6.
6. Holladay JT, Prager TC, Chandler TY, Musgrove KH, Lewis JW, Ruiz RS. A three-part system for refining intraocular lens power calculations. J Cataract Refract Surg. 1988;13:17.
7. Sarver EJ, Sanders DR. Astigmatic power calculations for intraocular lenses in the phakic and aphakic eye. J Refract Surg. 2004;20:472–7.
8. Bennett AG, Rabbetts RB. Clinical visual optics. 3rd ed. Woburn, MA: Butterworth-Heinemann; 1994. p. 88–9.

9. MacKenzie GE, Harris WF. Determining the power of a thin toric intraocular lens in an astigmatic eye. Optom Vis Sci. 2002;79:667–71.

10. Langenbucher A, Szentmary N, Seitz B. Calculating the power of toric phakic intraocular lenses. Ophthal Physiol Opt. 2007;27:373–80.

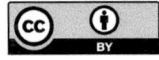

Part V

Toric IOL Calculations

Kristian Næser

Net astigmatisms and spherocylinders are complex formats with magnitudes in diopters (D) and directions in degrees (°). These entities represent individual keratometries or refractions, but must be converted to vectors to allow for calculations of surgically induced astigmatism (SIA), toric intraocular lens (IOL) power, averages, spreads, etc. Several methods for reporting surgically induced astigmatism (SIA) have been reported during the last 40 years [1–16]. However, this issue has remained contested up till this day due to the continued use of nonvector methods [17–23].

This chapter describes the principles for conversion of refractive data to dioptric vectors. Næser's polar value dioptric vectors are detailed [3, 7, 11, 16, 22], other dioptric vector formats are reviewed, their statistical assessments are described, a terminology is suggested, and practical calculations are demonstrated.

Spherocylinder Formats

Spheres and cylinders are lower-order (LO) aberrations, correctable with spectacle glasses or contact lenses. Higher-order aberrations are not part of this discussion. In an optimal spherical (*stigmatic* or point-like) optical system, a point in the object space is focused as a point image (Fig. 59.1) [16]. In a regular *astigmatic* optical system, an object point is focused as two mutually perpendicular line segments (Fig. 59.2) [16]. The optical effects of ocular astigmatism are blur in all fixation distances due to lack of point focus and distortion caused by unequal (differential) magnification of the retinal image in the various meridians. The blurs generated from a 1.0 D cylinder and a 0.5 D sphere are equivalent.

K. Næser (✉)
Department of Ophthalmology, Randers Regional Hospital, Randers, Denmark
e-mail: kristian.naeser@dadlnet.dk

J. Aramberri et al. (eds.), *Intraocular Lens Calculations*, Essentials in Ophthalmology,
https://doi.org/10.1007/978-3-031-50666-6_59

Fig. 59.1 A stigmatic ocular optical system. In the absence of diffraction, aberration, and scatter, a point in object space is focused as a point image. An object located in the far point is focused on the retina. Objects from any other position are defocused and blur circles are projected on the retina. (Reproduced with permission from John Wiley and Sons publishers)

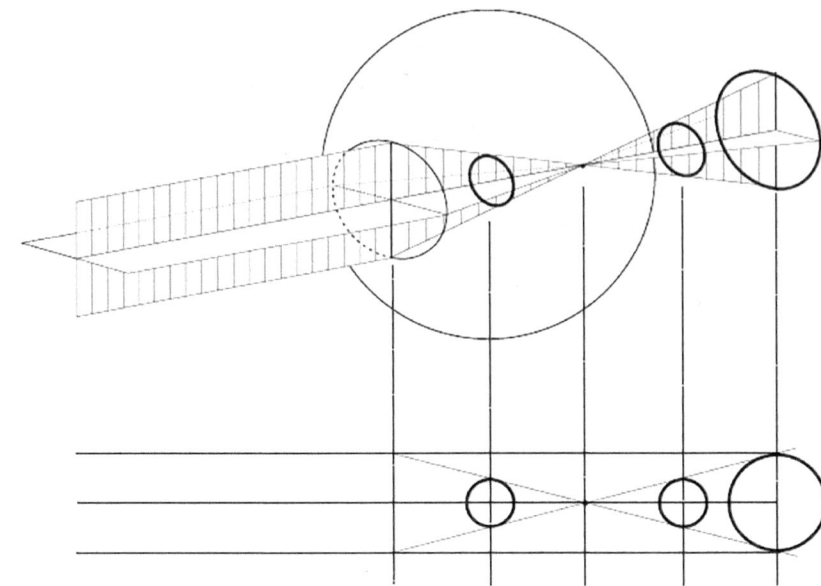

Fig. 59.2 An astigmatic with-the-rule ocular optical system. The mutually perpendicular focal lines delineate Sturm's interval. The position of the circle of least confusion is the dioptric average between the two focal lines and determines the spherical equivalent power. No point focus is formed. The image projected on the retina is always blurred due to its variable shapes and directions. (Reproduced with permission from John Wiley and Sons publishers)

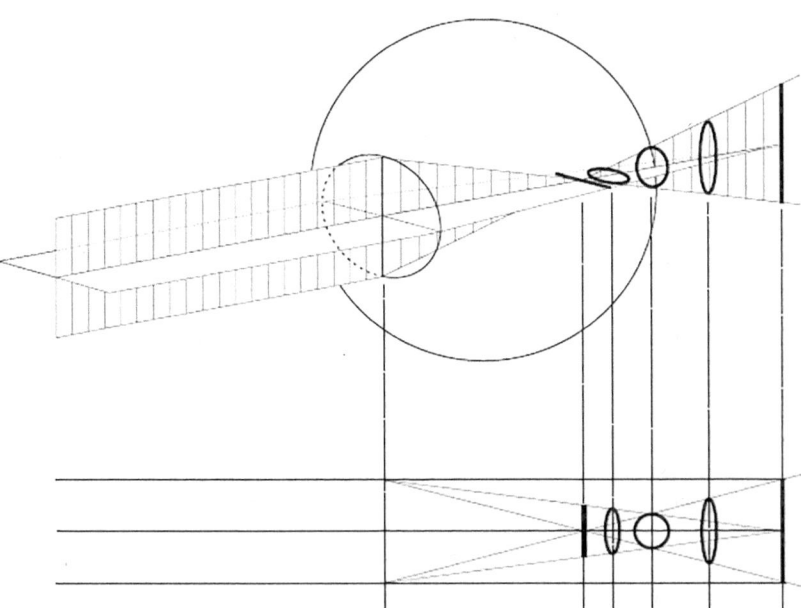

Corneal Spherocylinder Formats

Keratometry, topography, and tomography should be based on independent measurements, employing stationary (not handheld) devices. A single autokeratometry is inadequate, but the vector average of three measurements is sufficient for precise assessment. (Fig. 59.3) [24–26].

Corneal measurements identify the radii of curvature ($R1$ and $R2$ in mm) and meridians along the two orthogonal principal meridians. The *curvature C* with units in D is the reciprocal of the radius of curvature [16]:

$$C = 1/R \qquad (59.1)$$

The radii of curvature in mm ($R1$ and $R2$) are converted to powers ($K1$ and $K2$) in diopters with the paraxial formula:

Fig. 59.3 Individual differences in astigmatism between paired Nidek Tonoref II autokeratometries with their 95% tolerance [24, 25] ellipses for observations in various measurement modalities. Bivariate plot. Units in diopters. Differences based on one measurement (blue) produced the largest (least precise) tolerance ellipse, while the ellipses for three (black) and five (violet) measurements were overlapping as a sign of approximately similar precision. Also note the reduction in outliers with increasing number of measurements

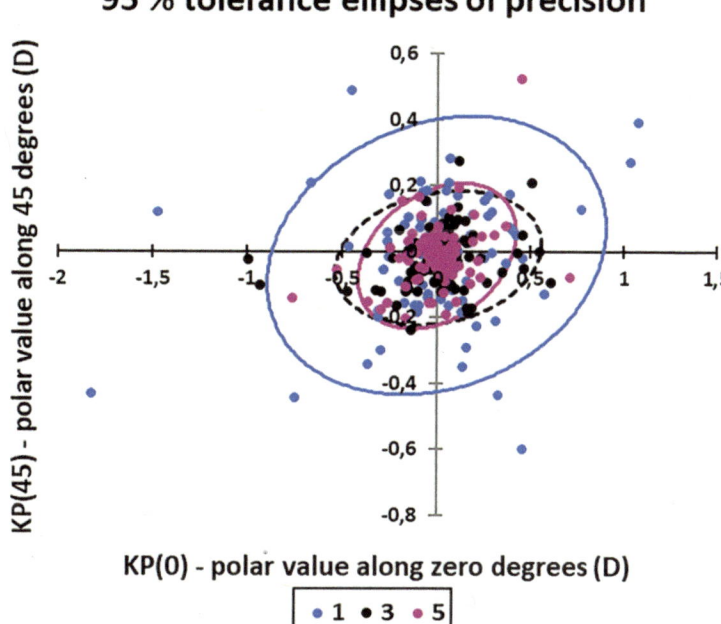

95 % tolerance ellipses of precision

KP(45) - polar value along 45 degrees (D)

KP(0) - polar value along zero degrees (D)

• 1 • 3 • 5

$$K = (n_2 - n_1) / R = \Delta n / R, \qquad (59.2)$$

where n_1 and n_2 are the refractive indices of the first and second medium along the optical pathway. The refractive index (n_1) of air = 1.0 is used in assessment of anterior corneal surfaces:

- *KA: Keratometric astigmatism* is based on measurement of the anterior surface only and employs an effective (or fictitious) refractive index n_2 of 1.3315 to 1.3375 to account for the average (but not measured) negative posterior corneal power (Fig. 59.4).
- *ACA: Anterior corneal astigmatism* also relies on measurement of the anterior surface and employs the actual refractive index of corneal tissue n_2 of 1.376.
- *PCA: Posterior corneal astigmatism* uses the corneal ($n_1 = 1.376$) and aqueous ($n_2 = 1.336$) refractive indices. The posterior corneal power is negative, because Δn (1.336–1.376 = −0.04) is negative (Fig. 59.5).
- *TCA: Total corneal astigmatism* employs tomographic measurements of both surfaces

and of corneal thickness to allow thick lens optics or ray tracing with various methods. To date, such direct measurement of PCA has failed to outperform methods based on various mathematical modulations of KA magnitude and direction.

The spherical equivalent is the average of any orthogonal principal powers:

$$SE = 0.5 \times (K1 + K2). \qquad (59.3)$$

The astigmatism magnitude M ($M \geq 0$) in diopters is the absolute difference between these two powers of maximal difference. For Næser's polar value system, a *plus power format* is selected. The astigmatic direction α in degrees is therefore defined as the *meridian* of *most positive* (or *least negative*) power. The net astigmatism M along the meridian α is symbolized as ($M @ \alpha$). Corneal astigmatisms are subgrouped as with-the-rule (WTR), oblique, and against-the rule (ATR) according to the direction of the steep anterior meridian (Fig. 59.6).

Angular directions are given as values between zero and 180°. However, regular astigmatism is a

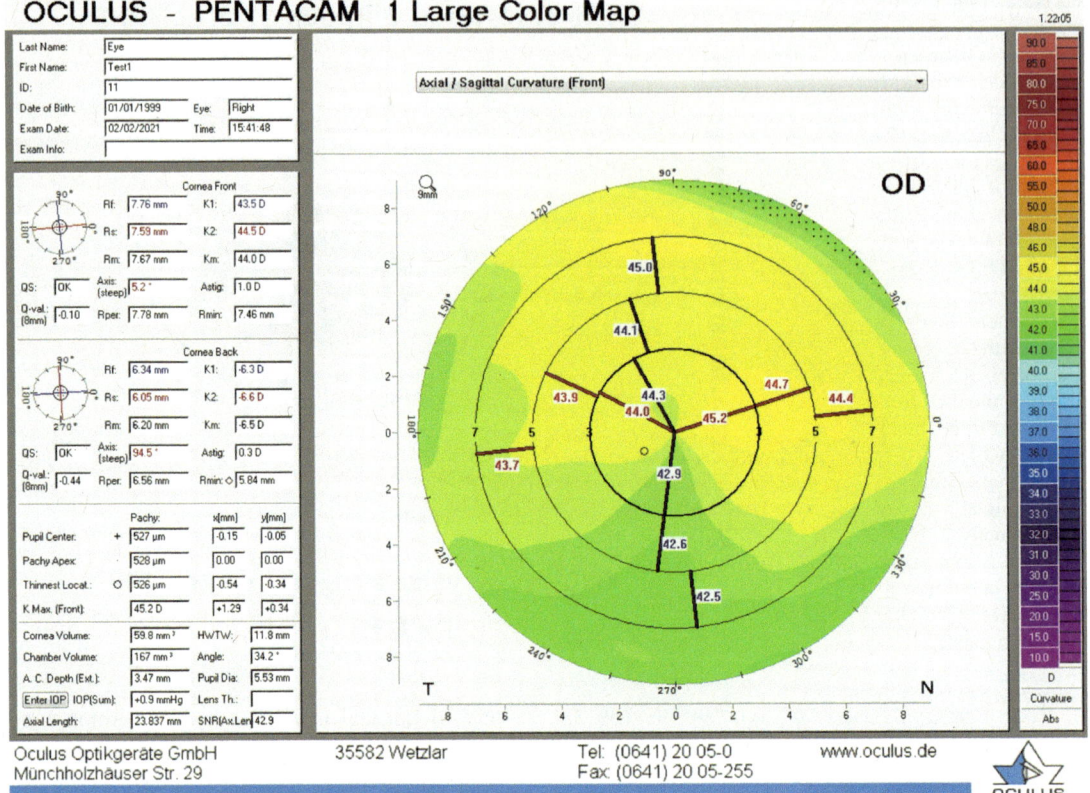

Fig. 59.4 Pentacam measurement of the anterior corneal surface. Simulated keratometry (top, left column) displays the steep meridian of (44.5 D @ 5.2°) and the flat merid-

ian (43.5 D @ 95.2°). This is written in spherocylinder plus format as 43.5 D () 1.0 D @ 5.2°

periodic function, with a period of 180°. A direction of, for instance, 150° may be indicated as −30 or 330° for any practical and calculational purposes.

This correlation is described below, where p is an integer:

$$(M @ \alpha) = (M @ (\alpha + p \times 180)) \quad (59.4)$$

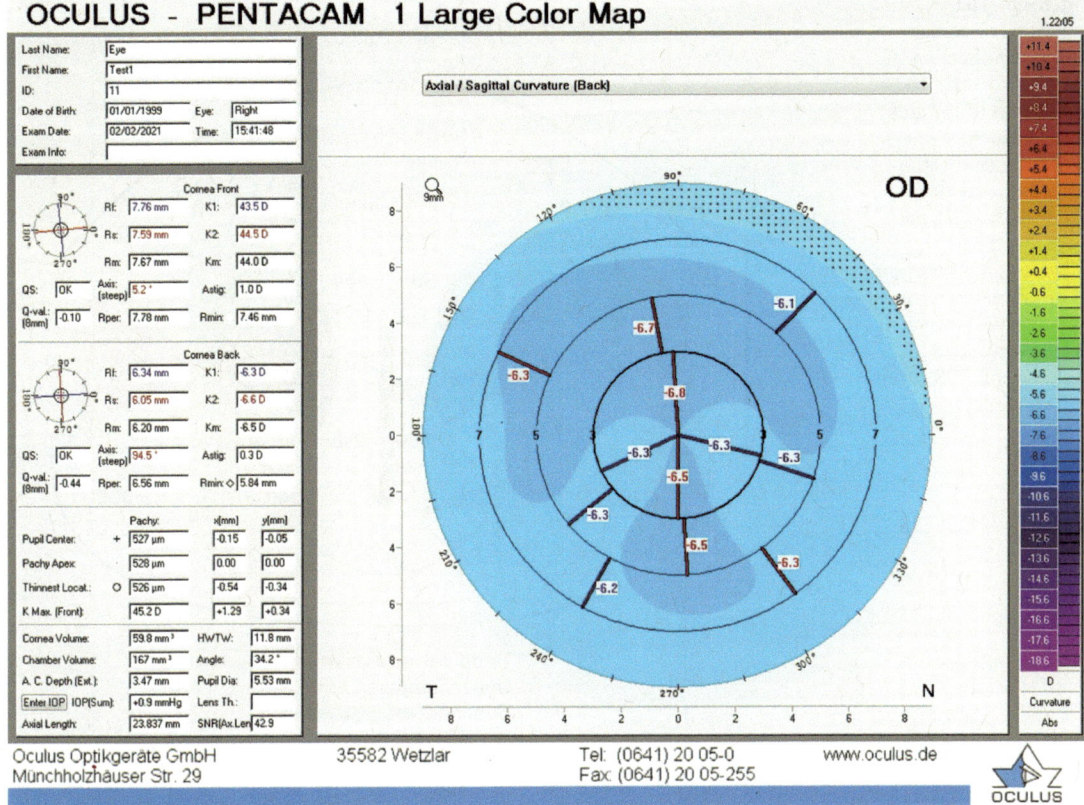

Fig. 59.5 Pentacam measurement of the posterior corneal surface (left column, middle) demonstrating a steep meridian of (−6.6 D @ 94.5°) and a flat meridian of (−6.3 D @ 4.5°). The spherocylinder plus format is (−6.6 D () 0.3 D @ 4.5°)

Fig. 59.6 The indication of corneal astigmatic direction is identical for right and left eyes as 0° towards the left ear, 90° superiorly, and 180° towards the right ear. Corneal astigmatisms are divided into subgroups as a function of the steep meridian direction; WTR (green), oblique (blue and yellow), and ATR (deep red and violet)

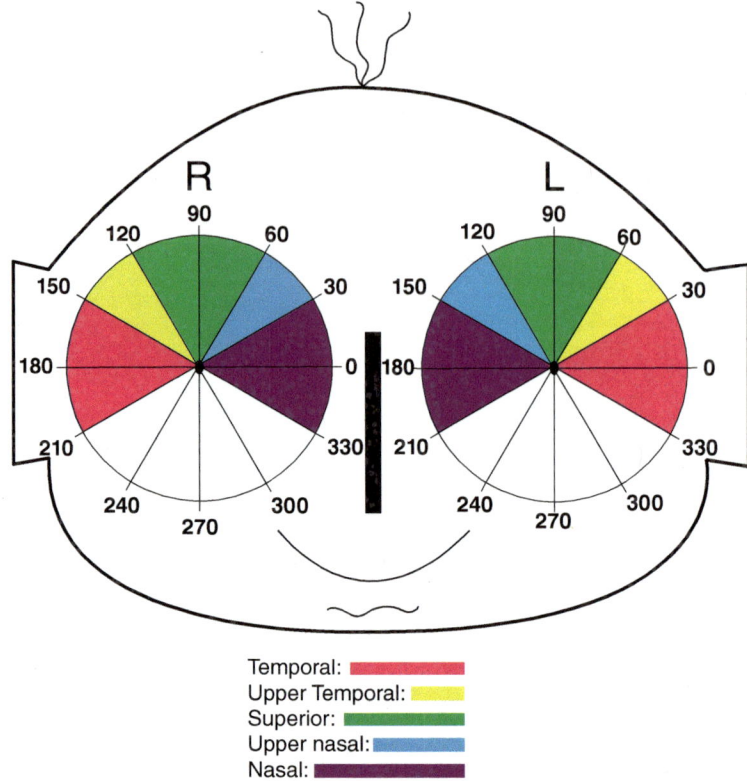

Temporal: ▬▬▬
Upper Temporal: ▬▬▬
Superior: ▬▬▬
Upper nasal: ▬▬▬
Nasal: ▬▬▬

Refractive Spherocylinder Formats

Refraction is optimally based on autorefraction using a stationary (not handheld) device, but always finalized by a meticulous subjective (manifest) refraction in 0.25 D steps for sphere and cylinder, and in ≤5° steps for the axis. To compensate for differences in chart distance and thereby assure uniform reporting of distance refractions, measured refractions may be adjusted to infinity. The formula for this is:

$$\text{Refraction}_{\text{infinity}} = \text{Refraction}_{\text{actual}} - \left(1/\left(\text{chart distance in meters}\right)\right) \qquad (59.5)$$

The spherocylinder prescription is given as: S () $(M \times \alpha)$; where S is the sphere (D), M is the astigmatic magnitude (D), and x is the astigmatic axis (°). The SE is given as:

$$\text{SE} = S + 0.5 \times M \qquad (59.6)$$

Both corneal and refractive spherocylinder data may be registered in a *plus* or *minus* cylinder format (Fig. 59.7). However, Næser's polar value system requires transformation to a plus format for both corneal and refractive data.

A *cross-cylinder* or *combined cylinder* format provides the cylinders along the orthogonal main axes. The cross-cylinders of the spherocylinder from Fig. 59.7 are written as $(-4.75 \text{ D} \times 53°)$ and $(-2.75 \text{ D} \times 143°)$. This format is used for conversion of each cross-cylinder from the vertex or spectacle plane (P_v) to the corneal surface (P_C), using the distance formula [9, 27]:

$$P_C = P_v / \left(1 - \left(P_v \times V / 1000\right)\right), \qquad (59.7)$$

where V is the vertex distance in mm.

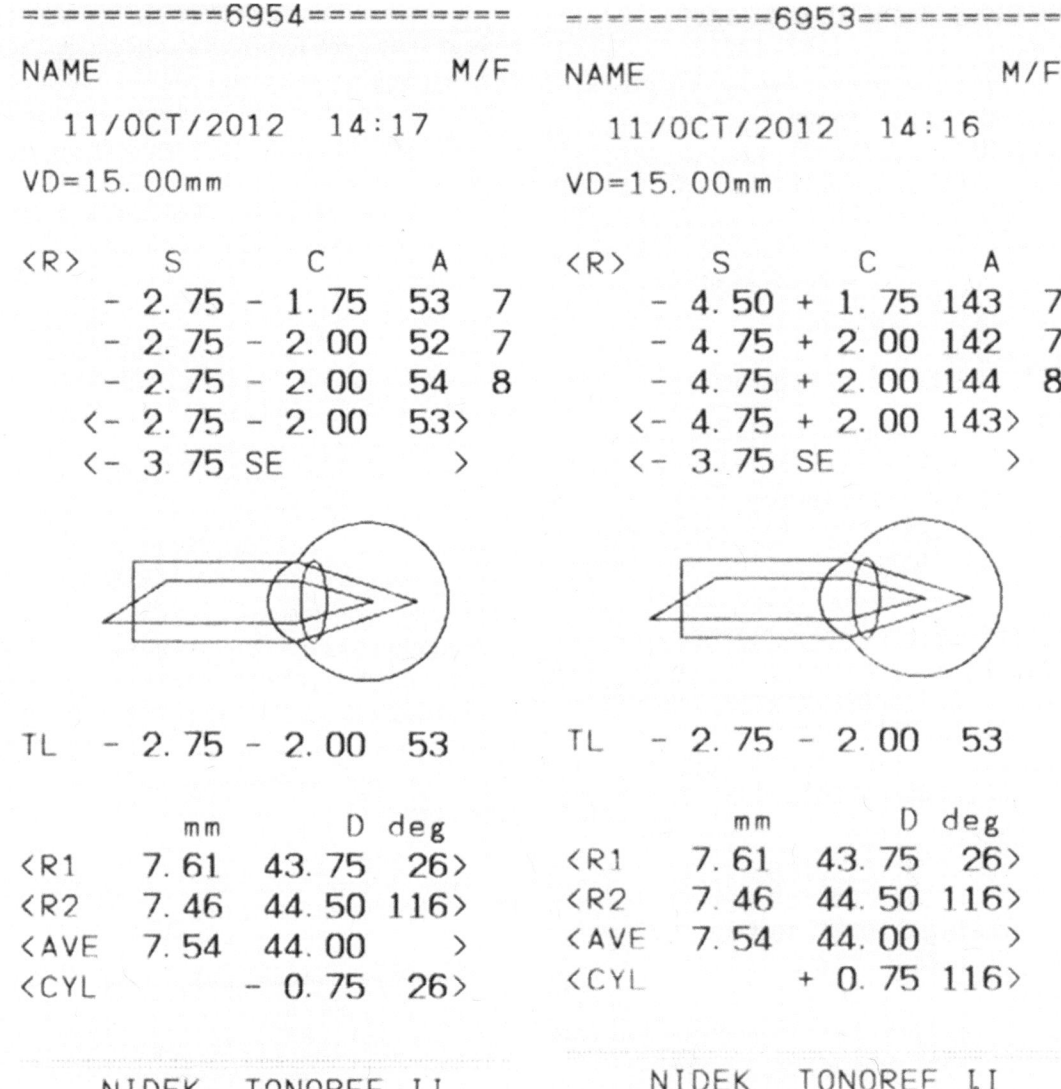

Fig. 59.7 Plus and minus formats for refractive and corneal measurements. Astigmatic directions are traditionally indicated by the *axes* for refractions and by the *meridians* for corneal measurements. The refractive spherical equivalent (SE) and the principle corneal meridians (here shown as *R*1 and *R*2) are always identical irrespective of the chosen plus or minus cylinder format

Cross cylinders are reconverted to the traditional plus or minus spherocylinder format in the corneal plane.

A similar *cross-cylinder* approach is employed for converting toric IOL toricity from the capsular to the anterior corneal plane.

Refractions and Aberrations

Consider a wavefront emanating from the eye. This is the total ocular aberration, generated by the ocular refractive surfaces and distances. The optical correction is the spherocylinder neutralizing the total ocular aberration. The refraction and the total ocular aberration at a given plane are therefore identical, but of opposite signs [16, 28]:

$$\text{Aberration} = -\text{Refraction} \qquad (59.8)$$

This is well-known in clinical practise. A myopic eye is corrected with a minus sphere, because the refractive surfaces are too powerful relative to the vitreous length, hereby focusing parallel incident light in front of the retina. The meridian of a minus spectacle cylinder is aligned with the most powerful refractive meridian. Alternatively, correction may be conceived as a plus meridian cylinder aligned with the orthogonal less powerful meridian. As Næser's polar value system requires plus cylinder formats for calculations, the latter approach will be used in the following.

Comparing Corneal and Refractive Astigmatisms

These subtle correlations are not widely appreciated, but come out neatly [27, 28]. So, hang on!

Comparison of corneal and refractive data requires common plane, format, and angular definition. We choose the anterior corneal astigmatism as reference, here given as the net cylinder (M_C @ α_C).

The common plane is therefore the anterior corneal vertex, the format is aberration, and the direction is given by the plus power meridian.

Refractive data are transformed from vertex to corneal plane with Eq. (59.7) and subsequently reconverted to a plus axis format, symbolized as ($M_R \times \alpha_R$). The refraction is converted to aberration format by adding 90° to the direction (rather than chancing sign, hereby maintaining plus power format), as indicated in Eq. (59.8), yielding the net cylinder $M_R \times (\alpha_R + 90)$. Axis is changed to meridional direction by further addition (or subtraction) of 90°, changing the net cylinder to $M_R \times (\alpha_R + 180)$, which—according to Eq. (59.4)—is identical to ($M_R \times \alpha_R$). The entered refractive cylinder in axis format is therefore identical to the intended aberrational data in power format, and no further modifications are required for comparison! [27, 28]

Astigmatism directions are given as meridians for corneal measurements and as axes for refractions. Refractions are converted from the vertex to the anterior corneal plane to allow for comparison with corneal measurements.

Dioptric Vector Formats

Spherocylinders are converted to vectors in diopters by using meridional powers. Consider a spherocylinder in plus power format, S () (M @ α), with minimal power S along ($\alpha + 90$)° and maximal power ($M + S$) along α. According to the sine-squared correlation, the meridional power along an oblique plane Φ is given as [16]:

$$\text{Meridional power along the plane } \Phi = S + M \times \cos^2(\alpha - \Phi) \qquad (59.9)$$

Meridional powers along additional three planes are required (Figs. 59.8 and 59.9):

$$\text{Orthogonal plane along}(\Phi + 90) = S + M \times \cos^2(\alpha - (\Phi + 90)) = S + M \times \sin^2(\alpha - \Phi) \qquad (59.10)$$

$$\text{Oblique plane along}(\Phi + 45), \text{counter} - \text{clockwise to} \Phi = S + M \times \cos^2(\alpha - (\Phi + 45)) \qquad (59.11)$$

$$\text{Oblique plane along}(\Phi - 45), \text{clockwise to} \Phi = S + M \times \sin^2(\alpha - (\Phi + 45)) \qquad (59.12)$$

All vector systems provide correct results, but vary with respect to reference meridians. Some systems use meridional powers directly, others

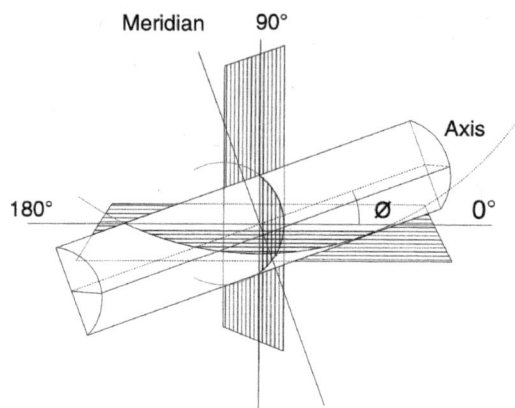

Fig. 59.8 A plano-cylinder in an oblique meridian. The meridional powers along 0 and 90° are illustrated by the radii of curvature in the hatched planes. KP(0), the polar value along the reference meridian Φ in 0°, is the dioptric difference between these meridional powers. (Reproduced with permission from Wolters Kluwer Health Inc.)

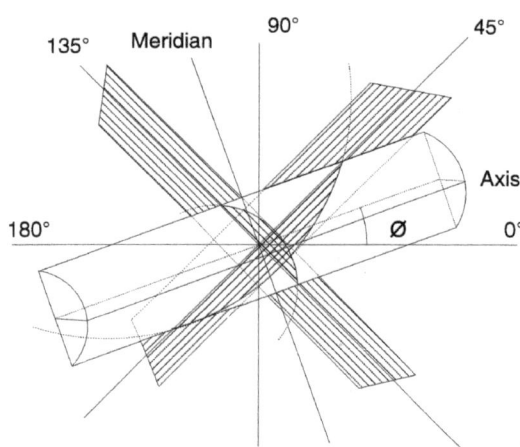

Fig. 59.9 The meridional powers along 45 and 135° are illustrated by the radii of curvature in the hatched planes. KP(45), the polar value along 45°, is the dioptric difference between these meridional powers. (Reproduced with permission from Wolters Kluwer Health Inc.)

rely on the difference between orthogonal meridional powers.

Næser's Polar Value System

The objective of refractive surgery is to flatten the steeper and/or to steepen the flatter corneal meridian or refractive wavefront, while simultaneously avoiding rotation of the cylinder direction. Næser's polar valuer system was designed for description of SIA by quantitating the flattening, steepening, and rotation of the surgical meridian.

A spherocylinder may be converted to a dioptric vector in the form of a SE power and two polar values, separated by an arch of 45° [3, 7, 11, 16, 22]. Optically, the polar values are cross cylinders in 45° inclinations. The three variables describe the spherocylinder completely, are mathematically independent, and allow for all types of algebraic operations.

The SE for corneal and refractive powers are reported in Eqs. (59.3) and (59.6). The astigmatism is completely characterized by the meridional and torsional polar values, with units in diopters [16]:

For the net cylinder ($M @ \alpha$), the meridional polar value KP(Φ) along the (surgical) plane Φ is the difference in meridional powers along Φ and (Φ + 90), as reported in Eqs. (59.9) and (59.10) [16]:

$$\text{Meridional polar value} = M \times \cos\left(2 \times \left(\alpha - \Phi\right)\right) \tag{59.13}$$

The torsional polar value is the difference in meridional powers along the planes (Φ + 45) and (Φ − 45)), given in Eqs. (59.11) and (59.12):

$$\text{Torsional polar value} \, KP\left(\Phi + 45\right) = M \times \sin\left(2 \times \left(\alpha - \Phi\right)\right) = 2M \times \sin\left(\alpha - \Phi\right) \times \cos\left(\alpha - \Phi\right) \tag{59.14}$$

The magnitude of the torsional relative to the meridional power determines the angle and direction of cylinder relative to the reference plane Φ.

The polar value system always reports the change in astigmatism along the chosen meridian. This plane is usually the surgical meridian.

The investigator chooses a *variable* or *fixed* reference plane Φ, for analysis of various clinical situations.

1. A *variable* reference plane along the preoperatively measured most powerful direction

for each eye is most useful for analysis of SIA. This direction varies for each eye, and Φ = preoperative value for α. *All* changes in astigmatism are referred to the preoperatively measured highest power of either the meridian (for cornea) or axis (for refraction). In this way, one can easily ascertain the refractive result, whether perfect or under- or overcorrected. For a preoperative astigmatic magnitude M and a target postoperative astigmatism of zero, the surgically induced meridional and torsional powers should be exactly $-M$ (for elimination of M) and zero (securing no axis rotation), respectively. For the SE and the meridional power, a power reduction or an overcorrection is indicated by a negative value, while an increase in power/under correction is given by a positive value. For the torsional power, a positive value indicates a counterclockwise and a negative value clockwise rotation of the cylinder meridian.

Recommended reference meridians for standard surgery:

Corneal incisional surgery: Variable reference meridians along the preoperative steep corneal meridians for on-median corneal incisional or fixed meridians (usually zero or 90°) for standard incisions.

Toric IOLs: The toric IOL axis = the predicted postoperative steep TCA meridian.

Corneal laser surgery: The plane of the preoperative refractive cylinder in plus format.

2. A *fixed* value for the reference plane of Φ = zero is used for analysis of temporal corneal incisions placed exactly in 0°. It may also be employed for interim calculations and population statistics within a with-the-rule (WTR) and against-the-rule (ATR) concept. By inserting Φ = zero in Eqs. (59.13) and (59.14), we obtain:

$$KP(0) = M \times \cos(2 \times \alpha) \qquad (59.15)$$

$$KP(45) = M \times \sin(2 \times \alpha) \qquad (59.16)$$

KP(0) is positive for ATR astigmatism and negative for WTR astigmatism. KP(45) is positive for oblique angular direction from 1 to 89°, and negative in angular directions between 90 and 180°.

3. Analysis of SIA following any other *fixed* direction is constructed similarly. For instance, in a right-handed surgeon consistently using a main corneal phacoemulsification incision in 100°, meridional and torsional powers emerge as:

$$KP(100) = M \times \cos(2 \times (\alpha - 100)) \qquad (59.17)$$

$$KP(145) = M \times \sin(2 \times (\alpha - 100)) \qquad (59.18)$$

The dynamics of SIA are best understood by remaining in the vector space and conceptually visualizing any surgically induced change in the terms of variation in SE and the meridional and torsional vectors. However, any single astigmatism and any compilation of astigmatisms may be converted to traditional cylinder format with the following equations: [16]

The astigmatic magnitude M in diopters:

$$M = \sqrt{KP(\Phi)^2 + KP(\Phi + 45)^2} \qquad (59.19)$$

The astigmatic direction α in degrees:

$$\alpha = \arctan\left(\frac{M - KP(\Phi)}{KP(\Phi + 45)}\right) \qquad (59.20)$$

The direction is given relative to the chosen reference meridian.

Other Vector Formats

Most dioptric power formats employ a SE power, combined with two cross cylinders in fixed directions along 0 and 45°, as described in Eqs. (59.15) and (59.16) [4, 6, 9, 10, 13, 14]. This analysis is correct within a WTR/ATR context, but cannot generally be interpreted as over- or under-correction for any surgical meridian. Signs may vary due to different definitions of direction. Thibos'

J0 and J45 use the half value of the astigmatic magnitude [14]. The equations reported by Holladay [4] for with-the-wound (incision) and Against-the-wound change are identical to the meridional powers in Eqs. (59.9) and (59.10).

Long's power matrix [29] relies on meridional powers with *axes* along zero and 90° (Eqs. 59.9 and 59.10) together with a torsional component (Eq. 59.16) and takes the following general formats:

$$f_{11} = S + M \times \sin^2(\alpha); f_{22} = S + M \times \cos^2(\alpha); f_{21} = f_{12} = -M \times \sin(\alpha) \times \cos(\alpha) \qquad (59.21)$$

This vector format was used by Kaye [12] and Harris [15] for analysis of SIA.

Statistical Analysis

Descriptive and analytical statistical analyses of univariate SE, meridional, and torsional powers are performed with Excel or other database facilities [22]. Bivariate [24, 25] (simultaneous) statistical analysis of meridional and torsional powers may require data transfer to designated statistical programs. In double-angled plots, the "centroid" is the combined, bivariate mean of the individual distributions, while the extension of the confidence ellipse reflects the variability [16, 21, 24, 25]. *Accurate* surgical procedures are characterized by average differences in refraction close to zero. Univariate average means are assessed with a Student's t-test, bivariate means with Hotelling's T [24, 25]. Univariate and bivariate averages of multiple procedures are compared with analysis of variance (ANOVA) and multiple analysis of variance (MANOVA), respectively. *Precise* procedures have small standard deviations and variances, narrow confidence limits, and small confidence ellipses [24–26]. Bivariate analyses are based on the averages and standard deviations of and the correlation between *both* polar values and are therefore more reliable than univariate assessments. The total variance (TV) for an astigmatism entity is the sum of the meridional and torsion variances [24, 25]. The total standard deviation, TSD, is the square root of TV. Two variances may be compared with an F-test and multiple variances with Levene's or similar homogeneity test. All procedures mentioned assume normally distributed data.

Univariate non-normal data may be assessed with nonparametric statistics.

The mean absolute error (MAE) for astigmatism is the average of individually calculated magnitudes without consideration of directions, calculated with Eq. (59.19). The MAE relies on both the bias from the average error and from the variability of the individual observations. After conversion to this reduced scalar, directional data regarding over- or under-correction are irretrievably lost.

Terminology

The clinician *measures* the *preoperative* and a *postoperative* corneal and refractive power. The clinician *chooses* the *target refraction*. All other results are derived from these variables.

The terminology is identical for corneal and refractive measurements and include the Preoperative, Postoperative, Target, Surgically Induced, Target Induced, and the Error in *spherical equivalent* and *astigmatism*. Each astigmatism is further characterized by its meridional and torsional polar values. Abbreviations are listed in Table 59.1. The **SISE** and **SIA** are calculated as the **vector** differences between the postoperative and the preoperative measurements. The Target Induced Spherical Equivalent (**TISE**) and astigmatism (**TIA**) are defined as the **vector** differences between the target and the preoperative variables. The errors in spherical equivalent (**EISE**) and astigmatism (**EIA**) are calculated as the **vector** differences between the postoperative and the target values [22].

Dioptric power vectors are based on meridional powers. All vector systems provide correct calculations. They differ by the choice of reference meridians and definitions of direction. Some systems use meridional powers

Table 59.1 (Næser). Terminology with abbreviations [22]. All units in diopters (D). The astigmatism is further fully characterized by its meridional and torsional polar values. (Reproduced with permission from Wolters Kluwer Health Inc.)

Terminology	Spherical equivalent	Astigmatism
Preoperative	PRESE	PREA
Postoperative	POSE	POA
Target	TSE	TA
Surgically induced	SISE	SIA
Target induced	TISE	TIA
Error in	EISE	EIA

directly, others rely on the difference between orthogonal meridional powers.

Practical Calculation of Surgically Induced Refractive Change

Clinicians may copy the described formulas for their own use. A number of commercial and free web-based programs for calculating corneal and refractive changes are available. See for example: https://www.researchgate.net/publication/324106602_Surgically_induced_astigmatism_SIA_calculator_using_dr_Naesers_polar_value_system_Version_10_Free_software http://links.lww.com/JRS/A281.

Abulafia and Koch's double-angled plots for corneal and refractive SIA are freely available on the American Society of Cataract and Refractive Surgery and the Journal of Cataract and Refractive Surgery homepages.

Calculating the Corneal SIA for a Temporal Incision

The error in astigmatism (**EIA**) for toric IOL calculation is the vector difference between the corneal plane postoperative refractive astigmatism (**POA**) and the calculated target astigmatism (**TA**). The TA is the vector sum of the preoperative total corneal astigmatism (**TCA**), corneal **SIA**, and corneal plane **IOL toricity**. Vector calculation of corneal **SIA** is demonstrated in the following as an example.

We performed Nidek Tonoref II autokeratometry once before and 6 weeks after 2.4 mm clear corneal phakoemulcification incisions in 99 right eyes. All incisions were placed temporally in 180°. For SIA analysis, we therefore chose a fixed reference meridian in zero (=180) degrees. Autokeratometries were converted to SE power and the meridional (KP(0)) and torsional (KP(45)) polar values. The surgically induced change was calculated as the vector differences between the preoperative and postoperative values.

Data are summarized in Tables 59.2 and 59.3 and in Fig. 59.10. The three variables were normally distributed with a Kolmogorov-Smirnov test. The corneal incisions induced a statistically significant 0.09 D flattening and a nonsignificant 0.06 D counterclockwise torsion. The bivariate mean ("centroid") differed significantly from zero (Hotelling's $T^2 = 0.008$). Both average surgically induced polar values should be used for

Table 59.2 Key values for univariate description of the surgically induced refractive change. **SISE** is the surgically induced spherical equivalent power. The deviation of the average values from zero was tested with a two-tailed, univariate t-test (right column)

Univariate data		
Spherical equivalent (SE) power	Mean (SD); min–max value (D)	t-test
SISE	0.07 (0.30); −1.26–1.04	0.03
ASTIGMATISM (SIA)		
Meridional power (KP (0))	−0.09 (0.44); −1.36–1.52	0.03
Torsional power (KP(45))	−0.06 (0.32); −0.93–0.91	0.06

Table 59.3 Metrics for bivariate SIA analysis. Some metrics may be recognized from Fig. 59.10. The total variance (TV) is the sum of meridional and torsional univariate variances. The TSD is the square root of TV

SIA bivariate data	
"Centroid" as combined mean polar values (D)	(−0.09, −0.06)
"Centroid" as net astigmatism	0.11 D @ 107°
Pearson correlation	−0.19
Hotelling T^2 p-value	0.008
Total variance (TV)	0.29
Total standard deviation (TSD)	0.54
Mean absolute error (MAE)	0.46 D

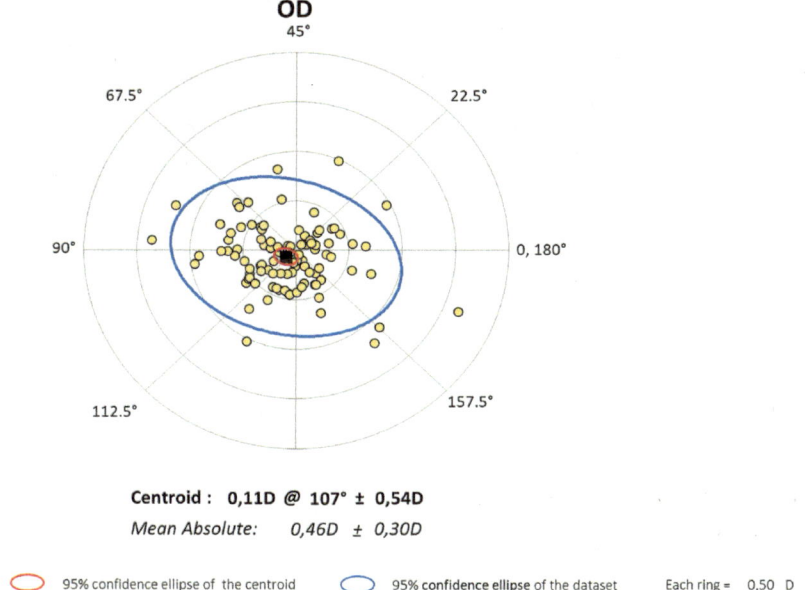

Centroid : 0,11D @ 107° ± 0,54D

Mean Absolute: 0,46D ± 0,30D

■ Centroid ⬭ 95% confidence ellipse of the centroid ⬭ 95% **confidence ellipse** of the dataset Each ring = 0,50 D

Fig. 59.10 Individual measurements and confidence ellipses for corneal SIA following temporal 2.4 mm phakoemulcification incisions in 99 right eyes. Each ring represents 0.5 D. Abscissa: meridional polar value KP(90. Ordinate: torsional polar value KP(45). Large black dot represents the bivariate mean ("centroid") in (−0.09 D, −0.06 D) = the net astigmatism (0.11 D @ 107°). Red line: 95% confidence ellipse of the mean. The bivariate mean differed statistically significantly from zero, as the origin (0,0) was outside this confidence ellipse. Blue line: 95% confidence ellipse for observations (also called tolerance ellipse). The two ellipses are congruent, and their relative axes length is the square root of the number of observations, or approximately ten in this example

future toric IOL calculations with similar corneal incisions. However, in contemporary web-based toric IOL calculation, only the flattening effect is considered. This is not entirely correct, but in this case a flattening of 0.1 D for "SIA" should be used for enhanced future average accuracy.

The spread is considerable in Fig. 59.10. Is this spread caused by the surgery or by the corneal measurements? The confidence ellipses for observations in Fig. 59.3 were constructed on a different data set of non-operated eyes, but with the same autokeratometer. The standard deviations for the paired difference between two single autokeratometries (blue confidence ellipse) amounted to 0.37 and 0.17 for KP(0) and KP(45). An F-test comparison of variances between Fig. 59.3 (blue ellipse) and the surgical case in Fig. 59.10 revealed a statistically significant ($p < 0.001$) difference for KP(45), but no ($p = 0.10$) difference for KP(0). A proportion of the spread in Fig. 59.10 may therefore be caused

by the measurements. In Fig. 59.3, the variances based on three to five measurements were reduced to a third. Using the vector average of at least three autokeratometries will tend to enhance the precision of toric IOL calculation.

After transformation of corneal and refractive data to dioptric vectors, all calculations and statistical analyses may be performed in a univariate or a bivariate manner.

References

1. Jaffe NS, Clayman HM. The pathophysiology of corneal astigmatism after cataract extraction. Trans Am Acad Ophthalmol Otolaryngol. 1975;79:615–30.
2. Cravy TV. Calculation of the change in corneal astigmatism following cataract extraction. Ophthalmic Surg. 1979;10:38–49.
3. Naeser K. Conversion of keratometer readings to polar values. J Cataract Refract Surg. 1990;16:741–5.
4. Holladay JT, Cravy TV, Koch DD. Calculating the surgically induced refractive change following ocular surgery. J Cataract Refract Surg. 1992;18:429–43.

5. Kaye SB, Campbell SH, Davey K, Patterson A. A method for assessing the accuracy of surgical technique in the correction of astigmatism. Br J Ophthalmol. 1992;76:738–40.

6. Alpins NA. A new method of analyzing vectors for changes in astigmatism. J Cataract Refract Surg. 1993;19:524–33.

7. Naeser K, Behrens JK, Næser EV. Quantitative assessment of corneal astigmatic surgery: expanding the polar values concept. J Cataract Refract Surg. 1994;20:162–8.

8. Olsen T, Dam-Johansen M. Evaluating surgically induced astigmatism. J Cataract Refract Surg. 1994;20:517–22.

9. Holladay JT, Dudeja DR, Koch DD. Evaluating and reporting astigmatism for individual and aggregate data. J Cataract Refract Surg. 1998;24:57–65.

10. Alpins N. Astigmatism analysis by the Alpins method. J Cataract Refract Surg. 2001;27:31–49.

11. Naeser K, Hjortdal J. Polar value analysis of refractive data. J Cataract Refract Surg. 2001;27:86–94.

12. Kaye SB, Patterson A. Analyzing refractive changes after anterior segment surgery. J Cataract Refract Surg. 2001;27:50–60.

13. Holladay JT, Moran JR, Kezirian GM. Analysis of aggregate surgically induced refractive change, prediction error, and intraocular astigmatism. J Cataract Refract Surg. 2001;27:61–79.

14. Thibos LN, Horner D. Power vector analysis of the optical outcome of refractive surgery. J Cataract Refract Surg. 2001;27:80–5.

15. Harris WF. Analysis of astigmatism in anterior segment surgery. J Cataract Refract Surg. 2001;27:107–28.

16. Næser K. Assessment and statistics of surgically induced an astigmatism. Acta Ophthalmol. 2008 (Issue Thesis 1);86:1–28.

17. Reinstein DZ, Archer TJ, Randleman JB. JRS standard for reporting astigmatism outcomes of refractive surgery. J Refract Surg. 2014;30:654–9.

18. Næser K. Surgically induced astigmatism: distinguishing between vectors and non-vectors. J Refract Surg. 2015;31:349–50.

19. Næser K. Surgically induced astigmatism is characterized by optical vectors, not by ratios. J Cataract Refract Surg. 2016;43:347–8.

20. Reinstein DZ, Archer TJ, Srinivasan S, Mamalis N, Kohnen T, Dupps WJ Jr, Randleman JB. Standard for reporting refractive outcomes of intraocular lens-based refractive surgery. J Cataract Refract Surg. 2017;43:435–9.

21. Abulafia A, Koch DD, Holladay JT, Wang L, Hill W. Pursuing perfection in intraocular lens calculations. IV. Rethinking astigmatism analysis for intraocular lens-based surgery: suggested terminology, analysis, and standards for outcome. J Cataract Refract Surg. 2018;44:1169–74.

22. Næser K. Surgically induced astigmatism made easy: calculating the surgically induced change in sphere and cylinder for corneal incisional, corneal laser, and intraocular lens–based surgery. J Cataract Refract Surgery. 2021;47:118–22.

23. Koch DD, Wang L, Abulafia A, Holladay JT, Hill W. Rethinking the optimal methods for vector analysis of astigmatism. J Cataract Refract Surgery. 2021;47:100–5.

24. Naeser K, Hjortdal J. Bivariate analysis of surgically induced regular astigmatism. Mathematical analysis and graphical display. Ophthal Physiol Opt. 1999;19:50–61.

25. Naeser K. Hjortdal: multivariate analysis of refractive data. Mathematics and statistics of spherocylinders. J Cataract Refract Surg. 2001;27:129–42.

26. Javadi-Ottosen S, Næser K. Precision of the Nidek Tonoref II autokeratometer: how many repeated measurements are required? Acta Ophthalmol. 2021;99:611–5.

27. Bregnhøj JF, Mataji P, Næser K. Refractive, anterior corneal and internal astigmatism in the pseudophakic eye. Acta Ophthalmol. 2015;93:33–40.

28. Næser K. Combining refractive and topographic data in corneal refractive surgery for astigmatism. A new method based on polar value analysis and mathematical optimization. Acta Ophthalmol. 2012;90:768–72.

29. Long WF. A matrix formalism for decentration problems. Am J Optom Physiol Optic. 1976;53:27–33.

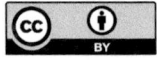

Astigmatism of the Cornea

60

Li Wang and Douglas D. Koch

Accurate measurement of total corneal astigmatism is a critical element in correcting astigmatism during cataract surgery. The prevalence of anterior corneal astigmatism ≥1.0 D has been reported to range from 32 to 41% [1–4]. Using partial coherence interferometry (IOLMaster), in 23,239 eyes, Hoffmann and Hütz [5] reported that 73.7% of eyes had anterior corneal astigmatism ≥0.5 D, and 36.1% had anterior corneal astigmatism ≥1.0 D.

Traditionally, corneal astigmatism has been calculated based on anterior corneal measurements only. The magnitude of posterior corneal astigmatism was thought to be clinically negligible because of the small difference in refractive indices between the cornea and aqueous. This chapter will discuss corneal astigmatism calculated based on anterior corneal measurement, the contribution of posterior corneal astigmatism to total corneal astigmatism, corneal astigmatism changes with aging, and higher-order aberrations of the cornea.

Corneal Astigmatism Based on Anterior Corneal Measurement

Until recently, we could only measure the anterior corneal surface. Technologies used to measure the anterior corneal surface include manual

and automated keratometers, Placido disk corneal topographers, and reflection-based topographers or biometers.

To compensate for the negative power of the posterior surface, a corneal index of refraction (1.3375) is typically used to estimate the refractive power of the entire cornea. The origin of 1.3375 as the keratometric index of refraction is Gullstrand's corneal model with anterior and posterior radii of curvature of 7.7 mm and 6.8 mm, respectively [6, 7]. The ratio of posterior-to-anterior radii of curvature is 6.8/7.7 = 0.883, which is higher than those reported recently using the Scheimpflug devices. Using the Pentacam, Dubbelman et al. [8] reported the posterior/anterior ratio to be on average 0.813. Using the Galilei Dual Scheimpflug Analyzer (Ziemer Ophthalmic System AG, Port, Switzerland) [9], we found that the average ratio of posterior/anterior radii of curvature (P/A ratio) was 0.82 in normal eyes, ranging from 0.73 to 0.87. We have found a mean P/A ratio of 0.76 (range 0.69–0.83) in myopic-LASIK/PRK eyes, 0.86 (range 0.82–0.91) in hyperopic-LASIK/PRK eyes [9], and 0.93 (but with a huge range of 0.67–1.25) in post-radial keratotomy eyes (unpublished data). In addition, various types of keratoplasty can alter the P/A ratio, as can corneal scarring or any other process that alters only anterior corneal curvature. This indicates that the estimation of total corneal power using anterior corneal curvature measurements and the standard refractive index of 1.3375 is often inaccurate, par-

L. Wang · D. D. Koch (✉)
Cullen Eye Institute, Baylor College of Medicine, Houston, TX, USA
e-mail: liw@bcm.edu; dkoch@bcm.edu

© The Author(s) 2024
J. Aramberri et al. (eds.), *Intraocular Lens Calculations*, Essentials in Ophthalmology,
https://doi.org/10.1007/978-3-031-50666-6_60

ticularly in nonvirgin corneas. As we discuss below, this also has important implications for estimating the contribution of the posterior cornea to total corneal astigmatism.

Contribution of Posterior Corneal Astigmatism to Total Corneal Astigmatism

The disparity between refractive and anterior corneal astigmatism was first noted by Javal [10]. The potential cause was felt by many to be lenticular astigmatism, but Tscherning surmised that it could be due to posterior corneal astigmatism [11]. However, only recently have clinical devices capable of measuring posterior corneal astigmatism become available. The measurement modalities include slit-scanning imaging, Scheimpflug imaging, optical coherence tomography (OCT), and detection of the second Purkinje images.

Several studies have evaluated posterior corneal astigmatism using different methodologies. The main findings of posterior corneal astigmatism and its contribution to the total corneal astigmatism are summarized as follows [12–15]:

- The mean magnitude of posterior corneal astigmatism is around −0.20 to −0.30 D, but there is wide variability.
- In the majority of corneas, the steepest meridian of the posterior corneal surface is aligned vertically (Fig. 60.1). Since the posterior corneal surface has negative power, a steeper curvature at the 90° meridian creates net refractive power horizontally. This results in most corneas having more net against-the-rule (ATR) astigmatic refractive power than is measured from the anterior corneal surface. Thus, posterior corneal astigmatism partially compensates for anterior corneal astigmatism in corneas that have with-the-rule (WTR) astigmatism on the anterior corneal surface, but it increases total corneal astigmatism in corneas that have ATR anterior astigmatism.
- In corneas with WTR astigmatism on the anterior corneal surfaces, the magnitude of posterior corneal astigmatism increases with increasing amount of anterior corneal astigmatism, ranging up to over 1 D in eyes with anterior WTR of 4 D or more (Fig. 60.2 top). This indicates that compared to the total corneal astigmatism calculated using a fixed corneal refractive index based on the ante-

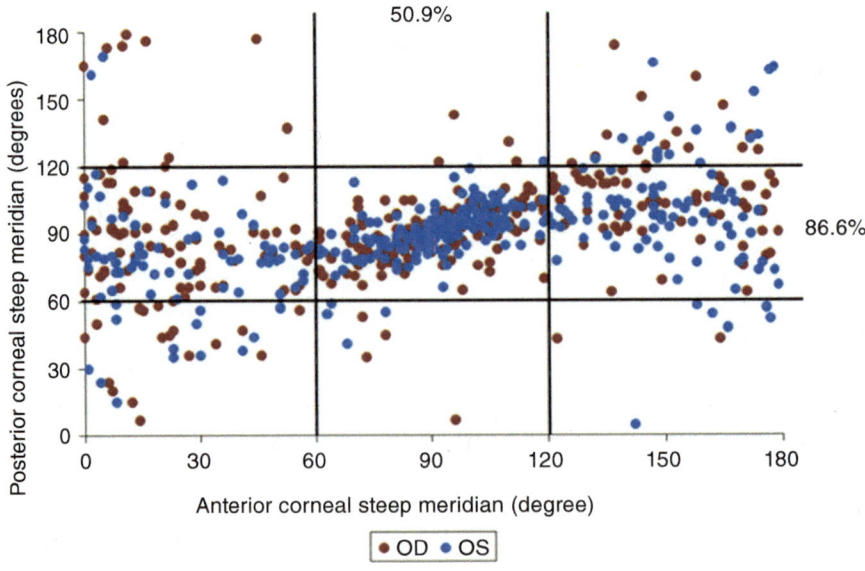

Fig. 60.1 Location of the steep meridian on anterior and posterior corneal surfaces. (Adopted from [12])

Fig. 60.2 Magnitude of astigmatism on the anterior corneal surface and posterior corneal surface in eyes with with-the-rule (top) and against-the-rule (bottom) astigmatism on the anterior cornea. (Adopted from [12])

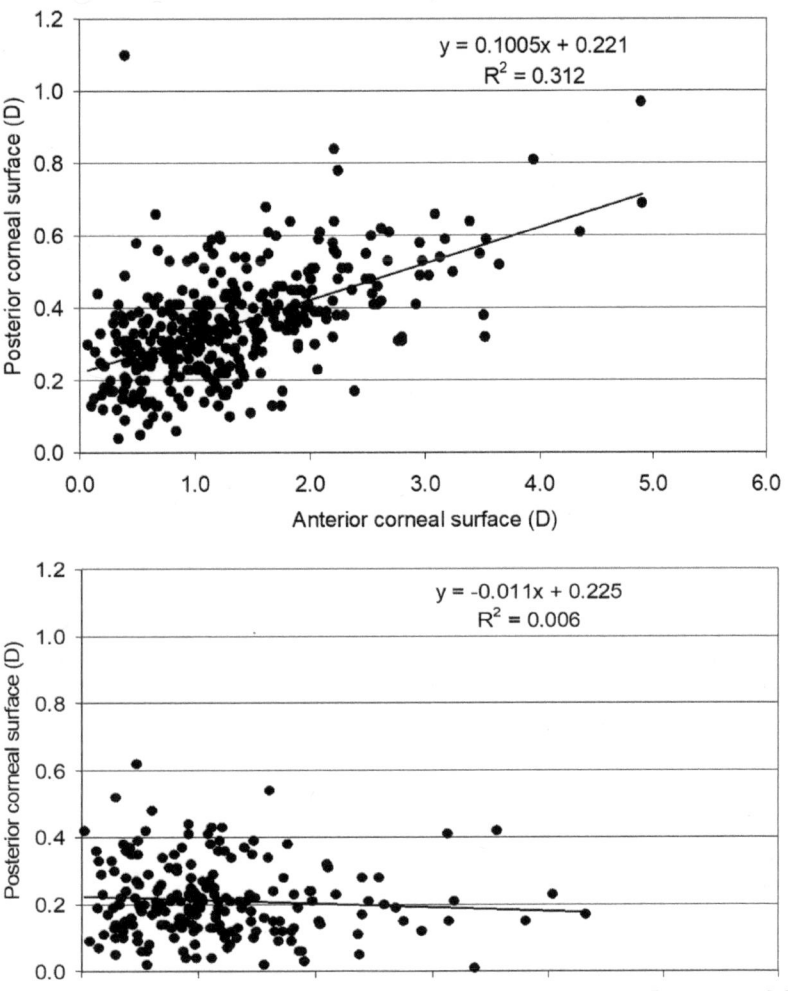

rior corneal surface only, the total corneal astigmatism magnitude is smaller, and more so in eyes with large amounts of anterior corneal astigmatism. If the posterior corneal astigmatism is ignored, overcorrection can occur when correcting astigmatism with toric IOLs.

- In corneas with ATR astigmatism on the anterior corneal surfaces, posterior corneal astigmatism is relatively constant around 0.3 D and does not increase with increasing amount of anterior corneal astigmatism (Fig. 60.2 bottom). If the posterior corneal astigmatism is ignored, undercorrection can occur.

- However, the location of the steep meridian of the posterior corneal surface is more variable in eyes that have oblique and ATR astigmatism, as can be seen in Fig. 60.1. In addition, in a study of 3818 corneas measured with the Pentacam, Tonn et al. [14] reported the variability of the location of the steep posterior corneal meridian as a function of the steep anterior corneal meridian.

  - As Fig. 60.3 shows, the percentage of corneas with the posterior surface steepest vertically decreases as a function of the change in anterior corneal astigmatism from WTR to oblique to ATR.

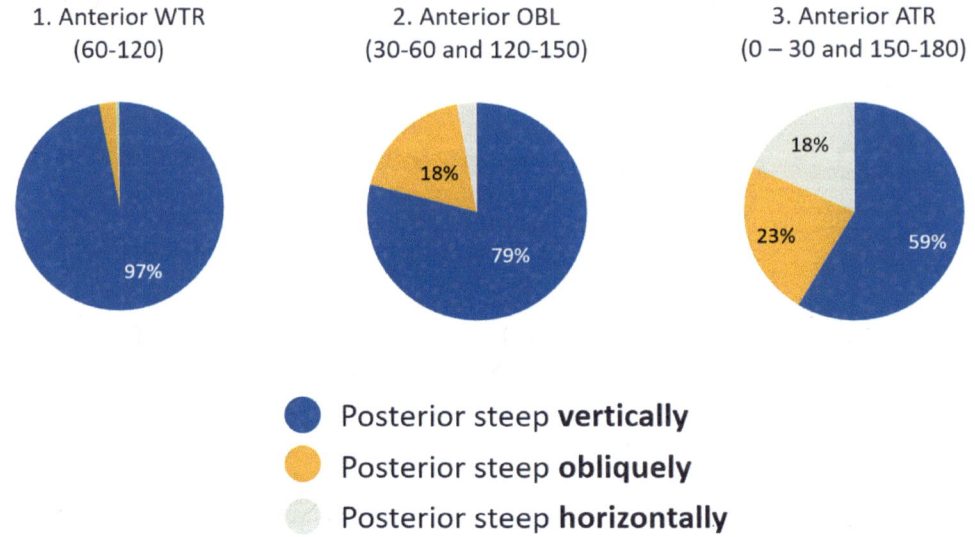

Fig. 60.3 Percentage of eyes with vertical, oblique, and horizontal steep meridian on the posterior corneal surface in eyes with anterior with-the-rule (WTR), oblique (OBL), and against-the-rule (ATR) astigmatism. (Adopted from [14])

- These studies highlight the impact and variability of posterior corneal astigmatism and the need to get reliable measurements in patients undergoing cataract surgery.
- There are two ways to factor posterior corneal astigmatism into toric IOL calculations: (1) mathematical models based on prior toric IOL outcomes and (2) direct measurement of posterior corneal curvature.
  - Studies to date largely suggest that the former are more accurate for determining IOL toricity [16], perhaps due to the inaccuracy of our devices and/or the fact that other factors such as IOL tilt contribute to refractive astigmatism.

In summary, ignoring posterior corneal astigmatism may yield an incorrect estimation of total corneal astigmatism. In general, selecting toric intraocular lenses based on anterior corneal measurements could lead to overcorrection in eyes that have WTR astigmatism and undercorrection in eyes that have ATR astigmatism. More accurate methods of measuring posterior corneal astigmatism may be needed, and optimal toric IOL formulas will incorporate this as one of several elements in postoperative refractive astigmatism.

Corneal Astigmatism Changes with Aging

In case series studies using Scheimpflug technology, studies reported that, with increasing age, the steep anterior corneal meridian tends to change from vertical to horizontal, while there is minimal change in the steep posterior corneal meridian [12, 14].

Hayashi and colleagues [17] investigated long-term changes in anterior corneal astigmatism with aging, comparing eyes that underwent sutureless cataract surgery and those that did not undergo surgery. They evaluated the keratometric cylinder between baseline and 5 years after baseline and between 5 and 10 years. Corneal astigmatism after cataract surgery showed a long-term ATR change with aging, and this change was similar to that of normal cornea without surgery. In another study, Hayashi et al. [18] examined how corneal astigmatism changes with age over 20 years after cataract surgery and again assessed whether the changes differ from those in eyes that did not have surgery. They found that the corneal astigmatism continued to change toward ATR astigmatism over 20 years after cataract surgery, and this change was similar in eyes that did not have surgery. The mean ATR change over

20 years is approximately 0.65 D, with a 0.30–0.35 D of change over each 10-year period.

These findings suggest that the against-the-rule change that occurs with aging should be taken into consideration at the time of cataract surgery and that a reasonable astigmatic target is a small amount of WTR astigmatism [13].

Higher-Order Aberrations of the Cornea

In addition to astigmatism, the cornea also has higher-order aberrations and irregular astigmatism. In a previous study [19], we found that the anterior corneal wavefront aberrations varied greatly among subjects, with higher-order Zernike coefficient values ranging from −0.579 to +0.572 μm. Higher-order aberration root-mean-square and coma root-mean-square values increased with aging (Fig. 60.4). Nearly all virgin corneas had positive fourth-order spherical aberration, but these values did not change with aging. Similarly, Oshika et al. [20] reported that spherical-like aberrations did not vary significantly with aging, whereas comalike aberrations of the cornea correlated with age, implying that the corneas become less symmetrical along with aging.

Of relevance to astigmatism correction, corneal higher-order aberrations, particularly coma, can impact the patient's perception of astigmatism during refraction and thereby contribute to refractive astigmatism [21]. How this affects toric IOL outcomes remains to be elucidated.

Future Directions/Needs

We often encounter clinically significant differences in corneal astigmatism values obtained from different devices. Although this may be caused by different areas of the astigmatic cornea measured and different algorithms employed by different devices, accuracy, repeatability, and reproducibility of corneal astigmatism measurements by these devices may also need improvements.

In a recent study [15], we compared corneal astigmatism obtained from an OCT-based biometer and a Dual Scheimpflug Analyzer (Galilei, DSA). Comparing the total corneal astigmatism values from these two devices, 84.3 and 98.9% of eyes had differences in magnitude of ≤0.50 and ≤1.0 D, and in eyes with OCT total keratometry astigmatism of ≥0.5 D, 34.5% and 60.1% of eyes had differences in the steep meridian of ≤5 and ≤10°, respectively; 52.8–63.5% of eyes had vec-

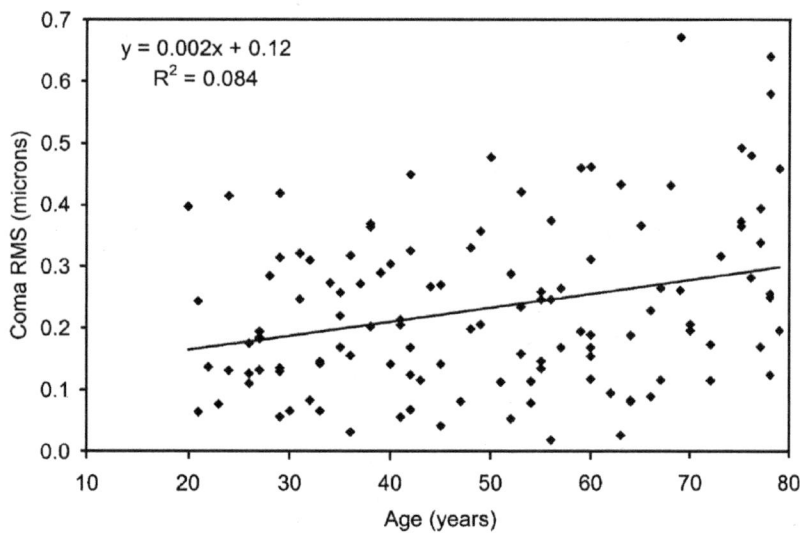

Fig. 60.4 Scattergram of corneal coma root-mean-square values as a function of age (Pearson's correlation coefficient $r = 0.290$, $P < 0.001$). (Adopted from [19])

$y = 0.002x + 0.12$
$R^2 = 0.084$

tor differences of ≤0.50 D. These results indicate that there were clinically significant differences in total corneal astigmatism obtained from OCT and DSA devices.

The future direction is the evolution of current devices and possibly the development of new ones that will enable us to more accurately measure total corneal astigmatism.

Conclusion

Total corneal astigmatism is determined by both the anterior and posterior corneal surfaces. Ignoring posterior corneal astigmatism may yield an incorrect estimation of total corneal astigmatism. Correcting corneal astigmatism based on anterior corneal measurements only could lead to overcorrection in eyes that have WTR astigmatism and undercorrection in eyes that have ATR astigmatism. The ATR change that occurs with aging should be taken into consideration at the time of cataract surgery. Devices with more accurate and repeatable anterior and posterior corneal measurements are desirable.

References

1. Ferrer-Blasco T, Montés-Micó R, Peixoto-de-Matos SC, González-Méijome JM, Cerviño A. Prevalence of corneal astigmatism before cataract surgery. J Cataract Refract Surg. 2009;35(1):70–5.
2. Prasher P, Sandhu JS. Prevalence of corneal astigmatism before cataract surgery in Indian population. Int Ophthalmol. 2017;37(3):683–9.
3. Curragh DS, Hassett P. Prevalence of corneal astigmatism in an NHS cataract surgery practice in Northern Ireland. Ulster Med J. 2017;86(1):25–7.
4. Sharma A, Phulke S, Agrawal A, Kapoor I, Bansal RK. Prevalence of astigmatism in patients undergoing cataract surgery at a tertiary Care Center in North India. Clin Ophthalmol. 2021;15:617–22.
5. Hoffmann PC, Hütz WW. Analysis of biometry and prevalence data for corneal astigmatism in 23,239 eyes. J Cataract Refract Surg. 2010;36(9):1479–85.
6. Norrby S. Unfortunate discrepancies. J Cataract Refract Surg. 1998;24:433–4.
7. Norrby S. Pentacam keratometry and IOL power calculation. J Cataract Refract Surg. 2008;34:3.
8. Dubbelman M, Van der Heijde GL, Weeber HA, Vrensen GF. Radius and asphericity of the posterior corneal surface determined by corrected Scheimpflug photography. Acta Ophthalmol Scand. 2002;80:379–83.
9. Wang L, Mahmoud A, Anderson B, Koch D, Roberts C. Total corneal power estimation: ray tracing method versus Gaussian optics formula. Invest Ophthalmol Vis Sci. 2011;52(3):1716–22.
10. Javal E. Memoires d'Ophtalmom_etrie: Annotés et Précédés d'une Introduction. Paris, France: G. Masson; 1890. p. 131.
11. Tscherning MHE. Encycl Franç Ophtal. 1904;3:105.
12. Koch DD, Ali SF, Weikert MP, Shirayama M, Jenkins R, Wang L. Contribution of posterior corneal astigmatism to total corneal astigmatism. J Cataract Refract Surg. 2012;38(12):2080–7.
13. Koch DD, Jenkins RB, Weikert MP, Yeu E, Wang L. Correcting astigmatism with toric intraocular lenses: effect of posterior corneal astigmatism. J Cataract Refract Surg. 2013;39(12):1803–9.
14. Tonn B, Klaproth OK, Kohnen T. Anterior surface-based keratometry compared with Scheimpflug tomography-based total corneal astigmatism. Invest Ophthalmol Vis Sci. 2014;56(1):291–8.
15. Wang L, Cao D, Vilar C, Koch DD. Posterior and total corneal astigmatism measured with optical coherence tomography-based biometer and dual Scheimpflug analyzer. J Cataract Refract Surg. 2020;46(12):1652–8.
16. Abulafia A, Hill WE, Franchina M, Barrett GD. Comparison of methods to predict residual astigmatism after intraocular lens implantation. J Refract Surg. 2015;31:565.
17. Hayashi K, Hirata A, Manabe S, Hayashi H. Long-term change in corneal astigmatism after sutureless cataract surgery. Am J Ophthalmol. 2011;151:858–65.
18. Hayashi K, Manabe SI, Hirata A, Yoshimura K. Changes in corneal astigmatism during 20 years after cataract surgery. J Cataract Refract Surg. 2017;43(5):615–21.
19. Wang L, Dai E, Koch DD, Nathoo A. Optical aberrations of the human anterior cornea. J Cataract Refract Surg. 2003;29(8):1514–21.
20. Oshika T, Klyce SD, Applegate RA, Howland HC. Changes in corneal wavefront aberrations with aging. Invest Ophthalmol Vis Sci. 1999;40:1351–5.
21. Zhou W, Stojanovic A, Utheim TP. Assessment of refractive astigmatism and simulated therapeutic refractive surgery strategies in coma-like-aberrations-dominant corneal optics. Eye Vis (Lond). 2016;3:13.

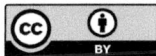

Lens and IOL Tilt

61

Nino Hirnschall and Oliver Findl

Tilt and Visual Quality

A tilt of an intraocular lens (IOL) reduces optical quality due to an increase of lower [1, 2] and higher order aberrations [3]. The impact of tilt on positive and negative dysphotopsia as well as chromatic aberrations appears to be uncertain [4, 5]. Aberrations are a problem for any kind of IOL, but especially for aspheric [6–9], toric [10, 11], extended depth of focus [12, 13], and multifocal IOLs [3].

In the case of an aspherical IOL, tilt leads to a reduction of the aspherical effect up to a worse performance compared to a spherical IOL [6–9]. A "common" amount of tilt (up to 5°) was not shown to have a relevant influence on the performance of the Strehl ratio in a randomized trial (spherical versus aspherical IOL) [14, 15]. Higher amounts of tilt increase coma (which can mimic astigmatism) [16] and reduce the effect of asphe-

ricity [10]. Comparing aspherical, aberration neutral and spherical IOLs in the presence of tilt showed that an aberration neutral IOL outperforms an aspherical IOL [17, 18].

For toric IOLs, tilt has a direct and indirect impact on post-operative astigmatism [10, 11] and it explains approximately 11% of the residual astigmatism error or up to 20% if angle kappa is also taken into account [19].

Multifocal IOLs show a reduced optical quality if tilted. Although this accounts for any type of multifocal IOL, especially the performance of rotationally asymmetric multifocal IOLs decreases with tilt [20, 21].

Measurement of Tilt

Severe tilt may be detected at the slit lamp, although it does not allow any quantification of tilt and the measurement is not reliable.

In general, there are two principal methods to quantify tilt:

1. Cross-sectional scans of the anterior segment
   - Scheimpflug imaging or rotating slit lamp images
   - Optical coherence tomography (OCT)
   - Ultrasound biomicroscopy (UBM)
2. Assessing the Purkinje reflexes

N. Hirnschall
Department for Ophthalmology and Optometry, Kepler University Hospital GmbH and Medical Department Johannes Kepler University Linz, Linz, Austria
e-mail: nino@hirnschall.at

O. Findl (✉)
Vienna Institute for Research in Ocular Surgery (VIROS), A Karl Landsteiner Institute, Hanusch Hospital, Vienna, Austria
e-mail: oliver@findl.at

© The Author(s) 2024
J. Aramberri et al. (eds.), *Intraocular Lens Calculations*, Essentials in Ophthalmology, https://doi.org/10.1007/978-3-031-50666-6_61

Cross Section-Based Imaging

Tilt quantification with cross-sectional images was introduced in the 1980s [22]. Due to the fact that conventional imaging techniques (except ultrasound) use a light source, imaging behind the iris is not possible. Therefore, this type of tilt quantification uses a fitting concept, where the visible parts of the anterior and posterior lens surfaces are fitted using curved lines (Fig. 61.1). The point of contact is then the estimated equator of the lens. This kind of measurement needs to be performed with a well-dilated pupil in order to assess as much surface of the IOL as possible. In some cases, it is also difficult to identify the anatomical structures of the eye that are necessary to align the points of the reference axis [23].

More recently, OCT devices have been used to quantify tilt. This concept was shown to be successful for older concepts, such as the time domain OCT [24], but also for more modern devices, such as longitudinal B scans using a swept source OCT [25], or anterior segment swept source OCT devices [26]. Fig. 61.1

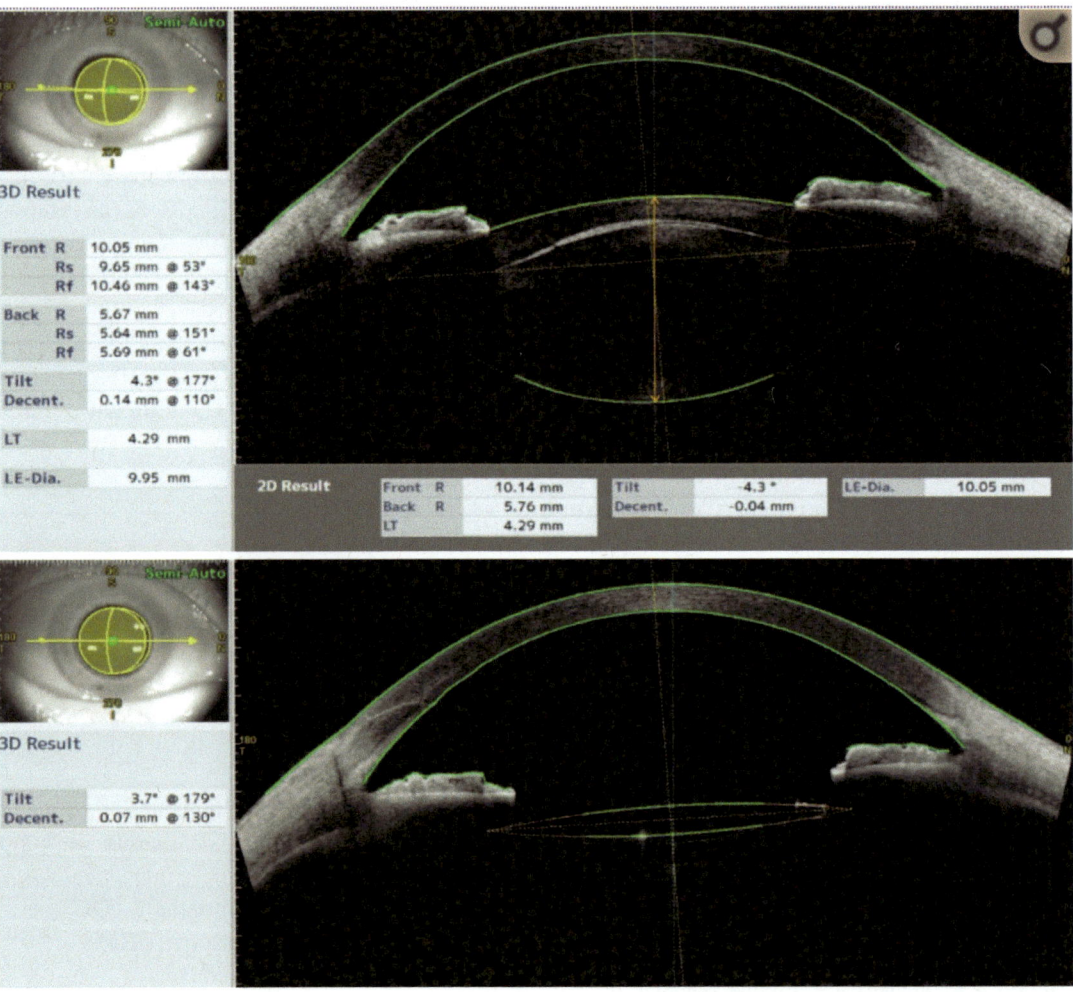

Fig. 61.1 ssOCT images of the phakic (above) and pseudophakic eye (below). The anterior/posterior surfaces of the cornea and the lens are automatically detected [27]

shows the large imaging range of up to 13 mm width that allows to measure the region between the epithelium of the cornea and the posterior lens capsule in a single scan [27]. Additionally, tilt was also quantified using a 3-dimensional approach [28–30] and a deep learning approach was introduced that allowed to automatically quantify tilt using the scleral spur as a reference [31].

Another possibility is to use a high resolution ultrasound device, often referred to as ultrasound biomicroscopy (UBM), which allows measurements behind the iris [32]. A disadvantage of UBM is that a probe is needed and while the eye is in contact with the probe, the patient cannot fixate on a target. However, it is a good approach for cases where low compliance levels are expected [33]. Although it is more difficult to define the reference axis for UBM scans, it was shown to be beneficial for quantification of out of the bag IOL implantation [34–37].

Purkinje Reflexes

Purkinje reflexes are another possibility to assess tilt. This concept was already used in the early 1980s [38–40]. Since light is reflected at all interfaces of media with a difference in refractive index, these reflections, called Purkinje reflexes, may be used to assess tilt of IOLs.

Two different clinically applicable Purkinje meter systems have been used for the measurement of IOL decentration and tilt [3, 41]. These Purkinje meters use a different algorithm for the analysis. A video camera-based photograph of the reflections from the cornea and the IOL is performed in both devices and with the help of a dedicated software, tilt is calculated [3]. The technique is a non-contact technique which is quick and easy to perform. The improvement and advancement of both systems have been shown to be accurate to measure IOL alignment and to evaluate the effect of IOL misalignment on optical performance [42].

Tabernero et al. [41] improved the measureability of tilt by using a semicircular ring of light emitting diodes. These semicircles are captured

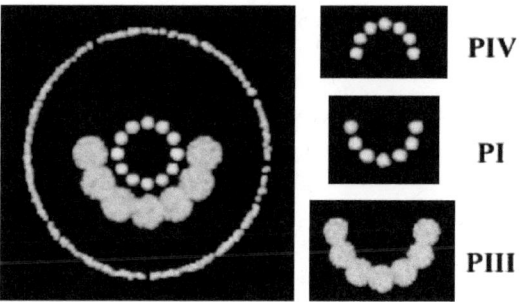

Fig. 61.2 Purkinje imaging of a perfectly aligned ophthalmic system—the outer circle represents the pupillary margin, the inner complete dotted circle the first and second (lower half) and the fourth (upper half) Purkinje reflex. The third Purkinje reflex representing the anterior surface of the lens is reflected as a thick dotted half circle [43]

and analysed according to their size and distance to each other as well as their position within the pupil (Fig. 61.2).

As shown in Fig. 61.2, only three semicircles are visible, because the first and second Purkinje reflex (anterior and posterior surface of the cornea) overlap. The distances between the reflexes and the position within the pupil are then plotted as an angular fixation function, where the fixation angle correspondences with the overlapping point of the third (anterior surface of the lens) and the fourth (posterior surface of the lens) Purkinje reflexes. Due to the fact that the patient fixates a central target, IOL tilt and decentration can be measured. This idea was previously described by Guyton et al. [44] in a more manual fashion that was also confirmed in a later study [45].

Another Purkinje meter was developed by Schaeffel [43] and differs from Tabernero's Purkinje meter in terms of the light source (single LED instead of a semicircle) and the patient has to fixate on an LED target at different positions instead of one central fixation target (Fig. 61.3).

In a direct comparison between both Purkinje meters including 30 eyes and inviting both inventors to assist with the measurements, a higher feasibility for the Purkinje meter developed by Tabernero and Artal was found [46]. Comparing only the successfully measured cases, both devices should not be used interchangeably.

Fig. 61.3 Purkinje meter using dots instead of half circles and an audio system to evaluate the quality of the image [43]

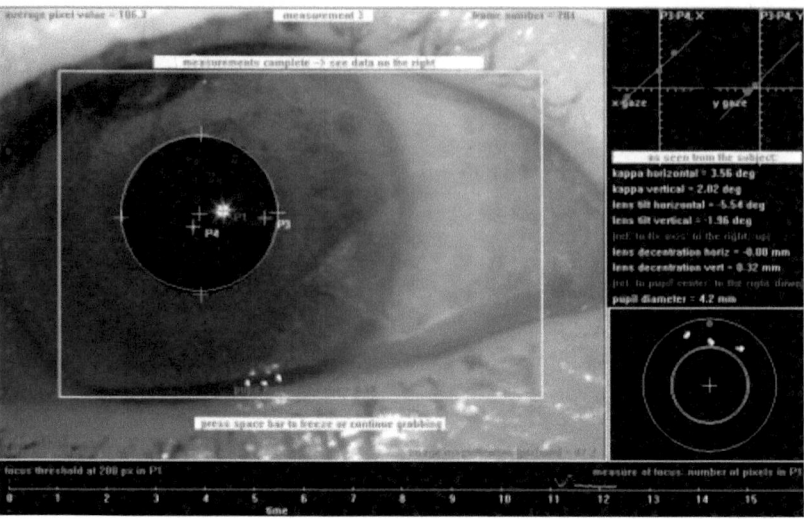

In a direct comparison of Scheimpflug imaging and Purkinje meter measurements, both were shown to be reproducible, but the accuracy was higher for the Purkinje meter measurements [47].

Physiological Tilt

A certain amount of tilt is beneficial, as it compensates for horizontal coma [48]. The mean amount of tilt of the crystalline lens was shown to range between 4.3° [49], 4.6° [43], 4.9° [27], and 5.2° [50]. Furthermore, there is a correlation between axial eye length and tilt with shorter eyes having a higher amount of tilt [25, 51]. This should be kept in mind and the term "physiological tilt" should be introduced. There is evidence that the physiological tilt is inferotemporal (the fovea is slightly temporal to the pupillary axis) [49–51] and that there is a mirror-symmetry between the eyes [49]. Furthermore, tilt slightly increases (on average less than 0.5°) in the presence of mydriasis [50].

For IOLs, there is a variety of studies assessing the amount of tilt ranging from 2.7° [52], 2.9° [53], 2.9° [28], 3.9° [54], 4.1° [55], 4.8° [51] to 6.2° [49]. Although this list is not complete, it shows the range of tilt. The amount of tilt depends on several factors, such as axial eye length, different measurement and analysis systems, and differences in reference axes. Unfortunately, there is no standardization and different authors have used different definitions and different reference axes so that they cannot be used interchangeably (Fig. 61.4) [56]. This is relevant as some reference axes include angle kappa, whereas others do not [56].

Fig. 61.4 Graphical definition of pupillary axis and line of sight and the angle kappa [41]

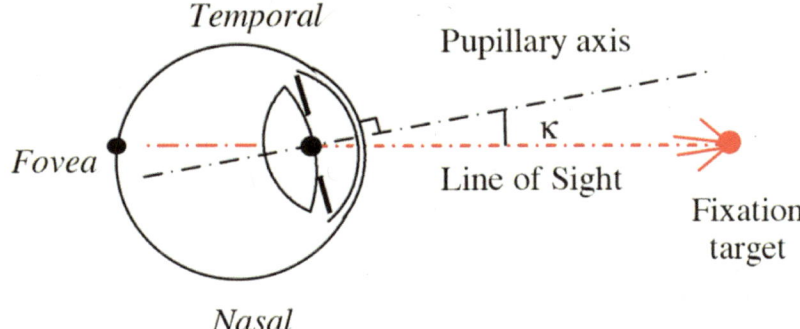

Fig. 61.5 Swept source OCT imaging at three different meridians of the same eye in the phakic state (left) and the pseudophakic state (right) [49]

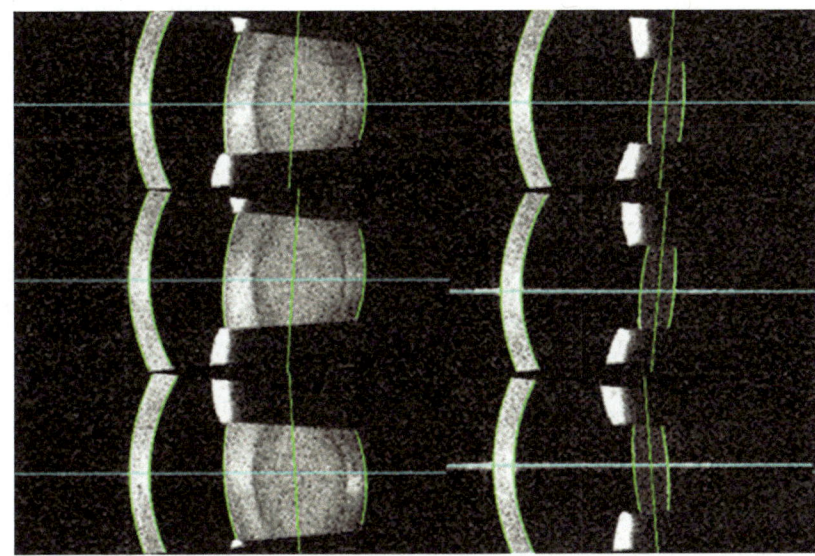

Prediction of Post-operative Tilt

As mentioned above, tilt accounts for more than 10° of the error in toric IOL power calculation and this value increases to almost 20%, if combined with angle kappa [57]. Therefore, predicting tilt and taking it into account would significantly improve toric IOL power calculation [49, 57, 58].

Although prediction of the post-operative amount of tilt is more difficult (correlation of $r = 0.4$) [49], it was shown that the orientation of tilt can be predicted quite well with a correlation of $r = 0.7$ (Fig. 61.5) [49]. The average orientation before and after cataract surgery is approximately 16–17° and the predictive power is high [49]. The correlation for the pre- to post-operative amount of tilt was found to be higher ($r = 0.5$–0.7) in two other studies (Table 61.1) [25, 27]. Axial eye length was not found to be a good predictor of post-operative tilt ($r = 0.2$) [25].

Table 61.1 Data of pre-operative and post-operative amount of tilt in three different studies. * data not in the paper, but calculated from the associated online .xls file

	Mean Crystalline tilt in ° (SD)	Mean IOL tilt in ° (SD)
Gu et al. [27]	4.9 (1.8)	4.75 (1.66)
Kimura et al. [50]	5.15 (1.4 *)	4.31 (1.7 *)
Wang [25]	3.7 (1.1)	4.9 (1.8)
Hirnschall et al. [49]	4.3 (0.9)	6.2 (1.3)

Factors Influencing Tilt

Although there is currently no good prediction algorithm on which eye will have severe IOL tilt after cataract surgery, several risk factors were discussed.

Capsulorrhexis

Different aspects of the capsulorrhexis were evaluated concerning their impact on IOL tilt. There is good evidence that the size of the capsulorrhexis has no influence on IOL tilt [55, 59]. Shape and centration of the rhexis were also not found to be clinically relevant in the same two studies. However, an incomplete capsulorrhexis overlap (probably less than 50% overlap—estimation) was found to be a risk factor for tilt [55, 59, 60]. Older techniques used before the introduction of the continuous curvilinear capsulorrhexis, such as the envelop technique, resulted in significantly higher tilt values and should be avoided [61].

As the size and shape of the capsulorrhexis were not shown to have a relevant impact on tilt with modern single-piece IOLs (except for a severe missing overlap), it is likely that femtosecond laser-assisted cataract surgery (FLACS) does not reduce post-operative tilt either. However, it should be mentioned that this was not confirmed in all studies [62].

The bag-in-the-lens IOLs, where the IOL is connected to the anterior and posterior capsulorrhexis edges, were shown to have small amounts of tilt [63, 64]. Although this type of IOL may be used with a meticulously made manual capsulorrhexis, it may be easier to be used with a FLACS made capsulotomy, as the shape and the size of the capsular opening are crucial for the position of the IOL. Incision size was not found to be a relevant factor for predicting tilt [65, 66].

Pseudoexfoliation

Pseudoexfoliation was found to be a relevant risk factor for a post-operative forward tilting of the superior haptic [24, 67, 68] as well as a long-term risk factor for IOL dislocation [69, 70]. Furthermore, pseudoexfoliation is associated with anterior capsule contraction syndrome, which may also result in a tilted IOL [71].

In another study, there was a tendency that a capsular tension ring prevents tilt to a certain degree [72]. This could be beneficial in eyes with pseudoexfoliation, but evidence is scarce and further studies would be necessary for confirmation.

IOL Material and Design

There is general agreement that the influence of IOL material has no or only a minor impact on IOL tilt [73–75]. Walkow et al. [76] observed similar results, when assessing the reason for IOL explantation due to decentration or subluxation.

On the other side, the design of the haptics was found to be relevant [73]. This leads to the question, if there is a difference between 1-piece and 3-piece IOLs. A large randomized bilateral comparison found significant differences with the 3-piece IOL showing a significantly higher amount of tilt [53]. This was also confirmed by another randomized trial [53]. Two other studies did not confirm this finding [52, 77]. Although the design of the haptics potentially has an effect on the amount of tilt, the orientation of the haptic position was not found to be relevant [53].

Possibly, the higher tilt in 3-piece designs is a consequence of a slight kinking or bending of the haptic during the implantation process since the haptics have a limited memory compared to the thicker single-piece haptics used.

After-Cataract

Although only mild in extent, posterior capsule opacification, or after-cataract, potentially increases tilt and may be relieved with a posterior Nd:YAG capsulotomy which was shown to decrease tilt back to normal levels [78, 79].

IOL Implantation Outside the Capsular Bag

Three piece IOLs in the sulcus tend to have higher tilt levels (horizontal tilt on average 7.7°) compared to those in the bag IOLs [80]. If this is due to the position in the sulcus itself, or due to the typically compromised posterior capsule has not been identified. Another explanation could be that in the case of sulcus IOLs sometimes one of the haptics unintentionally is positioned in the bag instead of being in the sulcus [37].

For scleral fixated IOLs, slightly higher tilt values were observed compared to those in the bag IOL implantation. For scleral fixated IOLs with a Z-suture, relevant tilt was found in 72% of all cases [81], whereas intrascleral fixation showed lower tilt values of little more than 3°, even though 8% of all cases had an iris capture [82]. Low tilt values were also confirmed for self-sealing scleral pockets measured with UBM [34–36] and OCT technology [35] and for long-term results using glue [83].

Furthermore, scleral fixated IOLs showed less tilt, if the sclerectomy was performed with 24 gauge compared to 30 gauge [84]. In the case of relevant post-operative tilt shortening, the length of the haptics was found to be useful to reduce tilt in some cases [85]. There is little information comparing tilt data of scleral fixated IOLs versus iris claw IOLs. One study performed in children showed higher tilt values for scleral fixated IOLs [86].

Combined Surgery

For phacotrabeculectomy, there is no evidence for an increased risk of clinically relevant IOL tilt [87]. Phacovitrectomy potentially increases the risk of IOL tilt, depending on the vitreous tamponade [51]. If air or gas is used, there is evidence for an increased tilt compared to no tamponade [26, 88, 89]. However, this difference was not found to have a significant influence on lower or higher order aberrations and the clinical effect is questionable [88]. It should also be mentioned that a randomized study directly comparing combined phacovitrectomy including endotamponade versus cataract surgery as a stand-alone procedure did not confirm these findings and no difference in tilt was observed [90].

Effect of Tilt on Refraction

The effect of tilt on the induced astigmatism in an aspherical toric IOL depends on several variables:

– Power of the IOL (spherical equivalent and astigmatism if the lens is toric)
– Amount and orientation of tilt

As shown by Weikert et al. [10], a non-toric aspheric IOL tilted horizontally (nasal border more anterior, like physiological tilt) will induce against the rule astigmatism. A horizontal tilt of 10° of a 16D and a 28D IOL would result in an induced against the rule astigmatism of 0.33D and 0.56D, respectively (Fig. 61.6).

In the case of a toric IOL oriented at 90°, the horizontal tilt resulted in increased against the rule astigmatism, resulting in overcorrection. If the IOL was oriented at 180°, the consequence would be an undercorrection. It's curious to observe that this against the rule trend is similar to the effect of the posterior corneal surface astigmatism.

Fig. 61.6 Simulated against the rule astigmatism induced by tilt in an eye with an aspheric IOL for three different IOL powers [10]

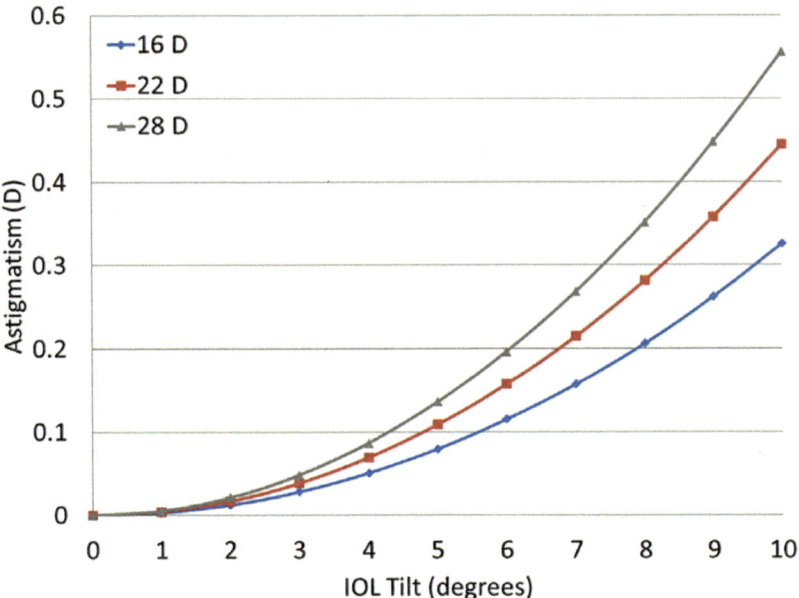

Marcos presented a method to estimate the effect of tilt on astigmatism (in air) using a thin lens formula (Eq. 61.1).

$$A = P\left\{1 + \frac{(\sin\alpha)^2}{3}\right\} * (\tan\alpha)^2 \quad (61.1)$$

Estimating the effect of tilt on astigmatism (A = astigmatism in D, P = power of the IOL in D, α = amount of tilt [91].

A more complex approach would be to use a model with a thin spherical lens. Simplifying the model by neglecting all effects above the second order of aberrations, the Coddington formula may be used [92]. The effect of tilt has to be explained for each order of aberration. Atchison published a thin lens calculation for the effect of tilt on first- and second-order aberrations [92]. According to the Coddington formula, a finite principal ray is sent from an object through a spherical lens and another neighboured ray is sent from the same object through the same lens, where these two rays intersect after refraction [93]. This intersection point consists of focal lines. The two main focal lines are usually called tangential (V_T) and sagittal (V_S) (Eq. 61.2).

$$V_S : \frac{n'}{s'} = \frac{n}{s} + (n'\cos I' - n\cos I)c_S$$

$$V_T : \frac{n'\cos^2 I'}{t'} = \frac{n\cos^2 I}{t} + \frac{n'\cos I' - n\cos I}{r}$$

$$(61.2)$$

Vergence for tangential (V_T) and sagittal (V_S) focal lines [93].

s and t = distance from the incident point of the ray to the sagittal and tangential point of the image.

c_S = curvature of the anterior lens surface.

I and I' = angles of incidence and refraction.

n and n' = refractive indices of the object and image spaces (n represents the refractive index of the object side medium and n' represents the refractive index of the image side medium).

In a very similar fashion, V_T' can be calculated using the Coddington formula for V_T, as shown in Eq. (61.3).

$$V_T' = V + \left(1 + \delta^2 + \frac{n\delta^2}{2\delta}\right)F \quad (61.3)$$

Vergence for the transversally misaligned focal line [92] (modified).

As for the longitudinal displacement, the formula for the effective lens power can be used (Eq. 61.4).

$$V_{CS} = \frac{V_s'}{1 + \dfrac{dV_s'}{n}} \text{ and } V_{CT} = \frac{V_T'}{1 + \dfrac{dV_T'}{n}} \quad (61.4)$$

Converted using the effective lens power [92] (modified) V_{CS}=Vergence of the sagittally misaligned lens on the corneal plane.

V_{CT} = Vergence of the transversally misaligned lens on the corneal plane.

The refractive error is, similar to the longitudinal displacement, the difference between the correct position of the lens and the displaced image of the lens ($V_C - V_{CS}$; $V_C - V_{CT}$).

In a next step, these estimations of the refractive error can be combined to explain the spherical equivalent of the refractive error due to lens displacement (Eq. 61.5).

$$\Delta F_{SE} = \Delta F + \Delta F_S + \frac{\Delta F_T}{2} \quad (61.5)$$

Effect of longitudinal misalignment and tilt on the spherical equivalent.

This concept [92] was evaluated using tilt, pseudophakic ACD and refraction data of 100 eyes. The correlation between the theoretically predicted refractive error and the actually measured refractive error using subjective and objective refraction was found to be only moderate ($r^2 = 0.42$ (not published)). The most likely reason is the low accuracy of the post-operative manifest refraction.

Summary

Physiological tilt shows a mirror symmetry between both eyes, depends on the axial eye length, is orientated inferotemporally, and does not exceed 5°. Tilt above this physiological level has a significant impact on visual quality, especially for aspheric, toric, and multifocal IOLs. Predicting post-operative tilt was shown to be successful and to improve toric IOL power calculation. There are two concepts for tilt measurements, cross-sectional-based scans (Scheimpflug, OCT, UBM) and imaging of the Purkinje reflexes of the eye. Risk factors for tilt are pseudoexfoliation syndrome, 3-piece IOLs, after cataract, and potentially phacovitrectomy with endotamponade. The capsulorrhexis was found to have a minor influence on tilt.

References

1. Hoffer KJ. Astigmatism from lens tilt. J Am Intraocul Implant Soc. 1985;11(1):67.
2. Schroder S, Schrecker J, Daas L, Eppig T, Langenbucher A. Impact of intraocular lens displacement on the fixation axis. J Opt Soc Am A Opt Image Sci Vis. 2018;35(4):561–6.
3. Tabernero J, Piers P, Benito A, Redondo M, Artal P. Predicting the optical performance of eyes implanted with IOLs to correct spherical aberration. Invest Ophthalmol Vis Sci. 2006;47(10):4651–8.
4. Ashena Z, Maqsood S, Ahmed SN, Nanavaty MA. Effect of intraocular lens tilt and decentration on visual acuity, Dysphotopsia and Wavefront aberrations. Vision (Basel). 2020;4(3).
5. Marcos S, Burns SA, Prieto PM, Navarro R, Baraibar B. Investigating sources of variability of monochromatic and transverse chromatic aberrations across eyes. Vis Res. 2001;41(28):3861–71.
6. Lawu T, Mukai K, Matsushima H, Senoo T. Effects of decentration and tilt on the optical performance of 6 aspheric intraocular lens designs in a model eye. J Cataract Refract Surg. 2019;45(5):662–8.
7. Madrid-Costa D, Ruiz-Alcocer J, Perez-Vives C, Ferrer-Blasco T, Lopez-Gil N, Montes-Mico R. Visual simulation through different intraocular lenses using adaptive optics: effect of tilt and decentration. J Cataract Refract Surg. 2012;38(6):947–58.
8. McKelvie J, McArdle B, McGhee C. The influence of tilt, decentration, and pupil size on the higher-order aberration profile of aspheric intraocular lenses. Ophthalmology. 2011;118(9):1724–31.
9. Fisus AD, Hirnschall ND, Maedel S, Fichtenbaum M, Draschl P, Findl O. Capsular bag performance of a novel hydrophobic acrylic single-piece intraocular lens: two-year results of a randomised controlled trial. Eur J Ophthalmol. 2020;31:1120672120960591.
10. Weikert MP, Golla A, Wang L. Astigmatism induced by intraocular lens tilt evaluated via ray tracing. J Cataract Refract Surg. 2018;44(6):745–9.
11. Felipe A, Artigas JM, Diez-Ajenjo A, Garcia-Domene C, Peris C. Modulation transfer function of a toric intraocular lens: evaluation of the changes produced by rotation and tilt. J Refract Surg. 2012;28(5):335–40.
12. Georgiev S, Palkovits S, Hirnschall N, Doller B, Draschl P, Findl O. Visual performance after bilat-

eral toric extended depth-of-focus intraocular lens exchange targeted for micro-monovison. J Cataract Refract Surg. 2020;46:1346.

13. Georgiev S, Palkovits S, Hirnschall N, Doller B, Draschl P, Findl O. Visual performance after bilateral toric extended depth-of-focus IOL exchange targeted for micromonovision. J Cataract Refract Surg. 2020;46(10):1346–52.

14. Baumeister M, Buhren J, Kohnen T. Tilt and decentration of spherical and aspheric intraocular lenses: effect on higher-order aberrations. J Cataract Refract Surg. 2009;35(6):1006–12.

15. Rosales P, De Castro A, Jimenez-Alfaro I, Marcos S. Intraocular lens alignment from purkinje and Scheimpflug imaging. Clin Exp Optom. 2010;93(6):400–8.

16. Perez-Gracia J, Varea A, Ares J, Valles JA, Remon L. Evaluation of the optical performance for aspheric intraocular lenses in relation with tilt and decenter errors. PLoS One. 2020;15(5):e0232546.

17. Eppig T, Scholz K, Loffler A, Messner A, Langenbucher A. Effect of decentration and tilt on the image quality of aspheric intraocular lens designs in a model eye. J Cataract Refract Surg. 2009;35(6):1091–100.

18. Pieh S, Fiala W, Malz A, Stork W. In vitro strehl ratios with spherical, aberration-free, average, and customized spherical aberration-correcting intraocular lenses. Invest Ophthalmol Vis Sci. 2009;50(3):1264–70.

19. Hirnschall N, Findl O, Bayer N, Leisser C, Norrby S, Zimper E, Hoffmann P. Sources of error in toric intraocular lens power calculation. J Refract Surg. 2020;36:646.

20. Liu X, Xie L, Huang Y. Effects of decentration and tilt at different orientations on the optical performance of a rotationally asymmetric multifocal intraocular lens. J Cataract Refract Surg. 2019;45(4):507–14.

21. Montes-Mico R, Lopez-Gil N, Perez-Vives C, Bonaque S, Ferrer-Blasco T. In vitro optical performance of nonrotational symmetric and refractive-diffractive aspheric multifocal intraocular lenses: impact of tilt and decentration. J Cataract Refract Surg. 2012;38(9):1657–63.

22. Sasaki K, Sakamoto Y, Shibata T, Nakaizumi H, Emori Y. Measurement of postoperative intraocular lens tilting and decentration using Scheimpflug images. J Cataract Refract Surg. 1989;15(4):454–7.

23. Baumeister M, Neidhardt B, Strobel J, Kohnen T. Tilt and decentration of three-piece foldable high-refractive silicone and hydrophobic acrylic intraocular lenses with 6-mm optics in an intraindividual comparison. Am J Ophthalmol. 2005;140(6):1051–8.

24. Burgmuller M, Mihaltz K, Schutze C, Angermann B, Vecsei-Marlovits V. Assessment of long-term intraocular lens (IOL) decentration and tilt in eyes with pseudoexfoliation syndrome (PES) following cataract surgery. Graefes Arch Clin Exp Ophthalmol. 2018;256(12):2361–7.

25. Wang L, Guimaraes de Souza R, Weikert MP, Koch DD. Evaluation of crystalline lens and intraocular lens tilt using a swept-source optical coherence tomography biometer. J Cataract Refract Surg. 2019;45(1):35–40.

26. Sato T, Korehisa H, Shibata S, Hayashi K. Prospective comparison of intraocular lens dynamics and refractive error between phacovitrectomy and phacoemulsification alone. Ophthalmol Retina. 2020;4(7):700–7.

27. Gu X, Chen X, Yang G, et al. Determinants of intraocular lens tilt and decentration after cataract surgery. Ann Transl Med. 2020;8(15):921.

28. Wang X, Dong J, Wang X, Wu Q. IOL tilt and decentration estimation from 3 dimensional reconstruction of OCT image. PLoS One. 2013;8(3):e59109.

29. Ding X, Wang Q, Chang P, et al. The repeatability assessment of three-dimensional capsule-intraocular lens complex measurements by means of high-speed swept-source optical coherence tomography. PLoS One. 2015;10(11):e0142556.

30. Li L, Wang K, Yan Y, Song X, Liu Z. Research on calculation of the IOL tilt and decentration based on surface fitting. Comput Math Methods Med. 2013;2013:572530.

31. Xin C, Bian GB, Zhang H, Liu W, Dong Z. Optical coherence tomography-based deep learning algorithm for quantification of the location of the intraocular lens. Ann Transl Med. 2020;8(14):872.

32. Ang GS, Duncan L, Atta HR. Ultrasound biomicroscopic study of the stability of intraocular lens implants after phacoemulsification cataract surgery. Acta Ophthalmol. 2012;90(2):168–72.

33. Zhao YE, Gong XH, Zhu XN, et al. Long-term outcomes of ciliary sulcus versus capsular bag fixation of intraocular lenses in children: an ultrasound biomicroscopy study. PLoS One. 2017;12(3):e0172979.

34. Marianelli BF, Mendes TS, de Almeida Manzano RP, Garcia PN, Teixeira IC. Observational study of intraocular lens tilt in sutureless intrascleral fixation versus standard transscleral suture fixation determined by ultrasound biomicroscopy. Int J Retina Vitreous. 2019;5:33.

35. Boral SK, Agarwal D. A simple modified way of Glueless, Sutureless scleral fixation of an IOL: a retrospective case series. Am J Ophthalmol. 2020;218:314–9.

36. Mura JJ, Pavlin CJ, Condon GP, et al. Ultrasound biomicroscopic analysis of iris-sutured foldable posterior chamber intraocular lenses. Am J Ophthalmol. 2010;149(2):245–52 e2.

37. Vasavada AR, Raj SM, Karve S, Vasavada V, Vasavada V, Theoulakis P. Retrospective ultrasound biomicroscopic analysis of single-piece sulcus-fixated acrylic intraocular lenses. J Cataract Refract Surg. 2010;36(5):771–7.

38. Phillips P, Perez-Emmanuelli J, Rosskothen HD, Koester CJ. Measurement of intraocular lens decentration and tilt in vivo. J Cataract Refract Surg. 1988;14(2):129–35.

39. Auran JD, Koester CJ, Donn A. In vivo measurement of posterior chamber intraocular lens decentration and tilt. Arch Ophthalmol. 1990;108(1):75–9.

40. Kirschkamp T, Dunne M, Barry JC. Phakometric measurement of ocular surface radii of curvature, axial separations and alignment in relaxed and accommodated human eyes. Ophthalmic Physiol Opt. 2004;24(2):65–73.

41. Tabernero J, Benito A, Nourrit V, Artal P. Instrument for measuring the misalignments of ocular surfaces. Opt Express. 2006;14(22):10945–56.

42. Nishi Y, Hirnschall N, Crnej A, et al. Reproducibility of intraocular lens decentration and tilt measurement using a clinical Purkinje meter. J Cataract Refract Surg. 2010;36(9):1529–35.

43. Schaeffel F. Binocular lens tilt and decentration measurements in healthy subjects with phakic eyes. Invest Ophthalmol Vis Sci. 2008;49(5):2216–22.

44. Guyton DL, Uozato H, Wisnicki HJ. Rapid determination of intraocular lens tilt and decentration through the undilated pupil. Ophthalmology. 1990;97(10):1259–64.

45. Wu M, Li H, Cheng W. Determination of intraocular lens tilt and decentration using simple and rapid method. Yan Ke Xue Bao. 1998;14(1):13–6, 26.

46. Maedel S, Hirnschall N, Bayer N, et al. Comparison of intraocular lens decentration and tilt measurements using 2 Purkinje meter systems. J Cataract Refract Surg. 2017;43(5):648–55.

47. de Castro A, Rosales P, Marcos S. Tilt and decentration of intraocular lenses in vivo from Purkinje and Scheimpflug imaging. Validation study. J Cataract Refract Surg. 2007;33(3):418–29.

48. Marcos S, Rosales P, Llorente L, Barbero S, Jimenez-Alfaro I. Balance of corneal horizontal coma by internal optics in eyes with intraocular artificial lenses: evidence of a passive mechanism. Vis Res. 2008;48(1):70–9.

49. Hirnschall N, Buehren T, Bajramovic F, Trost M, Teuber T, Findl O. Prediction of postoperative intraocular lens tilt using swept-source optical coherence tomography. J Cataract Refract Surg. 2017;43(6):732–6.

50. Kimura S, Morizane Y, Shiode Y, et al. Assessment of tilt and decentration of crystalline lens and intraocular lens relative to the corneal topographic axis using anterior segment optical coherence tomography. PLoS One. 2017;12(9):e0184066.

51. Chen X, Gu X, Wang W, et al. Characteristics and factors associated with intraocular lens tilt and decentration after cataract surgery. J Cataract Refract Surg. 2020;46(8):1126–31.

52. Mutlu FM, Erdurman C, Sobaci G, Bayraktar MZ. Comparison of tilt and decentration of 1-piece and 3-piece hydrophobic acrylic intraocular lenses. J Cataract Refract Surg. 2005;31(2):343–7.

53. Crnej A, Hirnschall N, Nishi Y, et al. Impact of intraocular lens haptic design and orientation on decentration and tilt. J Cataract Refract Surg. 2011;37(10):1768–74.

54. Harrer A, Hirnschall N, Tabernero J, et al. Variability in angle kappa and its influence on higher-order aberrations in pseudophakic eyes. J Cataract Refract Surg. 2017;43(8):1015–9.

55. Findl O, Hirnschall N, Draschl P, Wiesinger J. Effect of manual capsulorhexis size and position on intraocular lens tilt, centration, and axial position. J Cataract Refract Surg. 2017;43(7):902–8.

56. Zhang F, Zhang J, Li W, et al. Correlative comparison of three ocular axes to tilt and Decentration of intraocular lens and their effects on visual acuity. Ophthalmic Res. 2020;63(2):165–73.

57. Hirnschall N, Findl O, Bayer N, et al. Sources of error in Toric intraocular lens power calculation. J Refract Surg. 2020;36(10):646–52.

58. Hirnschall N, Buehren T, Trost M, Findl O. Pilot evaluation of refractive prediction errors associated with a new method for ray-tracing-based intraocular lens power calculation. J Cataract Refract Surg. 2019;45(6):738–44.

59. Cornaggia A, Clerici LM, Felizietti M, Rossi T, Pandolfi A. A numerical model of capsulorhexis to assess the relevance of size and position of the rhexis on the IOL decentering and tilt. J Mech Behav Biomed Mater. 2021;114:104170.

60. Ding X, Wang Q, Xiang L, Chang P, Huang S, Zhao YE. Three-dimensional assessments of intraocular lens stability with high-speed swept-source optical coherence tomography. J Refract Surg. 2020;36(6):388–94.

61. Akkin C, Ozler SA, Mentes J. Tilt and decentration of bag-fixated intraocular lenses: a comparative study between capsulorhexis and envelope techniques. Doc Ophthalmol. 1994;87(3):199–209.

62. Kranitz K, Mihaltz K, Sandor GL, Takacs A, Knorz MC, Nagy ZZ. Intraocular lens tilt and decentration measured by Scheimpflug camera following manual or femtosecond laser-created continuous circular capsulotomy. J Refract Surg. 2012;28(4):259–63.

63. Auffarth GU, Friedmann E, Breyer D, et al. Stability and visual outcomes of the capsulotomy-fixated FEMTIS-IOL after automated femtosecond laser-assisted anterior capsulotomy. Am J Ophthalmol. 2021;225:27.

64. Holland D, Rufer F. [New intraocular lens designs for femtosecond laser-assisted cataract operations: chances and benefits]. Ophthalmologe. 2020;117(5):424–30.

65. Gangwani V, Hirnschall N, Koshy J, et al. Posterior capsule opacification and capsular bag performance of a microincision intraocular lens. J Cataract Refract Surg. 2011;37(11):1988–92.

66. Chen YA, Hirnschall N, Maedel S, Findl O. Misalignment of a novel single-piece acrylic intraocular lens in the first three months after surgery. Ophthalmic Res. 2014;51(2):104–8.

67. Petrovic MJ, Vulovic TS, Vulovic D, Janicijevic K, Petrovic M, Vujic D. Cataract surgery in patients with ocular pseudoexfoliation. Ann Ital Chir. 2013;84(6):611–5.

68. Maedel S, Hirnschall N, Chen YA, Findl O. Effect of heparin coating of a foldable intraocular lens

on inflammation and capsular bag performance after cataract surgery. J Cataract Refract Surg. 2013;39(12):1810–7.

69. Mayer CF, Hirnschall N, Wackernagel W, et al. Late dislocation of a hydrophilic intraocular lens: risk ratios for predisposing factors and incidence rates. Acta Ophthalmol. 2018;96(7):e897–e8.

70. Mayer-Xanthaki CF, Pregartner G, Hirnschall N, et al. Impact of intraocular lens characteristics on intraocular lens dislocation after cataract surgery. Br J Ophthalmol. 2020;105:1510.

71. Hayashi H, Hayashi K, Nakao F, Hayashi F. Anterior capsule contraction and intraocular lens dislocation in eyes with pseudoexfoliation syndrome. Br J Ophthalmol. 1998;82(12):1429–32.

72. Miyoshi T, Fujie S, Yoshida H, Iwamoto H, Tsukamoto H, Oshika T. Effects of capsular tension ring on surgical outcomes of premium intraocular lens in patients with suspected zonular weakness. PLoS One. 2020;15(2):e0228999.

73. Remon L, Siedlecki D, Cabeza-Gil I, Calvo B. Influence of material and haptic design on the mechanical stability of intraocular lenses by means of finite-element modeling. J Biomed Opt. 2018;23(3):1–10.

74. Hayashi K, Harada M, Hayashi H, Nakao F, Hayashi F. Decentration and tilt of polymethyl methacrylate, silicone, and acrylic soft intraocular lenses. Ophthalmology. 1997;104(5):793–8.

75. Auffarth GU, McCabe C, Wilcox M, Sims JC, Wesendahl TA, Apple DJ. Centration and fixation of silicone intraocular lenses: clinicopathological findings in human autopsy eyes. J Cataract Refract Surg. 1996;22(Suppl 2):1281–5.

76. Walkow T, Anders N, Pham DT, Wollensak J. Causes of severe decentration and subluxation of intraocular lenses. Graefes Arch Clin Exp Ophthalmol. 1998;236(1):9–12.

77. Sato T, Shibata S, Yoshida M, Hayashi K. Short-term dynamics after single- and three-piece acrylic intraocular lens implantation: a swept-source anterior segment optical coherence tomography study. Sci Rep. 2018;8(1):10230.

78. Uzel MM, Ozates S, Koc M, Taslipinar Uzel AG, Yilmazbas P. Decentration and tilt of intraocular lens after posterior capsulotomy. Semin Ophthalmol. 2018;33(6):766–71.

79. Cinar E, Yuce B, Aslan F, Erbakan G, Kucukerdonmez C. Intraocular lens tilt and decentration after Nd:YAG laser posterior capsulotomy: femtosecond laser capsulorhexis versus manual capsulorhexis. J Cataract Refract Surg. 2019;45(11):1637–44.

80. Sauer T, Mester U. Tilt and decentration of an intraocular lens implanted in the ciliary sulcus after capsular

bag defect during cataract surgery. Graefes Arch Clin Exp Ophthalmol. 2013;251(1):89–93.

81. Kemer Atik B, Altan C, Agca A, et al. The effect of intraocular lens tilt on visual outcomes in scleral-fixated intraocular lens implantation. Int Ophthalmol. 2020;40(3):717–24.

82. Yamane S, Sato S, Maruyama-Inoue M, Kadonosono K. Flanged Intrascleral intraocular lens fixation with double-needle technique. Ophthalmology. 2017;124(8):1136–42.

83. Kumar DA, Agarwal A, Agarwal A, Chandrasekar R, Priyanka V. Long-term assessment of tilt of glued intraocular lenses: an optical coherence tomography analysis 5 years after surgery. Ophthalmology. 2015;122(1):48–55.

84. Matsumura T, Takamura Y, Makita J, Kobori A, Inatani M. Influence of sclerotomy size on intraocular lens tilt after intrascleral intraocular lens fixation. J Cataract Refract Surg. 2019;45(10):1446–51.

85. Kurimori HY, Inoue M, Hirakata A. Adjustments of haptics length for tilted intraocular lens after intrascleral fixation. Am J Ophthalmol Case Rep. 2018;10:180–4.

86. Shuaib AM, El Sayed Y, Kamal A, El Sanabary Z, Elhilali H. Transscleral sutureless intraocular lens versus retropupillary iris-claw lens fixation for paediatric aphakia without capsular support: a randomized study. Acta Ophthalmol. 2019;97(6):e850–e9.

87. Mutlu FM, Bayer A, Erduman C, Bayraktar MZ. Comparison of tilt and decentration between phacoemulsification and phacotrabeculectomy. Ophthalmologica. 2005;219(1):26–9.

88. Iwama Y, Maeda N, Ikeda T, Nakashima H, Emi K. Impact of vitrectomy and air tamponade on aspheric intraocular lens tilt and decentration and ocular higher-order aberrations: phacovitrectomy versus cataract surgery. Jpn J Ophthalmol. 2020;64(4):359–66.

89. Ozates S, Kiziltoprak H, Koc M, Uzel MM, Teke MY. Intraocular lens position in combined phacoemulsification and vitreoretinal surgery. Retina. 2018;38(11):2207–13.

90. Leisser C, Hirnschall N, Findl O. Effect of air tamponade on tilt of the intraocular lens after Phacovitrectomy. Ophthalmologica. 2019;242(2):118–22.

91. Marcos S. Chapter 40: Slack incorporated. In: Hoffer K, editor. IOL power. 1st ed; 2011. p. 224.

92. Atchison DA. Refractive errors induced by displacement of intraocular lenses within the pseudophakic eye. Optom Vis Sci. 1989;66(3):146–52.

93. Kingslake R. Who? Discovered Coddington's equations? Opt Photonics News. 1994;5(8):20–3.

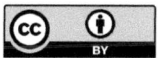

Toric Calculations

62

Giacomo Savini and Adi Abulafia

Calculators for toric intraocular lenses (IOLs) have undergone a remarkable development over the last decade. Until around 2015, most calculators were directly developed by IOL manufacturers and suffered from two main limitations: (1) they were based on anterior keratometric values of corneal astigmatism, without taking posterior corneal astigmatism into account and (2) they assumed a fixed ratio between the cylinder of the IOL and the cylinder effect at the corneal plane (usually 1.46), based on the average pseudophakic eye [1].

Keratometric Astigmatism and Total Corneal Astigmatism

The clinical relevance of posterior corneal astigmatism (PCA) and its influence on total corneal astigmatism (TCA) was described by Ho et al. in 2009 and highlighted by Koch et al. in 2012 [2, 3]. These and other studies demonstrated that the posterior corneal surface has on average the steepest meridian vertically aligned and thus generates an against-the-rule (ATR) astigmatism [3–5]. As a consequence, if PCA is not accounted for, keratometric astigmatism (KA) usually overestimates TCA in eyes with with-the-rule (WTR) astigmatism and underestimates it in eyes with ATR astigmatism. For the same reason, studies comparing KA to TCA found the latter to predict more accurately the postoperative refractive astigmatism in eyes receiving toric and non-toric IOLs [6, 7]. Savini and Næser, for example, reported that using TCA leads to a mean prediction error (ERA, error in refractive astigmatism) close to zero, i.e., -0.13 ± 0.42 diopters (D) in eyes with WTR astigmatism and $+0.07 \pm 0.59$ D in eyes with ATR astigmatism; on the contrary, using KA provided a mean overcorrection of the cylinder (-0.59 ± 0.34 D) in WTR eyes and a mean undercorrection (0.32 ± 0.42 D) in ATR eyes [6]. For surgeons who could not measure PCA and TCA, Koch et al. developed the first method used to predict TCA: the Baylor toric IOL nomogram. This took into account the mean values of PCA that they found (ATR astigmatism) and aimed to leave eyes after the toric IOL implantation with small amounts of WTR refractive astigmatism. It was required to manually perform the calculation following the guidelines indicated in some tables [8]. Shortly after the Barrett Toric Calculator was released, which was somehow revolutionary, it was the first to adjust the KA provided by keratometers included in the optical biometers in order to take PCA into

G. Savini (✉)
IRCCS Bietti Foundation, Rome, Italy

Studio Oculistico d'Azeglio, Bologna, Italy
e-mail: giacomo.savini@startmail.com

A. Abulafia
Department of Ophthalmology, Shaare Zedek Medical Center and the Hebrew University-Hadassah Medical School, Jerusalem, Israel

© The Author(s) 2024
J. Aramberri et al. (eds.), *Intraocular Lens Calculations*, Essentials in Ophthalmology,
https://doi.org/10.1007/978-3-031-50666-6_62

account. Barrett Toric Calculator was followed by several calculators that shared the same purpose: optimize the KA and eliminate the fixed ratio between the cylinder at the IOL and at the corneal plane. Different studies have shown that toric calculators estimating TCA are more accurate than toric calculators using direct TCA measurements: the percentage of eyes with an absolute prediction error within 0.50 D increases from around 40% to around 60% [9, 10]. This apparently nonsense finding is likely to depend on the fact that estimating algorithms, in addition to posterior corneal astigmatism, take other sources of error into account (e.g., IOL tilt).

Solving the ACD Issue

Back in 2011, Goggin et al. pointed out that the Alcon web-based toric IOL calculator did not take into consideration the distance between the corneal and IOL planes when calculating the corneal plane cylinder equivalent power of the IOL [11]. They described an improved method to calculate the corneal plane cylinder equivalent power of the IOL by means of a thick lens vertex power formula, which contains the data of anterior chamber depth (ACD) and corneal pachymetry. However, different authors felt that his method had some limitations [12–14]. In order to take the ACD into account, we preferred to rely on the method previously described by Fam et al., who based their calculation on a thin-lens formula for IOL power calculation, the Holladay 1 formula [15]. Their method, known as meridional analysis, calculates the IOL power for the steep and flat meridians separately: the difference between the two values is the required IOL toricity for that eye, on condition that the postoperative ACD is separately calculated using the mean corneal power [16]. Using this method in a theoretical model, we found that the above mentioned ratio depends on the predicted ACD and can range from 1.29 in short eyes with shallow ACD to 1.86 in long eyes with deep ACD [17]. Today this issue has just a historical interest, since almost all calculators have fixed it.

The Influence of IOL Tilt

Both the natural crystalline lens and the IOL are known to be physiologically tilted towards the inferotemporal direction by a mean value of about 4–5° [18, 19]. This means that they are tilted horizontally around the vertical meridian with anterior displacement of the nasal portion. In a ray-tracing eye model, it has been shown that IOL tilting around the vertical meridian induces ATR astigmatism, which can be as high as 0.56 D with a 28.0 D IOL tilted 10° [20]. Consistently, Hirnschall et al. reported that IOL tilt is a relevant source of error in toric IOL calculation [21]. None of the currently available toric calculators enable direct input of IOL tilt, probably because optical biometers do not provide this value and it is difficult to develop a calculator including a parameter that is not readily available. However, the effect of tilt is indirectly taken into account by all toric calculators estimating TCA and this is one of the most likely reasons why such calculators are, on average, more accurate with respect to those using measured TCA values.

Current Toric Calculators

Abulafia-Koch Toric Calculator

This calculator uses the first published mathematical model that used a seperate regression formula for the X and Y vector components of anterior-based corneal astigmatism. This formula is aiming to compensate for the effect of posterior corneal astigmatism and any other physiological factors (e.g., IOL tilt) since it is derived from the differences between the postoperative anterior-based corneal astigmatism measurements and the calculated refractive astigmatism of the pseudophakic eye [22]. With minor andjusments from the original published formula, and the use of Fams' method to calculate the cylinder effect of a toric IOL at the corneal plane, it has been incorporated into several toric calculators such as the Hill-RBF, Hoya, Medicontur, Ophtec,

Physiol, and Veracity surgical software. Its results are similar to those obtained with Barrett's calculator [22, 23].

Barrett Toric Calculator

Barrett's has been the first toric calculator (Figs. 62.1 and 62.2) to change the cylinder obtained as the keratometric astigmatism into a new value defined "net astigmatism". With respect to keratometric astigmatism, net astigmatism is lower in eyes with with-the-rule astigmatism and higher in eyes with against-the-rule astigmatism. The mathematics behind Barrett's calculator have never been published. However, it can be easily observed that net astigmatism also depends on the ACD and axial length values. Moreover, the version available on several biometry devices (e.g., IOLMaster700, Lenstar, etc.) and on the ASCRS (https://ascrs.org/tools/barrett-toric-calculator) and the APACRS website (https://calc.apacrs.org/toric_calculator20/Toric%20Calculator.aspx) does not only calculate the cylinder, but also the spherical equivalent power of the IOL.

Several papers have demonstrated that Barrett's toric calculator is one of the most accurate options to calculate the power of toric IOLs

[24, 25]. Recently, 2 new features have been added to the online calculator.

1. An option to utilize direct measurements of the posterior cornea instead of using its standard mathematical model. This option incorporates an additional algorithem to compensate for the estimated effect of IOL tilt.
2. The K calculator which allows the user to select the keratometry measurements of up to three devices and provides integrated K values using vector-based calcultions.

Barrett True-K Toric Calculator

This toric calculator is designed for toric IOL power calculation for eyes following corneal ablation refractive surgery (myopic and hyperopic) and radial keratotomy. It is based on the Barrett True-K formula with an adjusted algorithm for toric IOL power calculation.

EVO 2.0 Toric Calculator

This unpublished toric calculator (Fig. 62.3), developed by Tun Kuan Yeo, MD, is available at the same website of the EVO 2.0 formula (https://www.evoiolcalculator.com/toric.aspx).

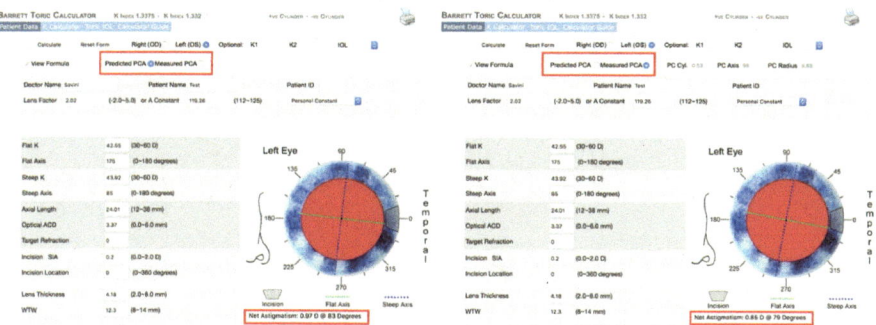

Fig. 62.1 Barrett toric calculator using posterior corneal astigmatism reduces the keratometric astigmatism by the IOLMaster 700 (1.37 D @ 85°) to a net astigmatism of 0.78 D @ 82° (not shown), which is increased up to 0.97 D @ 83° after including SIA. Right:

Barrett toric calculator using measured posterior corneal astigmatism reduces the keratometric astigmatism to a net astigmatism of 0.67 D @ 76° (not shown), which is increased up to 0.85 D @ 79° after including SIA

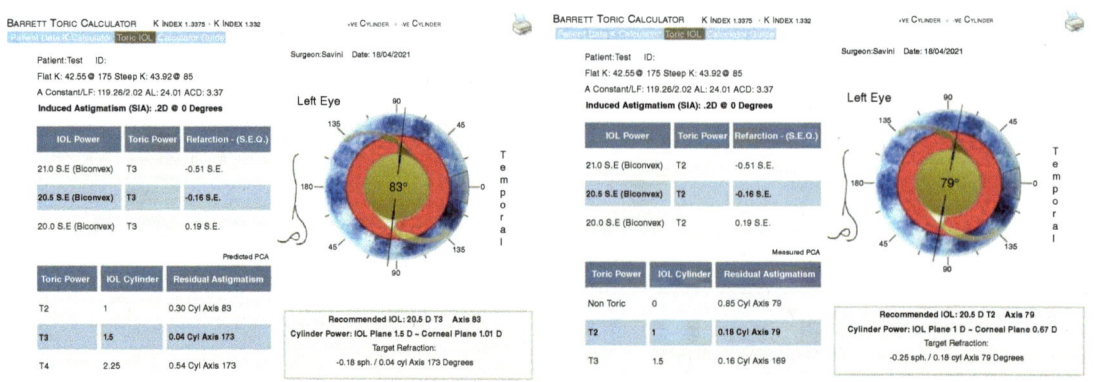

Fig. 62.2 Results of Barrett toric calculator with predicted posterior corneal astigmatism (left) and measured posterior corneal astigmatism (right). The predicted residual astigmatism with the implanted toric IOL (T3) is slightly different, as in the first case it is 0.04 D @ 173° and in the second case it is 0.16 D @ 169°

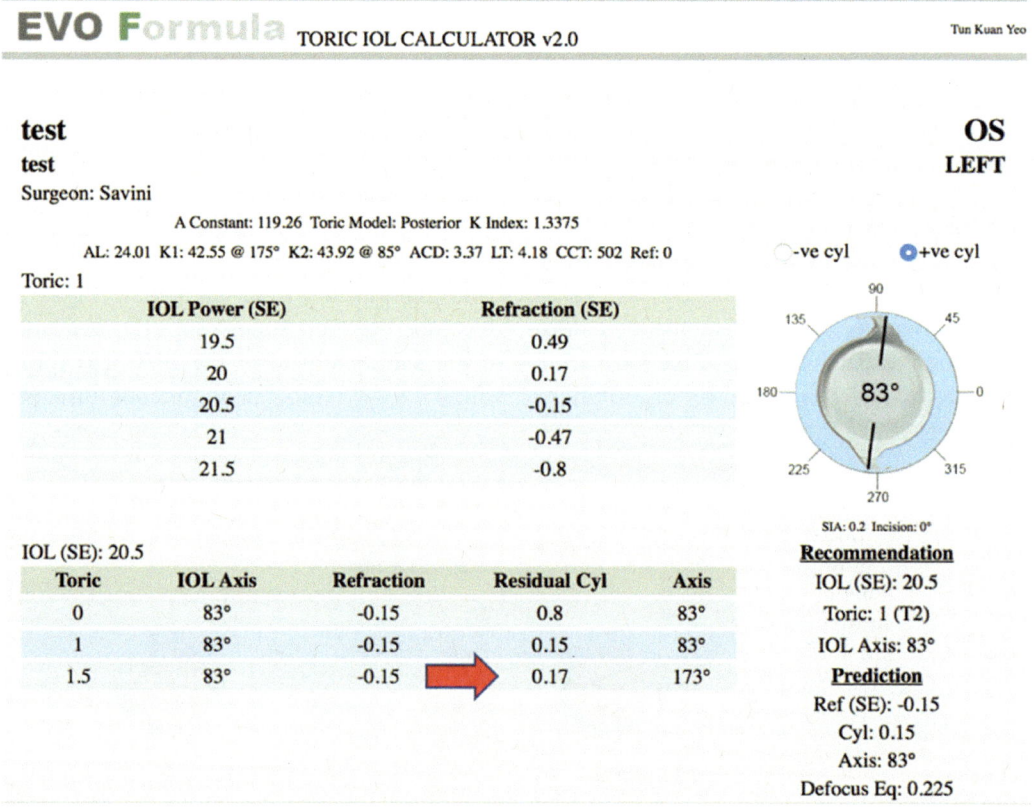

Fig. 62.3 EVO toric calculator directly provides the residual cylinder (0.17 D @ 173°)

The accuracy is close to that of the other toric calculators [26]. The online version provides the predicted SE based on the EVO 2.0 formula and has an additional feature for toric IOL power calculation for eyes following myopic corneal ablation refractive procedures.

Goggin Keratometry Adjustor Calculator

This calculator is different with respect to the other in this chapter, as it does not calculate the toric power of the IOL, but only adjusts the KA according to the coefficient published by Goggin et al. [27] The adjusted KA readings must be entered into a toric calculator that does not modify KA. Moreover, it is suggested that KA adjustments are unnecessary in eyes with KA > 2.0 D. The calculator is available at http://goggin-toric.com.

Holladay Toric Calculator

This calculator has been released in 2019 following a publication by the author and is available at http://www.hicsoap.com/pro-description.php [28]. The Holladay toric calculator is based on the concept of the back-calculated SIA, which accounts for all factors that contribute to the difference between the preoperative K-reading and the ideal, back-calculated K-reading based on the actual postoperative refraction. The total SIA is calculated using the Gaussian vergence formula. It is worth mentioning that as opposed to other toric calculators, the corneal SIA is incorporated within the mathematical algorithem of this calculator and that it applies for surgeons who utilize temporal main corneal incisions (0/180°).

Johnson & Johnson Toric Calculator

Some manufacturers developed their own toric calculator. Johnson & Johnson uses a specific algorithm that can incorporate the effect of PCA, thus improving the refractive accuracy when compared to calculations based solely on KA [29]. The details of this PCA algorithm are unpublished, but it can be easily applied to any eye on the online toric calculator (https://tecnis-toriccalc.com) by selecting the option "Include Posterior Corneal Astigmatism".

Kane Toric Calculator

This calculator is available at https://www.iolformula.com (Fig. 62.4). Like for the Barrett and the EVO Toric Calculators, the Kane toric formula is unpublished. The author states that it "uses the Kane formula to calculate an ELP before using an advanced algorithm incorporating regression, theoretical optics, and artificial intelligence techniques to calculate the total corneal astigmatism". The results published by Kane et al. show the most accurate prediction with respect to the other calculators in this chapter [26]. The online version provide the SE prediction based on the Kane formula and it also has an option for toric IOL power calculation for eyes with keratoconus.

Næser-Savini Toric Calculator

The calculator developed by Drs. Kristian Næser and Giacomo Savini (Figs. 62.5 and 62.6) is based on the concept of optimized keratometry, a modification of the keratometric astigmatism that zeroes out the mean prediction, i.e., the difference between the predicted and the achieved refractive astigmatism [9]. Like for Barrett's calculator, also Næser-Savini toric calculator reduces the magnitude of the corneal astigmatism in eyes with a with-the-rule astigmatism and increases it in eyes with against-the-rule astigmatism. The new cylinder is calculated according to the following equation:

$$\text{Optimal keratometric astigmatism} = 0.103 + 0.836 \times \text{Measured keratometric astigmatism} + 0.457 \times \cos(2 \times \alpha).$$

This calculator takes ACD and axial length into consideration, according to meridional analysis as described by Fam [7]. It is available in its original version on the website of the Italian

Fig. 62.4 Kane toric calculator directly provides the calculated toric IOL and the predicted residual cylinder (0.01 D @ 85°)

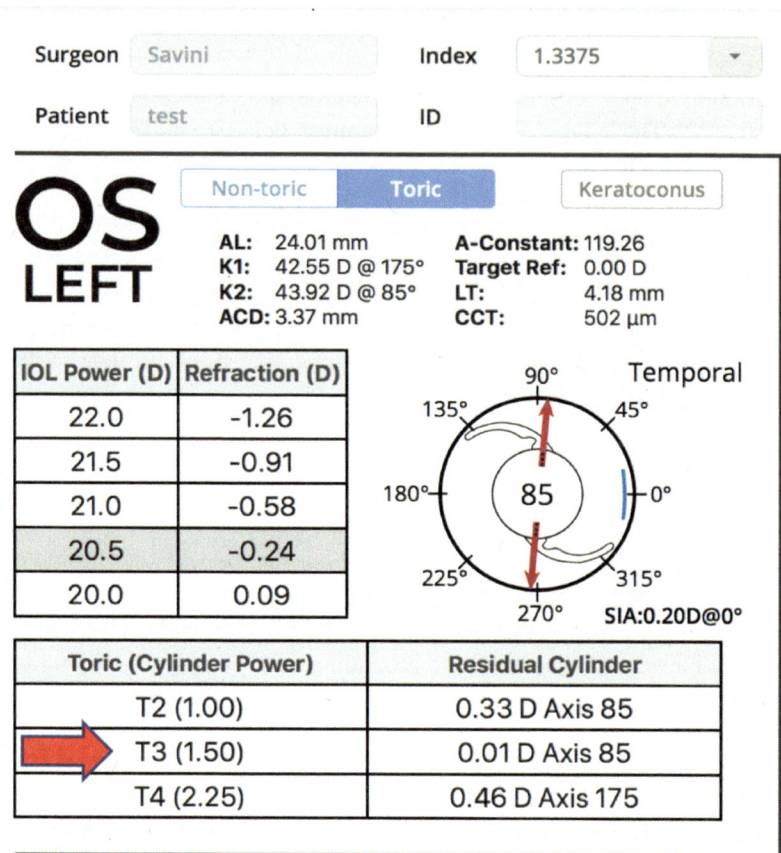

Ophthalmology Society (https://www.soiweb.com/toric-calculator/), where calculations are performed also with TCA by Scheimpflug cameras or anterior segment OCT for comparative purposes. The latest version is available on the Hoffer QST website (www.hofferqst.com). The published results are close to those obtained with the other calculators [9, 26].

Rayner Toric Calculator

Ray*trace* 3.5 is Rayner's proprietary online calculator for premium IOLs (available at, https://rayner.com/en/raytrace/). Ray*trace* 3.5 utilizes a combination of regression formulas, applying the recommended formula based on the patient's biometry input. PCA is an optional consideration, the mathematical method for which is unpublished.

Zeiss Toric Calculator

Calculations for Zeiss toric IOLs are performed by means of a proprietary online calculator (Z CALC 2.0, available at https://zcalc.meditec.zeiss.com) that offers two alternative options to include the PCA: (1) using Total Keratometry values directly measured by the IOLMaster 700

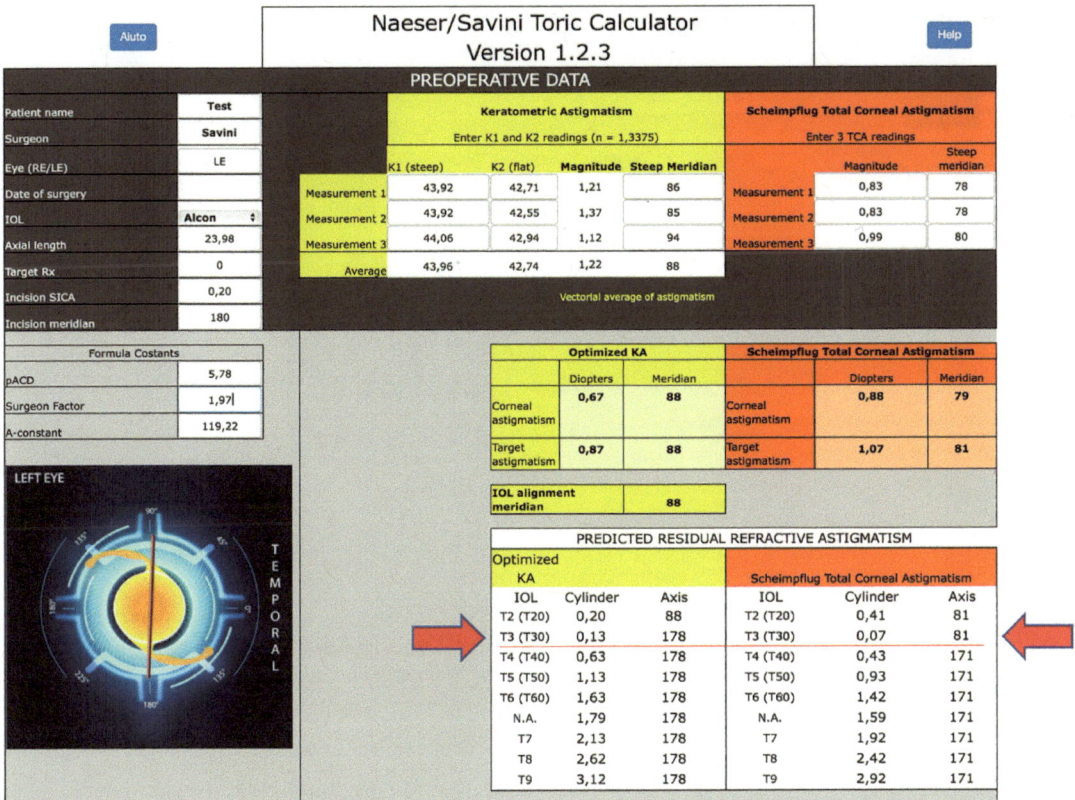

Fig. 62.5 Næser-Savini calculator (https://www.sedesoi.com/toric-2020/) suggests a T3/T30 Alcon IOL with both calculations. In the yellow section, the optimized keratometry, which takes posterior corneal astigmatism and IOL tilt into account, is derived from 3 keratometric measurements of corneal astigmatism: measurement 1 from Aladdin (Topcon), measurement 2 from IOLMaster 700 (Zeiss), and measurement 3 from OA-2000 (Tomey). The vectorial average of these three measurements is 1.22 D @ 88°. Optimization reduces corneal astigmatism to 0.67 D @ 88°. Addition of surgically induced corneal astigmatism (SICA) increases it up to 0.87 D @ 88°, which is the final target. In the orange section, three measurements of total corneal astigmatism by a Scheimpflug camera are entered: their vectorial average (0.88 D @ 79°) is lower than the mean non-optimized keratometric astigmatism (1.22 D @ 88°). Target astigmatism, including the effect of SICA, is 1.07 D @ 81°. The predicted residual refractive astigmatism is 0.13 D @ 178° with the optimized keratometric astigmatism and 0.07 D @ 81° with measured total corneal astigmatism

and (2) using an estimated TCA, which is based on measured KA and a mathematical model of PCA derived from clinical data (defined as Z CALC nomogram). The latter is recommended for post-refractive surgery eyes. So far, there are no studies showing which approach (Total Keratometry versus estimated TCA) is more accurate. On the other hand, Z CALC 2.0 with estimated TCA has been shown to be more accurate with respect to the previous version of the same calculator [30].

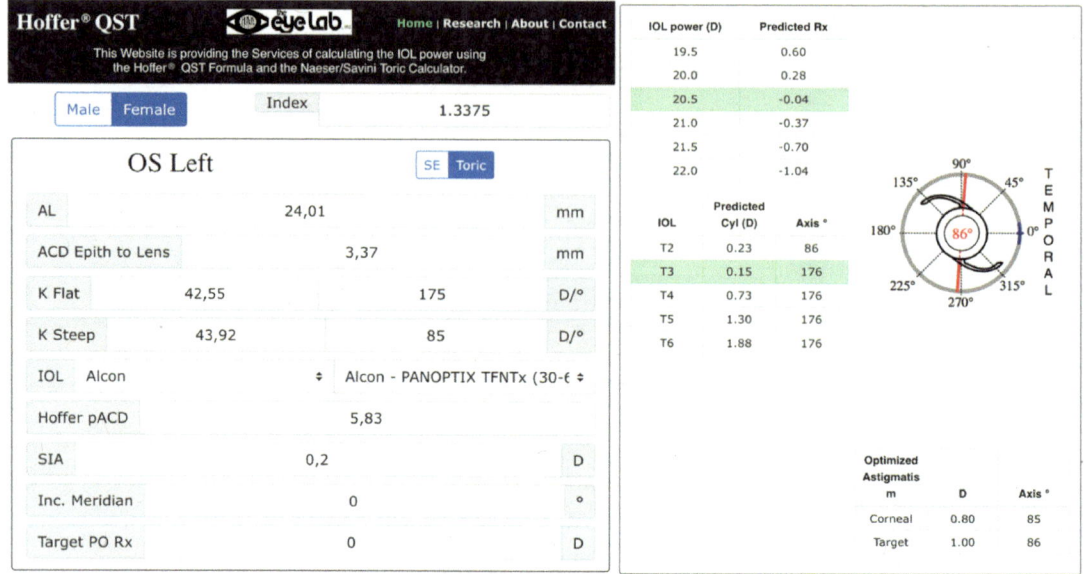

Fig. 62.6 The Næser-Savini calculator version available on the website of the Hoffer QST formula (https://hoffer-qst.com) reduces the keratometric astigmatism by the IOLMaster 700 (1.37 D @ 85°) to an optimized value of 0.80 D @ 85°, which is increased up to 1.00 D @ 86° after including the surgically induced astigmatism. The predicted cylinder with the T3 IOL is 0.15 D @ 176°

Results

Refractive results of toric calculators have remarkably improved over the last decade, although they are still far from perfection, as some amount or residual refractive astigmatism is often observed. Like for calculation of non-toric IOLs, the main outcome is the prediction error, which—in the case of toric IOLs—is the difference between the postoperative refractive astigmatism and the predicted refractive astigmatism. This analysis should consider the actual orientation of the toric IOL, evaluated at the slit lamp under pupil dilation, and not just the planned orientation.

When analyzing such results, we should look at two main outcomes: the centroid prediction error and the percentage of eyes with an absolute prediction error within 0.50 D. The former is the vectorial average of all prediction errors and provides us with an estimation of the systematic deviation from the predicted refractive astigmatism, so that values closer to zero reveal a better performance of a given calculator; its standard deviation is a measure of the spread of the results. The latter is a useful metric to understand what we can expect, from a clinical point of view, in our patients, as it explains in how many cases we are able to reach an absolute prediction error within 0.50 D, which can be arbitrarily selected as a very good result.

All current calculators lead to a mean centroid prediction error close to zero (Table 62.1) [9, 10, 22, 26]. On the contrary, older calculators based on standard keratometric values (with no optimization to take the PCA into consideration) lead to a systematic overcorrection in eyes with WTR astigmatism and undercorrection in eyes with ATR astigmatism [9, 22]. Calculators based on TCA measurements, such as those provided by Scheimpflug cameras, usually provide intermediate outcomes, as they are better than those based on KA and—on average—are less accurate than those estimating TCA [9, 10, 25].

The percentage of eyes with an absolute prediction error within 0.50 D ranges between 55 and 79% with calculators estimating TCA,

Table 62.1 Refractive outcomes obtained with current toric calculators

	Centroid Prediction Error (D @ angle) + standard deviation	Percentage of eyes with an absolute prediction within 0.50 D
Abulafia-Koch [10]	0.07 ± 0.26 @ 172°	72.0%
Abulafia-Koch [26]	0.11 ± 0.65 @ 110°	59.5%
Abulafia-Koch [9]	0.17 ± 0.77 @ 70°	54.7%
Abulafia-Koch [22]	0.04 ± 0.31 @ 176°	78.2%
Barrett [10]	0.13 ± 0.37 @ 174°	67.0%
Barrett [26]	0.10 ± 0.64 @ 111°	59.9%
Barrett [9]	0.11 ± 0.63 @ 56°	57.2%
Barrett [22]	0.05 ± 0.30 @ 176°	79.5%
EVO 2.0 [26]	0.16 ± 0.63 @ 100°	58.9%
Holladay [26]	0.13 ± 0.66 @ 168°	53.9%
Johnson & Johnson [29]	0.19 ± 0.41 @ 3°	53.0%
Kane [26]	0.03 ± 0.60 @ 163°	65.6%
Næser-Savini [9]	0.11 ± 0.61 @ 47°	57.8%
Næser-Savini [26]	0.01 ± 0.67 @ 150°	56.7%

whereas it is close to 40% with calculators using measured TCA and around 25–30% with calculators using KA [9, 10, 22, 25, 26].

Example of the results obtained from different toric calculators in a patient with WTR astigmatism who ended up with plano refraction after implantation of toric 20.5 D Panoptix TFNT30 oriented at 88°.

References

1. Savini G, Hoffer KJ, Ducoli P. A new slant on toric intraocular lenses power calculation. J Refract Surg. 2013;29:348–54.
2. Ho JD, Tsai CY, Liou SW. Accuracy of corneal astigmatism estimation by neglecting the posterior corneal surface measurement. Am J Ophthalmol. 2009;147:788–95.
3. Koch DD, Ali SF, Weikert MP, et al. Contribution of posterior corneal astigmatism to total corneal astigmatism. J Cataract Refract Surg. 2012;38:2020–87.
4. Tonn B, Klaproth OK, Kohnen T. Anterior surface-based keratometry compared with Scheimpflug tomography-based total corneal astigmatism. Invest Ophthalmol Vis Sci. 2015;56:291–8.
5. Savini G, Versaci F, Vestri G, Ducoli P, Næser K. Influence of posterior corneal astigmatism on total corneal astigmatism in eyes with moderate to high astigmatism. J Cataract Refract Surg. 2014;40:1645–53.
6. Savini G, Næser K. An analysis of the factors influencing the residual refractive astigmatism after cataract surgery with toric intraocular lenses. Invest Ophthalmol Vis Sci. 2015;56:827–35.
7. Klijn S, Reus NJ, Van Der Sommen CM, et al. Accuracy of total corneal astigmatism measurements with a Scheimpflug imager and a color light-emitted diode corneal topographer. Am J Ophthalmol. 2016;167:72–8.
8. Koch DD, Jenkins RB, Weikert MP, et al. Correcting astigmatism with toric intraocular lenses: effect of posterior corneal astigmatism. J Cataract Refract Surg. 2013;39:1803–9.
9. Savini G, Næser K, Schiano-Lomoriello D, Ducoli P. Optimized keratometry and total corneal astigmatism for toric intraocular lens calculation. J Cataract Refract Surg. 2017;43:1140–8.
10. Ferreira TB, Ribeiro P, Ribeiro FJ, OO'Neill JG. Comparison of methodologies using estimated or measured values of total corneal astigmatism for toric intraocular lens power calculation. J Refract Surg. 2017;33:794–800.
11. Goggin M, Moore S, Easterman A. Outcome of toric intraocular lens implantation after adjusting for anterior chamber depth and intraocular lens sphere equivalent power effects. Arch Ophthalmol. 2011;129:998–1003.
12. Simpson MJ. Refractive outcomes for toric intraocular lenses. Arch Ophthalmol. 2012;130:945–6.
13. Holladay JT. Exact toric intraocular lens calculations using currently available lens constants. Arch Ophthalmol. 2012;130:946–7.
14. Savini G, Hoffer KJ. Toric intraocular lens calculations. Arch Ophthalmol. 2012;130:947–8.
15. Holladay JT, Prager TC, Chandler TY, et al. A three-part system for refining intraocular lens power calculations. J Cataract Refract Surg. 1988;14:17–24.
16. Fam HB, Lim KL. Meridional analysis for calculating the expected spherocylindrical refraction in eyes with toric intraocular lenses. J Cataract Refract Surg. 2007;33:2072–6.
17. Savini G, Hoffer KJ, Carbonelli M, Ducoli P, Barboni P. Influence of axial length and corneal power on the astigmatic power of toric intraocular lenses. J Cataract Refract Surg. 2013;39:1900–3.
18. Kimura S, Morizane Y, Shiode Y, Hirano M, Doi S, Toshima S, Fuijiwara A, Shiraga F. Assessment of tilt and decentration of crystalline lens and intraocular

lens relative to the topographic axis using anterior segment optical coherence tomography. PlosOne. 2017;12(9):e01184066.

19. Wang L, Guimaraes de Souza R, Weikert MP, Koch DD. Evaluation of crystalline lens and intraocular lens tilt using a swept-source optical coherence tomography biometer. J Cataract Refract Surg. 2019;45:35–40.

20. Weikert MP, Golla A, Wang L. Astigmatism induced by intraocular lens tilt evaluated via ray tracing. J Cataract Refract Surg. 2018;44:745–9.

21. Hirnschall N, Findl O, Bayer N, Leisser C, Norrby S, Zimper E, Hoffmann P. Sources of error in toric intraocular lens power calculation. J Refract Surg. 2020;36:646–52.

22. Abulafia A, Koch DD, Wang L, Hill WE, Assia EI, Franchina M, Barrett GD. New regression formula for toric intraocular lens calculations. J Cataract Refract Surg. 2016;42:663–71.

23. Ribeiro FJ, Ferreira TB, Relha C, Esteves C, Gaspar S. Predictability of different calculators in the minimization of postoperative astigmatism after implantation of a toric intraocular lens. Clin Ophthalmol. 2019;13:1649–56.

24. Reitblat O, Levy A, Kleinmann G, Abulafia A, Assia EI. Effect of posterior corneal astigmatism on power calculation and alignment of toric intraocular lenses: comparison of methodologies. J Cataract Refract Surg. 2016;42:217–25.

25. Abulafia A, Hill WE, Franchina M, Barrett GD. Comparison of methods to predict residual astigmatism after intraocular lens implantation. J Refract Surg. 2015;31:699–707.

26. Kane JX, Connell B. A comparison of the accuracy of 6 modern toric intraocular lenses formulas. Ophthalmology. 2020;127:1472–86.

27. Goggin M, Zamora-Alejo K, Easterman A, van Zyl L. Adjustment of anterior corneal astigmatism values to incorporate the likely effect of posterior corneal curvature for toric intraocular lens calculation. J Refract Surg. 2015;31:98–102.

28. Holladay JT, Pettit G. Improving toric intraocular lens calculations using total surgically induced astigmatism for a 2.5 mm temporal incision. J Cataract Refract Surg. 2019;45:272–83.

29. Canovas C, Alarcon A, Rosén R, Kasthurirangan S, Ma JK, Koch DD, Piers P. New algorithm for toric intraocular lens power calculation considering the posterior corneal astigmatism. J Cataract Refract Surg. 2018;44:168–74.

30. Lesieur G. Microincision cataract surgery with implantation of a bitoric intraocular lens using an enhanced program for intraocular lens power calculation. Eur J Ophthalmol. 2020;30:1308–13.

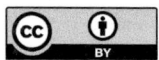

Part VI

Special Situations

IOL Power Calculation in Long Eye

63

Li Wang, Rachel Lopes Franke Bezerra, and Douglas D. Koch

In long axial length (AL) eyes, traditional intraocular lens (IOL) power formulas tend to select IOLs of insufficient power, leaving patients with postoperative hyperopia. To reduce the chances for hyperopic surprises, surgeons used to empirically aim for a more myopic postoperative outcome by targeting a postoperative refraction of −1.00 to −2.00 diopter (D). Norrby [1] reported that the largest contributor of error in IOL power calculation was the estimation of effective lens position (ELP) (35%), followed by the postoperative refraction determination (27%) and AL measurement (17%). In long eyes, the required IOL powers are low, and errors in ELP produce low refractive effect. This indicates that accuracy of ELP estimation in long eyes is not as important as in normal and short eyes in which higher IOL powers are required. In this chapter, we will discuss the factors contributing to challenges in IOL power prediction in long eyes, the formulas appropriate for use in these eyes, and the refractive outcomes with these formulas.

L. Wang (✉) · D. D. Koch
Cullen Eye Institute, Baylor College of Medicine, Houston, TX, USA
e-mail: liw@bcm.edu; dkoch@bcm.edu

R. L. F. Bezerra
Cullen Eye Institute, Baylor College of Medicine, Houston, TX, USA

Hospital de Olhos do Paraná, Paraná, Brazil

Factors Contributing to Challenges in IOL Power Calculation in Long Eyes

Inaccurate measurement of preoperative AL has been reported to be the main reason for postoperative refractive error in axial high myopia [2]. There are three factors that primarily contribute to challenges in IOL power calculations in long eyes.

Posterior Staphyloma

The incidence of posterior staphyloma increases with increasing AL, and it is likely that nearly all eyes with pathologic myopia have some form of posterior staphyloma. Ultrasonic biometric methods can produce errors in the presence of a posterior staphyloma by giving falsely long AL.

An immersion A/B-scan approach for AL measurement has been described in the setting of posterior staphyloma [3]. Using a horizontal axial B-scan, an immersion echogram through the posterior fundus is obtained with the cornea and lens echoes centered while simultaneously displaying the optic nerve void. The A-scan vector is then adjusted to pass through the middle of the cornea as well as the anterior and posterior lens echoes to ensure that the vector will intersect the retina in the region of the fovea. Optical biometry with appropriate patient fixation may solve this problem of identifying the fovea and

© The Author(s) 2024
J. Aramberri et al. (eds.), *Intraocular Lens Calculations*, Essentials in Ophthalmology,
https://doi.org/10.1007/978-3-031-50666-6_63

has improved outcomes in long eyes with a posterior staphyloma.

Calculation of Axial Length Matching US Data: The IOL Master Calibration

Theoretically, optical biometry permits more accurate measurements when a posterior staphyloma is present. However, in a study investigating the accuracy of SRK/T formula in eyes with negative and zero-powered IOLs, MacLaren and colleagues [4] reported consistent hyperopic errors across all three methods of biometry (A-scan, B-scan, and optical). This indicates that eliminating or minimizing the adverse impact of posterior staphylomata on IOL calculations does not prevent hyperopic surprises in long eyes.

During the development of the first optical biometer (Carl Zeiss Meditec, Jena, Germany), first, the OPL data were transformed to geometrical path length (GPL) data using a group refractive index calculated theoretically from the Gullstand eye model ($n = 1.3549$). Then regression analysis produced the definitive conversion formula programmed in the commercial version of the first IOL Master model: GPL (OPL/1.3549) = $AL_{GBS} \times 0.9571 + 1.3033$, where AL_{GBS} is the AXL measured by immersion US. There were two main reasons for this transformation: (1) to avoid the bias produced in the extremes of the AXL range that would have occurred if only an average refractive index was used for the calculation from measured OPL and (2) to adjust the retinal plane reference from PCI to the internal limiting membrane for US. In the PCI instrument, the main retinal signal is produced in the retinal pigment epithelium, which produces systematically longer measurements.

With the IOL Master calibration, the same IOL constants could be used when surgeons moved from immersion US to optical biometry, which, of course, made this transition easier. All optical biometers developed thereafter, except the Argos biometer (Movu, Komaki, Japan), are all calibrated to provide an AL equivalent or similar to the first optical biometer. However, in long eyes, the relative lengths of the ocular segments

may differ from those in eyes with normal ALs, and the use of a fixed group refractive index for the entire eye may yield incorrect values for AL.

We proposed a segmented AL that is calculated by summing the GPL of individual ocular segments converted from their respective OPLs using specific refractive indices for each ocular medium: cornea, aqueous depth (AD), lens thickness (LT), and vitreous chamber depth [6]. Theoretically, the segmented AL may provide more accurate AL measurements in eyes with unusual ocular segment proportions. We found that the segmented ALs were shorter in long eyes compared with the AL calculated with the IOL Master calibration in an OLCR instrument. The refractive accuracy with segmented ALs was improved in long eyes with the Barrett, Haigis, Hoffer Q, Holladay 1, and SRK/T formulas [6]. Cooke and Cooke [7] compared prediction accuracy with the AL calculation method of the Lenstar biometer (transitional AL) and that of the Argos biometer (sum-of-segments AL). They found that using sum-of-segments AL, instead of traditional AL, improved predictions for formulas designed on ultrasound data (SRK/T, Holladay 1, Holladay 2, Hoffer Q, and Haigis), although it worsened the Barrett and Olsen formulas. Further studies are desirable in this regard.

Extrapolation Issue in Extreme Long Eyes

The dataset used in the study by Haigis et al that developed regression formula by converting the OPL data to GPL in millimeters, eyes with AL up to 27.45 mm were included [5]. When this conversion method is used in eyes longer than 27.45 mm, extrapolation is introduced and errors may presumably occur.

Principal Plane Shift in Negative-Power IOLs

There are differences in geometries of positive-diopter IOLs and negative-diopter IOLs. The optic principle plane shifts in negative-power

IOLs, compared to the principle plane in positive-power IOLs. Petermeier and colleagues [8] proposed seperate constants optimization for eyes with negative IOL powers.

IOL Power Calculation Formulas for Long Eyes

Axial Length Adjustment Methods (Wang-Koch Adjustment)

We assume that the hyperopic error seen in long eyes is in the measurement of AL or in the way that formulas use this value. In a previous study, we proposed a method of optimizing AL in long eyes (Wang-Koch adjustment) [9]. Our results showed that this method significantly improved the accuracy of IOL power calculation in eyes with IOL powers ≤5 D, and significantly reduced the percentage of eyes that would be left hyperopic.

In a more recent study [10], we modified the original AL adjustment formulas by using ULIB (User Group for Laser Interference Biometry) lens constants and manifested refraction converted to 6 meters. The modified AL adjustment formulas are less aggressive (less myopic outcomes) than the original AL adjustment formulas. AL adjustment is required in eyes with an AL > 26.5 mm for the modified Holladay 1 formula and AL > 27.0 mm for the modified SRK/T formula. The modified equations for optimizing the AL are as follows:

- Modified Holladay 1 optimized AL = 0.817 × (measured AL) + 4.7013.
- Modified SRK/T optimized AL = 0.8453 × (measured AL) + 4.0773.

Based on the formula, the optimized AL is calculated from the measured optical or ultrasonic AL. Then, the optimized AL is entered into the IOLMaster or Lenstar, and the calculation is performed again. We recommend selecting the IOL power that predicts a minus prediction error close to zero (−0.1 to −0.2 D), since slight myopic results may occur with this approach of optimiz-

ing AL. Figure 63.1 shows that an 8.0 D SN6ATT was suggested using the Holladay 1 with original AL of 28.41 mm. Recalculation with the optimized AL of 27.81 mm produced a 9.5 D IOL with predicted refraction of −0.06 D. A 9.5 D SN6AT3 was implanted and, at 3 weeks postoperatively, the uncorrected visual acuity was 20/15 and the manifest refraction was plano.

We also developed an AL adjustment equation for Holladay 2 formula [11]. The polynomial optimization equation is as follows:

- Holladay 2 optimized AL = $0.0001154786 \times$ (measured AL)^3 + $0.0032939472 \times$ (measured AL)^2 + $1.001040305 \times$ (measured AL) − 0.3270056564.

With the Holladay IOL Consultant Software, users have the option to select the AL adjustment method, and IOL power calculations will be performed automatically using the optimized AL in long eyes.

It should be noted that the AL adjustment method should be used with combination of the Holladay 1, Holladay 2, and SRK/T formulas. The newer IOL power calculation formulas already have the AL optimized or adjusted empirically by their authors and the AL adjustment method should not be used.

Super Formula

This formula is a combination of the Hoffer Q, Holladay 1, Holladay 2, and SRK/T formulas and also has a small component of artificial intelligence [12]. In long eyes, the Wang-Koch AL adjustment is used. In 2019, the formula was revised using the postoperative data as component of artificial intelligence. It is available at www.iolcalc.com.

Barrett Universal II Formula

The Barrett Universal II (BUII) formula is the evolution of the Barrett Universal I, which was published in 1987 as a thick-lens paraxial for-

IOLMaster AL

OD right	AL: 28.41 mm (*) K1: 41.77 D / 8.08 mm @ 179° K2: 42.94 D / 7.86 mm @ 89° R / SE: 7.97 mm (SD = 42.36 mm) Cyl.: 1.17 D @ 89° opt. ACD: 3.50 mm Refraction: -14.00 D +0.00 D Visual Acuity: 20/70 Eye Status: phakic

SN60WF-REV		ZCB00-OPT	
SF:	1.95	SF:	2.11
IOL (D)	REF (D)	IOL (D)	REF (D)
9.0	−0.82	9.5	−1.07
8.5	−0.49	9.0	−0.74
8.0	−0.16	8.5	−0.42
7.5	**0.16**	**8.0**	**−0.09**
7.0	0.48	7.5	0.22
6.5	0.80	7.0	0.54
6.0	1.11	6.5	0.85

SN6ATT		Softec HD	
SF:	1.96	SF:	1.48
IOL (D)	REF (D)	IOL (D)	REF (D)
9.5	−1.15	8.25	−0.54
9.0	−0.82	8.0	−0.37
8.5	−0.49	7.75	−0.20
8.0	−0.16	7.5	−0.03
7.5	0.16	7.25	0.14
7.0	0.48	7.0	0.30
6.5	0.80	6.75	0.47

Optimized AL

OD right	AL: 27.81 mm (*) K1: 41.77 D / 8.08 mm @ 179° K2: 42.94 D / 7.86 mm @ 89° R / SE: 7.97 mm (SD = 42.36 mm) Cyl.: 1.17 D @ 89° opt. ACD: 3.50 mm Refraction: -14.00 D +0.00 D Visual Acuity: 20/70 Eye Status: phakic

SN60WF-REV		ZCB00-OPT	
SF:	1.95	SF:	2.11
IOL (D)	REF (D)	IOL (D)	REF (D)
11.0	−1.06	11.0	−0.96
10.5	−0.73	10.5	−0.63
10.0	−0.40	10.0	−0.31
9.5	**−0.07**	**9.5**	**0.01**
9.0	0.25	9.0	0.33
8.5	0.57	8.5	0.65
8.0	0.89	8.0	0.96

SN6ATT		Softec HD	
SF:	1.96	SF:	1.48
IOL (D)	REF (D)	IOL (D)	REF (D)
11.0	−1.05	9.75	−0.49
10.5	−0.72	9.5	−0.32
10.0	−0.39	9.25	−0.15
9.5	−0.06	9.0	0.02
9.0	0.26	8.75	0.19
8.5	0.58	8.5	0.35
8.0	0.89	8.25	0.52

Fig. 63.1 A sample of IOL power calculation using the original IOLMaster axial length (AL) (left) and the optimized AL with the Holladay 1 Wang-Koch AL adjustment (right)

mula [13]. It uses AL, keratometry, anterior chamber depth (ACD), LT, and corneal diameter (CD) values. The detailed prediction approach for effective lens position (ELP) is not published. This formula has been refined to improve outcomes in long eyes.

Hill-RBF Formula

The Hill-RBF (Radial Basis Function) calculator is an artificial intelligence-based, self-validating method for IOL power selection employing pattern recognition and a sophisticated form of data interpolation [14]. Based on artificial intelligence, this methodology is entirely data-driven. This approach also employs a validating boundary model, indicating to the user when it is performing within a defined area of accuracy. The

Hill-RBF 3.0 was recently released based on significantly expanded datasets for short and long eyes. Additionally, it has increased the number of parameters used for IOL power selection by adding central corneal thickness (CCT), LT, CD, and gender to the existing parameters of AL, keratometry, ACD, and the desired postoperative spherical equivalent refraction.

Olsen Formula

With the Olsen formula, IOL power is calculated based on exact ray tracing (Snell's law of refraction) and paraxial ray tracing (Gaussian Optics). This formula incorporates the latest generation ACD prediction algorithms based on the complex relationship between the preoperative ocular dimensions (in particular ACD and LT) and the postoperative position of the IOL (the postoperative ACD) [15]. Measurements of the anterior and posterior corneal curvatures as well as conic coefficients (Q-values) obtained by modern anterior segment imaging systems can be used directly by the PhacoOptics program developed by Thomas Olsen (www.phacooptics.net).

Kane Formula

The Kane formula was developed by Jack X. Kane. It uses theoretical optics with artificial intelligence and regression-based components to refine the predictions (www.iolformula.com). It utilizes K, AL, ACD, and gender to predict the IOL position, with LT and CCT being optional factors.

EVO Formula

The Emmetropia Verifying Optical (EVO) formula was developed by Tun Kuan Yeo in Singapore (www.evoiolcalculator.com). It is a thick lens formula based on the theory of emmetropization. It uses AL, K, and ACD as the predictors, and LT and CCT are optional.

Panacea IOL Calculator

The Panacea IOL calculator was developed by David Flikier (www.panaceaiolandtoriccalculator.com). It is a vergence formula. In addition to the AL, keratometry, ACD, and LT, it also uses additional variables, such as ratio of posterior to anterior corneal radius of curvature for corneal value adjustment, and corneal asphericity in the IOL power calculation.

Pearl-DGS Calculator

The PEARL stands for Prediction Enhanced by ARtificial Intelligence and output Linearization, and DGS is named after the formula developers: Debellemanière, Gatinel, and Saad. This formula

is based on artificial intelligence and optics (www.iolsolver.com). It uses several machine learning models that are selected according to the inputs entered by the surgeon and can adjust its prediction using the postoperative data of the contralateral eye if it is available.

Refractive Accuracy of IOL Formulas in Long Eyes

Table 63.1 shows the refractive accuracy of IOL power prediction in long eyes using different formulas reported in the literature over the past 10 years.

IOL Power Prediction Accuracy

Axial length adjustment methods ((Wang-Koch Adjustment): With the AL adjustment method, 64–82.4% of eyes have accuracy of refractive prediction errors ±0.5 D using Holladay 1 formula, 60–76.22% using SRK/T formula, and 71–84.21% using Holladay 2 formula. In an independent dataset of 1664 eyes with $AL \geq 25$ mm used for the Hill-RBF formula development from Dr. Warren Hill, 93% of eyes had prediction errors of ±0.5 D using the modified AL adjustment Holladay 1 formula (unpublished data).

Super formula: With the Super formula, 55.3–83.33% of eyes have accuracy of refractive prediction errors ±0.5 D.

Barrett Universal II formula: The BUII formula is refined/optimized constantly. There are many studies that evaluated the accuracy of the BUII formula in long eyes, and 57.14–89.5% of eyes have accuracy of refractive prediction errors ±0.5 D.

Hill-RBF formula: The Hill-RBF 3.0 version was just released recently, and no study has yet reported its outcomes in long eyes. Several studies evaluated its accuracy in long eyes using the Hill-RBF 2.0 version, and 51.79–94.74% % of eyes had accuracy of refractive prediction errors ±0.5 D.

Table 63.1 Percentage of eyes with refractive prediction errors (RPE) within ±0.50 D, percentage of eyes with hyperopic RPE, refractive mean absolute error (MAE), and median absolute error (MedAE) in long eyes using various formulas reported in studies over the past 10 years

Studies with various formulas	No. of eyes	AL (mm)	RPE ± 0.50 D (%)	Hyperopic RPE (%)	MAE (D)	MedAE (D)
Axial length adjustment methods						
Original AL adjustment Holladay 1						
Cheng et al. [21]	370	≥26	NA	27.8, 52.4	0.39, 0.34	0.32, 0.27
Zhang et al. [26]	164	≥26	74.39	NA	0.35	0.27
Zhang et al. [22]	108	>26	74.07	NA	0.40	0.34
Liu et al. [19]	136	≥26	72	15	0.37	0.34
Popovic et al. [23]	262	>25	62–82.4	NA	0.35–0.56	0.24–0.40
Hill et al. [20]	51	>28	82.4, 81.6	49.0, 47.4	NA	NA
Cooke et al. [24]	54	>25	75.9, 72.2	NA	0.348, 0.335	0.291, 0.278
Abulafia et al. [25]	106	≥26	69.7, 80.0	NA	0.36, 0.32	0.33, 0.29
Modified AL adjustment Holladay 1						
Cheng et al. [21]	370	>26	NA	45.7, 50.5	0.35, 0.34	0.27, 0.28
Liu et al. [19]	136	≥26	64	33	0.39	0.38
Zhang et al. [22]	108	≥26	75.51	NA	0.36	0.34
Original AL adjustment SRK/T						
Cheng et al. [21]	370	>26	NA	25.9, 52.7	0.46, 0.39	0.34, 0.32
Zhang et al. [26]	164	≥26	76.22	NA	0.38	0.29
Liu et al. [19]	136	≥26	63	18	0.46	0.40
Zhang et al. [22]	108	≥26	67.59	NA	0.45	0.37
Abulafia et al. [25]	106	>26	65.8, 66.7	NA	0.41, 0.39	0.39, 0.34
Modified AL adjustment SRK/T						
Cheng et al. [21]	370	>26	NA	39.7, 51.9	0.41, 0.39	0.33, 0.32
Zhang et al. [26]	164	≥26	69.51	NA	0.42	0.36
Liu et al. [19]	136	≥26	60	28	0.47	0.43
Zhang et al. [22]	108	≥26	69.41	NA	0.41	0.33
AL adjustment Holladay 2						
Savini et al. [27]	19	>26	84.21	NA	0.296	0.265
Darcy et al. [28]	637	≥26	71.0	NA	0.352	NA
Super formula						
Gonzalez et al. [29]	115	>25	83.33	NA	0.29	0.22
Kane et al. [30]	47	≥26	55.3	NA	0.503	0.435
Cooke et al. [24]	54	≥26	75.9, 72.2	NA	0.348, 0.335	0.291, 0.278

Table 63.1 (continued)

Studies with various formulas	No. of eyes	AL (mm)	RPE ± 0.50 D (%)	Hyperopic RPE (%)	MAE (D)	MedAE (D)
Barrett universal II formula						
Cheng et al. [21]	370	≥26	NA	63.8, 47.6	0.39, 0.37	0.33, 0.31
Ji et al. [31]	56	>26	57.14	NA	0.53	0.46
Savini et al. [27]	19	>26	84.21	NA	0.253	0.22, 0.25
Gonzalez et al. [29]	115	≥25	88.60	NA	0.26	0.24
Omoto et al. [32]	44,87	≥26	84.1, 83.9	NA	0.22, 0.25	NA
Zhang et al. [26]	164	≥26	73.17	NA	0.38	0.28
Tang et al. [33]	125	>25	62.9	NA	0.507	0.355
Fernandes et al. [34]	51	≥26	NA	NA	0.319	NA
Darcy et al. [28]	637	≥26	70.7	NA	0.338	NA
Liu et al. [19]	136	≥26	78	36	0.32	0.27
Zhang et al. [22]	108	>26	71.56	NA	0.42	0.33
Zhou et al. [35]	43, 23	≥27	NA	NA	0.29, 0.55	NA
Wan et al. [36]	127	≥26	86.61	NA	NA	0.21
Rong et al. [37]	108	>26	70	NA	0.36–0.45	0.34–0.40
Wang et al. [10]	310	≥26	75, 82	NA	0.37, 0.32	0.31, 0.26
Roberts et al. [38]	90	>24.5	NA	NA	0.507	NA
Connell et al. [39]	44	≥26	NA	NA	0.331	NA
Kane et al. [30]	47	≥26	76.6	NA	0.375	0.325
Hill et al. [20]	51	>25	73.9, 79.4	76.1, 73.5	NA	NA
Kane et al. [40]	77	≥26	62.7	NA	0.435	0.37
Cooke et al. [24]	54	≥26	75.9, 83.3	NA	0.303, 0.274	0.255, 0.218
Abulafia et al. [25]	106	>26	89.5, 83.3	NA	0.28, 0.30	0.26, 0.21
Hill-RBF calculator 2.0						
Cheng et al. [21]	370	≥26	NA	72.4, 49.5	0.46, 0.38	0.38, 0.30
Ji et al. [31]	56	>26	51.79	NA	0.58	0.47
Gonzalez et al. [29]	115	≥25	81.58	NA	0.29	0.22
Tang et al. [33]	125	>25	62.5	NA	0.474	0.335
Savini et al. [27]	19	>26	94.74	NA	0.244	0.230
Darcy et al. [28]	637	≥26	71.2	NA	0.352	NA
Liu et al. [19]	136	≥26	76	54	0.37	0.33
Wan et al. [36]	127	≥26	86.61	NA	NA	0.20
Roberts et al. [38]	90	>24.5	NA	NA	0.32	NA
Connell et al. [39]	44	≥26	NA	NA	0.358	NA
Kane et al. [30]	47	≥26	66.0	NA	0.373	0.310
Hill et al. [20]	51	>25	76.7, 78.8	74.4, 69.7	NA	NA
Olsen formula						
Savini et al. [27]	19	>26	84.21, 89.47	NA	0.338, 0.256	0.205, 0.209
Gonzalez et al. [29]	115	≥25	85.96	NA	0.27	0.22
Darcy et al. [28]	637	≥26	70.6	NA	0.352	NA
Rong et al. [37]	108	>26	65	NA	0.34–0.53	0.32–0.43
Wang et al. [10]	310	≥26	77, 273	NA	0.36, 0.35	0.28, 0.31
Connell et al. [39]	44	≥26	NA	NA	0.352	NA
Cooke et al. [24]	54	≥26	83.3, 85.2	NA	0.290, 0.249	0.198, 0.218
Abulafia et al. [25]	106	>26	88.6, 57.1	NA	0.26, 0.49	0.21, 0.37
Kane formula						
Cheng et al. [21]	370	≥26	NA	54.1, 50.3	0.34, 0.34	0.27, 0.26
Savini et al. [27]	19	>26	94.74	NA	0.220	0.200
Gonzalez et al. [26]	115	≥25	86.84	NA	0.27	0.22
Fenandes et al. [34]	51	≥26	NA	NA	0.301	NA
Darcy et al. [28]	637	≥26	72.0	NA	0.329	NA
Connell et al. [39]	44	≥26	NA	NA	0.326	NA

(continued)

Table 63.1 (continued)

Studies with various formulas	No. of eyes	AL (mm)	RPE ± 0.50 D (%)	Hyperopic RPE (%)	MAE (D)	MedAE (D)
EVO formula						
Cheng et al. [21]	370	≥26	NA	56.5, 49.7	0.41, 0.40	0.32, 0.31
Savini et al. [27]	19	>26	89.47	NA	0.211	0.168
Gonzalez et al. [29]	115	≥25	85.96	NA	0.28	0.24
Zhang et al. [26]	164	≥26	79.27	NA	0.35	0.27
Fernandes et al. [34]	51	≥26	NA	NA	0.308	NA
Panacea IOL calculator						
Savini et al. [27]	19	>26	63.16	NA	0.415	0.345

D diopter; *AL* axial length; *NA* not available

Olsen formula: Several studies evaluated the accuracy of Olsen formula in long eyes, and 65–89.47% of eyes had refractive prediction errors ±0.5 D.

Kane formula: A few studies evaluated the accuracy of Kane formula in long eyes, and 72–94.74% of eyes had refractive prediction errors ±0.5 D.

EVO formula: A few studies evaluated the accuracy of EVO formula in long eyes, and 79.27–89.47% of eyes had refractive prediction errors ±0.5 D.

Panacea IOL Calculator: One study evaluated the accuracy of Panacea IOL calculator in long eyes, and 63.16% of eyes had refractive prediction errors ±0.5 D.

Pearl-DGS Calculator: The Pearl-DGS calculator was introduced recently and there is no report of its accuracy in long eyes yet.

Comparison of Refractive Accuracy Among Formulas

The majority of studies reported that the performances of the above formulas were comparable in long eyes [16–18]. In general, studies have reported that the BUII, Kane, Hill-RBF, and Olsen formulas produced the best results or the lowest prediction errors, with no significant differences among those formulas.

The incidence of hyperopic outcomes (hyperopic relative to the predicted refraction) with the AL adjustment formulas was significantly lower than the BUII and Hill-RBF 2.0 (15–33% vs. 36–54%) [19]. Hill and colleagues [20] reported

that the AL adjusted Holladay 1 produced less eyes with hyperopic outcomes (47.4–49%) than did the BUII and Hill-RBF 1.0 formulas (69.7–76.1%). Using the ULIB lens constants, Cheng et al. [21] found that the original AL adjustment Holladay 1 and SRK/T formulas produced significantly lower percentages of eyes (25.9–27.8%) with hyperopic outcomes than did the Kane, Hill-EBF 2.0, EVO, and BUII formulas (54.1–72.4%).

Conclusion

Due to the low IOL powers required in long eyes, accuracy of ELP estimation is not as important as in normal and short eyes. By adjusting the AL values used in Holladay 1, Holladay 2, and SRK/T formulas, excellent outcomes can be achieved. The refractive accuracy can be improved in long eyes with segmented ALs using specific refractive indices for each ocular medium. For IOL power calculation, based on the findings in the literature, any of the following formulas is a reasonable choice in long eyes: modified AL adjustment Holladay 1, BUII, Hill-RBF, Olsen, Kane, and EVO formulas.

References

1. Norrby S. Sources of error in intraocular lens power calculation. J Cataract Refract Surg. 2008;34(3):368–76.
2. Kora Y, Koike M, Suzuki Y, Inatomi M, Fukado Y, Ozawa T. Errors in IOL power calculations for axial high myopia. Ophthalmic Surg. 1991;22(2):78–81.

3. Zaldivar R, Shultz MC, Davidorf JM, et al. Intraocular lens power calculations in patients with extreme myopia. J Cataract Refract Surg. 2000;26(5):668–74.

4. MacLaren RE, Sagoo MS, Restori M, Allan BD. Biometry accuracy using zero- and negative-powered intraocular lenses. J Cataract Refract Surg. 2005;31(2):280–90.

5. Haigis W, Lege B, Miller N, Schneider B. Comparison of immersion ultrasound biometry and partial coherence interferometry for intraocular lens calculation according to Haigis. Graefes Arch Clin Exp Ophthalmol. 2000;238(9):765–73.

6. Wang L, Cao D, Weikert MP, Koch DD. Calculation of axial length using a single group refractive index versus using different refractive indices for each ocular segment: theoretical study and refractive outcomes. Ophthalmology. 2019;126(5):663–70.

7. Cooke DL, Cooke TL. A comparison of two methods to calculate axial length. J Cataract Refract Surg. 2019;45(3):284–92.

8. Petermeier K, Gekeler F, Messias A, Spitzer MS, Haigis W, Szurman P. Intraocular lens power calculation and optimized constants for highly myopic eyes. J Cataract Refract Surg. 2009;35(9):1575–81.

9. Wang L, Shirayama M, Ma XJ, Kohnen T, Koch DD. Optimizing intraocular lens power calculations in eyes with axial lengths above 25.0 mm. J Cataract Refract Surg. 2011;37(11):2018–27.

10. Wang L, Koch DD. Modified axial length adjustment formulas in long eyes. J Cataract Refract Surg. 2018;44(11):1396–7.

11. Wang L, Holladay JT, Koch DD. Wang-Koch axial length adjustment for the Holladay 2 formula in long eyes. J Cataract Refract Surg. 2018;44(10):1291–2.

12. Ladas JG, Siddiqui AA, Devgan U, Jun AS. A 3-D "super surface" combining modern intraocular lens formulas to generate a "super formula" and maximize accuracy. JAMA Ophthalmol. 2015;133(12):1431–6.

13. Barrett GD. Intraocular lens calculation formulas for new intraocular lens implants. J Cataract Refract Surg. 1987;13:389–96.

14. Hill WE. IOL power selection: think different. In: 11th annual Charles D. Kelman Lecture AAO, Las Vegas, Nevada; 2015.

15. Olsen T, Hoffmann P. C constant: new concept for ray tracing-assisted intraocular lens power calculation. J Cataract Refract Surg. 2014;40(5):764–73.

16. Melles RB, Holladay JT, Chang WJ. Accuracy of intraocular lens calculation formulas. Ophthalmology. 2018;125:169–78.

17. Melles RB, Kane JX, Olsen T, Chang WJ. Update on intraocular lens calculation formulas. Ophthalmology. 2019;126(9):1335.

18. Kane JX, Chang DF. Intraocular lens power formulas, biometry, and intraoperative aberrometry: a review. Ophthalmology. 2020;128(11):e94–e114.

19. Liu J, Wang L, Chai F, Han Y, Qian S, Koch DD, Weikert MP. Comparison of intraocular lens power calculation formulas in Chinese eyes with axial myopia. J Cataract Refract Surg. 2019;45(6):725–31.

20. Hill DC, Sudhakar S, Hill CS, King TS, Scott IU, Ernst BB, Pantanelli SM. Intraoperative aberrometry versus preoperative biometry for intraocular lens power selection in axial myopia. J Cataract Refract Surg. 2017;43(4):505–10.

21. Cheng H, Wang L, Kane JX, Li J, Liu L, Wu M. Accuracy of artificial intelligence formulas and axial length adjustments for highly myopic eyes. Am J Ophthalmol. 2020;223:100–7.

22. Zhang JQ, Zou XY, Zheng DY, Chen WR, Sun A, Luo LX. Effect of lens constants optimization on the accuracy of intraocular lens power calculation formulas for highly myopic eyes. Int J Ophthalmol. 2019;12(6):943–8.

23. Popovic M, Schlenker MB, Campos-Möller X, Pereira A, Ahmed IIK. Wang-Koch formula for optimization of intraocular lens power calculation: evaluation at a Canadian center. J Cataract Refract Surg. 2018;44(1):17–22.

24. Cooke DL, Cooke TL. Comparison of 9 intraocular lens power calculation formulas. J Cataract Refract Surg. 2016;42(8):1157–64.

25. Abulafia A, Barrett GD, Rotenberg M, Kleinmann G, Levy A, Reitblat O, Koch DD, Wang L, Assia EI. Intraocular lens power calculation for eyes with an axial length greater than 26.0 mm: comparison of formulas and methods. Cataract Refract Surg. 2015;41(3):548–56.

26. Zhang J, Tan X, Wang W, Yang G, Xu J, Ruan X, Gu X, Luo L. Effect of axial length adjustment methods on intraocular lens power calculation in highly myopic eyes. Am J Ophthalmol. 2020;214:110–8.

27. Savini G, Hoffer KJ, Balducci N, Barboni P, Schiano-Lomoriello D. Comparison of formula accuracy for intraocular lens power calculation based on measurements by a swept-source optical coherence tomography optical biometer. J Cataract Refract Surg. 2020;46(1):27–33.

28. Darcy K, Gunn D, Tavassoli S, Sparrow J, Kane JX. Assessment of the accuracy of new and updated intraocular lens power calculation formulas in 10930 eyes from the UK National Health Service. J Cataract Refract Surg. 2020;46(1):2–7.

29. Carmona-González D, Castillo-Gómez A, Palomino-Bautista C, Romero-Domínguez M, Gutiérrez-Moreno MÁ. Comparison of the accuracy of 11 intraocular lens power calculation formulas. Eur J Ophthalmol. 2020;31(5):2370–6.

30. Kane JX, Van Heerden A, Atik A, Petsoglou C. Accuracy of 3 new methods for intraocular lens power selection. J Cataract Refract Surg. 2017;43(3):333–9.

31. Ji J, Liu Y, Zhang J, Wu X, Shao W, Ma B, Luo M. Comparison of six methods for the intraocular lens power calculation in high myopic eyes. Eur J Ophthalmol. 2021;31(1):96–102.

32. Omoto MK, Torii H, Hayashi K, Ayaki M, Tsubota K, Negishi K. Ratio of axial length to corneal radius in Japanese patients and accuracy of intraocular lens

power calculation based on biometric data. Am J Ophthalmol. 2020;218:320–9.

33. Tang KS, Tran EM, Chen AJ, Rivera DR, Rivera JJ, Greenberg PB. Accuracy of biometric formulae for intraocular lens power calculation in a teaching hospital. Int J Ophthalmol. 2020;13(1):61–5.

34. Hipólito-Fernandes D, Elisa Luís M, Gil P, Maduro V, Feijão J, Yeo TK, Voytsekhivskyy O, Alves N. VRF-G, a new intraocular lens power calculation formula: a 13-formulas comparison study. Clin Ophthalmol. 2020;14:4395–402.

35. Zhou D, Sun Z, Deng G. Accuracy of the refractive prediction determined by intraocular lens power calculation formulas in high myopia. Indian J Ophthalmol. 2019;67(4):484–9.

36. Wan KH, Lam TCH, Yu MCY, Chan TCY. Accuracy and precision of intraocular lens calculations using the New Hill-RBF version 2.0 in eyes with high axial myopia. Am J Ophthalmol. 2019;205:66–73.

37. Rong X, He W, Zhu Q, Qian D, Lu Y, Zhu X. Intraocular lens power calculation in eyes with extreme myopia: comparison of Barrett universal II, Haigis, and Olsen formulas. J Cataract Refract Surg. 2019;45(6):732–7.

38. Roberts TV, Hodge C, Sutton G, Lawless M, contributors to the Vision Eye Institute IOL outcomes registry. Comparison of Hill-radial basis function, Barrett universal and current third generation formulas for the calculation of intraocular lens power during cataract surgery. Clin Exp Ophthalmol. 2018;46(3):240–6.

39. Connell BJ, Kane JX. Comparison of the Kane formula with existing formulas for intraocular lens power selection. BMJ Open Ophthalmol. 2019;4(1):e000251.

40. Kane JX, Van Heerden A, Atik A, Petsoglou C. Intraocular lens power formula accuracy: comparison of 7 formulas. J Cataract Refract Surg. 2016;42(10):1490–500.

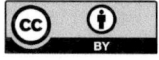

IOL Power Calculation in the Short Eye

64

David Flikier

Introduction

Cataract extraction surgery with the intraocular lens implant in a short or small eye is one of the most complex interventions for the anterior segment surgeon, [1, 2] and its biometrical difficulty is inversely proportional to the axial length [3].

With the improvement of surgical techniques, instruments, equipment, design, and intraocular lens material, both outcome optimization and patients' expectations have increased for these difficult cases. The success of the final visual outcome, obtained with emmetropia, is still one of the critical issues to resolve. The great variability of dimensions of the internal ocular structures and the difficulty in the estimation of the effective lens position are the culprits for the errors in the calculation formulas, even for the latest generation ones.

Definition

What constitutes a short eye? The diagnostic parameters include: **the axial length, the corneal diameter, and the anterior chamber depth.** The existence of different eye patterns, which include variable corneal diameters and

D. Flikier (✉)
Instituto de Cirugía Ocular, San José, Costa Rica

normal or narrow anterior chambers, can aid us in classifying a short eye and to anticipate modifications in their pre, trans, and postoperatory management, in order to avoid complications.

The median axial length oscillates between 22.76–23.55 mm ± 1.17–1.49 mm [4–9], which is why a standard deviation below that threshold would get closer to 22.0 D and two standard deviations, would remain within the 20.5 D range. These values have generally been used as starting points in order to describe short eye classifications. In Melles et al.'s [10] work, they studied 27,191 eyes and considered small eyes whose axial length was shorter than 22.5 mm, where they included the lowest 10% of the population under study.

Short Eye Classification

The axial hyperopic eye is a short eye, which has a length shorter than 22.0 mm and up to 20.5 mm, placing it outside of the first standard deviation, but within the second one; they are considered normal short eyes, due to their anatomical characteristics and difficulties in their calculation of the intraocular eye. (see Fig. 64.1.)

The clinical spectrum of the short eye varies in a phenotypical range, according to the relative sizes for the anterior and posterior segments, and it is classified in [2, 12–16] (see Fig. 64.2):

© The Author(s) 2024
J. Aramberri et al. (eds.), *Intraocular Lens Calculations*, Essentials in Ophthalmology,
https://doi.org/10.1007/978-3-031-50666-6_64

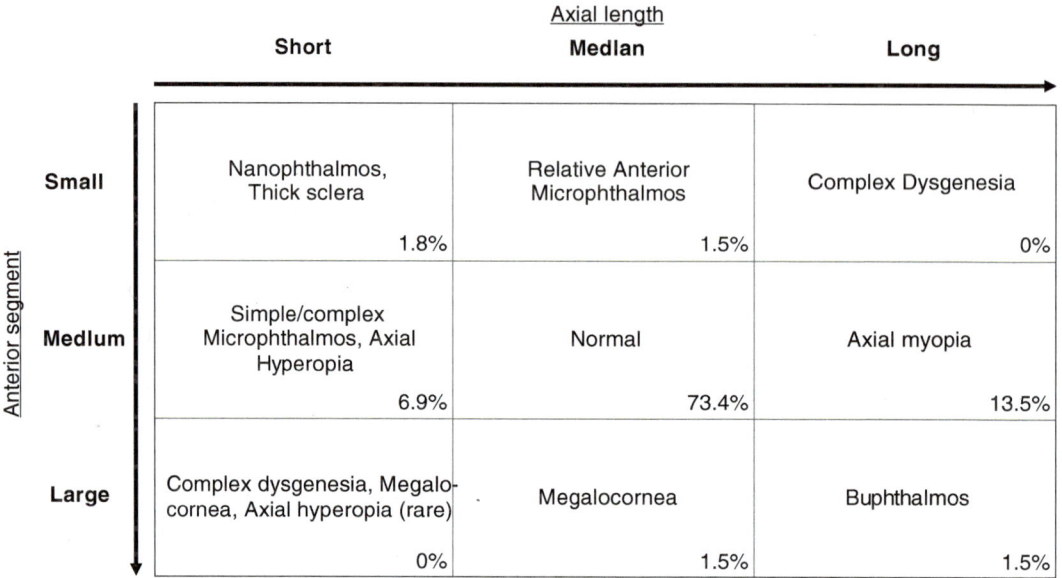

	Axial length		
Anterior segment	**Short**	**Median**	**Long**
Small	Nanophthalmos, Thick sclera 1.8%	Relative Anterior Microphthalmos 1.5%	Complex Dysgenesia 0%
Medium	Simple/complex Microphthalmos, Axial Hyperopia 6.9%	Normal 73.4%	Axial myopia 13.5%
Large	Complex dysgenesia, Megalocornea, Axial hyperopia (rare) 0%	Megalocornea 1.5%	Buphthalmos 1.5%

Fig. 64.1 Eye classification according to anatomical characteristics, axial length vs. size of the anterior segment. (Modified from Holladay's diagram [11])

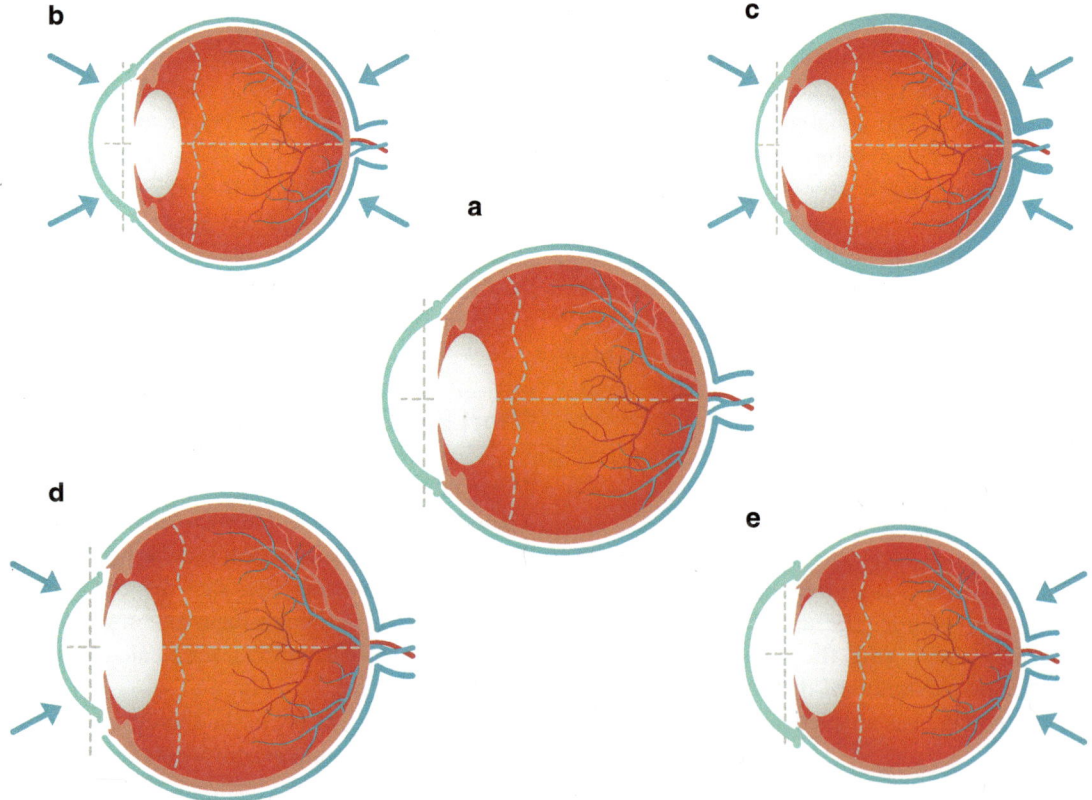

Fig. 64.2 Representation of short eye variants, comparing the axial length, anterior chamber depth, corneal diameter, crystalline lens thickness, and scleral thickness. (**a**) Eye with normal parameters, (**b**) Microphthalmos, with axial length reduction, (**c**) Nanophthalmos, with axial length reduction, anterior segment, crystalline lens thickness, and an increase in scleral thickness, (**d**) relative anterior Microphthalmos, with its reduced anterior segment, (**e**) Posterior Microphthalmos with axial length reduction, by a reduction of the posterior pole

(a) Simple Microphthalmos.

(b) Complex Microphthalmos.

(c) Nanophthalmos.

(d) Relative anterior Microphthalmos.

(e) Posterior Microphthalmos.

Microphthalmos corresponds to an eye with short axial length and is classified into two types: *Simple* and *Complex*, based on the presence of ocular anatomical malformations.

1. **Simple Microphthalmos:** is an eye with short axial length, without ocular malformations. As short, we mean two standard deviations (2 SD) shorter than normal for the age group. Historically, it has been reported as shorter than 20.5 mm in adults and shorter than 17.8 mm in children up to one year of age. Other epidemiological studies have defined this value at 21.0 mm for the adult [17], present in 0.046–0.11% of ophthalmological patients. These eyes are hyperopic, but they have a normal anterior chamber and normal scleral thickness. They are not at risk for angle-closure glaucoma.

2. Complex **Microphthalmos:** It is an eye with small axial length and anatomical malformations. As in the simple microphthalmos, the axial length is more than two standard deviations shorter than its age group. Besides, they can present with marked ocular anatomical malformations, such as coloboma of the iris, chorioretinal coloboma, persistent fetal vasculature, and retinal dysplasia. They also have normal scleral thickness.

3. **Nanophthalmos:** It is a condition where there is also a short eye, with a small anterior segment, and a thick choroid and sclerotic [2]. There is no consensus for the axial length, which defines the nanophthalmos, but there are reports that range from less than 20.5 mm [18], 20.0 mm [19], 18.0 mm [16], and 17.0 mm [20], though accepting those at 20.0 and 20.5 mm as the most recent ones [1, 3, 21–24]. These eyes are constituted by:

   (a) **Anterior chambers** that keep narrowing, as the crystalline grows with age.

   (b) **Convex iris** with propension towards painless angle-closure chronic glaucoma.

   (c) **Scleral and choroid thickness increase**, larger than 1.7 mm [18, 25] predisposing to uveal effusion.

   Also, in 2016, Guo et al. [25] described the characteristic features of ciliary body ultrasonic biomicroscopy, iris, and the eye angle with Nanophthalmos, both for chronic primary angle-closure glaucoma and for chronic secondary angle-closure glaucoma. The typical feature for Nanophthalmos is a small eye, with a narrow anterior chamber, and where the growth of the crystalline lens is the cause for the development of chronic secondary angle-closure glaucoma, with symptoms comparable to primary angle-closure.

   They may have associated microcorneas with shorter diameters than 11 mm [26]. The microcornea is a distortion that can be observed in any of the short eyes: *simple microphthalmos, complex microphthalmos, nanophthalmos, and anterior relative microphthalmos.*

4. **Relative anterior Microphthalmos**: name coined by Naumann [27], it is an eye with a normal axial length, but with a small anterior segment, with an axial length longer than 20.5 mm, but with an ACD equal or lesser than 2.2 mm and a corneal diameter shorter than 11 mm [12, 28]. They have no other ocular anatomical malformations, nor any associated increase in scleral growth. It is sub-diagnosed before cataract surgery due to its normal axial length. However, it is crucial to differentiate, due to the high incidence of angle-closure glaucoma, cornea guttata, and pseudoexfoliation association.

5. **Posterior Microphthalmos:** It is an extremely rare condition, typically recessive, with an anterior segment at normal dimensions, but with a posterior shortening, from a reduction of the growth of the posterior segment that results in high hyperopia [29–31]. Due to the scleral thickening, the choroidal and pigment epithelial growth is limited, but with normal neuroretinal development, inducing the development of papillomacular folds [32] including the retina without pigment epithelium or choroidal tissue. They may be

associated to several pathologies such as: esotropia, peripheral avascular zones without vascular crest formation, uveal effusion syndrome [28], pigment retinopathy, retinoschisis, and retinal dialysis [14, 33–36].

Kaderli et al. [37] reported in 2018, in a normal and short eye study, using an EDI-OCT test, that the thickness of the choroids and the diameter of large-sized choroid vessels in the posterior pole increases are inversely proportional to the axial length, regardless of sex or patient's gender.

It is important to understand that this complex of anatomical characteristics for nanophthalmos and posterior microphthalmos is associated with a symmetrical reduction of the axial length and high hyperopia, such as a variable phenotypical spectrum, but could also be the expression of the same genetic mutation, usually variable biallelic in MFRP [38] and PRSS56 [39, 40] and rare monoallelic in TMEM98 [41, 42] and MYRF. Variable expressions of the gene can be found in a same family, with nanophthalmos in some members and microphthalmos of different magnitude in others. In the case of PRSS56, the production of a soluble protease stimulating the axial length was found, through a function gain mechanism, also implicated in the development of myopia [43]. In a near future, we could think about treatments through protease inhibitors or monoclonal antibodies.

The genetic origin of these entities is polygenic; and the axial length is raised as associated to the degree of involvement by deep intronic or regulatory variants in the four known genes [43, 44].

Characteristic Features of Short Eyes

Achieving a precise refractive outcome in the short eye is a real challenge, and often enough, simple axial length, keratometry, and ACD parameters become insufficient.

The best calculation formulas are those that can predict the *effective lens position (ELPo)* in

a more exact manner, but even so, the standard deviation is high.

The three main variables in the calculation of the intraocular lens are:

1. **The power of the cornea.**
2. **The axial length.**
3. **The effective lens position**.

In any eye, the main challenge will always be the estimation of the final lens position, based on preoperatory measurements. In the large eye with high myopia and a low power intraocular lens, the ELPo is **not** critical; a small anteroposterior movement would produce a very small refractive deviation. In contrast, the short eye, with the combination of certain variables such as narrow chambers, thick crystalline, steep corneas, and higher powers, produces the ideal mix to derail the prediction algorithms for the effective lens position, severely affecting the final refraction.

Third-generation formulas use only two variables for ELPo prediction: *Keratometry and axial length*. They assume that the greater corneal curvatures have a deeper chamber, but in reality, in short eyes, the anterior chambers tend to be narrow, and therefore the outcome estimates a lens position more posterior than the desired one.

With the formulas that use ACD (anterior chamber depth) to calculate the effective lens position, such as the Haigis formula, the opposite happens, by neglecting to take the thickness of the crystalline lens into account. In the short eye, chambers are narrow and therefore Haigis formula estimates a very anterior position, but since the thickness of the crystalline is large, the position ends up being a little more posterior.

Due to the introduction of new variables, in *fourth-generation formulas such as*: **Corneal Diameter: CD, Lens thickness: LT, and the Anterior Chamber Depth: ACD** associated to the keratometry and axial length, the estimation of the effective lens has improved, and therefore the calculation power for the lens.

As it was previously mentioned, according to the classification of the short eye, each type of eye will have its own specific characteristics, but as a general rule, and as an average data (taken from the Kane et al. study [45]), we find:

1. A reduction of the axial length.
2. A relative increase in the percentage of the ratio between the anterior and posterior segments, due to an **increase in the thickness of the crystalline lens**; in average 4.7 mm and ±0.42 mm SD.
3. Narrow anterior chambers, with a median 2.61 mm and ±0.39 mm SD.
4. Steep keratometries, with a median 43.81 D ±1.76.
5. Some smaller corneas.

In the year 2008, Erdol et al. [34] reported a couple of cases of posterior microphthalmos with an apparent normal anterior segment, where ultrasonic biomicroscopy was performed, demonstrating a thickened and anteriorized ciliary body [34]. These data increase the possibility that the equator of the crystalline lens is not in normal relationship with the other measurements (Axial length, Keratometry, ACD, LT, CD, age, etc.) usually considered in order to estimate the position of the intraocular lens. Therefore, the theory is introduced; when dealing with short eyes, the placement of the equator of the crystalline lens, the position of the ciliary body and sulcus, could be of greater value to improve the estimation for the effective positioning of the intraocular lens.

In the year 2016, Goto et al. [46] conducted a study in search for other variables in order to improve the estimation of the postoperative ACD. They found that the depth of the angle to angle, measured with AS OCT from the angular recess, and introduced as a regression coefficient in a prediction formula for the ELPo for the postoperative ACD, along with the preoperatory ACD and the axial length, using Haigis and SRK/T formulas, increased predictions for the IOL power in a significant manner and reduced the residual postoperatory defect (98.7% ± 0.50 D). As interesting data, the study demonstrated that the anterior segment in the nanophthalmos is

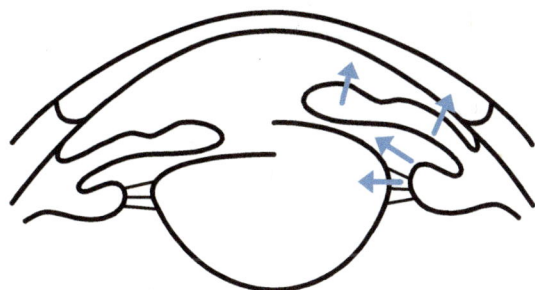

Fig. 64.3 Representation of the normal eye vs. variants of short eyes, reduction of the ciliary ring (diameter of the ciliary body, CBD), the anterior rotation of the ciliary processes against the equator of the crystalline lens, and the vault of the crystalline lens (in a more anterior position)

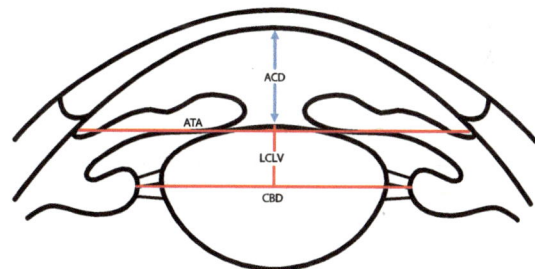

Fig. 64.4 Representation for short eyes, reduction of the ciliary body (Ciliary Body Diameter, CBD), anterior chamber (ACD), lens-ciliary body-lenticular vault (LCLV), angle to angle distance (ATA)

more crowded, *due to the reduction of the ciliary ring (ciliary body diameter, CBD), the anterior rotation of the ciliary processes against the equator of the crystalline, and the vault of the crystalline (in a more anterior position);* all of them risk factors for developing malignant glaucoma.

For the topic at hand in this chapter, the proposal rests on the fact where the crystalline lens anteriorization, the modification of the position of the equator, and the ciliary body, with regard to the anatomic positions used as baselines to calculate the ELPo, are the origin of the calculation error for the IOL power. Therefore, these three variables: the position of the ciliary body, the position of the equator, and the vault of the crystalline lens, must be considered in order to help define the effective lens' position (see Figs. 64.3, 64.4, and 64.5).

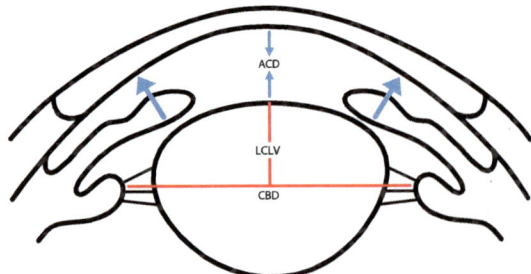

Fig. 64.5 Representation of short eyes, reduction of the ciliary ring (Ciliary Body Diameter, CBD), crystalline lens with greater thickness, with reduction of the anterior chamber (ACD), lens-ciliary body-lenticular vault (LCLV)

Biometry in the Short Eye

A small error on the axial length, ACD, and crystalline lens thickness measurements will result in a greater refractive error in the patient with short eye. This is why we require equipment to measure the axial length and the different intraocular structures in a very precise manner.

From the beginnings of optical biometry by partial coherence interferometry (PCI), its manufacturers decided to use a group refractive index and a calibration function to calculate the geometrical axial length from the measured optical path length (OPL) in spite of the differences in the refraction indexes for each of the structures in the eye and the travel speed difference when crossing them [47–50]. Using this calibration, the axial length measurements are accurate only for average eyes. The problem arises in extreme eyes, and especially in the case of short eyes, where proportionally, the crystalline lens occupies a greater percentage of the anterior segment and the eye.

Wang et al. [50] reported higher axial length measurements in short eyes, when segmentation with correction for refractive indexes for each segment was done. This difference with the real axial length, measured with the sum of the segments, versus the measurements by the biometers, explains in part the myopization observed with the calculation of the majority of the third-generation short eye formulas [47, 50].

Cooke et al. [47] described the method to modify the axial length, with a regression formula (Cooke-modified AL), in the Hoffer Q, SRK/T and Holladay 1 and 2 formulas, noticeably improving the results, both for long eyes and for short eyes. The separation of the segments can be achieved through automatic detection with the Spike Finder developed by David Cooke. Being able to measure each structure with its real refractive index and obtaining the precise measurements leads to better results with the IOL power calculation, specifically in short eyes with the Holladay 1 and 2, Hoffer Q, and SRK/T; with the Haigis formula only if the constants were optimized. The results did not improve or were worse with Barrett and Olsen formulas; and with OKULIX, only improved in the study of short eyes [47–50].

Since the internal limiting membrane is hardly identified by the optic biometers, detecting the interface between the retina and the pigment epithelium, the length of the optic trajectory of the vitreous really becomes the vitreous and retinal one. In order to determine the length of the vitreous, the retina is given a theoretical thickness, which will then be subtracted from the vitreous-retinal thickness in the segmentation or sum of segments [49]. This retinal theoretic value has been generally calculated according to the axial length, accepting that long eyes have a thinner thickness and short eyes a thicker one. With the emergence of OCT, a precise measurement of the foveal thickness will be accomplished to incorporate this real measurement in calculation programs.

Another important consideration in biometric variants is the relative size of the anterior chamber in comparison with the axial length. The calculation for the power of the IOL tends to be more precise in a short eye with a proportionally smaller anterior chamber than with a deep chamber. Holladay et al. [11, 51] discovered that approximately 20% of eyes with short axial length have a small anterior segment and are classified as nanophthalmics and the remaining 80% have a normal anterior segment (see Fig. 64.3). Eyes with a flat ACD tend to require IOLs with +30.0 D or less, whereas those with normal ACDs require IOLs with more than +40.0 D [13], which entails Piggy-back lens systems and wider anterior segments.

The closer to the retina the IOL is, the greater the transcendence will be for a small change on ELPo and in its refractive result. The A constant used in the IOL power calculations depends on multiple factors, including: the type of lens used, the refractive index of the material, the geometry, the variance of the biometric equipment, the surgical technique, and factors affecting ELPo. This is why in a small eye, the A constant must be **personalized.**

Results in Short Eyes

In normal eyes, 90–98% of the cases reach their final refraction between ±1.00 D, whereas in eyes with nanophthalmos, with shorter lengths than 20.5 mm, only 46–66% achieve theirs [3].

Third-generation formulas only use the axial length and the corneal curvature (keratometry). **Fourth-generation** formulas such as Haigis and Holladay 2 and other more modern ones like Barrett Universal II and others include a greater number of parameters [52], mainly the **depth of the anterior chamber ACD** [21, 53], increasing the quality of the results. Eom et al. found that Haigis formula has better results than the Hoffer Q formula, in short eyes with narrow chambers, ACD < 2.4 mm [54].

It should be made clear that in the studies the median axial length for short eyes is very variable and oscillates between 19.53 and 21.69 mm. However, for the very small eye with simple microphthalmos group, there is no comparative statistic study for formulas, rather isolated case reports [22–24].

In the Melles and colleagues study [10] also with short or small eyes, shorter than 22.5 mm (between 21.0 and 22.5 mm), several interesting conclusions were found:

1. Barrett and Olsen's formulas had the best behavior.
2. Hoffer Q tends towards a myopic outcome, by reducing the axial length.

3. Haigis and SRK/T tend towards the hyperopic defect in very flat anterior chambers.
4. Hoffer Q and Holladay 1 tend towards myopia.
5. Olsen and Haigis tend towards hyperopia.

Other more recent studies such as Shivastava and colleagues [55], also in short eyes, but not as small, between 20.76 and 21.96 mm, found no statistically significant differences when comparing the Barrett Universal, the Hill RBF method, Haigis, Hoffer Q, and Holladay 2, with an outcome that coincides with two previous studies by Kane and cols. [56] and by Gokce et al. [57]. It is interesting to highlight that in the study by Shivastava [57], the median absolute error found within the ±0.50 D range oscillates between 46 and 56%, and ±1.00 D between 76 and 80%.

In the year 2018, Wang et al. [58] conducted a meta-analysis with 1161 cases, in order to compare Haigis, Holladay 2, Hoffer Q, SRK/T, and SRK II formulas. In short eyes, a frank superiority was found for the Haigis formula over the other ones. More recently, Melles et al. [59] found better performances in the formulas by Kane, Olsen (with 4 factors), and Barrett, followed by EVO and Hill RBF 2, over Holladay 2, Haigis, Hoffer Q, and SRK/T.

Sudhakar et al. [55] in 2019, in a study of hyperopic eyes (19.77–22.06 mm), compared the intra-operatory aberrometry, the Hill RBF method, and several formulas: Barrett Universal, Holladay, Haigis, and Hoffer Q. Among their conclusions, it is interesting to see that they didn't find the aberrometer to be superior to the studied formulas, in the cases where the difference in the predictions was higher than 0.50 D. Taking the value of the aberrometer as final value, they only estimated it as adequately in half of the cases, and none of the methods obtained a result superior to ±0.50 D in more than 60% of patients.

The most recent report, from Kane and Melles [45], for 270 eyes from 182 patients including smaller eyes, with axial lengths starting at 18.86 mm up to 22.46 mm, intraocular lenses with 30 D or more, found mean absolute errors oscillating between 0.838 and 0.533, with SD ±0.812–0.707 and median absolute errors oscil-

Short axial length sub analysis (≤22.0 mm)

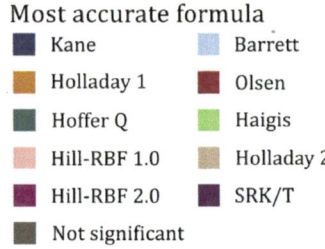

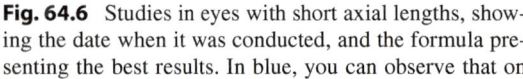

All studies

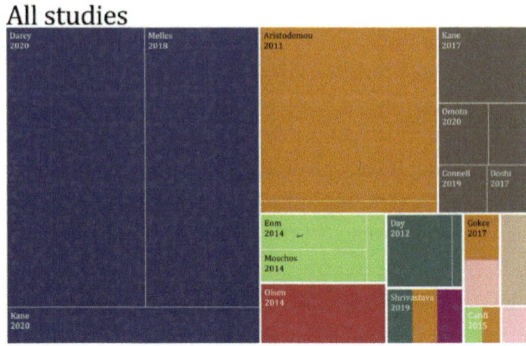

Fig. 64.6 Studies in eyes with short axial lengths, showing the date when it was conducted, and the formula presenting the best results. In blue, you can observe that on the most recent studies, with the greatest number of patients (table sizes), the predominant formula is Kane's [61]

lating between 0.696 and 0.371. Continues with less than 60% of patients having a final refraction between ±0.50 D, with better statistic results in Kane and EVO 2.0 formulas, followed by Haigis, Holladay 2, Olsen, and Hill RBF 2 and finally Barrett y Hoffer Q.

Confirming these latest data, Hipólito-Fernandes et al. [60] conducted a study where they compared 13 formulas in several eye sizes. In the short eye group (20.82–22.0 mm), they found the best results with the VRF-G, EVO 2.0, and Kane formulas.

In the year 2020, Kane along with Chang [61] conducted a very complex review of the literature of the last 10 years and concluded that currently the best results are obtained with Kane's formula, followed by good results with the Olsen formulas (4-factors), Haigis, and Hill-RBF (see Fig. 64.6.).

Poly-pseudophakia: Piggy-Back Lens

The piggy-back lens option was described for the first time by Gayton and Sanders [62] in the year 1990, in a 31-year patient with microphthalmos, requiring an approximate lens with 46 D for both eyes. For the surgery in the first eye, the second lens implanted in the sulcus left a residual hyperopic defect at +8.00 D, requiring its replacement. For the second eye, an empirical calculation allowed for a closer emmetropic result.

This report was the beginning of the correction of high refractive defects with two lenses, where the residual correction for the second lens can be left for a second intervention according to the residual defect, and not to the biometrical characteristics.

Due to the possibility of opacification and inter-lenticular membrane formation as a result of the implantation of two lenses in the capsular bag, it is recommended to place the greater power IOL in the capsular bag and the second IOL in the ciliary sulcus. Ideally, this lens must be low-powered, angulated, with rounded edges in order to reduce the risk for iris touch and UGH syndrome or pigment dispersion. The sulcus lens could be implanted on a second surgical time, after the stability of the second postoperatory graduation, so as to increase the refractive success possibilities, even though the additional risks for a new intervention must be considered.

In order to calculate the power of the Piggy-back lens, there are different options:

(a) Primary poly-pseudophakia, when the implantation of the IOL will be made both in the capsular bag and in the sulcus in the same act. The total calculation for the value of the lens to be placed in the plane of the capsular bag, according to the ELPo, trying to correct the greatest amount of the defect as possible at this level, according to the lenses available by the various commercial companies. The remaining defect will be corrected by the second lens, which will be implanted at the ciliary sulcus level, adjusting the power due to its more anterior position. When a lens is placed more anteriorly, it requires less power in order to have the same effect, and this reduction is proportional to the power of the intraocular lens. The lens at the sulcus must be adjusted, according to the Holladay 1997 table [11] for poly-pseudophakia in hypermetropy, in the following way:

1. From +1.00 to +8.00 does not require adjustment.
2. From +8.50 to +15.00 subtract 0.5 D to the value of the IOL.
3. From +15.5 to +25.5 D subtract 1.0 D to the value of the IOL.
4. From +25.5 D to +30.0 D subtract 1.5 D to the value of the IOL.

(b) The second option is used when the lens will be implanted in another surgical act, once the residual defect is stable. To calculate it, this residual hyperopic defect is multiplied by 1.5, in lower defects smaller than +6.00 D [63].

For other cases, it is advisable to use optical vergence formulas which take the keratometry into account, the ELPo for the sulcus, and the residual defect, used as ACD value, the value of the manufacturer −0.65 in order to adapt it to the sulcus.

The new lenses that have surfaced, specific for placement on the sulcus, and for the correction of residual defects, have specific optic vergency programs in the web pages for their companies [64]. We are attaching some examples. Sulcoflex: https://www.ray-trace.rayner.com/, Add-On: https://www.1stq.de/en/34-addoncalculator, ICL: https://ocos.starag.ch/.

High-Power Intraocular Lenses

The ideal in short eyes is to achieve optical correction with a high-power intraocular lens which will allow for poly-pseudophakia in case of an unexpected high residual defect. These are hard to get and sometimes do require special orders.

Even with the highest standards, and lots of care in the biometry, the biometric results may be affected by the variability in tolerance when manufacturing intraocular lenses [54]. In high power ranges of IOLs (>30.0 D) that are usually required in this high hyperopic eyes, the real dioptric power may vary as much as ±1.0 D, according to the International Organization of Standards [65].

The three problems with high power lenses are:

1. Values for the International Organization for Standardization allowing for a tolerance of ±1.0 D in IOL at >+30.0 D, and ±0.50 in IOL <+30 D [65, 66]
2. Increase in spherical aberration by increasing the power for the IOL [64]. Important in high power lenses free from spherical aberration such as Aspira-aAY
3. The rarity of this cases makes lens manufacturers to lose the appeal for their mass production and therefore there is scarce global availability.

Visual Acuities Obtained

Corrected visual acuities in nanophthalmic eyes tend to be considerably worse in normal eyes, with a range of +0.55 logMAR to +0.41 logMAR [1, 3, 21, 24].

This is in part due to the relative effect of optic minification or reduced image magnification in comparison with distant correction for glasses or contact lenses in such high hyperopic cases and for amblyopia inherent to the refractive defect.

These possible optic results alongside the risks for complications must be discussed with the patients ahead of time in the preoperatory, as well as the limitations in the calculation prediction for the IOL. Even with these risks, the potential for improvement is significant for the quality of life of these nanophthalmos cases, by reducing the preoperatory refractive error and by eliminating dependence in glasses or contact lenses.

Conclusions

The short eye is a phenotypical spectrum for genetic abnormalities, leading to anatomical conditions of the ocular structures, producing not only clinical-pathological consequences, which increase pre, trans, and postoperatory comorbidities in cataract surgery, but they also pose a significant challenge for the physician when calculating the intraocular lens. There is a marked variability for the estimate of the effective lens position, even when using the new calculation formulas, with unprecise and unexpected refractive results in some cases.

According to the latest reports, the recommendation is to use multiple formulas and to compare at least three formulas, such as Kane, Olsen, EVO2, Haigis, and Hill RBF v3.0, especially in eyes with lengths shorter than 21.5 mm. Even so, you must explain to the patients the possibility of getting unexpected results, with >40% outside ±0.50 D, and visual acuities, according to preoperative amblyopia and a possible optic effect from the degree of image reduced magnification, in the case of prior corrections with glasses or contact lenses.

References

1. Lemos JA, Rodrigues P, Resende RA, Menezes C, Goncalves RS, Coelho P. Cataract surgery in patients with nanophthalmos: results and complications. Eur J Ophthalmol. 2016;26(2):103–6.
2. Singh OS, Simmons RJ, Brockhurst RJ, Trempe CL. Nanophthalmos: a perspective on identification and therapy. Ophthalmology. 1982;89(9):1006–12.
3. Jung KI, Yang JW, Lee YC, Kim SY. Cataract surgery in eyes with nanophthalmos and relative anterior microphthalmos. Am J Ophthalmol. 2012;153(6):1161–8.e1.
4. Cao X, Hou X, Bao Y. The ocular biometry of adult cataract patients on lifeline express hospital eye-train in rural China. J Ophthalmol. 2015;2015:171564.
5. Fotedar R, Wang JJ, Burlutsky G, Morgan IG, Rose K, Wong TY, et al. Distribution of axial length and ocular biometry measured using partial coherence laser interferometry (IOL Master) in an older white population. Ophthalmology. 2010;117(3):417–23.
6. Lim LS, Saw SM, Jeganathan VS, Tay WT, Aung T, Tong L, et al. Distribution and determinants of ocular biometric parameters in an Asian population: the Singapore Malay Eye Study. Invest Ophthalmol Vis Sci. 2010;51(1):103–9.
7. Pan CW, Wong TY, Chang L, Lin XY, Lavanya R, Zheng YF, et al. Ocular biometry in an urban Indian population: the Singapore Indian Eye Study (SINDI). Invest Ophthalmol Vis Sci. 2011;52(9):6636–42.
8. Shufelt C, Fraser-Bell S, Ying-Lai M, Torres M, Varma R, Los Angeles Latino Eye Study Group. Refractive error, ocular biometry, and lens opalescence in an adult population: the Los Angeles Latino Eye Study. Invest Ophthalmol Vis Sci. 2005;46(12):4450–60.
9. Warrier S, Wu HM, Newland HS, Muecke J, Selva D, Aung T, et al. Ocular biometry and determinants of refractive error in rural Myanmar: the Meiktila Eye Study. Br J Ophthalmol. 2008;92(12):1591–4.
10. Melles RB, Holladay JT, Chang WJ. Accuracy of intraocular lens calculation formulas. Ophthalmology. 2018;125(2):169–78.
11. Holladay JT. Standardizing constants for ultrasonic biometry, keratometry, and intraocular lens power calculations. J Cataract Refract Surg. 1997;23(9):1356–70.
12. Auffarth GU, Blum M, Faller U, Tetz MR, Volcker HE. Relative anterior microphthalmos: morphometric analysis and its implications for cataract surgery. Ophthalmology. 2000;107(8):1555–60.
13. Hoffman RS, Vasavada AR, Allen QB, Snyder ME, Devgan U, Braga-Mele R, et al. Cataract surgery in the small eye. J Cataract Refract Surg. 2015;41(11):2565–75.
14. Khairallah M, Messaoud R, Zaouali S, Ben Yahia S, Ladjimi A, Jenzri S. Posterior segment changes associated with posterior microphthalmos. Ophthalmology. 2002;109(3):569–74.
15. Vingolo EM, Steindl K, Forte R, Zompatori L, Iannaccone A, Sciarra A, et al. Autosomal dominant simple microphthalmos. J Med Genet. 1994;31(9):721–5.
16. Weiss AH, Kousseff BG, Ross EA, Longbottom J. Simple microphthalmos. Arch Ophthalmol. 1989;107(11):1625–30.
17. Foster PJ, Broadway DC, Hayat S, Luben R, Dalzell N, Bingham S, et al. Refractive error, axial length and anterior chamber depth of the eye in British adults: the EPIC-Norfolk Eye Study. Br J Ophthalmol. 2010;94(7):827–30.
18. Wu W, Dawson DG, Sugar A, Elner SG, Meyer KA, McKey JB, et al. Cataract surgery in patients with nanophthalmos: results and complications. J Cataract Refract Surg. 2004;30(3):584–90.
19. Yuzbasioglu E, Artunay O, Agachan A, Bilen H. Phacoemulsification in patients with nanophthalmos. Can J Ophthalmol. 2009;44(5):534–9.
20. Faucher A, Hasanee K, Rootman DS. Phacoemulsification and intraocular lens implantation in nanophthalmic eyes: report of a medium-size series. J Cataract Refract Surg. 2002;28(5):837–42.
21. Day AC, MacLaren RE, Bunce C, Stevens JD, Foster PJ. Outcomes of phacoemulsification and intraocular

lens implantation in microphthalmos and nanophthalmos. J Cataract Refract Surg. 2013;39(1):87–96.

22. Naujokaitis T, Scharf D, Baur I, Khoramnia R, Auffarth GU. Bilateral implantation of +56 and +58 diopter custom-made intraocular lenses in patient with extreme nanophthalmos. Am J Ophthalmol Case Rep. 2020;20:100963.

23. Singh H, Wang JC, Desjardins DC, Baig K, Gagne S, Ahmed II. Refractive results in nanophthalmic eyes after phacoemulsification and implantation of a high-refractive-power foldable intraocular lens. J Cataract Refract Surg. 2015;41(11):2394–402.

24. Zheng T, Chen Z, Xu J, Tang Y, Fan Q, Lu Y. Outcomes and prognostic factors of cataract surgery in adult extreme microphthalmos with axial length <18 mm or corneal diameter <8 mm. Am J Ophthalmol. 2017;184:84–96.

25. Guo C, Zhao Z, Zhang D, Liu J, Li J, Zhang J, et al. Anterior segment features in nanophthalmos with secondary chronic angle closure glaucoma: an ultrasound biomicroscopy study. Invest Ophthalmol Vis Sci. 2019;60(6):2248–56.

26. Jackson TL, Hussain A, Salisbury J, Sherwood R, Sullivan PM, Marshall J. Transscleral albumin diffusion and suprachoroidal albumin concentration in uveal effusion syndrome. Retina. 2012;32(1):177–82.

27. Bartke TU, Auffarth GU, Uhl JC, Volcker HE. Reliability of intraocular lens power calculation after cataract surgery in patients with relative anterior microphthalmos. Graefes Arch Clin Exp Ophthalmol. 2000;238(2):138–42.

28. Nihalani BR, Jani UD, Vasavada AR, Auffarth GU. Cataract surgery in relative anterior microphthalmos. Ophthalmology. 2005;112(8):1360–7.

29. Khan AO. Recognizing posterior microphthalmos. Ophthalmology. 2006;113(4):718.

30. Khan AO. Posterior microphthalmos versus nanophthalmos. Ophthalmic Genet. 2008;29(4):189.

31. Spitznas M, Gerke E, Bateman JB. Hereditary posterior microphthalmos with papillomacular fold and high hyperopia. Arch Ophthalmol. 1983;101(3):413–7.

32. Alkin Z, Ozkaya A, Karakucuk Y, Demirok A. Detailed ophthalmologic evaluation of posterior microphthalmos. Middle East Afr J Ophthalmol. 2014;21(2):186–8.

33. Boynton JR, Purnell EW. Bilateral microphthalmos without microcornea associated with unusual papillomacular retinal folds and high hyperopia. Am J Ophthalmol. 1975;79(5):820–6.

34. Erdol H, Kola M, Turk A, Akyol N. Ultrasound biomicroscopy and OCT findings in posterior microphthalmos. Eur J Ophthalmol. 2008;18(3):479–82.

35. Kim JW, Boes DA, Kinyoun JL. Optical coherence tomography of bilateral posterior microphthalmos with papillomacular fold and novel features of retinoschisis and dialysis. Am J Ophthalmol. 2004;138(3):480–1.

36. Kiratli H, Tumer B, Kadayifcilar S. Bilateral papillomacular retinal folds and posterior microphthalmus: new features of a recently established disease. Ophthalmic Genet. 2000;21(3):181–4.

37. Kaderli A, Acar MA, Unlu N, Uney GO, Ornek F. The correlation of hyperopia and choroidal thickness, vessel diameter and area. Int Ophthalmol. 2018;38(2):645–53.

38. Sundin OH, Leppert GS, Silva ED, Yang JM, Dharmaraj S, Maumenee IH, et al. Extreme hyperopia is the result of null mutations in MFRP, which encodes a frizzled-related protein. Proc Natl Acad Sci U S A. 2005;102(27):9553–8.

39. Gal A, Rau I, El Matri L, Kreienkamp HJ, Fehr S, Baklouti K, et al. Autosomal-recessive posterior microphthalmos is caused by mutations in PRSS56, a gene encoding a trypsin-like serine protease. Am J Hum Genet. 2011;88(3):382–90.

40. Nair KS, Hmani-Aifa M, Ali Z, Kearney AL, Ben Salem S, Macalinao DG, et al. Alteration of the serine protease PRSS56 causes angle-closure glaucoma in mice and posterior microphthalmia in humans and mice. Nat Genet. 2011;43(6):579–84.

41. Awadalla MS, Burdon KP, Souzeau E, Landers J, Hewitt AW, Sharma S, et al. Mutation in TMEM98 in a large white kindred with autosomal dominant nanophthalmos linked to 17p12-q12. JAMA Ophthalmol. 2014;132(8):970–7.

42. Khorram D, Choi M, Roos BR, Stone EM, Kopel T, Allen R, et al. Novel TMEM98 mutations in pedigrees with autosomal dominant nanophthalmos. Mol Vis. 2015;21:1017–23.

43. Tedja MS, Wojciechowski R, Hysi PG, Eriksson N, Furlotte NA, Verhoeven VJM, et al. Genome-wide association meta-analysis highlights light-induced signaling as a driver for refractive error. Nat Genet. 2018;50(6):834–48.

44. Siggs OM, Awadalla MS, Souzeau E, Staffieri SE, Kearns LS, Laurie K, et al. The genetic and clinical landscape of nanophthalmos and posterior microphthalmos in an Australian cohort. Clin Genet. 2020;97(5):764–9.

45. Kane JX, Melles RB. Intraocular lens formula comparison in axial hyperopia with a high-power intraocular lens of 30 or more diopters. J Cataract Refract Surg. 2020;46(9):1236–9.

46. Goto S, Maeda N, Koh S, Ohnuma K, Hayashi K, Iehisa I, et al. Prediction of postoperative intraocular lens position with angle-to-angle depth using anterior segment optical coherence tomography. Ophthalmology. 2016;123(12):2474–80.

47. Cooke DL, Cooke TL. Approximating sum-of-segments axial length from a traditional optical low-coherence reflectometry measurement. J Cataract Refract Surg. 2019;45(3):351–4.

48. Cooke DL, Cooke TL. A comparison of two methods to calculate axial length. J Cataract Refract Surg. 2019;45(3):284–92.

49. Cooke DL, Cooke TL, Suheimat M, Atchison DA. Standardizing sum-of-segments axial length using refractive index models. Biomed Opt Express. 2020;11(10):5860–70.

50. Wang L, Cao D, Weikert MP, Koch DD. Calculation of axial length using a single group refractive index versus using different refractive indices for each ocular segment: theoretical study and refractive outcomes. Ophthalmology. 2019;126(5):663–70.

51. Holladay JT, Gills JP, Leidlein J, Cherchio M. Achieving emmetropia in extremely short eyes with two piggyback posterior chamber intraocular lenses. Ophthalmology. 1996;103(7):1118–23.

52. Gokce SE, Zeiter JH, Weikert MP, Koch DD, Hill W, Wang L. Intraocular lens power calculations in short eyes using 7 formulas. J Cataract Refract Surg. 2017;43(7):892–7.

53. Carifi G, Aiello F, Zygoura V, Kopsachilis N, Maurino V. Accuracy of the refractive prediction determined by multiple currently available intraocular lens power calculation formulas in small eyes. Am J Ophthalmol. 2015;159(3):577–83.

54. Eom Y, Kang SY, Song JS, Kim YY, Kim HM. Comparison of Hoffer Q and Haigis formulae for intraocular lens power calculation according to the anterior chamber depth in short eyes. Am J Ophthalmol. 2014;157(4):818–24.e2.

55. Sudhakar S, Hill DC, King TS, Scott IU, Mishra G, Ernst BB, et al. Intraoperative aberrometry versus preoperative biometry for intraocular lens power selection in short eyes. J Cataract Refract Surg. 2019;45(6):719–24.

56. Kane JX, Van Heerden A, Atik A, Petsoglou C. Intraocular lens power formula accuracy: comparison of 7 formulas. J Cataract Refract Surg. 2016;42(10):1490–500.

57. Shrivastava AK, Behera P, Kumar B, Nanda S. Precision of intraocular lens power prediction in eyes shorter than 22 mm: an analysis of 6 formulas. J Cataract Refract Surg. 2018;44(11):1317–20.

58. Wang Q, Jiang W, Lin T, Wu X, Lin H, Chen W. Meta-analysis of accuracy of intraocular lens power calculation formulas in short eyes. Clin Exp Ophthalmol. 2018;46(4):356–63.

59. Melles RB, Kane JX, Olsen T, Chang WJ. Update on intraocular lens calculation formulas. Ophthalmology. 2019;126(9):1334–5.

60. Hipolito-Fernandes D, Elisa Luis M, Gil P, Maduro V, Feijao J, Yeo TK, et al. VRF-G, a new intraocular lens power calculation formula: a 13-formulas comparison study. Clin Ophthalmol. 2020;14:4395–402.

61. Kane JX, Chang DF. Intraocular lens power formulas, biometry, and intraoperative aberrometry: a review. Ophthalmology. 2020;128:e94.

62. Gayton JL, Sanders VN. Implanting two posterior chamber intraocular lenses in a case of microphthalmos. J Cataract Refract Surg. 1993;19(6):776–7.

63. Levinger E, Mimouni M, Finkelman Y, Yatziv Y, Shahar J, Trivizki O. Outcomes of refractive error correction in pseudophakic patients using a sulcus piggyback intraocular lens. Eur J Ophthalmol. 2021;31(2):422.

64. Barbero S, Marcos S, Jimenez-Alfaro I. Optical aberrations of intraocular lenses measured in vivo and in vitro. J Opt Soc Am A Opt Image Sci Vis. 2003;20(10):1841–51.

65. Hoffer KJ, Calogero D, Faaland RW, Ilev IK. Testing the dioptric power accuracy of exact-power-labeled intraocular lenses. J Cataract Refract Surg. 2009;35(11):1995–9.

66. Hoffer KJ, Savini G. IOL power calculation in short and long eyes. Asia Pac J Ophthalmol (Phila). 2017;6(4):330–1.

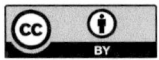

IOL Power Calculation After Corneal Refractive Surgery

65

Jaime Aramberri, Giacomo Savini, and Kenneth J. Hoffer

Introduction

Central corneal curvature is a fundamental variable in the intraocular lens (IOL) power calculation process. Its modification by corneal refractive surgery (CRS) will affect both measurement accuracy and measurement performance within calculation formulas, leading to an IOL power prediction error. The residual refractive error is usually hyperopic after myopic refractive surgery and myopic after hyperopic refractive surgery [1]. The calculation process needs to be adjusted to reduce or eliminate the induced error.

Corneal Refractive Surgery

The cataract surgeon must know the different techniques that have been performed through the years and their impact on corneal anatomy and optical properties. Many of them are no longer used, but the patients who underwent them demand now refractive lensectomy or cataract surgery. These techniques modify, by definition, the anterior corneal surface: flattening to correct myopia and steepening to correct hyperopia. The effect will be asymmetrically applied in two orthogonal meridians to correct astigmatism.

- LASIK and PRK: Excimer laser is used to eliminate tissue from the cornea by photoablation. In LASIK, a lamellar flap is cut and lifted, giving access to the stromal layer where the ablation is performed. In PRK, there is no need for corneal cutting as the laser is applied directly on the stromal surface after epithelium removal. Posterior corneal surface is not affected by surgery.
- SMILE: Tissue is eliminated by intrastromal resection by means of a femtosecond laser. Posterior corneal surface is not affected as well as in excimer techniques.
- RADIAL KERATOTOMY (RK): A variable number of radial cuts performed with a diamond knife produce central anterior and posterior corneal flattening with the aim of correcting myopia. A relevant feature is effect progression many years after surgery in certain cases.
- HEXAGONAL KERATOTOMY: Similar to the previous technique, but with an hexagonal pattern instead of a radial one, in order to

J. Aramberri
Clínica Miranza Begitek, Donostia-San Sebastian, Spain

Clínica Miranza ÓKULAR, Vitoria-Gasteiz, Spain

G. Savini (✉)
IRCCS Bietti Foundation, Rome, Italy
e-mail: giacomo.savini@startmail.com

K. J. Hoffer
St. Mary's Eye Center, Santa Monica, CA, USA

Stein Eye Institute, UCLA, Los Angeles, CA, USA
e-mail: KHofferMD@StartMail.com

J. Aramberri et al. (eds.), *Intraocular Lens Calculations*, Essentials in Ophthalmology,
https://doi.org/10.1007/978-3-031-50666-6_65

induce central anterior and posterior corneal steepening to correct hyperopia.

- THERMOKERATOPLASTY AND CONDUCTIVE KERATOPLASTY: Both techniques were used to correct hyperopia. Heat was delivered focally to portions of cornea producing central anterior corneal steepening
- INTRACORNEAL RING SEGMENTS (ICRS): Two ring segments were implanted in the corneal stroma to produce central corneal flattening to correct myopia. There might be some alterations of posterior corneal surface.
- CORNEAL INLAYS: Synthetic intracorneal lenticular implants that steepen the anterior corneal surface to correct hyperopia.
- INTRACOR: This technique produced a central anterior corneal slight steepening to correct presbyopia by means of intrastromal annular cuts with a femtosecond laser.

The effect of these surgeries on the anterior and posterior corneal surfaces must be known in order to calculate properly the IOL power (Fig. 65.1). The keratometric power can be different despite similar topographic patterns (Fig. 65.1a and b).

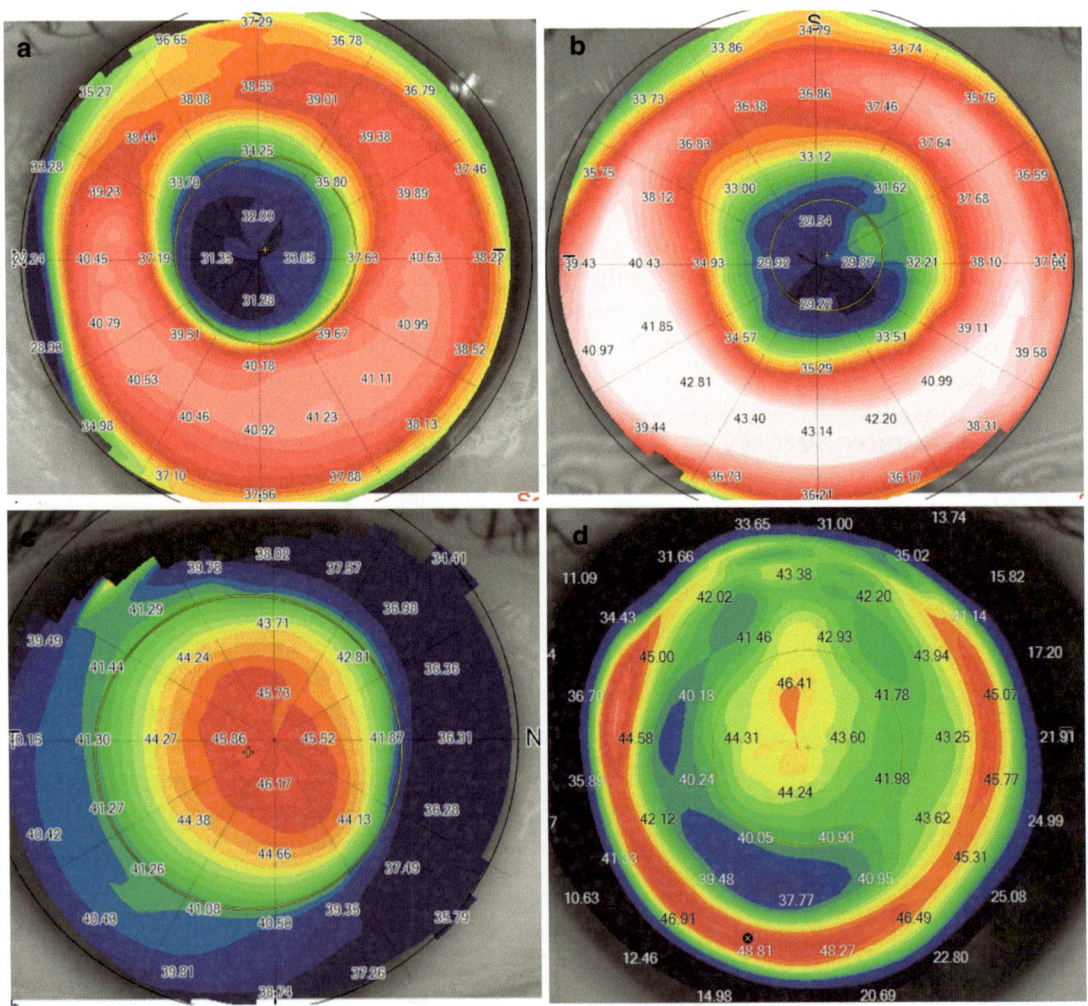

Fig. 65.1 (**a**) LASIK-M. (**b**) RK. (**c**) LASIK-H. (**d**) Intracorneal ring segments (Intacs)

Sources of Error

Three different sources of error can be identified in the IOL power calculation process after CRS. Sometimes they shift the refraction in the same direction and sometime signs cancel out: Effective lens position (ELP) prediction error, corneal radius measurement error, and corneal power calculation error [2].

- **ELP prediction after corneal refractive surgery:**

  After CRS K value has been modified while anterior segment anatomical dimensions remain unchanged. Therefore, the physical position of the implant after IOL surgery, distance to cornea and retina, is not affected by CRS and ELP value should be the same as without CRS. However, IOL power formulas that use K value as predictor of ELP will be driven to error: after any cornea flattening surgery, e.g., LASIK-M, PRK-M, and RK, the formula will underestimate ELP with a subsequent underestimation of IOL power. This will shift postoperative refraction towards hyperopia. After any cornea steepening surgery, e.g., LASIK-H or PRK-H, the formula will overestimate ELP and IOL power, producing a myopic effect on refraction (Fig. 65.2).

  Well-known formulas that use K in this way: Holladay 1 and 2, Hoffer Q, SRK/T,

Olsen, Barrett Universal II, Kane, and EVO. It must be highlighted that Haigis formula is not affected by this problem since K is not used as ELP predicting variable (Table 65.1).

It should be pointed out that not all algorithms are equally affected. Hoffer Q formula bases the ELP prediction on a curve formula and decreases the ELP shortening effect as a function of K, leading to a lower ELP underestimation than SRK/T and Holladay 1 [3]. That's why this formula produces less hyperopia after myopic CRS as several authors have proved [4, 5] (Fig. 65.3).

The induced error magnitude is proportional to the dioptric correction of the CRS, potentially achieving up to 2–2.50 D of IOL power error (approximately 1.4–1.75 D in spectacle plane) after 10–12 D myopic corrections.

- **Corneal power calculation error:**

  Most theoretical IOL power calculation formulas are thin lens analytical vergence formulas. Corneal total power (K or Sim K) is an essential variable calculated from the anterior corneal radius of curvature measured by keratometry or topography applying the formula

$$K = \frac{n2 - n1}{r}$$

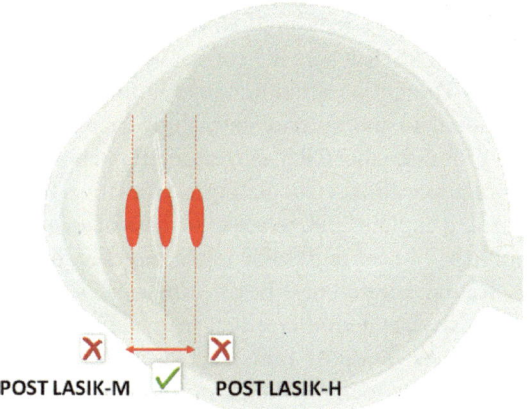

Fig. 65.2 After myopic laser, ELP is underestimated, smaller cornea-IOL distance, and after hyperopic laser ELP is overestimated

POST LASIK-M ✓ POST LASIK-H

Table 65.1 ELP predicting variables of different theoretical formulas

Formula	K	AL	ACD	Lens thickness	Others
SRK/T	Yes	Yes	No	No	No
Hoffer Q	Yes	Yes	No	No	No
Holladay 1	Yes	Yes	No	No	No
Holladay 2	Yes	Yes	Yes	Yes	Rx; age HCD
Haigis	No	Yes	Yes	No	No
Olsen	Yes/No	Yes	Yes	Yes	No
Barrett UII	Yes	Yes	Yes	Yes	HCD
Okulix	No	Yes	Yes	Yes	No
Kane	Yes	Yes	Yes	Yes	Gender
EVO	Yes	Yes	Yes	No	

K Mean keratometry, *AL* Axial length, *ACD* Anterior chamber depth, *Rx* Preoperative refraction, *HCD* Horizontal corneal diameter distance

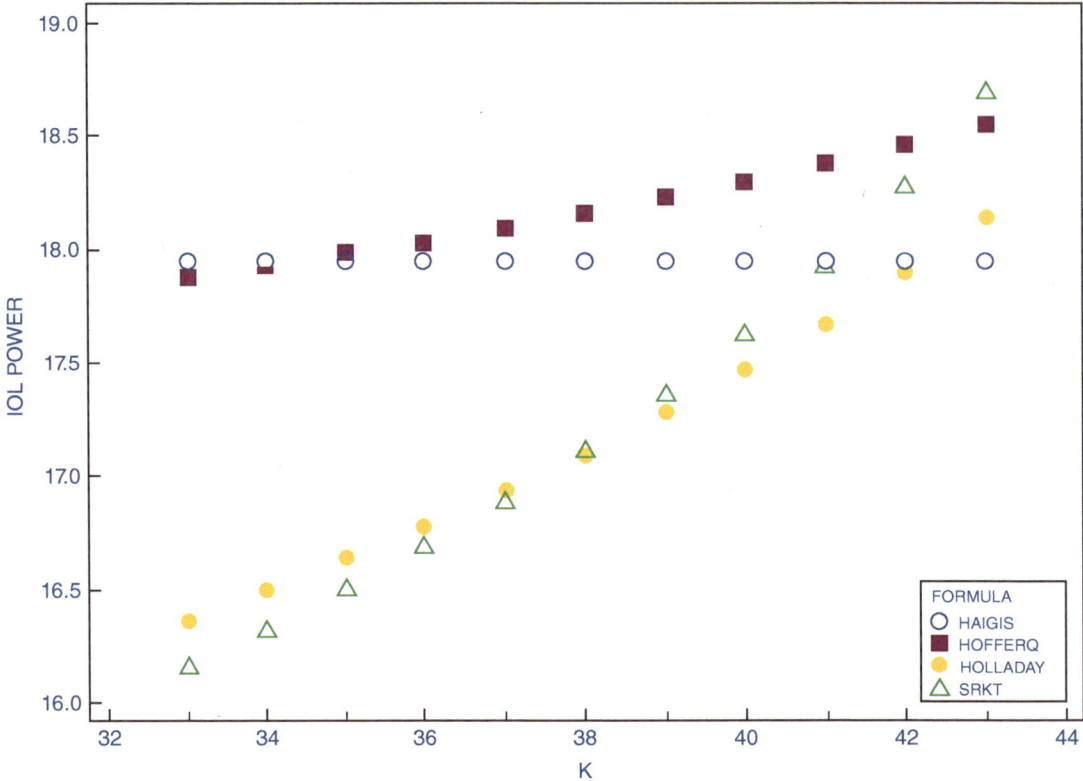

Fig. 65.3 IOL power prediction with different K pre values. SRK/T, Holladay 1, and Hoffer Q are programmed in Double K mode. In X axis different values of K pre, from 32 to 44 D. K post is always 38 D. AL is 27 mm. Haigis is not affected as K is not used to predict ELP

where $n2$ is 1.3375 (standard keratometric index of refraction, SKIR), $n1$ is 1 (index of refraction of air), and r is the corneal radius of curvature. The first is an arbitrary value to account for the unmeasured posterior corneal power effect. Each formula will internally recalculate this "total power" applying different corneal indices of refraction values: 1.3330 (SRK/T), 4/3 (Holladay 1), 1.3315 (Haigis), etc. [6]. The accuracy of SKIR depends on the normality of anterior/posterior surface proportion. The population mean value for anterior radius/posterior radius is around 1.21 ± 0.02. Many papers present the inverse ratio, posterior r/anterior r, with a mean value around 0.82 ± 0.02 [7].

After ablational laser CRS, either LASIK or PRK, there is a selective anterior flattening or steepening that doesn't change the posterior surface significantly [8]. This alters the anterior/posterior ratio and leads to a miscalculation of total corneal power by keratometers and topographers: overestimation of K after a myopic laser treatment and underestimation after a hyperopic laser treatment. E.g., measured K value is 37 D after myopic LASIK where the correct value should be 36 D. The ant/post ratio change is linearly proportional to the anterior curvature change, and therefore, to the CRS corrected diopters. This correlation allows calculating a predictive function and explains the, relative, success of so many published linear regression equations (Fig. 65.4).

Radial keratotomy, being a myopic surgery, curiously has a similar effect to hyperopic laser techniques: ant/post ratio decreases due to the simultaneous central flattening of both anterior and posterior surfaces. Camellin described a mean value of 1.12 ± 0.07 in a sample of 29 eyes measured with Pentacam [9]. Jaime Aramberri

Fig. 65.4 Anterior curvature/posterior curvature ratio: Increases after LASIK/PRK-M and decreases after LASIK/PRK-H and RK

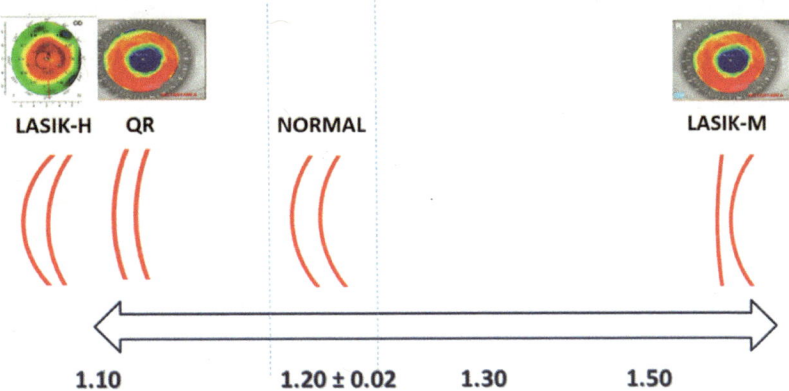

LASIK-H   QR   NORMAL   LASIK-M

1.10   1.20 ± 0.02   1.30   1.50

K is underestimated   **K is overestimated**

presented a series of 59 eyes in the annual meeting of the IPC in Haarlem 2013 where the average value was very similar: 1.15 ± 0.09. Measurements were performed with Pentacam and Sirius. The variance was high, even between both eyes of same subjects with identical number of cuts. This fact can be attributed to the manual nature of the technique and, opposed to laser surgeries, makes it difficult to calculate a predicting function based on anterior curvature.

– **Corneal radius of curvature measurement error:**

In normal corneas, K and Sim K values are calculated from radii of curvature measured in an annular paracentral zone of around 3 mm of diameter. But this value depends on the curvature and asphericity of the central cornea. Regarding curvature the bigger the measurement area gets, the flatter the cornea is and vice versa [10]. A high asphericity level means that the gradient of curvature, and power, is high. A combination of both factors will determine the sign and magnitude of radius of curvature measurement error. After myopic surgery, either laser or RK, the area of measurement is larger than normal and the curvature is measured in a more peripheral steeper zone. The flatter and more oblate the cornea is, the larger overestimation of K occurs (Fig. 65.5). This effect can be very relevant after high corrections, 6–12 D, which are very

prevalent. After hyperopic laser, the effect is more variable, so in a very steep and prolate cornea there will be an overestimation of K if the measurement area is very small and central. However, it's more frequent to see a neutral or even K underestimation error if the central cornea is not very steep (e.g., 46 D) and the cornea is very prolate (topographic image of small optical zone), where the measurement is taken in a curvature changing area (Fig. 65.6).

Keratometric error after CRS will result from the combination of the previously exposed sources of error and will depend on the type of refractive surgery (Fig. 65.7):

– After myopic LASIK and PRK: Both the ant/post ratio change and the increase of measurement area produce an overestimation of K value.
– After hyperopic LASIK and PRK: The ant/post ratio change induces underestimation of K. The radius of curvature measurement sometimes shows underestimation but in very steep corneas there can be some overestimation. The net effect is normally underestimation of K value.
– After RK: The ant/post ratio change induces underestimation of K. But this is compensated by the peripheral measurement of steeper values whenever the cornea is very flat and

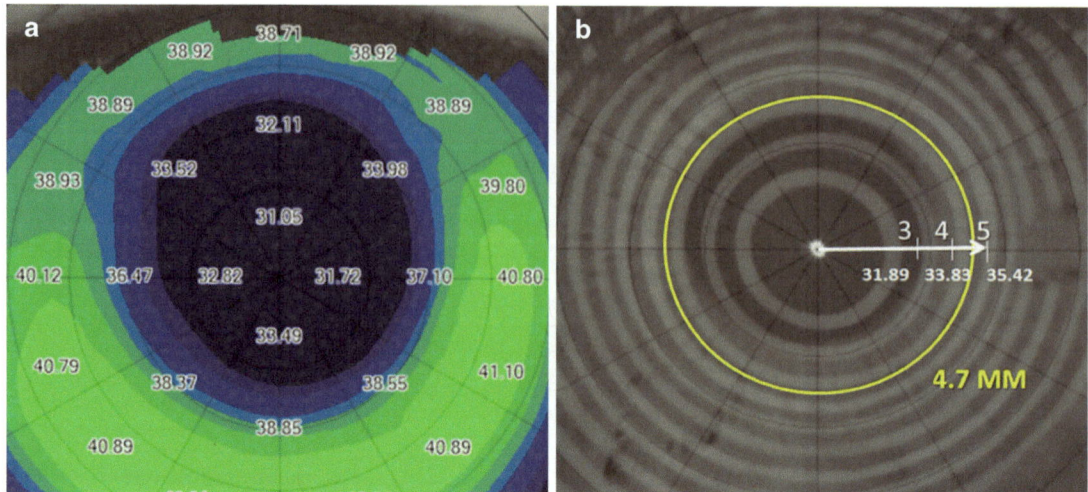

Fig. 65.5 Corneal reflection topography after LASIK-M. Sim K measurement area has become 4.7 mm due to corneal flattening. Corneal shape (oblate) deter- mines a high power gradient as it can be seen by the val- ues at 3, 4, and 5 mm of diameter

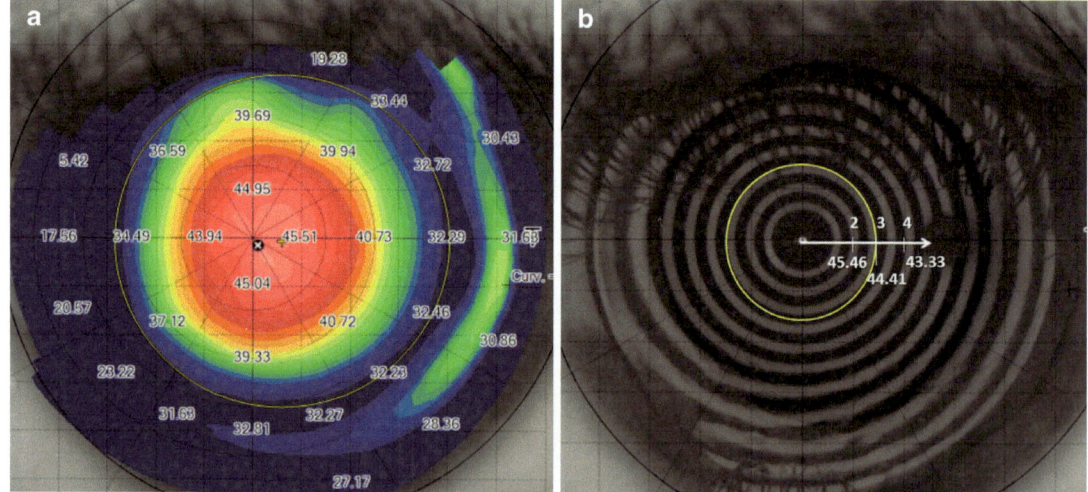

Fig. 65.6 Hyperopic LASIK cornea: Central curvature is not very steep and measurement area diameter is 2.98 mm. But asphericity is high (Q (4 mm): −1.15) and K value is underestimated (**a**) corneal map after hyperopic LASIK (**b**) Placido disc rings after hyperopic LASIK

prolate. The net effect depends on the curva- ture and asphericity of the cornea.

It is a frequent observation after myopic laser and RK that K value measured by autokeratome- ters is flatter than Sim K measured by corneal topographers due to the fact that in the former the measurement area is smaller. The opposite trend is seen after hyperopic laser surgery. However, this phenomenon will finally depend on the mea- surement method of each device.

The keratometric error has been estimated to account for 14–30% of the corrected refraction amount by the refractive surgery after myopic laser surgery [11, 12]. E.g., this means that if K value is 37 D and the refractive surgery has cor- rected 10 D, assuming a 15% correcting factor, the corrected K value will be 37 − 1.5 = 35.5 D.

SURGERY	TOPOGRAPHY	CENTRAL CURVATURE	SHAPE	ANT/POST RATIO	KERATOMETRY ERROR
LASIK-M	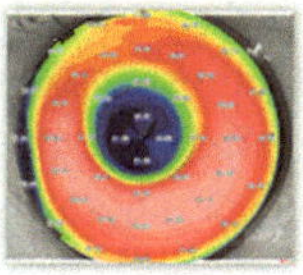	FLAT	OBLATE	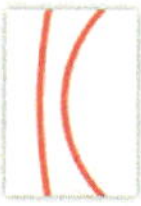 INCREASE	OVERESTIMATION
RK	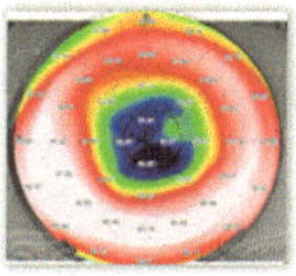	FLAT	OBLATE	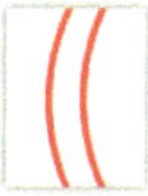 DECREASE	OVERESTIMATION UNDERESTIMATION
LASIK-H	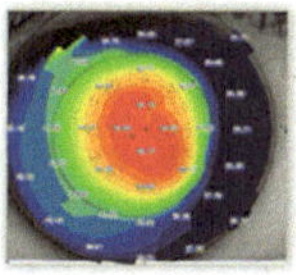	STEEP	PROLATE	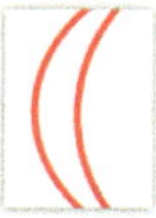 DECREASE	UNDERESTIMATION

Fig. 65.7 Keratometric error after CRS. Topographic and keratometric changes vary depending on the type of surgery

The effect of higher order aberrations (HOA) in the optical performance of these eyes shouldn't be overlooked. It is a heterogeneous population of corneas with a high prevalence of HOA, spherical aberration and coma being the most frequent. There is an evident difference between old treatments, where small optical zones and decentrations are common, and modern treatments where optimized profiles and effective eye trackers render good optical quality. Very aberrated corneas are multifocal and can't be represented by a paraxial parameter as the K value. Even postoperative refraction in terms of sphere-cylinder diopters is inadequate as outcome metrics. This probably explains the variability in reported results among the published multiple studies.

Another issue is corneal power change after IOL surgery. This is particularly noticeable after RK, where there is some corneal flattening in the first postoperative months with a variable regression that can end in a different final K value. The reason is transitory incisional epithelial edema

that increases the incisional flattening effect of radial cuts [13]. Moreover, there can be a hyperopic refractive shift through the years in some of these eyes.

Solutions

In order to get an accurate prediction, the IOL power calculation method must be adjusted providing solutions to the different problems:

Correct ELP Calculation

The easiest solution is to use a calculation formula that doesn't use K to predict the IOL position within the eye. Haigis formula uses ACD and AL to predict ELP and is quite accurate as long as the 3 IOL constants (a0,a1 and a2) are correctly optimized. Olsen formula should be used with the C-constant algorithm, which uses ACD and LT to estimate the ELP. Okulix software uses AL,

ACD, and LT for this task and can be used with no specific correction. Shammas PL formula doesn't use K to predict ELP.

Any formula that uses corneal power to predict ELP can be used with a modification that allows a sequential use of two different K values: The pre CRS K value will be used in the ELP calculation algorithm and the post-CRS K value will be used in the final optical calculation of IOL power. This procedure has been called Double-K method [14]. At present time, most IOL calculators apply this method once the post-CRS calculation mode has been selected. The Holladay IOL Consultant software only applies it within the Holladay 2 formula. The online ASCRS IOL calculator (https://iolcalc.ascrs.org/) uses this method with the Holladay 1 and Barrett formulas. The Barrett true K formula is programmed in Double K manner. It can be accessed in the APACRS website (http://calc.apacrs.org/Barrett_True_K_Universal_2105/). Another option is to perform a regular calculation (single K) and then modify the result following some conversion tables as published by Koch [15].

If K pre-CRS is not available, and this is quite usual, an average number like 43.5 D can be used (Holladay 2 and ASCRS online calculator use 43.86 D). An alternative and probably more adequate recourse is to measure corneal posterior radius of curvature with a Scheimpflug or OCT tomographer, and applying the average post/ant ratio, 0.82 ± 0.02 [8], calculates the pre CRS radius of curvature: e.g., posterior radius 6.15 mm means a preCRS anterior radius of 7.5 mm (6.15/0.82 = 7.5). With the formula $\frac{n2-1}{r}$ being $n2 = 1.3375$, Kpre = 337.5/7.5 = 45 D.

It shouldn't be assumed that these third-generation double K formulas will keep the same accuracy as in the normal range of biometric variables. There are intrinsic biases that can express more, or differently, in this extreme K values combined with low or high AL values. E.g., In low K values, Haigis formula tends to overestimate IOL power while SRK/T tends to the opposite. In very high K values, SRK/T tends to overestimate ELP. Hoffer Q formula tends to overestimate ELP with K values lower than 42.

Some of these trends are more notorious after myopic surgery because IOL power has increased while in non-operated eyes they were concealed by the low power of the implant.

Another K pre CRS choice is to select an arbitrary number that compensates the blindness of SRK/T, Hoffer Q, and Holladay 1 to the anterior segment size in cases where this is very long or short. This is frequent after myopic surgery where a deep anterior segment can lead to an underestimation of ELP that will have more effect than that before CRS as the IOL power is higher. One of the authors (JA) has recommended to neglect the actual Kpre (if known) and to choose 45 when the anterior segment depth parameter (ACD + 0.5*LT) is higher than 5.85 mm and 42 when it is lower than 4.9 mm.

The Double K formulas are quite tolerant to Kpre error: in an average eye 1 D of error in Kpre (the value used exclusively in ELP prediction) induces 0.50 D of error in IOL power, which means around 0.35 D in spectacle plane.

The Double K method, not using the measured K in IOL position prediction, should be used in any clinical situation where an abnormal K value can induce ELP calculation error: severe keratoconus, corneal scar, keratoplasty, etc.

Correct Keratometry Calculation

Each IOL power calculation formula is designed to admit corneal power in a certain way: most of them use K value calculated with the SKIR (1.3375). Any adjusted value must be referenced to the same optical plane.

- CRS correction-based calculation: The simplest way to calculate Kpost is to add the effect of the CRS to Kpre. This is the basis of the so-called Clinical History Method [16]. However, it seldom can be used for two usual issues: lack of preoperative information and difficulty to determine if any posterior refractive change was due to corneal or lens change.
- Modified K: a myriad of methods have been proposed to modify the measured K value, either keratometric or topographic, after

CRS. In the oldest papers, the keratometric error was not distinguished from the ELP estimation error and therefore in many cases overcorrecting the former compensated the latter as well. Among the most cited methods, these can be remarked: prepupillary area power (with or without Styles-Crawford effect) [10, 17]; K adjustment by 1 D subtraction [18]; linear regression formulas with a constant value for the posterior surface. Seitz first proposed a posterior corneal power of 5.9 D [1]. The Maloney method became popular later with a posterior value of 6.1 D [19]; empirical adjustment with a linear regression function by Shammas [20]; radius of curvature correction as a function of the CRS dioptric correction and AL [21]. Two methods that correct the anterior radius of curvature empirically still in use by many surgeons are the Haigis-L and the Barrett True K formulas [22, 23].

A method that consisted in averaging the K value calculated by different methods was called the consensus K method by Randleman. Included methods for this calculation were: refractive history, contact lens, manual K, Hamed, Shammas, and Maloney and corneal topography. Extreme values were eliminated (1.5 D off the mean) and the consensus K was averaged from a group located in the central 0.75 D range. The reported error with the Holladay 2 formula was 0.23 ± 0.61 D [24].

- K calculated from posterior surface measurement:

The development of technologies that can measure the corneal thickness and posterior curvature has allowed the calculation of total corneal power based in actual measurements getting rid of assumptions or any dependence on clinical history information. These technologies are scanning slit, Scheimpflug photography, OCT, and posterior surface reflection keratometry. However, it must be highlighted that central total corneal power calculated by numerical ray tracing or analytical vergence formulas with the Gullstrand refraction indices, 1.376 for cornea and 1.336 for aqueous, can't be used, at least with the same IOL constants, in the regular formulas because the ref-

erence plane will be more anterior than the one used by K. This parameter receives different names in the commercially available tomographers: TCRP in Pentacam, TCP in Galilei and Anterion, RP in Casia 2, MPP in Sirius and MS39, etc.

Holladay described a total corneal power value converted to the K (1.3375) reference plane that could be used in regular IOL power calculations: The equivalent K reading (EKR) [25]. In his paper, a conversion factor was calculated once the anterior radius of curvature was deduced from the normal anterior to posterior corneal ratio. In the Pentacam software, EKR can be calculated for different diameters. The 4.5 mm diameter value showed the best equivalency with the regular K. EKR can also be found in the Cassini topographer. However, the use of Pentacam EKR is in controversy as reported results have not satisfied expectations. Recently, Seo has proposed a new EKR value adding 0.7 to the Pentacam 4 mm TCRP (total corneal refractive power) getting better results than those with Holladay EKR [26]. One of the authors, JA, found good results in a series of 26 eyes after myopic LASIK/PRK with Cassini EKR and the Haigis formula with a predictive error of −0.16 ± 0.73 D.

Zeiss IOL Master 700 has included a similar parameter: Total Keratometry (TK). Both anterior and posterior surfaces are measured with SS-OCT which probably yields better image quality than Scheimpflug. Savini has reported excellent repeatability in normal and post-CRS eyes, with a Sw value of 0.07 D and 0.09 D, respectively [27]. This value can be used in any regular formula without further adjustments. On the contrary, formulas that already corrected K in eyes after CRS like Haigis-L and Barret True K shouldn't work with this value. Barrett true K allows introducing the posterior measured corneal power in order to perform calculation with actual values bypassing its K correcting empirical algorithm. This is called Barrett True K TK, and good results have been published [28].

There are several programs and formulas using thick lens pseudophakic eye models where the corneal radii of curvature are input avoiding any power- (K) related issues like incorrect anterior/posterior ratio or erroneous K equivalent value calculation. Some are based on ray tracing, like Olsen, Okulix, and Barret True K TK. The EVO formula performs the optical calculations with analytical vergence formulas. Corneal asphericity can be input in the Olsen formula taking account of the spherical aberration effect, sometimes high in these eyes. In certain topographers, exact ray tracing calculations can be done with these formulas: Olsen, Okulix, CSO proprietary software (MS39 and Sirius tomographers), and ExactIOL. The advantage is that the effect of HOA is computed and the IOL that produces the best visual quality can be selected going beyond the paraxial concept of spectacle refraction. This can be relevant in very irregular corneas.

Calculation Methods

Many methods have been published in the last 20 years since these eyes were identified as being problematic for IOL power calculation. Some have been abandoned and some are still in use. In this section, a list of still relevant methods will be presented. A practical classification is to distinguish between methods that require clinical history data and methods that don't.

Methods Requiring Clinical History Data (Original Keratometry and/or Refractive Change)

– PreLASIK/PRK calculation method

It has been used by many surgeons since long time and published as AS technique [29] and corneal power bypass [30]. The IOL power is calculated with the original K value aiming for the refraction corrected by the CRS in the spectacle plane. Attractive for its simplicity, it usually faces the limitations of unavailability of the Clinical History and/or the error induced by any unknown K change in the time after CRS.

– Barrett True-K formula:

This unpublished formula is a modification of the Barrett Universal II where the ELP estimation error is avoided using the Double K method and, on the other hand, the keratometric error is fixed using an internal regression formula that modifies the prediction in a different way for myopic laser, hyperopic laser, and radial keratotomy. The "history" version of the Barrett True-K formula requires the surgically induced refractive change (SIRC) and has been found to be an accurate option for IOL power calculation, as the prediction error (PE) is within ±0.50 D in 64–67% of eyes [23, 31, 32]. Its results are further improved by adding the posterior corneal curvature data measured by Scheimpflug or OCT. Savini reported that this was the best method with 70% of eyes within ±0.50 D of prediction error [31].

This formula is available on the websites of the Asia-Pacific Association of Cataract & Refractive Surgeons (www.apacrs.org), the American Society of Cataract and Refractive Surgery (https://ascrs.org/tools/iol-calculator), and on several optical biometers and tomographers.

– Masket formula:

In this commonly used formula, available at https://ascrs.org/tools/iol-calculator, the IOL power is calculated as if the eye had not undergone previous excimer laser surgery. The IOL power by Single-K SRK/T (in the case of myopia) or Single-K Hoffer Q (in the case of hyperopia) is then adjusted according to the following equation [33]:

$$\text{IOL power adjustment} = \text{SIRC} * (-0.326) + 0.101$$

In the ASCRS website, a modification of this formula by Warren Hill can also be found:

$$\text{IOL power adjustment} = \text{SIRC} * (-0.4385) + 0.0295.$$

This formula should be used using the Holladay 1 for AL > 23 mm and the Hoffer Q for AL < 23 mm [34].

Several studies have shown that this method is quite accurate (up to more than 70% of eyes with a PE within ±0.50 D), although it may give slightly hyperopic results [32, 35, 36].

– Savini's method:
– With this method, the keratometric index of 1.3375, which is no longer valid after LASIK or PRK, is decreased as the amount of myopic correction increases, according to the formula:

$$\text{Post CRS index of refraction} = \text{SIRC} * 0.0009856 + 1.338$$

Once the adjusted keratometric index has been calculated, the corneal power is calculated using the usual formula $P = (n-1)/R$ [37]. This method has been proven to give reliable results when combined with the Double-K SRK/T formula, as the percentage of eyes with a PE within ±0.50 D ranges between 64 and 73% [35, 38, 39]. The high accuracy of this method when the refractive change is known is offset by a high sensitivity to bad clinical data.

Similar methods have been developed by Camellin and Calossi and Jarade [40, 41].

– Seitz/Speicher's method:

This method, which has been described independently by Speicher and Seitz between 2000 and 2001 [42, 43], relies on preoperative keratometry and does not require the SIRC. It assumes that the total dioptric power of the cornea (P) can be calculated by adding the power of the anterior (P_a) and posterior (P_p) corneal surfaces:

$$P = P_a + P_p = (n_2 - n_1)/r_1 + (n_3 - n_2)/r_2$$

where n_1 is the refractive index of air (= 1), n_2 is the refractive index of the cornea (= 1.376), and n_3 is the refractive index of the aqueous humor (= 1.336). Both preoperatively and postoperatively, the power of the anterior corneal surface (P_a) can be obtained using the refractive index of the cornea (1.376) rather than the keratometric index (1.3375). This means that the keratometric power (K) provided by the corneal topographer or optical biometer has to be multiplied by 1.114 (corresponding to 376/337.5). Hence:

$$P_a = K \times 1.114$$

Before LASIK or PRK, knowing the power of the anterior corneal surface enables us to estimate the power of the posterior corneal surface (Pp) according to the formula:

$$P_p = P_a - P = (K \times 1.114) - K$$

After LASIK or PRK, the power of the anterior corneal surface can then be added to that of the posterior corneal surface (which is assumed to be unchanged), as expressed by the formula:

$$P = \text{postop} P_a + P_p = \text{postop} K \times 1.114 + (\text{preop} K \times 1.114 - \text{preop} K)$$

This method has been shown to provide excellent results when combined with the Double-K SRK/T formula [35, 39, 44]. The main advantage of this method is that it does not require perioperative refractive data, as the preoperative K readings are sufficient.

Methods Not Requiring Clinical History Data (Original Keratometry and/or Refractive Change)

Perioperative data, i.e., the pre-LASIK/PRK keratometry and the surgically induced refractive change, are often not available. Therefore, No-History methods represent the only solution in many cases. It is interesting to distinguish between methods that use the posterior corneal power measured by Scheimpflug or OCT and methods that don't. It could be thought a priori that IOL power calculation based on measurements should be more accurate than one based on empirical estimations.

Methods that Don't Use Posterior Corneal Measurement

- Barrett True-K No History formula:

    This formula can work without historical data correcting the calculation as a function of the measured K and AL with an empirical algorithm. It can be accessed in the previously reported websites. The results are good (56–63% of eyes with a PE within ±0.50 D) [23, 31, 32] and can be improved by adding the posterior corneal curvature (up to 70% of eyes with a PE within ±0.50 D) [31, 45]. Compared to other No-History formulas, it appears to be the most accurate choice in eyes with axial length (AL) <28 mm [46].

- Haigis-L formula:

    This is a modification of the Haigis formula where the anterior radius of curvature measured by the IOL Master is corrected with a formula empirically calculated from a series of cases. This is done separately for eyes with previous myopic and hyperopic corrections. In the case of myopia, the formula is

$$rcorr = \frac{331.5}{-5.1625 * rmeas + 82.2603 - 0.35}$$

where rmeas is the measured radius of curvature and rcorr is the corrected radius of curvature that will be input in the Haigis formula.

With this formula, there is no need for ELP calculation correction (e.g., Double K method) as K is not used for this task [22].

The results reported have been good but not outstanding (34–61% of eyes with a PE within ±0.50 D), with a trend towards myopic outcomes [22, 23, 32, 45].

- Shammas-PL and PHL (for previously myopic and hyperopic eyes)

    These formulas calculate the corneal power by means of the following equation:

$$\text{Corneal power} = 1.14\,K\text{post} - 6.8$$

where Kpost is the post-refractive surgery keratometry [20].

The calculated corneal power value has to be entered into the original Shammas formula, which does not need the Double-K adjustment as it does not depend on corneal curvature to estimate the ELP (so called Shammas-PL formula) [47]. Several studies reported good results not only in eyes without historical data, but also in those with perioperative data available, as the PE was within ±0.50 D in 46–60% of eyes [32, 35, 36, 39]. Compared to other No-History methods, Shammas PL-formula provided the highest accuracy in eyes longer than 30 mm, but was inferior to Barrett True-K and Triple-S in eyes with shorter AL [46]. A specific version (Shammas-PHL formula) can be used for eyes with previous hyperopic LASIK [48]:

$$\text{Corneal power} = 1.0457\,K\text{post} - 1.9538$$

- Triple-S method (Seitz/Speicher/Savini):

    This method is a modification of Seitz/Speicher method that does not require pre-LASIK/PRK keratometry. The K measured by the keratometer is converted into the sum of the anterior power and a mean value of −4.98 diopters (D) for the posterior corneal surface empirically calculated from a series of cases [44]:

$$K = \text{measured}\,K \times 1.114 - 4.98D$$

Here, the preoperative unknown K must still be entered into the Double-K formula and several options are available to estimate it: an average value may be used (e.g., 43.50 D), the preoperative K may be obtained by adding the refractive change at the corneal plane to the modified postoperative K value, or it may be calculated from the posterior corneal surface parameters [49]. The results have been among the best for No-History formulas, as the PE was within ±0.50 D in 53–70% of eyes [35, 38, 46]. It has also been reported to be the best No-History formula in eyes with AL between 28 and 30 mm (compared to Barrett True-K, Haigis-L and Shammas PL) [46].

– Maloney and Wang-Koch-Maloney methods:

A very similar option is Maloney's method. The main difference lies in the choice of the topographic value, which in Maloney's method is not the SimK but rather the single power at the center of the axial map (Atlas topographer) and a posterior corneal power of −4.90 D rather than −4.98D.

Hence, corneal power according to Maloney's method reads as:

$$K = \text{measured } K\ 1.114 - 4.90$$

Wang proposed a change for the posterior corneal value to −6.1 D and later further changed it to −5.59 D [19]. This modified K can be used in a Double K formula or in one that doesn't use K as ELP predictor (e.g., ASCRS online calculator uses Shammas-PL).

– Intraoperative aberrometry:

This method calculates the IOL power from the intraoperative aphakic refraction. The first reference was based in automatic refractometry [50], but it later evolved to using a Talbot-Moiré aberrometer (ORA System, Alcon, Fort Worth, TX) to get the measurement. The IOL power is calculated with a refractive vergence formula statistically optimized with a large database of thousands of cases. Ianchulev reported a PE of 67% of eyes within ±0.5 D in a sample of 246 eyes [51] and

Fram a similar figure, 74%, in a simple of 39 eyes [52]. This method has a significant economic cost and time requirement during surgery to be considered when compared to other methods.

Methods that Use Posterior Corneal Measurement

– IOL Master Total Keratometry (TK):

This new parameter has been included recently in the IOL Master 700 biometer and follows the EKR concept introduced by Holladay in the Pentacam. TK is calculated from the OCT measured anterior and posterior corneal radii referenced to the same plane as K (1.3375). Therefore, it can be used in any standard formula. In normal eyes, TK should be very similar to K, with some difference explained by the anterior/posterior corneal ratio variability [27, 53]. After CRS, it can be used in any formula that doesn't use K to predict ELP, e.g., Haigis, or in any Double K formula as K post. In these cases, TK will be lower than K after myopic laser surgery, with a difference proportional to the surgery-induced anterior flattening, and it will be higher after hyperopic laser. After RK, it might be higher, similar, or lower. Wang reported a difference between TK and K of -0.39 ± 0.26 D, 0.06 ± 0.17 D, and 0.15 ± 0.32 D, in 53 eyes post-M-laser, 32 eyes post-H-laser, and 44 eyes post-RK [54]. PE after LASIK/PRK-M with 3[a] generation formulas is around 60% of eyes within ±0.50 D. With Haigis formula, Wang reported 58.5%, Lawless 60%, and Yeo 64%. With Double K Holladay 1, Lawless reported 60% and Yeo 54.69%. With the Double K SRK/T, Yeo found 57.81% [28, 45, 54].

The Barrett True K formula has been modified to use the TK value taking the name Barrett True K TK. The algorithm that corrects the K value is disabled and measured anterior and posterior radii are used instead. Reported outcomes suggest an improved PE: Lawless reports 75% of eyes within ±0.5 D and Yeo 64% [28, 45].

The EVO 2.0 formula has been modified in a similar way, EVO TK, with a first paper by its author reporting 68.75% of cases within ±0.50 D of the target [45]. This is a thick lens vergence formula where the posterior corneal radii measured with IOL Master 700 can be input. The normal corneal posterior/anterior ratio (0.883) is used to calculate the pre-CRS K value in order to apply the Double-K method in the ELP algorithm.

- OCT-based calculation:

Tang published a method based in the corneal measurements of the SD-OCT RTvue where the total corneal power was calculated using a Gaussian equivalent power formula and later used in a thin lens vergence formula. IOL position was estimated using ACD, LT, and AL as predicting variables. Results in 16 eyes after LASIK-M were similar to Haigis-L formula: MAE 0.50 and 0.76, respectively [55, 56].

- Ray tracing models:

Numerical ray tracing models perform optical calculations tracing rays surface by surface applying Snell's law. In the paraxial mode, the main advantage over thin lens analytical formulas is that cornea is defined by anterior and posterior radii of curvature, both of which can be measured skipping power calculation issues. In the exact mode, the effect of HOA is also considered, and this can be significant in many of these cases where corneas can be very irregular: small optical zones, decentration, etc.

Okulix and Phacooptics are two commercial programs where IOL calculations are based on thick lens ray tracing. If only corneal radii are input, the calculation will be paraxial. If asphericity is added, spherical aberration effect will also be calculated. If cornea is defined by a topographic data matrix, then exact ray tracing will take account of HOA.

Okulix software uses AL, ACD, and LT for IOL position estimation and published results with anterior and posterior corneal measurements are fairly good: 63.6% of cases within ±0.50 D of the target [57]. Results might be even better if measurements are obtained with a SS-OCT device: Gjerdrum has reported excellent results with Anterion and Okulix: PE within ±0.5 D in 88% of eyes [58].

Phacooptics software is programmed with the Olsen formula. In post-CRS cases, the C constant method should be used to calculate the ELP. Only ACD and LT will take part in the IOL position calculation [59].

The Italian Company CSO has included an IOL power calculation program based on exact ray tracing in the AS-tomographers Sirius (Scheimpflug) and MS 39 (SD-OCT). ELP is calculated with a proprietary algorithm that doesn't use corneal parameters. Savini reported 71% of eyes with a PE within ±0.50 D with the Sirius [60] and 75% of eyes in a non-published series with the MS 39 instrument using optical segmented AL.

- Total corneal power:

All AS-tomographers provide some central corneal power parameter calculated by ray tracing from the measured anterior and posterior radii of curvatures. The name will be different for each device (Table 65.2):

These values can be used in regular formulas only if the IOL constant is adjusted ad hoc because the reference plane is different from the K calculated with the SKIR (1.3375). Then results are correct in normal eyes [61, 62]. After CRS, the values should be used in a formula that doesn't use cornea to predict ELP, e.g., Haigis, or in a Double-K formula: Savini

Table 65.2 AS-tomographers and central total corneal power

Instrument	Technology	Total K parameter
Galilei	Placido + Scheimpflug	Total corneal power
Pentacam	Scheimpflug	Total corneal refractive power
Sirius	Placido + Scheimpflug	Mean pupil power
Anterion	Swept source OCT	Total corneal power
Casia 2	Swept source OCT	Real power
MS 39	Placido + Spectral OCT	Mean pupil power
Revo NX	Spectral OCT	Real power

reported 70% of eyes within ±0.50 D of target with Total corneal power of Galilei and Double-K SRK/T formula [57].

– Fórmula Stop:

In this method, the calculation of Holladay 1 and SRK/T formulas is modified by the posterior/anterior corneal ratio. It was originally developed from a series of 61 eyes that had myopic and hyperopic laser surgery, measured with Pentacam and IOL Master [63]. These are the adjustment formulas

$$Holladay1 = \left(5.73 - 8.69^* \, r\text{post} / r\text{ant} - 0.69^* \, r\text{ant} + 0.29^* \, AL\right) \times 1.5$$

$$SRK / T = \left(9.11 - 10.81^* \, r\text{post} / r\text{ant}\right) * 1.5$$

The obtained number must be added to the IOL power calculated by each formula. Savini reported fair results, comparable to other no-history methods: 60% and 62% of eyes within ±0.5 D of the target [38].

Calculation After Radial Keratotomy

After RK corneal topography has a similar shape after myopic laser surgery, LASIK or PRK, cornea. But there is a relevant geometrical and optical difference due to the fact that posterior cornea has flattened as well, decreasing the anterior/posterior corneal ratio in a similar way to a post-hyperopic LASIK cornea. This leads to an underestimation of K. This effect is very variable and doesn't correlate well with the number of cuts, probably due to the manual character of this surgical technique. However, the magnitude of anterior/posterior ratio change is not as intense as in laser surgery (for a similar refractive correction) and therefore the induced error is lower. Moreover, there is some compensation from the measured area enlargement produced by the corneal curvature and shape change. Hence, the net keratometric error is variable, under or overestimation, depending on the surgery effect. The flatter the cornea, the higher the trend toward K overestimation and vice versa. All this variability makes inaccurate any correcting regression function based on the anterior keratometry, differently to post-laser situation.

Another issue is the frequent temporal fluctuation of keratometry, and thus refraction, some-times following a circadian cycle. Target refraction in these eyes is many times a moving target.

The first proposed calculation methods, based on Placido topography, substituted Sim K by central measurements like ACCP(3 mm) of the TMS device or Effective Refractive Power (EffRP) of EyeSys topographer [64, 65]. These values should be used in the adequate formulas to avoid the ELP error. Potvin didn't find a significant difference using several corneal parameters of Pentacam, with and without posterior curvature, in the Double K Holladay 1 formula, with a similar result to Placido topography: around 40% of eyes within ±0.50 D and 75% of eyes within ±1.00 D of target refraction [66]. Ma et al. reported similar results with Double K Holladay 1 with IOL Master K, OCT corneal power, and Barrett true K. They found a hyperopic early postoperative refraction that decreased in 4 months. Results were very variable and 27% of eyes had a final predictive error >1 D [67]. Curado compared different methods: ORA system, IOL Master K and Haigis, Holladay 2, and Barrett true K, with a predictive error ≤0.50 D in 48.1%, 53.8%, 57.7%, and 63.5% of eyes, respectively [68].

Recently, Turnbull has found better results with Barrett true K with historical data, 76.6%, than Barrett true K without data, 69.2%, Haigis, 69.2%, and Double K Holladay 1, 50%. Predictive error >1 D incidence in this series is lower than others [69].

Our experience with calculations based on ray tracing and posterior corneal measurement by OCT is positive with more than 60% of cases with ±0.50 D of target and few errors over 1 D.

Availability of These Methods

– Software of biometers and topo/tomographers:

All biometers in the marker have specific formulas for these calculations. 3° generation formulas are programmed applying the Double-K method, Shammas-PL and Barrett true K. Ray tracing software like Okulix and Phacooptics are optional in some devices and can be linked to the measuring software.

– Online calculators (free access):

(a) ASCRS: Different methods are used depending on the inputs. Average calculation is also calculated (https://iolcalc.ascrs.org/wbfrmCalculator.aspx).

(b) APACRS: Barrett True K formula is used (http://calc.apacrs.org/Barrett_True_K_Universal_2105/).

(c) EVO formula: (https://www.evoiolcalculator.com/calculator.aspx).

(d) IOL Power Club: An excel file programmed by Giacomo Savini and Ken Hoffer with different methods can be downloaded (https://www.iolpowerclub.org/post-surgical-iol-calc).

– Commercial software:

Phacooptics and Okulix ray tracing software can be acquired in their respective websites.

References

1. Seitz B, Langenbucher A, Nguyen NX, et al. Underestimation of intraocular lens power for cataract surgery after myopic photorefractive keratectomy. Ophthalmology. 1999;106:693–702.

2. Aramberri J. Cálculo de la potencia de la LIO tras cirugía refractiva. Facoemulsificación y emetropía. Monografía SECOIR. Madrid: SECOIR; 2001. p. 55–65.

3. Hoffer KJ. The Hoffer Q formula: a comparison of theoretic and regression formulas. J Cataract Refract Surg. 1993;19:700–12 Errata 1994;20:677, 2007;33(1):2–3.

4. Odenthal MTP, Eggink CA, Melles G, et al. Clinical and theoretical results of intraocular lens power calculation for cataract surgery after photorefrac-

tive keratectomy for myopia. Arch Ophthalmol. 2002;120:431–8.

5. Stakheev A. Intraocular lens calculation for cataract after previous radial keratotomy. Ophthalmic Physiol Opt. 2002;22:289–95.

6. W Haigis. The Haigis formula. [aut. libro] H. John Shammas. Intraocular lens power calculations. Thorofare: Slack; 2004. p. 41–57.

7. Ho JD, Tsai CY, Tsai RJ, Kuo LL, Tsai IL, Liou SW. Validity of the keratometric index: evaluation by the Pentacam rotating Scheimpflug camera. J Cataract Refract Surg. 2008;34:137–45.

8. Smadja D, Santhiago MR, Mello GR, et al. Response of the posterior corneal surface to myopic laser in situ keratomileusis with different ablation depths. J Cataract Refract Surg. 2012;38:1222–31.

9. Camellin M, Savini G, Hoffer K, et al. Scheimpflug camera measurement of anterior and posterior corneal curvature in eyes with previous radial keratotomy. J Refract Surg. 2012;28:275–9.

10. Maeda N, Klyce SD, Smolek MK, et al. Disparity between Keratometry-style readings and corneal power within the pupil after refractive surgery for myopia. Cornea. 1997;16:517–24.

11. Kalski RS, Danjoux JP, Fraenkel GE, et al. Intraocular lens power calculation for cataract surgery after photorefractive keratectomy for high myopia. J Refract Surg. 1997;13:362–6.

12. Gobbi PG, Carones F, Brancato R. Keratometric index, videokeratography and refractive surgery. J Cataract Refract Surg. 1998;24:202–11.

13. Koch DD, Liu JF, Hyde LL, Rock RL, Emery JM. Refractive complications of cataract surgery after radial keratotomy. Am J Ophthalmol. 1989;108:676–82.

14. Aramberri J. Intraocular lens power calculation after corneal refractive surgery: double-K method. J Cataract Refract Surg. 2003;29:2063–8.

15. Koch L, Wang DD. Calculating IOL power in eyes that have undergone refractive surgery. J Cataract Refract Surg. 2003;29:2039–42.

16. Holladay JT. Consultations in refractive surgery. IOL calculations following radial keratotomy surgery. Refract Corneal Surg. 1989;5:203.

17. Celikkol L, Pavlopoulos G, Weinstein B, et al. Calculation of intraocular lens power after radial keratotomy with computerized videokeratography. Am J Ophthalmol. 1995;120:739–50.

18. Lyle WA, Jin GJ. Intraocular lens power prediction in patients who undergo cataract surgery following previous radial keratotomy. Arch Ophthalmol. 1997;115:457–61.

19. Wang L, Booth MA, Koch DD. Comparison of intraocular lens power calculations methods in eyes that have undergone LASIK. Ophthalmology. 2004;111:1825–31.

20. Shammas HJ, Shammas MC, Garabet A, et al. Correcting the corneal power measurements for intraocular lens power calculations after myo-

pic laser in situ keratomileusis. Am J Ophthalmol. 2003;136:426–32.

21. Rosa N, Capasso L, Romano A. A new method of calculating intraocular lens power after photorefractive keratectomy. J Refract Surg. 2002;18:720–4.

22. Haigis W. Intraocular lens calculation after refractive surgery for myopia: Haigis-L formula. J Cataract Refract Surg. 2008;34:1658–63.

23. Abulafia A, Hill WE, Koch DD, Wang L, Barrett GD. Accuracy of the Barrett True-K formula for intraocular lens power prediction after laser in situ keratomileusis or photorefractive keratectomy for myopia. J Cataract Refract Surg. 2016;42:363–9.

24. Randleman JB, Foster BJ, Loupe DN, et al. Intraocular lens power calculations after refractive surgery: consensus-K technique. J Cataract Refract Surg. 2007;33:1892–8.

25. Holladay JT, Hill WE, Steinmueller A. Corneal power measurements using Scheimpflug imaging in eyes with prior corneal refractive surgery. J Refract Surg. 2009;25:862–8.

26. Seo KY, Im CY, Yang H, et al. New equivalent keratometry reading calculation with a rotating Scheimpflug camera for intraocular lens power calculation after myopic corneal surgery. J Cataract Refract Surg. 2014;11:1834–42.

27. Savini G, Taroni L, Schiano-Lomoriello D, Hoffer KJ. Repeatability of total keratometry and standard keratometry by the IOLMaster 700 and comparison to total corneal astigmatism by Scheimpflug imaging. Eye. 35:307–15.

28. Lawless M, Jiang JY, Hodge C, Sutton G, Roberts TV, Barrett G. Total keratometry in intraocular lens power calculations in eyes with previous laser refractive surgery. Clin Exp Ophthalmol. 2020;48:749–56.

29. Sambare C, Naroo S, Shah S, et al. The AS biometry technique to aid accurate intraocular lens power calculation after corneal laser refractive surgery. Contact Lens Anterior Eye. 2006;29:81–3.

30. Walter KA, Gagnon MR, Hoopes PC, et al. Accurate intraocular lens power calculation alter myopic laser in situ keratomileusis, bypassing corneal power. J Cataract Refract Surg. 2006;32:425–9.

31. Savini G, Hoffer KJ, Barrett GD. Results of the Barrett True-K formula for IOL power calculation based on Scheimpflug camera measurements in eyes with previous myopic excimer laser surgery. J Cataract Refract Surg. 2020;46:1016–9.

32. Wang L, Tang M, Huang D, Weikert MP, Koch DD. Comparison of newer intraocular lens power calculation methods for eyes after corneal refractive surgery. Ophthalmology. 2015;122:2443–9.

33. Masket S, Masket SE. Simple regression formula for intraocular lens power adjustment in eyes requiring cataract surgery after excimer laser photoablation. J Cataract Refract Surg. 2006;32:430–4.

34. https://www.doctor-hill.com/iol-main/modified_masket_method.htm. Acceso on Jan 10, 2021.

35. Savini G, Barboni P, Carbonelli M, Ducoli P, Hoffer KJ. Intraocular lens power calculation after myopic excimer laser surgery: selecting the best method using available clinical data. J Cataract Refract Surg. 2015;41:1880–8.

36. McCarthy M, Gavanski GM, Paton KE, Holland SP. Intraocular lens power calculations after myopic laser refractive surgery: a comparison of methods in 173 eyes. Ophthalmology. 2011;118:940–4.

37. Savini G, Barboni P, Zanini M. Correlation between attempted correction and keratometric refractive index after myopic excimer laser surgery. J Refract Surg. 2007;23:461–6.

38. Savini G, Hoffer KJ, Barboni P, Balducci N, Schiano-Lomoriello D. Validation of the SToP formula for calculating intraocular lens power in eyes with previous myopic excimer laser surgery. J Cataract Refract Surg. 2019;45:1562–7.

39. Savini G, Hoffer KJ, Carbonelli M, Barboni P. Intraocular lens power calculation after myopic excimer laser surgery: clinical comparison of published methods. J Cataract Refract Surg. 2010;36:1455–65.

40. Camellin M, Calossi A. A new formula for intraocular lens power calculation after refractive corneal surgery. J Refract Surg. 2006;22:187–9.

41. Jarade EF, Abi Nader FC, Tabbara KF. Intraocular lens power calculation following LASIK: determination of the new effective index of refraction. J Refract Surg. 2006;22:75–80.

42. Seitz B, Langenbucher A. Intraocular lens power calculation in eyes after corneal refractive surgery. J Refract Surg. 2000;16:349–61.

43. Speicher L. Intra-ocular lens calculation status after corneal refractive surgery. Curr Opin Ophthalmol. 2001;12:17–29.

44. Savini G, Barboni P, Zanini M. Intraocular lens power calculation after myopic refractive surgery: theoretical comparison of different methods. Ophthalmology. 2006;113:1271–82.

45. Yeo K, Heng WJ, Pek D, Wong J, Fam HB. Accuracy of intraocular lens formulas using total keratometry in eyes with previous myopic laser refractive surgery. Eye (Lond). 2021;35(6):1705–11.

46. Whang WJ, Hoffer KJ, Kim SJ, Chung SSH, Savini G. Comparison of intraocular lens power formulas according to axial length after myopic corneal laser refractive surgery. J Cataract Refract Surg. 2021, 47(3):297–303.

47. Shammas HJ, Shammas MC. No-history method of intraocular lens power calculation for cataract surgery after myopic laser in situ keratomileusis. J Cataract Refract Surg. 2007;33:31–6.

48. Shammas HJ, Shammas MC, Hill WE. Intraocular lens power calculation in eyes with previous hyperopic laser in situ keratomileusis. J Cataract Refract Surg. 2013;39:739–44.

49. Savini G, Hoffer KJ, Schiano-Lomoriello D, Ducoli P. Estimating the preoperative corneal power with

Scheimpflug imaging in eyes that have undergone myopic LASIK. J Refract Surg. 2016;32:332–6.

50. Ianchulev T, Salz J, Hoffer K, et al. Intraoperative optical refractive biometry for intraocular lens power estimation without axial length and keratometry measurements. J Cataract Refract Surg. 2005;31:1530–6.

51. Ianchulev T, Hoffer KJ, Yoo SH, Chang DF, Breen M, Padrick T, Tran DB. Intraoperative refractive biometry for predicting intraocular lens power calculation after prior myopic refractive surgery. Ophthalmology. 2014;121:56–60.

52. Fram NR, Masket S, Wang L. Comparison of intraoperative aberrometry, OCT-based IOL formula, Haigis-L, and Masket formulae for IOL power calculation after laser vision correction. Ophthalmology. 2015;122:1096–101.

53. Srivannaboon S, Chirapapaisan C. Comparison of refractive outcomes using conventional keratometry or total keratometry for IOL power calculation in cataract surgery. Graefes Arch Clin Exp Ophthalmol. 2019;257:2677–82.

54. Wang L, Spektor T, de Souza RG, Koch DD. Evaluation of total keratometry and its accuracy for intraocular lens power calculation in eyes after corneal refractive surgery. J Cataract Refract Surg. 2019;45:1416–21.

55. Tang M, Li Y, Huang D. An intraocular lens power calculation formula based on optical coherence tomography: a pilot study. J Refract Surg. 2010;26:430–7.

56. Tang M, Wang L, Koch DD, Li Y, Huang D. Intraocular lens power calculation after previous myopic laser vision correction based on corneal power measured by Fourier-domain optical coherence tomography. J Cataract Refract Surg. 2012;38:589–94.

57. Savini G, Hoffer KJ, Schiano-Lomoriello D, Barboni P. Intraocular lens power calculation using a Placido disk-Scheimpflug tomographer in eyes that had previous myopic corneal excimer laser surgery. J Cataract Refract Surg. 2018;44(8):935–41.

58. Gjerdrum B, Gundersen KG, Lundmark PO, Aakre BM. Refractive precision of ray tracing IOL calculations based on OCT data versus traditional IOL calculation formulas based on reflectometry in patients with a history of laser vision correction for myopia. Clin Ophthalmol. 2021;15:845–57.

59. Olsen T, Hoffmann P. C constant: new concept for ray tracing-assisted intraocular lens power calculation. J Cataract Refract Surg. 2014;40:764–73.

60. Savini G, Bedei A, Barboni P, Ducoli P, Hoffer KJ. Intraocular lens power calculation by ray-tracing after myopic excimer laser surgery. Am J Ophthalmol. 2014;157:150–3.

61. Savini G, Barboni P, Carbonelli M, Hoffer KJ. Accuracy of a dual Scheimpflug analyzer and a corneal topography system for intraocular lens power calculation in unoperated eyes. J Cataract Refract Surg. 2011;37:72–6.

62. Savini G, Negishi K, Hoffer KJ, Schiano-Lomoriello D. Refractive outcomes of intraocular lens power calculation using different corneal power measurements with a new optical biometer. J Cataract Refract Surg. 2018;44:701–8.

63. Schuster AK, Schanzlin DJ, Thomas KE, Heichel CW, Purcell TL, Barker PD. Intraocular lens calculation adjustment after laser refractive surgery using Scheimpflug imaging. J Cataract Refract Surg. 2016;42:226–31.

64. Kim SH, Lee JH. Videokeratography to calculate intraocular lens power after radial keratotomy. J Refract Surg. 2004;20:284–6.

65. Awwad ST, Dwarakanathan S, Bowman W, et al. Intraocular lens power calculation after radial keratotomy: estimating the corneal power. J Cataract Refract Surg. 2007;33:1045–50.

66. Potvin R, Hill W. New algorithm for post-radial keratotomy intraocular lens power calculations based on rotating Scheimpflug camera data. J Cataract Refract Surg. 2013;39(3):358–65.

67. Ma JX, Tang M, Wang L, Weikert MP, Huang D, Koch DD. Comparison of newer IOL power calculation methods for eyes with previous radial keratotomy. Invest Ophthalmol Vis Sci. 2016;57(9):OCT162–8.

68. Curado SX, Hida WT, Vilar CMC, Ordones VL, Chaves MAP, Tzelikis PF. Intraoperative aberrometry versus preoperative biometry for IOL power selection after radial keratotomy: a prospective study. J Refract Surg. 2019;35:656–61.

69. Turnbull AMJ, Crawford GJ, Barrett GD. Methods for intraocular lens power calculation in cataract surgery after radial keratotomy. Ophthalmology. 2020;127(1):45–51.

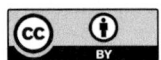

66

IOL Power Calculation in Keratoconus

Jack X Kane

Keratoconus is a progressive disorder characterised by central or paracentral corneal thinning and ectasia. The changes in the keratoconic cornea affect multiple aspects of IOL power calculation and keratoconus remains one of the last major challenges existing in IOL power calculation. There are several factors which, when combined, lead to inaccurate results including the following:

1. **Corneal Power Measurement Issues**

   The keratometry value that is displayed on biometry devices is based on an assumed ratio of the anterior to the posterior cornea. For most eyes, this anterior-to-posterior ratio remains reasonably accurate; however, in keratoconus, this is not the case. The change in shape of the cornea means that the assumed ratio is incorrect which leads to an incorrect keratometry value as "measured" by corneal biometry.

   Additionally, biometry devices have difficulty in producing repeatable measurements of keratoconic corneas which worsens with the degree of keratoconus [1].

2. **IOL Formula Calculation Errors**

   The error in the keratometry values in keratoconus patients is propagated in two ways in the majority of IOL formulas. Most formulas use keratometry values as one of the factors in predicting the effective lens position (ELP), and hence, any error in keratometry leads to an error in the ELP. Given the importance of ELP to IOL power calculation, this leads to significant errors.

   Additionally, the keratometry error is also included in the vergence/thick lens equation, so even if the ELP is calculated entirely independently of the keratometry value, the remainder of the equation will still require use of the erroneous keratometry, thus leading to errors in IOL power calculation.

3. **Difficulty in Refraction**

   Keratoconus patients are notoriously difficult to refract with a study showing a 6× higher difference in test-retest refractions in keratoconus patients compared to normal myopes [2]. This difficulty in refraction makes it difficult to create keratoconus specific adjustments for IOL formulas as the target is not as well defined as in other difficult-to-predict conditions such as post-LASIK.

4. **Other Issues**

   Other issues which contribute to the lack of understanding on IOL power calculation in keratoconus include small sample sizes of published studies and difficulty defining which patients have true keratoconus rather than form fruste keratoconus.

J. X. Kane (✉)
Northern Health Ophthalmology,
Melbourne, VIC, Australia

© The Author(s) 2024
J. Aramberri et al. (eds.), *Intraocular Lens Calculations*, Essentials in Ophthalmology,
https://doi.org/10.1007/978-3-031-50666-6_66

Approaches to IOL Power Calculation in Keratoconus

The significant barriers to accuracy in keratoconus patients, poor understanding on how to conduct IOL power studies, and small patient sample sizes have limited the refractive outcomes in keratoconus patients.

Keratoconus leads to a hyperopic prediction error which has been well established in studies by Watson et al. [3] and Hashemi et al. [1] However, these early studies into IOL power calculation often had significant issues such as measuring with a mixture of optical biometry, contact ultrasound, and immersion ultrasound or calculating the prediction error using target refraction rather than the predicted refraction for each formula. Although the issues with keratoconus patients were somewhat understood, the evidence available to guide decision making was lacking—the general consensus being to use the SRK II or SRK/T [4] and to use standard keratometry values if the average corneal power became too excessive [3]. The introduction of clear guidelines and detailed instruction on how to properly conduct an IOL power study [5] as well as the widened availability of optical biometry and increased availability of larger datasets from electronic medical record systems has allowed researchers to significantly improve our understanding of keratoconus patients including which IOL power formula is the most accurate in these patients.

The first paper in keratoconus patients to follow the correct guidelines on IOL power calculation studies was done by Savini et al. in JCRS [6]. They used optical biometry in 41 eyes of 41 patients and demonstrated that the SRK/T formula was the most accurate of all formulas and that there was no additional benefit of using the Barrett Universal 2 formula in keratoconus patients. The study additionally splits patients into the Krumeich classification based on average keratometry (stage 1: less than or equal to 48.0 dioptres [D]; stage 2: 48.01–53.0 D, and stage 3: greater than 53 D). This split was used in early studies [3] and has continued to be used in the largest keratoconus IOL power studies. Savini

demonstrated that the amount of hyperopic error worsened with the stage of keratoconus (+0.44 D in stage 1 up to +3.01 D in stage 3 for the SRK/T formula) and that the accuracy of IOL power calculation worsened with an increasing stage of keratoconus (the SRK/T having 61.9% within 0.50 D in stage 1, 30.8% in stage 2, and 14.3% in stage 3, whereas the Barrett had 42.9% in stage 1, 15% in stage 2, and 0% in stage 3).

Another recent paper by Wang et al. [7] in the AJO in 73 eyes of 73 patients confirmed these initial results found by Savini. The hyperopic errors worsened with the stage of keratoconus (+0.12 for stage 1 to +2.51 for stage 3 when using the SRK/T formula). They used the same classification system as Savini; however, in stage 1 and 2 patients, they found that the Barrett was more accurate than the SRK/T. In stage 3 patients, they were unable to calculate many patients using the Barrett as the keratometry values exceeded the limits of the online calculator. The SRK/T was more accurate than the other formulas studied. Again, the accuracy of the formulas worsened with increasing keratoconus (48% within 0.50 D in stage 1; 18% in stage 2; and 0% in stage 3 for the SRK/T formula).

New Methods for IOL Power Calculation in Keratoconus

Although the issues with IOL power calculation in keratoconus have been known for a long time, only very recently specific adjustments to IOL formulas have been made to improve results. This is a significant contrast to post-refractive IOL formulas of which there are numerous.

The Kane keratoconus formula utilises modified anterior corneal radii of curvature that better represents the true anterior/posterior ratio in keratoconic eyes while also minimising the effect of corneal power on the ELP calculation. It works using standard IOLMaster biometry and requires only the variables used in the standard Kane formula (AL, K, ACD and patient gender with optional variables LT and CCT). The Kane keratoconus formula is designed to be used with the same IOL constant, given the impossibility of a surgeon obtaining a large enough sample of post-operative eyes with keratoconus for a specific IOL to perform optimisation.

This formula was first presented at the 15th IPC meeting in Napa with an article in *Ophthalmology* in 2020 [8]. This article described the largest cohort of keratoconus patients with 146 eyes of 146 patients who all had IOLMaster biometry. This study confirmed the findings of Savini et al. [6] and Wang et al. [7] with hyperopic refractive errors that worsened with the stage of keratoconus for the conventional formulas. The paper demonstrated the similar performance of the SRK/T and the Barrett Universal 2 in keratoconus patients with no significant difference found between the SRK/T and the Barrett in this patient population. The study found that the SRK/T (but not the Barrett) was better than all other conventional formulas studied. The Kane keratoconus formula had the best results achieving 8.3% more patients within 0.50 than the SRK/T and 7.1% more within 0.50 D than the Barrett in stage 1 eyes. In stage 2, it demonstrated as additional 5.4% for Barrett and 13.5% for SRK/T within 0.50 D. In stage 3 eyes, it achieved 20% more within 0.50 D compared with the Barrett and 12% more than the SRK/T. In stage 3,

it had 32% more within 1.00 D compared with the Barrett and 28% more than the SRK/T. The study demonstrated a slight hyperopic refractive surprise in stage 2 patients +0.53 D but no significant hyperopic refractive surprise in stage 3 patients (+0.02 D for the Kane keratoconus formula compared with +1.72 D for Barrett and +1.86 D for the SRK/T) (Fig. 66.1).

The Barrett True K formula for keratoconus was first published in 2021. The formula incorporates the posterior corneal power and central corneal thickness to improve post-operative prediction in keratoconus. The formula uses the posterior corneal astigmatism either predicted or measured if available. There is only one study on the accuracy of the formula by Ton and Barrett et al. [9] in JCRS which used 32 eyes of 23 patients. The Barrett True-K formula for keratoconus was created based on some of the cases that were used in this study which makes it difficult to accurately assess the results of the study for the Barrett True-K formula for keratoconus. As expected, the study demonstrated good results with Barrett True K formula for keratoconus with 96.9% of patients within 1.00 D with the predicted PCA. The Barrett True-K formula for keratoconus with measured PCA and Kane

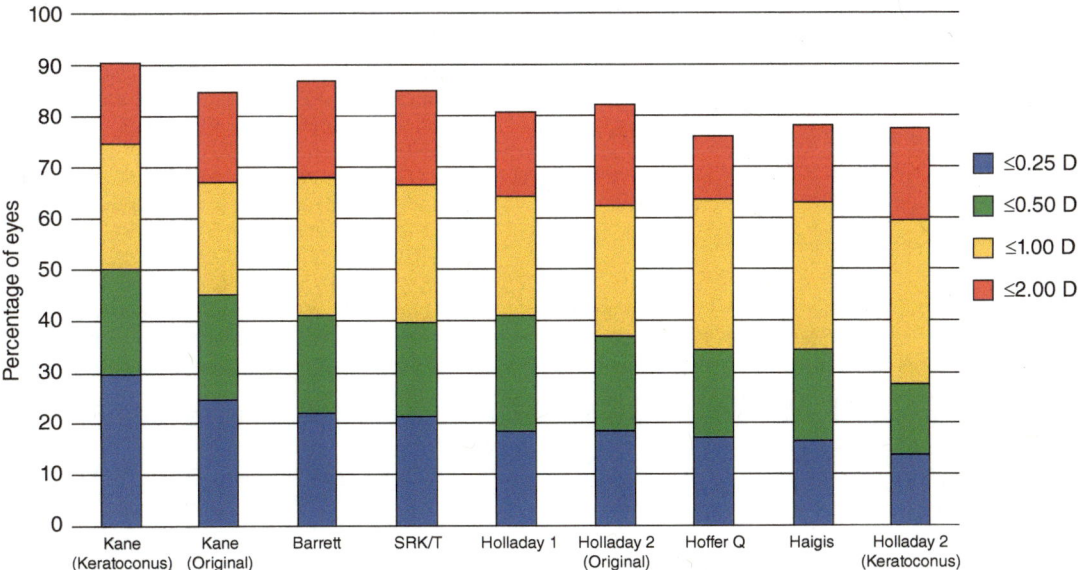

Fig. 66.1 Stacked histograms comparing the percentage of cases within a given diopter range of predicted spherical equivalent refraction outcome for the entire data set (adapted from Kane et al. [8] with permission)

keratoconus formula has the same number of eyes within 1.00 D (90.6%). The number of patients in the study was inadequate to allow subgroup analysis. Excluding the Barrett True-K formula (which was created using some of the patients in the study), the Kane keratoconus formula had the lowest standard deviation, lowest MAE, and the mean error closest to zero confirming the findings of the largest keratoconus IOL power study. The study included eight eyes with an average keratometry reading over 48 D. Comparing the Kane versus the Kane keratoconus formula in these eyes showed a reduction in the mean absolute error from 1.54 for the original Kane formula to 0.54 D for the Kane keratoconus formula as well as change from a high hyperopic prediction error +1.11 D to a low myopic prediction error −0.15 D.

Conclusion

After many years of little progress in IOL power calculation in keratoconus, attention in this important field has now increased. For surgeons aiming to select a target refraction for their keratoconus patient, Table 66.1 can give guidance on the appropriate refractive aim for the three most accurate IOL formulas for keratoconus patients to reduce the risk of an undesirable hyperopic refractive outcome. A myopic refractive outcome is preferred especially if the patient will require a contact lens as a myopic lens has greater flexibility in terms of vault and lens diameter compared with hyperopic lenses. The Kane keratoconus formula should be used in keratoconus patients with

Table 66.1 Refractive aim based on average keratometry to avoid hyperopic refractive surprise for the 3 most accurate IOL formulas in keratoconus

	≤48 D	48–53 D	53–59 D	>59 D
Kane keratoconus formula	Plano	−0.50 DS	−1.00 DS	−1.50 to 2.00 DS
Barrett		−0.50 DS	−1.00 DS	−2.50 DS	−3.00 to 4.00 DS
SRK/T		−0.50 DS	−1.00 DS	−2.50 DS	−3.00 to 4.00 DS

either the Barrett or SRK/T formulas being the next most accurate. There is currently not enough available evidence to recommend the Barrett True-K formula for keratoconus. The management of patient expectation should be central to the informed consent of these patients and reasonable figures to discuss with patients (when using the Kane keratoconus formula) are: 60% within 0.50 D if the average keratometry is <48 dioptres; 40% if the average keratometry is 48–53; and 25% if the average keratometry is >53 D.

References

1. Hashemi H, Yekta A, Khabazkhoob M. Effect of keratoconus grades on repeatability of keratometry readings: comparison of 5 devices. J Cataract Refract Surg. 2015;41(5):1065–72. https://doi.org/10.1016/j.jcrs.2014.08.043.
2. Raasch TW, Schechtman KB, Davis LJ, Zadnik K. Repeatability of subjective refraction in myopic and keratoconic subjects: results of vector analysis. Ophthalmic Physiol Opt. 2001;21(5):376–83. https://doi.org/10.1046/j.1475-1313.2001.00596.x.
3. Watson MP, Anand S, Bhogal M, et al. Cataract surgery outcome in eyes with keratoconus. Br J Ophthalmol. 2014;98(3):361–4. https://doi.org/10.1136/bjophthalmol-2013-303829.
4. Kamiya K, Iijima K, Nobuyuki S, et al. Predictability of intraocular lens power calculation for cataract with keratoconus: a multicenter study. Sci Rep. 2018;8(1):1312. https://doi.org/10.1038/s41598-018-20040-w.
5. Hoffer KJ, Aramberri J, Haigis W, et al. Protocols for studies of intraocular lens formula accuracy. Am J Ophthalmol. 2015;160(3):403–405.e1. https://doi.org/10.1016/j.ajo.2015.05.029.
6. Savini G, Abbate R, Hoffer KJ, et al. Intraocular lens power calculation in eyes with keratoconus. J Cataract Refract Surg. 2019;45(5):576–81. https://doi.org/10.1016/j.jcrs.2018.11.029.
7. Wang KM, Jun AS, Ladas JG, Siddiqui AA, Woreta F, Srikumaran D. Accuracy of intraocular lens formulas in eyes with keratoconus. Am J Ophthalmol. 2020;212:26–33. https://doi.org/10.1016/j.ajo.2019.11.019.
8. Kane JX, Connell B, Yip H, et al. Accuracy of intraocular lens power formulas modified for patients with keratoconus. Ophthalmology. 2020;127(8):1037–42. https://doi.org/10.1016/j.ophtha.2020.02.008.
9. Ton Y, Barrett GD, Kleinmann G, Levy A, Assia EI. Toric intraocular lens power calculation in cataract patients with keratoconus. J Cataract Refract Surg. 2021;47(11):1389–97. https://doi.org/10.1097/j.jcrs.0000000000000638.

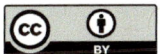

Patient-Specific Eye Models for Intraocular Lens Power Calculation in Irregular Corneas

67

Pablo Pérez-Merino

Cataract surgery is the most common procedure performed by the ophthalmic surgeon, with more than nine million procedures executed annually worldwide. The exceptional collection of high-resolution imaging techniques to acquire precise biometric data along with the constant improvement of intraocular lens (IOL) power formulas has clearly enhanced the prediction of the refractive outcome. Although paraxial-based formulas typically offer the desired emmetropic results for patients with regular corneal surfaces and average ocular dimensions (22.5–25.5 mm of axial length), they have their own downfalls in patients with an abnormal corneal topography, such as keratoconus or eyes with previous corneal refractive surgery.

The irregular corneal surface pattern in keratoconus and the reshaping of the corneal surface after corneal refractive surgery (1) modifies the anterior-posterior corneal ratio and (2) induces significant amounts of corneal high-order aberrations (mainly, vertical coma—in keratoconus—and spherical aberration—after corneal refractive surgery). This introduces a source of error in the corneal power data input and an incorrect effective lens position (ELP) prediction for the IOL power calculation, producing a post-operative refractive surprise in most cases. Therefore, there is considerable debate about which IOL power formula and methodology match the refractive prediction in these scenarios.

The Current Landscape for IOL Power Calculation in Keratoconus

Keratoconus derives from the Greek words *Kerato* (cornea) and *Konos* (cone), and it is caused by the progressive and asymmetric weakening of the corneal tissue, in which gradual thinning lead to a cone-like appearance of the cornea, manifesting irregular astigmatism, myopia, and high levels of high-order aberrations. Symptoms of keratoconus vary and depend on its stage: from forme fruste keratoconus, with very little visual impact, to advanced stages, in which the distorted corneal surfaces severely increase astigmatism and high-order aberrations [1–7]. For these patients, cataract surgery planning presents innumerable challenges in IOL calculation due to the abnormal corneal curvature, the irregular surface pattern, an unusual anterior chamber depth, a longer axial length, and the option to combine the cataract surgery with other corneal treatments that stabilize or delay the progression of keratoconus (e.g., intracorneal ring segments [ICRS] or corneal cross-linking).

Previous studies showed that IOL power calculation in eyes with keratoconus is considerably

P. Pérez-Merino (✉)
Centre for Microsystems Technology, Ghent University and imec, Ghent, Belgium
e-mail: pablo.perezmerino@ugent.be

© The Author(s) 2024
J. Aramberri et al. (eds.), *Intraocular Lens Calculations*, Essentials in Ophthalmology,
https://doi.org/10.1007/978-3-031-50666-6_67

Table 67.1 Refractive prediction error in eyes with three stages of keratoconus

| Formula | Mean prediction error ± standard deviation (range) | | |
	Stage I	Stage II	Stage III
Barret	+0.63 ± 0.86 (−0.91, +2.23)	+1.32 ± 2.00 (−3.47, +5.09)	+2.64 ± 2.14 (−0.79, +6.28)
Haigis	+0.54 ± 0.79 (−0.61, +2.25)	+1.66 ± 2.05 (−2.97, +5.69)	+3.26 ± 2.38 (−0.62, +7.17)
Holladay 1	+0.75 ± 0.83 (−0.55, +2.58)	+1.54 ± 2.52 (−3.70, +3.17)	+3.77 ± 2.48 (−0.27, +7.50)
Hoffer Q	+0.90 ± 0.85 (−0.59, +2.47)	+1.63 ± 2.17 (−2.97, +6.23)	+3.46 ± 2.29 (−0.38, +6.78)
SRK/T	+0.44 ± 0.79 (−0.55, +2.32)	+0.54 ± 2.40 (−4.40, +6.09)	+3.01 ± 2.97 (−1.35, +7.17)

less accurate than for patients with regular corneal surfaces and average ocular dimensions [8–13]. In two recent publications comprising a sufficient number of series of eyes, Kamiya et al. [12] and Savini et al. [13] compared the accuracy of different conventional IOL formulas: Barret Universal 2, Haigis, Holladay 1, Hoffer Q, and SRK/T. Both studies reported that the tested formulas resulted in a hyperopic refractive outcome and found that the SRK/T was the most accurate formula with 36% and 43.9% of eyes within 0.5 diopters (D) of the final predicted refraction, respectively. However, these outcomes were much lower than that reported for normal eyes (with 75% [14] and 83% [15] of eyes within 0.5 D) and worsened noticeably in advanced stages of the disease, as we can observe in Table 67.1 (reproduced from Savini et al. [13]).

The SRK/T formula showed the highest accuracy for refractive prediction error in early and moderate stages compared with the other conventional IOL formulas; however, the post-operative refractive error was manifestly unpredictable in advanced stages for all the analyzed approaches. Melles et al. [14] described a tendency of the SRK/T formula towards myopic prediction errors with higher corneal powers in non-keratoconus eyes. This phenomenon might counterbalance the hyperopic tendency observed in early and moderate keratoconic stages (stages I and II), where the amount of high-order aberrations is relatively low; however, the refractive prediction with the SRK/T clearly failed in eyes with a higher magnitude of corneal aberrations, as keratoconic corneas in stage III, indicating that most of the assumptions made during calculations with the formula might not be valid in eyes with keratoconus and high levels of corneal aberrations.

To improve the refractive prediction in these patients, two formulas have developed specific adjustments: Kane keratoconus [16] and Holladay 2 with keratoconus adjustment [17]. The Kane keratoconus formula focuses on reducing the influence of corneal power on ELP prediction, whereas the Holladay 2 keratoconus aims to differentiate a steep keratometry reading and a small anterior segment from a patient with keratoconus, presumably to ensure that the ELP is not too affected by the high corneal power reading. Although the Kane keratoconus formula resulted in more accurate predictions compared with the Holladay 2 with keratoconus adjustment (50%-Kane vs. 27.4%-Holladay of eyes within 0.5 D), the predictability of the formula is still lower compared with patients without keratoconus and needs further refinement for IOL power calculation in keratoconus eyes, particularly in moderate and advanced stages with high levels of corneal aberrations.

IOL Power Calculation After Keratoplasty (Penetrating or Posterior Lamellar)

As in keratoconus, post-penetrating keratoplasty and posterior lamellar keratoplasty eyes are frequently associated with high refractive errors due to regular or irregular graft astigmatism and high levels of corneal aberrations, coupled with uncertain posterior corneal values and a relevant change in the anterior to posterior corneal curvature ratio [18–20]. Therefore, high unpredictability and a hyperopic refractive surprise are expected using the traditional formulas for IOL power calculation, with the SRK/T formula showing the best refractive prediction.

Present-Day Strategies for IOL Power Calculation After Corneal Refractive Surgery

The IOL power calculation after corneal refractive surgery also represents an on-going concern for surgeons and is specially challenging because the ablation profile in laser-assisted in situ keratomileusis (LASIK) or photorefractive keratectomy (PRK) modifies the anterior corneal surface (modifying the normal anterior to posterior curvature ratio) [21], changes its asphericity (e.g., more oblate cornea in a myopic treatment) [22] and induces different amounts of corneal high-order aberrations (e.g., spherical aberration) [23, 24]. In general, there are three major sources of error for the patients who have had LASIK or PRK for the treatment of myopia or hyperopia: (1) corneal power measurement, (2) keratometric index, and (3) ELP estimation [25, 26]. Actually, the proportion of eyes within 0.5 D of the final manifest refraction calculated with traditional IOL formulas (e.g., Haigis [27], Hoffer Q [28], or SRK/T [29]) was categorically low, ranging between 8.1 and 40.3% and showing again a post-operative hyperopia as a norm [26].

Therefore, numerous calculation methods, recommendations (e.g., the American Society of Cataract and Refractive Surgery (ASCRS) IOL calculation website), and modifications in the formulas have been introduced in the last years to compensate the source of errors in surgically modified eyes with LASIK or PRK. They can be classified based on a priori knowledge: (1) pre-refractive surgery keratometry and the change in the manifest refraction (pre-refractive vs. post-refractive): for example, Feiz-Mannis [30] or corneal bypass [31]; (2) change in the manifest refraction (pre-refractive vs. post-refractive): Adjusted EffRP [32], Masket's [33] and Barret True K [34], among others; and (3) no historical clinical data: Shammas [35], Awwad [36], Potvin-Hill [37], Wang-Koch-Maloney [38], Haigis-L [39], Barret True K no history or derived methods from specific equipment (e.g., Optovue RTVue and Oculus pentacam HR) [26], among others.

The methods that use pre-refractive surgery keratometry showed the poorest outcomes, with 26–44% of eyes within 0.5 D of target and significant variability; whereas, the Barret True K demonstrated the highest performance of the methods that only require the change in the manifest refraction before and after corneal refractive surgery, with 67.4% falling within 0.5 D of the final manifest refraction. The online ASCRS calculator includes most of the no historical clinical data formulas and allows simultaneous calculation using multiple formulas [40]. For example, averaging three of the included formulas (Barret True K no history, Haigis-L, and OCT-RTVue), the ASCRS calculator showed that the proportion of eyes within 0.5 D was 65.4%. Although the Barret True K and the ASCRS website meet the standards of the British National Health Service (55–85% of eyes within 0.5 D and 1.0 D, respectively) [41], the predictability of these formulas is still lower than that of an IOL power calculation for a normal eye with regular corneas and there is real need of prospective studies with larger sample sizes ($n > 40$) [26] .

Behind the Need for Change in Odd-Corneas: Three-Dimensional Corneal Shape

Corneal power is a critical variable for IOL power calculation. The options for its estimation have progressed from keratometers to topographic methods using "correction" factors of the cornea to account for the contribution of the posterior corneal curvature. On average, the radius of the curvature has a magnitude of 7.8 mm and 6.5 mm for the anterior and posterior corneal surfaces, respectively. Assuming the cornea as a single refractive surface with the anterior corneal radius and the keratometric index ($n = 1.3375$), the K-reading for a 7.8 mm radius would be 43.27 D. However, although the anterior corneal surface supposes the dominant factor to corneal power, the posterior cornea also has a remarkable implication. Thus, considering the refractive index of the cornea ($n = 1.376$), the dioptric power of the corneal surfaces would be 48.20 D (anterior) and −6.15 D (posterior) with a total corneal power of 42.05 D; therefore, it shows a refractive discrepancy of about 1.2 D with the value obtained from the common keratometer index .

In addition, these average values (7.8 mm and 6.5 mm for the anterior and posterior corneal surfaces, respectively) show a ratio between surfaces of approximately 1.2. But, this ratio is not constant along the corneal radius range of an average eye with regular surfaces (7.5–8.0 mm: anterior surface; 5.9–6.7 mm: posterior surface) and can vary between 1.11 and 1.35 [42]. This variability is even greater in patients with keratoconus and patients with surgically modified corneas, in which there is an abnormal curvature and an irregular corneal pattern. In most keratoconic patients, the corneal topography map is characterized by focal steepening (the cone vertex is typically displaced toward the lower midperipheral region), and there is usually a vertical asymmetry with a certain diagonal angle, resulting in irregular astigmatism and a high magnitude of high-order aberrations (in particular, vertical coma) [1, 2, 6, 7, 43]. While the ablation profile in standard refractive surgery modifies the topographic pattern and induces a shift in the anterior corneal asphericity, toward more positive values after myopic ablation and more negative values after hyperopic ablation and the consequence of higher corneal spherical aberration (increased positive spherical aberration, in myopia correction; increased negative spherical aberration, in hyperopia correction) [22–24, 44, 45]. Figure 67.1 shows an illustration of the anterior and posterior surface pattern for a normal cornea with astigmatism, a post-LASIK cornea and a keratoconic cornea .

There is evidence that the topography pattern (toricity, asphericity, and irregularities; i.e., astigmatism, spherical aberration, and non-rotationally symmetric high-order aberrations) of both corneal surfaces, anterior and posterior, influences the refractive outcomes in the IOL power calculation [43–47]. Therefore, it is expected that the customization for the exact IOL power in all these scenarios could benefit from the inclusion of the anterior and posterior elevation corneal data in the calculation methods, instead of simplified corneal parameters such as the corneal power with their innumerable assumptions .

To date, there is a huge variety of commercial systems to measure corneal topography that can be classified based on the imaging principle: specular reflection, scattered light, Scheimpflug imaging, and optical coherence tomography (OCT) [48]. Scheimpflug and OCT are the only imaging techniques that generate true elevation points with micron-resolution of both corneal surfaces, anterior and posterior [3, 49–51]. Figure 67.2 shows an illustration of three-dimensional OCT corneal analysis and representation.

Assuming that the corneal surface is given by $z = f(x,y)$ in a Cartesian system with first and second derivatives continuous at any point, there are three ways of representing corneal topography [52]:

Fig. 67.1 Anterior and posterior corneal surface pattern for a normal cornea with regular astigmatism, a post-LASIK cornea with higher amounts of spherical aberration and a keratoconic cornea with irregular surfaces and higher levels of astigmatism and high-order aberrations (*denotes the different vertex locations in the posterior corneal surface)

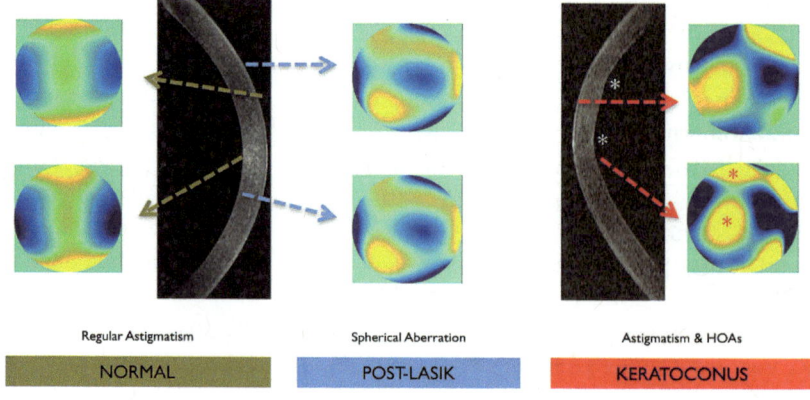

Fig. 67.2 Illustration of the OCT segmentation process and calculation of the topographic map from direct subtraction of the elevation data minus the best fitted-sphere

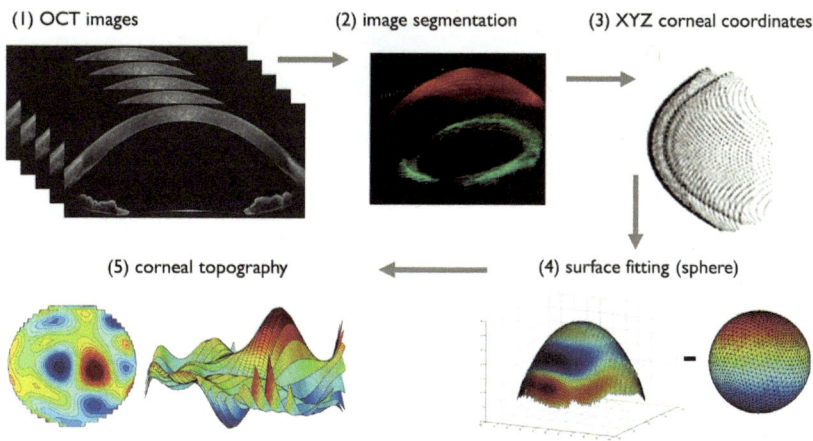

(1) OCT images

(2) image segmentation

(3) XYZ corneal coordinates

(5) corneal topography

(4) surface fitting (sphere)

- By *surface elevation f(x,y)* with respect to a reference surface (e.g., sphere). A typical reference sphere is one with the minimum standard deviation with respect to the corneal surface and with the same optical axis. The best-fit sphere to evaluate the topography of the cornea is calculated using a least squares method.
- By *local slopes* with respect to the reference sphere, since at any point on the surface, the slope is a function of the direction.
- By *local curvature*, for a given point, there is a maximum value in a certain direction and a minimum value in the perpendicular direction.

The corneal surface data is commonly expressed in Euclidean coordinates, and it is fitted by standard functions: sphere (from the sphere we obtain the radius and the center of the sphere), ellipsoid (from the ellipsoid we obtain three radii of curvature and the center of the ellipsoid), conicoid (the fitting parameters of the conicoid are the radius and the conic constant), or Zernike polynomial expansions (note that these are fits to surface elevations, not corneal wave aberrations).

Patient-Specific IOL Power Calculation: Ray Tracing

Patient-specific IOL selection by virtual ray-tracing eye modeling is gaining awareness amongst IOL manufacturing companies and the ophthalmology community since this methodology:

1. Exploits the complete information of the corneal topography for IOL power calculation, considering the anterior and posterior surface pattern of the cornea (XYZ surface coordinates or Zernike polynomial expansions of the anterior and posterior surfaces) instead of simplified corneal parameters
2. Allows realistic individual simulations of defocus, astigmatism, and high-order aberrations and any associated change in retinal image quality, i.e., influence of patient's corneal topography (avoiding, for example, the keratometry error of an aspheric cornea), IOL design (monofocal, toric, and multifocal), IOL positioning (including tolerance to tilt and decentration), impact of the corneal incision, decentered pupil, and foveal misalignment

Geometric optics assumes that the wavelength of the light is sufficiently small, so light propagation can be described in terms of rays and it is calculated by applying the Snell's law. Analyzing the optical system by tracing many rays through multiple analytical surfaces is therefore known as ray tracing, and in terms of geometrical optics every deviation from a perfect optical system can be quantified as optical aberrations.

Most of the current generic eye modeling requires the assistance of ray tracing computational programs, optical optimization by integrating a merit function in order to approach the specific targets (e.g., best focal position and optical quality metrics) and the definition of different

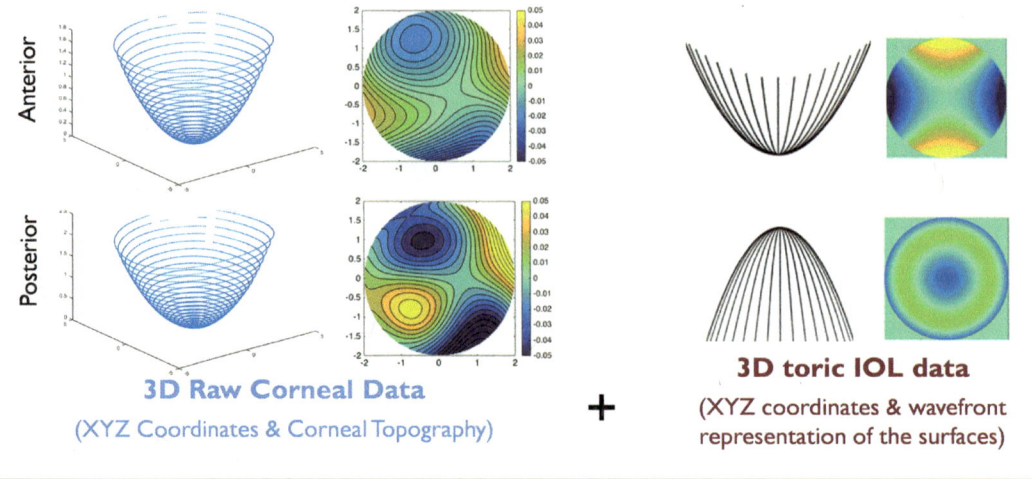

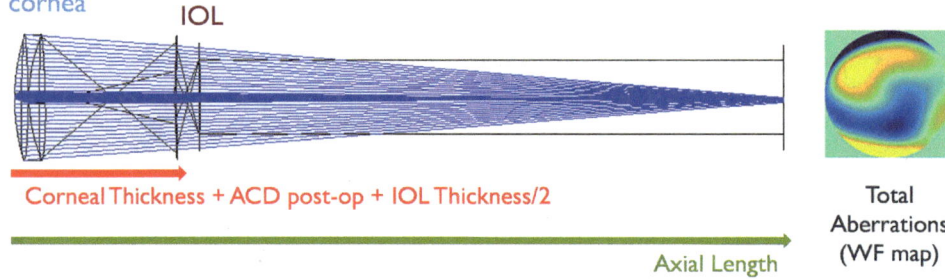

Fig. 67.3 Ray-tracing personalized eye model in ZEMAX. Three-dimensional corneal (Sirius, CSO, Firenze, Italy) and IOL data (Precizon Toric, OPHTEC BV, Groningen, The Netherlands)

variables: (1) position of the object point, (2) position and shape of the image surface (normally a plane), (3) stop surface and diameter, which defines the entrance-exit pupil size and position, and (4) wavelength. The most common programs to generate ray-tracing eye models are as follows: ZEMAX (Radiant ZEMAX; Focus software, Tucson, AZ), Code V (Optical Research Associates, Pasadena, CA), ASAP (Breault Research Organization, Inc., Tucson, AZ) and OSLO (Lambda Research Corporation, Littleton, MA) [46, 53–62]. Furthermore, examples of ray tracing modules for IOL power calculation found on commercially available corneal topographers are Olsen's PhacoOptics (IOL Innovations ApS, Aarhus, Denmark) and Okulix (Okulix, Dortmund, Germany). In these modules, following determination of the anterior and posterior corneal surfaces, thicknesses and refractive indices, the IOL is mod-

elled to determine the effective focal length that matches the axial length, i.e., the IOL power and cylinder is calculated to minimize the refractive error (with zero defocus and astigmatism as the final refractive target) [63]. Figure 67.3 illustrates the computation of ocular aberrations in the pseudophakic eye model using ZEMAX.

One key issue is the ELP, a very sensitive variable in IOL selection and also challenging to precisely estimate from the data of pre-operative measurements [64]. Most of paraxial-based IOL power formulas typically correlated the ELP with one or more pre-surgery biometry measurements, including anterior chamber depth (ACD), anterior corneal curvature, and axial length. However, these parameters are unrelated to the crystalline lens, and therefore, some uncertainty in the prediction is expected, since the IOL position will depend on the individual shrinkage of the capsular bag.

Recent improvements in biometry imaging techniques and image processing tools for accurate three-dimensional quantification of the anterior segment, especially with OCT technology in the spectral domain configuration, have opened the possibility of considering different crystalline lens variables [65–68]. Latest ELP approaches included three-dimensional crystalline lens parameters (lens volume, surface area, diameter, and equatorial plane position) and found in the pre- and postoperative measurements a strong correlation between the geometry of the crystalline lens and the IOL position [69]. Therefore, it would be possible to create patient-specific eye models (i.e., anterior and posterior corneal topography, accurate axial distances, IOL nominal values, and ray tracing) that include an accurate ELP based on the pre-operative shape of the crystalline lens.

Redefining the Refractive Target: Matching the Ideal IOL in Keratoconus and Surgically Modified Patients

To date, IOL power calculation methodologies, including ray tracing, estimate the IOL power by minimizing the refractive error, with zero defocus and astigmatism as the optimum postoperative target in all the scenarios. However, it has been demonstrated that the optical quality could be improved by adding certain amounts of spherical aberration to a given level of defocus, as well as specific amounts of astigmatism and coma can interact favourably to increase the visual performance (Fig. 67.4) [70–72]. As a consequence, the contribution of spherical aberration, coma, and other high-order aberrations to the target refraction needs to be considered.

Therefore, a specific magnitude of defocus and astigmatism in combination with the natural corneal high-order aberrations might improve the visual performance and enhance the prediction of the refractive outcome. Under this premise, the online calculator *https://www.exactiol.com* proposes a novel methodology for a patient-specific IOL selection based on exact ray tracing, simulated visual performance at different light conditions and through-focus optimization. The program uses the anterior and posterior corneal elevation maps and artificial neural networks to accurately calculate the IOL power and cylinder.

The results of the exactiol calculator in different group of patients are shown in the following figures (Figs. 67.5, 67.6, 67.7, and 67.8). Figure 67.5 illustrates the simulated visual performance (Snellen E letter) of a patient with keratoconus (Fig. 67.5a) and two post-LASIK patients (Fig. 67.5b, myopic-LASIK; Fig. 67.5c, hyperopic-LASIK). This figure shows the visual performance for a 4-mm pupil diameter in (1) the pre-operative condition with the values of astigmatism, spherical and high-order aberrations of the cornea: −4.5D at 85 degrees of astigmatism, −0.24 µm of spherical aberrations and the root mean square of high-order aberrations (RMS HOAs) of 0.53 µm (keratoconus); −1.00D at 120 degrees of astigmatism, +0.20 µm of spherical aberrations and the RMS HOAs of 0.42 µm (post-LASIK myopia); −0.75D at 120 degrees of astigmatism, −0.05 µm of spherical aberrations and the RMS HOAs of 0.28 µm (post-LASIK hyperopia). (2) Zero defocus and astigmatism in combination with the natural corneal aberrations. (3) The ideal defocus and astigmatism for this amount of high-order corneal aberrations: +1.5D −0.75D at 125° (keratoconus); −1.25D −0.75D at 180° (post-LASIK myopia); +0.25D −0.50 D at 160 degrees (post-LASIK hyperopia). As we can see, there is an ideal combination of defocus and astigmatism that produces the highest visual performance.

Specifically, plotting the through-focus curve in the representative keratoconus example (Fig. 67.6), we appreciate the visual benefit of the optimization process in which a certain magnitude of defocus and astigmatism lead to an increase in peak Visual Strehl values. For this example, the comparison of the traditional formula SRK/T vs. exactiol showed a difference in power and cylinder in the final IOL calculation of 1D, in power, and 1D −5°, in cylinder (SRK/T: Power: 14D; cylinder: 5.5D at 85°. Exactiol: Power: 13D; cylinder: 6.5D at 80°).

In Fig. 67.7, we can see how eyes with low visual quality have most to gain in terms of visual

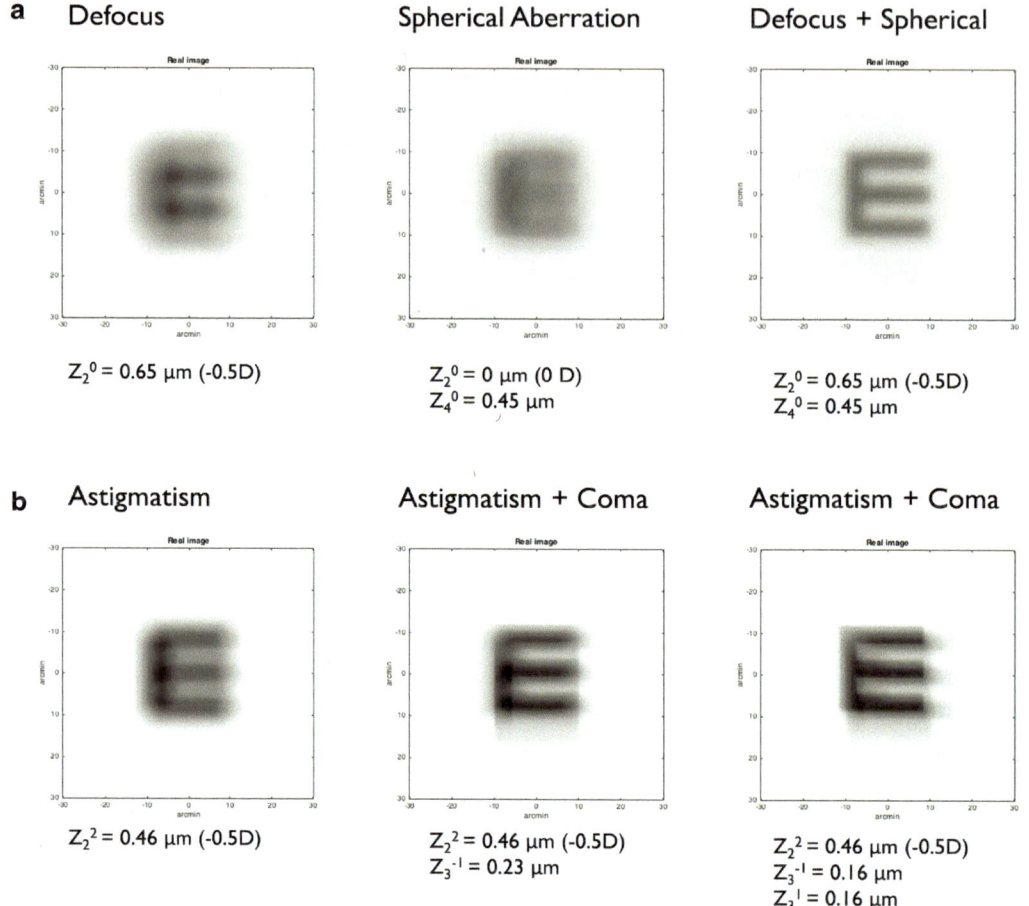

Fig. 67.4 Simulated visual acuity of the Snellen E-letter of 20 arc-min for 6-mm pupil diameter. (**a**) −0.5 D of defocus—left panel; +0.45 microns of spherical aberration—center panel; −0.5 D of defocus with +0.45 microns of spherical aberration—right panel. (**b**): −0.5 D of astigmatism at 0°—left panel; −0.5 D of astigmatism at 0° with 0.23 microns of coma at 45°—center panel; −0.5 D of astigmatism at 0° with 0.23 microns of coma at 90°—right panel (reproduced from de Gracia et al. [72])

benefit, that means, corneas with higher levels of corneal aberrations presented greater visual improvement with an optimized refractive target. On average, the ideal post-operative astigmatism target would be around 1 D for a cornea with a RMS HOAs of 0.3 microns, while the astigmatism target would be around 2 D for a cornea with a RMS HOAs of 0.6 microns (this analysis included 184 irregular corneas; pupil diameter: 4-mm).

Finally, Fig. 67.8 plots the post-operative defocus target as a function of the pre-operative spherical aberration (left) and as a function of spherical aberration, astigmatism, and high-order aberrations (right). As expected, in addition to the amount of spherical aberration (i.e., asphericity), the levels of corneal astigmatism and high-order aberrations have a manifest impact in the final IOL power calculation, offering us a unique opportunity for an accurate IOL selection.

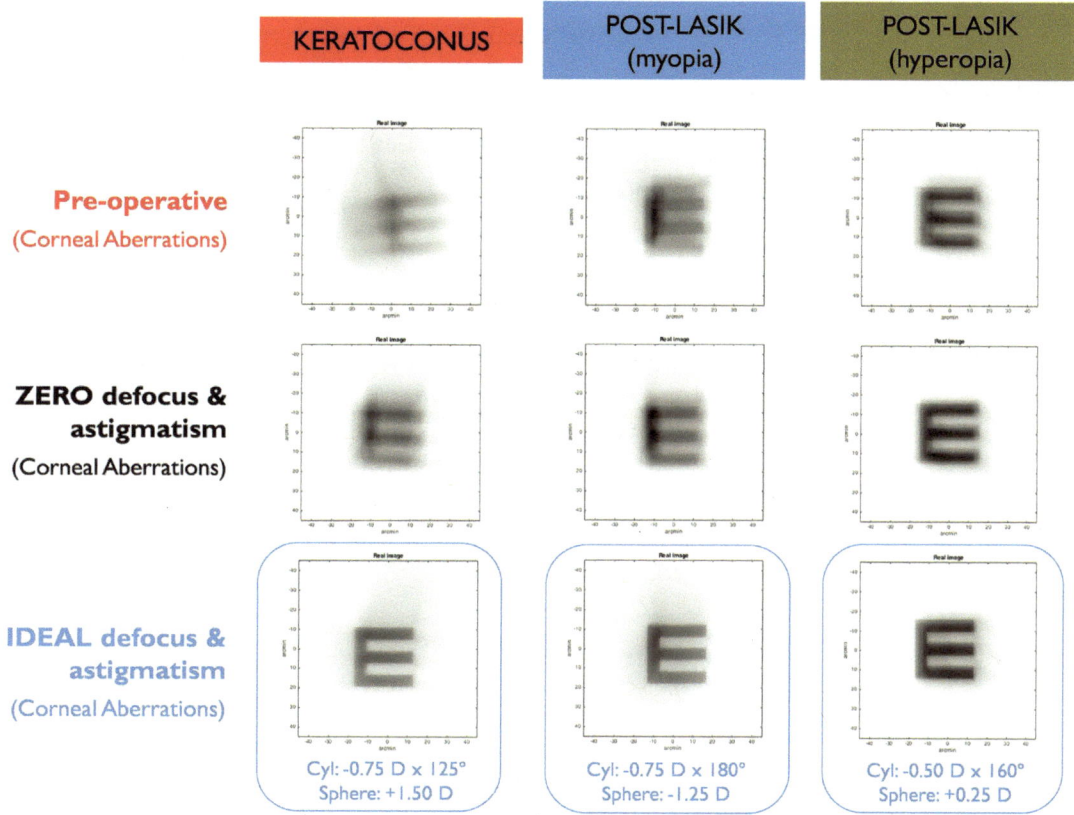

Fig. 67.5 Theoretical simulations of the Snellen E-letter of 30 arc-min for 4-mm pupil diameter in different patients with odd-corneas: keratoconus and surgically modified (post-LASIK myopia and post-LASIK hyperopia). Top: convolved letter with the pre-operative amount of astigmatism and high-order aberrations. Center: con-volved letter with the natural corneal high-order aberrations (cancelling defocus and astigmatism). Bottom: convolved letter with the natural corneal high-order aberrations and the amount of defocus and astigmatism that produced the best optical quality

Fig. 67.6 Through-focus Visual Strehl for the keratonic eye and the corresponding convolved images: pre-operative (red), zero astigmatism (grey), and 0.75 D of astigmatism at 125° (light blue)

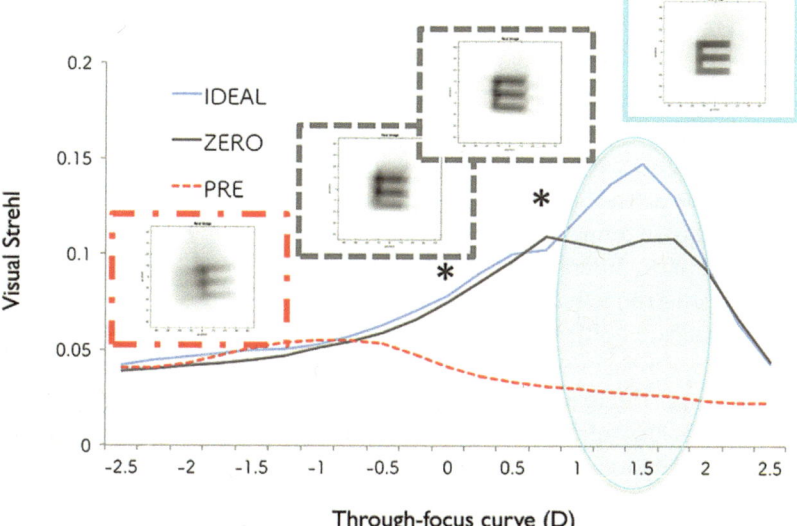

Fig. 67.7 Visual benefit of considering the natural corneal aberrations and astigmatism for the IOL power calculation

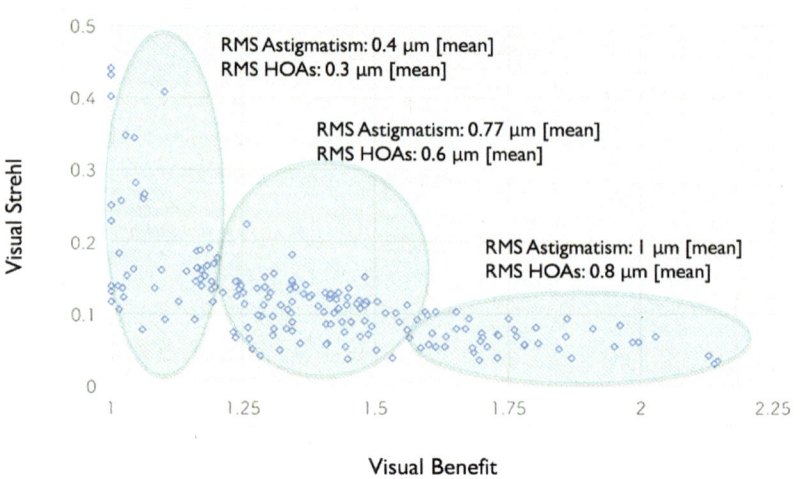

Fig. 67.8 IOL power prediction as a function of the corneal astigmatism and high-order aberrations. Left: Defocus vs. Spherical aberration. Right: Defocus vs. Spherical aberration, astigmatism, and HOAs

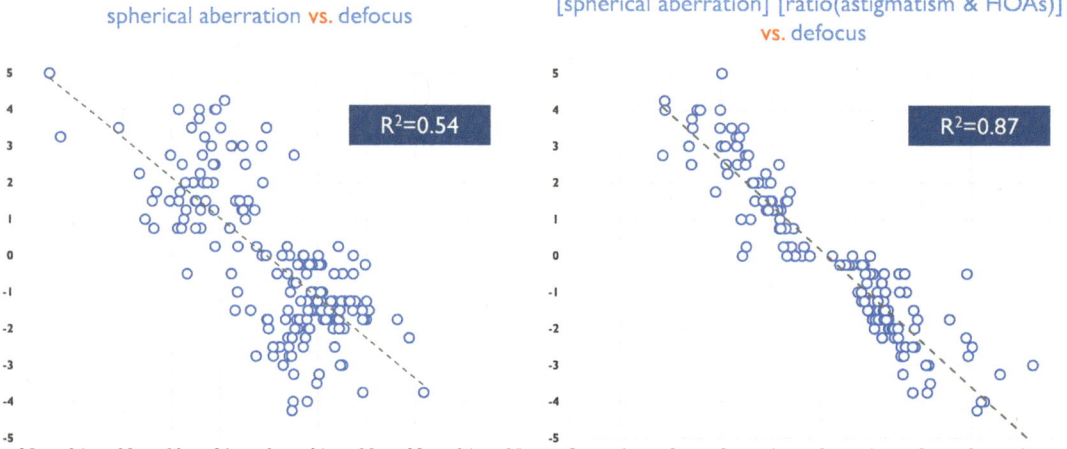

Personalized Surgical Planning

Another area of discussion in these patients is the selection of the IOL type: monofocal vs. toric vs. multifocal. Toric IOL implantation has been shown to be a feasible option for patients with non-progressive forme fruste or moderate keratoconus. However, different studies showed that the post-operative refractive astigmatism after a toric IOL implantation differed from the planned target of zero astigmatism from 0.8 to 6.9 D using the traditional formulas [10, 12, 73]. Besides, a key issue is the tolerance to decentration and rotational stability of the toric design, since

decentration and/or rotation results in an induction of astigmatism and coma [74]. Regarding the IOL selection in post-LASIK eyes, state-of-the-art monofocal IOLs have aspheric surfaces with the aim at reducing the positive spherical aberration of the average cornea, mimicking the spherical aberration balance between the cornea and crystalline lens in the young eye. However, some caution is needed with the aspheric IOL design and the spherical aberration compensation, since patients who had myopic LASIK/PRK had increased positive spherical aberration values, whereas those who had hyperopic LASIK/PRK had increased the magnitude of negative corneal spherical aberration [45]. Moreover, in these groups of patients, a contraindication for the implantation of a multifocal IOL is the level of high-order aberrations; but, to date, there are no guidelines about the cut-off values of corneal aberrations in the implantation of multifocal IOLs. So, there is a critical window of opportunity to harness IOL selection and surgical planning with patient-specific eye models:

1. Cataract surgery tends to render defocus and astigmatism neutral but minimizing the refractive error (with zero defocus and astigmatism as the final refractive target) is not the best strategy for keratoconus and surgically modified corneas, since the position of best focus is highly influenced by the presence of corneal astigmatism and high-order aberrations.

2. Centration and rotational stability is more critical with the increasing complexity of toric and multifocal IOL designs; thus, it is essential to incorporate the three-dimensional IOL design to evaluate the simulated visual performance and tolerance to decentration and multifocality of a specific cornea. With the incorporation of the three-dimensional corneal geometry and the IOL design in the eye models, it would possibly design a customized strategy to define the cut-off values of astigmatism and high-order aberrations in the implantation of toric and multifocal IOLs.

3. Even with small corneal incisions and fixed meridians, not only surgically induced astigmatism (SIA) is highly variably but also there is lack of evidence about the surgically induced coma (SIC) and/or trefoil (SIT). The three-dimensional analysis of the corneal surfaces and different refractive corneal parameters (i.e., power vectors of astigmatism, coma and trefoil) might open new avenues to predict the impact of the surgical induced changes in the corneal surfaces.

$$\text{Pupil function } g\left(x',y'\right) = p\left(x',y'\right)\exp\left(i\frac{2\pi}{\lambda}W\left(x,y\right)\right)$$
(67.1)

where $p(x',y')$ is a circle that defines the aperture of the eye, $w(x',y')$ is the wavefront aberration of the subject and λ the wavelength used for calculations (550 nm).

$$PSF = \left|FT\left(g\left(x',y'\right)\right)\right|^2 \qquad (67.2)$$

$$OTF = FT\left(PSF\right) \qquad (67.3)$$

$$MTF \text{ \# } OTF\text{\#} \qquad (67.4)$$

$$\text{Strehl Ratio} = \frac{PSF_{\text{aberrated}}\left(x',y'\right)}{PSF_{\text{ideal}}\left(x',y'\right)} \qquad (67.5)$$

$$CSF = MTF_{\text{optical}} * MTF_{\text{neural}} \qquad (67.6)$$

$$\text{VSOTF} = \frac{\int_{-\infty}^{\infty}\int_{-\infty}^{\infty} \text{CSF}_N\left(f_x,f_y\right)\text{\#}\,\text{Re}\left\{\text{OTF}\left(f_x,f_y\right)\right\}\text{\#}\,df_x\,df_y}{\int_{-\infty}^{\infty}\int_{-\infty}^{\infty} \text{CSF}_N\left(f_x,f_y\right)*\left\{\text{OTF}\left(f_x,f_y\right)\right\}df_x\,df_y} \qquad (67.7)$$

where $OTF(f_x,f_y)$ denotes the diffraction-limited OTF, $CSF_N(f_x,f_y)$ is the neural contrast sensitivity function, and (f_x,f_y) are the spatial frequency coordinates. Here, the VSOTF was based on calculated OTF across all spatial frequencies.

Appendix 1 Patient-Specific Ray-Tracing Eye Model (ZEMAX)

The commercial software of most corneal topographers allows the extraction of the raw elevation points of the anterior and posterior corneal surfaces and corneal thickness. For example, in Pentacam (OCULUS Optikgeräte GmbH, Wetzlar, Germany): the [Export] button in the Patient Data Management exports the chosen examinations directly to the folder Pentacam.exp (PatientID_Eye_Date_Hour.ELE and PatientID_Eye_Date_Hour.PAC; .ELE and .PAC contains the XYZ coordinates of the surfaces), while in Sirius and MS39 (CSO, Firenze, Italy): the Phoenix v2.1 software from CSO permits to export the following data from the tomographer: PatientID.csv and PatientID.xyX). The Pentacam raw data consists of the elevation value for every corneal point sampled in a Cartesian grid (from −7 to +7 mm, nasal-temporal, superior-inferior) in 100 μm steps. The Sirius and MS-39 raw data comprises 7937 anterior and posterior elevation points over a polar grid with 256 meridians (from −6 to +6 mm, nasal-temporal, superior-inferior).

One key issue is to convert the data format used by the instrument into a suitable structure for the ray-tracing in ZEMAX. For example, the corneal elevation data file could be fitted with Zernike polynomial expansions and imported into ZEMAX using the *Zernike sag surface* type (note that *Zernike sag surface* in ZEMAX is in Noll's format; hence, previous conversion is needed since Noll's notation differs from the OSA standards).

Regarding the IOL, a *standard* ZEMAX surface type (radius, asphericity, thickness, and refractive index) is acceptable to calculate the ocular aberrations (cornea and IOL) and predict the refractive error of a monofocal IOL. Although the *Zernike sag surface* could be also used if the three-dimensional design of the IOL is available.

For ray-tracing in ZEMAX, the object (light source) is set at infinity. The point source at infinity will be best focused on the retinal surface after iteration (for example, the best focus position as is the position that minimizes the root-mean-square wavefront error). Refractive indices of 1.376 and 1.336 are commonly used for the cornea and aqueous humor, respectively. Wave aberrations for the defined pupil diameter (e.g., 4-mm pupil diameter) are calculated for the defined wavelenght (e.g., monochromatic light at

555 nm), by tracing an array of 64 × 64 rays collimated through a 2-surface model (anterior and posterior cornea, separated by corneal thickness) and 4-surface model (adding to the corneal surfaces: the nominal values of the IOL, the estimated lens position (e.g., anterior chamber depth post-op+IOL thickness/2), and the axial length. Pseudophakic eyes are simpler than phakic eye models to analyze the optical quality, as the refractive index of the IOL is constant and the surfaces curvature are known.

The optical performance of the pseudophakic eye model is evaluated with the three-dimensional representation (*3D Layout*), the *Spot Diagram,* and the Zernike wavefront aberrations (*Zernike Standard Coefficients*). Figure 67.3 shows an illustration of a personalized eye model in ZEMAX using three-dimensional corneal and IOL data.

Appendix 2 Optical Aberrations and Image Quality Metrics

The image-forming properties of any optical system can be described in terms of wave aberration. Light can be considered as a series of waves coming from a source. In aberrations-free optical systems, all the parallel rays will intersect the retina at the same point, or equivalently, all the imaging wavefronts will be spherical and centered in the image point. However, an imperfect lens will impose phase distortions on the plane waves, there is no longer a focal point and the different rays will intersect the image plane at different points (the wavefronts will no longer be spherical). The difference between the distorted waves and the ideal waves is the wavefront aberration, representing the distortions of the wavefront (surface containing points with the same phase and orthogonal to the propagation axis) in the pupil plane as it goes through the optical system.

The *wave aberration* of a general optical system can be described mathematically by a polynomial series. Zernike polynomial expansion has become the standard for representing wave aberration data because they form an orthogonal set over a circle of unit radius, and aberrations are usually referred to circular pupils. An interesting feature of the Zernike polynomials is that some terms are directly related to commonly known ocular aberrations. For example, structural abnormalities of the eye, such as myopia, hyperopia and astigmatism, appear in the second order of this expansion. Further, Zernike terms represent higher-order aberrations such as spherical aberration (arising from the asphericity of the optical surfaces) and coma (mainly associated to local irregularities, tilt, and decentration of the surfaces of the optical system).

From the wave aberration coefficients, different optical quality descriptors can be directly derived after mathematical operations [71, 75–80]. The two classic descriptors are the *Modulation Transfer Function (MTF)* and the *Point Spread Function (PSF)*. The MTF quantifies the loss in contrast associated to each spatial frequency, the higher the MTF, the better the image provided by the system. The PSF is the impulse response of the system, i.e., the degraded image of an ideal point as imaged by the system. The PSF is calculated as the squared magnitude of the inverse Fourier transform of the pupil function (the pupil function defines how light passes through the pupil). The *Root Mean Square (RMS)* is also a common descriptor; it is defined as the root square of the variance of the wave aberration and is typically used as the global metric for the optical quality. The *Strehl ratio* is a scalar metric used to describe the quality of the PSF in an eye. As the Strehl ratio includes in the calculation regions of the MTF with spatial frequencies beyond those relevant to the visual system, a new metric is introduced to adapt the definition to visual optics (Visual Strehl). The *Visual Strehl* has been shown to hold the highest correlation variance against subjective acuity. It is computed as the volume under the visual MTF, obtained from the overlapping of the MTF with the inverse of a general neural transfer function, normalized to diffraction limit. The neural sensitivity, function of the spatial frequency, is a common measurement of the neural performance. In a similar way as the optical MTF, it is possible to define and measure the neural MTF, and the product of the neural and optical MTFs gives the Contrast Sensitivity Function (CSF) of the eye.

References

1. Nordan LT. Keratoconus: diagnosis and treatment. Int Ophthalmol Clin. 1997;37(1):51–63.
2. Rabinowitz YS. Keratoconus. Surv Ophthalmol. 1998;42(4):297–319.
3. Tomidokoro A, Oshika T, Amano S, et al. Changes in anterior and posterior corneal curvatures in keratoconus. Ophthalmology. 2000;107(7):1328–32.
4. Saad A, Gatinel D. Topographic and tomographic properties of forme frustre keratoconus corneas. Invest Ophthalmol Vis Sci. 2010;51(11):5546–55.
5. Alio JL, Shabayek MH. Corneal higher order aberrations: a method to grade keratoconus. J Refract Surg. 2006;22(6):539–45.
6. Barbero S, Marcos S, Merayo-Lloves J, et al. Validation of the estimation of corneal aberrations from videokeratography in keratoconus. J Refract Surg. 2002;18:263–70.
7. Maeda N, Fujikado T, Kuroda T, et al. Wavefront aberrations measured with Hartmann-Shack sensor in patients with keratoconus. Ophthalmology. 2002;109(11):1996–2003.
8. Navas A, Suárez R. One-year follow-up of toric intraocular lens implantation in forme fruste keratoconus. J Cataract Refract Surg. 2009;35:2024–7.
9. Nanavaty MA, Lake DB, Daya SM. Outcomes of pseudophakic toric intraocular lens implantation in keratoconic eyes with cataract. J Refract Surg. 2012;28:884–9.
10. Hashemi H, Heidarian S, Seyedian MA, Yekta A, Khabazkhoob M. Evaluation of the results of using toric IOL in the cataract surgery of keratoconus patients. Eye Contact Lens. 2015;41:354–8.
11. Kamiya K, Shimizu K, Miyake T. Changes in astigmatism and corneal higher-order aberrations after phacoemulsification with toric intraocular lens implantation for mild keratoconus with cataract. Jpn J Ophthalmol. 2016;60:302–8.
12. Kamiya K, Iijima K, Nobuyuki S, Mori Y, Miyata K, Yamaguchi T, Shimazaki J, Watanabe S, Maeda N. Predictability of intraocular lens power calculation for cataract with keratoconus: a multicenter study. Sci Rep. 2018;8(1):1312.
13. Savini G, Abbate R, Hoffer KJ, Mularoni A, Imburgia A, Avoni L, D'Eliseo D, Schiano-Lomoriello D. Intraocular lens power calculation in eyes with keratoconus. J Cataract Refract Surg. 2019;45(5):576–81.
14. Melles RB, Holladay JT, Chang WJ. Accuracy of intraocular lens calculation formulas. Ophthalmology. 2018;125:169–78.
15. Melles RB, Kane JX, Olsen T, Chang WJ. Update on intraocular lens calculation formulas. Ophthalmology. 2019;126:1334–5.
16. Kane JX, Connell B, Yip H, McAlister JC, Beckingsale P, Snibson GR, Chan E. Accuracy of intraocular lens power formulas modified for patients with keratoconus. Ophthalmology. 2020;127(8):1037–42.

17. Holladay JT. Holladay IOL Consultant software and surgical outcomes assessment. 1105.2019 ed. Bellaire: Holladay Consulting; 2019.

18. Koch DD. The enigmatic cornea and intraocular lens calculations: the LXXIII Edward Jackson memorial lecture. Am J Ophthalmol. 2016;171:xv–xxx.

19. Lockington D, Wang EF, Patel DV, Moore SP, McGhee CN. Effectiveness of cataract phacoemulsification with toric intraocular lenses in addressing astigmatism after keratoplasty. J Cataract Refract Surg. 2014;40(12):2044–9.

20. Wade M, Steinert RF, Garg S, Farid M, Gaster R. Results of toric intraocular lenses for post-penetrating keratoplasty astigmatism. Ophthalmology. 2014;121(3):771–7.

21. Aramberri J. Intraocular lens power calculation after corneal refractive surgery: double-K method. J Cataract Refract Surg. 2003;29(11):2063–8.

22. Anera RG, Jiménez JR, Jiménez del Barco L, Bermudez J, Hita H. Changes in corneal asphericity after laser in situ keratomileusis. J Cataract Refract Surg. 2003;29(4):762–8.

23. Marcos S, Barbero S, Llorente L, Merayo-Lloves J. Optical response to LASIK surgery for myopia from total and corneal aberration measurements. Invest Ophthalmol Vis Sci. 2001;42(13):3349–56.

24. Moreno-Barriuso E, Lloves JM, Marcos S, Navarro R, Llorente L, Barbero S. Ocular aberrations before and after myopic corneal refractive surgery: LASIK-induced changes measured with laser ray tracing. Invest Ophthalmol Vis Sci. 2001;42(6):1396–403.

25. Hoffer KF. Intraocular lens power calculation after previous laser refractive surgery. J Cataract Refract Surg. 2009;35(4):759–65.

26. Pantanelli SM, Lin CC, Al-Mohtaseb Z, Rose-Nussbaumer JR, Santhiago MR, Steigleman WA 3rd, Schallhorn JM. Intraocular lens power calculation in eyes with previous excimer laser surgery for myopia: a report by the American Academy of Ophthalmology. Ophthalmology. 2021;128(5):781–92.

27. Haigis W, Lege B, Miller N, Schneider B. Comparison of immersion ultrasound biometry and partial coherence interferometry for intraocular lens calculation according to Haigis. Graefes Arch Clin Exp Ophthalmol. 2000;238(9):765–73.

28. Hoffer KJ. The Hoffer Q formula: a comparison of theoretic and regression formulas. J Cataract Refract Surg. 1993;19(6):700–12.

29. Retzlaff JA, Sanders DR, Kraff MC. Development of the SRK/T intraocular lens implant power calculation formula. J Cataract Refract Surg. 1990;16(3):333–40.

30. Feiz V, Mannis MJ, Garcia-Ferrer F, Kandavel G, Darlington JK, Kim E, Caspar J, Wang JL, Wang W. Intraocular lens power calculation after laser in situ keratomileusis for myopia and hyperopia: a standardized approach. Cornea. 2001;20(8):792–7.

31. Walter KA, Gagnon MR, Hoopes PC Jr, Dickinson PJ. Accurate intraocular lens power calculation after myopic laser in situ keratomileusis, bypassing corneal power. J Cataract Refract Surg. 2006;32(3):425–9.

32. Hamed AM, Wang L, Misra M, Koch DD. A comparative analysis of five methods of determining corneal refractive power in eyes that have undergone myopic laser in situ keratomileusis. Ophthalmology. 2002;109(4):651–8.

33. Masket S, Masket SE. Simple regression formula for intraocular lens power adjustment in eyes requiring cataract surgery after excimer laser photoablation. J Cataract Refract Surg. 2006;32(3):430–4.

34. Abulafia A, Hill WE, Koch DD, Wang L, Barrett GD. Accuracy of the Barrett True-K formula for intraocular lens power prediction after laser in situ keratomileusis or photorefractive keratectomy for myopia. J Cataract Refract Surg. 2016;42(3):363–9.

35. Shammas HJ, Shammas MC. No-history method of intraocular lens power calculation for cataract surgery after myopic laser in situ keratomileusis. J Cataract Refract Surg. 2007;33(1):31–6.

36. Awwad ST, Manasseh C, Bowman RW, Cavanagh HD, Verity S, Mootha V, McCulley JP. Intraocular lens power calculation after myopic laser in situ keratomileusis: estimating the corneal refractive power. J Cataract Refract Surg. 2008;34(7):1070–6.

37. Potvin R, Hill W. New algorithm for intraocular lens power calculations after myopic laser in situ keratomileusis based on rotating Scheimpflug camera data. J Cataract Refract Surg. 2015;41(2):339–47.

38. Wang L, Hill WE, Koch DD. Evaluation of IOL power prediction methods using the ASCRS post-keratorefractive IOL power calculator. J Cataract Refract Surg. 2010;36:1466–73.

39. Haigis W. Intraocular lens calculation after refractive surgery for myopia: Haigis-L formula. J Cataract Refract Surg. 2008;34:1658–63.

40. Hill W, Wang L, Koch DD. IOL power calculation in eyes that have undergone LASIK/PRK/RK. https://iolcalc.ascrs.org.

41. Gale RP, Saldana M, Johnston RL, Zuberbuhler B, McKibbin M. Benchmark standards for refractive outcomes after NHS cataract surgery. Eye. 2009;23:149–52.

42. Olsen T. Calculation of intraocular lens power: a review. Acta Ophthalmol Scand. 2007;85(5):472–85.

43. Goto S, Maeda N. Corneal topography for intraocular lens selection in refractive cataract surgery. Ophthalmology. 2021;128:e142–52. S0161-6420(20)31108-1108.

44. Holladay JT. Effect of corneal asphericity and spherical aberration on intraocular lens power calculations. J Cataract Refract Surg. 2015;41(7):1553–4.

45. Canovas C, Abenza S, Alcon E, Villegas EA, Marin JM, Artal P. Effect of corneal aberrations on intraocular lens power calculations. J Cataract Refract Surg. 2012;38(8):1325–32.

46. Canovas C, Artal P. Customized eye models for determining optimized intraocular lenses power. Biomed Opt Express. 2011;2(6):1649–62.

47. Wang L, Koch DD. Intraocular lens power calculations in eyes with previous corneal refractive sur-

gery: review and expert opinion. Ophthalmology. 2021;128(11):e121–31. S0161-6420(20)30625-4.

48. Mejia-Barbosa Y, Malacara-Hernandez D. A review of methods for measuring corneal topography. Optom Vis Sci. 2001;78:240–53.

49. Ortiz S, Siedlecki D, Perez-Merino P, Chia N, de Castro A, Szkulmowski M, Wojtkowski M, Marcos S. Corneal topography from spectral optical coherence tomography (sOCT). Biomed Opt Express. 2011;2:3232–47.

50. Pérez-Merino P, Ortiz S, Alejandre N, de Castro A, Jimenez-Alfaro I, Marcos S. Ocular and optical coherence tomography-based corneal aberrometry in keratoconic eyes treated by intracorneal ring segments. Am J Ophthalmol. 2014;157:116–27.

51. Pérez-Merino P, Ortiz S, Alejandre N, Jimenez-Alfaro I, Marcos S. Quantitative OCT-based longitudinal evaluation of intracorneal ring segment implantation in keratoconus. Invest Ophthalmol Vis Sci. 2013;54:6040–51.

52. Sicam V, Van der Heijde RGL. Topographer reconstruction of the nonrotation-symmetric anterior corneal surface features. Optom Vis Sci. 2006;83(12):910–8.

53. Zhu Z, Janunts E, Eppig T, Sauer T, Langenbucher A. Tomography-based customized IOL calculation model. Curr Eye Res. 2011;36(6):579–89.

54. Preussner PR, Wahl J, Lahdo H, Dick B, Findl O. Ray tracing for intraocular lens calculation. J Cataract Refract Surg. 2002;28(8):1412–9.

55. Preussner PR, Wahl J, Weitzel D. Topography-based intraocular lens power selection. J Cataract Refract Surg. 2005;31(3):525–33.

56. Preussner PR, Olsen T, Hoffmann P, Findl O. Intraocular lens calculation accuracy limits in normal eyes. J Cataract Refract Surg. 2008;34(5):802–8.

57. Hoffmann P, Wahl J, Preussner PR. Accuracy of intraocular lens calculation with ray tracing. J Refract Surg. 2012;28(9):650–5.

58. Olsen T, Hoffmann P. C constant: new concept for ray tracing-assisted intraocular lens power calculation. J Cataract Refract Surg. 2014;40(5):764–73.

59. Hoffmann PC, Wahl J, Hütz WW, Preußner PR. A ray tracing approach to calculate toric intraocular lenses. J Refract Surg. 2013;29(6):402–8.

60. Sun M, Pérez-Merino P, Martinez-Enriquez E, Velasco-Ocana M, Marcos S. Full 3-D OCT-based pseudophakic custom computer eye model. Biomed Opt Express. 2016;7(3):1074–88.

61. Rosales P, Marcos S. Customized computer models of eyes with intraocular lenses. Opt Express. 2007;15(5):2204–18.

62. Tabernero J, Piers P, Benito A, Redondo M, Artal P. Predicting the optical performance of eyes implanted with IOLs to correct spherical aberration. Invest Ophthalmol Vis Sci. 2006;47(10):4651–8.

63. Hoffmann PC, Lindemann CR. Intraocular lens calculation for aspheric intraocular lenses. J Cataract Refract Surg. 2013;39(6):867–72.

64. Norrby S. Sources of error in intraocular lens power calculation. J Cataract Refract Surg. 2008;34:368–76.

65. Ortiz S, Perez-Merino P, Gambra E, de Castro A, Marcos S. In vivo human crystalline lens topography. Biomed Opt Express. 2012;3:2471–88.

66. Pérez-Merino P, Velasco-Ocana M, Martinez-Enriquez E, Marcos S. OCT-based crystalline lens topography in accommodating eyes. Biomed Opt Express. 2015;6:5039–54.

67. Martinez-Enriquez E, Sun M, Velasco-Ocana M, Birkenfeld J, Pérez-Merino P, Marcos S. Optical coherence tomography based estimates of crystalline lens volume, equatorial diameter, and plane position. Invest Ophthalmol Vis Sci. 2016;57(9):OCT600–10.

68. Martinez-Enriquez E, Pérez-Merino P, Velasco-Ocana M, Marcos S. OCT-based full crystalline lens shape change during accommodation in vivo. Biomed Opt Express. 2017;8(2):918–33.

69. Martinez-Enriquez E, Pérez-Merino P, Durán-Poveda S, Jiménez-Alfaro I, Marcos S. Estimation of intraocular lens position from full crystalline lens geometry: towards a new generation of intraocular lens power calculation formulas. Sci Rep. 2018;8(1):9829.

70. Applegate RA, Ballentine C, Gross H, Sarver EJ, Sarver CA. Visual acuity as a function of Zernike mode and level of root mean square error. Optom Vis Sci. 2003;80(2):97–105.

71. Cheng X, Bradley A, Thibos LN. Predicting subjective judgment of best focus with objective image quality metrics. J Vis. 2004;4:310–21.

72. de Gracia P, Dorronsoro C, Gambra E, Marin G, Hernández M, Marcos S. Combining coma with astigmatism can improve retinal image over astigmatism alone. Vision Res. 2010;50(19):2008–14.

73. Alió JL, Peña-García P, Abdulla Guliyeva F, Soria FA, Zein G, Abu-Mustafa SK. MICS with toric intraocular lenses in keratoconus: outcomes and predictability analysis of postoperative refraction. Br J Ophthalmol. 2014;98(3):365–70.

74. Pérez-Merino P, Marcos S. Effect of intraocular lens decentration on image quality tested in a custom model eye. J Cataract Refract Surg. 2018;44(7):889–96.

75. Applegate RA, Marsack JD, Thibos LN. Metrics of retinal image quality predict visual performance in eyes with 20/17 or better visual acuity. Optom Vis Sci. 2006;83(9):635–40.

76. Cheng X, Bradley A, Hong X, Thibos L. Relationship between refractive error and monochromatic aberrations of the eye. Optom Vis Sci. 2003;80:43–9.

77. Cheng X, Thibos L, Bradley A. Estimating visual quality from wavefront aberration measurements. J Refract Surg. 2003;19:579–84.

78. Watson AB. Computing human optical point spread functions. J Vis. 2015;15(2):26.

79. Águila-Carrasco AJ, Read SA, Montés-Micó R, Iskander DR. The effect of aberrations on objectively assessed image quality and depth of focus. J Vis. 2017;17(2):2.

80. Iskander DR. Computational aspects of the visual Strehl ratio. Optom Vis Sci. 2006;83(1):57–9.

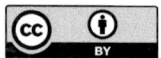

IOL Calculation in Vitreoretinal Pathology and Surgery

68

Jaime Aramberri

Introduction

Pars plana vitrectomy (PPV) has become a frequent surgery indicated in the treatment of many vitreoretinal pathologies: retinal detachment (RD), epiretinal membrane (ERM), macular hole (MH), vitreous hemorrhage, etc. Cataract surgery will soon be needed in 1–2 years as up to 80% of cases will develop this condition [1]. In the Eurequo database, December 2018, from 1,715,348 reported cataract surgeries, 1.1% had previous PPV [2]. Moreover, the combined cataract and PPV procedure, phacovitrectomy, has proved to be a very safe and effective procedure and is being performed as their primary technique by many vitreoretinal surgeons [3, 4].

These eyes present unique challenges to the IOL calculation process that have to be recognized and corrected especially in this era of high demand of accurate refractive predictions motivated by the good functional outcomes of cataract and PPV surgeries plus the introduction of new EDOF and multifocal IOLs, where success depends directly on an emmetropic refractive result.

J. Aramberri (✉)
Miranza Ókular Clinic, Vitoria-Gasteiz, Spain

Miranza Begitek Clinic,
Donostia-San Sebastian, Spain

Axial Length Measurement

Axial length (AL) measurement is more prone to present some error in eyes with macular pathology and when the vitreous cavity's content differs from the natural vitreous humor. These factors will affect ultrasound (US) and optical measurements differently.

In US biometry, a probe containing a transducer is manually aligned with the eye by the operator and a 10 MHz sound beam is emitted through the globe generating echo spikes at each boundary of media with different acoustic densities: anterior and posterior cornea, anterior and posterior lens capsule and retina. The device measures the time between spikes that limit each eye compartment and multiplies by the US velocity of the medium to calculate the linear distance. The higher the medium material density, the higher the US velocity is. Usual values are 1532 m/s for the anterior and vitreous chambers and 1641 m/s for the cornea and lens [5]. The retinal echo spike is generated by the internal limiting membrane (ILM) which is around 0.2 mm before the photoreceptors (Fig. 68.1). This distance is compensated by the IOL formulas. There are two different techniques, applanation and immersion US biometry, with differences in AL up to 0.2 mm shorter with applanation [6] due most probably to corneal compression and thus not affected by any vitreoretinal condition. However, if any retinal tam-

© The Author(s) 2024
J. Aramberri et al. (eds.), *Intraocular Lens Calculations*, Essentials in Ophthalmology,
https://doi.org/10.1007/978-3-031-50666-6_68

Fig. 68.1 The retinal reflection plane is different for ultrasound (US) and for optical biometry (OPT). Internal limiting membrane for the US and pigment epithelium for the OPT

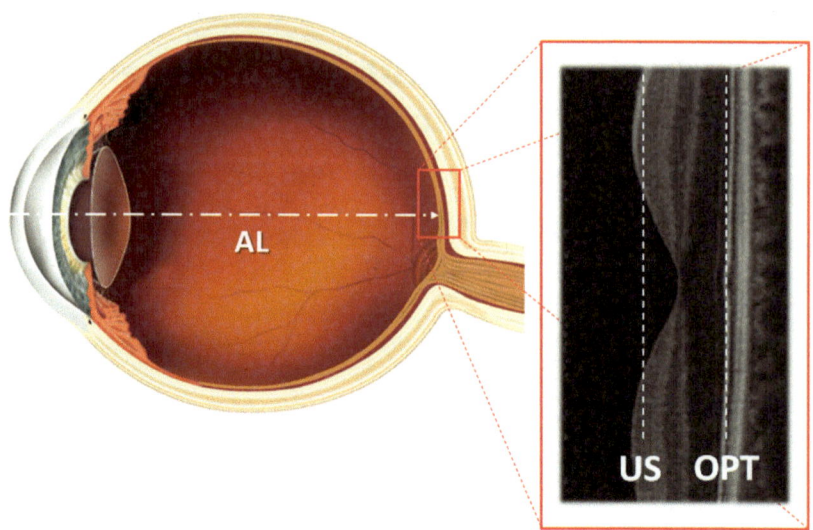

ponade agent, gas or silicone oil, is in the vitreous cavity the exploring patient position, upright in contact and supine in immersion, might have an effect on the measurement.

In optical biometry, a beam of infrared light is projected into the eye and the reflected light generates an A-scan with spikes at the boundaries of media with different optical densities in the case of Time-domain interferometry (partial coherence interferometry (PCI) and optical low coherence reflectometry (OLCR)) and a B-scan image in the case of Swept Source-OCT (SS-OCT) [7]. The speed of light cannot be measured in the way it is done in the US biometry, but interferometry allows measuring the optical path length (OPL), also called air-distance, that is finally converted to linear distance following this formula:

$$AL = OPL / n \qquad (68.1)$$

where n is the index of refraction of the measured medium.

In the first PCI device, The IOLMaster® (Carl Zeiss-Meditec), the lens position could not be measured and thus segmental biometry could not be done. Another source of difficulty was that the retinal spike was generated in the retinal pigment epithelium (RPE), around 200 µm posterior to the US biometry retinal reference plane. In order to achieve an agreement with the gold standard at that time, the US immersion biometry, the IOLMaster was calibrated to match that technique's measurements with a regression equation [8]:

$$AL = \left(OPL / 1.3549 - 1.3033 \right) / 0.9571 \qquad (68.2)$$

Since then, this calibration has been the standard in optical biometry. Even with the evolution of new technologies that could finally measure the lens capsular positions allowing segmental biometry, like OLCR and SS-OCT devices, this standard has continued in order to keep the *Status Quo* with formulas and IOL constants developed for the original IOLMaster calibration. Recently, the debate has been opened and there is one SS-OCT biometer, Argos® (Movu), performing segmental biometry where the length of each eye segment is calculated using Eq. 68.1. Obviously, formulas will have to adapt if this becomes a new standard [9].

The optical biometry is clearly superior to US biometry in terms of accuracy and precision: The resolution is two orders of magnitude higher, the repeatability is one order of magnitude higher and the fixation light targeting ensures the visual axis is being measured [7, 10]. The only advantage of US biometry is that all cataracts can be measured, while optical biometry fails in certain cases due to opaque media.

Macular Thickening

In the case of macular thickening, US biometry will underestimate optical AL, overestimating IOL power and leading to a myopic result with a magnitude of 0.10–0.70 D as reported [11]. Kovacs et al. described a mean macular thickening of 142 µm and a decrease in AL of 0.20 mm in a series of macular edema and epiretinal membrane (ERM) cases. The observed prediction error was 0.72 D [12]. In a similar study, Sun et al. reported a macular thickening of 129 µm with an AL decrease of 0.13 µm [13]. This problem should not be found in optical biometry as the retinal reflection originates in the pigment epithelium, and therefore, it is not affected by macular thickening. However, there are several reports of similar measurement errors. Falkner-Radler et al. presented a myopic predictive error of 0.37 D in 40 eyes with macular disease. The error was higher in the case of ERM than in the case of macular hole. It was also higher in cases of gas tamponade [14]. Kojima et al. described a plausible reason for AL error with the old IOL Master: 18.9% of cases presented a double peak in the retina, where it seems logical that the anterior peak corresponds to the ILM-ERM and the posterior to the RPE, as the distance showed good correlation with the OCT measured macular thickness [15]. Kitaguchi defined a "hidden double-peak" also with the IOL Master 5.4 in a case with myopic predictive error. The analysis of all the A-scans showed a double-peak in 8 of 20 scans. The distance between peaks was 0.6 mm, and the attributed refractive error was 0.32 D [16]. We have found similar cases of ERM with Lenstar®, Haag Streit, where a double-peak can be identified in the A-scan image. The software can automatically set the retinal gate at the first peak underestimating the AL (Fig. 68.2).

The magnitude of this refractive error is small and will depend on the AL and IOL power: 0.1 mm of AL error will produce 0.35 D of refractive error in the spectacle plane in a short eye (21 mm) while it will only induce 0.15 D error in a long eye (30 mm) (Fig. 68.3). There is some variability in the reported macular thickening in the case of ERM as there is no standard method

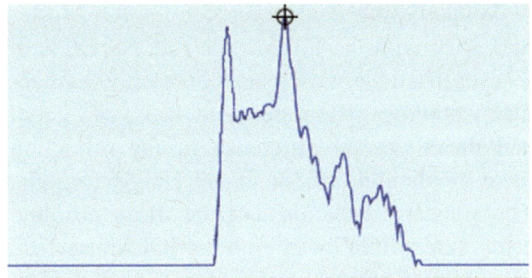

Fig. 68.2 Magnification of the retinal peak. Double-peak produced by ERM. The reference has been manually moved to the posterior peak

0.1 mm AL error

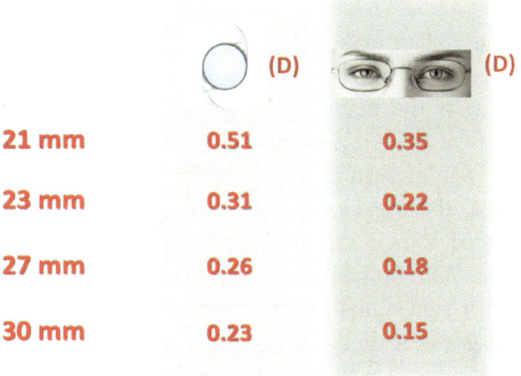

	(D)	(D)
21 mm	0.51	0.35
23 mm	0.31	0.22
27 mm	0.26	0.18
30 mm	0.23	0.15

Fig. 68.3 Paraxial calculation of the effect of 0.1 mm AL error in the IOL and spectacle planes for 4 different AL values. IOL position is adapted to the AL and K = 43.5 D

to measure the OCT image. In a metanalysis by Huang et al. (535 eyes from 8 studies), the macular thinning after vitrectomy ranged between 68.6 µm and 179 µm [17]. Considering an average 123 µm error, the refraction error would be 0.42 D in a 21-mm eye and 0.18 D in a 30-mm eye.

The proposed solution to correct this error is to add the thickened macular value to the measured AL. If there are two clear peaks in the A-scan, the gate that determines the retinal plane should be manually moved to the posterior peak. This value can be checked with a retinal OCT image; as an alternative option, Sun proposes using the macular thickness of the normal eye [13].

Vounotrypidis et al. compared the IOLMaster 500, PCI, with the IOLMaster 700, SS-OCT, in 79 eyes that underwent phacovitrectomy for macular pathology. The agreement was very good, and there was no difference in the refraction mean prediction error with the Haigis formula. The standard deviation and the mean absolute error were a little lower with the IOLMaster 700 ($p < 0.05$). Curiously, a difference was found in the eyes with ERM and macular hole, while in the eyes with vitreomacular traction syndrome, there was no significant difference [18].

Macula-Off Retinal Detachment

In case of retinal detachment (RD), the macular state will affect the accuracy of the AL measurement. If the macula is detached (macula-off), both the US A-scan and the optic biometry will tend to underestimate the AL (Fig. 68.4). In both cases, the signal reflected from the anteriorly located retinal internal surface will cause this error. With optical biometry, this can occur even with a high signal-to-noise ratio (SNR) as shown by Lege et al. in the first years of the IOLMaster. In a case of macula-off RD, they obtained a measurement with a SNR of 6.5 where the AL was 1.30 mm shorter than the one measured with B-scan US [19]. Optical biometry will more often fail to measure AL and the other biometric parameters than in normal eyes. Even with the new SS-OCT, the failure rate is significant. Liu et al. reported 28.6%, 22.2%, and 14.3% failure rate for AL, anterior chamber depth (ACD), and lens thickness (LT) in 63 eyes with macula-off RD measured with IOLMaster 700 [20].

The most reliable method in such cases is the vector-A/B-scan US biometry. A horizontal B-scan is taken imaging simultaneously the cornea, anterior and posterior lens capsules, and the optic nerve. Then, a vector is overlaid intersecting the central cornea, lens, and macular area. With this technique, Abou-Shousha et al. reported similar measurements to postoperative (PO) IOLMaster numbers in 100 eyes. The mean difference with preoperative applanation vector-A/B-scan US biometry was 0.08 mm. On the other hand, both preoperative A-scan US biometry and IOLMaster biometry measured a shorter AL; 0.82 mm with the former and 0.79 mm with the latter. Depending on the AL used for the IOL power calculation, the PO refraction would have been within ±1.00 D of prediction in 50% of cases with US A-scan, 57% with the IOLMaster, and 83% with applanation vector-A/B-scan US biometry [21]. Rahman

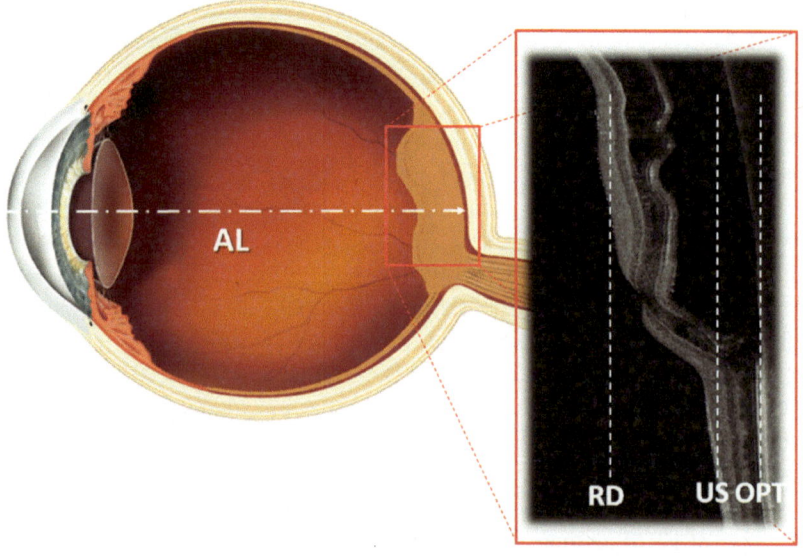

Fig. 68.4 Both US and PCI will measure a shorter AL if the detached retinal signal is used as reference for the retinal plane

et al. reported similar results in 54 cases of macula-off RD where the optical biometry with the IOLMaster (v.5.4) underestimated the AL value by 0.98 ± 1.55 mm as compared to US biometry. They noticed some correlation between bullous RD and a higher level of AL underestimation [22]. In 2016, Rahman et al. proposed a solution by selecting a more posterior peak in the IOLMaster display. With this method, they achieved equaling the preoperative measurement to the PO measurement with a mean difference of 0.049 ± 0.144 mm in 13 eyes [23].

If immersion US is done in supine position, the error might be smaller as the retina sinks closer to its natural position by gravity. This probably explains the lack of difference, 0.03 ± 0.63 mm, between preop and PO measurements reported by Pongsachareonnont et al. in 16 cases of macula-off RD with immersion US biometry, while the IOLMaster presented a difference of 0.98 ± 1.02 mm [24].

Another option is to use the AL of the fellow-eye if there is refractive symmetry. El-Khayat et al. reported a refraction prediction error of −0.01 ± 1.09 D in contrast to the actually measured AL with a value of −1.22 ± 2.32 D. In the first group, 71.4% of eyes where within ±1.00 D of error while in the second group, this was 58.5% [25].

Scleral Buckling

Although PPV is the most common technique for the treatment of RD, scleral buckling with scleral implants is still a popular procedure with a high success rate, especially in developing countries due to a lower cost. The indentation of the eye wall layers beneath the retinal break, and the drainage of subretinal fluid will close the defect and reduce the vitreoretinal traction, leading to the resolution of the RD. This anatomical modification will change several biometric parameters affecting refraction: The encircling circumferential buckling will elongate the eyeball with an AL increase between 0.44 and 1.20 mm in the short term. This variability can be explained by differences in surgical techniques and analyzed population samples [26, 27]. Lee et al. reported a long-term AL increase, 26.05 ± 11.39 months follow-up, of 1.28 mm in low myopes and 1.40 mm in high myopes. An AL threshold value of 26.5 mm was used to define these two groups [26]. Albanese et al. studied 34 eyes phakic eyes with a mean follow-up of 50.9 ± 21.9 months reporting an AL increase of 0.83 mm (95% CI 0.72–0.95). The myopic shift was 1.35 D. The fellow eye experienced an AL increase of 0.08 mm (95% CI 0.00–0.16) in the same period of time [28].

The optical effect of this AL increase will depend on the AL of the eye: 1 mm will change refraction around 2.60 D in an average eye (AL = 23.75 mm), 3.5 D in a short eye (AL = 21.00 mm), and 1.5 D in a long eye (AL = 30.00 mm).

The ACD will decrease after scleral buckling surgery with some variability in the magnitude: from 0.09 to 0.52 mm. It has been argued that this change can be attributed to the anterior movement of the iris-lens diaphragm due to some choroidal effusion [27]. It is not clear if this will have any effect on the IOL position after cataract surgery.

Astigmatism is reported to increase after this surgery, especially if radial buckles are in use [29]. The induced astigmatism seems to be much variable, probably depending on the size and position of the scleral implant. The effect decreases through the first PO year. This should be considered if a toric IOL is planned shortly after retinal surgery.

Vitrectomized Eyes

After vitrectomy, the vitreous cavity is filled with aqueous humor. This will not affect US biometry as US speed seems to be similar in both elements. The water content of the vitreous humor is very high, with a value around 1532 m/s [30], and hence, there is no need to adjust this parameter for the vitreous compartment using US. However, light speed could experience some difference: it is not clear if there is a change in the index of refraction of vitreous after vitrectomy, but if the

IOLMaster calibration works under the assumption of equal indices and the actual index decreases after vitrectomy, there might be an error in the optical biometry measurement of the vitreous segment which is around 70% of the total length. The AL will be underestimated because the biometer is not aware of this index of refraction difference. More research is needed to clarify this point. This error will add to the model error as later explained below.

Silicone Oil

The use of silicone oil as tamponade agent has expanded from the initial indication of complex RD (such as RD with proliferative vitreoretinopathy and diabetic tractional RD) to other retinal conditions like macular hole, myopic foveoschisis, optic disk pit, uveitis, etc. [31]. There are various silicone oils with different physico-chemical properties (Table 68.1): The most frequently used ones are polydimethylsiloxanes (PDMS), that float within the vitreous cavity as they are lighter than water (specific gravity 0.97 g/cm³). The reported index of refraction is 1.4.

Cataracts are frequently developed after vitrectomy with silicone oil endotamponade, and therefore, biometry must be performed after they are used. The presence of this material will affect this measurement as both US and light speed are different from the vitreous humor.

The induced error will be higher in US biometry, where the acoustic density of the silicone oil will determines a US speed lower than vitreous:

972–980 m/s in the 1000 cSt and 978.5–1040 m/s in the 5000 cSt silicone oil [33]. If the normal measuring mode is used with the regular 1532 m/s US velocity for the vitreous compartment, the AL will be overestimated. The simplest solution is to adjust the vitreous humor speed correcting the value. If the software cannot be accessed, the corresponding segment can be recalculated with the following formula:

$$VC\,correct = VC(1532) * (US\,speed\,SO\,/\,1532)$$

where VC correct is the correct vitreous chamber length, VC(1532) is the vitreous chamber length measured with the regular US speed, and US speed SO is the US speed of the silicone oil within the eye. E.g. If the measured vitreous length is 22 mm and the silicone oil speed is 980 m/s: VC correct = 22(980/1532) = 14.07 mm.

Sometimes, there are different fluid segments within the vitreous chamber if the anterior vitreous has not been completely removed or if the silicon oil only partially fills the cavity, leaving a so-called retrosilicone space, which will be especially manifest if the biometry is done in supine position. This problem can be overcome by measuring the eye in the upright position, so that the silicone oil occupies the whole antero-posterior axis (Fig. 68.5).

Another issue can be the emulsification of silicone oil that occurs typically with low viscosity oils: Multiple oil drops will generate decreasing echo spikes not allowing the identification of the retinal signal. This adds to the fact that silicone oil sound absorption is high and the signal is attenuated as it travels through the fluid.

Table 68.1 Physico-chemical characteristics of silicone oils

Silicone oil tamponades	Chemical composition	Viscosity (centistoke)	Specific gravity (g/cm³)	Interfacial tensión (mN/m)	Refractive index
Conventional SO					
1000 cSt SO	100% PDMS	1000	0.97	35	1.4
5000 cSt SO	100% PDMS	5000	0.97	35	1.4
Heavy SO					
Oxane HD	88.1% 5700 cSt	3300	1.02	45	1.4
Densiron 68	Oxane/11.9% RMN-3 69.5% 5000 cSt PDMS/30.5% F₆H₈	1400	1.06	41	1.4

SO silicone oil, *RMN-3* a partially fluorinated olefin, *PDMS* polydimethylsiloxane [32]

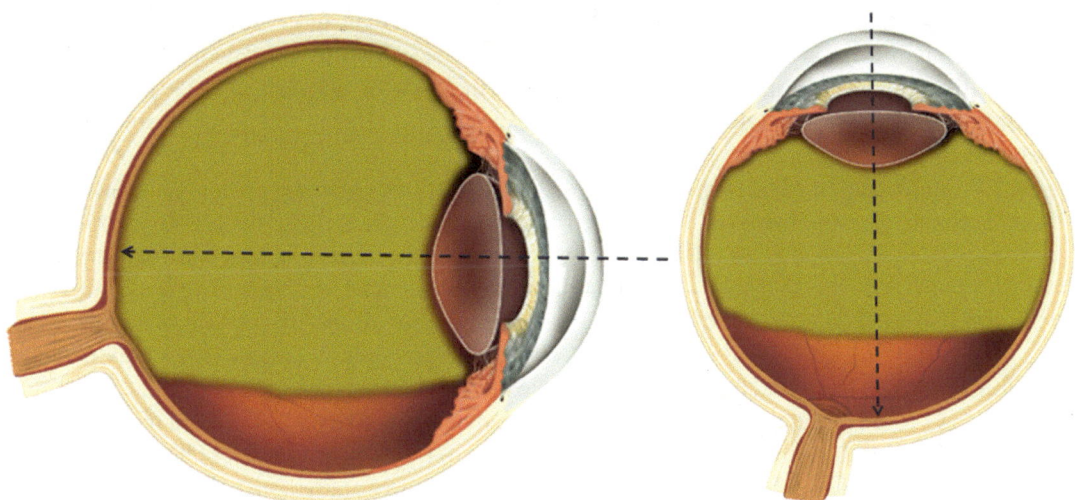

Fig. 68.5 Silicone oil filled eye US biometry: In supine position (left), a retrosilicone space will affect the measurement. This error will be avoided if the measurement is done in the upright position (right)

In a retrospective study, Madanagopalan et al. compared refractive results with US biometry between one group where cataract surgery and silicone oil removal was done the same day and another group where biometry was done after silicone oil removal in a two-step approach. Three months after surgery, the refractive error was higher in the silicone oil biometry group: -1.73 ± 2.04 vs. -0.64 ± 1.59 [34].

Optical biometry is less affected due to the lower relative impact of index of refraction change: from 1.336 to 1.4 (Densiron 68 has 1.387). If AL is measured in the normal phakic mode, the necessary correction is around -0.75 mm.

Since the first IOLMaster, all optical biometers have a silicone oil mode where a correction is applied. Reported results are good with no significant difference before and after silicone oil removal and low refraction prediction error [35, 36]. There might be some differences among different devices. Kulikov et al. found a slight underestimation of AL in shorter eyes (<23.63 mm) and an overestimation in longer eyes (<23.63 mm) when measurements with and without silicone oil were compared using Lenstar 900 and IOLMaster. The former had a difference of 0.09 mm and 0.23 mm in short and long eyes,

respectively. The same values were 0.12 mm and 0.28 mm for the IOLMaster [37].

Several studies report higher accuracy with optical biometry than with US biometry. Tayyab et al. compared IOL Master (version 5) and US A-scan before and after silicone oil removal: There was no significant difference with IOL Master while the US biometry showed a mean underestimation of AL of 0.63 mm. Postoperative refractive error was 0.70 ± 0.32 D with IOL Master and 1.55 ± 0.98 D with US biometry [38].

It can be concluded that adjusted optical biometry is quite accurate in these eyes, while adjusted US biometry is more affected by factors that decrease its precision.

It will be interesting to analyze the performance of new Swept Source biometers that measure segmental AL (e.g., Argos) where simply changing the index of refraction of the vitreous chamber should provide more correct measurements.

In order to avoid all these biometry inaccuracies, it is highly recommended that any eye undergoing PPV has measurements done before the surgery. It must be taken into account if the pathology itself can lead to a mismeasurement, e.g., macula-off RD, or if any other procedure that can alter the AL is performed, e.g., scleral buckling. The AL of the fellow eye can be used as a reference only if there is refraction and biometry symmetry. Another alternative is to perform intraoperative biometry (e.g., ORA system) once the silicone oil has been removed. Finally, delaying the IOL implantation can always be considered until reliable measurements can be obtained.

Bad Fixation and Macular Screening

The IOLMaster 700® has a unique feature among all biometers. It displays a 1 mm horizontal cross-sectional scan of the macular region where the foveal pit can be identified. It uses a wavelength of 1055 nm and has a scan depth of 44 mm and a scan width of 6 mm. Its resolution in tissue is 22 μm, and its measurement speed is 2000 A-scans per second [39]. This macular scan helps identifying the fixation status of the eye even in cases of low visual acuity due to retinal pathology.

Another benefit is the possibility of detecting unknown macular pathologies at the time of biometry. Even if the resolution of the image is much lower than in conventional retinal OCTs, foveal anatomy is usually recognized (Fig. 68.6).

Hirnshall et al. studied 125 eyes by three examiners and reported a moderate sensitivity (0.42–0.68) and high specificity (0.89–0.98) in the detection of macular pathologies. The interobserver reproducibility was 78.3–86.7%. Some diseases like mild-moderate macular atrophy or ERM were more difficult to detect than others probably due to the low resolution of the image [40]. Tognetto et al. studied 1089 eyes by seven examiners. In the detection of macular pathology, the mean sensitivity was 0.81 and the mean specificity 0.84. The positive predictive value was 0.78, and the negative predictive value was 0.86. Similarly to the previous study, the detection rate was higher for the macular hole and other pathologies involving retinal inner layer and lower for geographic atrophies, small drusen, and pigmented epithelium detachments [41].

The conclusion is that it is a valuable tool for macular screening but it cannot substitute for macular FD-OCT that performs better and provides information from a wider macular area.

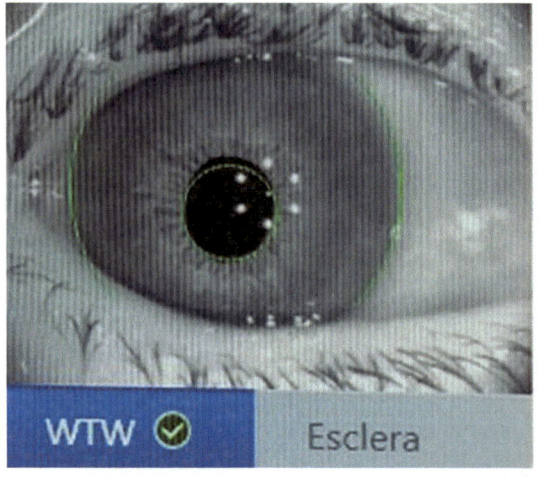 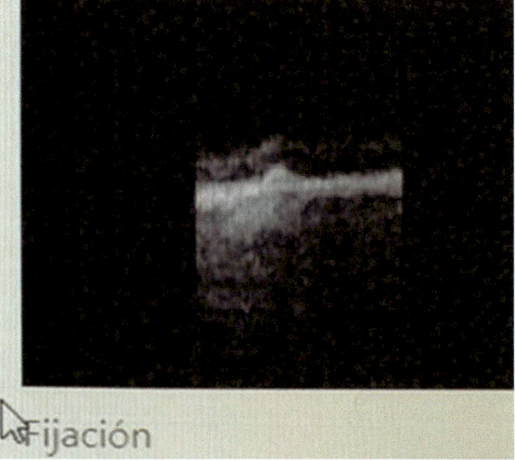

Fig. 68.6 Macular scar with IOLMaster 700 SS-OCT biometer

Vitreous Humor Optics

The vitreous humor is composed of 98–99% water and a framework of collagen fibers and hyaluronic acid. Hitzenberger calculated the group refractive index of these media from the dispersion values of water: 1.3459 and 1.3445 (for $\lambda = 780$ nm). There is some variability in the scientific literature about measurements of actual values with reported differences up to 0.009 [42].

All IOL power calculation formulas are pseudophakic eye models. Most of them are thin lens vergence formulas and some are thick lens exact raytracing models. But all of them assume that the index of refraction of vitreous and aqueous humors are equal (usually 1.336). This is also what can be found in the best known schematic eyes (Table 68.2) [43]. All of them show a very small difference between these two values (around 0.001).

Table 68.2 Refractive index of ocular humors in schematic eyes [43]

	Aqueous humor	Vitreous humor
Gullstrand exact #1	1.336	1.336
Le Grand	1.3374	1.336
Navarro	1.3374	1.336
Liou-Brennan	1.336	1.336

If the vitreous/aqueous index of refraction ratio of the vitrectomized eye is different from the model (formula), there will be a consequent error in the calculation. This will depend mainly on the IOL power and to a lesser extent, on its shape. If the index of refraction decreases, the optical effective power increases with a myopic shift in refraction. This might explain some of the refractive changes found after vitrectomy but more research is needed to clarify this point.

In Fig. 68.7, there is a plot of the refraction shift on the spectacle plane as a function of IOL power for a 0.005 change of vitreous index of refraction. The calculation was done for a biconvex IOL (Acrysof® SA60AT model).

This might be the explanation for the myopic refractive shift that has been reported in pseudophakic eyes undergoing vitrectomy. Sharma reported 0.85 D myopic shift in 25 RD eyes [44]. Hamoudi found 0.26 D myopic change in 28 eyes with ERM. ACD change was not analyzed in either of these studies [45]. Byrne studied 84 eyes and reported a myopic shift of 0.45 D. This was higher than 0.50 D in 52% of eyes. The ACD was unchanged [46]. Other potential factors of myopic shift, e.g., AL increase, were not investigated.

Fig. 68.7 Refraction shift as a function of IOL power for a vitreous index of refraction change of 0.005 with a biconvex IOL. Paraxial calculation. K = 43.5, corneal anterior/posterior ratio = 1.21; n cornea = 1.376; n aqueous = 1.336

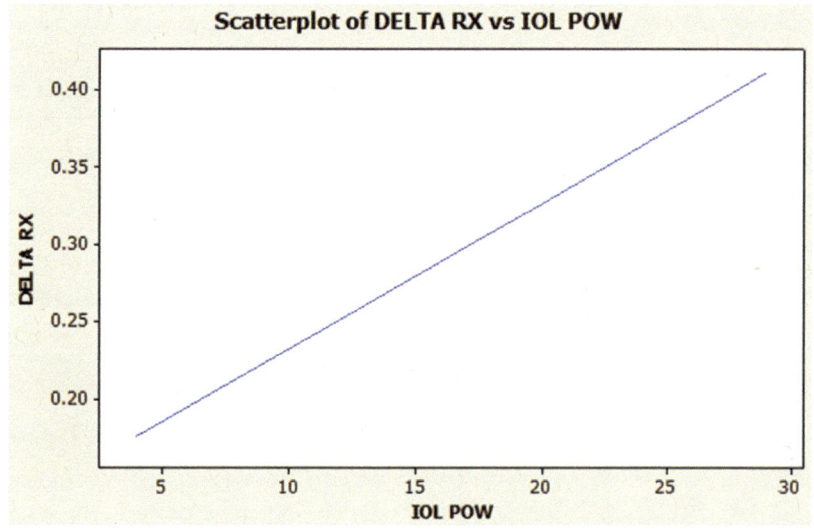

Silicone Oil and Refraction

In certain complicated cases, the silicone oil will not be removed from the eye and the induced refractive effect must be taken into account to achieve the desired refractive target. The increased index of refraction within the vitreous segment will affect the IOL-vitreous interface refraction, producing a decrease in the IOL effective power leading to a hyperopic spectacle plane refraction in which magnitude depends on the IOL index of refraction, IOL shape, and IOL power. The main factor is the IOL shape: The more convex the posterior surface is, the higher

Table 68.3 Refractions produced by different IOL shapes and powers [46]

	IOL power	Refraction
Plano Convex	13	6.27
	18	7.93
	23	9.59
Biconvex	13	5.36
	18	5.41
	23	5.45
Convex-Plano	13	2.47
	18	2.70
	23	2.95
Meniscus	13	−0.19
	18	0.06
	23	0.44

the refractive shift will be. McCartney et al. calculated this effect theoretically on different IOL shapes. For a biconvex IOL, the effect was around 5.50 D. On the contrary, a meniscus IOL had a negligible refractive change (Table 68.3) [47]. In Fig. 68.8, the refractive change as a function of IOL power is plotted for a silicone oil with the index of refraction value of 1.4 . The calculations are done by paraxial raytracing for a biconvex IOL (Acrysof® SA60AT).

Grinbaum reported a mean PO hyperopia of 4 D, with a wide 4.40 D range in a series of eight cases [48]. Fang et al. studied 27 eyes with a mean AL of 25.84 ± 3.28 mm. The silicone oil induced a refractive shift of 3.90 ± 1.74D, which was correlated with IOL power and with ACD [49]. Song et al. reported a myopic shift of −4.51 ± 1.79 D when the silicone oil was removed from the eyes of 26 eyes [50].

The refractive target will depend on the power and shape of the IOL that will be implanted. It must be remembered than for 0.35 D spectacle plane refraction change, approximately 0.50 D of labeled IOL power change is needed. For example, if 4.5 D of hyperopia are expected, the amount needed to be added to the calculated IOL for emmetropia is 6.43 D.

An alternative that minimizes this source of error is to implant a meniscus or a convex-plano IOL to minimize the induced refractive change.

Fig. 68.8 Silicone oil (*n* = 1.4) induced refractive change is directly proportional to IOL power. Paraxial calculations for a biconvex IOL. K = 43.5 and ELP is adjusted for AXL

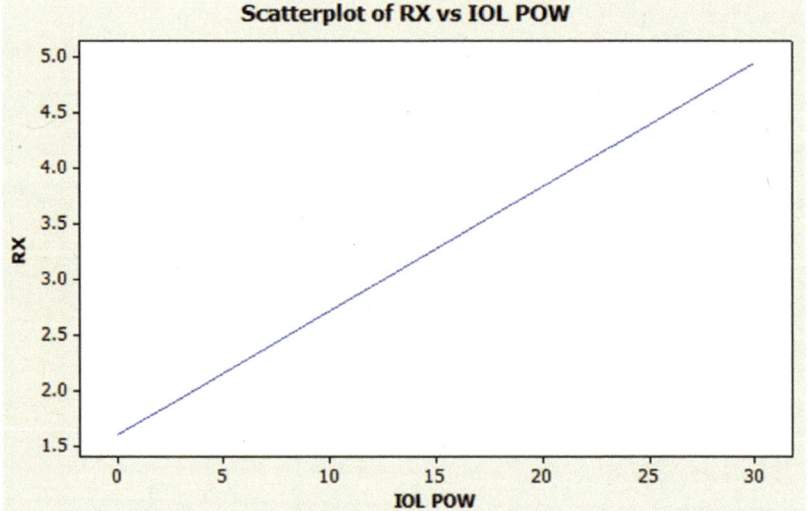

IOL Position, Tilt and Centration

The IOL power calculation formulas predict the position of the IOL using different algorithms based on a data series. Linear and non-linear regression functions, and lately machine learning algorithms, have been used to accomplish this task. After vitrectomy, this might be a source of error in refraction prediction, as some differences in IOL position have been reported.

Any change in the axial IOL position within the eye will affect the effective refractive power of the IOL. If the IOL sits posterior to the predicted plane, i.e., deeper in the eye, a hyperopic error will occur while the inverse situation will produce a myopic error. The refractive error magnitude will depend mainly on the ACD error and on the IOL power. Figure 68.9 shows how a small (0.10 mm) and a mid-level (0.50 mm) error will affect the refraction in the IOL plane and in the spectacle plane in eyes of four different ALs.

Many studies have measured this parameter usually comparing a sample undergoing phacovitrectomy and a matched sample of phacoemulsification without vitrectomy as control. Contradictory results have been published: deeper, shallower, and unchanged ACD after vitrectomy. Recently, very accurate SS-OCT devices are probably reporting the most reliable numbers: Three papers using Casia 2 (Tomey) SS-OCT found no significant differences between phacovitrectomy and control groups [51–53]. One study found a shallower ACD in a group that had had gas tamponade [53]. Mijnsbrugge et al. described a deeper ACD after phacovitrectomy in 20 eyes using the IOLMaster 700. This is the only published paper where the control group was composed of the other 20 fellow eyes that underwent phacoemulsification. The difference was 0.16 mm [54].

Even in the papers where there is no difference, it can be seen that in eyes without gas tamponade, there is a trend towards a deeper ACD. It has been proposed that the use of any tamponade after surgery (air, gas, or silicone oil) can alter the zonular fibers and induce an anteriorization of the IOL-bag complex. But more evidence is needed to support this concept and to calculate any predicting function.

IOL tilt and decentration affect the optical performance of the IOL inducing astigmatism and higher-order aberrations [55]. It can be expected that these eyes have a higher incidence due to zonular and IOL instability, the use of

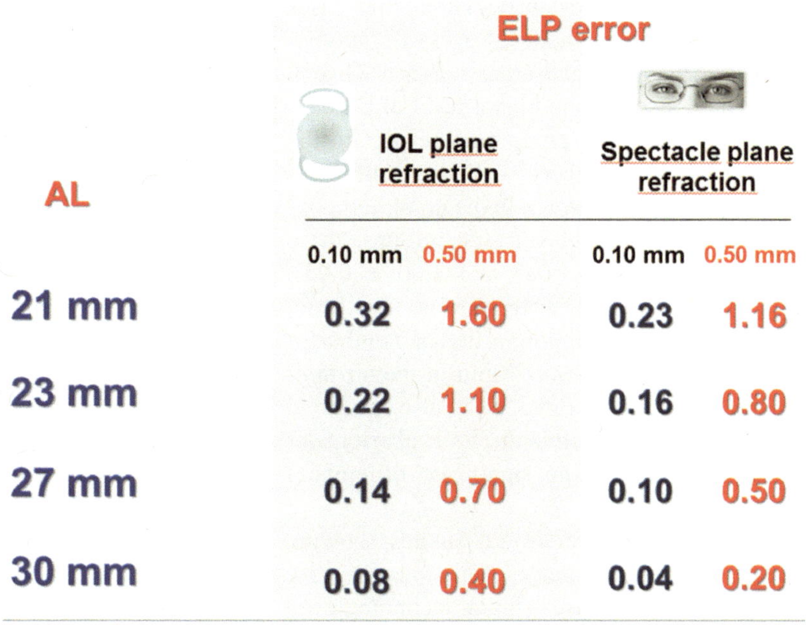

Fig. 68.9 Refractive effect in the IOL plane and the spectacle plane refraction of two different effective lens position (ELP) errors: 0.10 and 0.50 mm. Calculations are done for four different ALs. Paraxial calculations with K = 44 D

ELP error

AL	IOL plane refraction		Spectacle plane refraction	
	0.10 mm	0.50 mm	0.10 mm	0.50 mm
21 mm	0.32	1.60	0.23	1.16
23 mm	0.22	1.10	0.16	0.80
27 mm	0.14	0.70	0.10	0.50
30 mm	0.08	0.40	0.04	0.20

endotamponades, and increased capsular fibrosis. This knowledge is valuable in order to calculate the effect on toric IOLs and to help in the selection of the IOL model. Highly aspheric IOLs can induce HOAs if tilt and decentration are significant. Holladay et al. calculated on a theoretical model some threshold values beyond which the performance (in terms of MTF) of an aspheric IOL is affected: 7° for tilt and 0.4 mm for decentration [56].

There are a few papers studying this issue, and again, they yielded contradictory conclusions. Tan et al. found an increase of tilt and decentration when they compared 104 eyes with the previous vitrectomy and 104 eyes without any previous surgery using SS-OCT AS-tomography. Tilt was 5.36° ± 2.50° and 4.54° ± 1.46°, respectively. Decentration was 0.27 ± 0.17 mm and 0.19 ± 0.12 mm. In the vitrectomy group, tilt was >7° in 18.27% of cases vs 5.77% of cases in the control group. In a similar way, decentration >0.4 mm occurred in 21.25% of cases in the vitrectomy group and only in 6.73% of cases in the control group. Ocular aberrometry measured a significantly higher level of HOA in the vitrectomy group: 0.64 ± 0.51 μm vs 0.31 ± 0.17 μm. Risk factors for tilt were silicone oil use in the PPV and a hydrophilic IOL. The only risk factor for decentration was diabetes mellitus [52]. Iwama et al. compared phacovitrectomy cases with (24 eyes) and without (21 eyes) air tamponade, and regular cataract surgery cases (18 eyes). They found a significant higher level of tilt only in the air tamponade group with respect to the normal group. Surgery induced tilt was 1.89° ± 1.32° in this group. In the no-air tamponade and the phacoemulsification groups, these values were 1.54 ± 1.08° and 1.00 ± 0.95°, respectively. Although there were no significant differences in decentration, a higher number of eyes with decentration >0.4 mm in the air tamponade group was reported. They also measured the HOAs with a Hartmann-Shack aberrometer finding that there is no significant differences among groups [57].

However, there are several studies showing non or minimal differences. This was the case with Sato et al. who used similar technologies to compare a group of 60 eyes that underwent phacovitrectomy and 60 eyes of a control group with only phacoemulsification surgery. Three months after surgery, there were no significant differences neither in tilt (4.33° ± 1.47° and 4.84° ± 1.43°, respectively) nor in decentration (0.19 ± 0.12 mm and 0.18 ± 0.09 mm, respectively) [51]. Leisser et al. compared tilt and decentration in two groups that underwent phacovitrectomy using air tamponade in one of them and balanced salt solution in the other. There were no significant differences in either of the variables. Average values were 4.33° ± 1.47° for tilt and for 0.18 ± 0.09 mm decentration. These values look similar to non-vitrectomized eyes [58].

As new SS-OCT tomographers and biometers expand and become the standard of use, more studies will be performed and hopefully all issues related to IOL positioning after PPV will be clearly described.

IOL Calculation in the Vitrectomized Eye

Cataract surgery in a previously vitrectomized eye is technically more challenging due to several anatomical factors produced by the removal of the vitreous and the use of tamponade agents: deep and variable ACD, posterior capsule damage and fluctuations, zonular weakness, and intraoperative miosis, etc.

The IOL power calculation is also more difficult in these eyes: There is a high prevalence of very long eyes with their intrinsic challenges, the IOL position prediction might be affected by the absence of vitreous and the effect of the vitrectomy on the zonular apparatus, the presence of silicone oil can affect the biometric measurements, and finally, the reliability of PO refraction is certainly worse due to the lower visual acuity of these eyes affecting the analysis of outcomes. There are very few papers analyzing these calculations in the last 15 years. Most of them reported some hyperopic shift in the refraction after surgery if the normal IOL constants are used. The most plausible reason is a combination of IOL position prediction error (the IOL is more poste-rior than predicted) and a formula error if AL is longer than average.

The newer generation formulas predict the IOL position using four or more variables: In addition to AL and K, they normally get direct information about the anterior segment depth from ACD and LT. Moreover, they have corrected the AL bias related to the IOLMaster calibration method [8]. Many papers have shown a real accu-racy improvement over the third-generation for-mulas [59].

Regarding vitrectomized eyes, Tan et al. stud-ied 111 eyes and found some hyperopic shift with the normal IOL constants in all formulas (Barrett UII, EVO, Ladas, Haigis, SRK/T, Hoffer Q and Holladay 1) except the Kane formula that had a mean PE of only 0.09 D. Haigis had the highest hyperopic shift (0.46 D) This error was AL related as it was higher in a subgroup with AL > 26 mm. When the IOL constants were opti-mized, the results of the new formulas were a little better, although there was no statistically significant differences in prediction accuracy among them and Haigis and Hoffer Q. Refractions were within ±0.50 D of prediction in a range of 49.53–60.75%. Formula results from best to worst were EVO, Kane, Haigis, Barrett UII, Hoffer Q, SRK/T, Holladay 1 and Ladas SF. In long eyes (33 eyes with AL > 26 mm), the Wang-Koch AL optimization improved the results of the third-generation formulas, and there was no significant difference among all formulas in the study [60]. Lamson et al. studied 61 eyes and found some hyperopic prediction error for all for-mulas. IOL constants were not optimized. The standard deviation of all prediction error was similar for all formulas: 0.72–0.82. A small sub-group of eyes calculated with Holladay 1 and SRK/T and the Wang-Koch adjustment showed a nil prediction error. Refractions were within ±0.5D of prediction in a range of 45–60.42%. Formulas from best to worst were Holladay 2, Holladay 1, SRK/T, Barrett UII, RBF and Ladas [61]. In 2009, Lee et al. studied 45 eyes where AL had been measured with US biometry. The calculation formulas were SRK/T for eyes with Al > 25 mm and SRK II. This group had a hyper-

opic prediction error of +0.40 ± 1.07 D while a control group had +0.19 ± 0.82 D [62].

From these studies, it can be concluded that there is some hyperopic prediction error in the IOL power calculation on vitrectomized eyes that should be considered in the preoperative assess-ment. There is no clear explanation for this, although a plausible hypothesis is a more poste-rior IOL location within the eye attributable to the lack of vitreous support and/or higher zonular laxity.

IOL Calculation in Phacovitrectomy

Combined phacoemulsification and PPV (phaco-vitrectomy) has become a routine procedure for the retinal surgeon. IOL calculation and refrac-tive results have been extensively analyzed in multiple studies where a phacovitrectomy group is compared with a regular phacoemulsification control group. The vast majority of them report either a myopic prediction error [13, 18, 53, 63–66] or a neutral effect with no difference between groups [51, 53, 67–70].

Myopic shift was first related to incorrect AL measurement in certain pathologies like macula off RD, where both the US and the PCI biometry tend to get the retinal signal from the anteriorized vitreoretinal interface underestimating the AL value [19, 21]. This can also occur in macular pucker where the PCI can identify the thick epiretinal membrane as the retina displaying a double peak in the A-scan [15]. This point has been discussed above. However, there are studies with the same pathologies and no myopic shift. Shiraki et al. report no refractive error in a group of 20 ERM eyes and a myopic shift (−0.82 ± 0.64 D) in a group of 22 eyes that had macular hole and RD. They explain the myopic shift by the use of gas tamponade in the second group [53]. Hötte et al. reported similar results in a group of macu-lar pathology, where the eyes that had gas tam-ponade (macular holes) had a myopic prediction error (−0.31) and those who had not showed nil prediction error (ERM and floaters) [66]. On the contrary, Van der Geest found no prediction error in an analogous sample, macular pathology, with no difference between gas use or not [68]. Ercan also reported no prediction error in 100 eyes with macular pathology with gas tamponade. Prediction accuracy was very good with 80–84% of eyes with MAE < 0.50 D [67].

Biometry technology analysis does not clarify this controversy: There are studies on both sides with all biometers: US, PCI, and SS-OCT. The same can be said about IOL calculation formulas. Modern formulas with new ELP algorithms and AL bias correction render accurate results in some cases and myopic errors in others: Sato et al. [51] and Shiraki et al. (no gas eyes) [53] found no error with Barrett UII, while Vounotrypidis et al. reported myopic shift with modern formulas, Barrett UII included [63]. In this last study, where only ERM cases were included, the calculation was done after IOL constants were optimized in the phacoemulsification group. With these "normal" IOL constants, there was a myopic predictive error in all formulas: −0.14 to −0.21 D. When the constants were optimized for the phacovitrectomy group, results were similarly accurate for all formulas: 65.6% −73.4% of eyes with MAE < 0.50 D. Formulas from best to worst were Holladay 2, Kane, Haigis, SRK/T, Barrett UII, Hoffer Q, RBF, and Holladay 1. Eyes longer than 27 mm were not included in this study, and this might have biased results in detriment to newer generation formulas.

AL has been related to the degree of myopic error: Jee et al. studied 91 eyes that had surgery for macular hole where AL was measured with PCI. In 73 eyes with AL < 26 mm, the prediction error was lower (−0.43 ± 0.63 D) than in 18 eyes with AL > 26 mm (−1.08 ± 0.87 D) [64]. In US biometry, it has been argued that there is some IOP effect leading to the underestimation of AL: Cho et al. found myopic prediction error (−0.43 ± 0.67 D) in 25 eyes that had macula-on RD and no prediction error in 30 eyes with other pathologies [71].

In conclusion, biometric measurements must be carefully checked in this surgical technique, looking for any incorrect retinal identification in the scan. There might be some myopic refractive error that can only be addressed optimizing the IOL constant for phacovitrectomy eyes. Newer generation formulas will address AL induced bias with outcomes slightly worse than those obtained in normal eyes.

References

1. Hsuan JD, Brown NA, Bron AJ, Patel CK, Rosen PH. Posterior subcapsular and nuclear cataract after vitrectomy. J Cataract Refract Surg. 2001;27(3):437–44.
2. Lundström M, Dickman M, Henry Y, Manning S, Rosen P, Tassignon MJ, Young D, Stenevi U. Cataract surgery of eyes with previous vitrectomy: risks and benefits as reflected in the European Registry of Quality Outcomes for Cataract and Refractive Surgery. J Cataract Refract Surg. 2020;46(10):1402–7.
3. Sisk RA, Murray TG. Combined phacoemulsification and sutureless 23-gauge pars plana vitrectomy for complex vitreoretinal diseases. Br J Ophthalmol. 2010;94(8):1028–32.
4. Savastano A, Savastano MC, Barca F, Petrarchini F, Mariotti C, Rizzo S. Combining cataract surgery with 25-gauge high-speed pars plana vitrectomy. Ophthalmology. 2014;121:299–304.
5. Shammas HJ. A-scan biometry. Intraocular lens power calculations. Thorofare: Slack Incorporated; 2004. p. 95–104.
6. Ademola-Popoola DS, Nzeh DA, Saka SE, Olokoba LB, Obajolowo TS. Comparison of ocular biometry measurements by applanation and immersion A-scan techniques. J Curr Ophthalmol. 2016;27(3–4):110–4.
7. Hitzenberger CK, Drexler W, Leitgeb RA, Findl O, Fercher AF. Key developments for partial coherence biometry and optical coherence tomography in the human eye made in Vienna. Invest Ophthalmol Vis Sci. 2016;57(9):460–74.
8. Haigis W, Lege B, Miller N, Schneider B. Comparison of immersion ultrasound biometry and partial coherence interferometry for intraocular lens calculation according to Haigis. Graefes Arch Clin Exp Ophthalmol. 2000;238:765–73.
9. Cooke DL, Cooke TL. A comparison of two methods to calculate axial length. J Cataract Refract Surg. 2019;45(3):284–92.
10. Vogel A, Dick HB, Krummenauer F. Reproducibility of optical biometry using partial coherence interferometry : intraobserver and interobserver reliability. J Cataract Refract Surg. 2001;27(12):1961–8.
11. Hamoudi H, La Cour M. Refractive changes after vitrectomy and phacovitrectomy for macular hole and epiretinal membrane. J Cataract Refract Surg. 2013;39:942–7.
12. Kovacs I, Ferencz M, Nemes J, Somfai G, Salacz G. Intraocular lens power calculation for combined cataract surgery vitrectomy and peeling of epiretinal membranes for macular oedema. Acta Ophthalmol Scand. 2007;85:88–91.

13. Sun HJ, Choi KS. Improving intraocular lens power prediction in combined phacoemulsification and vitrectomy in eyes with macular oedema. Acta Ophthalmol. 2011;89:575–8.

14. Falkner-Radler CI, Benesch T, Binder S. Accuracy of preoperative biometry in vitrectomy combined with cataract surgery for patients with epiretinal membranes and macular holes; results of a prospective controlled clinical trial. J Cataract Refract Surg. 2008;34:1754–60.

15. Kojima T, Tamaoki A, Yoshida N, Kaga T, Suto C, Ichikawa K. Evaluation of axial length measurement of the eye using partial coherence interferometry and ultrasound in cases of macular disease. Ophthalmology. 2010;117(9):1750–4.

16. Kitaguchi Y, Yano S, Gomi F. Axial length estimation error caused by hidden double-peak on partial coherence interferometry in an eye with epiretinal membrane: a case report. Clin Ophthalmol. 2014;8:555–9.

17. Huang Q, Li J. With or without internal limiting membrane peeling during idiopathic epiretinal membrane surgery: a meta-analysis. PLoS One. 2021;16(1):e0245459.

18. Vounotrypidis E, Haralanova V, Muth DR, Wertheimer C, Shajari M, Wolf A, Priglinger S, Mayer WJ. Accuracy of SS-OCT biometry compared with partial coherence interferometry biometry for combined phacovitrectomy with internal limiting membrane peeling. J Cataract Refract Surg. 2019;45(1):48–53.

19. Lege BA, Haigis W. Laser interference biometry versus ultrasound biometry in certain clinical conditions. Graefes Arch Clin Exp Ophthalmol. 2004;242(1):8–12.

20. Liu R, Li Q. Changes in ocular biometric measurements after vitrectomy with silicone oil tamponade for rhegmatogenous retinal detachment repair. BMC Ophthalmol. 2020;20(1):360.

21. Abou-Shousha M, Helaly HA, Osman IM. The accuracy of axial length measurements in cases of macula-off retinal detachment. Can J Ophthalmol. 2016;51(2):108–12.

22. Rahman R, Bong CX, Stephenson J. Accuracy of intraocular lens power estimation in eyes having phacovitrectomy for rhegmatogenous retinal detachment. Retina. 2014;34(7):1415–20.

23. Rahman R, Kolb S, Bong CX, Stephenson J. Accuracy of user-adjusted axial length measurements with optical biometry in eyes having combined phacovitrectomy for macular-off rhegmatogenous retinal detachment. J Cataract Refract Surg. 2016;42(7):1009–14.

24. Pongsachareonnont P, Tangjanyatam S. Accuracy of axial length measurements obtained by optical biometry and acoustic biometry in rhegmatogenous retinal detachment: a prospective study. Clin Ophthalmol. 2018;12:973–80.

25. El-Khayat AR, Brent AJ, Peart SAM, Chaudhuri PR. Accuracy of intraocular lens calculations based on fellow-eye biometry for phacovitrectomy for macula-off rhegmatogenous retinal detachments. Eye. 2019;33(11):1756–61.

26. Lee DH, Han JW, Kim SS, Byeon SH, Koh HJ, Lee SC, Kim M. Long-term effect of scleral encircling on axial elongation. Am J Ophthalmol. 2018;189:139–45.

27. Wong CW, Ang M, Tsai A, Phua V, Lee SY. A prospective study of biometric stability after scleral buckling surgery. Am J Ophthalmol. 2016;165:47–53.

28. Albanese GM, Cerini A, Visioli G, Marenco M, Gharbiya M. Long-term ocular biometric variations after scleral buckling surgery in macula-on rhegmatogenous retinal detachment. BMC Ophthalmol. 2021;21(1):172.

29. Malukiewicz-Wiśniewska G, Stafiej J. Changes in axial length after retinal detachment surgery. Eur J Ophthalmol. 1999;9(2):115–9.

30. Van der Heijde GL, Weber. Accommodation used to determine ultrasound velocity in the human lens. J Optom Vis Sci. 1989;66:830–3.

31. Stappler T, Morphis G, Irigoyen C, Heimann H. Is there a role for long-term silicone oil tamponade for more than twelve months in vitreoretinal surgery? Ophthalmologica. 2011;226 Suppl 1:36–41.

32. Vaziri K, Schwartz SG, Kishor KS, Flynn HW Jr. Tamponade in the surgical management of retinal detachment. Clin Ophthalmol. 2016;10:471–6.

33. Kanclerz P, Grzybowski A. Accuracy of intraocular lens power calculation in eyes filled with silicone oil. Semin Ophthalmol. 2019;34(5):392–7.

34. Madanagopalan VG, Susvar P, Arthi M. Refractive outcomes of a single-step and a two-step approach for silicone oil removal and cataract surgery. Indian J Ophthalmol. 2019;67(5):625–9.

35. Habibabadi HF, Hashemi H, Jalali KH, Amini A, Esfahani MR. Refractive outcome of silicone oil removal and intraocular lens implantation using laser interferometry. Retina. 2005;25:162–6.

36. Parravano M, Oddone F, Sampalmieri M, Gazzaniga D. Reliability of the IOLMaster in axial length evaluation in silicone oil-filled eyes. Eye (Lond). 2007;21(7):909–11.

37. Kulikov AN, Kokareva EV, Kuznetsov AR. Optical biometry features in silicon oil filled eye. Ophthalmol J. 2018;11:15–20.

38. Tayyab H, Ali HM, Jahangir T. Intraocular lens power calculation in silicone oil filled eye: IOL master versus A-mode acoustic biometry. Pak J Ophthalmol. 2017;33(1):4–8.

39. Hirnschall N, Varsits R, Doeller B, Findl O. Enhanced penetration for axial length measurement of eyes with dense cataracts using swept source optical coherence tomography: a consecutive observational study. Ophthalmol Ther. 2018;7(1):119–24.

40. Hirnschall N, Leisser C, Radda S, Maedel S, Findl O. Macular disease detection with a swept-source optical coherence tomography-based biometry device in patients scheduled for cataract surgery. J Cataract Refract Surg. 2016;42(4):530–6.

41. Tognetto D, Pastore MR, De Giacinto C, Merli R, Franzon M, D'Aloisio R, Belfanti L, Giglio R,

Cirigliano G. Swept-source optical coherence tomography biometer as screening strategy for macular disease in patients scheduled for cataract surgery. Sci Rep. 2019;9(1):9912.

42. Sardar DK, Swanland GY, Yow RM, Thomas RJ, Tsin AT. Optical properties of ocular tissues in the near infrared region. Lasers Med Sci. 2007;22(1):46–52.

43. Atchison D. Schemetic eyes. [aut. libro] Artal P. Handbook of visual optics. Boca Raton: CRC Press; 2017. p. 235–248.

44. Sharma YR, Karunanithi S, Azad RV, Vohra R, Pal N, Singh DV, Chandra P. Functional and anatomic outcome of scleral buckling versus primary vitrectomy in pseudophakic retinal detachment. Acta Ophthalmol Scand. 2005;83:293–7.

45. Hamoudi H, Kofod M, La Cour M. Refractive change after vitrectomy for epiretinal membrane in pseudophakic eyes. Acta Ophthalmol. 2013;91:434–6.

46. Byrne S, Ng J, Hildreth A, Danjoux JP, Steel DH. Refractive change following pseudophakic vitrectomy. BMC Ophthalmol. 2008;8:19.

47. McCartney DL, Millar KM, Stara WJ, et al. Intraocular lens style and refraction in eyes treated with silicone oil. Arch Ophthalmol. 1987;71:898–902.

48. Grinbaum A, Tresiter G, Moisseiev J. Predicted and actual refraction alter intraocular lens implantation in eyes with silicone oil. J Cataract Refract Surg. 1996;22:726–9.

49. Fang W, Li J, Jin X, Zhai J, Dai Y, Li Y. Refractive shift of silicone oil tamponade in pseudophakic eye. BMC Ophthalmol. 2016;16:144.

50. Song WK, Kim SS, Kim SE, Lee SC. Refractive status and visual acuity changes after oil removal in eyes following phacovitrectomy, intraocular lens implantation, and silicone oil tamponade. Can J Ophthalmol. 2010;45(6):616–20.

51. Sato T, Korehisa H, Shibata S, Hayashi K. Prospective comparison of intraocular lens dynamics and refractive error between phacovitrectomy and phacoemulsification alone. Ophthalmol Retina. 2020;4(7):700–7.

52. Tan X, Liu Z, Chen X, Zhu Y, Xu J, Qiu X, Yang G, Peng L, Gu X, Zhang J, Luo L, Liu Y. Characteristics and risk factors of intraocular lens tilt and decentration of phacoemulsification after pars plana vitrectomy. Transl Vis Sci Technol. 2021;10(3):26.

53. Shiraki N, Wakabayashi T, Sakaguchi H, Nishida K. Effect of gas tamponade on the intraocular lens position and refractive error after phacovitrectomy: a swept-source anterior segment OCT analysis. Ophthalmology. 2020;127(4):511–5.

54. Mijnsbrugge JV, Fils JF, Jansen J, Hua MT, Stalmans P. The role of the vitreous body in effective IOL positioning. Graefes Arch Clin Exp Ophthalmol. 2018;256(8):1517–20.

55. de Castro A, Rosales P, Marcos S. Tilt and decentration of intraocular lenses in vivo from Purkinje and Scheimpflug imaging. Validation study. J Cataract Refract Surg. 2007;33:418–29.

56. Holladay JT, Piers PA, Koranyi G, van der Mooren M, Norrby NE. A new intraocular lens design to reduce spherical aberration of pseudophakic eyes. J Refract Surg. 2002;18:683–91.

57. Iwama Y, Maeda N, Ikeda T, Nakashima H, Emi K. Impact of vitrectomy and air tamponade on aspheric intraocular lens tilt and decentration and ocular higher-order aberrations: phacovitrectomy versus cataract surgery. Jpn J Ophthalmol. 2020;64(4):359–66.

58. Leisser C, Hirnschall N, Findl O. Effect of air tamponade on tilt of the intraocular lens after phacovitrectomy. Ophthalmologica. 2019;242(2):118–22.

59. Melles RB, Kane JX, Olsen T, Chang WJ. Update on intraocular lens calculation formulas. Ophthalmology. 2019;126(9):1334–5.

60. Tan X, Zhang J, Zhu Y, Xu J, Qiu X, Yang G, Liu Z, Luo L, Liu Y. Accuracy of new generation intraocular lens calculation formulas in vitrectomized eyes. Am J Ophthalmol. 2020;217:81–90.

61. Lamson TL, Song J, Abazari A, Weissbart SB. Refractive outcomes of phacoemulsification after pars plana vitrectomy using traditional and new intraocular lens calculation formulas. J Cataract Refract Surg. 2019;45(3):293–7.

62. Lee NY, Park SH, Joo CK. Refractive outcomes of phacoemulsification and intraocular lens implantation after pars plana vitrectomy. Retina. 2009;29(4):487–91.

63. Vounotrypidis E, Shajari M, Muth DR, Hirnschall N, Findl O, Priglinger S, Mayer WJ. Refractive outcomes of 8 biometric formulas in combined phacovitrectomy with internal limiting membrane peeling for epiretinal membrane. J Cataract Refract Surg. 2020;46(4):591–7.

64. Jee D, Park YR, Jung KI, Kim E, La TY. Refractive errors in high myopic eyes after phacovitrectomy for macular hole. Int J Ophthalmol. 2015;8(2):369–73.

65. Sakamoto M, Yoshida I, Sodeno T, Sakai A, Masahara H, Maeno T. Postoperative refractive prediction error measured by optical and acoustic biometry after phacovitrectomy for Rhegmatogenous retinal detachment without macular involvement. J Ophthalmol. 2019;2:5964127.

66. Hötte GJ, de Bruyn DP, de Hoog J. Post-operative refractive prediction error after phacovitrectomy: a retrospective study. Ophthalmol Ther. 2018;7(1):83–94.

67. Ercan ZE, Akkoyun İ, Yaman Pınarcı E, Yılmaz G, Topçu H. Refractive outcome comparison between vitreomacular interface disorders after phacovitrectomy. J Cataract Refract Surg. 2017;43(8):1068–71.

68. Van der Geest LJ, Siemerink MJ, Mura M, Mourits MP, Lapid-Gortzak R. Refractive outcomes after phacovitrectomy surgery. J Cataract Refract Surg. 2016;42(6):840–5.

69. Manvikar SR, Allen D, Steel DH. Optical biometry in combined phacovitrectomy. J Cataract Refract Surg. 2009;35(1):64–9.

70. Jeoung JW, Chung H, Yu HG. Factors influencing refractive outcomes after combined phacoemulsification and pars plana vitrectomy: results of a prospective study. J Cataract Refract Surg. 2007;33(1):108–14.

71. Cho KH, Park IW, Kwon SI. Changes in postoperative refractive outcomes following combined phacoemulsification and pars plana vitrectomy for rhegmatogenous retinal detachment. Am J Ophthalmol. 2014;158(2):251–6.

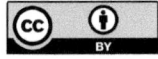

IOL Power Calculation in Keratoplasty

Edmondo Borasio

In the last 20 years or so, giant steps have been made in the transition from full thickness (penetrating) to partial thickness (lamellar) corneal grafts, where only the diseased layer is replaced. This has led to safer, less invasive procedures and faster vision recovery. The improvement in the results has also increased the importance of accurate IOL power calculations in these cases.

The most commonly used techniques are **Penetrating Keratoplasty (PK)** (Fig. 69.1e), where all layers of the cornea are replaced and kept in place by several sutures; **Deep Anterior Lamellar Keratoplasty (DALK)** (Fig. 69.1f), where the front layers are removed, only leaving the Descemet membrane and the corneal endothelium (in some cases, a fine layer of the posterior corneal stroma is also left in place); **Descemet Stripping Automated Keratoplasty (DSAEK)** (Fig. 69.1c), where only the endothelium and the Descemet membrane are removed and replaced with a lamella comprising posterior stroma, Descemet membrane and corneal endothelium, held in place with an air bubble. It is called "automated" because the donor lamella is harvested from the eye by means of a mechanical microkeratome; **Endothelial Keratoplasty (EK)** (Fig. 69.1d), where only the endothelium and the Descemet membrane are removed and replaced by Descemet and endothelium carefully stripped from the donor with a manual technique.

For the purpose of IOL power calculations, it is important to understand the changes that the different procedures produce to the anterior and posterior corneal curvature and on the other parameters (Table 69.1).

E. Borasio (✉)
EYE PRO Studio Oculistico
e-mail: dr@edmondoborasio.com;
http://www.edmondoborasio.com

J. Aramberri et al. (eds.), *Intraocular Lens Calculations*, Essentials in Ophthalmology,
https://doi.org/10.1007/978-3-031-50666-6_69

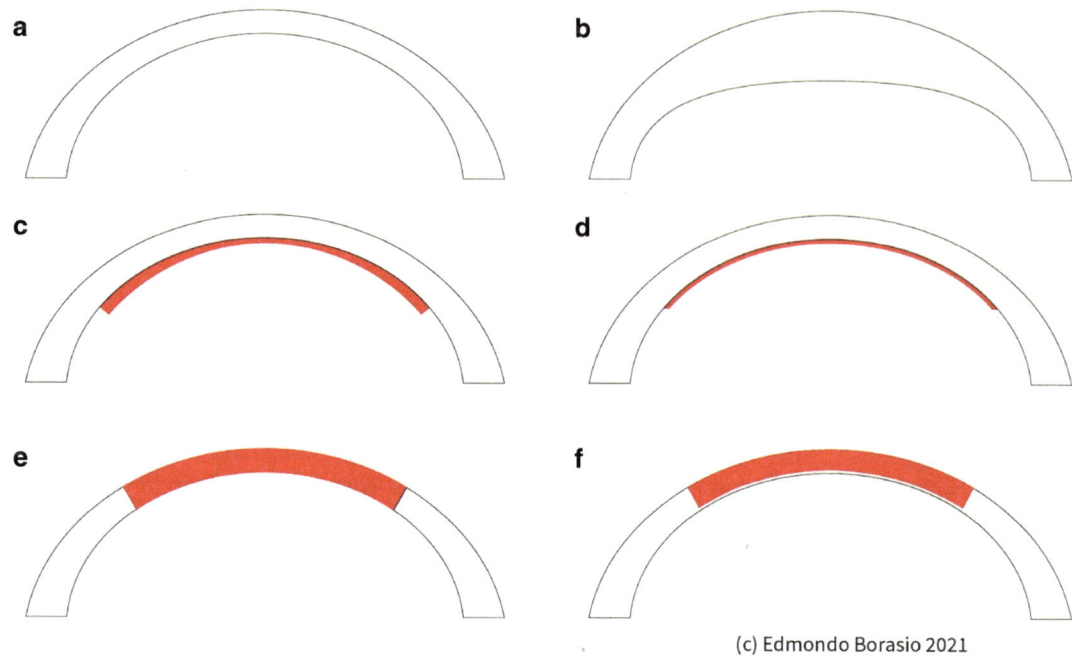

Fig. 69.1 Keratoplasty techniques. **a**) Normal corneal anatomy. **b**) Altered posterior corneal curvature due to endothelial failure such as in Fuch's corneal endothelial dystrophy or bullous keratopathy from any cause. **c**) Status post DSAEK. **d**) Status post DMEK. **e**) Status post PK. **f**) Status post DALK

Table 69.1 Corneal changes induced by keratoplasty techniques

	Changes in anterior corneal curvature	Changes in posterior corneal curvature	Changes in axial length	Changes in ant/post corneal ratio	Changes in central corneal thickness	Changes in ACD
PK	Yes	Possible	Yes	Possible	Yes	Possible
DALK	Yes	Possible	Yes	Possible	Yes	Posssible
DSAEK	No[a]	Yes—marked[b]	No	Yes	Yes—marked	No
EK	No[a]	Yes[b]	No	Yes	Yes—marked	No

[a] No significant changes unless presence of massive bullae in the decompensated cornea

[b] The changes in the posterior corneal curvature are not only due to the actual anatomy of the donor lamella as in the case of DSAEK, but also due to the resolving edema (Fig. 69.1b), in the weeks following a successful DSAEK or EK procedure

Factors Limiting IOL Power Calculation Accuracy in Eyes Undergoing Simultaneous Cataract Surgery and Corneal Transplantation (Triple Procedure)

IOL power calculation in eyes undergoing simultaneous keratoplasty and cataract surgery is intrinsically inaccurate and unpredictable due to the fact that the parameters used in the calculation get altered during the procedure itself [1, 2]. In particular:

- **Anterior corneal curvature (K readings, or Sim Ks)** gets significantly affected after Penetrating Keratoplasty (PK) or Deep Anterior Lamellar Keratoplasty (DALK) as a result of: (a) Disparity between donor corneal button size and host cornea trephination size (undersized grafts leading to central corneal flattening while oversized grafts leading to central corneal steepening) and (b) differences in corneal graft suture tension (the higher the tension, the flatter the central corneal curvature postoperatively).

$$IOL\ power\ formulas\ affected: \boldsymbol{all\ formulas} \begin{pmatrix} both\ those\ based\ on\ regression \\ and\ those\ based\ on\ ray tracing \end{pmatrix}.$$

- **Axial length (AL)** can change after PK/DALK as a result of: (a) Different corneal thickness and corneal architecture between diseased excised cornea and healthy donor cornea and (b) variable corneal graft suture tension.

$$IOL\ power\ formulas\ affected: \boldsymbol{all\ formulas} \begin{pmatrix} both\ those\ based\ on\ regression \\ and\ those\ based\ on\ ray tracing \end{pmatrix}.$$

- **Anterior/posterior corneal radius ratio** gets altered after endothelial procedures such as Descemet Stripping (Automated) Endothelial Keratoplasty (DSAEK/DSEK) and Descemet Membrane Endothelial Keratoplasty (DMEK).
- In endothelial dysfunction such as in Fuchs' corneal endothelial dystrophy, the cornea becomes edematous. Unless large bullae are present, anterior corneal curvature and axial length remain constant, whereas posterior corneal curvature decreases (becomes flatter) as the cornea becomes more edematous. This progressive edema causes a myopic shift. After endothelial keratoplasty is performed, as the corneal edema resolves, the posterior corneal curvature increases (it goes back towards its normal curvature) and this induces the commonly reported postoperative hyperopic shift [3–9]. This hyperopic shift has been reported both after DSAEK [10–18] and after DMEK [4–9], which demonstrates that the refractive shift is not simply the consequence of the negative lenticule shape of the DSAEK donor lamella as it was previously postulated [14, 16, 19, 20].

*IOL power formulas affected : **all formulas**.*

- *Third-generation formulas (SRK/T, HofferQ, Holladay, Haigis) are all affected because they assume a fixed anterior/posterior corneal radius ratio. Raytracing methods are also affected because the corneal curvature measurements are taken preoperatively when the cornea is still edematous and hence with a flatter posterior curvature compared to the postoperative status in which the edema has resolved, and the posterior curvature has increased.*
- **Central corneal thickness (CCT)** gets altered following endothelial procedures such as DSAEK, DSEK and DMEK due to the fact that corneal edema reduces after endothelial transplantation.

$$IOL\ power\ formulas\ affected: \boldsymbol{ray\ tracing}\ formulas\ only$$
$$(3rd\ generation\ formulas\ do\ not\ require\ CCT\ as\ an\ input\ parameter).$$

The only biometric factor that does not get altered following keratoplasty is the **actual position of the IOL inside the capsular bag**. This position however cannot be accurately predicted before the operation. The "constants" used in its place as predictors of IOL position are the A constant (for SRK/T formula), SF (for Holladay formula), pACD (for HofferQ formula), a0, a1, a2 (for Haigis formula). These constants are derived empirically from back calculations starting from the postoperative refractive outcome and a given set of inputs, including the same ones that get altered during the corneal transplantation itself (mainly K readings). Hence, also these constants are no longer reliable after the procedure and for this reason, **they should ideally be customized for each combination of corneal graft type (penetrating, anterior lamellar, and endothelial graft), surgical technique (extent of donor graft oversizing, suture tension), IOL model implanted, and operating surgeon**. This however is not practical and probably only feasible in centers where a large number of corneal grafts are performed each year.

Further sources of possible error to consider:

- Donor corneas that have previously undergone laser refractive surgery
- Donor corneas with undetected keratoconous
- Mislabeled IOL power (as in normal eyes undergoing cataract surgery)

With the growing number of laser refractive procedures being done worldwide and the technical difficulties of performing corneal topography on either the cadaver eye or on the harvested corneo-scleral rim (main difficulty being the altered epithelium after death), it is becoming increasingly more likely that a donor cornea could have undergone some refractive procedure in the past, with the risk, generally speaking, of a hyperopic outcome following a myopic procedure and the risk of a myopic outcome following a hyperopic procedure, if not detected. A keratoconic donor cornea could also make the IOL power calculations unreliable.

Methods Available to Limit Refractive Surprises

Triple Procedures (Simultaneous Keratoplasty + Cataract Extraction + IOL Implantation)

- **PK/DALK**
  - Using estimated postoperative, **K values taken from previous cases series done by the same surgeon,** ideally using a **similar suturing** technique **and with a similar graft/donor size disparity.**
  - Using **average estimated postoperative K values** taken from the literature involving cases done with a similar technique. Postoperative average K values vary greatly and are summarized in Table 69.2, ranked in ascending order [1, 21–26].
  - Using **K readings taken from the fellow (unoperated or already transplanted) cornea**.
  - Ideally, one should use the predicted K values taken after suture removal, as sutures can cause a significant flattening especially in the first few months after the operation. In any case, it is always advisable aiming for a mild residual myopia (>−0.75 D),

Table 69.2 Postoperative average K values in keratoplasty techniques

Technique	Pathology	Postop Average K (D)	Author	References
PK (same size)	KC	42.25	Duran	[21]
DMEK	Fuchs'	43.11	Alnawaiseh	[22]
PK	Various but not KC	44.71	Abd Elaziz	[23]
PK	KC	44.80	Raecker	[24]
PK	Various	45.06	Geerards	[25]
PK (oversized graft)	KC	45.16	Duran	[21]
PK	Keratopathy	45.34	Duran	[21]
PK	Keratopathy with vascularization	45.34	Duran	[21]
DALK	KC	45.54	Schiano Lomoriello	[26]
PK (oversized graft)	Various	45.70	Javadi	[1]
PK	Fuchs'	46.10	Raecker	[24]

Table 69.3 Postoperative hyperopic shift: DSAEK vs DMEK

Technique	Postop hyperopic shift (D)	References
DSAEK	From 0.70 to 1.50	[12–18]
DMEK	0.33, 0.43, 0.73, 0.90	[4, 5, 8, 9]

given the fact that a hyperopic result is never a desirable outcome for the patient.

- **DSAEK/DSEK/DMEK**
  - Using third-generation formulas and aiming for a myopic target of around −0.75 to **−1.00 D** [3–9]. Studies show a greater hyperopic shift after DSAEK compared to DMEK (Table 69.3), and therefore, more myopia should be targeted in DSAEK. It has been shown that the most affected formula after endothelial keratoplasty is the Haigis, formula, while the SRK/T is the least affected one [9].
  - **Raytracing**
  - Some studies have shown a reduction of the hyperopic error using raytracing techniques (0.24 D hyperopic error) compared to standard third-generation formulas; however, it should be noted that posterior corneal curvature measurements taken preoperatively differ from the final postoperative measurements, and hence, the scientific validity of this method is limited [5, 27].

- **All Cases**

  - Of all the preoperative parameters, axial length (AL) is the one having the largest impact on IOL power calculation accuracy, and therefore, it should always be measured by means of optical biometry whenever possible in order to minimize the errors [2].

Aphakic Eyes (Eyes Which Have Undergone Keratoplasty and Cataract Surgery and Have Been Left Aphakic)

One option is performing keratoplasty with simultaneous cataract extraction leaving the eye aphakic in order to plan for a secondary IOL implantation at a later stage. Typically, the secondary IOL is placed in the ciliary sulcus as the capsular bag layers soon coalesce after surgery, not allowing in-bag implantation. The power of the secondary IOL can be calculated in different ways:

- Aphakic Refraction Using the Refractive Vergence Formula [28]

$$IOL_e = \frac{1336}{\dfrac{1336}{\dfrac{1000}{\dfrac{1000}{PreRx} - V} + K_o} - ELP_o} - \frac{1336}{\dfrac{1336}{\dfrac{1000}{\dfrac{1000}{DPostRx} - V} + K_o} - ELP_o}$$

With this formula by J Holladay, for a given pre-operative refractive error (**PreRx**) [e.g., +2.25 D] measured at a specific vertex distance (**V**) [e.g., 12 mm] in an eye with a given corneal true net power (**Ko**) [e.g., 41.98 D], it is possible to calculate the IOL power required (**IOLe**) to achieve the desired post-operative refraction (**DPostRx**) [e.g., 0.00 D]. The formula requires a value to be entered for the effective lens position (**ELPo**). This is the distance from the secondary corneal principal plane to the IOL principal plane in thin-lens equivalent terms and it varies according to the position of the IOL (typically 4.80 mm is used for the sulcus, 5.55 mm for the capsular bag, and 3.50 mm for the anterior chamber). Corneal true net power (**Ko**) can be taken from devices that are able to measure both the anterior and the posterior corneal curvature, such as Pentacam (Oculus), Sirius or MS-39 (CSO), Galilei G6 (Ziemer), Anterion (Heidelberg), or alternatively, it can be approximated from K1 and K2 with the following equation:

$$0.5^* (K1 + K2) * 0.98765431$$

In the example above, a 3.24 D sulcus IOL would be required to achieve emmetropia. A more advanced version of this formula is present in the Holladay IOL Consultant software.

- **Raytracing**

Raytracing allows corneal and IOL power calculations from objective anterior and posterior corneal curvature measurements and axial length and, differently from third- and fourth-generation formulas, does not require any adjustment or regression for special cases such as post-laser refractive surgery eyes which assume a constant anterior/posterior corneal curvature ratio [29, 30]. Good results, comparable to those using the SRK/T and HofferQ formula, have been shown with this technique in normal eyes and the method has also been used successfully in post-laser refractive surgery eyes, especially after myopic laser vision correction [31–34]. Raytracing can also be used to accurately back-calculate IOL power in pseudophakic eyes provided that the IOL position can be accurately measured [35]. A single paper describes the use of raytracing in keratoconus [36]. To our knowledge, publications are lacking on raytracing IOL power calculations after corneal transplantation. This is a pity, because theoretically, the cases that would benefit the most from raytracing would indeed be post-keratoplasty eyes, especially those with irregular corneal graft curvature or those with tilted/eccentric grafts or distorted/eccentric pupils. More studies are needed on this subject.

- **Intraoperative aberrometry**

The validity of this method has been proven in studies involving both normal eyes [37–41] and eyes that had undergone laser refractive surgery [42–46]; however, no data is available for post-keratoplasty eyes.

In theory also, this method should be able to provide accurate results, provided that the transplanted cornea is clear and it is possible to scan it well. Its main limitation however, cost aside, is the need of a large stock of IOLs with different powers directly on the premises in order to be able to choose the exact power required. Having a complete stock of IOLs is already an issue for standard spherical IOLs, and it is even more so in the case of corneal grafts because they often require a toric IOL to correct high residual astigmatism. In most clinical settings, it is probably better to perform biometry well ahead of surgery.

The following ones are the main drawbacks of implanting the IOL via an additional procedure at a later date after the initial keratoplasty:

- The patient has to cope with poor vision for several months (in the case of a PK, sutures are removed after 12 months and it would take another couple of months for the cornea to stabilize before an accurate biometry can be done).
- It is often not possible to wear a contact lens immediately after surgery to cope with being aphakic.
- Aphakic glasses may be unbearable due to anisometropia.
- The secondary IOL implantation procedure may trigger a corneal graft rejection.
- The secondary IOL implantation procedure may further damage the weak corneal graft endothelium.
- Extended usage of steroid drops prescribed to reduce the risk of graft rejection may cause a raised IOP (steroid response).

For these reasons, although leaving the eye aphakic on purpose would seem to be the best method in terms of IOL power calculation, this is not clinically safe and therefore it is not advised.

Pseudophakic Eyes (Eyes Which Have Undergone Keratoplasty and Have Been Left Pseudophakic with a Significant Residual Refractive Error)

The same principles (and drawbacks) of the aphakic method above apply with the sole difference being the fact that the correcting IOL can either be implanted as a piggyback IOL in the ciliary sulcus or in the capsular bag, or as as a single new primary IOL as in the cases of IOL exchanges.

To prevent interlenticular opacification, lab studies suggest that it would be advisable not to implant two hydrophobic acrylic IOLs in contact with each other, but rather combining an acrylic IOL with a silicon IOL, or using two silicon IOLs [47].

Recently, implantable collamer lenses (Visian ICL, Staar) have been used as alternative sulcus piggyback lenses to standard 3-piece IOLs with good results in children [48]. Their advantage is the minimal incision size required and the ease of explantation whenever needed.

Transplanted Corneas Which Still Have Cataract (Eyes Which Have Undergone Keratoplasty But Still Have to Undergo Cataract Surgery)

When planning cataract surgery in an eye that has previously undergone keratoplasty, it is essential that corneal curvature measurements are taken when the refraction has fully stabilized. This occurs after at least 2–3 months following complete suture removal.

In eyes that have undergone DSAEK and where the donor corneal lenticule is particularly thick and negative-meniscus shaped, it is advisable **to aim for a mild residual myopia** and comparing standard IOL power calculations results with those of **raytracing**.

In eyes that have undergone PK or DALK and in which there are no major corneal irregularities, third-generation formulas can generally be used as in normal eyes with fairly accurate results. In very irregular corneas, raytracing may provide better clues.

In corneal grafts where the final corneal anatomy is similar to that of a normal cornea (such as after either DMEK or after an extremely thin DSEK or after a shallow femtolaser ALK), standard third-generation formulas can be used without any major adjustments.

To reduce the risk of triggering a graft rejection, the operation should be done when the eye is completely quiet. Postoperative treatment with cortisone eye drops should be tapered slowly over several weeks or months, especially after PK/DALK.

Management of Refractive Surprises

1. Glasses or contact lenses
2. Femto LASIK or PRK with Mitomycin C
3. IOL Exchange or piggyback IOL implantation using vergence formula

Small errors on the myopic side are usually fairly well tolerated and may be corrected with glasses or contact lenses. Hybrid or gas-permeable contact lenses or scleral lenses are sometimes required in grafts with unusual curvatures or in irregular graft-host interfaces.

Enhancements by means of Femto LASIK or PRK (always with the application of Mitomycin C 0.02% for >30 s in order to prevent the onset of corneal haze) have shown to give excellent results with a low risk of triggering a graft rejection. This should always be followed by several weeks of cortisone drops treatment on a tapering regime to prevent graft rejection.

For severe refractive errors, the best approach is either replacing the IOL or placing a piggyback IOL in the ciliary sulcus after calculating the power using the refractive vergence formula or raytracing.

Summary

1. Accurate IOL power prediction at the same time of cataract surgery is not possible.
2. Leaving the eye aphakic on purpose after corneal transplantation and aiming for accurate IOL power calculation for a secondary IOL implantation later on theoretically would provide the most accurate results; however, it is very debilitating for the patient and poses a serious risk of triggering a corneal graft rejection or damaging the corneal endothelium, and therefore, it is not advisable.
3. Implanting an IOL at the same time of keratoplasty is by far the best option and K values should ideally be taken from individual case series done with a similar surgical technique (similar corneal graft type; surgical and suturing technique; donor-host cornea size disparity) and always aiming for a mild residual myopia. In endothelial transplants, a myopic target of at least -0.75 D should always be targeted due to the expected postoperative hyperopic shift.
4. Residual refractive errors can be well managed by means of glasses/contact lenses or by means of laser refractive surgery (such as PRK + Mitomycin C or Femto LASIK) and in extreme cases by means of IOL exchange or piggyback IOL implantation using the refractive vergence formula or raytracing.

References

1. Javadi MA, Feizi S, Moein HR. Simultaneous penetrating keratoplasty and cataract surgery. J Ophthalmic Vis Res. 2013;8(1):39–46. PMID: 23825711; PMCID: PMC3691977.
2. Norrby S. Sources of error in intraocular lens power calculation. J Cataract Refract Surg. 2008;34(3):368–76. https://doi.org/10.1016/j.jcrs.2007.10.031. PMID: 18299059.
3. Price MO, Price FW Jr. Descemet membrane endothelial keratoplasty. Int Ophthalmol Clin. 2010;50(3):137–47. https://doi.org/10.1097/IIO.0b013e3181e21a6f. PMID: 20611024.
4. Schoenberg ED, Price FW Jr, Miller J, McKee Y, Price MO. Refractive outcomes of Descemet membrane endothelial keratoplasty triple procedures (combined with cataract surgery). J Cataract Refract Surg. 2015;41(6):1182–9. https://doi.org/10.1016/j.jcrs.2014.09.042. Epub 2015 Jun 19. PMID: 26096520.
5. Diener R, Treder M, Lauermann JL, Eter N, Alnawaiseh M. Assessing the validity of corneal power estimation using conventional keratometry for intraocular lens power calculation in eyes with Fuch's dystrophy undergoing Descemet membrane endothelial keratoplasty. Graefes Arch Clin Exp Ophthalmol. 2021;259(4):1061–70. https://doi.org/10.1007/s00417-020-04998-w. Epub 2020 Nov 13. PMID: 33185732; PMCID: PMC8016760.
6. Alnawaiseh M, Rosentreter A, Eter N, Zumhagen L. Changes in corneal refractive power for patients with Fuchs endothelial dystrophy after DMEK. Cornea. 2016;35(8):1073–7. https://doi.org/10.1097/ICO.0000000000000842. PMID: 27055217.
7. Ham L, Dapena I, Moutsouris K, Balachandran C, Frank LE, van Dijk K, Melles GR. Refractive change and stability after Descemet membrane endothelial keratoplasty. Effect of corneal dehydration-induced hyperopic shift on intraocular lens power calculation. J Cataract Refract Surg. 2011;37(8):1455–64. https://doi.org/10.1016/j.jcrs.2011.02.033. PMID: 21782088.
8. Korine van Dijk K, Ham L, Tse WH, Liarakos VS, Quilendrino R, Yeh RY, Melles GR. Near complete visual recovery and refractive stability in modern corneal transplantation: Descemet membrane endothelial keratoplasty (DMEK). Cont Lens Anterior Eye. 2013;36(1):13–21. https://doi.org/10.1016/j.clae.2012.10.066. Epub 2012 Oct 26. PMID: 23108011.
9. Alnawaiseh M, Zumhagen L, Rosentreter A, Eter N. Intraocular lens power calculation using standard formulas and ray tracing after DMEK in patients with Fuchs endothelial dystrophy. BMC Ophthalmol. 2017;17(1):152. https://doi.org/10.1186/s12886-017-0547-7. PMID: 28835226; PMCID: PMC5569506.
10. Kim SE, Lim SA, Byun YS, Joo CK. Comparison of long-term clinical outcomes between Descemet's stripping automated endothelial keratoplasty and penetrating keratoplasty in patients with bullous keratopathy. Korean J Ophthalmol. 2016;30(6):443–50. https://doi.org/10.3341/kjo.2016.30.6.443. Epub 2016 Dec 6. PMID: 27980363; PMCID: PMC5156618.
11. Koenig SB, Covert DJ, Dupps WJ Jr, Meisler DM. Visual acuity, refractive error, and endothelial cell density six months after Descemet stripping and automated endothelial keratoplasty (DSAEK). Cornea. 2007;26(6):670–4. https://doi.org/10.1097/ICO.0b013e3180544902. PMID: 17592314.
12. Gorovoy MS. Descemet-stripping automated endothelial keratoplasty. Cornea. 2006;25(8):886–9. https://doi.org/10.1097/01.ico.0000214224.90743.01. PMID: 17102661.
13. Koenig SB, Covert DJ. Early results of small-incision Descemet's stripping and automated endothelial keratoplasty. Ophthalmology. 2007;114(2):221–6. https://doi.org/10.1016/j.ophtha.2006.07.056. Epub 2006 Dec 5. PMID: 17156845.

14. Scorcia V, Matteoni S, Scorcia GB, Scorcia G, Busin M. Pentacam assessment of posterior lamellar grafts to explain hyperopization after Descemet's stripping automated endothelial keratoplasty. Ophthalmology. 2009;116(9):1651–5. https://doi.org/10.1016/j.ophtha.2009.04.035. Epub 2009 Jul 29. PMID: 19643500.

15. Lee WB, Jacobs DS, Musch DC, Kaufman SC, Reinhart WJ, Shtein RM. Descemet's stripping endothelial keratoplasty: safety and outcomes: a report by the American Academy of Ophthalmology. Ophthalmology. 2009;116(9):1818–30. https://doi.org/10.1016/j.ophtha.2009.06.021. Epub 2009 Jul 30. PMID: 19643492.

16. Holz HA, Meyer JJ, Espandar L, Tabin GC, Mifflin MD, Moshirfar M. Corneal profile analysis after Descemet stripping endothelial keratoplasty and its relationship to postoperative hyperopic shift. J Cataract Refract Surg. 2008;34(2):211–4. https://doi.org/10.1016/j.jcrs.2007.09.030. PMID: 18242442.

17. Xu K, Qi H, Peng R, Xiao G, Hong J, Hao Y, Ma B. Keratometric measurements and IOL calculations in pseudophakic post-DSAEK patients. BMC Ophthalmol. 2018;18(1):268. https://doi.org/10.1186/s12886-018-0931-y. PMID: 30332995; PMCID: PMC6192275.

18. Dupps WJ Jr, Qian Y, Meisler DM. Multivariate model of refractive shift in Descemet-stripping automated endothelial keratoplasty. J Cataract Refract Surg. 2008;34(4):578–84. https://doi.org/10.1016/j.jcrs.2007.11.045. PMID: 18361978; PMCID: PMC2796246.

19. Rao SK, Leung CK, Cheung CY, Li EY, Cheng AC, Lam PT, Lam DS. Descemet stripping endothelial keratoplasty: effect of the surgical procedure on corneal optics. Am J Ophthalmol. 2008;145(6):991–6. https://doi.org/10.1016/j.ajo.2008.01.017. Epub 2008 Mar 14. PMID: 18342831.

20. Bahar I, Kaiserman I, McAllum P, Slomovic A, Rootman D. Comparison of posterior lamellar keratoplasty techniques to penetrating keratoplasty. Ophthalmology. 2008;115(9):1525–33. https://doi.org/10.1016/j.ophtha.2008.02.010. Epub 2008 Apr 28. PMID: 18440638.

21. Duran JA, Malvar A, Diez E. Corneal dioptric power after penetrating keratoplasty. Br J Ophthalmol. 1989;73(8):657–60. https://doi.org/10.1136/bjo.73.8.657. PMID: 2669941; PMCID: PMC1041840.

22. Alnawaiseh M, Zumhagen L, Rosentreter A, Eter N. Changes in anterior, posterior, and total corneal astigmatism after Descemet membrane endothelial keratoplasty. J Ophthalmol. 2017;2017:4068963. https://doi.org/10.1155/2017/4068963. Epub 2017 May 2. PMID: 28553547; PMCID: PMC5434235.

23. Abd Elaziz MS, Elsobky HM, Zaky AG, Hassan EAM, KhalafAllah MT. Corneal biomechanics and intraocular pressure assessment after penetrating keratoplasty for non keratoconic patients, long term results. BMC Ophthalmol. 2019;19(1):172. https://doi.org/10.1186/s12886-019-1186-y. PMID: 31391006; PMCID: PMC6686420.

24. Raecker ME, Erie JC, Patel SV, McLaren JW, Hodge DO, Bourne WM. Long-term keratometric changes after penetrating keratoplasty for keratoconus and Fuchs endothelial dystrophy. Am J Ophthalmol. 2009;147(2):227–33. https://doi.org/10.1016/j.ajo.2008.08.001. Epub 2008 Oct 2. PMID: 18834579; PMCID: PMC3783204.

25. Geerards AJ, Hassmann E, Beekhuis WH, Remeyer L, van Rij G, Rijneveld WJ. Triple procedure; analysis of outcome, refraction, and intraocular lens power calculation. Br J Ophthalmol. 1997;81(9):774–7. https://doi.org/10.1136/bjo.81.9.774. PMID: 9422932; PMCID: PMC1722304.

26. Schiano Lomoriello D, Savini G, Naeser K, Colabelli-Gisoldi RM, Bono V, Pocobelli A. Customized toric intraocular lens implantation in eyes with cataract and corneal astigmatism after deep anterior lamellar keratoplasty: a prospective study. J Ophthalmol. 2018;(2018):1649576. https://doi.org/10.1155/2018/1649576. PMID: 30057802; PMCID: PMC6051070.

27. Olsen T. On the calculation of power from curvature of the cornea. Br J Ophthalmol. 1986;70(2):152–4. https://doi.org/10.1136/bjo.70.2.152. PMID: 3947615; PMCID: PMC1040942.

28. Holladay JT. Refractive power calculations for intraocular lenses in the phakic eye. Am J Ophthalmol. 1993;116(1):63–6. https://doi.org/10.1016/s0002-9394(14)71745-3. PMID: 8328545.

29. Olsen T, Jeppesen P. Ray-tracing analysis of the corneal power from Scheimpflug data. J Refract Surg. 2018;34(1):45–50. https://doi.org/10.3928/1081597X-20171102-01. PMID: 29315441.

30. Langenbucher A, Szentmáry N, Weisensee J, Wendelstein J, Cayless A, Menapace R, Hoffmann P. Prediction model for best focus, power, and spherical aberration of the cornea: raytracing on a large dataset of OCT data. PLoS One. 2021;16(2):e0247048. https://doi.org/10.1371/journal.pone.0247048. PMID: 33617531; PMCID: PMC7899355.

31. Miyata K, Otani S, Honbou N, Minami K. Use of Scheimpflug corneal anterior-posterior imaging in ray-tracing intraocular lens power calculation. Acta Ophthalmol. 2013;91(7):e546–9. https://doi.org/10.1111/aos.12139. Epub 2013 Jul 26. PMID: 23890181.

32. Minami K, Kataoka Y, Matsunaga J, Ohtani S, Honbou M, Miyata K. Ray-tracing intraocular lens power calculation using anterior segment optical coherence tomography measurements. J Cataract Refract Surg. 2012;38(10):1758–63. https://doi.org/10.1016/j.jcrs.2012.05.035. Epub 2012 Aug 1. PMID: 22857986.

33. Ghoreyshi M, Khalilian A, Peyman M, Mohammadinia M, Peyman A. Comparison of OKULIX ray-tracing software with SRK-T and Hoffer-Q formula in intraocular lens power calcula-

tion. J Curr Ophthalmol. 2017;30(1):63–7. https://doi.org/10.1016/j.joco.2017.06.008. PMID: 29564411; PMCID: PMC5859630.

34. Savini G, Bedei A, Barboni P, Ducoli P, Hoffer KJ. Intraocular lens power calculation by ray-tracing after myopic excimer laser surgery. Am J Ophthalmol. 2014;157(1):150–153.e1. https://doi.org/10.1016/j.ajo.2013.08.006. Epub 2013 Oct 5. PMID: 24099275.

35. Olsen T, Funding M. Ray-tracing analysis of intraocular lens power in situ. J Cataract Refract Surg. 2012;38(4):641–7. https://doi.org/10.1016/j.jcrs.2011.10.035. Epub 2012 Feb 18. PMID: 22342009.

36. Schedin S, Hallberg P, Behndig A. Three-dimensional ray-tracing model for the study of advanced refractive errors in keratoconus. Appl Opt. 2016;55(3):507–14. https://doi.org/10.1364/AO.55.000507. PMID: 26835925.

37. Davison JA, Potvin R. Preoperative measurement vs intraoperative aberrometry for the selection of intraocular lens sphere power in normal eyes. Clin Ophthalmol. 2017;11:923–9. https://doi.org/10.2147/OPTH.S135659. PMID: 28553072; PMCID: PMC5440073.

38. Zhang Z, Thomas LW, Leu SY, Carter S, Garg S. Refractive outcomes of intraoperative wavefront aberrometry versus optical biometry alone for intraocular lens power calculation. Indian J Ophthalmol. 2017;65(9):813–7. https://doi.org/10.4103/ijo.IJO_163_17. PMID: 28905823; PMCID: PMC5621262.

39. Cionni RJ, Dimalanta R, Breen M, Hamilton C. A large retrospective database analysis comparing outcomes of intraoperative aberrometry with conventional preoperative planning. J Cataract Refract Surg. 2018;44(10):1230–5. https://doi.org/10.1016/j.jcrs.2018.07.016. Epub 2018 Aug 10. PMID: 30104081.

40. Sudhakar S, Hill DC, King TS, Scott IU, Mishra G, Ernst BB, Pantanelli SM. Intraoperative aberrometry versus preoperative biometry for intraocular lens power selection in short eyes. J Cataract Refract Surg. 2019;45(6):719–24. https://doi.org/10.1016/j.jcrs.2018.12.016. Epub 2019 Mar 8. PMID: 30853316.

41. Cionni RJ, Breen M, Hamilton C, Williams R. Retrospective analysis of an intraoperative aberrometry database: a study investigating absolute prediction in eyes implanted with low cylinder power toric intraocular lenses. Clin Ophthalmol.

2019;13:1485–92. https://doi.org/10.2147/OPTH.S191887. PMID: 31496639; PMCID: PMC6689545.

42. Raufi N, James C, Kuo A, Vann R. Intraoperative aberrometry vs modern preoperative formulas in predicting intraocular lens power. J Cataract Refract Surg. 2020;46(6):857–61. https://doi.org/10.1097/j.jcrs.0000000000000173. PMID: 32176162.

43. Canto AP, Chhadva P, Cabot F, Galor A, Yoo SH, Vaddavalli PK, Culbertson WW. Comparison of IOL power calculation methods and intraoperative wavefront aberrometer in eyes after refractive surgery. J Refract Surg. 2013;29(7):484–9. https://doi.org/10.3928/1081597X-20130617-07. PMID: 23820231.

44. Ianchulev T, Hoffer KJ, Yoo SH, Chang DF, Breen M, Padrick T, Tran DB. Intraoperative refractive biometry for predicting intraocular lens power calculation after prior myopic refractive surgery. Ophthalmology. 2014;121(1):56–60. https://doi.org/10.1016/j.ophtha.2013.08.041. Epub 2013 Oct 30. PMID: 24183339.

45. Fram NR, Masket S, Wang L. Comparison of intraoperative aberrometry, OCT-based IOL formula, Haigis-L, and Masket formulae for IOL power calculation after laser vision correction. Ophthalmology. 2015;122(6):1096–101. https://doi.org/10.1016/j.ophtha.2015.01.027. Epub 2015 Mar 10. PMID: 25766733.

46. Fisher B, Potvin R. Clinical outcomes with distance-dominant multifocal and monofocal intraocular lenses in post-LASIK cataract surgery planned using an intraoperative aberrometer. Clin Exp Ophthalmol. 2018;46(6):630–6. https://doi.org/10.1111/ceo.13153. Epub 2018 Feb 23. PMID: 29360197; PMCID: PMC6100005.

47. Werner L, Mamalis N, Stevens S, Hunter B, Chew JJ, Vargas LG. Interlenticular opacification: dual- optic versus piggyback intraocular lenses. J Cataract Refract Surg. 2006;32(4):655–61. https://doi.org/10.1016/j.jcrs.2006.01.022. PMID: 16698490.

48. Eissa SA. Management of pseudophakic myopic anisometropic amblyopia with piggyback Visian® implantable collamer lens. Acta Ophthalmol. 2017;95(2):188–93. https://doi.org/10.1111/aos.13203. Epub 2016 Sep 29. PMID: 27681455.

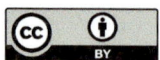

Scott K. McClatchey and Thaddeus S. McClatchey

When one of my children had cataract surgery and IOL implantation in 25 years ago at the age of 3, the optics of the growing eye and the pattern of growth were poorly understood. He received an IOL power of +25 D in the eye that had surgery, with an intended initial postoperative refraction of +2.5 D.

During fellowship, I studied the patterns of long-term refractive change in hundreds of aphakic pediatric eyes from the practice of Marshall M. Parks, M.D. The pattern of ocular growth was

We have no conflicts of interest.

The opinions expressed in this presentation are solely those of the authors, and do not reflect the official policy or position of the Department of the Navy, the Department of the Defense, or the US Government.

I am an employee of the U.S. Government. This work was prepared as part of my official duties. Title 17, U.S.C. §105 provides that copyright protection under this title is not available for any work of the U.S. Government. Title 17, U.S.C., §101 defines a U.S. Government work as a work prepared by a military service member or employee of the U.S. Government as part of that person's official duties.

S. K. McClatchey (✉)
Naval Medical Center San Diego,
San Diego, CA, USA

Uniformed Services University of the Health Sciences, Bethesda, MD, USA

T. S. McClatchey
Nassau University Medical Center,
East Meadow, NY, USA

clear: on average, there was a myopic shift that was greatest early in life and declined with age [1]. Subsequently, others and I studied the long-term refractive change in a large number of pseudophakic pediatric eyes, and found the same pattern [2–4]. The aphakic or pseudophakic refractive error follows a semi-logarithmic decline with age through at least 20 years of age. Notably, there is a large variance in the rate of this refractive growth, and there is no way to precisely predict future refractions for a particular child [5].

Great emphasis has been placed on which IOL formula is most accurate in children's eyes. However, the fact is that these pseudophakic pediatric eyes grow, and with ocular growth comes a large and highly variable quantity of myopic shift. Seeking the most accurate formula for initial postop refraction with a goal of long-term refractive prediction is analogous to the parent who tries to predict her young child's future adult weight by using an accurate scale at age 3. Instead, the choice of IOL power for a child should take into consideration the myopic shift that results from ocular growth with age.

Although the goal of IOL power choice in adults is usually emmetropia, the goal of cataract surgery in children is twofold: optimal management of vision in childhood and emmetropia in adult life. The former requires spectacles to manage the changing refractive error in the growing eye, as well as often-intensive treatment for

J. Aramberri et al. (eds.), *Intraocular Lens Calculations*, Essentials in Ophthalmology,
https://doi.org/10.1007/978-3-031-50666-6_70

amblyopia. The latter requires a combination of careful choice of the initial postoperative refraction (based primarily on age), with a goal of achieving an adult refractive error that can be easily managed with spectacles or contact lenses. In some cases, due to the large variance in the rate of refractive growth, resulting high refractive errors in adults may require refractive surgery or IOL exchange.

IOL Formula Accuracy

Studies of the accuracy of IOL formulas find that the prediction error is worse in children than in adults, especially for children less than 3 years of age [6, 7]. This is primarily due to the current limits of biometry in a child, and to the limits of measuring post-operative pseudophakic refractions in children.

Errors with biometry in children are primarily driven by errors in axial length (AL) measurements. As very young children require general anesthesia for biometry, currently ultrasound is used to measure AL. The surgeon or ultrasonographer must be careful to center the probe on the cornea, and align the beam to the axis of the eye. Ideally the A-scan is done using immersion, but contact A-scan is commonly used by pediatric ophthalmologists [8]. When the tip of the contact A-scan probe touches the soft cornea, it tends to depress the corneal apex, resulting in a shorter measurement of AL by 0.27 [9] to 1 mm [10], increasing the calculated IOL power for emmetropia by 1 to 3 D. There can be a greater variance in measurements of AL when using a contact probe: a prospective study of 50 eyes (mean age: 3.87 years) found the absolute prediction error of <0.5 D in 50% of eyes when AL was measured using immersion, vs 23% when using a contact probe [9], although a retrospective study found no difference in absolute prediction error (APE) between a recent group of 65 eyes measured using immersion, vs 138 historical controls measured using contact A-scan [11].

The surgeon should also account for the speed of ultrasound in an infant eye: the speed of sound in a 20-mm eye is 1561 m/s, vs. 1555 m/s for a 23.5 mm phakic eye [8]. Because the child's eye is small, the same quantity of power prediction error is greater in proportion to that in an adult eye: a 1 mm AL error in an adult eye could result in a 2.5 D IOL power change, but in a child's eye, this same error could change the IOL power by 4 D.

Hand-held keratometers measure corneal power (K) with an accuracy equivalent to mounted keratometers. However, under supine general anesthesia, the supple nature of an infant eye can lead to flatter Ks [10].

With optimal biometry, these errors can be reduced, depending on age. Younger children have a shorter axial length, require a higher power IOL, and their refraction is measured with less precision: because of these factors, the measured and expected postop refractive error goes up substantially in infants. In a study of children with a median age of 3.56 years, Trivedi et al. found a median absolute error of 0.53–0.67 D using common theoretical IOL formulas (Holladay 1 & 2, Hoffer Q and SRK-T) [12]. By my calculations, this is close to the theoretic minimum postop error for this age (unpublished data). In the Infant Aphakia Treatment Study (IATS), where cataract surgery with IOL implantation was performed on much younger children (<7 months of age), the median APE was 1.2 D using the Holladay 1 formula, and was worse for eyes with AL < 18 mm [13].

We compiled the results of several recent studies of formula accuracy in children, with the results for absolute prediction error (APE) shown in Tables 70.1 and 70.2. APE is the most indicative of the accuracy of the formula; medians are preferred to means because APE does not follow a Gaussian curve.

Eibschitz-Tsimhoni et al. studied the sensitivity of errors in axial length and corneal power for a variety of IOL formulas (HofferQ, Holladay, SRK-T, Haigis and SRK II) on the IOL power

Table 70.1 Study population characteristics for recent studies of IOL formula accuracy in pediatric patients, in order of mean age at surgery

Study reference	N	Mean age (std dev), years	Axial length measurement technique
[13]	43	0.2 (0.1)	Immersion A-scan for most
[6]	68	2.8 (2.1)	A-scan for very young (no mention of immersion vs. applanation); Lenstar if cooperative
[12]	45	3.9 (2.9)	Immersion A-scan
[7]	377	4.6 (2.3)	Applanation A-scan
[14]	64	5.9 (3.6)	Immersion A-scan
[15]	135	6.4	Applanation A-scan

Table 70.3 Calculated initial pseudophakic refractions for IOL implantation in children of 0–20 years of age, for three commonly used IOL formulas

Age (years)	AL (mm)	K (D)	IOL (D)	SRK-T	HofferQ	Holladay
0.0	16.8	51.3	29.0	8.01	10.50	7.96
0.3	18.5	47.9	29.0	4.36	5.68	4.68
0.8	19.2	45.3	28.0	4.55	5.61	5.00
1.5	20.2	45.0	26.0	3.20	3.87	3.53
2.5	21.4	44.2	23.0	2.63	3.01	2.85
4.0	22.4	43.8	22.0	1.21	1.42	1.35
20.0	23.6	43.2	21.0	−0.30	−0.27	−0.25

Table 70.2 Median absolute prediction error (APE, in diopters) for recent studies of IOL formula accuracy in pediatric patients, in order of mean age at surgery

Ref	SRK II	SRK-T	Hoffer Q	Holladay 1	Holladay 2	Haigis	Barrett U II	Olsen	T2	Super	Notes
[13]	2.2	1.3	2.1	1.2	1.4						
[6]	0.83	0.75	0.83	0.88	1.00	0.74	0.89	0.89			*1
[12]		0.67	0.56	0.58	0.53						
[7]	0.95	0.81	0.68	0.70					0.76	0.73	*1
[14]		0.86	0.88		0.81		0.79				
[15]	0.90	0.71	0.61	0.64							*2

Ref = study reference number
*1: much greater scatter in APE for eyes before the age of 3 years
*2 biometry done in office resulted in better APE than when done under anesthesia; e.g., 0.83 vs. 0.60 D using the Holladay 1 formula

calculated to give emmetropia [16]. They found the calculated IOL power to be relatively insensitive to a +1 D error in K (0.5 to 1.4 D). However, a +1 mm error in AL resulted in large differences in calculated IOL powers, especially in infancy (ranging from −6.7 D for the SRK-T formula to −14.2 D for HofferQ).

However, we think that this analysis can be improved in two significant ways. Axial length errors in children are most commonly underestimates, especially if AL is measured by contact A-scan or the A-scan is off axis. In addition, the important outcome for the child and surgeon is the refractive outcome rather than the IOL

power. Therefore, we calculated the resulting error in a different way from Eibschitz-Tsimhoni et al.: we calculated the resulting refractive error due to a −1 mm error in axial length measurement for a similar group of patients, given a combination of age, AL, K, and IOL power likely to be chosen by the surgeon who wishes to leave the child with initial hyperopia that is greater at younger ages. The results are shown in Tables 70.3 and 70.4. Although the error in IOL power for emmetropia is especially large for the HofferQ formula, the resulting error in refraction is less sensitive to errors in axial length for IOL powers typically implanted in children.

Table 70.4 The resulting error when there is an underestimate of axial length by 1 mm, for three common formulas. The errors are shown for the IOL power for emmetropia, or the resulting pseudophakic refraction for the specific IOL choice stated in Table 70.3

| | Error in IOL power (D) for emmetropia | | | Error in refraction (D) for chosen IOL power | | |
Age (years)	SRK-T	HofferQ	Holladay	SRK-T	HofferQ	Holladay
0.0	6.34	12.44	6.81	3.61	4.21	3.87
0.3	5.11	7.23	5.48	3.27	3.95	3.43
0.8	4.67	6.04	5.01	3.05	3.54	3.17
1.5	4.21	5.05	4.50	2.83	3.15	2.94
2.5	3.75	4.27	3.99	2.53	2.75	2.64
4.0	3.43	3.84	3.65	2.37	2.57	2.47
20.0	3.10	3.47	3.29	2.18	2.38	2.28

Fig. 70.1 In a normal child's eye, the optical components of the eye grow in approximate proportion

Why is the adult natural lens power lesser than that of a child?

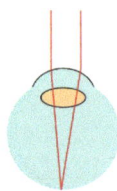 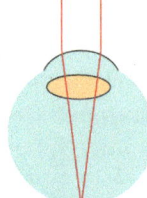

Small child's eye
Small lens has **high** power
Focus is on the retina

Large adult eye
Large lens has **lower** power
Focus is *still* on the retina

Answer: because everything grows in proportion

The Growth of the Eye

For young children, the large and variable growth of the eye is far more important than the initial biometric errors.

The growth of the eye follows a logarithmic curve with age. The eye grows as the child grows, rapidly at first, then slowing down over time. The components of the eye that determine its refractive error consist of the cornea, lens, and axial length. In a normal child, the nearly proportional growth of all optical elements of the eye results in the maintenance of near-constant refraction from birth through adult life (Fig. 70.1), although there is a trend in modern societies towards disproportionate growth of AL, resulting in myopia in many, and there are individual variations.

If an eye is rendered aphakic in infancy, the crystalline lens is removed and the aphakic eye has a high hyperopic refractive error, typically about +21 D. If the aphakic eye grows normally,

the increased axial length results in greatly reduced hyperopia, while the flattening of the cornea increases hyperopia but to a lesser degree. The overall result is a myopic shift with age (Fig. 70.2). Just like the growth of the eye itself, this myopic shift is rapid at first and then slows with age.

Gordon and Donzis first described this changing growth of the eye [17]. They measured the axial length and keratometry of otherwise normal children. Other authors based their cataract surgery IOL power choice on the growth of the eye. For example, Enyedi et al. recommended initial postoperative refraction goal by age: +6 at 1 year, +5 at 2 years, +4 at 3 years, +3 at 4 years, +2 at 5 years, +1 at 6 years, 0 for 7 years, and −1 to −2 for ≥8 years of age [18].

Some authors have described limited or segmented ocular growth with age. Nyström et al. described 49 eyes with surgery at an average of 2.8 months: the refraction in aphakic eyes fol-

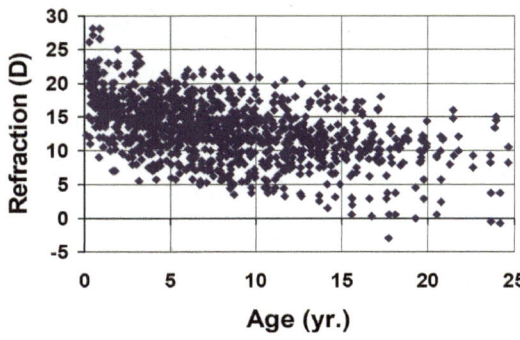

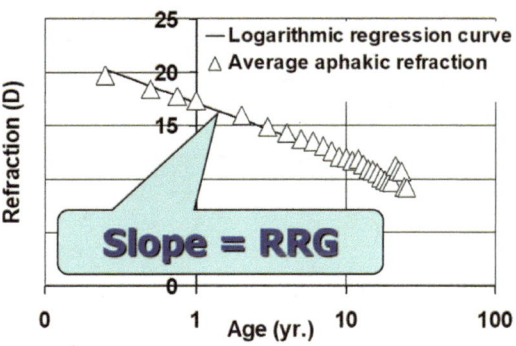

Fig. 70.2 Longitudinal refraction data from 281 aphakic pediatric eyes [1]

Fig. 70.3 Refraction vs. log of age for aphakic eyes [1]

lowed a logarithmic change in refraction in the first 3 years of life [19]. Wilson and Trivedi noted three phases of ocular growth, from birth to 6-months, 6–18 months, and >18 months [8]. Ohara noted that the cornea steepness stabilizes in the first 18 months of life; axial length increases dramatically in first 2 years of life, then grows at a slower rate into the second decade of life [20]. Even at the age of 10 years, the globe has not stopped growing. Wilson et al. studied 98 eyes with two AL measurements in the second decade of life [21]. A theoretical eye with an AL at the age of 10 years of 23.11 mm would grow to 24.41 mm by the age of 20 (with a wide variance), resulting in a 4-diopter difference between IOL powers needed for emmetropia at the two ages. This implies that a surgeon who implants multifocal IOLs in this age range should consider the continuing ocular growth.

Instead of thinking of the child's eye growing in phases, or until a certain age, we have found that a simpler approach is to recognize the semi-logarithmic growth of the eye from infancy through at least 20 years of age. In a group of 156 aphakic pediatric eyes followed for a mean of 8.8 years, a plot of average refraction vs. log of age was a straight line (Fig. 70.3).

The same plot (equivalent aphakic refraction vs. log of age) can be obtained for pseudophakic and normal eyes, by mathematically removing the effect of the IOL power (in the former case), or by calculation of aphakic refraction from AL and K taken from Gordon and Donzis study [17]. The slope of the straight line, called "Rate of

Refractive Growth" (RRG, or the preferred RRG2 or RRG3), is a measure of how fast the eye is growing. In data from aphakic, pseudophakic and normal eyes, the mean RRG2 is nearly the same in the three groups. A study by Tadros et al. backs this up: in 24 children with surgery at 2.6 months average and 8.4 years mean FU time, the growth of the AL and fellow eyes (4.1 vs 4.4 mm) was not statistically different [22]. In short, it appears that cataract surgery does not affect the growth of the eye. Applying Occam's razor, because it is simpler to work with a single description (rate of refractive growth) than one with several segments of varied growth rates, the semi-logarithmic model is preferred.

RRG2 is a characteristic parameter of each eye, correlating to how fast it grows. Data on mean RRG2 and its variance exists for aphakic and pseudophakic eyes [23]. The mean RRG2 and variance have been used to make calculators [24, 25] that predict the future refraction of any eye, whether aphakic or pseudophakic (Fig. 70.4).

There is a very large variance in RRG3 in both aphakic and pseudophakic eyes. This variance prevents precise prediction of future refractions, but has been included in pediatric IOL calculators to allow the surgeon to predict the approximate likely range of future refractions for any given child (Fig. 70.5). The variance in RRG3 is so large that it tends to overwhelm any initial errors in IOL power calculation.

Normal eyes also have a variance in the rate of refractive growth. However, a study of 103 subjects from the Infantile Aphakia Treatment Study (IATS) found that the variance in RRG3 in nor-

Fig. 70.4 The Pediatric
IOL Calculator
computer program.

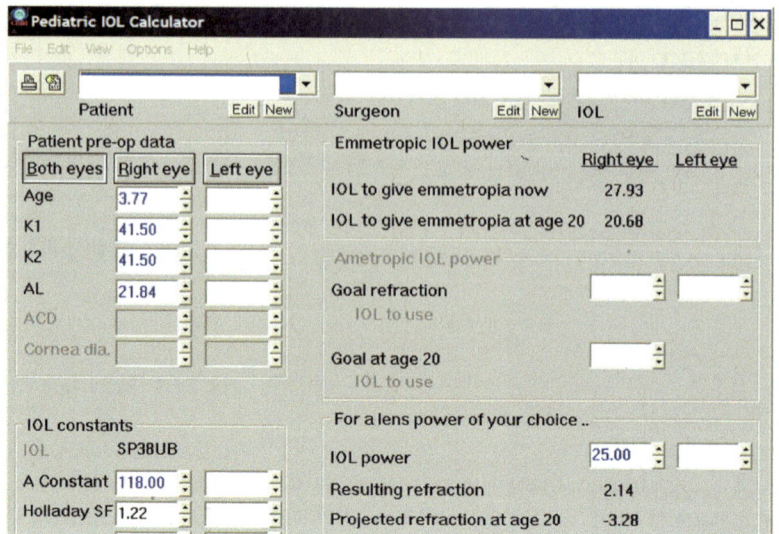

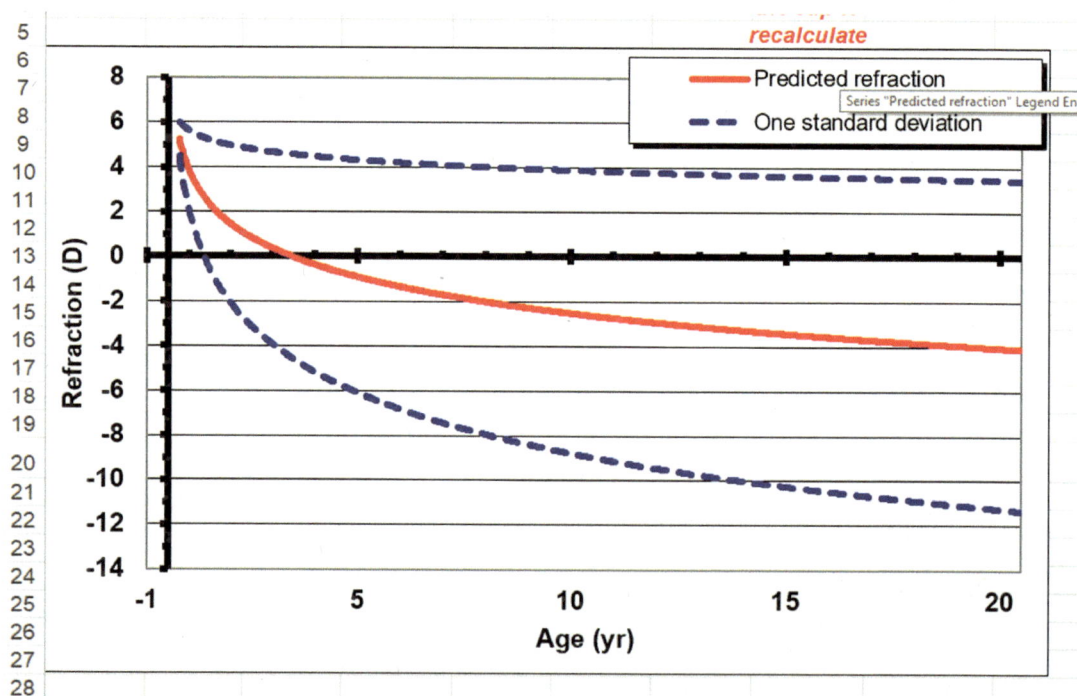

Fig. 70.5 A graph from the Pediatric Piggyback IOL Calculator spreadsheet, showing predicted refraction and standard deviation curves, of a child who has cataract removal with IOL implantation in infancy.

mal eyes was half that was seen in aphakic or pseudophakic eyes [26]. This study also found that RRG3 was greater in aphakic and pseudophakic eyes than the fellow, normal eyes. RRG3 for normal eyes was −15.0 (3.0) D (reported as mean (standard deviation)), for aphakic eyes −17.7 (6.2) D, and for pseudophakic eyes −16.7 (6.2) D.

The Choice of Initial Postoperative Refraction

There is no consensus on the choice of initial postoperative refraction in pseudophakic children. Most pediatric ophthalmologists prefer a moderate hyperopia that varies with age, and whether the IOLs are to be implanted uni- or bilaterally. Hiles in 1984 stated "…because of inaccuracies induced by the growth of the eye, a standard adult power lens is now routinely implanted" [27]. Eibschitz-Tsimhoni et al. noted in a Survey of Ophthalmology article that there are varied opinions: adult IOL power, myopia, emmetropia, and hyperopia. No study shows an advantage of one approach over another [28]. Nischal wrote, "Ideally, a child should be left as close as possible to emmetropia for visual rehabilitation" but it is recommended to under-correct to leave initial hypermetropia [29]. Indram et al. stated, "the goal is… to achieve emmetropia or a low level of myopia when the child is fully grown" [10]. A study by Lambert et al. of 24 children with unilateral cataract, age 2 to <6 years of age, divided into two groups: group 1 (full correction) and group 2 (undercorrection by ≥2 D). Neither the myopic shift nor the median final visual acuity differed significantly between the groups [30]. Lekskul et al. studied that 50 children were given initial undercorrection of IOL power (resulting in initial hyperopia) of between 10 and 30%, based on age at surgery for those between 0.5 and 5 years of age. In the children ≥7 years of age at last follow-up (quite varied length of follow-up), 45 of 74 eyes were myopic (up to −8.25 D, higher in those with surgery at younger ages); 21 eyes were hyperopic (up to +3.25 D). The authors propose to aim for a greater degree of undercorrection in future surgical cases [31].

My son's initial pseudophakic refraction was +1.5 D at the age of 3.77 years; it gradually shifted more towards myopia. As predicted, his myopic shift followed a semilogarithmic trajectory as he got older, though at a faster rate than average (Fig. 70.6). At the age of 20 years, he had

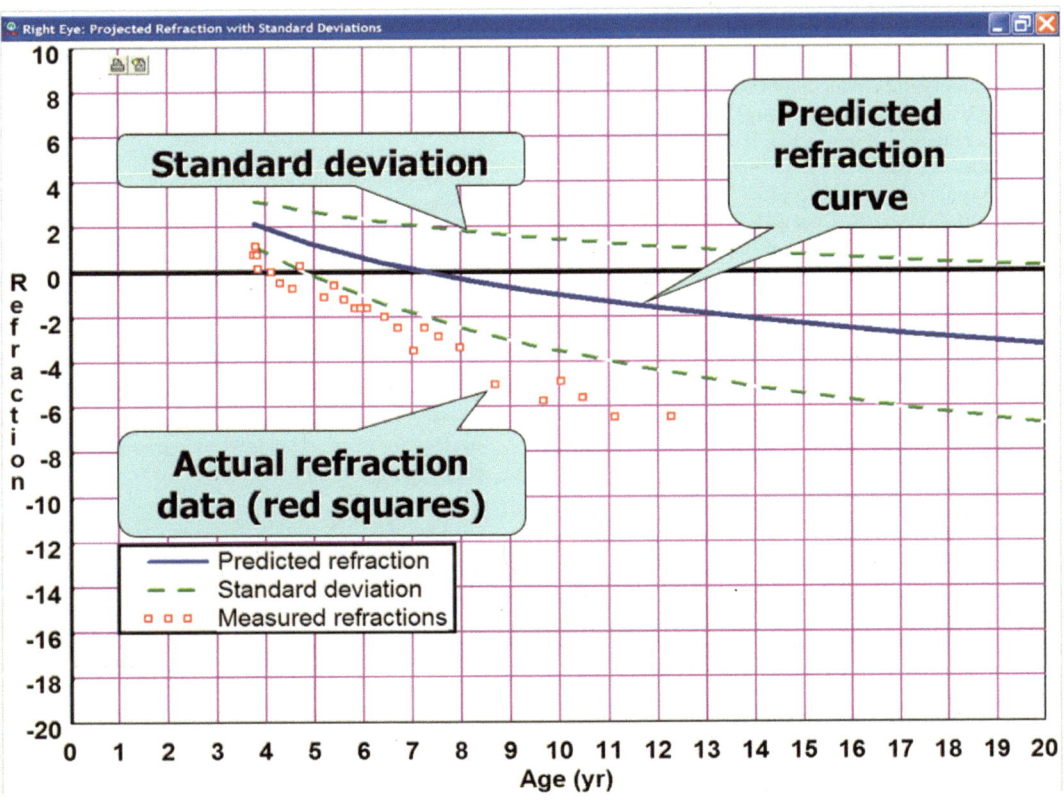

Fig. 70.6 Pseudophakic refraction, predicted vs. actual, for a child who had cataract surgery with a +25 D IOL implant at the age of 3.77 years

photorefractive keratectomy (PRK) for his refraction of −8 D. Now, several years later, he has a small amount of myopia, with 20/30 vision and good stereopsis. In retrospect, had we chosen an IOL power to result in initial myopia (say, −2.0 D), his refractive error at the age of 20 years would have required IOL exchange. Had we chosen an IOL power to result in greater initial hyperopia (say, +4 D), the PRK would could have removed less corneal stroma to achieve emmetropia.

References

1. McClatchey SK, Parks MM. Myopic shift after cataract removal in childhood. J Pediatr Ophthalmol Strabismus. 1997;34:88–95.
2. McClatchey SK, Parks MM. Theoretic refractive changes after lens implantation in childhood. Ophthalmology. 1997;104:1744–51.
3. McClatchey SK, Dahan E, Maselli E, et al. A comparison of the rate of refractive growth in pediatric aphakic and pseudophakic eyes. Ophthalmology. 2000;107:118–22.
4. McClatchey SK. Refractive changes after lens implantation in childhood: author's reply. Ophthalmology. 1998;105:1572–4.
5. McClatchey SK. Choosing IOL power in pediatric cataract surgery. Int Ophthalmol Clin. 2010;50:115–23.
6. Chang P, Lin L, Li Z, Wang L, Huang J, Zhao YE. Accuracy of 8 intraocular lens power calculation formulas in pediatric cataract patients. Graefes Arch Clin Exp Ophthalmol. 2020;258(5):1123–31.
7. Li J, Liu Z, Wang R, Cheng H, Zhao J, Liu L, Chen W, Wu M, Liu Y. Accuracy of intraocular lens power calculations in paediatric eyes. Clin Exp Ophthalmol. 2020;48(3):301–10.
8. Wilson ME, Trivedi RH. Axial length measurement techniques in pediatric eyes with cataract. Saudi J Ophthalmol. 2012;26(1):13–7.
9. Trivedi RH, Wilson ME. Axial length measurements by contact and immersion techniques in pediatric eyes with cataract. Ophthalmology. 2011;118:498–502.
10. Indaram M, VanderVeen DK. Postoperative refractive errors following pediatric cataract extraction with intraocular lens implantation. Semin Ophthalmol. 2018;33(1):51–8. Review. PMID: 29131702.
11. Ben-Zion I, Neely DE, Plager DA, Ofner S, Sprunger DT, Roberts GJ. Accuracy of IOL calculations in children: a comparison of immersion versus contact A-scan biometery. J AAPOS. 2008;12:440–4.
12. Trivedi RH, Wilson ME, Reardon W. Accuracy of the Holladay 2 intraocular lens formula for pediatric eyes in the absence of preoperative refraction. J Cataract Refract Surg. 2011;37:1239–43.
13. Vanderveen DK, Trivedi RH, Nizam A, Lynn MJ, Lambert SR, Infant Aphakia Treatment Study Group. Predictability of intraocular lens power calculation formulae in infantile eyes with unilateral congenital cataract: results from the Infant Aphakia Treatment Study. Am J Ophthalmol. 2013;156(6):1252–1260.e2.
14. Eppley SE, Arnold BF, Tadros D, Paricha N, de Alba Campomanes AG. Accuracy of a universal theoretical formula for lens power calculation in pediatric intraocular lens implantation. J Cataract Refract Surg. 2021;47:599.
15. Nihalani BR, VanderVeen DK. Comparison of intraocular lens power calculation formulae in pediatric eyes. Ophthalmology. 2010;117(8):1493–9.
16. Eibschitz-Tsimhoni M, Tsimhoni O, Archer SM, Del Monte MA. Effect of axial length and keratometry measurement error on intraocular lens implant power prediction formulas in pediatric patients. J AAPOS. 2008;12(2):173–6.
17. Gordon RA, Donzis PB. Refractive development of the human eye. Arch Ophthalmol. 1985;103(6):785–9.
18. Enyedi LB, Peterseim MW, Freedman SF, Buckley EG. Refractive changes after pediatric intraocular lens implantation. Am J Ophthalmol. 1998;126(6):772–81.
19. Nyström A, Lundqvist K, Sjöstrand J. Longitudinal change in aphakic refraction after early surgery for congenital cataract. J AAPOS. 2010;14(6):522–6.
20. O'Hara MA. Pediatric intraocular lens power calculations. Curr Opin Ophthalmol. 2012;23(5):388–93.
21. Wilson ME, Trivedi RH, Burger BM. Eye growth in the second decade of life: implications for the implantation of a multifocal intraocular lens. Trans Am Ophthalmol Soc. 2009;107:120–4.
22. Tadros D, Trivedi RH, Wilson ME, Davidson JD. Ocular axial growth in pseudophakic eyes of patients operated for monocular infantile cataract: a comparison of operated and fellow eyes measured at surgery and 5 or more years later. J AAPOS. 2016;20(3):210–3.
23. McClatchey SK, Hofmeister EM. The optics of aphakic and pseudophakic eyes in childhood. Surv Ophthalmol. 2010;55:174–82.
24. McClatchey SK. Intraocular lens calculator for childhood cataract. J Cataract Refract Surg. 1998;24:1125–9.
25. Boisvert C, Beverly DT, McClatchey SK. Theoretical strategy for choosing piggyback intraocular lens powers in young children. J AAPOS. 2009;13(6):555–7.
26. McClatchey SK, McClatchey TS, Cotsonis G, Nizam A, Lambert SR, Infant Aphakia Treatment Study Group. Refractive growth variability in the Infant Aphakia Treatment Study. J Cataract Refract Surg. 2021;47:512.
27. Hiles DA. Intraocular lens implantation in children with monocular cataracts. 1974-1983. Ophthalmology. 1984;91(10):1231–7.
28. Eibschitz-Tsimhoni M, Archer SM, Del Monte MA. Intraocular lens power calculation in children. Surv Ophthalmol. 2007;52:474–82.

29. Nischal KK. State of the art in pediatric cataract surgery. Dev Ophthalmol. 2016;57:15–28. Review.
30. Lambert SR, Archer SM, Wilson ME, Trivedi RH, del Monte MA, Lynn M. Long-term outcomes of undercorrection versus full correction after unilateral intraocular lens implantation in children. Am J Ophthalmol. 2012;153(4):602–8, 608.e1.
31. Lekskul A, Chuephanich P, Charoenkijkajorn C. Long-term outcomes of intended undercorrection intraocular lens implantation in pediatric cataract. Clin Ophthalmol. 2018;12:1905–11.

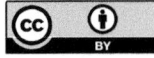

Out-of-the-Bag Implantation IOL Power

Jaime Aramberri

Introduction

The lens capsular bag offers an excellent position for the intraocular lens (IOL) in cataract surgery, providing a stable and predictable location within the eye. There is no direct contact with adjacent tissues, the optical plane is similar to the natural lens and the capsular fibrosis that occurs during the first year after surgery will set a permanent axial and rotational position [1]. The postoperative in-the-bag IOL plane has a relationship with some preoperative anatomic features of the eye such as the anterior chamber depth (ACD), the lens thickness (LT), and the axial length (AL), and therefore, a predicting function can be calculated to estimate this position before surgery and calculate the IOL power for a certain refraction using Optics theory or build a predictive model to directly calculate the IOL power from those variables.

However, in several clinical situations, in-the-bag implantation will not be possible due to a lack of safe capsular support. Depending on the circumstances, the IOL will be implanted in another anatomical plane: anterior chamber, iris, ciliary sulcus, or pars plana [2]. This will change the optical effective power of the IOL, and thus, the power calculation needs to be adjusted in order to achieve an accurate refractive prediction as all the usual IOL power calculation formulas assume an in-the-bag IOL location. Moreover, some IOL models are specifically designed for another anatomical location and the IOL formula must be aware of this and adapt the calculation usually through a different IOL constant.

The most frequent out-of-the-bag implant locations and IOL designs are as follows (Fig. 71.1):

- Anterior chamber: Angle supported and iris-claw (prepupillary) IOLs
- Ciliary sulcus: Iris-claw (retropupillary) and posterior chamber (PC) IOLs. The latter can be iris-sutured and sulcus supported
- Scleral fixation: PC IOL

J. Aramberri (✉)
Clínica Miranza Begitek,
Donostia-San Sebastian, Spain

Clínica Ókular, Vitoria-Gasteiz, Spain

© The Author(s) 2024
J. Aramberri et al. (eds.), *Intraocular Lens Calculations*, Essentials in Ophthalmology,
https://doi.org/10.1007/978-3-031-50666-6_71

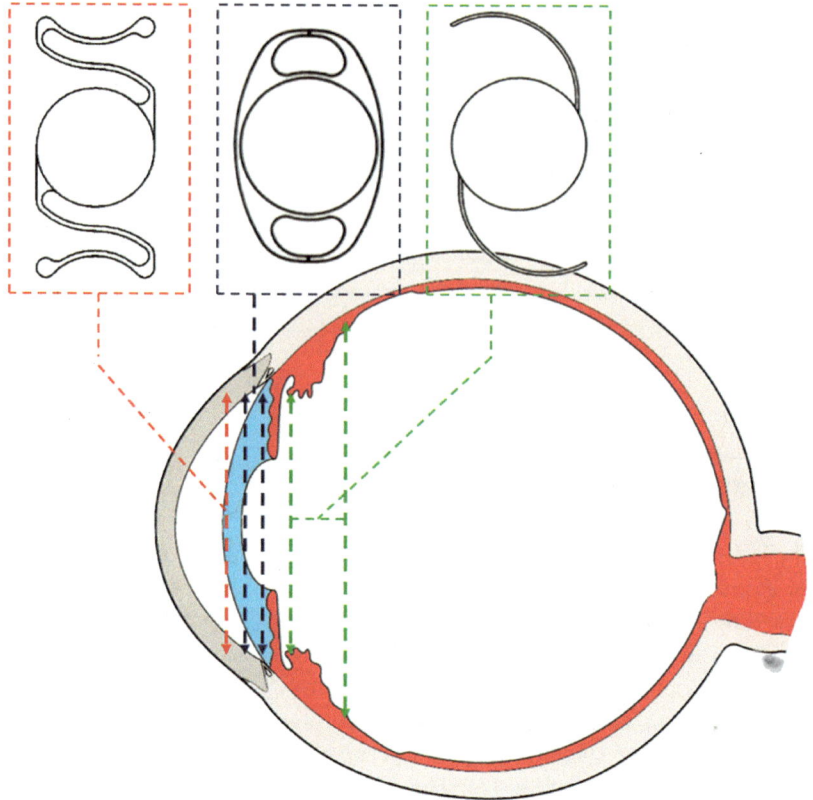

Fig. 71.1 IOL models for different out-of-the-bag implantation planes. From left to right: anterior chamber IOL, iris-claw IOL (anterior and posterior to iris), and posterior chamber IOL (iris-sutured, ciliary sulcus and pars plana fixated)

Clinical Situations

Insufficient capsular bag support can occur as a consequence of various clinical conditions. From a practical point of view, capsular and zonular damage should be distinguished.

Capsular Damage

The lens capsule can be injured in different degrees leaving some capsular support if the anterior capsule is still in place, where a PC IOL can be implanted over it, or no capsular support at all if the anterior capsule remnant is insufficient to hold the IOL in place and creating the need of an alternative IOL fixation technique.

The most usual clinical situations where the capsule is damaged are as follows:

– Capsular rupture during cataract surgery: This is a relatively frequent surgical complication with a reported incidence ranging between 0.1 and 5% depending on the series. A recent met-analysis reported 0.42% in Femto-second laser-assisted (FLACS) surgery and 0.27% in conventional phacoemulsification surgery [3]. Some related factors are surgeon's experience, cataract degree, pupil size, etc.

– Traumatic capsular rupture: It has been described in the context of blunt trauma, where the combined action of globe deformation and the shock wave can affect the capsular integrity [4], and also in perforating trauma.

Zonular Damage

Depending on the degree, there will be a partial or a total lens luxation:

– Simple ectopia lentis: Zonular damage due to genetic mutation, inherited in an autosomal dominant or recessive pattern.

– Ectopia lentis associated to systemic disease: There is a long list of associated pathologies being the most frequent: Marfan syndrome, Weill-Marchesani syndrome, sulfite oxidase deficiency, etc. [5].

- Ectopia lentis associated to ocular disease: Several ocular morbidities are associated to luxation and subluxation of the lens: pseudo-exfoliation syndrome, high myopia, congenital glaucoma, aniridia, syphilis, retinitis pigmentosa, etc. [5].
- In-the-bag IOL dislocation: An increasing trend for the incidence of this condition has been reported. The main associated factor is pseudoexfoliation syndrome, 31–83% of cases. Less frequent are previous vitreoretinal surgery, high myopia, uveitis, etc. [6].

Out-of-the-Bag IOL Implantation

Posterior Chamber

Posterior capsular tear or rupture is a frequent and unexpected complication during cataract surgery. The risk of IOL dislocation and/or tilt runs beyond a certain degree of capsular damage in-the-bag implantation, and therefore, an alternative IOL placement must be considered. If the anterior capsule is intact with maintained zonular tension, a PC IOL can be implanted over the anterior capsule with the haptics in the ciliary sulcus. The optic is sometimes captured with the capsulorrhexis to ensure centration and stability. If there isn't enough anterior capsular support, the IOL will have to be fixated to the sclera or to the iris. Scleral fixation can be done either in the sulcus or in the pars plana. Some techniques use non-absorbable sutures while others are sutureless.

PC IOLs are usually calculated with an IOL constant value optimized for in-the-bag IOL placement. Any axial offset will change the effective power of the IOL modifying the final refraction and turning the IOL power calculation inaccurate. There will be a myopic refraction shift if the IOL is more anterior (closer to the cornea) and a hyperopic refraction shift if the IOL is more posterior (closer to the retina).

Sulcus Support

This is the easiest situation for the surgeon both from the technical and calculation point of view. The IOL is positioned over the remaining anterior capsule, and the haptics will normally sit on the ciliary sulcus.

This anterior IOL location entails some pathophysiological and optical consequences:

- There will be more contact between the IOL and the iris and ciliary body tissue with risk of uveitis, glaucoma, and hyphema (UGH syndrome) [7]. The ideal PC IOL for sulcus should have thin haptics to avoid excessive contact with the iris root and an adequate design to leave as much space as possible between the optic and iris to minimize iris chaffing. This means posteriorly angulated haptics and a thin optic (material with high index of refraction), preferably with rounded and smooth edges. Some 3-piece hydrophobic IOL models meet these conditions and are the preferred designs for sulcus implantation. The overall IOL diameter must be sufficiently long to enhance centration and allow for stable fixation in the sulcus (minimum of 13.0 mm) [8].
- The IOL effective power will be higher and the refraction more myopic than the in-the-bag prediction. The surgeon must convert the IOL power calculation from the bag to the sulcus plane taking into account the expected distance change.

Several studies report a mean distance of around 0.75 mm between the bag and the sulcus position. Hayashi measured with a Scheimpflug camera a mean ACD of 4.27 ± 0.25 mm in 50 eyes with in-the-bag IOL, 3.54 ± 0.48 mm in 51 eyes with sulcus IOL and 3.59 ± 0.45 mm in 50 eyes with sulcus scleral-sutured IOL [9]. Suto measured with US biometry the same distances finding a mean ACD of 3.51 ± 0.25 mm in 30 eyes with sulcus IOL and 4.26 ± 0.29 mm in the fellow eye where the IOL was in-the-bag [10]. In one personal series (non-published study), we measured a mean difference of 0.69 ± 0.17 mm (0.40–0.86 mm) in 19 eyes using the fellow eye as reference in 17 eyes and the same eye where

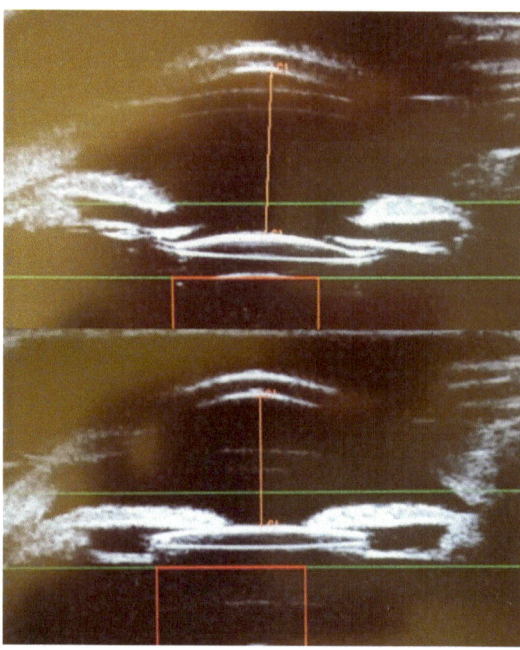

Fig. 71.2 IOL exchange in a case of negative dysphotopsia. The new IOL is implanted in the sulcus. The distance from the cornea to the anterior surface of the IOL changed from 4.35 to 3.49 mm (difference 0.86 mm)

Table 71.1 Refractive change (Rx) induced by 0.75 mm axial movement of a biconvex IOL. Output of a regression equation (see text) based on paraxial calculations in an eye model

IOL power	Rx	IOL power	Rx	IOL power	Rx
5	0.15	15	0.77	25	1.39
6	0.21	16	0.83	26	1.45
7	0.27	17	0.89	27	1.51
8	0.34	18	0.95	28	1.57
9	0.40	19	1.02	29	1.63
10	0.46	20	1.08	30	1.70
11	0.52	21	1.14	31	1.76
12	0.58	22	1.20	32	1.82
13	0.65	23	1.26	33	1.88
14	0.71	24	1.33	34	1.94

$$Rx = -0.158 + 0.0618 * \text{IOL power}$$

Table 71.1 contains the output of this equation for IOL power ranging from +6.00 D until +34.00 D. This can be a useful tool to estimate the refractive shift induced by 0.75 mm IOL axial movement (i.e., from in-the-bag to sulcus position).

Although there is some variability, the empirically observed refractive shift generally agrees with these calculations: Hayashi et al. report a lower value, -0.39 ± 0.71 D prediction error in 51 eyes with the IOL in the sulcus against 0.08 ± 0.54 D in 50 eyes with in-the-bag IOL [9]. Suto et al. compared 30 cases where the IOL was in the sulcus in one eye and in-the-bag in the other. The refraction prediction error was -0.78 ± 0.47 D [10]. Dubey et al. analyzed a group of 36 eyes where some surgeons had subtracted 0.5 D and others 1 D to the in-the-bag IOL power. Less prediction error was found in the latter group where in normal AL (22–25 mm), it was 0.38 ± 0.20 D and in short eyes (<22 mm), it was 1.01 ± 0.32 D. In the former group, the prediction error was 1.82 ± 0.47 D, 0.86 ± 0.29 D, and 0.42 ± 0.31 D in short (<22 mm), medium (22–25 mm), and long (>25 mm) eyes, respectively [12]. Eom et al. reported a prediction error of -0.91 ± 0.74 D and -0.93 ± 0.71 D with two different IOL models using the Haigis formula [13].

There is some difference when the IOL optic is captured with the capsulorrhexis. The IOL plane will be more posterior, and the effective power of

the IOL was moved for dysphotopsia treatment in 2 cases (Fig. 71.2).

The refractive shift induced by this axial distance will be directly proportional to the power of the IOL. It can be theoretically calculated using a human eye schematic model. Suto used a Gullstrand eye to calculate an IOL power difference of 0.67 D, 1.53 D, and 2.60 D for IOL powers of 10 D, 20 D, and 30 D, respectively. The refractive change in the spectacle plane would be 0.47 D, 1.07 D, and 1.82 D [11]. We obtained very similar figures using a ray tracing thick-lens paraxial model with a constant anterior corneal radius of 7.71 mm and posterior corneal radius of 6.38 mm. A biconvex IOL with known physical features was used (SA60AT, Alcon). The spectacle plane refraction for each IOL power (from +6.00 to +34.00 D) was calculated in two different IOL positions 0.75 mm apart. A regression equation for Spectacle refraction difference as dependent variable was calculated as follows:

the IOL will change less from the in-the-bag position. Millar et al. found a significant difference in a group of 58 eyes where 41% had optic capture and 59% had not. The prediction error was 0.34 ± 0.75 D and -0.40 ± 0.74 D respectively. They had subtracted 0.5, 1, and 1.5 D from the in-the-bag IOL power for long, medium, and short eyes, respectively [14]. Brunin et al. optimized the IOL constants and reported some better predictability in the optic capture group ($n = 29$) with a standard deviation (SD) of 0.75 D versus the non-optic-capture group ($n = 10$) where the SD was 0.82 D [15]. Both papers conclude that whenever it is possible, the sulcus implanted IOL optic should be captured with the capsulorrhexis because it provides a more stable and safe position.

Sulcus IOL Power

The most recommendable method would be to optimize the IOL constant for the same sulcus implanted IOL model based on the surgeon's own experience. Normally, this will not be possible except for very high volume centers. Eom et al. followed another approach modifiying the Haigis ELP prediction formula, adding the corneal radius as independent variable to the normally used AL and ACD. They found a correlation in a set of 132 eyes where the eyes with flatter corneas had more myopic error. They calculated new constants (b0, b1, b2, and b3) for this implantation plane. With this new equation, 68.1% of cases were within ± 0.5 D of the prediction [13]. The most suitable option will be to subtract some power from the in-the-bag IOL following what has been exposed in the above section. Table 71.1 can provide some reference values in this sense. Several authors recommend similar figures: Dubey et al. proposed subtracting 0.5 D in low powers (<18 D), 1 D in medium powers (18 D–25 D), and 1.5 D in high powers (>25 D) [12]. Knox-Cartwright et al. proposed reducing 5% the in-the-bag power for sulcus implantation. This number came out from the back-calculated IOL power change in a series of 24 eyes and it is an easy-to-remember rule. This means that the power should be reduced 0.5 D, 1 D, and 1.5 D in 10 D, 20 D, and 30 D in-the-bag IOL powers, respectively [16].

Scleral Fixation

Transscleral fixation of a PC IOL is a popular option in the management of IOL implantation with absence of capsular support. Its main advantage over the anterior chamber or the iris plane is that the IOL stands away from these structures avoiding endothelial and angular damage or uveal contact. In 1981, Girard first described a technique of pars plana scleral fixation with sutures [17]. Some years later, Malbran et al. proposed a similar one suturing the IOL at the sulcus plane [18]. Both ciliary sulcus and pars plana fixation have pros and cons. Pars plana fixation takes the risks of retinal injury and unstable IOL fixation, while sulcus fixation can produce corectopia, pupil capture, and UGH syndrome. At this moment, there is no consensus on which one is more effective or safe [19].

The refractive results of these techniques depend significantly on the fixation technique. There has been some evolution through the years that affect the reported results. In the beginning, *ab interno* sutured scleral fixation was more popular and it was related to some complications and high variability of haptics location. Later, *ab externo* scleral fixation with the knots covered by scleral flaps and a standard distance from the limbus (i.e., 2 mm) became the rule improving the refractive precision of the surgery. In recent years, several factors have increased the reproducibility of this technique: new IOLs with closed-loop haptics that allow four points of fixations, a trend to thicker sutures (7-0 Gore-Tex and 9-0 polypropylene) to provide extended safety, the improvement in surgical skills of the surgeons, and new vitrectomy technologies [20]. Lately, several sutureless techniques have been described to avoid some complications related to sutures like long-term suture erosion and breakage. The haptic ends are inserted into scleral tunnels with or without fibrin glue to secure the fixation [21, 22]. In another recently described technique, the haptic ends are melted and thickened with a cautery creating flanges to avoid slippage through the tunnels [23].

Fixation Point

The main disadvantage of these techniques is that scleral fixation is a blind maneuver as the ciliary sulcus and pars plana cannot be directly seen during surgery. In *ab externo* techniques, the needle is passed from outside the eye while in *ab interno* techniques, this is done from the inside. Normally, a certain distance from the surgical limbus is taken as reference for the entry/exit point. Most surgeons use 1–2 mm distance for sulcus and 3 mm for pars plana. Intermediate distances should be avoided not to injure the ciliary body (with the major arterial circle) and the ciliary processes. However, several studies have shown that the accuracy of these numbers is far from perfect and there is much variability in the anatomical location of the haptics which explains the higher refractive prediction error of these cases as compared to other techniques.

The ciliary sulcus has an oval shape with a higher diameter in the vertical meridian. Biermann studied a sample of phakic young adults and reported a difference of 0.35 mm in emmetropes and 0.30 mm in myopes [24]. Petermeier found a difference of 0.27 mm in 50 pseudophakic eyes with a mean age of 72.15 years. In this paper, the mean sulcus diameter was 11.10 mm [25]. Sulcus location using the surgical limbus as reference has a limited accuracy because the correlation between the corneal diameter (so-called corneal diameter distance) and the sulcus diameter is not very high and the previously mentioned vertical-horizontal sulcus diameter relationship suffers from some variability with 5–10% of cases where the horizontal diameter is higher than the vertical [24–26]. Duffey et al. found that a straight needle perpendicular to the sclera exits in the sulcus when the distance between the limbus and the entry point was 0.83 ± 0.10 mm in the vertical meridian and 0.46 ± 0.10 mm in the horizontal meridian [27]. From this paper, many surgeons adopted 1 mm behind the limbus as guide for sulcus fixation. However, Pavlin et al. reported several cases with entry point 1.5 mm behind the limbus and haptics anterior to the sulcus deforming the iris-angle and realized that in vivo, the situation might be different: The needle trajectory is normally parallel to the iris posterior surface and consequently the outer sclera exit will be more posterior than the inner sclera entry [28]. Sewelam et al. studied 20 eyes with ab externo scleral fixation placing the sutures 1 mm posterior to the limbus. With UBM, they found that only 55% of haptics were in sulcus, while 27.5% were anterior affecting the angle and 17.5% posterior to sulcus [29].

Some methods and devices have been proposed to improve the accuracy of scleral fixation: direct visualization of the sulcus with an endoscope [30], transillumination of the sulcus area using an intraoperative endo-illuminator [31], a needle injector with a tip that matches the shape of the sulcus for *ab interno* suture [32], etc.

Sugiura et al. estimated from UBM measurements that the distance from the surgical limbus to the exit point of a straight needle in the outer scleral wall would be 2.37 mm, assuming a trajectory parallel to the posterior surface of the iris. They found a similar value in 128 eyes where endoscopy confirmed the sulcus fixation with a straight needle: 2.50 mm from the posterior surgical limbus. In 28 eyes where a curved needle had been used, this distance was shorter: 2.00 mm (Fig. 71.3) [33].

Scleral Fixated IOL Power

Most of the scleral fixated IOLs are in-the-bag designs with IOL constants calculated for such position. The calculation must take into account the optical effect of the IOL plane difference from the regular location. In the last 25 years, there are dozens of published papers about IOL scleral fixation cases and techniques but most of them are retrospective, with very heterogeneous and small samples, merging different techniques within the same study as the surgeon's experience has evolved through time, using different IOL models and very few of them analyze refractive results with an adequate methodology. Moreover, these eyes have normally lower than normal BCVA making refractions less reliable. To make it worse, these surgical techniques are more surgeon dependent than regular phacoemulsification where in-the-bag implantation guarantees a reproducible IOL location for all

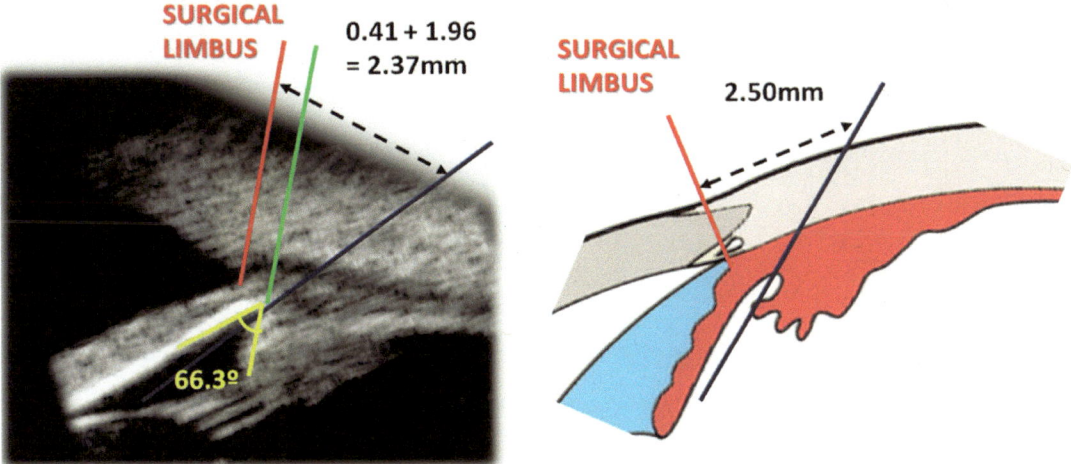

Fig. 71.3 Estimation of surgical limbus to scleral fixation straight needle exit point based on UBM image (left). In 128 eyes where the sulcus pass was checked by endoscopy, the actual distance with a straight needle was 2.50 mm [32]

cases and surgeons. Hence, the final IOL position will vary among different surgeons even for the same surgical technique and the same study. All this explains why the published results are contradictory to some extent, making it difficult to extract conclusions to provide precise recommendations.

As it has been described above, there are two main target locations: The ciliary sulcus and the pars plana. It seems logical that in the first case, the IOL position will be anterior to the in-the-bag plane and thus refraction will shift towards myopia in a similar way and magnitude to non-fixated sulcus implantation. While in the pars plana fixation, the IOL plane might be close to the in-the-bag one. There are very few studies reporting postoperative ACD values that allow comparison with the regular surgery: Hayashi et al. measured with a Scheimpflug camera a mean ACD of 4.27 ± 0.25 mm in 50 eyes with in-the-bag IOL, 3.54 ± 0.48 mm in 51 eyes with sulcus IOL, and 3.59 ± 0.45 mm in 50 eyes with sulcus scleral-sutured IOL [9]. Yamane et al. reported a higher number with a sutureless sulcus fixation technique in 100 eyes: 4.28 mm [23]. Muth et al. measured the ACD with three different sulcus fixation techniques: 3.67 ± 1.37 mm (Gore-tex suture), 4.01 ± 0.96 mm (Prolene suture), and 3.76 ± 1.08 mm (sutureless Yamane technique) [34]. Liu et al. used UBM to measure

4.31 ± 0.29 mm in 68 eyes where sutureless scleral fixation had been done 1.75 mm from limbus [35]. This variability makes it difficult to define a distance difference from in-the-bag plane in order to calculate the dioptric difference in the IOL power. However, all reported numbers are lower than the regular ones, so some myopic refractive shift would be expected.

Refractive Results

An analysis of the published refractive results with these procedures (Table 71.2) shows again some contradictory outcomes even for similar techniques. The distance to the surgical limbus determines the implantation plane of the IOL: 1.0–2.5 mm for sulcus and 3 mm for pars plana. Therefore, more myopic shift should be expected in the former case. However, this is not always the case in the published data. Some 1.5–2.5 mm series report hyperopic prediction error like McMillin et al. in 40 eyes operated with Yamane technique (YT) [36], Randerson et al. in 109 eyes with YT [37], and Abbey et al. in 23 eyes operated with sutureless scleral fixation with, paradoxically, more hyperopic error in the 1.5 mm distance (7 cases) than in the 2 mm (15 cases) distance [42]. In 100 eyes, Rocke et al. reported nil prediction error, −0.04 ± 0.88 D, with YT (2 mm to limbus) and Barrett formula [38]. Most of the sulcus fixation studies report some myopic

Table 71.2 Refraction prediction error with different scleral fixation techniques. Formulas are reported as third and fourth generation

First author	Year	N	Suture fixation	IOL model	Distance to limbus (mm)	Formula	Rx prediction error (D)
McMiliin [36]	2021	40	No	ZA9003 Lucia 602	2	Third and fourth gen.	+0.48 to +0.67
Randerson [37]	2020	109	No	Lucia 602	2	Third gen	0.18 ± 1.45
Rocke [38]	2020	100	No	ZA9003	2	Fourth gen	−0.04 ± 0.88
Ohr [39]	2020	20	Yes	A060	3	Third gen	0.16 ± 0.69
Sugiura [32]	2019	128	Yes	NR-81K	2.5	n.a.	−0.63
Su [40]	2019	13	Yes	A060 MX60	2–3	Third gen	−1.35 ± 1.32
Su [40]	2019	42	Yes	A060 MX60	3	Third gen	−0.43 ± 0.71
Botsford [41]	2019	31	Yes	A060 CZ70BD	3	Third and fourth gen.	−0.19 ± 0.72
Yamane [23]	2017	50	No	X70	2	Third gen	−0.41 ± 0.98
Yamane [23]	2017	32	No	ZA9003	2	Third gen	−0.02 ± 0.93
Brunin [15]	2017	24	Yes	n.a.	n.a.	Third gen	−0.23 ± 0.79
Abbey [42]	2014	15	No	MA60AC	2	n.a.	0.32
Abbey [42]	2014	7	No	MA60AC	1.5	n.a.	0.56
Huang [43]	2013	18	Yes	P366UV CZ708D	1	Third gen	−1.66 ± 0.94
Ma [44]	2011	38	Yes	MA60BM YA60BBR	1.5	n.a.	−1.03 ± 1.82
Ma [44]	2011	56	Yes	MA60BM YA60BBR	3	n.a.	−0.88 ± 2.15
Hayashi [9]	1999	52	Yes	S62UV P336UV	1	n.a.	−0.65 ± 1.11

n.a. not available

shift ranging from −0.19 to −1.66 D. In some cases, within the same study, results depended on the IOL model. Yamane found a prediction error of −0.41 ± 0.98 D with the X70 IOL and −0.02 ± 0.93, with the ZA9003 IOL model [23]. This might be related to factors like the IOL design, the accuracy of used IOL constant, etc.

The pars plana fixation techniques normally show less myopic refractions but there are significant exceptions like the study by Ma et al. that found a myopic prediction error of −0.88 ± 2.15 D with scleral sutures 3 mm from limbus [44] and the paper by Su et al. that reported −0.43 ± 0.71 D error at the same distance [40]. In both papers, another group with sulcus fixation had a higher myopic error.

In all these published studies, the variance of the refraction prediction error is quite variable as well. This is probably related to the heterogeneity of the samples but might have some relationship with the IOL models or with surgical technique. In a subgroup of studies with YT and similar IOL models, the standard deviation of the prediction error ranges from 0.67 to 1.45 D [23, 36–38].

The recommended strategy in scleral fixation should be to use an optimized constant calculated for the same surgeon, same IOL model, and surgical technique. Randerson et al. calculated the refractive results with third-generation formulas using optimized constants for the YT and one IOL model and surgeon: They reported 32–46% of eyes with an absolute PE <0.50 D and 63.30–64.22% of eyes with an absolute PE <1.00 D [37]. Due to the fact that in many of these eyes, ACD and LT will not be available in the preoperative study, fourth-generation formulas that use these parameters will be less useful and more difficult to get enough eyes for constant optimization.

In an average volume, clinic IOL constants optimization will probably take years as these cases are not so frequent. Meanwhile, the expected refraction with in-the-bag IOL constants will be assumed to be −0.5 to −1.00 in sulcus fixation and 0.00 to −0.50 in pars plana fixation.

Sulcus Fixation IOL

Recently, a new IOL specifically designed for sutureless sulcus fixation has been marketed: FIL SSF Carlevale (Soleko Inc). It is a 1-piece foldable acrylic IOL with T-shaped haptics that will be externalized through the sclera with a forceps at two points 180° apart and 2 mm from limbus. Therefore, it can be defined as sutureless sulcus transcleral fixation.

The IOL constant is calculated for this implantation site and therefore should be quite accurate. The manufacturer provided IOL constants for optical biometry are A constant = 119.1 for SRK/T, SF = 1.9 for Holladay 1, a0 = 0.051, a1 = 0.140 and a2 = 0.197 for Haigis and pACD = 5.68 for Hoffer Q and Holladay 2. With this, A constant two different studies found very similar prediction errors, both in terms of mean and SD values: Rouhette et al. reported −0.30 ± 0.70 in 70 cases [45] and Barca et al. found −0.24 ± 0.81 D in 32 cases [46]. Vaiano et al. optimized the IOL constants for the third-generation formulas using a selected sample of 25 cases: values for SRK/T, Hoffer Q, and Holladay 1 were 118.92, 5.48, and 1.75, respectively. The SD of the prediction error with these constants was 0.89 for SRK/T, 0.94 for Holladay 1, and 0.95 for Hoffer Q. The percentage of eyes within ±0.50 D and ±1.00 D were 56% and 72% for SRK/T, 64% and 68% for Holladay 1 and 60% and 72% for the Hoffer Q formula [47].

Iris Plane

The iris can be used as a IOL supporting anatomical structure in the case of absence of capsular support. There are two different options: The iris-claw IOL design which is specifically designed for iris fixation and a PC IOL with the haptics sutured to the mid-perypheral iris.

Iris Claw IOL

The first iris claw IOL was designed by Jan Worst in 1978 to optically correct aphakia after intracapsular surgery [48]. A later evolution of that lens is still in use today: The Artisan aphakia 205 IOL (Ophtec). This is a 1-piece PMMA IOL 8.5 mm long (7.5 mm for pediatric patients) with an optical zone of 5.0 mm. The haptics have a claw shape design in order to pull a small section of iris through it securing the lens to the mid-peripheral iris. It can be implanted in the anterior chamber with a posterior to anterior iris enclavation maneuver or in the posterior chamber enclavating the iris in the opposite sense. Both techniques are considered to be safe and effective but the last years, the retropupilar implantation seems to be more popular, especially in younger patients, due to a lower endothelial damage risk [49].

Iris Claw IOL Power

The Artisan IOL power is calculated as any pseudophakic IOL using normally a third-generation theoretical formula. Most of the published studies use the SRK/T formula. These formulas employ the AL and K value as effective lens position predictors. This could be considered to be senseless as there is no in-the-bag IOL position to predict. The manufacturer recommended A constant values are: 116.8 (US) and 116.9 (optical) for retropupillary (RP) placement and 115.0 (US) and 115.7 (optical) for prepupillary (PP) implantation (Table 71.3).

The reported outcomes can be generally considered better than those obtained with scleral fixated IOLs, and this is probably one of the reasons that explains the increasing popularity of this surgical technique in the correction of aphakia. Very few papers report the refraction prediction error (PE): Choi et al. studied 103 eyes with RP position and found a PE of −0.56 ± 0.98 D. 71.8% of eyes had <0.50 D absolute PE [50]. Gonnermann et al. analyzed 137 eyes calculated with the SRK/T formula. The final refraction was 0.00 ± 1.21 D. At last visit, 75.9% of eyes where within ±1.00 D [51].

Table 71.3 Manufacturer recommended IOL constants for Artisan aphakia 205 IOL

	Constants	Prepupillary	Retropupillary
US biometry	SRK/T	115.0	116.8
Optic biometry	SRK/T (A)	115.7	116.9
	Holladay 1 (SF)	−0.08	0.54
	Hoffer Q (pACD)	3.62	4.34
	Haigis a0	−0.16	−0.25
	Haigis a1	0.4	0.4
	Haigis a2	0.1	0.1
	Barrett (LF)	0.15	0.78

https://es.ophtec.com/productos/cirugia-de-cataratas/lios/artisan-afaquia. Accessed 9 Sept. 2021

Vounotrypidis et al. studied 40 eyes and reported a PE of −0.11 ± 1.06 D. The eyes that were aphakic preoperatively had slightly lower PE than those who were pseudophakic: −0.09 ± 1.18 D and −0.12 ± 0.98 D, respectively. However, 36% of eyes were within ±0.50 D of prediction and 52% within ±1.00 D [52]. In a prospective randomized study of IOL reposition vs exchange with RP iris claw implantation, Dalby et al. reported a PE of +0.29 ± 0.86 D in 50 eyes [53]. Baykara et al. studied 32 eyes operated by one surgeon and reported a PE of −0.13 ± 0.28 D [54]. Choragiewicz et al. analyzed 47 eyes with RP Artisan/Verysyse. They used the Haigis formula with these constants: a0: −0.25, a1: 0.4 and a2: 0.1. The prediction error was −0.27 ± 1.28 D and 61% of eyes where within ±1.00 D of the prediction [55].

There is some variability in these mean values and their variances than can be explained, as in other aphakia treatment modalities, by the difference among treated clinical conditions.

The main drawback of this IOL is that it is non-foldable, and therefore, it demands a large wound size which will induce more astigmatism than other techniques where foldable IOLs are implanted. This can be improved using a tunneled scleral incision instead of a corneal one. Lajoie et al. report a surgically induced astigmatism (SIA) of 1.67 D × 176° in 21 cases of PP implantation and 1.19 D × 11° in 51 cases of RP IOL placement. This difference was not significant [56]. Seknazi et al. found higher induced astigmatism with the Artisan, 1.72 ± 0.96 D than with the Carlevale, 0.72 ± 0.52 D, in 22 and 20 cases ,respectively [57].

Iris Sutured

A PC IOL can be suturede to the mid-perypheral iris with 10/0 polypropylene sutures. The IOL is implanted in the anterior chamber placing the haptics posteriorly in the sulcus, and then, two sutures are passed from limbus to limbus engaging the haptics and the iris. Finally, the optic is gently pushed behind the pupil. This technique was first proposed by McCannel in 1976 and gained quick popularity especially when combined with penetrating keratoplasty as it was easy to perform in sky-open surgery [58, 59]. When performed with a closed chamber, first McCannel suturing was used tying the knot from a paracentesis located above the haptic but Condon related the incidence of haptic slippage and IOL dislocation to the intrinsic difficulty of this technique in cinching correctly the knot and defended the Siepser technique tying the knot outside a lateral paracentesis and then sliding it by opposite pulling without any haptic countertraction [60]. Chang reported eight cases of successful iris sutured IOLs using the Siepser knot [61].

In this technique, the IOL optic will be located in the sulcus plane, maybe slightly more anterior than the sulcus supported IOL, but probably with no significant optical effect. Mura et al. reported a mean ACD of 3.84 ± 0.36 mm (range 3.17–4.5 mm) in 15 cases measured with UBM. The haptics were found to be in sulcus in 53.3%, over the ciliary processes in 30% and over pars plana in 16.7% of the cases. No haptic was found anteriorly placed pushing the iris root [62].

The IOL model selection should follow the same recommendations for any iris-touching model: 3-piece IOL with thin haptics and optic and haptic-optic posterior angulation if only to release some pressure on the iris.

Iris Sutured IOL Power

There are very few reports regarding IOL power calculation in PC IOL sutured to iris. Most of them focus on technique and safety and outcomes are normally expressed in terms of number of eyes over certain UCVA and BCVA. There is no paper with a detailed IOL power calculation methodology description. Dzhaber et al. studied 117 eyes operated by one surgeon with the same IOL model and found a myopic refraction of −1.3 ± 1.4 D ($n = 43$) with a prediction error of 0.8 ± 0.7 D ($n = 38$) (sic) [63]. Soiberman et al. reported a postoperative refraction of −0.88 ± 1.91 D in 27 eyes operated by one surgeon with the same IOL model [64]. Condon et al. found −0.36 ± 1.00 D final refraction in 46 eyes, but again with no calculation method description [65].

The recommended IOL power calculation method therefore is not based on data supported evidence but on the knowledge of the produced IOL plane shift. The guidelines have been described above in this chapter for sulcus supported IOLs: Conversion of the in-the-bag IOL power taking into account the IOL power value and the distance shift from in-the-bag to sulcus plane. The figures should be very similar, and therefore, the suggested methods should apply similarly for iris sutured PC IOLs. As soon as experience provides actual outcomes, these calculations can be fine-tuned optimizing an adequate IOL constant for this plane.

Anterior Chamber

Anterior chamber (AC) IOLs can be angle supported or iris supported. As the iris supported IOLs (iris claw) have been covered in a previous section of this chapter, here we will refer exclusively to angle supported IOL models.

After a long evolution since the first AC implantation in 1952 (Baron), the present day models are 1-piece lenses with open-loop flexible haptics. Most designs are based on the Kelman Multiflex IOL with 5.5 mm optic and different

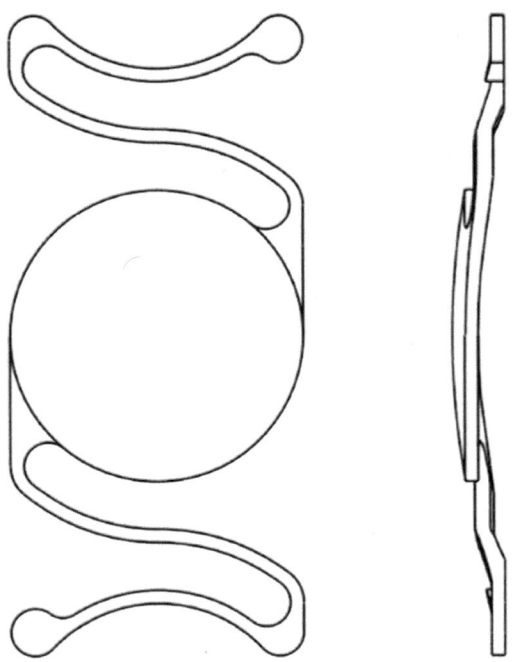

Fig. 71.4 Anterior chamber angle supported IOL. Open-loop haptics with some anterior angulation to provide anterior vaulting of the optic. Model Kelman Multiflex III (Alcon)

longitudinal sizes where selection will depend on the horizontal corneal diameter. The recommended rule is to add 1 mm to the measured horizontal corneal diameter distance. Correctly sized, there will be some anterior optic vaulting avoiding contact with the iris and decreasing the risk of endothelial damage (Fig. 71.4). Most of these IOLs are PMMA made and hence non-foldable. Thus, the large incision size will induce more astigmatism than other techniques where foldable IOLs can be implanted.

The implantation technique is simple and the learning curve is short. A protocoled surgery will allow a safe procedure. There are several complications that have been traditionally associated to angle supported IOLs: corneal decompensation, glaucoma, pupil ovalization, uveitis, etc. [66]. However, the incidence decreased since the first closed-looped IOLs and a recent report by the American Academy of Ophthalmology concluded that the evidence shows no superiority of any single implantation technique in the absence of capsular support [2].

Anterior Chamber IOL Power

Angle supported IOLs are calculated by means of an IOL power calculation formula and a model-specific IOL constant that will take into account the IOL features and the IOL position within the eye, which is much closer to the cornea than any other IOL type. As it happens with the iris fixated IOLs, it is not logical to use a formula that estimates the IOL position with an algorithm calculated for the in-the-bag IOL plane. A lower outcomes spread could be expected with an anterior chamber specific IOL position algorithm. The IOL constant adjusts the calculation to this new IOL plane with a lower value. Cooke et al. calculated an optimized A constant of 115.7 ± 0.39 D for the MT*UO IOL model (Alcon) and the SRK/T formula with a dataset of 52 eyes. They highlighted that this was an increase of 0.4 over the manufacturer's labeled value, just as the median A constant increase of optimized values of most IOLs in ULIB website [67].

The published results suggest better accuracy than scleral fixated IOLs but it should be remarked that nearly all studies are retrospective, with small samples, without detailed calculation methodology description and significant differences in the clinical context: primary vs secondary implantation, aphakia, IOL exchange, etc.: Gore et al. studied 41 eyes and reported a refraction prediction error of 0.37 ± 0.89 D. 71.2% and 40.4% of the eyes were within ±1.00 D and ±0.50 D of the target, respectively [68]. Negretti et al. report a prediction error of −0.23 ± 1.31 D in a sample of 271 eyes [69]. Brunin et al. found a similar value in their series where 30 eyes with anterior chamber IOLs were analyzed: −0.22 ± 0.86 D. After IOL constant optimization, the mean absolute prediction error was 0.62 ± 0.58 D [15]. Harrison et al. studied 35 eyes and reported a prediction error of 0.31 ± 1.00 D. However, 69% and 37% of the eyes were within ±1.00 D and ±0.50 D of the target, respectively [70].

References

1. Oetting TA, Hilary Beaver H, Johnson T. Intraocular lens design, material and delivery. [aut. libro] Henderson BA. Essentials of cataract surgery. Thorofare: Slack Incorporated. pp. 167–182.
2. Shen JF, Deng S, Hammersmith KM, Kuo AN, Li JY, Weikert MP, Shtein RM. Intraocular lens implantation in the absence of zonular support: an outcomes and safety update: a report by the American Academy of Ophthalmology. Ophthalmology. 2020;127(9):1234–1.
3. Kolb CM, Shajari M, Mathys L, Herrmann E, Petermann K, Mayer WJ, Priglinger S, Kohnen T. Comparison of femtosecond laser-assisted cataract surgery and conventional cataract surgery: a meta-analysis and systematic review. J Cataract Refract Surg. 2020;46(8):1075–85.
4. Liu X, Wang L, Du C, Li D, Fan Y. Mechanism of lens capsular rupture following blunt trauma: a finite element study. Comput Methods Biomech Biomed Engin. 2015;18(8):914–21.
5. Nelson LB, Maumenee IH. Ectopia lentis. Surv Ophthalmol. 1982;27(3):143–60.
6. Kristianslund O, Dalby M, Drolsum L. Late in-the-bag intraocular lens dislocation. J Cataract Refract Surg. 2021;47(7):942–54.
7. Chang DF, Masket S, Miller KM, Braga-Mele R, Little BC, Mamalis N, Oetting TA, Packer M, ASCRS Cataract Clinical Committee. Complications of sulcus placement of single-piece crylic intraocular lenses: recommendations for backup IOL implantation following crylic intraocular lenses: recommendations for backup IOL implantation following. J Cataract Refract Surg. 2009;35(8):1445.
8. Werner L. Intraocular lenses: overview of designs, materials, and pathophysiologic features. Ophthalmology. 2021;128(11):e74–93, S0161-6420(20)30626-6.
9. Hayashi K, Hayashi H, Nakao F, Hayashi F. Intraocular lens tilt and decentration, anterior chamber depth and refractive error after trans-scleral suture fixation surgery. Ophthalmology. 1999;106:878–82.
10. Suto C, Hori S, Fukuyama E, Akura J. Adjusting intraocular lens power for sulcus fixation. J Cataract Refract Surg. 2003;29:1913–7.
11. Suto C. Sliding scale of IOL power for sulcus fixation using computer simulation. J Cataract Refract Surg. 2004;30(11):2452–4.
12. Dubey R, Birchall W, Grigg J. Improved refractive outcome for ciliary sulcus-implanted intraocular lenses. Ophthalmology. 2012;119(2):261–5.
13. Eom Y, Song JS, Kim HM. Modified Haigis formula effective lens position equation for ciliary sulcus-

implanted intraocular lenses. Am J Ophthalmol. 2016;161:142–9.

14. Millar ER, Allen D, Steel DH. Effect of anterior capsulorhexis optic capture of a sulcus-fixated intraocular lens on refractive outcomes. J Cataract Refract Surg. 2013;39(6):841–4.

15. Brunin G, Sajjad A, Kim EJ, Montes de Oca I, Weikert MP, Wang L, Koch DD, Al-Mohtaseb Z. Secondary intraocular lens implantation: complication rates, visual acuity, and refractive outcomes. J Cataract Refract Surg. 2017;43(3):369–76.

16. Knox Cartwright NE, Aristodemou P, Sparrow JM, Johnston RL. Adjustment of intraocular lens power for sulcus implantation. J Cataract Refract Surg. 2011;37(4):798–9.

17. Girard LJ. Pars plana phacoprosthesis (aphakic intraocular implant): a preliminary report. Ophthalmic Surg. 1991;109:1754–8.

18. Malbran ES, Malbran E Jr, Negri I. Lens guide suture for transport and fixation in secondary IOL implantation after intracapsular extraction. Int Ophthalmol. 1986;9(2–3):151–60.

19. Forlini M, Bedi R. Intraocular lens implantation in the absence of capsular support: scleral-fixated vs retropupillary iris-claw intraocular lenses. J Cataract Refract Surg. 2021;47(6):792–801.

20. Stem MS, Todorich B, Woodward MA, Hsu J, Wolfe JD. Scleral-fixated intraocular lenses: past and present. J Vitreoretin Dis. 2017;1(2):144–52.

21. Prenner JL, Feiner L, Wheatley HM, Connors D. A novel approach for posterior chamber intraocular lens placement or rescue via a sutureless scleral fixation technique. Retina. 2012;32(4):853–5.

22. Agarwal A, Kumar DA, Jacob S, Baid C, Agarwal A, Srinivasan S. Fibrin glue-assisted sutureless posterior chamber intraocular lens implantation in eyes with deficient posterior capsules. J Cataract Refract Surg. 2008;34(9):1433–8.

23. Yamane S, Sato S, Maruyama-Inoue M, Kadonosono K. Flanged Intrascleral intraocular lens fixation with double-needle technique. Ophthalmology. 2017;124(8):1136–42.

24. Biermann J, Bredow L, Boehringer D, Reinhard T. Evaluation of ciliary sulcus diameter using ultrasound biomicroscopy in emmetropic eyes and myopic eyes. J Cataract Refract Surg. 2011;37:1686–93.

25. Petermeier K, Suesskind D, Altpeter E, Schatz A, Messias A, Gekeler F, Szurman P. Sulcus anatomy and diameter in pseudophakic eyes and correlation with biometric data: evaluation with a 50 MHz ultrasound biomicroscope. J Cataract Refract Surg. 2012;38(6):986–91.

26. Reinstein DZ, Archer TJ, Silverman RH, Rondeau MJ, Coleman DJ. Correlation of anterior chamber angle and ciliary sulcus diameters with white-to-white corneal diameter in high myopes using Artemis VHF digital ultrasound. J Refract Surg. 2009;25:185–94.

27. Duffey RJ, Holland EJ, Agapitos PJ, Lindstrom RL. Anatomic study of transsclerally sutured intraocular lens implantation. Am J Ophthalmol. 1989;108:300–9.

28. Pavlin CJ, Rootman D, Arshinoff S, Harasiewicz K, Foster FS. Determination of haptic position of transsclerally fixated posterior chamber intraocular lenses by ultrasound biomicroscopy. J Cataract Refract Surg. 1993;19(5):573–7.

29. Sewelam A, Ismail AM, El Serogy H. Ultrasound biomicroscopy of haptic position after transscleral fixation of posterior chamber intraocular lenses. J Cataract Refract Surg. 2001;27(9):418–22.

30. Jürgens I, Lillo J, Buil JA, Castilla M. Endoscope-assisted transscleral suture fixation of intraocular lenses. J Cataract Refract Surg. 1996;22(7):879–81.

31. Horiguchi M, Hirose H, Koura T, Satou M. Identifying the ciliary sulcus for suturing a posterior chamber intraocular lens by transillumination. Arch Ophthalmol. 1993;111(12):1693–5.

32. Sugiura T, Kaji Y, Tanaka Y. Ciliary sulcus suture fixation of intraocular lens using an auxiliary device. J Cataract Refract Surg. 2019;45(6):711–8.

33. Sugiura T, Kaji Y, Tanaka Y. Anatomy of the ciliary sulcus and the optimum site of needle passage for intraocular lens suture fixation in the living eye. J Cataract Refract Surg. 2018;44(10):1247–53.

34. Muth DR, Wolf A, Kreutzer T, Shajari M, Vounotrypidis E, Priglinger S, Mayer WJ. Safety and efficacy of current sclera fixation methods for intraocular lenses and literature overview. Klin Monatsbl Augenheilkd. 2021;238(8):868–74.

35. Liu J, Fan W, Lu X, Peng S. Sutureless Intrascleral posterior chamber intraocular lens fixation: analysis of clinical outcomes and postoperative complications. J Ophthalmol. 2021;16:8857715.

36. McMillin J, Wang L, Wang MY, Al-Mohtaseb Z, Khandelwal S, Weikert M, Hamill MB. Accuracy of intraocular lens calculation formulas for flanged intrascleral intraocular lens fixation with double-needle technique. J Cataract Refract Surg. 2021;47(7):855–8.

37. Randerson EL, Bogaard JD, Koenig LR, Hwang ES, Warren CC, Koenig SB. Clinical outcomes and lens constant optimization of the Zeiss CT Lucia 602 lens using a modified Yamane technique. Clin Ophthalmol. 2020;14:3903–12.

38. Rocke JR, McGuinness MB, Atkins WK, Fry LE, Kane JX, Fabinyi DCA, Yeoh J, Chiu D, Essex MBiostat RW, Roufail E, Sheridan AM, Allen PJ, Edwards TL. Refractive outcomes of the Yamane flanged Intrascleral haptic fixation technique. Ophthalmology. 2020;127(10):1429–31.

39. Ohr MP, Wisely CE. Refractive outcomes and accuracy of IOL power calculation with the SRK/T formula for sutured, scleral-fixated Akreos AO60 intraocular lenses. Graefes Arch Clin Exp Ophthalmol. 2020;258(10):2125–9.

40. Su D, Stephens JD, Obeid A, Borkar D, Storey PP, Khan MA, Hsu J, Garg SJ, Gupta O. Refractive outcomes after pars plana vitrectomy and scleral fixated intraocular lens with Gore-Tex suture. Ophthalmol Retina. 2019;3(7):548–52.

41. Botsford BW, Williams AM, Conner IP, Martel JN, Eller AW. Scleral fixation of intraocular lenses with Gore-Tex suture: refractive outcomes and comparison of lens power formulas. Ophthalmol Retina. 2019;3(6):468–72.

42. Abbey AM, Hussain RM, Shah AR, Faia LJ, Wolfe JD, Williams GA. Sutureless scleral fixation of intraocular lenses: outcomes of two approaches. The 2014 Yasuo Tano Memorial Lecture. Graefes Arch Clin Exp Ophthalmol. 2015;253(1):1–5.

43. Huang YC, Tseng CC, Lin CP. Myopic shift of sulcus suture-fixated posterior chamber intraocular lenses. Taiwan J Ophthalmol. 2013;3(9):95–7.

44. Ma DJ, Choi HJ, Kim MK, Wee WR. Clinical comparison of ciliary sulcus and pars plana locations for posterior chamber intraocular lens transscleral fixation. J Cataract Refract Surg. 2011;37(8):1439–46.

45. Rouhette H, Meyer F, Pommier S, Benzerroug M, Denion E, Guigou S, Lorenzi U, Mazit C, Mérité PY, Rebollo O. FIL-SSF Carlevale intraocular lens for sutureless scleral fixation: 7 recommendations from a serie of 72 cases. MICA study (Multicentric Study of the Carlevale IOL). J Fr Ophtalmol. 2021;44(7):1038–46.

46. Barca F, Caporossi T, de Angelis L, Giansanti F, Savastano A, Di Leo L, Rizzo S. Trans-scleral plugs fixated IOL: a new paradigm for sutureless scleral fixation. J Cataract Refract Surg. 2020;46(5):716–20.

47. Vaiano AS, Hoffer KJ, Greco A, Greco A, D'Amico G, Pasqualitto V, Carlevale C, Savini G. Accuracy of IOL power calculation using the new carlevale sutureless scleral fixation posterior chamber IOL. J Refract Surg. 2021;37(7):472–6.

48. Worst JGF. Iris claw lens [letter]. Am Intraocular Implant Soc J. 1980;6:166–167.

49. Liang IC, Chang YH, Hernández Martínez A, Hung CF. Iris-Claw intraocular lens: anterior chamber or retropupillary implantation? A systematic review and meta-analysis. Medicina (Kaunas). 2021;57(8):785.

50. Choi EY, Lee CH, Kang HG, Han JY, Byeon SH, Kim SS, Koh HJ, Kim M. Long-term surgical outcomes of primary retropupillary iris claw intraocular lens implantation for the treatment of intraocular lens dislocation. Sci Rep. 2021;11(1):726.

51. Gonnermann J, Klamann MK, Maier AK, Rjasanow J, Joussen AM, Bertelmann E, Rieck PW, Torun N. Visual outcome and complications after posterior iris-claw aphakic intraocular lens implantation. J Cataract Refract Surg. 2012;38(12):2139–43.

52. Vounotrypidis E, Schuster I, Mackert MJ, Kook D, Priglinger S, Wolf A. Secondary intraocular lens implantation: a large retrospective analysis. Graefes Arch Clin Exp Ophthalmol. 2019;257(1):125–34.

53. Dalby M, Kristianslund O, Drolsum L. Long-term outcomes after surgery for late in-the-bag intraocular lens dislocation: a randomized clinical trial. Am J Ophthalmol. 2019;207:184–94.

54. Baykara M, Ozcetin H, Yilmaz S, Timuçin OB. Posterior iris fixation of the iris-claw intraocular lens implantation through a scleral tunnel incision. Am J Ophthalmol. 2007;144(4):586–91.

55. Choragiewicz T, Rejdak R, Grzybowski A, Nowomiejska K, Moneta-Wielgoś J, Ozimek M, Jünemann AG. Outcomes of sutureless Iris-Claw lens implantation. J Ophthalmol. 2016;2016:7013709.

56. Lajoie J, Glimois V, Petit T, Amelie R, Varenne F, Fournie P, Pagot Mathis V, Malecaze F, Wargny M, Gallini A, Soler V. Assessment of astigmatism associated with the iris-fixated ARTISAN aphakia implant: anterior fixation versus posterior fixation, study of postoperative follow-up at one year. J Fr Ophtalmol. 2018;41(8):696–707.

57. Seknazi D, Colantuono D, Tahiri R, Amoroso F, Miere A, Souied EH. Secondary sutureless posterior chamber lens implantation with two specifically designed IOLs: Iris Claw lens versus sutureless trans-scleral plugs fixated lens. J Clin Med. 2021;10(1):2216.

58. McCannel MA. A retrievable suture idea for anterior uveal problems. Ophthalmic Surg. 1976;7(2):98–103.

59. Price FW Jr, Whitson WE. Visual results of suture-fixated posterior chamber lenses during penetrating keratoplasty. Ophthalmology. 1989;96(8):1234–9.

60. Condon GP. Iris-fixated posterior chamber intraocular lenses. J Cataract Refract Surg. 2006;32(9):1409.

61. Chang DF. Siepser slipknot for McCannel iris-suture fixation of subluxated intraocular lenses. J Cataract Refract Surg. 2004;30(6):1170–6.

62. Mura JJ, Pavlin CJ, Condon GP, Belovay GW, Kranemann CF, Ishikawa H, Ahmed II. Ultrasound biomicroscopic analysis of iris-sutured foldable posterior chamber intraocular lenses. Am J Ophthalmol. 2010;149(2):245–52.

63. Dzhaber D, Mustafa OM, Tian J, Cox JT, Daoud YJ. Outcomes and complications of iris-fixated intraocular lenses in cases with inadequate capsular support and complex ophthalmic history. Eye (Lond). 2020;34(10):1875–82.

64. Soiberman U, Pan Q, Daoud Y, Murakami P, Stark WJ. Iris suture fixation of subluxated intraocular lenses. Am J Ophthalmol. 2015;159(2):353–9.

65. Condon GP, Masket S, Kranemann C, Crandall AS, Ahmed II. Small-incision iris fixation of foldable intraocular lenses in the absence of capsule support. Ophthalmology. 2007;114(7):1311–8.

66. Por YM, Lavin MJ. Techniques of intraocular lens suspension in the absence of capsular/zonular support. Surv Ophthalmol. 2005;50(5):429–62.

67. Cooke DL, Otto B. Lens constants for anterior chamber intraocular lenses. J Cataract Refract Surg. 2021;47(8):1094–5.

68. Gore DM, Wilkins MR. Refractive outcomes in anterior chamber intraocular lenses. Int Ophthalmol. 2013;33(5):453–4.

69. Negretti GS, Lai M, Petrou P, Walker R, Charteris D. Anterior chamber lens implantation in vitrectomised eyes. Eye (Lond). 2018;32(3):597–601.

70. Harrison BM, Idrees S, DiLoreto D, Chung M, Ramchandran R, Kuriyan AE. Refractive outcomes of anterior chamber intraocular lens implantation. Invest Ophthalmol Vis Sci. 2020;61(7):1683.

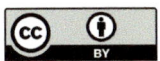

Fellow Eye Calculation

Thomas Olsen

Fellow Eye Calculation

Many surgeons have asked the question: "When I see this prediction error of the first eye, how can I use this information for the calculation of the second eye?" For a meaningful discussion, it is important to distinguish between a statistical error and a refractive surprise. As is the case with any refractive surprise, it is important to rule out any measurement gross errors (not just statistical), recording errors, IOL constant, IOL power label error, or other obvious mistakes. Gross errors can usually be identified by a repeat biometry of the pseudophakia eye to ensure the input variables were valid.

Having ruled out any mistakes or obvious input errors, we are left with a statistical error that has to do with the residual errors of the system as was described in the error propagation model. The idea of a fellow eye correction stems from the high symmetry that we often see between the right and left eye. In a way, the fellow eye surgery can be regarded as a repeat operation of the first eye. The symmetry is also apparent from the fact that the prediction error in the first eye correlates with that of the second eye. What does it mean? This means that no formula is perfect and that some factor related to the person is not picked up by the formula.

Case Study

To illustrate the fellow eye correlations and possible corrections, a study was performed on a series of 654 IOL implantations in 327 patients with two types of IOL: Alcon SA60AT or Abbott Tecnis ZCB00 implanted in both eyes using small incision phacoemulsification and in-the-bag placement of the IOL. The cases were collected some years ago while working at the University Clinic of Aarhus, Denmark. Preoperatively, the patients had Lenstar biometry of all intraocular distances which was necessary for the Olsen formula. The refractive outcome was recorded 1–3 weeks after surgery, and at that time, the biometry was repeated including measurement of the postop IOL position (pseudophakic, postoperative ACD).

The IOL power calculation was performed using the SRK/T as well as with the Olsen formula and the prediction error (defined as the observed mines the predicted refraction) calculated for the right and left eye in each case.

A significant correlation and regression coefficient was found between the prediction error of the right and left eye for both the SRK/T formula and the Olsen formula (Figs. 72.1 and 72.2, respectively). The regression coefficients were 0.52 and 0.38 for the SRK/T and the Olsen formula, respectively ($p < 0.001$).

T. Olsen (✉)
Aros Private Hospital, Aarhus, Denmark

© The Author(s) 2024
J. Aramberri et al. (eds.), *Intraocular Lens Calculations*, Essentials in Ophthalmology,
https://doi.org/10.1007/978-3-031-50666-6_72

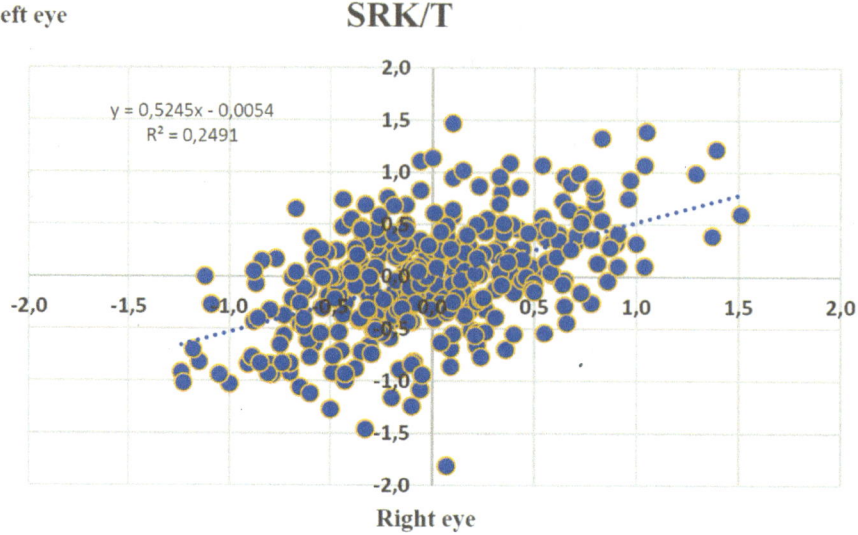

Fig. 72.1 Inter-eye correction of prediction error with the SRK/T formula in 345 cases

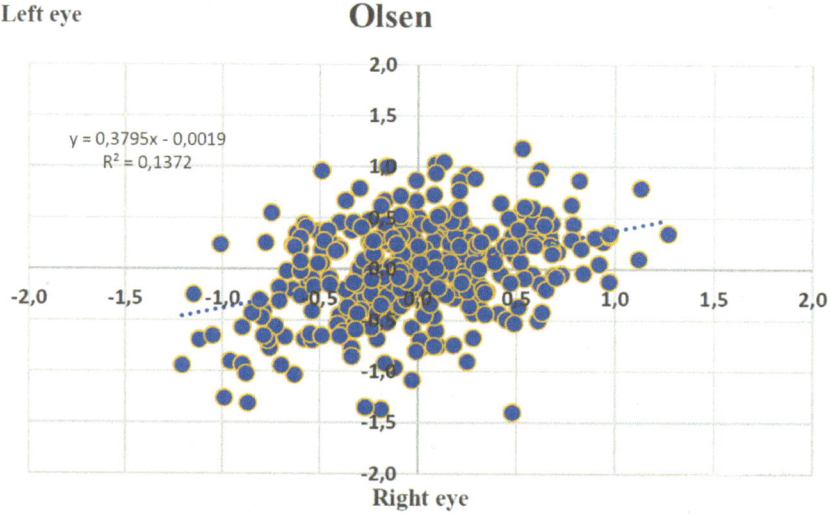

Fig. 72.2 Inter-eye correction of prediction error with the Olsen formula in 345 cases

Based on the observed inter-eye correlation, the prediction of one eye could be corrected according to a regression formula

$$Rx_{cor} = Rx_{exp} + \beta^* Px_{err} \qquad (72.1)$$

where Rx_{cor} and Rx_{exp} are the corrected and the uncorrected refractive prediction, respectively; Px_{err} is the observed error of the first eye; and β is the formula specific regression coefficient. The

method based on the refractive prediction error has fully described a previous publication [1].

A highly significant correlation between the IOL position of the right and left eye was found (Fig. 72.3). The mean difference (±SD) between the postoperative ACD of the left and right eye was found to be 0.0 ± 0.13 mm. This corresponds to 94.5% of the cases within ±0.25 mm difference. With the Olsen formula, you have the

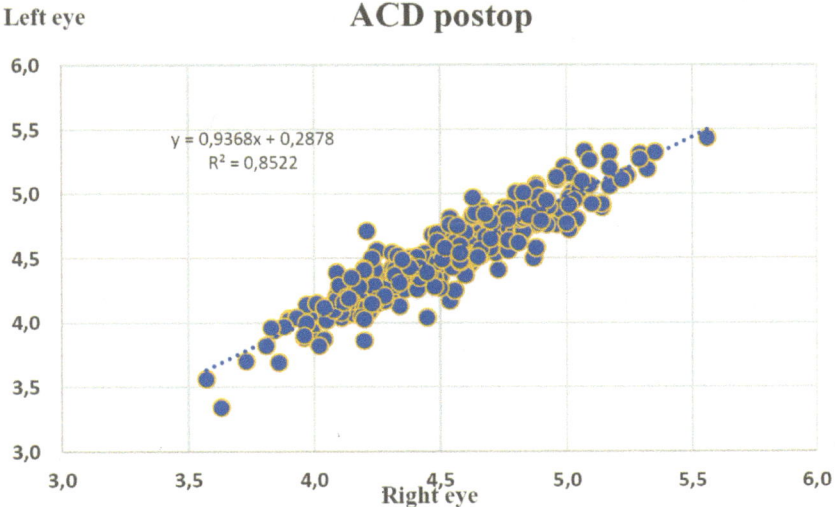

Fig. 72.3 Inter-eye correction of prediction error with the Olsen formula in 345 cases

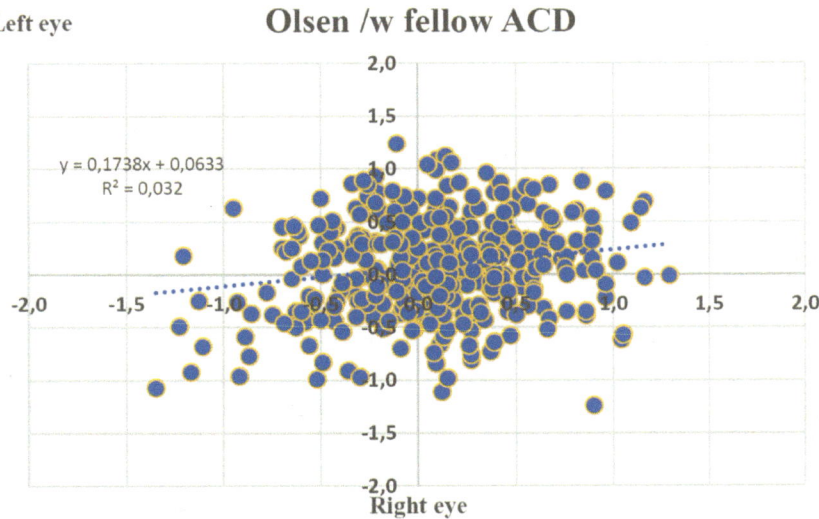

Fig. 72.4 Inter-eye correction of prediction error with the Olsen formula in 345 cases when the fellow postop ACD was used in the predictions

option to use the observed IOL position of the first eye and use this value as the predicted IOL position of the second eye. This was done as shown in Fig. 72.4. The regression coefficient R dropped from 0.38 to 0.17.

The improvement in prediction error (MAE) with fellow eye correction has been summarized in Fig. 72.5. The MAE dropped 14.2% with the SRK/T formula and 7.6% with the Olsen formula, respectively.

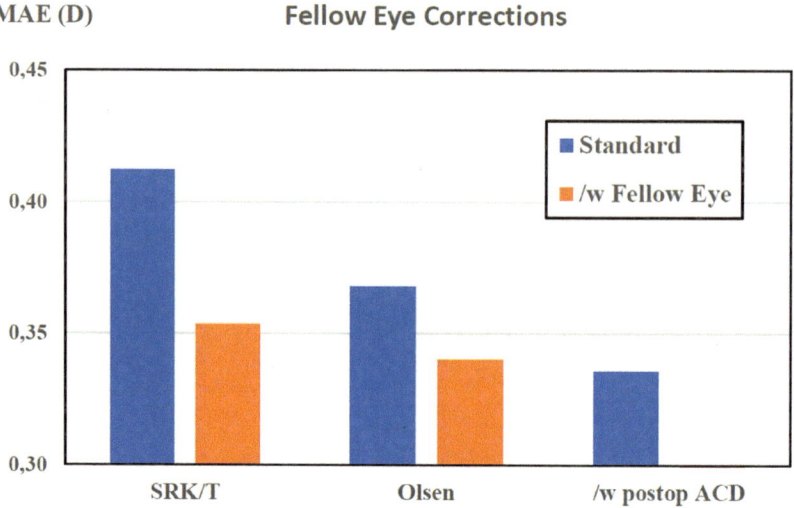

Fig. 72.5 Prediction error without and with fellow eye correction in 345 cases. For comparison is shown in the last column the prediction error when using the postoperative ACD in the 'predictions' with the Olsen formula

Comments

Several studies have now demonstrated a benefit of using the outcome of the first eye to improve the prediction of the second eye. Results vary according to the formula and the corresponding corrective term and hence also according to the improvement found after the fellow eye optimization.

Jabbour et al. [2] found no difference in adjusting for the full first-eye error in the second eye, whereas Covert et al. [3] found a statistically significant outcome by correcting 50% of the error from the first eye. The authors studied the Holladay and the SRK II formulas. This finding was largely supported by Aristodemou et al. [4] who likewise found a correction factor of 50% to be useful using the Hoffer Q, Holladay 1 and the SRK/T formulas.

Jivrajka et al. [5] demonstrated in a prospective study on 97 patients where the first eye prediction error exceeded 0.5 D (Haigis formula) that the refractive error of the second eye could be improved by modifying the IOL power to correct up to 50% of the error from the first eye. Turnbull and Barrett [6] found an improvement using a formula-specific correction factor ranging from 0.30 to 0.56 (Barrett Universal II 0.30;

Hoffer Q 0.56; Holladay I 0.53; SRK/T 0.48) based on 169 patients.

In a previous study by Olsen[46], it was shown that the correction factor was depending on the formula (formulas studied: Olsen, SRK/T and SRK II) so that the correction factor used to adjust the prediction was higher for the formula with the lowest accuracy. As it was also demonstrated in the present case series, an alternative method of optimization is to use the fellow eye pseudophakic ACD as the predicted ACD in the Olsen formula with a similar improvement. This observation underlines the fact that a large part of the error must be due to inaccurate ELP estimation. The fellow eye ACD method has several advantages: It is simple and directly aimed at the main source of error, namely, the ELP prediction. It is independent from the refractive prediction error, which may be influenced by biometric errors, abnormal K-readings, large inter-eye difference in axial length, staphylomas, or other asymmetries unrelated to the anatomy of the capsular bag holding the IOL. It can be used specifically to optimize those cases where a large prediction error is suspected, i.e., short eyes, post-LASIK, post-keratoplasty cases etc.

The fact that the IOL power calculation can be optimized based on the outcome of the fellow eye raises the question if this should be used in a wider scale. When we are comparing formula accuracy, we are often happy to see an improvement in MAE on the second decimal point. The fellow eye optimization has the potential to reduce the error considerably, depending on the formula (by 7–14% in the case study presented here). On the other hand, there is the question of cost. Waiting weeks to have the refraction of the first eye before doing the IOL power calculation and the surgery of the second eye adds substantial cost and time for the entire procedure. Moreover, many surgeons are now performing bilateral simultaneous cataract surgery to speed up recovery and reduce cost.

There is no question the future will demand accurate IOL power calculation in the first place.

References

1. Olsen T. Use of fellow eye data in the calculation of intraocular lens power for the second eye. Ophthalmology. 2011;118:1710–5.

2. Jabbour J, Irwig L, Macaskill P, Hennessy MP. Intraocular lens power in bilateral cataract surgery: whether adjusting for error of predicted refraction in the first eye improves prediction in the second eye. J Cataract Refract Surg. 2006;32:2091–7.

3. Covert DJ, Henry CR, Koenig SB. Intraocular lens power selection in the second eye of patients undergoing bilateral, sequential cataract extraction. Ophthalmology. 2010;117:49–54.

4. Aristodemou P, Cartwright NEK, Sparrow JM, Johnston RL. First eye prediction error improves second eye refractive outcome. Ophthalmology. 2011;118:1701–9.

5. Jivrajka RV, Jivrajka RV, Shammas MC, Shammas HJ. Improving the second-eye refractive error in patients undergoing bilateral sequential cataract surgery. Ophthalmology. 2012;119:1097–101.

6. Turnbull AMJ, Barrett GD. Using the first-eye prediction error in cataract surgery to refine the refractive outcome of the second eye. J Cataract Refract Surg. 2019;45:1239–45.

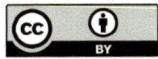

Index

© The Editor(s) (if applicable) and The Author(s) 2024
J. Aramberri et al. (eds.), *Intraocular Lens Calculations*, Essentials in Ophthalmology,
https://doi.org/10.1007/978-3-031-50666-6